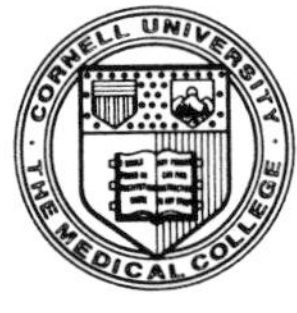
CORNELL UNIVERSITY
THE MEDICAL COLLEGE

D1400619

INTERNATIONAL ENCYCLOPEDIA OF
PHARMACOLOGY AND THERAPEUTICS

Executive Editor: W.C. BOWMAN, Glasgow

Section 130

PSYCHOTROPIC DRUGS OF ABUSE

Some Recent Volumes

MATSUMURA
Differential Toxicities of Insecticides and Halogenated Aromatics

BALFOUR
Nicotine and the Tobacco Smoking Habit

MITCHELL
The Modulation of Immunity

SHUGAR
Viral Chemotherapy, Volumes 1 & 2

De WIED, GISPEN and van WIMERSMA GREIDANUS
Neuropeptides and Behavior, Volumes 1 & 2

DENBOROUGH
The Role of Calcium in Drug Action

WEBBE
The Toxicology of Molluscicides

GRUNBERGER and GOFF
Mechanisms of Cellular Transformation by Carcinogenic Agents

TIPPER
Antibiotic Inhibitors of Bacterial Cell Wall Biosynthesis

CORY
Inhibitors of Ribonucleoside Diphosphate Reductase Activity

HAYASHI
Ornithine Decarboxylase: Biology, Enzymology, and Molecular Genetics

INTERNATIONAL ENCYCLOPEDIA OF
PHARMACOLOGY AND THERAPEUTICS

Section 130

PSYCHOTROPIC DRUGS OF ABUSE

SPECIALIST SUBJECT EDITOR

D. J. K. BALFOUR

Department of Pharmacology and Clinical Pharmacology
University of Dundee, Ninewells Hospital
Dundee, Scotland, U.K.

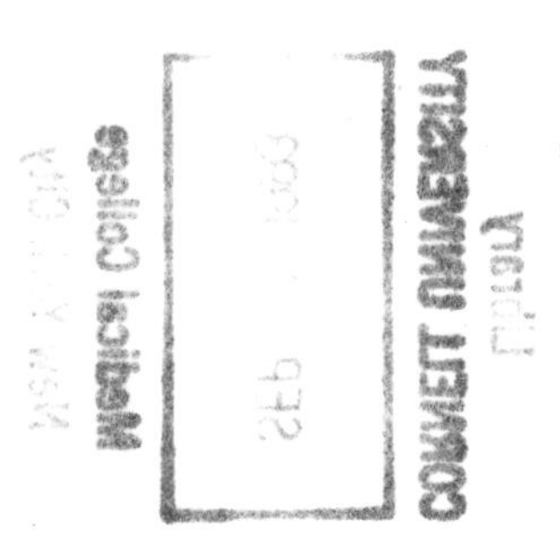

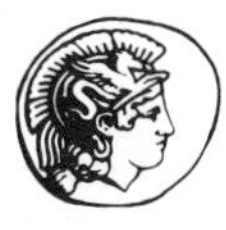

PERGAMON PRESS

Member of Maxwell Macmillan Pergamon Publishing Corporation
New York • Oxford • Beijing • Frankfurt
São Paulo • Sydney • Tokyo • Toronto

Pergamon Press Offices:

U.S.A.	Pergamon Press, Inc., Maxwell House, Fairview Park, Elmsford, New York 10523, U.S.A.
U.K.	Pergamon Press plc, Headington Hill Hall, Oxford OX3 0BW, England
PEOPLE'S REPUBLIC OF CHINA	Pergamon Press, Room 4037, Qianmen Hotel, Beijing, People's Republic of China
FEDERAL REPUBLIC OF GERMANY	Pergamon Press GmbH, Hammerweg 6, D-6242 Kronberg, Federal Republic of Germany
BRAZIL	Pergamon Editora Ltda, Rua Eça de Queiros, 346, CEP 04011, Paraiso, São Paulo, Brazil
AUSTRALIA	Pergamon Press Australia Pty Ltd., P.O. Box 544, Potts Point, NSW 2011, Australia
JAPAN	Pergamon Press, 8th Floor, Matsuoka Central Building, 1-7-1 Nishishinjuku, Shinjuku-ku, Tokyo 160, Japan
CANADA	Pergamon Press Canada Ltd., Suite 271, 253 College Street, Toronto, Ontario M5T 1R5, Canada

---

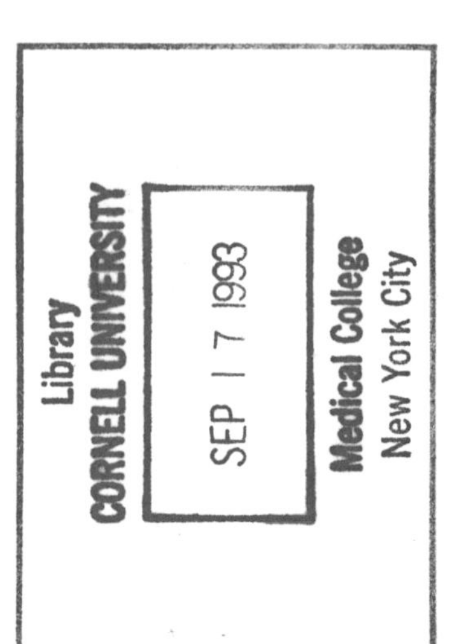

First printing 1990

Library of Congress Cataloging in Publication Data

Psychotropic drugs of abuse / specialist subject editor, D.J.K. Balfour.
p. cm. -- (International encyclopedia of pharmacology and therapeutics)
Includes bibliographies and index.
ISBN 0-08-036851-4 :
1. Psychotropic drugs--Side effects. 2. Drug abuse--Physiological aspects. 3. Molecular pharmacology. I. Balfour, D. J. K.
[DNLM: 1. Psychotropic Drugs--pharmacology. QV 77 P9753]
RM316.P79 1989
615'.788--dc20
DNLM/DLC 89-4003
for Library of Congress CIP

Printed in the United States of America

The paper used in this publication meets the minimum requirements of American National Standard for Information Sciences -- Permanence of Paper for Printed Library Materials, ANSI Z39.48-1984

CONTENTS

FOREWORD

The last few years have witnessed an explosion of concern with the problem of drug abuse in the community and the treatment of drug dependence. This period has also seen many new and exciting discoveries in the field of neuropharmacology, particularly with respect to the molecular aspects of the subject. One of the objectives of this volume of the encyclopedia is to seek to relate the recent advances in our understanding of the molecular basis of neuropharmacology to the current explanations for the behavioural and rewarding properties of "recreational" drugs. However, as one brought up in the molecular school of pharmacology, I have become increasingly aware of the fact that we do not, and may never, have convincing biochemical explanations for all of the effects of psychoactive drugs. The fields of experimental and clinical psychology can provide a different perspective on the problem which incorporates behavioural explanations for the responses to these drugs. A number of the reviews in this volume focus on this approach to the problem and, in particular, its value to the practical treatment of drug abuse. Thus the reviews included in this volume have been selected to try to demonstrate the wide and interdisciplinary nature of current studies on the mechanism of action of psychotropic drugs and I hope they have been presented in a way which emphasises the value of exploiting the interrelationship between molecular and behavioural neuroscience.

D. J. K. Balfour
July 1988

LIST OF CONTRIBUTORS

George K. Aghajanian
Connecticut Mental Health Center and the
Abraham Ribicoff Research Facilities
34 Park Street
New Haven, CT 06508

J.B. Appel
Behavioral Pharmacology Laboratory
Department of Psychology
University of South Carolina
Columbia, SC

John Brick
Rutgers-The State University
New Brunswick, NJ 08901

J. Broadbent
Behavioral Pharmacology Laboratory
Department of Psychology
University of South Carolina
Columbia, SC

J.L. Evenden
Department of Experimental Psychology
and Anatomy
University of Cambridge
Cambridge, UK

S.E. File
Psychopharmacology Research Unit
UMDS, University of London
Division of Pharmacology
Guy's Hospital
London SE1 9RT

Nick Heather
National Drug and Alcohol Research Centre
University of New South Wales
Australia

B.B. Johnston
Drug Dependence Service
Tayside Health Board and
Department of Psychiatry
University Medical School
Dundee, Scotland

Ian L. Martin
MRC Molecular Neurobiology Unit
MRC Centre
Hills Road
Cambridge CB2 2QH
United Kingdom

H.G. Morton
Department of Child and Family Psychiatry
Ninewells Teaching Hospital
and Medical School
Dundee, U.K.

S. Pellow
MRC Neuropharmacology Research Group
The School of Pharmacy
University of London
London WC1N 1AX
United Kingdom

R.G. Pertwee
Department of Pharmacology
Marischal College
University of Aberdeen
Aberdeen, AB9 1AS
Scotland

Larissa A. Pohorecky
Rutgers—The State University
New Brunswick, NJ 08901

Kurt Rasmussen
Departments of Psychiatry and Pharmacology
Yale University School of Medicine
New Haven, CT 06510-8066

C.N. Ryan
Department of Experimental Psychology
and Anatomy
University of Cambridge
Cambridge, UK

Shepard Siegel
Department of Psychology
McMaster University
Hamilton, Ontario L8S 4K1
Canada

P. Tyrer
St. Charles Hospital
London, W10 6DZ
United Kingdom

Roy A. Wise
Center for Studies in Behavioral Neurobiology
and Department of Psychology
Concordia University
Montreal, Quebec
Canada

CHAPTER 1

BEHAVIORAL RESPONSES TO PSYCHOMOTOR STIMULANT DRUGS: LOCALIZATION IN THE CENTRAL NERVOUS SYSTEM

J. L. EVENDEN and C. N. RYAN

Departments of Experimental Psychology and Anatomy, University of Cambridge, Cambridge, U.K.

ABBREVIATIONS

AMC	– anteromedial head of caudate	LH	– lateral hypothalamus
CR	– conditioned reinforcer	LI	– latent inhibition
CRF	– corticotropin releasing factor	LSD	– lysergic acid diethylamide
CTA	– conditioned taste aversion	MPFC	– medial prefrontal cortex
D1, D2	– dopamine receptor subtypes	MPTP	– *N*-methyl-4-phenyl-1,2,3,6-tetrahydropyridine
DA	– dopamine	NA	– noradrenaline
DLC	– dorsolateral head of caudate	N.acc.	– nucleus accumbens
DMC	– dorsomedial head of caudate	OT	– olfactory tubercle
DMI	– desmethylimipramine	6-OHDA	– 6-hydroxydopamine
DNAB	– dorsal noradrenergic bundle	beta-PEA	– beta-phenylethylamine
DRL	– differential reinforcement of low rates of responding	PFC	– prefrontal cortex
DSP4	– *N*-2-(chloroethyl)-*N*-ethyl-2-bromobenzylamine	(–)-3-PPP	– 3-(3-hydroxyphenyl)-*N*-n-propylpiperdine
FI	– fixed interval schedule of reinforcement	SIP	– schedule induced polydipsi
5-HT	– 5-hydropxytryptamine, serotonin	SNc	– substantia nigra, pars compacta
i.p.	– intra-peritoneal	SPFC	– suprarhinal prefrontal cortex
LA	– locomotor activity	VLC	– ventrolateral head of caudate
		VNAB	– ventral noradrenergic bundle
		VTA	– ventral tegmental area

1. INTRODUCTION

The definition of a drug as a psychomotor stimulant is based upon its effects on behavior, and the class consists of drugs that can increase locomotor activity or the frequency of occurrence of learned behaviors at doses well below those producing convulsions (Kelleher, 1977). Psychomotor stimulants should be differentiated from selective agonists of the excitatory amino acid neurotransmitter systems, or selective antagonists of inhibitory amino acid neurotransmitter systems. These drugs fall into the class of central nervous system stimulants which may produce convulsions but whose effects on behavior are relatively non-specific.

The effects of psychomotor stimulant drugs on behavior have been well documented over the years, and several up-to-date reviews exist (Creese, 1983). More recently, major advances have been made in localizing the effects of these drugs to specific systems in the brain, and this article will review this work.

In fact, most psychomotor stimulant drugs appear to function as direct or indirect dopamine agonists. Briefly, these two drugs enhance release of dopamine (DA) and inhibit its reuptake from the synaptic cleft. Kuczenski (1983) concludes that at DA neurones amphetamine primarily acts as a releaser. Cocaine, on the other hand, appears to block reuptake, and does not affect release.

Methylphenidate and its related compounds also affect DA neurotransmission, again by increasing release, and blocking reuptake, although they can be differentiated from amphetamine both in terms of potency (Robbins *et al.*, 1983) and because their effects may be blocked by reserpine (Scheel-Kruger, 1971). Psychomotor stimulant-like effects may also be obtained using direct DA receptor agonists such as apomorphine and DA itself. However, assessing the neural basis of the behavioral effects of stimulant drugs is complicated since many of them are not entirely specific to dopamine, and may also influence release and reuptake in the noradrenergic systems and, to a certain extent, serotonin.

Although these drugs all act in common as DA agonists, direct or indirect, the dopaminergic innervation of the brain is not, itself, unitary. Two types of division exist. The first is biochemical, in that DA receptors may be divided into different types. Two main types of receptor have been generally agreed, D1, linked to adenylate cyclase, and D2. At various times further sub-types of receptors have been suggested but these have not been generally accepted and may represent different states of D1 and D2 receptors (Seeman *et al.*, 1986). Direct receptor agonists and antagonists display different affinities for the two receptor types. DA receptors are also present on the presynaptic, dopamine neurones (Seeman, 1980). These receptors provide negative feedback, thus, stimulating DA autoreceptors results in a reduction in DA release by the neurone, and blocking the receptors results in a stimulation of DA release, so that, for example, apomorphine can inhibit behavior at low doses which it stimulates at higher doses (Costall *et al.*, 1985). These autoreceptors may have some similarity to the post-synaptic D2 receptors (Seeman *et al.*, 1986; Stahle and Ungerstedt, 1986) although autoreceptor specific drugs do exist, e.g. (−) 3-PPP (Hjorth *et al.*, 1983). DA receptors are also found in the dendrites and cell bodies of the DA neurones. These appear to function in a similar manner to the presynaptic receptors in the terminal areas.

The second division of the central dopamine systems is based upon neuroanatomy (see Bjorklund and Lindvall, 1984, for review). Whilst most of the dopamine-containing cell bodies lie within the mesencephalon, there are a number of dopamine-containing cell bodies originating in the thalamus and hypothalamus among other areas, which give rise to systems which appear to influence regulatory functions and hormonal control, and although affected by psychomotor stimulant drugs, do not appear to be important for the acute behavioral effects of these agents. The dopamine-containing cell bodies lying in the mesencephalon have primarily ascending projections to a wide range of forebrain areas, although there are some less well studied descending projections from this cell group. The ascending projections originate in the substantia nigra pars compacta (SNc) and the ventral tegmental area (VTA) and form a single topographically organized system which is classically divided, the nigrostriatal and mesolimbic dopamine systems (Fuxe, 1965). Since the discovery of the DA innervation of the prefrontal cortex to these has been added the mesocortical DA system. Because of their similarities, the nigrostriatal and mesolimbic systems may be classified as a single, mesostriatal system (Bjorklund and Lindvall, 1984). The mesolimbic system projects predominantly to the accumbens, the nigrostriatal system to the caudate, and the mesocortical system to the PFC. These systems, which may be grouped together to form the entire ascending DA projections from the mesencephalon, are called the mesotelencephalic DA system, and show roughly similar patterns of innervation in man, primates, and rodents. The contribution of these systems to the neurochemical basis of the behavioral effects of psychomotor stimulant drugs will form the basis of the remainder of this article.

The effects of psychomotor stimulant drugs on other systems should not be overlooked. For example, the locomotor-enhancing effects of caffeine and CRF appear to be mediated by a separate, non-dopaminergic system (Swerdlow *et al.*, 1986). Also, the effects of psychomotor stimulant drugs may be modulated by destruction of the NA systems (e.g. Braestrup, 1977; Archer *et al.*, 1986). However, although it may reasonably be assumed that this modulation is due to direct mediation of stimulant effects by NA, there are NA neurones which themselves modulate the DA systems (Herve *et al.*, 1982, 1986) so that changes in DA neurotransmission may also be mediated by an indirect mechanism.

2. TECHNIQUES

For practical reasons the study of the neurochemical basis of psychomotor stimulant drugs has been largely confined to the rodent species. There appear to be three reasons for this. The first is historical, in that initial interest in neuropsychology in animals occurred before selective neurotoxins were available and was aimed at drawing parallels between primates and human subjects who had had brain injuries or psycho-surgery. The appropriate human/animal comparison therefore involved ablation of the tissue regardless of neuroanatomical sub-structure or neurochemistry. The second reason is the lack of uniformity in species other than highly inbred rodent strains, with the result that stereotaxic surgery is less likely to be accurate. The third, it is almost needless to say, is cost.

There are three main methods for investigating the neural basis of the behavioral effects of stimulant drugs by manipulating DA systems. The first of these involves destroying the dopamine systems, either completely or selectively, and then treating the subject systemically with stimulant drugs to establish which components of the behavioral response have been altered. Selective destruction of the dopaminergic and noradrenergic systems can be achieved using a relatively specific neurotoxin, 6-hydroxydopamine (6-OHDA) which is taken up by and destroys dopaminergic and noradrenergic neurones, but has little or no effect on other neurotransmitter systems. By pretreating the subjects with a noradrenergic uptake blocker such as desmethylimipramine (DMI), damage can be restricted to dopamine neurones. This technique has been used successfully to destroy subcortical DA systems selectively, but with less success, to destroy the DA innervation of the cortex. Even with DMI pretreatment, infusions of 6-OHDA into this area inevitably lead to depletion of both dopamine and noradrenaline (NA) and these neurotransmitters may be depleted in the cortex when the neurotoxin is infused into the nucleus accumbens (N. acc.). Generally, it is assumed that the behavioral effects of these subcortical lesions, both spontaneous and drug-induced, result from damage to the mesolimbic DA system, rather than the mesocortical system, and are primarily related to DA loss in the N. acc. However, following VTA cell body lesions which deplete both N. acc. and PFC of DA, the behavioral deficits may be better correlated with DA loss in the PFC than in N. acc. (Tassin *et al.*, 1978). It is also possible, by infusing the toxin into the region of the ascending NA systems to destroy the NA innervation of hypothalamus, cortex, or hippocampus, leaving the DA systems intact.

Selective destruction of the DA and NA systems may also be achieved by neurotoxins which can be applied systemically, notably DSP4 and MPTP. DSP4 may be used to destroy the central NA systems in rats (Jaim-Etcheverry and Zeiher, 1980), because, although the toxin damages peripheral NA neurones, these appear to recover. However, the toxin is fatal in some species. MPTP may be used to destroy the central DA systems, particularly the nigrostriatal system (Burns *et al.*, 1983), although the mesocortical and mesolimbic DA systems and the ascending NA innervation may also be affected (Mitchell *et al.*, 1985). This drug is effective in primates, but relatively ineffective in rats.

The second method, which is less commonly used, involves the infusion of DA blocking agents into the terminal regions and, again, to examine which components of the response to systemically administered stimulants are affected. This approach is particularly effective for studying the receptor mediation of the effects of psychomotor stimulant drugs, since DA antagonists have been manufactured that are relatively selective to one or other DA receptor, and are thus more chemically specific than 6-OHDA. This method also has the advantage that the treatment is acute and there are no long-term problems of maintenance.

The third method, which is rather more common, is to infuse the stimulant drugs themselves into DA terminal areas. The behavior of the animals may then be compared with that of animals treated with systemic drugs. There are two major problems with this and the previous method. The first is anatomical specificity. Destruction of the DA systems using toxins can be measured independently of behavior *post mortem*. The degree of destruction of different DA terminal areas can be examined, and the extent of the loss of function or response attributed to the different systems can be estimated. However, there is no simple independent way of checking direct drug infusions, since there is no drug present when the subjects are killed and the infusion sites are verified histologically. The effects of a drug infusion may not necessarily be limited to the target site, particularly if high doses or large infusion volumes are used (Myers, 1974; Myers and Hoch, 1978). On the whole, concern can be reduced by using the minimum dose and volume practicable. However, while this may be appropriate for sensitive or densely innervated sites, such as the subcortical DA systems, it may be inappropriate for insensitive or sparsely innervated sites such as the prefrontal cortex. To an extent anatomical specificity can be verified in two ways. First, radiolabeled substances may be infused in the appropriate volume into the target site. Other sites can then be examined histologically for traces of labeled drug. Second, similar concentrations and volumes of drug may be infused into sites neighboring the target site. No behavioral response would be expected from the control sites.

Another problem is damage to the infusion site by multiple infusions, and damage to overlying tissue by the presence of a guide cannula and/or passage of the infusion cannula (Virjmoed-De Vries and Cools, 1986). Infusions into the brain inevitably damage the target tissue to some extent, although various methods have been developed to minimize this. However, for most practical purposes the maximum number of infusions appears to be limited to five or six unless the infusion volume is very small. This makes it difficult to study the effects of chronic infusions of drugs, interactions between drugs, and even limits the number of doses that may be included in a dose-response curve.

3. BEHAVIOR

A number of factors are important in determining the effects of drugs infused into the CNS, whether these have acute or permanent effects. These include such obvious factors as where the drug is infused, but as described in the previous section, the infusion volume and concentration are also important. However, for reasons of space and clarity full details of coordinates, dose and volume have been omitted. In work already published these may be found by consulting the original text. Otherwise, for more recent work, these will be provided when the results are published in full. The abbreviations used are summarized at the beginning of this article.

3.1. Locomotor Activity

As noted in the Section 1, one of the defining actions of psychomotor stimulant drugs is their ability to increase locomotor activity, although all doses of stimulant drugs do not increase locomotor activity in all circumstances. The effect of stimulant drugs on locomotor activity is one of the best examples of the inverted-U shaped function relating behavioral output to "arousal." At low doses of drug, as the dose is increased, so is locomotor activity, but after a certain point as the dose is increased further, locomotor activity (LA) declines. This does not mean, of course, that the animal is no longer activated, but rather that stereotyped, repetitive behavior becomes predominant (see Section 3.6).

Such inverted-U shaped functions complicate the interpretation of drug–lesion or drug–drug interactions unless a wide range of measures of behavior are recorded. A treatment which reduces the level of drug-induced locomotor activity may potentially represent a shift of the dose–response curve to the left (reduced activation), or to the right (increased activation) without independent behavioral or pharmacological verification.

The precise neural basis of the effects of stimulant drugs on LA has been the subject of much research. The deficits in spontaneous activity in Parkinson's disease suggest that complete loss of DA in the forebrain terminal areas, whether by 6-OHDA infused into the substantia nigra pars compacta (SNc), lateral hypothalamus (LH) or by systemically administered MPTP, leads to gross impairments, not only in locomotor activity, but in all forms of movement. These effects can be reduced by treatment with direct DA agonists and by L-DOPA. The effects of indirect agonists are largely blocked (Ljunberg and Ungerstedt, 1976).

Infusions of 6-OHDA directly into the terminal areas, selectively depleting DA in either the N. acc. or the caudate nucleus, produces differential motor effects depending upon the area of depletion (Kelly *et al.*, 1975). They found that destruction of the DA innervation of the N. acc. attenuated the amphetamine-induced increase in locomotor activity, and that conversely the LA response to apomorphine was greatly exaggerated. Loss of the DA innervation of the caudate nucleus left amphetamine-induced and apomorphine-induced LA unaffected. In support of the lesion data intra-accumbens infusions of haloperidol, a DA antagonist, block the locomotor stimulant effects of amphetamine, whereas injections into the caudate are ineffective (Pijnenburg *et al.*, 1975). In several studies, it has been found that 6-OHDA lesions of the caudate nucleus actually result in increased amphetamine-induced LA, perhaps as a result of a reduction in the competing stereotyped behavior. For example, Joyce and Iversen (1984) found dramatic increases in amphetamine-induced LA in rats which had received bilateral 6-OHDA lesions of anterior caudate, particularly at the highest dose which produced stereotyped behavior in unlesioned animals. To localize this behavioral competition more precisely, Dunnett (1981) made 6-OHDA lesions of either the anteromedial or ventrolateral caudate nucleus (AMC or VLC). In contrast to N. acc. lesioned rats (Koob *et al.*, 1977), neither group of rats in Dunnett's experiment showed any changes in spontaneous LA 10–16 days after surgery, but those rats with the VLC lesion showed a greater release of amphetamine-induced LA than those with lesions of AMC. Fink and Smith (1980) found that highly restricted N. acc. lesions alone did not attenuate amphetamine-induced LA unless DA depletion of AMC or VLC was included. An *increase* in amphetamine-induced locomotor activity has been reported following specific dopamine depletion by infusing 6-OHDA in DMI pretreated rats into the medial prefrontal cortex (Pycock *et al.*, 1980). Spontaneous increases in LA following 6-OHDA infusions into the PFC have also been found (Carter and Pycock, 1980; Pycock *et al.*, 1980; Morency *et al.*, 1985), but other studies have found no changes in LA following 6-OHDA infusions into the PFC (Joyce *et al.*, 1983; Dunn *et al.*, 1984; Ryan and Dunnett, 1985). It appears that whenever there is an increase in spontaneous LA following PFC DA depletion, the amphetamine-induced LA response is enhanced, and that where there is no change in spontaneous activity, rats with 6-OHDA infusions into the PFC show little change in responsiveness to amphetamine, although administration of high doses of this drug still significantly decrease amphetamine-induced locomotion (Koob *et al.*, 1984).

Lesions of the dorsal noradrenergic bundle (DNAB) also attenuate amphetamine-induced LA, whereas treatment with DSP4 or neonatal 6-OHDA treatment appear to reduce preferentially the rearing component, leaving locomotion, itself, unaffected (Archer *et al.*, 1986).

Increases in locomotor activity have also been obtained using central infusions of stimulant drugs. Pijnenburg *et al.* (1976) infused both d-amphetamine and DA itself into the N. acc. and found the locomotor activity of rats to be significantly increased. DA infused into the olfactory tubercles and amygdala had no reliable effect on LA (Jackson *et al.*, 1975). Although 6-OHDA lesions in the amygdala increased the LA response to systemic administration of amphetamine (Deminiere *et al.*, 1984).

Amphetamine, dopamine or longer-acting analogues do not stimulate LA when infused into the caudate nucleus (Jackson *et al.*, 1975; Elkhawad and Woodruff, 1976), although Dourish (1985) reported increased locomotion following intra-caudate beta-phenylethylamine (beta-PEA) infusions. Neill and Herndon (1978) obtained an increase in LA following application of crystalline amphetamine to the AMC but not the posterior caudate.

A similar anatomical dissociation was obtained by Annett *et al.* (1983) using microinfusions of amphetamine into N. acc. or caudate of marmosets, and by Dill *et al.* (1979) in rhesus and squirrel monkeys following DA infusions, in that increased activity occurs following intra-accumbens but not intra-caudate infusions. Recently, Cools (1986) found that infusions of apomorphine into the N. acc. also increased LA, but only after a time lag of an hour, suggesting that the effect might result from spread to an adjacent area. His suggested alternative was the olfactory tubercle, since he obtained a more rapid increase from this area. However, the effect from N. acc. infusions was larger and longer lasting than that seen in the OT. In primates the olfactory tubercle is smaller and lies lateral and caudal to the accumbens and it is unlikely that this structure is responsible for the effects attributed to the N. acc. (Dubach and Bowen, 1983).

Apomorphine infused into suprahinal prefrontal cortex reduced LA but increased exploratory activity measured by head poking and rearing (van der Gugten *et al.*, 1986). At higher doses head poking was also reduced. In contrast, systemic apomorphine reduces hole-poking, whereas systemic amphetamine increases hole-poking (Kelley *et al.*, 1986). The effects of infusions of DA agonists and antagonists on climbing in the mouse, a specific form of activity, were assessed by Costall *et al.* (1985). They found that low doses of apomorphine infused into subcortical areas increased inhibition of this response, presumably via autoreceptors, but the same doses had no effect when infused into cortical sites including the pregenual, supregenual and suprahinal prefrontal cortex. Infusion of higher doses into all areas increased climbing.

3.2. Asymmetry and Rotation

Unilateral lesions of the SNc or the caudate or unilateral infusions into the SNc or caudate produce asymmetries in motor behavior. Ungerstedt (1971) found transient ipsilateral rotational behavior in rats after unilateral destruction of the nigrostriatal DA system. After recovery, these could be reinstated by treatment with amphetamine. Such asymmetries are not produced by unilateral lesions of the N. acc., (Kelly, 1975), although rotation due to unilateral 6-OHDA lesions of the caudate may be blocked by 6-OHDA lesions of the nucleus accumbens (Kelly and Moore, 1976). In other words, the DA innervation of the N. acc. does not control the direction of the rotational response, but can influence the rate of rotation. The amphetamine-induced ipsilateral lesions of SNc may be *blocked* by transplants of foetal SNc neurones into or adjacent to the denervated striatum (Bjorklund *et al.*, 1980; Dunnett *et al.*, 1983; Freed *et al.*, 1983). More recently, behavioral overcompensation has been found following similar transplants (Herman *et al.*, 1985), in that transplanted rats showed spontaneous *contralateral* turns which were exaggerated by amphetamine and in some rats also by apomorphine. There was no correlation between the response to amphetamine and the response to apomorphine. The amphetamine-induced turns were abolished by haloperidol. In this case it seems likely that the response to amphetamine was being mediated by the transplanted DA neurones.

Rotation may also be seen, although to a much lesser extent, with peripheral administration of amphetamine or apomorphine in intact animal. This amphetamine- or apomorphine-induced asymmetry seems to be correlated with other spontaneous spatial asymmetries such as paw preference or choice of arm in a T-maze (Glick *et al.*, 1977). Zimmerberg *et al.* (1974) found elevated levels of dopamine in the striatum contralateral to the preferred side.

Circling may also be obtained following unilateral 6-OHDA lesions to the locus coeruleus (Pycock *et al.*, 1975). Following unilateral lesions, contralateral circling was seen in response to both amphetamine and apomorphine, particularly in rats where NA in the ipsilateral frontal cortex was low. Pycock *et al.* (1975) suggest that NA depletion in the frontal cortex results in an increase in DA in ipsilateral striatum, and hence to a subcortical asymmetry which is responsible for rotation.

Ungerstedt *et al.* (1969) infused DA or applied crystalline DA unilaterally into the caudate nucleus. They observed the opposite effects to the 6-OHDA lesions, DA stimulation producing contralateral turning. This effect was also seen after unilateral infusions of apomorphine. Unilateral infusions of neuroleptic drugs have an effect similar to lesions (Ungerstedt *et al.*, 1969). Costall *et al.* (1983) compared the ability of unilateral microinfusions of a number of DA antagonists to produce turning behavior. Only (−)-sulpiride did so when infused alone. However, ipsilateral asymmetry developed after infusions of all the drugs, with the exception of the enantiomers which are ineffective as DA antagonists, when the mice were treated with peripheral apomorphine. However, these effects consisted only of postural asymmetries and not fully-fledged rotation. Infusions of DA, itself, into the hemisphere contralateral to the neuroleptic infusions also produced postural asymmetries even when neither the doses of DA and neuroleptics used did so on their own. Joyce and Van Hartesveldt (1984) suggest that turning and postural asymmetries may be mediated by different areas of striatum, since infusions of DA into DLC stimulated postural deviation with an earlier onset than infusions into DMC, whereas DMC infusions stimulate rotation with more lateral placements having a relatively slower and smaller effect. This heterogeneity is also evident in the cell bodies as infusions of apomorphine into medial SNc produced ipsilateral circling, whereas there was no effect when the drug was infused into lateral SNc (Vaccarino and Franklin, 1984).

Infusions of DA antagonists unilaterally into the medial PFC in rats pretreated with systemic amphetamine produces ipsiversive circling suggesting that the mesocortical DA system is also involved in motor activity. Infusions of D2 receptor antagonists including sulpride (Morency *et al.*, 1985) and metoclopromide (Stewart *et al.*, 1985) produce ipsilateral circling. In contrast, contralateral circling has been induced by unilateral intraprefrontal infusions of DA agonists including amphetamine, and the D2 agonist LY 141865 (Stewart *et al.*, 1985).

3.3. Schedule-induced Behavior

Intermittent deliveries of a reinforcer, either contingent upon performance of a response or non-contingent may result in an increase in behavior unrelated to the schedule. The most widely studied of these adjunctive behaviors is schedule-induced polydipsia (SIP). SIP is attenuated by amphetamine whether it is generated by non-contingent (e.g. fixed time, Nieto *et al.*, 1979), or contingent (fixed interval, Wayner *et al.*, 1973) schedules of food delivery. Acquisition of SIP is attenuated by 6-OHDA lesions of the N. acc. (Robbins and Koob, 1980), and the PFC (Ryan and Dunnett, 1986). In contrast, 6-OHDA lesions of the septum increase SIP (Tagzhouti *et al.*, 1985a). Effects of amphetamine on pre-established SIP were attenuated by 6-OHDA lesions of the accumbens whereas the disruptive effects of apomorphine were markedly exaggerated (Robbins *et al.*, 1983). Replacement of the dopaminergic innervation of PFC by grafted tissue was not effective in restoring acquisition of SIP, and nigral transplants into intact PFC further reduced the acquisition of SIP (Ryan, 1987).

3.4. Response Disinhibition

The effects of stimulant drugs on activation may also be seen in changes in conditioned behavior. When subjects are required to withhold a response, amphetamine results in an increase in the performance of inappropriate, erroneous responses. This can be seen under schedules of reinforcement such as differential reinforcement of low rates of responding (DRL) or go/no-go discrimination performance (see Section 3.13). This does not generally reflect a breakdown of the control over behavior by the contingencies or discriminative stimuli, *d*, in signal detection theory terms, but a shift in response bias, *B*, reflecting an increase in the tendency to respond.

An intraventricular infusion of 6-OHDA, which depletes DA in the accumbens and caudate has been reported not to affect DRL performance *per se*, but attenuates the rate increasing effects of amphetamine (Levine *et al.*, 1980). In a more topographically specific study, Dunnett (1981) compared the effects of 6-OHDA and kainic acid lesions of the VLC and AMC on DRL performance. He found that rats made more premature responses following lesions with both neurotoxins in the VLC and efficiency correspondingly declined. Equivalent lesions to the AMC did not affect performance (Dunnett and Iversen, 1982).

Infusions of amphetamine into DA terminal areas also appear to have disinhibitory effects. Neill and Herndon (1978) examined the effects of applying crystalline amphetamine or infusing DA solution into AMC, dorsal globus pallidus and posterior caudate on DRL performance. They found a reduction in efficiency, produced by an increase in lever pressing only by infusion into AMC.

Carli *et al.* (1985) reported a method for examining the laterality of responding to visual stimuli in rats. Unilateral 6-OHDA lesions of mid ventral caudate resulted in a bias towards the lesioned side. In a further experiment, Carli and Robbins (personal communication) infused amphetamine unilaterally into the MVC or N. acc. When infused into the MVC, amongst other effects, the drug increased the number of responses made at inappropriate times contralateral to the infused side, thus resembling the effects of infusions on rotation. However, when the drug was infused *unilaterally* into the N. acc., a *bilateral* increase in erroneous responses was observed. In other words, a unilateral stimulation of the mesolimbic DA system resulted in bilateral behavioral activation. This explains the absence of rotation following N. acc. lesions or infusions, since there was no behavioral asymmetry.

3.5. Rate Dependent Effects

In addition to increasing the frequency of inappropriate responding, the stimulation of appropriate conditioned behavior, such as lever pressing, by amphetamine, cocaine and related drugs, has been well documented. This stimulation may be manifested in two ways, a stimulation of the rate of performance of a response, and an increase in the length of time that responding continues.

The effects of stimulant drugs on local rates of responding are complicated by the same factors that affect locomotor activity, that is, stimulation of competing behavior at higher doses results in a reduction in response rate. Indeed, high rates of responding may be reduced at the same dose of drug that stimulates low rates. Thus the effects of a stimulant drug on response rate may be said to depend upon the control rate of responding. This rate-dependent effect appears to hold across a range of species, responses and types of task (Dews and Wenger, 1977). One of the most widely used methods of studying the rate-dependent effects of drugs involves training animals under fixed-interval (FI) schedules of reinforcement. The rate of responding increases during the interval allowing the effects of the drug to be studied at a range of response rates. Peripheral administration of amphetamine increases the low rates at the start of the interval and leaves unaffected or reduces the high rates at the end. The effect of the drug is attenuated by 6-OHDA lesions of the N. acc. (Robbins *et al.*, 1983). The direct agonist, apomorphine, generally has weaker rate-dependent effects than amphetamine, but these were exaggerated following the lesions, presumably due to receptor supersensitivity. In a recent series of studies, we have infused amphetamine and apomorphine into a number of different sites in the DA terminal areas in the forebrain, including the accumbens, two sites in the caudate nucleus (Evenden, 1984, unpublished data), and three regions of the prefrontal cortex; the pregenual, supragenual and suprarhinal PFC (Ryan, 1987). Rate-dependent effects of directly infused amphetamine have been obtained from all sites except for the supragenual prefrontal cortex. However, the sites differed very much in their sensitivity to the drug. N. acc. was the site most sensitive to amphetamine, followed by the MVC, with a dramatic drop in sensitivity if a slightly more dorsal and posterior placement was used. Pregenual medial and suprarhinal PFC are less sensitive still. To obtain the same effect it was necessary to infuse 30 times the dose of drug into the PFC as into the N. acc.

However, a different picture holds for apomorphine, with PFC and N. acc. being roughly similar in sensitivity. With both drugs larger volumes were required for intracortical infusions, although preliminary autoradiographic studies indicate that, even so, after such infusions, little, if any, drug reached subcortical sites (Ryan, 1987).

3.6. Perseveration and Switching

In the context of the effects of stimulant drugs, perseveration refers to a tendency for subjects treated with a stimulant drug to continue responding when untreated subjects have stopped. One of the best examples of this has been provided by Poncelet *et al.* (1983). They used a progressive ratio schedule, in which as the rat makes more responses, so the number of responses required before food is delivered is increased. Under stimulant drugs, including amphetamine and methylphenidate, the number of responses made before giving up was dramatically increased. Apparently similar effects have been reported in human subjects, who are capable of performing at high levels of physical or cognitive load for longer after treatment with amphetamine (Laties and Weiss, 1966, 1981).

Conversely, Robbins and Watson (1981) and Evenden and Robbins (1983), have shown that amphetamine may increase switching between lever-press responses if the subjects have a history of switching, at the same doses at which perseveration of responding is increased. Increases in alternation under amphetamine in the Y-maze have been noted by Oades *et al.* (1985). However, Evenden (1984) found that neither the increase in switching nor the increase in perseveration produced by amphetamine were attenuated by 6-OHDA lesions to the N. acc. or MVC, although the lesions of the N. acc. themselves resulted in an increase in response switching, and the lesion of MVC resulted in increased perseveration. In contrast, Oades (1981) found that infusion of neuroleptics into VTA which increase mesolimbic DA activity increased the number of switches away from the preferred strategy in a hold-board search task. Some evidence, however, has been obtained for similar types of amphetamine effects in perseveration in primates. Ridley *et al.* (1981) found that marmosets treated with amphetamine would continue to respond to a previously reinforced stimulus when the discrimination was reversed. Since this perseveration involved responding to the left or right it could not be a simple motor perseveration alone. This effect could be blocked by haloperidol. Annett and Ridley (1985) found that marmosets treated with amphetamine infused directly into the N. acc. also showed increased perseveration on a successive reversal task where infusion into the caudate had no effect. In contrast, however, Kulig and Calhoun (1972) found that methamphetamine enhanced serial discrimination reversal in rats, although differences in procedure make direct comparison impossible.

Amphetamine-induced perseverative behavior in the radial-arm maze has been shown to depend, at least in part, on the noradrenergic system. Bruto *et al.* (1984) found that treatment with DSP4 enhanced amphetamine-induced perseveration, whereas intraventricular 6-OHDA attenuated this effect.

Effects of stimulant drugs which may be related to perseveration have also been found and studied in more detail in experiments primarily designed to examine the effects of the drugs on reinforcement (see Sections 3.8 and 3.9).

3.7. Stereotyped Behavior

At higher doses of psychomotor stimulant drugs, the perseverative behavior takes the form of stereotyped behavior, the repetition of seemingly purposeless acts. In the human or primate, stereotypes may be quite complex, but in the rat they generally consist of gnawing or sniffing in a restricted location. It is this stereotyped behavior that appears to be responsible for the reductions in locomotor activity at these doses of the drugs. The interaction between locomotor activity and stereotypy has already been discussed briefly above (Section 3.1). Kelly *et al.* (1975) found that 6-OHDA lesions to the caudate attenuated amphetamine-induced and enhanced apomorphine-induced stereotypy. Using 6-OHDA lesions localized to AMC or VLC, Dunnett (1981) found that both lesion groups showed attenuated amphetamine stereotypy, and did not differ from each other. In contrast, 6-OHDA induced lesions of the PFC enhance the stereotypic effects of amphetamine (Pycock *et al.*, 1980). These researchers have also shown that 6-OHDA localized in the PFC reduces apomorphine-induced stereotypy. Furthermore, direct infusions of fluphenazine into the PFC result in reduced systemic amphetamine-induced stereotypy.

Until recently, it has not been possible to demonstrate convincing stereotypy following central microinfusions of DA or stimulant drugs. Although increases in stereotypy rating have been recorded following intra-caudate but not intra-accumbens microinfusions (Staton and Solomon, 1984), these have generally been small compared with the effects seen with peripheral drug administration, and the average ratings do not correspond to true stereotyped behavior. For example, Dourish (1985) reported increased rearing and sniffing following intra-caudate infusions of beta-PEA. Nevertheless, in general, opinion is that stereotypy is indeed, mediated by the caudate, (Costall and Naylor, 1977), but that, as the lesion effects suggest, amphetamine stereotypy is mediated by the entire caudate and it may be difficult to achieve the same level of neurochemical stimulation over such a wide area with central administration than is possible with systemic drug. However, even with large doses of amphetamine simultaneously infused into both the caudate nucleus and the nucleus accumbens, Robbins *et al.* (1986a) were still only able to obtain moderate levels of stereotypy. The sensitivity of the post-synaptic DA receptors is increased following 6-OHDA lesions of caudate, and an augmentation of apomorphine stereotypy may be seen (Creese and Iversen, 1984). This was confirmed in a recent experiment by Hartgreaves and Randall (1986). They observed dramatic increases in stereotypy induced by peripherally administered apomorphine in rats given bilateral 6-OHDA into the caudate, and, additionally, similar stereotyped behavior could also be seen in the caudate lesioned animals after intracaudate infusions of DA agonists. This behavior was not seen after 6-OHDA lesions of the N. acc., either following peripheral or central administration of DA agonists, although 6-OHDA lesions of the caudate did affect the response to apomorphine infused into the N. acc.

As well as increases in the amount of stereotypy, Hartgreaves and Randall (1986) noted changes in the type of stereotyped behavior shown, particularly licking and grooming-like behavior. The neural substrate of the different elements of stereotypy may not necessarily lie in the caudate. For example, Costall *et al.* (1975) found that 6-OHDA induced lesions of the caudate reduced amphetamine-induced biting, but not sniffing, whereas 6-OHDA lesions of the N. acc. reduced amphetamine-induced sniffing but not biting. On the other hand, increases in apomorphine- and amphetamine-induced stereotyped licking have also been noted after 6-OHDA lesions of ascending noradrenergic neurones caudal to the site of origin of the DA systems (Braestrup, 1977).

In primates elevated levels of "look out" or "checking" behavior have been noted following both intra-accumbens and intra-caudate infusions of amphetamine (Dubach and Bowden, 1983; Annett *et al.*, 1983). These appear to be a form of stereotyped behavior since they are performed in a manner incompatible with appropriate visually-guided behavior (Ridley and Baker, 1983).

3.8. Conditioned Reinforcement

In explanation of the behavioral response to psychomotor stimulant drugs, Hill (1970) suggested that these drugs enhance the effectiveness of conditioned reinforcers. Since that time there has been considerable research linking brain dopamine to the effects of unconditioned reinforcers (see Section 3.9), but the importance of Hill's hypothesis is that enhancement of conditioned reinforcers results in behavior becoming independent of current contingencies of reinforcement. Hill's ideas were based upon the observation that perseveration of responding of a previously reinforced lever press response carried on for much longer in extinction if stimuli associated with the reinforcer, conditioned reinforcers (CRs), continued to be presented. This effect was exaggerated under the methylphenidate-like stimulant, pipradrol, since treated rats responded less than untreated rats in the absence of CRs (Hill, 1970). Subsequently, Robbins *et al.* (1983) trained animals on a visual CR-water association using classical conditioning, and only after the water had been removed, allowed the rats to press a lever reinforced by the CR alone. Pipradrol increased the amount of responding on the CR-reinforced lever but not on a control, unreinforced lever. However, the effects of amphetamine and cocaine were less reliable (Robbins *et al.*, 1983b). Taylor and Robbins (1984) repeated this experiment with infusions of amphetamine into the N. acc., caudate nucleus and thalamus. The enhanced preference for the CR lever was most marked after N. acc. infusions, present to a reduced extent after caudate infusions and entirely absent when the drug was infused into the thalamus. The effect of infusions into the N. acc. could be blocked by prior 6-OHDA lesions of the N. acc. but not by prior lesions of the MVC (Taylor and Robbins, 1986).

3.9. Reinforcement

Psychomotor stimulants have a long history of abuse in humans, and intravenous infusions of these drugs may be used as reinforcers in place of food and water in studies using animal subjects. Electrical stimulation of the brain may also act as a reinforcer, and appears to be dependent for expression on intact ascending DA systems. Such findings led to the suggestion that the ascending DA systems mediated reward (German and Bowden, 1974; Wise, 1982), and the actions of reinforcers in general, including natural reinforcers like food, and non-DAergic drugs such as morphine and heroin. To support this hypothesis, it has been found that 6-OHDA lesions of N. acc. permanently block intravenous administration of cocaine and amphetamine (Roberts *et al.*, 1977,1980; Lyness *et al.*, 1979) but do not affect responding reinforced by heroin, which may be mediated by post-synaptic peptidergic receptors (Pettit *et al.*, 1984). In direct contrast to this, 6-OHDA lesions of the amygdala increase intravenous self-administration of amphetamine (Deminiere *et al.*, 1984). 6-OHDA lesions of the PFC do not affect either the rate or the pattern of responding for intravenous cocaine (Martin-Iverson *et al.*, 1986). Spyraki *et al.* (1982a) reported a correlation between levels of amphetamine-conditioned place preference and DA levels following 6-OHDA lesions to the N. acc., but not to the caudate. However, neither of these lesions attenuated place preference to cocaine. Rats will prefer an environment associated with infusions of amphetamine into N. acc. but not infusions into the DLC (Carr and White, 1983), although 6-OHDA lesions of N. acc. did not affect cocaine-induced place preference (Spyraki *et al.*, 1982b). Infusions of amphetamine into the N. acc. will also reinforce lever responding (Hoebel *et al.*, 1984), as will infusions of morphine into the VTA mediated by peptidergic receptors on the DA neurones (Bozarth and Wise, 1984). In contrast, infusions of amphetamine into the PFC do not act as reinforcers, although infusions of cocaine do. The converse holds true for subcortical areas, in that cocaine will not act as a reinforcer when injected into either the accumbens or the VTA (Goeders and Smith, 1983). The reinforcing effects of cocaine in the PFC are furthermore blocked by 6-OHDA lesions of that structure (Goeders and Smith, 1983). Self-administration could be reinstated by substituting DA for cocaine, but not by substitution with serotonin and the effects of DA could be blocked by the D2 antagonist, sulpiride, all of which suggests that these reinforcing effects were mediated by DA (Goeders and Smith, 1986).

As well as acting as positive reinforcers, maintaining the responses on which they are contingent, stimulant drugs can also punish behavior. Wagner *et al.* (1981) administered methylamphetamine to rats after giving them access to a novel food which consisted of sweetened, condensed milk. Post-ingestive treatment with amphetamine leads to diminished intake of that food upon subsequent re-exposure, a conditioned taste aversion (CTA). This amphetamine CTA may be blocked by treatment with the DA antagonist, pimozide (Grupp, 1977). Wagner *et al.* (1981) demonstrated that treatment with intraventicular 6-OHDA, following DMI and pargyline pretreatments, blocked amphetamine CTA, but not lithium chloride CTA. However, there was widespread loss of DA following this treatment.

Carr and White (1986a) compared the effects of amphetamine infused into the PFC, accumbens, medial and lateral caudate, amygdala and area postrema as a positive reinforcer using place preference, and as a punisher using CTA. As in the earlier experiment noted above, they found a place preference only after accumbens infusions, and a significant CTA was only observed after area postrema infusions. However, although six anatomical locations were investigated, they used the same single dose of amphetamine in all six, apparently assuming equipotency of the drug at all sites, which may be mistaken (see Section 3.4). The possibility remains, therefore, that it might be possible to obtain either effect from other sites using a higher dose of the drug.

3.10. Drug Discrimination

In addition to acting as reinforcers or punishing stimuli, stimulant drugs can also act as discriminative stimuli. In the drug discrimination paradigm, animals are trained to choose one response when treated with vehicle and another equivalent response when treated with drug (usually right and left lever presses or key-peaks). Rats can be trained to discriminate amphetamine from saline, and then can be shown to generalize to cocaine, and, to a lesser extent, apomorphine (Stolerman and D'Mello, 1981). A similar generalization may be obtained from peripheral amphetamine to centrally infused amphetamine.

Neilen and Scheel-Kruger (1986) trained rats to discriminate systemically administered amphetamine from saline. A range of doses of amphetamine were then infused into the accumbens, AVL or ADM caudate on test days. Substantial choice of the drug lever was obtained after intra-accumbens but not after intra-caudate amphetamine. This effect could be blocked by co-infusion of sulpiride.

3.11. Anorectic and Feeding Effects

Aside from its effects on feeding behavior from CTA, amphetamine has a direct effect of suppressing food intake in hungry rats and in humans, its anorectic effect, which may actually result from competition between feeding and increases in activation, LA or stereotypy. Heffner *et al.* (1977) reported that this effect was attenuated by intra-ventricular 6-OHDA. Koob *et al.* (1977) reported that amphetamine-anorexia was unaffected by 6-OHDA lesions to the accumbens, suggesting that the effect of intra-ventricular 6-OHDA may be mediated by the nigrostriatal system, and not linked to increased LA. Indeed, Joyce and Iversen (1984), obtained attenuated anorexic effects following 6-OHDA lesions of anterior caudate even though amphetamine-induced locomotor activity was increased by the lesions. Leibowitz (1975) carried out a study which included amphetamine infusions into a wide range of mesencephalic, diencephalic and telencephalic sites. Insensitive sites were hippocampus, olfactory tubercle, caudate, accumbens, amygdala, septum, thalamus, medial and lateral midbrain tegmentum. The only reliably sensitive site was lateral hypothalamus. However, Carr and White (1986b) compared the anorexigenic effects of a single dose of amphetamine infused into the PFC, accumbens, medial and lateral caudate, amygdala and area postrema. Infusions into the accumbens and amygdala reduced feeding, but infusions into other areas had no effects. Carr and White (1986b) noted that the only agreement between themselves and Leibowitz (1975) was that infusions into the caudate have no anorexigenic effects. Chewing and swallowing result following peripheral and central administration of apomorphine (Ernst, 1967; Costall *et al.*, 1975). 6-OHDA lesions of the N. acc. result in deficits in tongue extension and lap volume (Brimley and Mogenson, 1979), and likewise intra-accumbens infusions of haloperidol disrupt oral motor responses (Jones and Mogenson, 1979). However, as noted in the introduction, 6-OHDA lesions of the nigrostriatal system themselves produce aphasia and adipsia (Ungerstedt, 1971). In fact, Winn *et al.* (1982) have shown that amphetamine infused into MVC actually increased feeding in rats allowed free access to food in the home cage. Such increases in feeding had previously been reported following systemic treatment with amphetamine and apomorphine (Eichler and Antelman, 1977; Blundell and Latham, 1978) but only in rats which had not been food-deprived, in contrast to the conditions required for amphetamine anorexia.

The hypothalamus receives a strong noradrenergic input, and it is this, rather than DA that has been implicated in the hypothalamic mediation of amphetamine-anorexia (Ahlskog, 1974). However, Sahakian *et al.* (1983) made separate 6-OHDA lesions of the dorsal and ventral noradrenergic bundle. They found that neither lesion attenuated amphetamine anorexia.

3.12. Cognitive Effects

Because psychomotor stimulant drugs produce changes in activation, perseveration, switching, and reinforcer effectiveness, it is difficult to demonstrate that apparent changes in cognitive performance are not secondary to changes in these more fundamental processes. Even if the experimental design includes elaborate procedures derived from learning theory such as those used by Solomon and Staton (1982), this possibility is not precluded.

Experiments reporting cognitive deficits following administration of stimulants often fail to ascertain the underlying cause of the deficit, which may not actually be cognitive.

One of the earliest studies involving central infusion of stimulus drugs was Khavari (1968), which compared the effects of intraventricular, intrahippocampal, intrahypothalamic and i.p. amphetamine on lever-press go/no-go alternation. Intraventricular, intrahypothalamic and i.p. amphetamine disrupted the task but intrahippocampal infusions did not. The changes produced by the central administrations resembled those produced by the peripheral drug. To try to rule out changes in locomotor activity, Khavari (1968) also concurrently measured wheel turning; there was no increase. Low doses of systemically administered amphetamine facilitate spontaneous alternation (see Taghzouti *et al.*, 1986), and alternation performance is also affected by catecholamine depletion. 6-OHDA injections into the medial septum facilitate spatial discrimination in a radial arm maze (Harrell *et al.*, 1984). 6-OHDA lesions in the lateral septum have been reported as either facilitating (Galey *et al.*, 1983) or impairing (Taghzouti *et al.*, 1986) performance of spontaneous alternation, and acquisition and reversal of spatial discrimination in a T-maze and impairing performance in the radial arm maze (Simon *et al.*, 1986). Changes in spatial alternation in the T-maze have been reported following 6-OHDA lesions to the accumbens (Taghzouti *et al.*, 1985b), VTA, anteromedial caudate, and PFC (Simon, 1981). Extensive depletion of both NA and DA in the PFC leads to impaired sequential delayed alternation in the operant chamber, although the effects in the T-maze appear less reliable (Ryan and Dunnett, 1985; Ryan, 1987). Ryan (1987) also examined the effects of central infusions of amphetamine, apomorphine or sulpiride into the PFC. These drugs all reduced the likelihood that the rats responded, but did not affect discrimination or memory in operant delayed alternation.

On the other hand, support for the hypothesis that the dopaminergic innervation of the prefrontal cortex plays a role in alternation comes from a study in the rhesus monkey, where selective dopamine depletion of the PFC results in impaired spatial delayed alternation (Brozoski *et al.*, 1979a). Lesions to the same area specifically depleting NA (with relatively little DA depletion) do not alter performance of this task. The dopamine-lesion induced deficit could be reversed following systemic administration of selective agonists including apomorphine or L-DOPA (Brozoski *et al.*, 1979a). Peripheral administration of amphetamine, however, was ineffective (Brozoski *et al.*, 1979b), whereas the NA agonist, clonidine improved all lesion groups (Brozoski *et al.*, 1979a; Arnsten and Goldman-Rakic, 1985). Systemic amphetamine or apomorphine did not alter the performance of controls.

Delayed alternation, as tested in the T-maze or operant chamber examines short-term memory. Long-term memory can be tested using procedures which give the subject a single training experience, following which recall is measured several days or weeks later. Passive avoidance is such a procedure. Martinez *et al.* (1980) investigated the effects of i.p. and intraventricular amphetamine on passive avoidance. They found that peripherally administered amphetamine facilitated retention, an effect which could be reduced by peripherally administered 6-OHDA. Intraventricular amphetamine had no effect. They concluded that the memory-enhancing effects of amphetamine were, like those of many other drugs, at least in part, mediated peripherally. However, Carr and White (1984) compared the effect of amphetamine either peripherally or infused into dorsolateral caudate. In both cases the drug was administered immediately after the establishment of a tone–shock association. Twenty-four hours later they tested memory for the association by measuring suppression of lick by the tone. In such procedures, the test drug is never present during either training or recall testing. Both treatments resulted in enhanced suppression in the test phase.

Post-training intrahippocampal infusions of apomorphine and ergometrine have also been reported as facilitating a discriminated active avoidance (Grecksch and Matthies, 1981), an effect which could be blocked by co-infusion of haloperidol and enhanced by prolonged pretreatment with haloperidol which led to receptor supersensitivity (Honza *et al.*, 1984).

The effects of amphetamine on discrimination performance *per se* are, in most circumstances, secondary to the effects on lower-level functions. The effects appear to be highly variable (Grilly *et al.*, 1980), depend upon the degree of stimulus control (Ksir, 1975; Ksir and Slifer, 1982) and are associated with generalized changes in response likelihood, (Milar, 1981; Spencer *et al.*, 1985), response repetition, (Koek and Slangen, 1983; Saghal and Clinke, 1986) and switching (Evenden and Robbins, 1985). The same also appears to be true for centrally administered amphetamine. Carli and Robbins (personal communication) could not separate changes in lateralized discrimination performance from changes in response bias following amphetamine infused into the MVC and N. acc. Cole and Robbins (1986) examined the effects of both amphetamine i.p. and intra-accumbens on a five choice visual discrimination task. They found that there was no effect of i.p. amphetamine on discrimination performance in intact rats, but an impairment at low doses of the drug following 6-OHDA lesions of the DNAB. A similar effect was observed when the drug was administered directly into the N. acc. This latter effect could be blocked by systemic administration of alpha-flupentixol demonstrating that it was mediated by DA. In contrast, the effects of the drug on premature responses, its activating effect (see Section 3.4), was equivalent in both sham and lesioned rats.

Evidence for a selective effect of amphetamine on discrimination performance has come from Robbins *et al.* (1986b). They used a visual discrimination task in which the rats were required to indicate which of two lights went off first. This has been used in humans as a test of attentional switching (Kristofferson, 1967). Amphetamine-impaired discrimination performance measured by accuracy and reaction time. The effect of the drug on reaction time was abolished by 6-OHDA lesions of the accumbens, but although the effects on choice were attenuated, there was not equivalent normalizing effect.

Further evidence for the involvement of accumbens in attention comes from Solomon and Staton (1982). They used the latent inhibition technique, in which the subjects are preexposed to a stimulus later to be conditioned. During this preconditioning stage, subjects come to ignore the stimulus leading to a retardation in the subsequent conditioning, known as latent inhibition (LI). Solomon and Staton (1982) demonstrated that LI was not present in rats treated with intra-accumbens amphetamine during the pre-conditioning stage. Intra-caudate infusions had no effect.

4. GENERAL DISCUSSION

Table 1 summarizes the cerebral localization of the effects of stimulant drugs described in Section 3. This table should be viewed with considerable caution on several grounds. First, not all areas which might be involved have been tested on all categories of behavior. Second, dose–response determinations have not been performed in many of the studies cited. For both of these reasons there may actually be involvement of the central dopaminergic or noradrenergic systems where none is listed above. Third, the table does not differentiate between the effects of the different stimulant drugs used. Fourth, assertions by the authors about the processes involved in a particular paradigm have not been critically examined. Fifth, many of the studies included in the table are the only ones that have investigated a particular behavior, and a number of these have not been formally published. Sixth, there are a few effects of stimulant drugs, for example the 'paradoxical' effects on punished behavior (Dews and Wenger, 1977) which have not yet been investigated using lesion or central administration techniques. Seventh, treatments used experimental controls such as implantation of infusion cannulae and/or infusions of vehicle, or implantation of grafted tissue into unlesioned animals can cause subjects to behave differently from untreated subjects.

Nevertheless, the overwhelming impression derived from the table is that the majority of the effects of peripherally administered stimulant drugs may be obtained by infusing the drug into the accumbens, or attenuated by lesions to that structure. The only notable departure from this is stimulant-induced stereotypy which may be mediated by the caudate nucleus. Nielsen and Scheel-Kruger (1986) suggest that the reason why the peripheral amphetamine cue may be mimicked by intra-accumbens amphetamine is that 'those aspects of the actions of amphetamine that are related to the 'net' experienced effect of the drug' may be mediated by the accumbens. On the basis of Table 1, it may be possible to go fur-

TABLE 1. *Summary*

Behavior	Involved	Not involved
Locomotor activity	N. acc., MPFC, SPFC, DNAB	Caudate
Asymmetry	Caudate, MPFC	N. acc.
Schedule-induced polydipsia	N. acc.	
Disinhibition	Caudate (lateralized) N. acc. (unlateralized)	
Rate-dependent effects	N. acc. > Caudate >PFC	Supragenual PFC
Perseveration	N. acc., DNAB	Caudate
Switching	N. acc	
Stereotypy	Caudate, D/VNAB	N. acc.
Conditioned reinforcement	N. acc. > Caudate	
Unconditioned reinforcement	N. acc., MPFC	Caudate, Amygdala Area Postrema
Conditioned taste aversion	Area Postrema	Caudate, N. acc. Amygdala
Drug cue	N. acc.	Caudate
Anorexia	LH, Amygdala, N. acc.	Caudate, DNAB, VNAB
Hyperphagia	Caudate	
Short-term memory	Lateral hypothalamus	Hippocampus, MPFC, SPFC
Long-term memory	Caudate, Hippocampus	
Attention	N. acc., DNAB	MVC

The first column in the table lists those aspects of behavior which have been studied using techniques which provide evidence of central localization. The center column lists those structures innervated by the ascending catecholamine systems for which evidence has been found of direct involvement in the central mediation of different aspects of the behavioral response to psychomotor stimulant drugs. The third column lists areas which have been examined experimentally, but which currently do not seem to be involved in the central response to psychomotor stimulants.

ther and suggest that at moderate doses, the observed response to peripherally administered stimulant drugs results solely from the actions of the drug in the accumbens.

In general, the actions of a systemically administered drug are assumed to result from the sum of its actions at many different sites in the central nervous system. However, for this to be true two corollaries must hold, (i) that the pharmacological efficacy of the drug is similar at the different sites, and (ii) that even if the pharmacological efficacy is similar, the relevance to behavior of the actions at the different sites is similar. Neither of these are necessarily true. The different types of dopamine receptors, the presence of autoreceptors, and the density of innervation will all change the pharmacological response to a particular drug at a particular site. Furthermore, modulation of the dopaminergic innervation of a brain area involved in cognitive performance is likely to affect behavior to a lesser extent than an area which is crucial to the motor performance necessary to demonstrate that cognitive performance and, in addition, other aspects of behavior. If the most pharmacologically sensitive site and the most behaviorally important site coincide, then the behavioral effects of a systemically administered drug will exclusively reflect the actions of the drug at that site, and the effects of the drug at other sites will at least be difficult to observe, and may, if ratio between the effective doses is too great, actually be impossible to see. This does not mean, of course, that the less effective sites are irrelevant to normal behavior, since under normal conditions the sites may be functionally independent. A simple example may be that the mesocortical DA system may be functionally independent of the mesolimbic system, and play an independent role in the organisation of behavior. However, because the accumbens is a prepotent site, that role will not be obviously reflected in the actions of systemic administration of DA agonists.

In addition to the localisation of the amphetamine cue, Nielsen and Scheel-Kruger (1986) also found evidence that the LSD cue is also primarily derived from its actions in the accumbens, probably through its actions on the serotonergic system (Nielsen *et al.*, 1985). This raises the possibility that the prepotent site of action of drugs acting on different neurotransmitter systems may be in the same area of the brain. If this is the case, similarities in the actions of apparently very different drugs may not reflect lack of specificity but a common site of action. For example, Ksir (1975) found similar actions of amphetamine and scopolamine on discrimination performance. He suggested that these resulted from non-specific actions of the drug on schedule controlled behavior. However, the similarity may in fact indicate that the predominant site of action for systemic scopolamine is also in the basal ganglia, perhaps in the mid-ventral caudate nucleus (these drugs have been used as antiparkinsonian agents) and that far from being non-specific the similar behavioral effects reflect similar actions of the drugs in the same area of the brain. The similarities found between peripherally administered amphetamine and scopolamine, and crystalline placements of the same drugs into anterior striatum by Neill and Herndon (1978) certainly support this point of view.

Nevertheless, it is also clear that there may be competition between sites of action. The clearest example of this presented here is the behavioral competition between locomotor activity and stereotyped behavior demonstrated by Joyce and Iversen (1984). Their study demonstrated that the expression of locomotor responses to amphetamine mediated by the accumbens is occluded at higher doses of the drug by the occurrence of stereotyped behavior mediated by the caudate nucleus. So, although the accumbens is more sensitive to amphetamine than the caudate, when the latter area is stimulated this prevents the expression of the nucleus accumbens mediated behavior. However, it is as yet unclear whether the competition is between locomotor activity and stereotypy, or between stereotyped locomotor behavior and stereotyped oral and grooming behavior (for discussion, see Lyon and Robbins, 1975).

There is also the possibility that different DA systems may have opposite effects on the same aspects of behavior. For example, at present it is unclear whether the dopaminergic innervation to PFC is inhibitory or excitatory on motor performance. The role of PFC dopamine on LA appears to be inhibitory, and thus contrary to the role played by DA subcortically. However, this conclusion is not supported by experiments on circling behavior, which suggest that the mesocortical DA system exerts an excitatory influence on motor activity similar to that exerted by the nigrostriatal DA system. If the dopaminergic innervation to the PFC was inhibitory, then DA antagonist infusions should result in circling towards the side of higher DA activity, i.e. contralateral circling should be seen rather than the observed ipsilateral circling.

Finally, it is remarkable how little of the behavioral response to psychomotor stimulant drugs can be related to their actions on noradrenaline and serotonin. It is clear from several experiments cited here that NA does have a modulatory effect on the behavioral responses to these drugs, but none of their actions appear to be mediated exclusively by NA or 5-HT, almost all have been obtained or altered by manipulations of the DA systems alone.

In conclusion, most of the diverse behavioral responses to amphetamine may be obtained by infusions into the accumbens. It is suggested that this is the prepotent site of action of this drug. Other stimulant drugs, such as cocaine and apomorphine are relatively less effective at this site, and the differences in behavioral effect between them and amphetamine may reflect this neuroanatomically shifted locus of action. At higher doses of the drugs, the effects at less sensitive sites, e.g. caudate nucleus, may occlude the effects of the drugs in the accumbens. Little if any of the behavioral response to psychomotor stimulants appears to be directly mediated by NA or 5-HT, these other neurotransmitter systems may be modulatory on the primary dopaminergic response.

Acknowledgments—We would like to thank T. W. Robbins and L. E. Annett for their comments on this manuscript, and M. Carli, B. J. Cole, S. B. Dunnett for allowing us to cite unpublished data. J. L. Evenden is supported by a grant from the Medical Research Council, and C. N. Ryan by a studentship from the Science and Engineering Research Council.

REFERENCES

AHLSKOG, J. E. (1974) Food intake and amphetamine anorexia after selective forebrain norepinephrine loss. *Brain Res.* **82**: 211–240.

ANNETT, L. E. and RIDLEY, R. M. (1985) Object discrimination reversal learning following intra-accumbens or caudate amphetamine in the marmoset. *Neurosci. Lett., Suppl.* **21**: 534.

ANNETT, L. E., RIDLEY, R. M., GAMBLE, S. J. and BAKER, H. F. (1983) Behavioural effects of intracerebral amphetamine in the marmoset. *Psychopharmacology* **81**: 18–23.

ARCHER, T., FREDRIKSSON, A., JONSSON, G., LEWANDER, T., MOHAMMED, A. K., ROSS, S.B. and SODERBERG, U. (1986) Central noradrenaline depletion antagonizes aspects of d-amphetamine-induced hyperactivity in the rat. *Psychopharmacology* **88**: 141–146.

ARNSTEN, A. F. T. and GOLDMAN-RAKIC, P. S. (1985) alpha-2-adrenergic mechanisms in prefrontal cortex associated with cognitive decline in aged nonhuman primates. *Science* **230**: 1273–1276.

BJORKLUND, A. and LINDVALL, O. (1984) Dopamine-containing cells in the CNS. In: *Handbook of Chemical Neuroanatomy*, pp. 55–122, BJORKLUND, A. and HOKFELT, T. (eds) Elsevier, Amsterdam.

BJORKLUND, A., DUNNETT, S. B., STENEVI, U., LEWIS, M. E. and IVERSEN, S. D. (1980) Reinnervation of the denervated striatum by substantia nigra transplants: Functional consequences as revealed by pharmacological and sensorimotor testing. *Brain Res.* **199**: 307–333.

BLUNDELL, J. E. and LATHAM, C. J. (1978) Pharmacological manipulation of feeding behavior: Possible influences of serotonin and dopamine on food intake. In: *Central Mechanisms of Anorectic Drugs*, pp. 83–109, GARATTINI, S. and SAMANIN, R. (eds) Raven Press, New York.

BOZARTH, M. A. and WISE, R. A. (1981) Intracranial self-administration of morphine into the ventral tegmental area. *Life Sci.* **28**: 551–558.

BRAESTRUP, C. (1977) Changes in drug-induced stereotyped behavior after 6-OHDA lesions in noradrenaline neurones. *Psychopharmacology* **51**: 199–204.

BRIMLEY, C. C. and MOGENSON, G. J. (1979) Oral motor deficits following lesions of the central nervous system in rats. *Am. J. Physiol.* **237**: R126–R131.

BROZOSKI, T. J., BROWN, R. M. ROSVOLD, H. E. and GOLDMAN, P. S. (1979a) Cognitive deficit caused by regional depletion of dopamine in prefrontal cortex of rhesus monkey. *Science* **205**: 929–932.

BROZOSKI, T. J., BROWN, R. M., PTAK, J. and GOLDMAN, P. S. (1979b) Dopamine in prefrontal cortex of rhesus monkeys: Evidence for a role in cognitive function. In: *Catecholamines: Basic and Clinical Frontiers*, pp. 1681–1683, USDIN, E., KOPIN, I. J. and BARCHAS, J. (eds) Pergamon Press, New York.

BRUTO, V., BEAUCHAMP, C., ZACHARKO, R. M. and ANISMAN, H. (1984) Amphetamine-induced perseverative behavior in a radial arm maze following DSP4 or 6-OHDA pretreatment. *Psychopharmacology* **83**: 62–69.

BURNS, R. S., CHIUEH, C. C., MARKEY, S. P., EBERT, M. H., JACOBOWITZ, D. M. and KOPIN, I. J. (1983) A primate model of parkinsonism: Selective destruction of dopaminergic neurones in the pars compacta of the substantia nigra by *N*-methyl-4-phenyl-1,2,3,6-tetrahydropyridine. *Proc. Natl. Acad. Sci. U.S.A.* **80**: 4546–4550.

CARLI, M., EVENDEN, J. L. and ROBBINS, T. W. (1985) Depletion of unilateral striatal dopamine impairs initiation of contralateral actions and not sensory attention. *Nature* **313**: 679–682.

CARR, G. D. and WHITE, M. N. (1983) Conditioned place preference from intra-accumbens but not intra-caudate amphetamine injections. *Life Sci.* **33**: 2551–2557.

CARR, G. D. and WHITE, N. M. (1984) The relationship between stereotypy and memory improvement produced by amphetamine. *Psychopharmacology* **82**: 203–209.

CARR, G. D. and WHITE, N. M. (1986a) Anatomical dissociation of amphetamine's rewarding and aversive effects: An intracranial microinjection study. *Psychopharmacology* **89**: 340–346.

CARR, G. D. and WHITE, M. N. (1986b) Contributions of dopamine terminal areas to amphetamine-induced anorexia. *Pharmacol. Biochem. Behav.* **25**: 17–22.

CARTER, C. J. and PYCOCK, C. J. (1980) Behavioral and biochemical effects of dopamine and noradrenaline depletion within the medial prefrontal cortex of the rat. *Brain Res.* **192**: 163–176.

COLE, B. J. and ROBBINS, T. W. (1986) Amphetamine impairs the discriminative performance of rats with dorsal noradrenergic bundle lesions on a 5-choice serial reaction time task: New evidence for central dopaminergic-noradrenergic interactions. *Behav. Neurosci.* (in press).

COOLS, A. R. (1986) Mesolimbic dopamine and its control of locomotor activity in rats: Differences in pharmacology and light/dark periodicity between the olfactory tubercle and the nucleus accumbens. *Psychopharmacology* **88**: 451–459.

COSTALL, B. and NAYLOR, R. J. (1977) Differentiation of the dopaminergic mechanisms mediating stereotyped behavior and hyperactivity in the nucleus accumbens and caudate putamen. *J. Pharm. Pharmacol.* **29**: 337–342.

COSTALL, B., NAYLOR, R. J. and NEIMEYER, J. L. (1975) Differences in the nature of the stereotyped behaviour induced by apomorphine derivatives in the rat and in their actions in extrapyramidal and mesolimbic brain areas. *Eur. J. Pharmacol.* **31**: 1–16.

COSTALL, B., KELLEY, M. E. and NAYLOR, R. J. (1983) The production of asymmetry and circling behaviour following unilateral, intrastriatal administration of neuroleptic agents: A comparison of abilities to antagonise striatal function. *Eur. J. Pharmacol.* **96**: 79–86.

COSTALL, B., ENIOJUKAN, J. F. and NAYLOR, R. J. (1985) Dopamine agonist action in mesolimbic, cortical and extrapyramidal areas to modify spontaneous climbing behaviour of the mouse. *Psychopharmacology* **86**: 452–457.

CREESE, I. (1983) *Stimulants: Neurochemical, Behavioral and Clinical Perspectives.* Raven Press, New York.

CREESE, I. and IVERSEN, S. D. (1984) The role of forebrain dopamine systems in amphetamine induced stereotyped behavior in the rat. *Psychopharmacologia* (*Berlin*) **39**: 345–357.

DEMINIERE, J. M., TAGHZOUTI, K., LE MOAL, M. and SIMON, H. (1984) Lesion of the meso-amygdala dopaminergic projection increases (+)-amphetamine self-administration and general activation in the rat. *Neurosci. Letts. S***18**, 202.

DEWS, P. B. and WENGER, G. R. (1977) Rate-dependency of the behavioral effects of amphetamine. In: *Advances in Behavioral Pharmacology*, Vol. 1, pp. 167–227, THOMPSON, T. and DEWS, P. B. (eds) Academic Press, New York.

DILL, R. E., JONES, D. L., GILLIN, C. and MURPHY, G. (1979) Comparison of behavioral effects of systemic L-DOPA and Intracranial dopamine in mesolimbic forebrain of non-human primates. *Pharmacol. Biochem. Behav.* **10**: 711–716.

DOURISH, C. T. (1985) Local application of beta-phenylethylamine to the caudate nucleus of the rat elicits locomotor stimulation. *Pharmacol. Biochem. Behav.* **22**: 159–162.

DUBACH, M. F. and BOWDEN, D. M. (1983) Response to intracerebral dopamine injection as a model of schizophrenic symptomatology. In: *Ethopharmacology: Primate Models of Neuropsychiatric Disorders*, pp. 157–184, MICZEK, K. (ed.) Alan R. Liss, New York.

DUNN, A. J., ALPERT, J. E. and IVERSEN, S. D. (1984) Dopamine denervation of frontal cortex or nucleus accumbens does not affect ACTH-induced grooming behaviour. *Behav. Brain Res.* **12**: 307–315.

DUNNETT, S. B. (1981) *Functional Organisation of the Neostriatum.* Unpublished doctoral dissertation, University of Cambridge.

DUNNETT, S. B. and IVERSEN, S. D. (1982) Neurotoxin lesions of ventrolateral but not anteriomedial neostriatum in rats impair differential reinforcement of low rates (DRL) performance. *Behav. Brain Res.* **6**: 213–226.

DUNNETT, S. B., BJORKLUND, A., SCHMIDT, R. H., STENEVI, U. and IVERSEN, S. D. (1983) Intracerebral grafting of neuronal cell suspensions. IV. Behavioural recovery in rats with unilateral implants of nigral cell suspensions in different forebrain sites. *Acta Physiol. Scand., Suppl.* **522**: 29–37.

EICHLER, A. J. and ANTELMAN, S. M. (1977) Apomorphine: Feeding or anorexia depending on internal state. *Commun. Psychopharmacol.* **1**: 533–540.

ELKHAWAD, A. O. and WOODRUFF, G. N. (1976) Studies on the behavioural pharmacology of a cyclic analogue of dopamine following its injection into the brains of conscious rats. *Br. J. Pharmacol.* **54**: 107–114.

ERNST, A. M. (1967) Mode of action of apomorphine and dexamphetamine on gnawing compulsions in rats. *Psychopharmacologia* **10**: 316–323.

EVENDEN, J. L. (1984) *A Behavioural and Pharmacological Analysis of Response Selection.* Unpublished doctoral dissertation, University of Cambridge.

EVENDEN, J. L. and ROBBINS, T. W. (1983) Increased response switching, perseveration and perseverative switching following d-amphetamine in the rat. *Psychopharmacology* **80**: 67–73.

EVENDEN, J. L. and ROBBINS, T. W. (1985) The effects of d-amphetamine, chlordiazepoxide and alpha-flupenthixol on food-reinforced tracking of a visual stimulus by rats. *Psychopharmacology* **85**: 361–366.

FINK, J. S. and SMITH, G. P. (1980) Relationships between selective denervation of dopamine terminal fields in the anterior forebrain and behavioral responses to amphetamine and apomorphine. *Brain Res.* **201**: 107–127.

FREED, W. J., KO, G. N., NIEHOFF, D. L., KUHAR M. J., HOFFER, B. J., OLSON, L., CANNON-SPOOR, H. E., MORIHISA, J. M. and WYATT, R. J. (1983) Normalisation of spiroperidol binding in denervated rat striatum by hologous grafts of substantia nigra. *Science* **222**: 937–939.

FUXE, K. (1965) Evidence for the existence of monoamine neurones in the central nervous system. IV. Distribution of monoamine nerve terminals in the central system. *Acta. Physiol. Scand.* **64** (Suppl. 247): 39–45.

GALEY, D., DURKIN, T., SIFAKIS, G., KEMPF, E. and JAFFARD, R. (1985) Facilitation of spontaneous and learned spatial behaviours following 6-hydroxydopamine lesions of the lateral septum: A cholinergic hypothesis. *Brain Res.* **340**: 171–174.

GERMAN, D. C. and BOWDEN, D. M. (1974) Catecholamine systems as the neural substrate for intra-cranial self-stimulation: A hypothesis. *Brain Res.* **73**: 381–419.

GLICK, S. D., JERUSSI, T. P. and ZIMMERBERG, B. (1977) Behavioral and neuropharmacological correlates of nigrostriatal dopamine asymmetry in the rat. In: *Lateralization in the Nervous System*, pp. 213–250, HARNAD, S., DOTY, R.W., GOLDSTEIN, L. JAYNES, J. and KRAUTHAMER, G. (eds) Academic Press, New York.

GOEDERS, N. E. and SMITH, J. E. (1983) Cortical dopaminergic involvement in cocaine reinforcement. *Science* **221**: 773–775.

GOEDERS, N. E. and SMITH, J.E. (1986) Reinforcing properties of cocaine in the media prefrontal cortex: Primary action on presynaptic dopaminergic terminals. *Pharmacol. Biochem. Behav.* **25**: 191–199.

GRECKSH, G. and MATTHIES, H. (1981) The role of dopaminergic mechanisms in the rat hippocampus for the consolidation in a brightness discrimination. *Psychopharmacology* **75**: 165–168.

GRILLY, D. M., GENOVESE, R. F., NOVAK, M. J. (1980) Effects of morphine, d-amphetamine and pentobarbital on shock and light discrimination performance in rats. *Psychopharmacology* **70**: 213–217.

GRUPP, L. A. (1977) Effects of pimozide on the acquisition, maintenance and extinction of an amphetamine-induced taste aversion. *Psychopharmacology* **53**: 235–242.

HARRELL, L. E., BARLOW, T. S., MILLER, M., HARING, J. H. and DAVIS, J. N. (1984) Facilitated reversal of a spatial memory task by medial septal injections of 6-hydroxydopamine. *Exp. Neurol.* **85**: 69–77.

HARTGREAVES, S. L. and RANDALL, P. K. (1986) Dopamine agonist-induced stereotypic grooming and self-mutilation following striatal dopamine depletion. *Psychopharmacology* **90**: 358–363.

HEFFNER, T. G., ZIGMOND, M. J. and STRICKER, E. M. (1977) Effects of dopaminergic agonists and antagonists on feeding in intact and 6-hydroxydopamine-treated rats. *J. Pharmacol. Exp. Therap.* **201**: 386–399.

HERMAN, J.-P., CHOULLI, K. and LE MOAL, M. (1985) Hyper-reactivity to amphetamine in rats with dopaminergic grafts. *Exp. Brain Res.* **60**: 521–526.

HERVE, D., BLANC, G., GLOWINSKI, J. and TASSIN, J.-P. (1982) Reduction of dopamine utilization in the prefrontal cortex but not in the nucleus accumbens after selective destruction of noradrenergic fibres innervating the ventral tegmental area. *Brain Res.* **237**: 510–516.

HERVE, D., STUDLER, J.-M., BLANC, G., GLOWINSKI, J. and TASSIN, J.-P. (1986) Partial protection by desmethylimipramine of the mesocortical dopamine neurones from the neurotoxic effect of 6-hydroxydopamine injected in ventral mesencephalic tegmentum. The role of noradrenergic innervation. *Brain Res* **383**:47–53.

HILL, R. T. (1970) Facilitation of conditioned reinforcement as a mechanism of psychomotor stimulation. In: *Amphetamine and Related Compounds*, pp. 781–795, COSTA, E. and GARATTINI, S. (eds) Raven Press, New York.

HJORTH, S., CARLSSON, A., CLARK, D., SVENSSON, K., WIKSTROM, H., SANCHEZ, D., LINDBERG, P., HACKSELL, U., ARVIDSSON, L.-E., JOHANSSON, A. and NILSSON, J. L. G. (1983) Central dopamine receptor agonist and antagonist actions of the enantiomers of 3-PPP. *Psychopharmacology* **81**: 89–99.

HOEBEL, B. G., MONACO, A. P., HERNANDEZ, L., AULISI, E. F., STANLEY, B. G. and LENARD, L. (1983) Self-injection of amphetamine directly into the brain. *Psychopharmacology* **81**: 158–163.

Honza, R., Schumacher, H., Klauck, A., Grecksch, G., and Matthies, H. (1984) Effect of apomorphine on retention of a brightness discrimination in dopamine supersensitive rats. *Behav. Neur. Biol.* **41**: 23–29.

Jackson, D. M., Anden, N.-E. and Dahlstrom, A. (1975) A functional effect of dopamine in the nucleus accumbens and in some other dopamine-rich parts of the rat brain. *Psychopharmacology* **45**: 139–149.

Jaim-Etcheverry, G. and Zeiher, L. M. (1980) DSP-4: A novel compound with neurotoxic effects on noradrenaline neurones of adult and developing rats. *Brain Res.* **188**: 513–523.

Jones, D. L. and Mogenson, G. J. (1979) Oral-motor performance following central dopamine receptor blockade. *Eur. J. Pharmacol.* **59**: 11–21.

Joyce, E. M. and Iversen, S. D. (1984) Dissociable effects of 6-OHDA-induced lesions of neostriatum on anorexia, locomotor activity and stereotypy: The role of behavioural competition. *Psychopharmacology* **83**: 363–366.

Joyce, J. N. and Van Hartesveldt, C. (1984) Rotation and postural deviation elicited by microinjections of dopamine into medial and lateral regions of dorsal striatum. *Pharmacol. Biochem. Behav.* **21**: 979–981.

Joyce, E. M., Stinus, L. and Iversen, S. D. (1983) Effects of injections of 6-OHDA into either nucleus accumbens septi or prefrontal cortex on spontaneous and drug-induced activity. *Neuropharmacology* **22**: 1141–1145.

Kelleher, R. T. (1977) Psychomotor stimulants. In: *Drug Abuse: The Clinical and Basic Aspects*, pp. 116–147, Pradhan, S. N. and Dutta, S. N. (eds) C. V. Mosby Company, St Louis, Missouri.

Kelley, A. E., Winnock, M. and Stinus, L. (1986) Amphetamine, apomorphine and investigatory behavior in the rat: Analysis of the structure and pattern of responses. *Psychopharmacology* **86**: 66–74.

Kelly, P. H. (1975) Unilateral 6-hydroxydopamine lesions of nigrostriatal or mesolimbic dopamine-containing terminals and the drug-induced rotation of rats. *Brain Res.* **100**: 163–169.

Kelly, P. H. and Moore, K. E. (1976) Mesolimbic dopamine neurones in the rotational model of nigrostriatal function. *Nature* **263**: 695–696.

Kelly, P. H., Seviour, P. W. and Iversen, S. D. (1975) Amphetamine and apomorphine responses in the rat following 6-OHDA lesions of the nucleus accumbens septi and corpus striatum. *Brain Res.* **94**: 507–522.

Khavari, K. A. (1968) Effects of central versus intraperitoneal d-amphetamine administration on learned behavior. *J. Comp. Physiol. Psychol.* **68**: 226–234.

Koek, W. and Slangen, J. L. (1983) Effects of d-amphetamine and morphine on discrimination: Signal detection analysis and assessment of response repetition in the performance deficits. *Psychopharmacology* **80**: 125–128.

Koob, G. F., Riley, S. J., Smith, C. and Robbins, T. W. (1977) Effects of 6-hydroxydopamine lesions of the nucleus accumbens septi and olfactory tubercle on feeding, locomotor activity and amphetamine anorexia in the rat. *J. Comp. Physiol. Psychol.* **92**: 917–927.

Koob, G. F., Simon, H., Herman, J. P. and Le Moal, M. (1984) Neuroleptic-like disruption of the conditioned avoidance response requires destruction of both the mesolimbic and nigrostriatal dopamine systems. *Brain Res.* **303**: 319–329.

Kristofferson, A. B. (1967) Attention and psychological time. *Acta Psychologica* **27**: 93–100.

Ksir, C. (1975) Scopolamine and amphetamine effects on discrimination: Interaction with stimulus control. *Psychopharmacology* **43**: 37–41.

Ksir, C. and Slifer, B. (1982) Drug effect on discrimination performance at two levels of stimulus control. *Psychopharmacology* **76**: 286–290.

Kuczenski, R. (1983) Biochemical actions of amphetamine and other stimulants. In: *Stimulants: Neurochemical, Behavioral and Clinical Perspectives*, pp. 31–61, Creese, I. (ed.) Raven Press, New York.

Kulig, B. M. and Calhoun, W. (1972) Enhancement of successive discrimination reversal learning by methamphetamine. *Psychopharmacology* **27**: 233–240.

Laties, V. G. and Weiss, B. (1966) Performance enhancement by the amphetamines: A new appraisal. *Excerpt Medica Int. Congr.* **129**: 800–808.

Laties, V. G. and Weiss, B. (1981) The amphetamine margin in sports. *Fed. Proc.* **40**: 2689–2692.

Leibowitz, S. F. (1975) Amphetamine: Possible site and mode of action for producing anorexia in the rat. *Brain Res.* **84**: 160–167.

Levine, T. E., Erinoff, L., Dregits, D. P. and Seiden, L. S. (1980) Effects of neonatal and adult 6-hydroxydopamine treatment on random interval behavior. *Pharmacol. Biochem. Behav.* **12**: 281–285.

Ljungberg, T. and Ungerstedt, U. (1976) Reinstatement of eating by dopamine agonists in aphagic dopamine denervated rats. *Physiol. Behav.* **16**: 277–283.

Lyness, W. H., Friedle, N. M. and Moore, K. E. (1979) Destruction of dopaminergic nerve terminals in nucleus accumbens: Effects of d-amphetamine self-stimulation. *Pharmacol. Biochem. Behav.* **11**: 553–556.

Lyon, M. and Robbins, T. W. (1975) The action of central nervous system stimulant drugs: A general theory concerning amphetamine effects. In: *Current Developments in Psychopharmacology*, Vol. 2, pp. 80–163, Essman, W. B. and Valzelli, L. (eds) Spectrum, New York.

Martin-Iverson, M. T., Szostak, C. and Fibiger, H. C. (1986) 6-Hydroxydopamine lesions of the medial prefrontal cortex fail to influence intravenous self-administration of cocaine. *Psychopharmacology* **88**: 310–314.

Martinez, J. L., Jensen, R. A., Messing, R. B., Vasquez, B. J., Soumireu-Mourat, B., Geddes, D., Liang, K. C. and McGaugh, J. L. (1980) Central and peripheral actions of amphetamine on memory storage. *Brain Res.* **182**: 157–166.

Milar, K. S. (1981) Cholinergic drug effects on visual discriminations: A signal detection analysis. *Psychopharmacology* **74**: 383–388.

Mitchell, I. J., Cross, A. J., Sambrook, M. A. and Crossman, A. R. (1985) Sites of the neurotoxic action of 1-methyl-4-phenyl-1,2,3,6-tetrahydropyridine in the macaque monkey include the ventral tegmental area and the locus coeruleus. *Neurosci. Lett.* **61**: 195–200.

Morency, M. A., Stewart, R. J. and Beninger, R. J. (1985) Effects of unilateral microinjection of sulpiride into the medial prefrontal cortex on circling behavior of rats. *Prog. Neuro-Psychopharmacol. Biol. Psychiat.* **9**: 735–738.

MYERS, R. D. (1974) *Handbook of Chemical Stimulation of the Brain*. Van Nostrand Rheinhold, New York.

MYERS, R. D. and HOCH, D. B. (1978) 14C-Dopamine microinjected into the brain stem of the rat: Dispersion kinetics, site content and functional dose. *Brain Res. Bull.* **3**: 601–609.

NEILL, D. B. and HERNDON, J. G. (1978) Anatomical specificity within rat striatum for dopaminergic modulation of DRL responding and activity. *Brain Res.* **153**: 529–538.

NIELSEN, E. B. and SCHEEL-KRUGER, J. (1986) Cueing effects of amphetamine and LSD: Elicitation by direct microinjection of the drugs into the nucleus accumbens. *Eur. J. Pharmacol.* **125**: 85–92.

NIELSEN, E. B., GINN, S. R., CUNNINGHAM, K. A. and APPEL, J. B. (1985) Antagonism of the LSD cue by putative serotonin antagonists: Relationship to inhibition of in vivo (^{3}H)Spiroperidol binding. *Behav. Brain Res.* **16**: 171–176.

NIETO, J., MAKLOUF, C. and RODRIGUEZ, R. (1979) d-Amphetamine effects on behavior produced by periodic food deliveries in the rat. *Pharmacol. Biochem. Behav.* **11**: 423–430.

OADES, R. D. (1981) Dopaminergic agonistic and antagonistic drugs in the ventral tegmentum inhibit and facilitate changes in food-search behaviour. *Neurosci. Lett.* **27**: 75–80.

OADES, R. D., TAGHZOUTI, K., SIMON, H. and LE MOAL, M. (1985) Dopamine-sensitive alternation and collateral behaviour in a Y-maze: Effects of d-amphetamine and haloperidol. *Psychopharmacology* **85**: 123–128.

PETTIT, H. O., ETTENBERG, A., BLOOM, F. E. and KOOB, G. F. (1984) Destruction of dopamine in the nucleus accumbens attenuates cocaine but not heroin self-administration in rat. *Psychopharmacology* **84**: 167–173.

PIJNENBURG, A. J. J., HONIG, W. M. M. and VAN ROSSUM, J. M. (1975) Effects of antagonists upon locomotor stimulation induced by injection of dopamine and noradrenaline into the nucleus accumbens of nialamide-pretreated rats. *Psychopharmacologia (Berlin)* **41**:175–180.

Pijnenburg, A. J. J., Honig, W. M. M., Van der Heyden, J. A. M. and VAN ROSSUM, J. M. (1976) Effects of chemical stimulation of the mesolimbic dopamine system on locomotor activity. *Eur. J. Pharmacol.* **35**: 45–58.

PONCELET, M., CHERMAT, R., SOUBRIE, P. and SIMON, P. (1983) The progressive ratio schedule as a model for studying the psychomotor stimulant activity of drugs in the rat. *Psychopharmacology* **80**: 184–189.

PYCOCK, C. J., DONALDSON, I. M. and MARSDEN, C. D. (1975) Circling behaviour produced by unilateral lesions in the region of the locus coeruleus in rats. *Brain Res.* **97**: 317–329.

PYCOCK, C. J., KERWIN, R. W. and CARTER, C. J. (1980) Effect of lesion of cortical dopamine terminals on subcortical dopamine receptors in rats. *Nature* **286**:74–76.

RIDLEY, R. M. and BAKER, H. F. (1983) Is there a relationship between social isolation, cognitive inflexibility and behavioral stereotypy? An analysis of the effects of amphetamine in the marmoset. In: *Ethopharmacology: Primate Models of Neuropsychiatric Disorders*, pp. 191–235, MICZEK, K. (ed.) Alan R. Liss, New York.

RIDLEY, R. M., HAYSTEAD, T. A. J. and BAKER, H. F. (1981) An involvement of dopamine in higher order choice mechanisms in the monkey. *Psychopharmacology* **72**: 173–177.

ROBBINS, T. W. and KOOB, G. F. (1980) Selective disruption of displacement behavior by lesions of the mesolimbic dopamine system. *Nature (London)* **285**: 409–412.

ROBBINS, T. W. and WATSON, B. A. (1981) Effects of d-amphetamine on response repetition and win-stay behaviour in the rat. In: *Quantification of Steady-State Operant Behaviour*, pp. 441–444, BRADSHAW, C. M., SZABADI, E. and LOWE, C. F. (eds) Elsevier-North Holland, Amsterdam.

ROBBINS, T. W., ROBERTS, D. C. S. and KOOB, G. F. (1983a) Effects of d-amphetamine and apomorphine upon operant behaviour and schedule-induced licking in rats with 6-hydroxydopamine induced lesions of the nucleus accumbens. *J. Pharmacol. Exp. Ther.* **222**: 662–673.

ROBBINS, T. W., WATSON, B. A., GASKIN, M. and ENNIS, C. (1983b) Contrasting interactions of pipradrol, d-amphetamine, cocaine, cocaine analogues, apomorphine and other drugs with conditioned reinforcement. *Psychopharmacology* **80**: 113–119.

ROBBINS, T. W., MITTLEMAN, G., O'BRIEN, J. and WINN, P. (1986a) The neuropsychological significance of stereotypy induced by stimulant drugs. In: *Neuropsychology of Stereotypy*, COOPER, S. J. and DOURISH, C. T. (eds) Oxford University Press, Oxford.

ROBBINS, T. W., EVENDEN, J. L., KSIR, C., READING, P., WOOD, S. and CARLI, M. (1986b) The effects of d-amphetamine, alpha-flupenthixol, and mesolimbic dopamine depletion on a test of attentional switching in the rat. *Psychopharmacology* **90**: 72–78.

ROBERTS, D. C. S., CORCORAN, M. E. and FIBIGER, H. C. (1977) On the role of the ascending catecholaminergic systems in intravenous self-administration of cocaine. *Pharmacol. Biochem. Behav.* **6**: 615–620.

ROBERTS, D. C. S., KOOB, G. F., KLONOFF, P. and FIBIGER, H. C. (1980) Extinction and recovery of cocaine self-administration following 6-OHDA lesions of nucleus accumbens. *Physiol. Biochem. Behav.* **12**: 781–787.

RYAN, C. N. (1987) *An Analysis of the Functional Role of the Mesocortical Dopamine System*. Unpublished doctoral dissertation, University of Cambridge.

RYAN, C. N. and DUNNETT, S. B. (1985) A comparison of 6-OHDA and aspirative lesions on alternation learning and locomotor activity tests in rats. *Neurosci. Letts. Suppl.* **22**: S601.

RYAN, C. N. and DUNNETT, S. B. (1986) Attenuated acquisition of schedule-induced polydipsia following 6-hydroxydopamine injections into the medial prefrontal cortex of rats. *Soc. Neurosci. Abs.* **12**: 309.3.

SAHAKIAN, B. J., WINN, P., ROBBINS, T. W., DEELEY, R. J., EVERITT, B. J., DUNN, L. T., WALLACE, M. and JAMES, W. P. T. (1983) Changes in body weight and food-related behaviour by destruction of the ventral or dorsal noradrenergic bundle in the rat. *Neuroscience* **10**: 1405–1420.

SAGHAL, A. and CLINCKE, G. H. C. (1986) A comparison of different methods of assessing patterns of responding in discrete trial choice procedures. *Psychopharmacology* **87**: 374–377.

SCHEEL-KRUGER, J. (1971) Comparative studies of various amphetamine analogues demonstrating different interactions with the metabolism of the catecholamines in the brain. *Eur. J. Pharmacol.* **14**: 47–59.

SEEMAN, P. (1980) Brain dopamine receptors. *Pharmacol. Rev.* **32**: 229–313.

SEEMAN, P., GRIGORADIS, D., GEORGE, S. R., WATANABE, M. and ULPIAN, C. (1986) Functional states of dopamine receptors. In: *Dopaminergic Systems and Their Regulation*, pp. 97–110, WOODRUFF, G. N., POAT, J. A. and ROBERTS, P. J. (eds) Macmillan, London.

SIMON, H. (1981) Neurones dopaminergiques A10 et système frontale. *J. Physiol. Paris* **77**: 81–95.

SIMON, H., TAGHZOUTI, K. and LE MOAL, M. (1986) Deficits in spatial memory tasks following lesions of septal dopaminergic terminals in the rat. *Behav. Brain Res.* **19**: 7–16.

SOLOMON, P. R. and STATON, D. M. (1982) Differential effects of microinjections of d-amphetamine into the nucleus accumbens or the caudate putamen on the rat's ability to ignore an irrelevant stimulus. *Biol. Psychi.* **17**: 743–756.

SPENCER, D. G., PONTECORVO, M. J. and HEISE, G. A. (1985) Central cholinergic involvement in working memory: Effects of scopolamine on continuous nonmatching and discrimination performance in the rat. *Behav. Neurosci.* **99**: 1049–1065.

SPYRAKI, C., FIBIGER, H. C. and PHILLIPS, A. G. (1982a) Dopaminergic substrates of amphetamine-induced place preference conditioning. *Brain Res.* **253**: 185–193.

SPYRAKI, C., FIBIGER, H. C. and PHILLIPS, A. G. (1982b) Cocaine-induced place preference conditioning: Lack of effects of neuroleptics and 6-hydroxydopamine lesions. *Brain Res.* **253**: 195–203.

STAHLE, L. and UNGERSTEDT, U. (1986) Effects of neuroleptic drugs on the inhibition of exploratory behavior induced by a low dose of apomorphine: Implications for the identity of dopamine receptors. *Pharmacol. Biochem. Behav.* **25**: 473–480.

STATON, D. M. and SOLOMON, P. R. (1984) Microinjections of d-amphetamine into the nucleus accumbens and caudate putamen differentially affect stereotypy and locomotion in the rat. *Physiol. Psychol.* **12**: 159–162.

STEWART, R. J., MORENCY, M. A. and BENINGER, R. J. (1985) Differential effects of intrafrontocortical microinjections of dopamine agonists and antagonists on circling behavior of rats. *Behav. Brain Res.* **17**: 67–72.

STOLERMAN, I. P. and D'MELLO, G. D. (1981) Role of training conditions in discrimination of central nervous system stimulants by rats. *Psychopharmacology* **73**: 295–303.

SWERDLOW, N. R., VACCARINO, F. J., AMALRIC, M. and KOOB, G. F. (1986) The neural substrates for the motor-activating properties of psychostimulants: A review of recent findings. *Pharmacol. Biochem. Behav.* **25**: 233–248.

TAGHZOUTI, K., SIMON, H., TAZI, A., DANTZER, R. and LE MOAL, M. (1985a) The effect of 6-OHDA lesions of the lateral septum on schedule-induced polydipsia. *Behav. Brain Res.* **15**: 1–8.

TAGHZOUTI, K., LOUILOT, A., HERMAN, J. P., LE MOAL, M. AND SIMON, H. (1985b) Alternation behavior, spatial discrimination, and reversal disturbances following 6-hydroxydopamine lesions in the nucleus accumbens of the rat. *Behav. Neural Biol.* **44**: 354–363.

TAGHZOUTI, K., SIMON, H. and LE MOAL, M. (1986) Disturbances in exploratory behavior and functional recovery in the Y and radial mazes following dopamine depletion of the lateral septum. *Behav. Neural Biol.* **45**: 48–56.

TASSIN, J. P., STINUS, L., SIMON, H., BLANC, G., THIERRY, A. M., LE MOAL, M., CARDO, B. and GLOWINSKI, J. (1978) Relationship between the locomotor activity induced by A10 lesions and the destruction of frontocortical dopaminergic innervation in the rat. *Brain Res.* **141**: 267–281.

TAYLOR, J. R. and ROBBINS, T. W. (1984) Enhanced behavioural control by conditioned reinforcers following microinjections of d-amphetamine into the nucleus accumbens. *Psychopharmacology* **84**: 405–412.

TAYLOR, J. R. and ROBBINS, T. W. (1986) 6-hydroxydopamine lesions of the nucleus accumbens, but not of the caudate nucleus, attenuate enhanced responding with reward-related stimuli produced by intra-accumbens d-amphetamine. *Psychopharmacology* **90**: 390–397.

UNGERSTEDT, U. (1971). Adipsia and aphagia after 6-hydroxydopamine induced degeneration of the nigro-striatal dopamine system. *Acta Physiol. Scand., Suppl.* **367**: 69–93.

UNGERSTEDT, U., BUTCHER, L. L., BUTCHER, S. G., ANDEN, N.-E. and FUXE, K. (1969) Direct chemical stimulation of dopaminergic mechanisms in the neostriatum of the rat. *Brain Res.* **14**: 461–471.

VACCARINO, F. J. and FRANKLIN, K. B. J. (1984) Opposite locomotor asymmetries elicited from the medial and lateral SN by modulation of SN DA receptors. *Pharmacol. Biochem. Behav.* **21**: 73–77.

VAN DER GUGTEN, J., DE BEUN, R., KOEK, W. and DE BRUIN, J. P. C. (1986) The prefrontal cortex and effects of dopaminergic agents on exploratory and locomotor activities in rats. *Psychopharmacology* **89**: S37.

VIRJMOED-DE VRIES, M. C. and COOLS, A. R. (1986) Differential effects of striatal injections of dopaminergic, cholinergic and GABAergic drugs upon swimming behavior of rats. *Brain Res.* **364**: 77–90.

WAGNER, G. C., FOLTIN, R. W., SEIDEN, L. S. and SCHUSTER, C. R. (1981) Dopamine depletion by 6-hydroxydopamine prevents conditioned taste aversion induced by methamphetamine but not by lithium chloride. *Pharmacol. Biochem. Behav.* **14**: 85–88.

WAYNER, M. J., GREENBERG, I. and TROWBRIDGE, J. (1973) Effects of d-amphetamine on schedule induced polydipsia. *Pharmacol. Biochem. Behav.* **1**: 109–111.

WINN, P., WILLIAMS, S. F. and HERBERG, L. J. (1982) Feeding stimulated by very low doses of d-amphetamine administered systemically or by microinjection into the striatum. *Psychopharmacology* **78**: 336–341.

WISE, R. A. (1982) Brain dopamine and reward. In: *Theory in Psychopharmacology*, Vol. 1, pp. 103–122, COOPER, S. J. (ed.) Academic Press, London.

WISE, R. A. (1978) *Pharmacol. Therap.* (in press).

ZIMMERBERG, B., GLICK, S. D. and JERUSSI, T. P. (1974) Neurochemical correlate of a spatial preference in rats. *Science* **185**: 623–625.

CHAPTER 2

THE ROLE OF REWARD PATHWAYS IN THE DEVELOPMENT OF DRUG DEPENDENCE

ROY A. WISE
Center for Studies in Behavioral Neurobiology and Department of Psychology, Concordia University, Montreal, Quebec, Canada

1. INTRODUCTION

Great progress in the understanding of the mechanisms by which drugs influence behavior has resulted from recent studies of the binding of drugs to receptors. While not all drugs have been identified with receptor-mediated actions, it seems clear that opiates (Goldstein *et al.*, 1971: Pert and Snyder, 1973; Simon *et al.*, 1973; Terenius, 1973), benzodiazepines (Mohler and Okada, 1977; Squires and Braestrup, 1977) and perhaps barbiturates (Dingemanse and Breimer, 1984; Haefely, 1984; Olsen, 1982; Ticku, 1983), amphetamine (Hauger *et al.*, 1984) and cocaine (Kennedy and Hanbauer, 1983; Pimoule *et al.*, 1983; Reith *et al.*, 1980), nicotine (Abood *et al.*, 1978; Martin and Aceto, 1981) and phencyclidine (Quirion *et al.*, 1981) have their central nervous system actions through receptor complexes that are embedded in the membranes of specific types of neurons.

The identification of the receptor molecule or complex which translates the presence of a drug into a change in neuronal activity is, however, only one of three critical steps in the understanding of the mechanism of a given drug action. The second step is to identify the neuronal "address" of the subset of receptors that is specific to the action in question, and the third step is to determine the normal function of the neuronal elements in which that subset of receptors is embedded. While the pharmacological specificity of a given drug is often due to the discrimination of that drug from others by receptors of specific molecular conformations, the fact that most drugs have multiple actions is due to the fact that most classes of drug receptors are found embedded in the neurons of more than one anatomical circuit. For example, morphine stimulates feeding or inhibits feeding depending on the relative concentration of morphine at two sets of mu-type opioid receptors: one set associated with feeding-inhibitory circuitry of the periaqueductal gray and another set associated with feeding-facilitory circuitry of the ventral tegmental area (Jenck *et al.*, 1986b).

Autoradiographic methods are being developed to localize the neuronal addresses of different classes of receptor within the brain. Both light and electron microscopy are being used to identify the neuronal elements in which drug receptors are embedded. On the basis of what has already been learned about some receptor types (Atweh and Kuhar, 1977; Clarke *et al.*, 1984), it seems unlikely that any class of receptor will be localized on cells of a single physiological mechanism; rather, it seems that the same receptor types are likely to be found on a variety of cell types and in a variety of brain regions. When drugs are taken orally, intravenously, intranasally, or, in short, through any of the current methods of human self-administration, they are distributed relatively homogeneously throughout the brain, presumably reaching all of the central circuits identified by a given class of receptor. The net behavioral effect of systemic drug administration is a composite of the actions of each of the independent circuits influenced by the drug. This is well illustrated by the opiates. The nausea associated with opiates derives from their effects on centers in the medulla; the increase in body temperature from effects in the medial preoptic area (Teasdale *et al.*, 1981); analgesia from effects at three different levels of the brain—the diencephalon (Cohen and Melzack, 1985), the midbrain (Yaksh and Rudy, 1978), and the spinal cord (Levine *et al.*, 1982; Yaksh and Rudy, 1979).

Where, among the dozens of nuclei containing drug receptors of different types, should we expect to find the subset involved in the rewarding or habit-forming action of opiates?

One approach to this question would be to proceed from molar considerations down, rather than from molecular considerations up. From molecular considerations we are faced with an overwhelming number of binding sites in an overwhelming number of brain regions. Only a fraction of these binding sites have relevance to any given function. For example, there are opiate receptors associated with dozens of anatomically distinct types of neuron (Atweh and Kuhar, 1977). From molecular considerations, there is no reason to think any of these to be more likely than another to play a given behavioral role. It is knowledge of the function of different anatomical regions or anatomical circuits or individual neurons that allows us to narrow the possibilities. It is unlikely that opiates are habit-forming because of actions in the gut or on peripheral neurons. It is unlikely that opiates are habit-forming because of actions in the pain mechanisms of the spinal cord. It is unlikely that opiates are habit-forming because of their effects in the temperature mechanisms of the preoptic area.

The present paper will explore a view generated by the discovery of endogenous opioid receptors and peptides. Goldstein (1976) has articulated this view as follows: "It seemed unlikely, a priori, that such highly stereospecific receptors should have been developed by nature to interact with alkaloids from the opium poppy" (p. 1081). Endogenous opioid peptide transmitters and opioid receptors appear to have evolved long before mammals had contact with the opium poppy. They are found in primitive portions of the nervous system (Barchas *et al.*, 1978; Bloom *et al.*, 1978; Watson *et al.*, 1982a,b) and in simple invertebrates (Kream *et al.*, 1980; Leung and Stefano, 1984; Stefano *et al.*, 1980). Stress induces feeding and analgesia in the slug (Kavaliers and Hirst, 1986), just as it does in mammals (Amir *et al.*, 1980; Terman *et al.*, 1984; Morley and Levin, 1980). As the discoverers of endogenous opioids and opiate receptors considered the implications of their findings, an important insight emerged: exogenous opiates have their various actions because they can activate the normal pathways serving a variety of normal brain functions.

This logic and the discovery of analgesic actions of the endogenous opioid peptides (Loh *et al.*, 1976; Tung and Yaksh, 1982; Wei *et al.*, 1977) gave support to the view (Melzack and Wall, 1965) that there were endogenous centrifugal, brainstem and spinal mechanisms for control of incoming pain signals. There are now multiple lines of evidence to support this view. First, pain perception is known to vary despite a constant pain stimulus; thus there must be some mechanism (central or peripheral) which is capable of pain modulation (Melzack, 1970; Melzack and Perry, 1975; Melzack *et al.*, 1977). Second, exogenous drugs can alter pain perception (Beecher, 1959), and opiates, at least, do so in proportion to their ability to cross the blood-brain barrier (Herz *et al.*, 1970; Oldendorf *et al.*, 1972); this suggests that the pain-modulation mechanism involves central circuitry. Third, alteration of pain perception can also be produced by direct electrical stimulation of specific brain regions (Mayer *et al.*, 1971; Reynolds, 1969); this confirms the presence of central pain-modulation pathways. Fourth, such analgesic stimulation summates with and shows cross-tolerance with analgesic effects of opiate drugs (Mayer and Hayes, 1975; Mayer and Murphin, 1976); this indicates that the same central mechanism mediates stimulation-produced and opiate-produced pain modulation. Fifth, synaptic sites of action have now been identified for analgesic effects of opiates (Yaksh and Rudy, 1978; Yeung and Rudy, 1980); thus a portion of the anatomy of the opioid pain-modulation mechanism is known. Sixth, endogenous transmitters have been found in neurons that terminate in the region of these synaptic mechanisms (Loh *et al.*, 1976; Tung and Yaksh, 1982; Wei *et al.*, 1977); thus it is clear that the receptors at which exogenous opiates initiate their analgesic actions are receptors that are part of intrinsic circuitry of the brain. Seventh, the opioid antagonists naloxone and naltrexone attenuate opiate analgesia, stimulation-produced analgesia, and some of the other analgesias that can be produced in the absence of exogenous opiates (Akil *et al.*, 1976; Watkins and Mayer, 1982). Thus the pathways of opiate analgesia are currently viewed as "endogenous pain-control" pathways, and opiate analgesia is seen as due to activation of such natural pathways by exogenous agents (Basbaum and Fields, 1978; Mayer and Price, 1976; Melzack and Wall, 1965).

The view explored in the present paper is that the habit-forming or "reinforcing" effects of opiates are similarly the result of the activation of endogenous brain mechanisms by an exogenous analogue of a natural transmitter. In this case, the endogenous mechanisms are not the mechanisms of pain modulation but rather presumed to be the mechanisms by which behavior is controlled by natural rewards or reinforcers. The evidence for this view is almost perfectly parallel to that just summarized for endogenous pain-control pathways. First, behavior is known to be controlled by natural rewards or reinforcers (Pavlov, 1927; Skinner, 1935). Second, exogenous drugs can exert a similar control (Weeks, 1962), due, at least in some cases, to central drug actions (Yokel and Pickens, 1974). Third, electrical stimulation of certain brain structures can be powerfully rewarding (Bishop *et al.*, 1963; Olds and Milner, 1954), confirming that the reward mechanism involves central brain circuitry. Fourth, there are facilitory interactions between drugs of abuse and rewarding brain stimulation (Adams *et al.*, 1972; Stein and Ray, 1960), suggesting overlapping or common mechanisms. Fifth, synaptic sites of rewarding action have been identified for at least some drugs of abuse (Bozarth and Wise, 1981b; Goeders *et al.*, 1984; Goeders and Smith, 1983; Hoebel *et al.*, 1983; Phillips and LePiane, 1980), and the implicated synapses are thought to play a role in the reinforcing effects of brain stimulation (Wise, 1980; Wise and Bozarth, 1984). Sixth, at least two classes of exogenous drug reward have been shown to depend on endogenous neurotransmitter systems (Glimcher *et al.*, 1984; Yokel and Wise, 1975). Seventh, receptor antagonists for the endogenous transmitter systems attenuate the rewarding effects of natural (Gerber *et al.*, 1981b; Sanger and McCarthy, 1982; Wise *et al.*, 1978a,b) and brain stimulation (Belluzzi and Stein, 1977; Fouriezos and Wise, 1976; Franklin, 1978) reward as well as drug reward (Davis and Smith, 1975; Goldberg *et al.*, 1971; Risner and Jones, 1976; Yokel and Wise, 1975, 1976). Thus it is as reasonable to search for the rewarding effects of drugs in the known components of endogenous reward mechanisms, as it is to search for the analgesic effects of drugs in the known components of endogenous pain control mechanisms. In the case of reward mechanisms, the endogenous mechanism has been a tool for understanding drug reward; in the case of pain control mechanisms, exogenous analgesics were the tool by which we have learned much about the endogenous mechanism.

2. FRAME OF REFERENCE

The notion to look for the biological mechanisms of drug habits or drug rewards in the endogenous mechanisms of habit or reward does not, by itself, advance our cause. We must know something about the endogenous mechanisms of habit or reward before we can use this knowledge as a tool for the understanding of the habits or rewards associated with exogenous drugs. Moreover, there is more than one kind of reward and there may be several mechanisms of reward. Thus, in order to use what is known about endogenous reward mechanisms to understand drug reward, we must make some selection from the available reward mechanisms. For this we must refine our notion of reward.

Rewards or "reinforcers" are, by definition, what establish and sustain habits. The term "reinforcer" is generally preferred by psychologists and behavioral pharmacologists, because it implies no motivational or affective valence. When we speak of positive or negative rewards, we are likely to associate them with pleasure or pain; Skinner (1935) has advocated the term "reinforcement" in an attempt to get away from attributing behavior to inferred affective states or "mental causes." It is difficult, however, even for the psychologist, not to associate pleasure and pain with reinforcement. At any rate, there are two major classes of reinforcers: positive reinforcers and negative reinforcers. Positive reinforcers establish and sustain habits because of central states that they cause; these are states we usually associate with the subjective feeling of pleasure. Negative reinforcers establish and sustain habits because of the central states that they alleviate; these states are usually associated with pain, distress, or aversion.

Drugs, like foods, appear to have the potential to serve as either positive or negative reinforcers. The drug effects that are initially sought by addicts are reported to be pleasant or euphoric, as are the tastes of needed foods and fluids; here they serve as positive reinforcers. However, once habits of intake have become established, deprivation of drugs of abuse, or of food or fluid produces an aversive condition the symptoms of which can be alleviated by the expected or desired substance; here they serve as negative reinforcers. Just as we are sometimes motivated to eat because of the expected pleasure of the taste of food, so may the addict be motivated to take a drug because of the expected euphoria it can produce. Just as we are, at other times, motivated to eat by the discomfort of hunger which food can alleviate, so may the addict be motivated to take a drug because of the distress which the drug can alleviate.

If we are to search for the mechanism of drug reward by considering what is known about endogenous reward mechanisms, we must thus consider, in turn, both positive reinforcement mechanisms and negative reinforcement mechanisms. In the physiological psychology of reward mechanisms, however, little is mentioned about negative reinforcement. What is known about reward pathways in the brain is, for the most part, related to positive reinforcement mechanisms—mechanisms associated with approach behaviors (Glickman and Schiff, 1967). Traditional theories of addiction, however, are negative reinforcement theories. Addiction is associated with notions of physical dependence, and the most overpowering motivation to take drug has traditionally been assumed to be motivation to relieve withdrawal discomfort. This assumption is fundamental to pharmacological treatments of addiction which involve medication of withdrawal distress (Dackis and Gold, 1985a; Dole and Nyswander, 1965; Gold *et al.*, 1978).

The two sections of this paper which follow deal with the two major views of reinforcement and addiction. The first deals with mechanisms of negative reinforcement and the view that drug self-administration represents self-medication of some form of distress symptoms. The second deals with the mechanisms of positive reinforcement and the view that drug self-administration is a form of pleasure-seeking or thrill-seeking which requires no pre-existing stress or dependence in order to establish compulsive drug-taking habits. While these two views are developed as alternatives to one another, there is good reason to assume that they each contribute significantly to the self-administration of at least some classes of abused drugs.

3. PATHWAYS OF NEGATIVE REINFORCEMENT

There are two kinds of distress that drugs have been suggested to relieve. First, there is the distress of their own withdrawal symptoms. The classic view of opiate dependence, prior to the discovery of endogenous opioid peptides, was that, whatever the motivation for initial drug intake, the compulsive drug self-administration of the addict became motivated primarily by the powerful need to alleviate withdrawal distress (Collier, 1968; Dole and Nyswander, 1967; Hebb, 1949; Himmelsbach, 1943; Lindsmith, 1947; Malmo, 1975; Martin, 1968; Wikler, 1952). Once opiate dependence is established, it is clear how negative reinforcement could serve to maintain drug self-administration. While the severity of opiate withdrawal symptoms may be exaggerated by addicts and in the minds of the public, they are certainly sufficiently severe as to motivate self-medication (Jaffe, 1980).

Second, there are forms of distress which can exist independently of those which result from exposure to exogenous opiates. Opiates can be used to self-medicate pain, and they might be used to self-medicate other forms of distress as well (Alexander and Hadaway, 1982; Chein *et al.*, 1964; Khantzian, 1974). In addition, with the realization that there are normally endogenous opioids in the brain, it became obvious that endogenous opioid dependence might develop; exogenous opiates might be used to medicate distress caused by shortage of endogenous opioids (Way, 1983). Since different mechanisms might be expected for these three possible forms of opioid negative reinforcement, each will be taken up in turn.

3.1. Physical Dependence and its Pathways

Whether it is considered a primary cause of addiction or merely a contributing factor, the question of importance for the present analysis is whether physical dependence has a mechanism common to all or only an important subset of drugs of abuse. If we can identify the anatomical pathways that are the central mechanism of physical dependence, then we can ask to what degree drug actions in these pathways participate in drug reward and to what degree they are influenced by drugs of different classes. Unfortunately, little is known about the anatomical pathways of physical dependence except in the case of the opiates. In general, the pathways of dependence are expected to be the pathways in which dependence-producing drugs have their direct pharmacological actions (Collier, 1968; Goldstein and Goldstein, 1961; Jaffe and Sharpless, 1968).

3.1.1. *Opiate Physical Dependence*

The strength of dependence theory is that objective signs of physical dependence can be identified independent of attempts of the animal to obtain drug. In the rat, the signs of opiate dependence include quiet but determined attempts to escape from the test box, tooth chattering, "wet-dog" shakes, ear blanching, diarrhea, ptosis, and swallowing movements (Wei *et al.*, 1973a). When chronic drug treatment is simply terminated, abstinence signs develop over a period of hours; when the effectiveness of circulating opiates are blocked pharmacologically in dependent animals, abstinence signs can be precipitated full-strength in a few minutes.

Physical dependence appears to reflect compensatory changes in the function of certain brain circuits and peripheral organs as a result of adaptation to a drug that is used on a chronic basis (Collier, 1968; Jaffe and Sharpless, 1968; Martin, 1967). In general, the withdrawal symptoms are opposite in direction to the direct pharmacological effect of the drug. Thus for drugs like opiates, barbiturates and ethanol, which generally depress behavior at high doses, the withdrawal state is characterized by the opposite: behavioral excitability. A direct effect of opiates is constipation; the associated withdrawal symptom is diarrhea (Wei *et al.*, 1973a). Thus the brain pathways of physical dependence are the brain pathways of the pharmacological agents that produced dependence. However, it is not clear whether all or only some of the pathways influenced by a drug contribute to dependence on that drug.

The localization of those anatomical pathways involved in opioid physical dependence has relied largely on the use of locally applied opioids and opiate antagonists. The location of the dependence mechanisms can be identified in several ways. Local injections of naloxone can be given to dependent rats; to the degree that naloxone remains localized near the injection site, only injections near the receptors involved in dependence precipitate abstinence symptoms. The effective sites are in the periaqueductal gray and medial thalamus; naloxone in limbic and cortical sites is much less effective (Wei *et al.*, 1973b). Another approach is to determine where morphine inhibits symptoms like wet-dog shakes elicited by natural stimuli such as an ice-bath; again, the periaqueductal gray proved an effective site. In addition, morphine injection into the preoptic area alleviates wet-dog shakes (Wei *et al.*, 1975). These findings are consistent with the notion that the sites of morphine's pharmacological actions are the sites of naloxone's precipitation of withdrawal reactions; wet-dog shakes are part of a thermoregulatory response (Wei *et al.*, 1973a; Wei, 1981a), and the preoptic area is involved in morphine's effects on thermoregulation (Teasdale *et al.*, 1981).

A third approach to localizing the dependence mechanisms is to give chronic morphine in a manner that restricts it to localized brain regions, and then to challenge with systemic naloxone. Wei and Loh (1976), Wei (1981b), and Laschka *et al.* (1976) used this method to demonstrate physical dependence on endogenous opioids chronically injected into the ventricular system. These studies implicated structures around the fourth ventricle and the aqueduct between the third and fourth ventricles in opioid dependence. The method was then extended to involve direct chronic infusions into the brain parenchyma (Bozarth and Wise, 1983, 1984); again, the periaqueductal gray stood out as a site of opioid dependence mechanisms. Animals given 72-hr infusions of morphine into the rostral or caudal periaqueductal gray showed pronounced escape responses and tooth chattering, whereas animals given similar infusions into the caudate, nucleus accumbens and the ventral tegmental area did not. Infusions into the rostal periventricular gray were associated with the strongest naloxone-precipitated escape; infusions into the caudal periventricular gray were associated with the strongest naloxone-precipitated tooth chattering (Bozarth and Wise, 1983).

Chronic infusions of morphine into specific brain regions did not result in the full syndrome of dependence signs seen when animals are given systemic morphine (Bozarth and Wise, 1984). For example, the periaqueductal gray injections that established dependence as indicated by tooth chattering and escape responses were not associated with weight loss or diarrhea. This and the differential association of tooth chattering and escape with rostral and caudal periaqueductal gray infusions indicate that the multiple signs of withdrawal distress associated with normal opiate dependence are signs reflecting multiple and independent physiological mechanisms. Thus the correlation between the various signs of opiate withdrawal results not from any unity of a single physiological mechanism, but rather from the correlated delivery of opiates by a common circulatory system to a number of independent mechanisms.

This means that we know very little about the physiological mechanisms of opiate dependence. We have strong reason to believe that dependence signs reflect rebound sensitization of those mechanisms that opiates inhibit and rebound desensitization of those mechanisms that opiates stimulate. The mechanism of the abstinence sign of diarrhea, for example, is probably the gut itself, where the direct action of opiates is constipation. The gut is likely to have nothing to do with restlessness or thermoregulatory responses; these are more likely to reflect central morphine effects and their after-effects. Escape responding appears to involve disinhibition of mechanisms of the periaqueductal gray, where morphine itself suppresses behavior (Broekkamp *et al.*, 1976; Jenck *et al.*, 1986b) and leads to freezing. Tooth chattering appears to involve mechanisms of the preoptic area and periaqueductal gray (Wei *et al.*, 1973a; Bozarth and Wise, 1983, 1984). Mechanisms of the other opiate withdrawal signs remain to be localized. None of the symptoms of opiate withdrawal are caused by chronic morphine infusions into the ventral tegmental area, nucleus accumbens, or caudate, so long as doses and routes of injection are used that prevent spread to adjacent areas (Bozarth and Wise, 1983, 1984). This fact will take on major significance when we take up the brain pathways of reward.

The question of interest is whether opioid actions in the periaqueductal gray pathways of dependence contribute negative reinforcement which contributes to the total rewarding impact of opiates; it will be argued below that such actions cannot be the only explanation of opiate reward. To the degree that dependence reflects a rebound excitation of neurons that are suppressed by opiates (Collier, 1968; Goldstein and Goldstein, 1961; Jaffe and Sharpless, 1968)—or, for that matter, a rebound depression of neurons that are excited by opiates—the ability of opiates to relieve opiate withdrawal symptoms derives from its direct action in the dependence pathways. To the degree that the relief of withdrawal symptoms contributes to the total rewarding impact of opiates, opiate actions in the dependence pathways should contribute to opiate reward. Thus, in dependent animals, local injections of morphine into the periaqueductal gray should have rewarding impact. To my knowledge, this obvious (Bozarth and Wise, 1984) possibility has not yet been successfully tested.

3.1.2. *Physical Dependence on other Depressant Drugs*

To the degree that the mechanisms of withdrawal symptoms are the physiological mechanisms through which drugs have their pharmacological actions, and to the degree that various drugs have common withdrawal symptoms, we must expect that different drugs will have common mechanisms of dependence. To the degree that withdrawal symptoms differ, we must assume that some aspects of the mechanisms of dependence will differ. There is, then, a prototypical set of withdrawal symptoms and mechanisms only if there is a prototypical addictive drug.

The withdrawal symptoms that come closest to deserving to be considered prototypical are symptoms shared, to some extent, by four very distinct classes of drug: opiates, barbiturates, benzodiazepines, and ethanol. These symptoms include restlessness, tremor, sleeplessness, anxiety, tachycardia and hyperthermia (Kalant, 1977). While there are commonalities between these drugs, there are also notable differences. These similarities and differences are of great importance for the question of whether a common dependence pathway is influenced by each of these agents.

Ethanol is particularly interesting in relation to opiates. The possibility was once seriously considered that ethanol dependence was a special case of opiate dependence, in which the presence of ethanol in the body causes abnormal metabolism of monoamines resulting in accumulation of opioid tetrahydroisoquinoline alkaloids, which might then be the mediators of some of ethanol's pharmacological actions (Cohen and Collins, 1970; Davis and Walsh, 1970). The possibility that such alkaloids played a critical role in ethanol's ability to produce physical dependence was tested by challenging ethanol-dependent mice with naloxone. If ethanol dependence were mediated by alkaloid metabolites through the opioid dependence mechanism, then blocking opioid receptors should precipitate ethanol dependence signs; it did not do so, and it was concluded that the mechanism of ethanol physical dependence was independent of that of any ethanol-induced opioid substance (Goldstein and Judson, 1971).

While this finding rules out the possibility that the mechanism of ethanol dependence involves pathways that cross the juncture where exogenous opiates interface with neural circuits—presumably an endogenous opioid peptide synapse—it does not rule out the possibility that ethanol and opiates have independent inputs to a common final dependence pathway. Other evidence, however, suggests that the mechanisms of ethanol dependence are largely independent of those of opiate dependence. The strongest evidence is that ethanol fails to relieve opiate withdrawal symptoms and opiates fail to relieve ethanol withdrawal symptoms (Kalant, 1977; Norton, 1970). As will be discussed below, ethanol does partially alleviate the symptoms of barbiturate and benzodiazepine withdrawal.

Little is known about the anatomical mechanisms of ethanol dependence, other than the obvious fact that they are connected to the organs in which the symptoms are seen. It has not been possible to isolate receptors at which ethanol's pharmacological actions are transduced; ethanol appears to have rather general interactions with the lipids and proteins of cell membranes throughout the nervous system (Chin and Goldstein, 1977; Rangaraj and Kalant, 1980; Seeman, 1972), which is thought to account for the large number of ethanol molecules—as compared with the case of opiates—needed to produce ethanol intoxication (Kalant, 1977). Moreover, since ethanol readily diffuses across the various barriers of the brain, ethanol cannot be restricted to a given region by local injection. Central injections of ethanol would quickly cross into blood and be diluted and carried to distal sites of potential action. Our knowledge of where in the brain ethanol initiates its action in the physiological mechanisms of dependence thus remains unknown.

Barbiturates and benzodiazepines also have dominant sedative effects and produce a dependence syndrome that is generally similar to that associated with ethanol. There is considerable cross-tolerance between ethanol and barbiturates, suggesting that these drugs have significant commonality of action (Lê *et al.*, 1986). There is also cross-dependence; ethanol can partially alleviate barbiturate withdrawal distress (Fraser *et al.*, 1957; Norton, 1970), and barbiturates can partially alleviate ethanol withdrawal symptoms (Essig *et al.*, 1969). This suggests that there is a major degree of overlap between the mechanisms of ethanol and barbiturate dependence (Kalant, 1977).

Benzodiazepines are thought to act through specific receptors (Mohler and Okada, 1977; Squires and Braestrup, 1977) which have been localized in various brain regions (Niehoff and Kuhar, 1983; Young and Kuhar, 1980). Barbiturates are thought to act at binding sites associated with those of benzodiazepines (Dingemanse and Breimer, 1984; Haefely, 1984; Olsen, 1982; Ticku, 1983); ethanol also interacts with benzodiazepine binding (Ticku and Davis, 1981). Thus there is good reason to expect that the mechanisms of action of, and thus the mechanisms of dependence on, ethanol, benzodiazepines and barbiturates may have a good deal of overlap and may be identified by some specific set of benzodiazepine receptors. While barbiturates have the same diffusion problems as ethanol, benzodiazepines could be restricted to local regions of the brain by central microinjection. However, the receptor populations associated with the benzodiazepine dependence syndrome have not yet been localized.

It has been argued that cannabis produces weak dependence symptoms of the depressant type (Jones, 1980), but nothing is known about the brain sites or mechanisms of this dependence.

3.1.3. *Stimulant Physical Dependence*

There are withdrawal symptoms associated with chronic use of the psychomotor stimulants cocaine and amphetamine (Jones, 1984); they are generally opposite in nature to those of depressant drugs. Nicotine also produces a physical dependence syndrome, but, like that of amphetamine and cocaine, nicotine withdrawal symptoms involve increased sleep and decreased arousal rather than the sleeplessness and restlessness associated with opiate, ethanol, barbiturate and benzodiazepine withdrawal symptoms (Shiffman, 1979). Thus there seems little question that the mechanisms of stimulant dependence and the mechanisms of sedative dependence differ in major ways. There has been no suggestion that a common "dependence pathway" might mediate the dependence syndromes of both stimulants and depressants. Indeed, since the psychomotor stimulants cause as their direct effects behaviors and organ responses similar to those seen during withdrawal from depressant drugs, the stimulants should exacerbate, rather than relieve, depressant drug withdrawal symptoms.

If this is true, however, then it may be the case that while the *mechanisms* of stimulant and depressant physical dependence are different, the *pathways* of physical dependence are largely the same. To the degree that the pathways of dependence are the pathways of the direct actions of various drugs, and to the degree that stimulants and depressants have opposite withdrawal symptoms, it may be that opposite effects in common pathways account for both classes of withdrawal distress. This would not implicate a common cause for stimulant and depressant addiction.

At the present time, however, there is little direct evidence on the pathways of stimulant physical dependence. Animal models of stimulant physical dependence have not yet been developed to the point where they might be used to examine the mechanisms involved.

3.2. Other Sources of Negative Reinforcement

3.2.1. *Situational Stress*

It is not clear how many forms of distress might be medicated by drugs of abuse. It seems unlikely that psychomotor stimulants medicate stress, since they amplify the actions of the autonomic catecholamines that are released by stress. Opiates, on the other hand, alleviate the stress of pain, and elevated opioid peptide levels are seen as a concomitant of various forms of pain-related stress (Csontos *et al.*, 1979; Guillemin *et al.*, 1977; Rossier *et al.*, 1977). It has also been suggested that opiates alleviate what might be called "psychological" pain or distress, such as is associated with emotional or economic suffering (Khantzian, 1974) or loss of a loved one (Peele and Brodsky, 1975). The major axes of motivational systems in the brain are approach and withdrawal (Schneirla, 1959); the pain control mechanism interacts with the pathways of the withdrawal system, attenuating withdrawal reflexes (Dewey *et al.*, 1969; Irwin *et al.*, 1951) which are common to a range of noxious stimuli that engage the distal as well as the proximal senses. Thus it is not unreasonable to consider opiates as alleviators of more than simply pain.

Several brain sites of opioid interaction with endogenous pathways of the suppression of withdrawal reflexes have been identified; they include sites at diencephalic (Cohen and Melzack, 1985), mesencephalic (Yaksh and Rudy, 1978; Yeung and Rudy, 1980), and spinal (Levine *et al.*, 1982; Yeung and Rudy, 1980) levels. The mesencephalic analgesia sites (Yaksh and Rudy, 1978; Yaksh *et al.*, 1976) are in close proximity to the pathways of opiate physical dependence (Bozarth and Wise, 1983, 1984; Laschka *et al.*, 1976; Wei *et al.*,

1973b). Thus it is possible that common periaqueductal gray pathways are involved in both opiate physical dependence and opiate suppression of the flexion reflexes of withdrawal. This view suggests a role of midline pathways of the mesencephalon as an important part of the mechanism of negative reinforcement. Such a suggestion fits well with the known anatomy of sites where electrical stimulation attenuates pain-associated withdrawal reflexes (Mayer and Price, 1976; Soper, 1976), and with the suggestion that withdrawal and negative feedback mechanisms are associated with periventricular pathways (Grossman, 1966; Margules and Stein, 1968; Olds and Olds, 1965). It is not clear, however, whether any addictive drugs other than opiates might interact with this system.

One form of distress other than pain-distress which opiates seem to alleviate is the distress of social isolation. It has been observed that the loss of a loved one produces (social) withdrawal symptoms in humans that are similar to the withdrawal symptoms associated with opiate physical dependence (Peele and Brodsky, 1975). In opiate-naive lower animals, opiate antagonists can increase isolation-distress vocalizations in individuals that are isolated (Herman and Panksepp, 1978), and can cause isolation-distress vocalizations even in individuals that are not isolated (Panksepp *et al.*, 1980a). Morphine alleviates the separation vocalizations of isolated animals (Panksepp *et al.*, 1978a), as do intracerebroventricular injections of β-endorphin and enkephalin (Panksepp *et al.*, 1978b, 1980b). In addition, social isolation increases the binding of diprenorphine to opioid receptors in drug-free animals (Panksepp and Bishop, 1981). The mechanism of these effects appears to overlap with the mechanism of opiate analgesia. Distress vocalizations can be elicited by stimulation of the dorsomedial (periventricular) thalamus in guinea pigs; these vocalizations are increased by naloxone and are inhibited by analgesic periventricular gray electrical stimulation but not by non-analgesic stimulation of nearby regions (Herman and Panksepp, 1981).

This raises the possibility that exogenous opiates could have negative reinforcing properties prior to the development of physical dependence. Exogenous opiates could relieve situational distress such as pain or social isolation distress in non-dependent animals. It has been suggested that the isolated housing conditions of most laboratories increases the susceptibility to negative reinforcement (Alexander *et al.*, 1978, 1981); indeed, it has been argued that laboratory animals would not self-administer opiates were it not for impoverished laboratory conditions (Alexander, 1984; Khantzian, 1974). If it is the case, however, that the pathways of suppression of separation distress are homologous with the pathways of pain suppression (Herman and Panksepp, 1981), then it would appear that negative reinforcement of this type does not account for the willingness of laboratory rats to learn responses for morphine (Weeks, 1962); non-dependent rats that will work for central injections of opioids into other brain regions (Bozarth and Wise, 1981b; Goeders *et al.*, 1984) will not work for similar injections at dependence (Bozarth and Wise, 1984) and analgesia (Yaksh and Rudy, 1978; Yaksh *et al.*, 1976) sites (Bozarth and Wise, 1983, 1984). Thus, if negative reinforcement plays a significant role in the rewarding effects of opiates in non-dependent animals, it would appear to involve pathways other than the ventral tegmental pathways of opiate dependence and analgesia.

3.2.2. *Endogenous Opioid Deficiency*

With the discovery of endogenous opioid peptides, it became obvious that opioid dependence could develop even without exposure to exogenous opiates (Way, 1983). The normal functioning of the endogenous opioid systems exposes the post-synaptic receptors to events comparable to those triggered by exogenous opiates. It is possible that some or all individuals develop some degree of opioid physical dependence from this exposure. There could be considerable variation in the degree of endogenous opioid dependence and the correlated susceptibility to exogenous opiate dependence, both across individuals and across times in the life of a given individual. Ground squirrels, for example, show seasonal variations in their susceptibility to opiate dependence, and this variation is presumed to reflect variation in the turnover of endogenous opioids across the hibernation cycle (Beckman *et al.*, 1982). If there developed a deficiency in endogenous opioids, such that their synpatic concentrations dropped below normal, symptoms would develop that parallel in nature, if not in degree, withdrawal from exogenous opiates. Again, this condition would establish the opportunity for negative reinforcement by exogenous opiates.

The anatomical pathways that could play a role in endogenous opioid dependence would be the same as are involved in exogenous opiate dependence. The major identified pathways are those of the periaqueductal gray (Bozarth and Wise, 1983, 1984; Laschka *et al.* 1976; Wei *et al.*, 1973b); again, these pathways do not appear to play a significant role in opiate negative reinforcement in non-dependent animals, since such animals do not work for periaqueductal gray injections of morphine which are rewarding when injected elsewhere (Bozarth and Wise, 1983, 1984).

4. PATHWAYS OF POSITIVE REINFORCEMENT

A variety of biologically significant rewards appear to control much of animal behavior. The animal is aware of these rewards through sensory mechanisms, and different rewards activate different sensory modalities. One of the rewarding qualities of food is sweet taste; hungry animals will work for solutions containing only non-nutritive saccharin (Sheffield and Roby, 1950), preferring it more and more to a bland but nutritive solution as the level of food deprivation is increased (Jacobs, 1967; Jacobs and Sharma, 1969). One of the rewarding qualities of water is its ability to cool the oral cavity; thirsty rats will lick at a stream of cool air (Mendelson and Chillag, 1970) or a stream of warm, dry air that will cause cooling by evaporating saliva from the oral cavity (Freed and Mendelson, 1974). In these cases, the animal is working for the sensation of sweetness or coolness; neither reinforcement reduces the physiological condition that motivates the behavior. Saccharin does not alleviate deficits in energy balance, and cool air does not alleviate the deficits in fluid balance. Thus these agents are positive reinforcers; they are substances that are rewarding in their own right, and not because they alleviate withdrawal symptoms. To the degree that it is the sweetness of caloric substances that establishes them as reinforcers for hungry animals, caloric substances are positive reinforcers above and beyond any negative reinforcing effect they may have; to the degree that it is coolness of water that establishes it as a reinforcer for thirsty animals, water is a positive reinforcer, above and beyond any negative reinforcing effects it may have.

Little is known as to how messages from the sensory nerves carrying sweetness and temperature information come to influence the messages to the musculature which execute goal-directed behavior. It is generally thought that motivational pathways of the medial forebrain bundle are activated, and that these motivational pathways are common to many positive reinforcers and to many forms of approach behavior (Glickman and Schiff, 1967; Olds and Olds, 1965). Most theorists who venture a speculation as to how this system might function suggest that it modifies, in some manner, the effectiveness of the ability of sensory stimuli (including the stimulus in question) to elicit approach, manipulatory and ingestive responses (Gallistel *et al.*, 1981; Glickman and Schiff, 1967; Huston, 1982; Milner, 1970; Olds and Olds, 1965).

What is known about the neural pathways assumed to be involved in the control of behavior by positive reinforcement is known largely from studies of the rewarding effects of electrical stimulation of the brain (German and Bowden, 1974; Glickman and Schiff, 1967; Olds and Milner, 1954). More recently, information as to the anatomy and pharmacology of these pathways has come from studies of drug reward (Fibiger, 1978; Wise, 1978b; Wise and Bozarth, 1984) and food reward (Wise, 1982). While this system was once referred to as a "pleasure center" in the brain (Olds, 1956), it was soon realized that multiple fiber systems, rather than a single integrative center, were involved (Olds, 1972). The number of circuit elements that feed into and out of the medial forebrain bundle system is not known (Gallistel *et al.*, 1981; Wise and Bozarth, 1984), nor is it known how many independent reward systems might exist in parallel with the medial forebrain system (Phillips, 1984).

4.1. The Substrate of Brain Stimulation Reward

4.1.1. *A Model System*

Several facts account for the attention received by the phenomenon of brain stimulation reward. First, stimulation can be a very powerful reward, preferred to food even by starving animals (Routtenberg, 1964). Second, stimulation activates motivational mechanisms of the association areas of the forebrain, where inputs from conventional reinforcers are difficult to trace. Conventional reinforcers activate sensory nerves, which influence central motivational mechanisms after one or more synaptic links, and electrophysiological attempts to identify the forebrain structures activated by conventional reinforcers have been fraught with difficulty (Olds, 1976). Third, the mechanisms of brain stimulation reward has anatomical specificity; the boundaries of the various regions where stimulation is reinforcing identify the approximate boundaries of at least some components of the reward mechanism. Fourth, it seems likely that the mechanism activated by brain stimulation reward is homologous with the mechanism of natural reinforcement, since the behavior that it supports is comparable, in various and subtle ways, to the behavior supported by conventional reinforcers (Trowill *et al.*, 1969; Beninger *et al.*, 1977).

4.1.2. *Pharmacology*

Of the two major axes along which reward mechanisms have been explored, it is the pharmacological axis, rather than the anatomical axis, which convincingly suggests involvement of a specific neurotransmitter system in reward mechanisms. While a number of drugs disrupt the behavior of animals working for brain stimulation reward, it is dopamine antagonists that disrupt the behavior in a manner which suggests degradation of the reinforcing efficacy of the stimulation and not simply degradation of the response capacity of the animal.

This generalization summarizes a decade of controversy, but it is now widely held that, above and beyond any motoric side effects they might cause, dopamine blockers reduce the rewarding effectiveness of stimulation. Several paradigms have been developed in order to be sure that no form of simple response impairment could account for the slowing or cessation of responding caused by these agents. Two paradigms that are generally accepted as convincing are the extinction paradigm and the curve-shift paradigm. Other paradigms that suggest the same conclusion include various threshold paradigms.

The extinction paradigm is a paradigm where the performance of well-trained, neuroleptic-treated animals is compared to that of well-trained, non-rewarded animals. When well-trained animals are tested under conditions of non-reward, they initiate responding normally, but slow and cease responding when they fail to receive the normal rewarding feedback for their efforts. When neuroleptic-treated rats are similarly tested, they too, respond normally at the beginning of sessions but slow and cease responding after a few minutes (lever-pressing task) or trials (runway task) (Fenton and Liebman, 1982; Fouriezos and Wise, 1976; Fouriezos *et al.*, 1978; Franklin and McCoy, 1979; Gallistel *et al.*, 1982). That the slowing of responding does not simply reflect some form of fatigue-like debilitation is shown by "spontaneous recovery" when stimuli previously paired with normal reinforcement are given (Fouriezos and Wise, 1976; Franklin and McCoy, 1979) and by normal performance in a second task following response cessation in the first (Gallistel *et al.*, 1982).

The curve-shift paradigm involves testing the animal over a range of stimulation intensities or frequencies, including low values that barely maintain minimal rates of responding and high values that maintain responding at high rates which do not improve with increases in reward. This paradigm was first developed by Edmonds and Gallistel (1974) who showed that altering the performance demands of the task or the performance capability of the animal altered the maximal level of responding of the animal, but did not alter the value of stimulation which was just sufficient to motivate maximal responding (see also: Stellar and Neeley, 1982). Alpha-methyl-para-tyrosine (in some but not all animals:

Edmonds, 1976) and decreased rewarding stimulation (Edmonds and Gallistel, 1974; Stellar and Neeley, 1982) increased the value of stimulation which was needed to motivate maximal responding, without altering the level of that responding. Neuroleptic treatment has similar effects; it increases the amount of stimulation necessary to produce a given level of responding, but with moderate doses it does not reduce the maximal level of responding (Franklin, 1978; Gallistel and Karras, 1984; Stellar *et al.*, 1983; Atalay, 1982, cited by Wise, 1985). Even when high doses are tested, and maximal rates of responding are reduced, it can be seen that abnormal amounts of stimulation are required to sustain responding at lower response rates that are well within the animals' demonstrated capacity (Stellar *et al.*, 1983; Atalay, 1982, cited by Wise, 1985).

Reduced rewarding efficacy of stimulation is also demonstrated in threshold paradigms, where it is the amount of stimulation the animal is willing to work for, rather than the rate of responding itself, that is the measured variable. Neuroleptic treated rats require higher than normal amounts of stimulation to sustain responding at minimal rates (Esposito *et al.*, 1979; Schaefer and Michael, 1980; Zarevics and Setler, 1979).

These studies, taken together, suggest that dopaminergic receptor blockade reduces the rewarding impact of brain stimulation (Liebman, 1983; Wise, 1978a,b). The ability of neuroleptics with mixed D-1 and D-2 actions to attenuate the rewarding effects of stimulation correlates with binding potency at the D-2 and not the D-1 receptor (Gallistel and Davis, 1983; Lynch and Wise, 1985), but SCH 23390, presumably selective for the D-1 receptor, is effective where sulpiride, presumably selective for the D-2 receptor, is not (Nakajima and McKenzie, 1986). Thus there remains some question as to which dopamine receptor class is involved. While the results summarized above come from studies where rewarding stimulation was applied at sites along the hypothalamic medial forebrain bundle, neuroleptics also attenuate self-stimulation when other stimulation sites are tested (dorsal tegmentum and olfactory bulb, unpublished observations; mesencephalic central gray, Miliaressis *et al.*, 1986; Rompré and Wise, unpublished observations).

4.1.3. *Anatomy*

Electrical stimulation of dozens of sites in the central nervous system has reinforcing effects (Olds and Olds, 1963; German and Bowden, 1974). It was initially thought that the lateral hypothalamic area was a center of integration of motivational signals from various structures (Olds, 1956, 1958; Olds and Olds, 1965), but this notion was soon supplanted by the view that catecholamine fibers of passage were activated by rewarding stimulation at a wide range of sites (Crow, 1972, 1973; German and Bowden, 1974; Lippa *et al.*, 1973; Stein, 1968, 1971; Stein and C. D. Wise, 1969).

Subsequent mapping revealed that the boundaries of the reward system did not correspond to the boundaries of the noradrenergic cells of locus coeruleus (Amaral and Routtenberg, 1975; Corbett and Wise, 1979; Simon *et al.*, 1975) or the noradrenergic fibers of the dorsal noradrenergic bundle (Corbett and Wise, 1979). Nor would animals work for stimulation near cells of origin of the ventral noradrenergic bundle (Clavier and Routtenberg, 1974). These studies shifted attention from the noradrenergic systems to the dopaminergic systems.

The boundaries of the reward system were found to correspond precisely to the region of the ventral tegmentum and substantia nigra which contains dopaminergic cell bodies (Corbett and Wise, 1980; Wise, 1981). Still, they did not correspond to the boundaries of the ascending dopaminergic fibers of the medial forebrain bundle (Gratton and Wise, 1983) or of the dopaminergic terminals of the caudate, nucleus accumbens, frontal, cingulate or entorhinal cortex, olfactory tubercle, or septal area (Prado-Alcala and Wise, 1984; Prado-Alcala *et al.*, 1984). The facts that the reward system had precisely the dorsal-ventral, medial-lateral, and caudal dispersion of the tegmental dopamine cell layer, but not the same dispersion of the axons or terminals of the dopaminergic cells themselves, were surprising, particularly when considered in light of the fact that dopaminergic function was critical for medial forebrain bundle reward. One suggestion which is consistent with all these facts is that the directly stimulated fibers of the reward system descends the medial forebrain bundle to synapse on the dopaminergic cells of that region (Wise, 1980; Yeomans, 1982), and that the dopaminergic fibers themselves are not directly activated by rewarding stimulation because their thresholds are too high (Shizgal *et al.*, 1980).

Other studies have converged to support this view. Yeomans (1979) estimated the refractory periods of the fibers activated by brain stimulation reward and found them to be much shorter than those estimated for catecholamine fibers. Gratton and Wise (1985) used a finer-grained analysis which suggested two sub-populations, one of which may be cholinergic, both of which have shorter refractory periods than those estimated for catecholamine fibers. Shizgal *et al.* (1980; Bielajew and Shizgal, 1982) estimated the conduction velocities of the medial forebrain bundle reward fibers, and found them to be much faster than those estimated for catecholamine fibers. The conduction velocity studies indicated that the medial forebrain bundle reward substrate involved fibers that span the ventral tegmental area and lateral hypothalamus, at least, without synaptic interruption. These workers also found evidence that a major component of those fibers carried information from the lateral hypothalamus to the ventral tegmental area—opposite to the direction of projection of the catecholamine fibers (Bielajew and Shizgal, 1986).

4.1.4. *Interaction with Drugs of Abuse*

A variety of drugs of abuse interact in a synergistic way with rewarding brain stimulation. The most extensively studied class is the opiates, which have biphasic effects on self-stimulation (Adams *et al.*, 1972) and a number of other functions (Babbini and Davis, 1972; Domino *et al.*, 1976; Eikelboom and Stewart, 1979; Sloan *et al.*, 1962). At moderate and high doses, morphine initially depresses lever-pressing for brain stimulation reward; this is followed, when the morphine is partially metabolized, by a period of responding at enhanced rates (Adams *et al.*, 1972; Esposito and Kornetsky, 1978; Lorens and Mitchell, 1973; Olds and Travis, 1960). With very low doses, the facilitory effect can be seen without any inhibitory effect (Gerber *et al.*, 1981a). The biphasic effects that are usually seen with systemic injections reflect independent suppressive and facilitating actions of opiates, rather than a dominant inhibitory effect followed by a rebound facilitation. This is evident from the facts that: (i) facilitation can be demonstrated with low doses which cause no inhibition (Gerber *et al.*, 1981a); (ii) the minimal current (threshold) which sustains lever-pressing decreases throughout the period of drug effectiveness, even during the period when high doses cause suppression of response rates (Esposito and Kornetsky, 1978); (iii) the sedative effects show tolerance across days, while the facilitory effects are unmasked and increase in strength (Bush *et al.*, 1976); (iv) pure facilitation can be seen in a shuttle-box task that makes minimal response demands on the animal (Levitt *et al.*, 1977); and (v) the facilitory and inhibitory effects on self-stimulation can be dissociated by microinjections of morphine into different brain regions (Broekkamp *et al.*, 1976).

The general findings summarized above refer to animals lever-pressing for stimulation of the medial forebrain bundle, usually at the level of the lateral hypothalamus or ventral tegmental area. In this case, it seems unlikely that an endogenous opioid peptide is a transmitter in the directly activated fibers at the electrode tip. While naloxone can cause major attenuation of lever-pressing for stimulation at some brain sites (Belluzzi and Stein, 1977; Collier and Routtenberg, 1984; Trujillo *et al.*, 1984; West and Wise, 1986) responding for medial forebrain bundle stimulation is only moderately influenced (Esposito *et al.*, 1980; Schaefer and Michael, 1981; Stapleton *et al.*, 1979; van der Kooy *et al.*, 1977; West *et al.*, 1983; West and Wise, 1986). This suggests that an endogenous opioid peptide pathway modulates the medial forebrain bundle reward pathway, but that it is not a critical component of that pathway and it is not a critical efferent of that pathway.

In the case of hippocampal self-stimulation, on the other hand, dynorphin-containing fibers appear to be a critical link in the effects of rewarding stimulation, and naloxone is capable of completely blocking the response at doses that have little effect on other behaviors or on lever-pressing for stimulation to other sites (Collier and Routtenberg, 1984). Responding for nucleus accumbens (Trujillo *et al.*, 1984; West and Wise, 1986) or central gray (Belluzzi and Stein, 1977) stimulation also seems more strongly influenced by naloxone than does medial forebrain bundle stimulation. Presumably, there are differential contributions of endogenous opioid pathways to rewarding stimulation at different sites.

Dynorphin or enkephalin pathways innervating the ventral tegmental area and substantia nigra (Vincent *et al.*, 1982; Watson *et al.*, 1982a,b; Zamir *et al.*, 1984) would appear to interact with medial forebrain bundle reward fibers, however, since morphine injections into the ventral tegmental area, where the descending fibers (Bielajew and Shizgal, 1986) are thought to synapse on dopaminergic neurons (Corbett and Wise, 1980; Wise, 1980; Yeomans, 1982), facilitate medial forebrain bundle reward (Broekkamp *et al.*, 1976). Similar doses injected into the nucleus accumbens and caudate nucleus fail to similarly facilitate medial forebrain bundle reward, suggesting the ventral tegmental area as the locus of the opiate receptor interfaces with reward pathways through which systemic opiates are most likely to influence brain stimulation reward (Broekkamp *et al.*, 1976, 1979).

The other major class of drugs of abuse which is known to act at identified sites in the brain reward pathways is the psychomotor stimulants. Amphetamine (J. Olds, 1972; Stein and Ray, 1960; C. D. Wise and Stein, 1970) and cocaine (Crow, 1970; Wauquier and Niemegeers, 1974) each facilitate medial forebrain bundle reward when moderate doses are used with moderate stimulation parameters (Stark *et al.*, 1969). Where opiates appear to facilitate medial forebrain bundle reward at the synapse between descending fibers and ventral tegmental dopamine cell bodies (Broekkamp *et al.*, 1976, 1979), amphetamine appears to interact at the next synapse in the system, at the dopamine terminals of nucleus accumbens (Broekkamp *et al.*, 1975; Colle and Wise, 1986); it is this site where local injections of amphetamine facilitate medial forebrain bundle self-stimulation.

Nicotine can facilitate brain stimulation reward, although like morphine, it interferes with behavior when high doses are given (Clarke and Kumar, 1984). Local injections of nicotine have not been given to animals working for brain stimulation reward, so the site of interaction of nicotine with the reward system is not known. It seems quite possible, however, that the site of action is the ventral tegmental area; there are nicotinic receptors on nigrostriatal and mesolimbic dopaminergic neurons (Clarke and Pert, 1985), and nicotine activates the dopamine systems (Clarke *et al.*, 1985; Lichtensteiger *et al.*, 1976, 1982; Svensson *et al.*, 1986; Yoon *et al.*, 1986).

Some other classes of drugs of abuse facilitate medial forebrain bundle brain stimulation reward, though the anatomical sites of their interactions are not yet known. Ethanol (De Witte and Bada, 1983; Lewis *et al.*, 1984; Lorens and Sainati, 1978; St Laurent and Olds, 1967), barbiturates (Mogenson, 1964; Reid *et al.*, 1964), benzodiazepines (Olds, 1966; Panksepp *et al.*, 1970), and nicotine (Clarke and Kumar, 1984) each appears to facilitate responding for brain stimulation reward when low doses are carefully selected; each suppresses responding at high doses. The sites of interaction of these substances with the reward pathways are unknown at the present time, though, as will be discussed below, ethanol is known to activate the dopamine system.

4.2. The Substrates of Food and Water Reward

A prediction of the theory that the mechanism of brain stimulation reward is an endogenous reward pathway that evolved in the service of more natural rewards involved the pharmacological challenge of lever-pressing for food and water. As it became clear that neuroleptics attenuate the rewarding impact of medial forebrain bundle stimulation (Fouriezos and Wise, 1976; Fouriezos *et al.*, 1978; Franklin, 1978; Wise, 1978b), the possibility was explored that the same drug would attenuate the rewarding impact of food and water. The initial studies suggested that the rewarding effects of food and water were each attenuated by neuroleptics (Gerber *et al.*, 1981b; Wise *et al.*, 1978a,b). As had been the case with studies of brain stimulation reward (Ettenberg *et al.*, 1979, 1981; Fibiger *et al.*, 1976; Wise, 1978b), the initial reaction to reports of neuroleptic-induced decreases in lever-pressing for food was the interpretation that the drug impaired only the performance capacity of the animal (Ahlenius, 1979; Ettenberg *et al.*, 1979; Gramling *et al.*, 1984; Koob, 1982; Mason *et al.*, 1980; Tombaugh *et al.*, 1979, 1980). As a result of newer and more sensitive paradigms, however, it became clear that neuroleptics do more than simply alter motoric capability. Indeed some of the authors that initially challenged the idea that neuroleptics interfered with reward pathways have now changed their view (Beninger, 1982; Ettenberg, 1982; Ettenberg and Camp, 1986a,b) and it is now widely accepted that neuroleptics inhibit mechanisms of food and water reinforcement (see discussion of Wise, 1982).

4.2.1. *Extinction Paradigm*

The first paradigm to suggest that neuroleptics attenuate the rewarding effects of food and water, and not merely the motoric capacity of the animal, were studies which compared the temporal pattern of neuroleptic effects to the temporal pattern of responding in non-rewarded animals (Gerber *et al.*, 1981b; Wise *et al.*, 1978a,b). In the first such study (Wise *et al.*, 1978a), the rats responded normally or near-normally at the beginning of the first test session, but slowed their rates of responding as the sessions proceeded. Doses were tested such that the within-session response-slowing of neuroleptic-treated rats was not significantly different from the slowing seen in non-rewarded rats or in non-drugged rats that were given normal food reinforcement; thus there was no obvious or significant motoric impairment under the conditions of this test. Neither was there any evidence, on the first day of testing, that the neuroleptic altered the reinforcing effects of food. However, on subsequent test days—separated from each other by two days of normal, drug-free testing—the neuroleptic-treated and non-rewarded rats responded progressively less; whereas normally rewarded rats responded on the order of 200 times per session, neuroleptic and non-rewarded rats responded fewer than 50 times by the fourth test session. The explanation of decreased "resistance to extinction" in the non-rewarded rats is that the animals learn, with repeated experience, to identify non-rewarded sessions and to cease responding earlier and earlier. A similar interpretation of the performance of the neuroleptic-treated animals suggests that neuroleptic treatment attenuates the rewarding impact of the food that the drug-treated rats earned for lever-pressing.

Two findings rule out the possibility that decreased responding reflects motoric impairment; first motoric performance was normal on the first test day, and, second animals that received neuroleptic treatment three times in their home cages, where they could not associate it with altered feedback from ingested food, responded normally on the day of the fourth injection, when they were tested under neuroleptic for the first time. The first finding indicates that the dose of neuroleptic did not seriously impair motor capacity by itself, and the second finding indicates that repeated dosing at three day intervals did not lead to a motorically impairing accumulation of drug. The day-to-day decline in responding has subsequently been replicated elsewhere (Mason *et al.*, 1980), and a similar day-to-day decline (but with lower initial performance) has been seen in animals trained under partial reinforcement (Tombaugh *et al.*, 1980).

The decline in response rate seen on the first day of testing might be attributed to extinction (response slowing associated with learning that reinforcement strength has been attenuated), or it might be attributed to satiation (since the neuroleptic-treated animals did eat the pellets). In another study, a non-nutritive saccharin solution was used; in this case normally rewarded control animals did not slow their response rate during the first session, whereas neuroleptic-treated rats did (Wise *et al.*, 1978b). The neuroleptic-treated rats responded at normal rates in the early minutes of the session, demonstrating that motoric incapacitation was not a factor in their slow responding at the end of the session.

Ettenberg and Camp (1986a,b) have taken the extinction paradigm one step further. In their experiment, rats were trained to run for access to food or water under various experimental conditions. The animals were then tested daily for three weeks in "extinction" conditions, where no reinforcement was offered. The number of responses made in the extinction tests was elevated in animals that were frustrated by non-reinforcement on $\frac{1}{3}$ of their training trials; this is the well-known "partial reinforcement extinction effect" (Robbins, 1971) in which animals trained with reinforcement on every trial persist in responding under non-reinforcement less than do animals trained with reinforcement on only a portion of the training trials.

In the Ettenberg and Camp studies, the group of interest was given neuroleptic treatment on every third day of training; performance in extinction was elevated as it was for animals with reinforcement withheld on every third day. This finding is very important. First, neuroleptic treatment on every third trial produced effects similar to the effects of reward-omission on every third trial. Second, the effect, in this paradigm, was an *increase* rather than the usual decrease in responding. The improvement in extinction performance caused by intermittent neuroleptic treatment during training cannot be attributed to neuroleptic-induced motoric impairment; thus this paradigm unambiguously points to neuroleptic actions above and beyond the "parkinsonian" side effects usually attributed to these drugs (Barbeau, 1974; Hornykiewicz, 1975). The most reasonable interpretation is that the neuroleptic treatment on every third day had the same effect as removing the reward on every third day; neuroleptics blocked the reinforcing efficacy of the food and water (Ettenberg and Camp, 1986a,b).

4.2.2. *Concentration Gradients*

Another approach is to study behavior under a number of reinforcement conditions, including some that normally establish high rates of responding and some that normally establish low rates of responding. If neuroleptics are tested across these conditions—as in the curve-shift paradigm for brain stimulation reward (Edmonds and Gallistel, 1974)—the high-rate conditions can establish an estimate of the response ceiling of the animal at a given neuroleptic dose. Performance under neuroleptics can then be compared to performance under normal reward and non-reward under reward parameters or reinforcement schedules that only require the animal to respond at rates well within its limitations under drug. Using this approach, Xenakis and Sclafani (1982) have demonstrated that neuroleptics attenuate drinking of weak concentrations of sweet solutions, and that the same animals were capable of much faster responding, as demonstrated with stronger concentrations of the same sweeteners. A similar demonstration has been made in a lever-pressing task (Bailey *et al.*, 1985).

An analogous demonstration has been made by Heyman *et al.* (1986); in this case different rates of water-reinforced responding were established by a variety of reinforcement ratios. Neuroleptics were shown to decrease responding under conditions of low reinforcement density (reinforcers per hour) to levels well below the rates of demonstrated response capability under high reinforcement density conditions. While parametric analysis of the data suggested here, as in other paradigms, that response capacity was impaired to some degree, the question of relevance was whether it was impaired to a sufficient degree to explain the response decrements observed. It clearly was not (Heyman *et al.*, 1986).

4.2.3. *Conditioned Place Preference*

Another approach to determining the effects of neuroleptics on the reinforcing efficacy of a natural reward involves the conditioned place preference paradigm. In this paradigm, animals are given experience with a reinforcer in a particular portion of the test box, and the strength of reinforcement is inferred by the degree to which the animal increases the percentage of time spent in that area. The advantage of this paradigm is that the reinforcing event occurs on one set of days ("conditioning" days, when the reinforcer is associated with the test environment) and the measure of reinforcement strength occurs on another set of days ("test" days). In testing the effects of a neuroleptic on reinforcing efficacy, the performance of the animal during testing is drug-free (since the neuroleptic is given on the conditioning days but not on the test days). Thus there is no question of motoric impairment by the neuroleptic on the test day. In this sense, the paradigm is similar to the runway paradigm of Ettenberg and Camp, 1986a,b). Neuroleptics have been shown to attenuate the reinforcing effects of food in this paradigm (Spyraki *et al.*, 1982).

These studies indicate that brain pathways containing dopamine as their neurotransmitter play an important role in the reinforcing effects of food and water, just as they play an important role in the reinforcing effects of brain stimulation. It is also the case that pathways containing endogenous opioid peptides seem implicated in food and water reward. Opiates and endogenous opioids stimulate free feeding and drinking (Ayhan and Randrup, 1973; Jalowiec *et al.*, 1981; Morley and Levine, 1981; Morley *et al.*, 1982, 1983; Sanger and McCarthy, 1980, 1981) and opiate antagonists decrease these behaviors (Holtzman, 1974, 1975; Maikel *et al.*, 1977) and lever-pressing for food and water (Mello *et al.*, 1981; Sanger and McCarthy, 1982). Opiate antagonists also inhibit the feeding which can be induced by electrical stimulation of medial forebrain bundle reward sites (Carr and Simon, 1983; Jenck *et al.*, 1986a). One site at which opiates facilitate both natural feeding and feeding induced by hypothalamic electrical stimulation is the ventral tegmental reward site (Jenck *et al.*, 1986b; Wise *et al.*, 1986). This suggests that opiate-facilitation of feeding is due to an interaction of opiates with reward pathways; opiates may facilitate food reward in the same way and at the same site as they facilitate brain stimulation reward (Broekkamp *et al.*, 1976).

4.3. The Substrate of Opiate Reward

4.3.1. *Ventral Tegmental Area*

A prediction of the theory that the mechanism of drug facilitation of brain stimulation reward would prove to be the mechanism of drug reward per se (Broekkamp *et al.*, 1975, 1976; Kornetsky *et al.*, 1979; Levitt *et al.*, 1977; C. D. Wise and Stein, 1970; Wise, 1980) was that local microinjections of morphine and amphetamine would be rewarding in their own right when injected into the sites where they facilitated brain stimulation reward. In the case of morphine, this prediction was borne out with the demonstration that ventral tegmental injections of opiates were rewarding (Bozarth and Wise, 1981b, 1984; Phillips and LePiane, 1980, 1982; van Ree and de Wied, 1980). The region where such injections were rewarding was bounded by the anterior and posterior (Bozarth and Wise, 1982) and dorsal (Bozarth and Wise, 1982; Phillips and LePiane, 1980) boundaries of the dopamine cell group, as predicted by Broekkamp (1975).

Several lines of study suggest that opiate injections in this region activate the dopaminergic neurons. First, bilateral injections into this region cause dopamine-dependent locomotion (Joyce and Iversen, 1979; Joyce *et al.*, 1981), while unilateral injections cause contraversive circling which is also dopamine-dependent (Holmes *et al.*, 1983; Holmes and Wise, 1985). Second, iontophoretic application of morphine to cells in this region causes an increase in cell firing (Hu and Wang, 1984; Matthews and German, 1984; Ostrowski *et al.*, 1982). Neuroleptics reduce intravenous heroin self-administration (Ettenberg *et al.*, 1982), and, while this effect is hard to interpret by itself, studies of heroin place preference conditioning indicate that neuroleptics interfere with the rewarding impact of heroin and not just the response capacity of the animal (Bozarth and Wise, 1981a; Spyraki *et al.*, 1983). Local injections of opiate antagonists in the ventral tegmental area decrease the rewarding impact of intravenous heroin (Britt and Wise, 1983; Vaccarino *et al.*, 1985). These studies, taken together, suggest the ventral tegmental area as one site at which opiates can interact with brain reward pathways.

4.3.2. *Nucleus Accumbens*

A second site at which opiates appear capable of interacting with the same circuit is at the next synaptic junction, in the nucleus accumbens. While morphine is not as effective as a reward or as a reward enhancer when injected into this region as it is when injected into the ventral tegmental area (Bozarth and Wise, 1981b, 1982; Broekkamp *et al.*, 1976), methionine enkephalin is readily self-administered directly into this nucleus (Goeders *et al.*, 1984). While diallyl-nor-morphinium bromide—a quaternary opiate mixed agonist-antagonist—is more effective in altering intravenous heroin self-administration when injected into the ventral tegmental area (Britt and Wise, 1983), methyl naloxonium chloride—a quaternary pure antagonist—is more effective when injected into nucleus accumbens (Vaccarino *et al.*, 1985). It may be that low doses of morphine are ineffective in nucleus accumbens (Bozarth and Wise, 1981b, 1982) because the drug must diffuse further from the cannula tip in this large nucleus, or because the affinity of nucleus accumbens receptors for morphine is lower than that of ventral tegmental receptors.

In addition, nucleus accumbens opiate receptors may exist in low numbers until the animal is challenged in certain ways. Opioids induce locomotor activity when injected either at the mesolimbic dopamine cell bodies (Joyce and Iversen, 1979; Joyce *et al.*, 1981) or at the nucleus accumbens dopamine terminals (Kalivas *et al.*, 1983; Pert and Sivit, 1977; Stinus *et al.*, 1985), but they are normally less effective in the nucleus accumbens (Kalivas *et al.*, 1983). When animals are treated with chronic neuroleptics or reserpine, marked increase is seen in the responsiveness to nucleus accumbens opioids (Stinus *et al.*, 1986). Since opiates themselves share some properties with neuroleptics (Kuschinsky and Hornykiewicz, 1974), chronic heroin self-administration may itself sensitize nucleus accumbens to opiates. A good deal of work is needed on this problem, since it appears possible that opiates interact with both pre- and post-synaptic opiate receptors in the nucleus accumbens (Kalivas and Bronson, 1985). It is important to determine whether the rewarding effects of intra-accumbens opioids is altered by chronic neuroleptic treatment or dopaminergic depletion.

Whether or not the sensitization produced by neuroleptics or dopamine depletion (Stinus *et al.*, 1985, 1986) is needed, it seems clear that opiates can activate the pathways involved in reward and locomotion at either the ventral tegmental area or the nucleus accumbens. The nucleus accumbens site of action is sufficient to maintain intravenous heroin self-administration in animals that have their mesolimbic dopamine system blocked with neuroleptics (Ettenberg *et al.*, 1982) or lesioned (Pettit *et al.*, 1984), and it is argued by some workers to be the major site of rewarding action of intravenous opiates (Ettenberg *et al.*, 1982). If sensitization of this structure by neuroleptics or dopamine depletion is not a prerequisite for its responsiveness to intravenous heroin, this would make good sense; all other things being equal, a drug should be most effective at the most efferent of several points of entry into a given neural pathway.

4.4. The Substrate of Psychomotor Stimulant Reward

The psychomotor stimulants owe their rewarding actions to their ability to increase concentrations of synaptic dopamine. Cocaine increases synaptic levels of catecholamines by blocking the reuptake mechanism which is the primary source of synaptic catecholamine inactivation (Heikkila *et al.*, 1975). Amphetamine also blocks reuptake; in addition it augments release of catecholamines (Axelrod, 1970; Carlsson, 1970). That it is the actions in dopamine synapses and not the actions in noradrenergic synapses which are essential for the reinforcing actions of amphetamine and cocaine is clear from a number of considerations. First, selective dopamine blockers attenuate the rewarding impact of intravenous amphetamine (Davis and Smith, 1975; Risner and Jones, 1976; Yokel and Wise, 1975, 1976) and cocaine (de Wit and Wise, 1977; Risner and Jones, 1980), while selective noradrenergic blockers do not (same studies). Second, while selective dopamine agonists have amphetamine-like rewarding properties (Baxter *et al.*, 1974; Davis and Smith, 1977; Wise *et al.*, 1976; Woolverton *et al.*, 1984; Yokel and Wise, 1978), selective noradrenergic agonists seem not to. The noradrenergic agonist clonidine is, over a narrow range of doses, self-administered by rats (Davis and Smith, 1977) and monkeys (Woolverton *et al.*, 1982), but it does not appear to have *amphetamine-like* rewarding properties (Yokel and Wise, 1978); rats self-administering clonidine resemble rats self-administering morphine more than they resemble rats self-administering amphetamine (Davis and Smith, 1977).

Lesion studies confirm that dopaminergic pathways are important for amphetamine and cocaine reward and that noradrenergic pathways are not. Lesions of noradrenergic systems have no effect on intravenous stimulant self-administration (Roberts and Zito, 1987) while selective neurotoxin (6-OHDA) lesions of nucleus accumbens block acquisition (Lyness *et al.*, 1979) and maintenance (Pettit *et al.*, 1984; Roberts *et al.*, 1977, 1980) of amphetamine self-administration as do neurotoxin lesions of the dopaminergic cell bodies of the ventral tegmental area (Bozarth and Wise, 1986; Roberts and Koob, 1982).

In addition, selective dopamine receptor blockade (Gunne *et al.*, 1972) and depletion (Jonsson *et al.*, 1971) attenuate the euphorigenic effect of intravenous amphetamines in humans, while selective noradrenergic blockade does not (Gunne, *et al.*, 1972).

4.4.1. *Nucleus accumbens*

Of the various dopamine pathways, the most strongly implicated in stimulant self-administration is the projection from the ventral tegmental area to the nucleus accumbens. In addition to the lesion studies already mentioned, rats will learn to lever-press for direct intracranial injections of amphetamine into the nucleus accumbens (Hoebel *et al.*, 1983). Rats will also lever-press for direct injections of dopamine into this region (Guerin *et al.*, 1984), though they are reported not to work for cocaine injections into this region (Goeders and Smith, 1983). This latter finding is surprising, since cocaine should block dopamine uptake in this nucleus (Heikkila *et al.*, 1975), and the post-synaptic neurons should not be able to discriminate increased dopamine caused by the presence of cocaine from increased dopamine caused by the presence of amphetamine. Moreover, nucleus accumbens injections of spiroperidol, a selective dopamine antagonist, block intravenous cocaine self-administration (Phillips *et al.*, 1983). Perhaps direct injection of cocaine into nucleus accumbens was not rewarding because the output neurons of that nucleus were inactivated by the local anesthetic effect of cocaine.

4.4.2. *Frontal Cortex*

Cocaine is self-administered into the dopamine terminal field of frontal cortex in rats (Goeders and Smith, 1983). Amphetamine is self-administered into dopamine-rich areas of orbitofrontal cortex in rhesus monkeys (Phillips *et al.*, 1981). These findings and the fact that injections of dopamine agonists into the frontal cortex of rats produce circling similar to that seen with striatal injections suggest that dopamine projections to different areas have common behavioral functions. Thus frontal cortex and nucleus accumbens may both receive dopaminergic pathways of reward. The caudate may similarly be involved; Phillips *et al.*, (1981) were able to train one monkey to panel-press for amphetamine injections into the caudate nucleus.

4.5. Other Drugs of Abuse

4.5.1. *Pathways of Direct Rewarding Actions*

Little is known about the pathways that are critical for the self-administration of other drugs of abuse. Intracranial self-administration has not been reported for other drugs, and lesion studies of animals responding for intravenous injections of other drugs have similarly not been done. Attempts to block self-administration of ethanol with neuroleptics have been restricted to an oral self-administration paradigm with no operant response requirement (Brown *et al.*, 1982); most rats (Sinclair, 1974) do not lever-press for oral ethanol (Lester, 1966; Lester and Freed, 1973; Mello, 1973) unless food deprivation and unusual training procedures (Meisch and Beardsley, 1975) are used.

4.5.2. *Psychomotor Stimulant Actions*

There may be something to be learned about shared actions of drugs of abuse from the study of unconditioned effects on unstructured behavior. While it has not been possible to find a common denominator in the physical dependence syndromes associated with psychomotor stimulants and opiates, these two seemingly different drug classes do have actions in common, and they relate to the pathways of positive reinforcement. Both stimulants and opiates activate or augment the dopaminergic input into the nucleus accumbens and frontal cortex. Three correlates of this common action are readily measured in animals that passively receive drugs, and there is evidence to suggest that other drugs of abuse have similar actions (Wise and Bozarth, 1987).

The common behavioral correlates of pyschomotor stimulant and opiate reward are psychomotor stimulant actions. The prototypical behavioral effects of self-administered doses of psychomotor stimulants are increased locomotion and stereotyped head movements (Pickens and Harris, 1968; Randrup and Munkvad, 1966, 1970). The locomotion and stereotypy appear to be mediated by independent and incompatible mechanisms; locomotion is seen at low doses and stereotypy replaces it at high doses (Randrup and Munkvad, 1970). The locomotor response is associated with dopaminergic activation in the nucleus accumbens and the stereotypy response is associated with dopaminergic activation in the striatum; dopamine-selective denervation of nucleus accumbens attenuates the locomotor response to amphetamine, while caudate denervation attenuates the stereotypy response (Keely *et al.*, 1975), and dopaminergic reinnervation of the dopamine-denervated accumbens reinstates locomotor responses, while reinnervation of the caudate reinstates stereotypy (Dunnett *et al.*, 1981, 1983). Reinnervation of the dopamine-denervated frontal cortex also reinstates locomotor responses to amphetamine, suggesting, again, common functions for dopamine projections to accumbens and frontal cortex (Dunnett *et al.*, 1984).

Opiates also increase locomotion and stereotypic head movements at self-administered doses. Stimulant effects of morphine, though paradoxical given the usual classification of opiates as depressants as narcotics and sedatives, are well-established (Ayhan and Randrup, 1973; Babbini and Davis, 1972; Browne and Segal, 1980; Iwamoto, 1981), and they are mediated by the activation of the ventral tegmental dopamine system (Joyce and Iversen, 1979; Joyce *et al.*, 1981; Stinus *et al.*, 1980). Indeed, it is the activation of this pathway that is presumed to account for the reinforcing effects of opiate injections into this area (Bozarth and Wise, 1981b; Phillips and LePiane, 1980, 1982).

Other sedative drugs also stimulate locomotor activity. As is the case with opiates, the effects are biphasic, with sedation predominating at higher dose levels and stimulation of locomotion becoming unmasked as the high-dose sedative effects wear off. Such effects are seen with barbiturates (Domino, 1962; Winters *et al.*, 1967), ethanol (Friedman *et al.*, 1980; Frye and Breese, 1981; Strombom and Liedman, 1982), benzodiazepines (Margules and Stein, 1968), cannabis (Glick and Milloy, 1972), and phencyclidine (Boren and Consroe, 1981; Castellani and Adams, 1981; Murray and Horita, 1979; Schlemmer *et al.*, 1978).

In the case of ethanol (Gessa *et al.*, 1985) and phencyclidine (Gerhardt and Rose, 1985; Vickroy and Johnson, 1982) the stimulation of locomotor activity is correlated with stimulation of dopamine turnover. Systemic benzodiazepines (Cheramy *et al.*, 1977; Weiner *et al.*, 1977; Wood, 1982) and barbiturates (Corrodi *et al.*, 1966), on the other hand, appear to inhibit dopamine turnover. Benzodiazepines and barbiturates are thought to interact with GABA receptors, however, and GABA is thought to interact with the locomotor and stereotypy pathways at a synapse efferent to the dopaminergic influence (Mogenson and Nielson, 1983; Redgrave *et al.*, 1980).

Other addictive drugs with psychomotor stimulant actions are nicotine and caffeine. Nicotine is self-administered by humans and lower animals (Cox *et al.*, 1984; Dougherty *et al.*, 1981; Henningfield and Goldberg, 1983; Spealman and Goldberg, 1982), and it causes increased locomotor activity and stereotypy in rats (Iwamoto, 1984). In drug discrimination studies, nicotine is more like amphetamine than saline (Henningfield and Jasinski, 1983; Schechter, 1981). Nicotine improves psychomotor performance in humans, particularly under conditions of fatigue or boredom (Wesnes and Warburton, 1983; Wesnes *et al.*, 1983). While the psychomotor stimulant properties of nicotine appear to be weak when the drug is given by injection (Iwamoto, 1984; Morrison and Stephenson, 1973; Pradhan, 1970; Schlatter and Battig, 1979), nicotine can activate the mesolimbic dopamine system (Arqueros *et al.*, 1978; Giorguieff-Chesselet *et al.*, 1979; Lichtensteiger *et al.*, 1982), and locomotor effects of nicotine can be induced by microinjections directly into the ventral tegmental area (Pert and Chiueh, 1986). Inasmuch as there are nicotinic receptors on the dopamine cell bodies of this region (Clarke and Pert, 1985), there is good reason to believe that this is the site of nicotine's stimulant action.

Caffeine is also compulsively self-administered by some humans (Gilbert, 1976), though it appears not to be a powerful reinforcer in lower animals (Deneau *et al.*, 1969). It does increase locomotor activity in rodents, and this effect is at least partially antagonized by dopamine receptor blockers (Estler, 1979; Waldeck, 1973). Caffeine increases mesolimbic dopamine turnover (Govoni *et al.*, 1984). Thus caffeine has weak amphetamine-like actions that probably involve activation of the mesolimbic reward pathways.

In addition, electrical stimulation of the medial forebrain bundle reward pathways has psychomotor stimulant properties (Glickman and Schiff, 1967). Such stimulation increases locomotor activity when animals are tested in an empty test box (Glickman and Schiff, 1967; Valenstein *et al.*, 1970), and it increases the approach and interaction with consummatory objects like food, water, sex partners, nesting material, and the like when such objects are present (Glickman and Schiff, 1967; Valenstein *et al.*, 1970). It has been suggested that approach responses are the common denominator of all positive reinforcers (Glickman and Schiff, 1967; Schneirla, 1959), and this view has recently been extended to the case of drugs of abuse (Wise and Bozarth, 1987). If this view is valid, then drugs of abuse, like rewarding medial forebrain bundle electrical stimulation, should increase the tendency to approach goal objects such as food or social partners.

The ability of drugs to stimulate appetite has been widely studied. Opiates stimulate appetite, as previously discussed, and this was recognized early as a stimulant action (Ayhan and Randrup, 1973). Barbiturates (Jacobs and Farel, 1971; Watson and Cox, 1976) and benzodiazepines (Cooper, 1980; Poschel, 1971; Randall *et al.*, 1960; Wise and Dawson, 1974) stimulate eating at the sub-sedative doses that stimulate locomotor activity. Ethanol has been reported to have a benzodiazepine-like stimulant effect on feeding in an open-field eating situation (Britton and Britton, 1981). Cannabis enhances feeding at low doses (Abel, 1971; Drewnowski and Grinker, 1978; Glick and Milloy, 1972; Hollister, 1971).

The nominal psychomotor stimulants, on the other hand, are thought to generally suppress appetite (Cole, 1967, 1970). However, just as the opiates have independent and opposite effects on locomotion, so do the amphetamines have opposite and seemingly independent effects on feeding. Amphetamine and the selective dopamine agonist apomorphine stimulate appetite in animals with experimental dopamine depletions (Ljungberg and Ungerstedt, 1976: Stricker and Zigmond, 1976; Wolgin *et al.*, 1976). Moreover, facilitory effects of amphetamine on feeding can be observed in intact animals (Blundell and Latham, 1978, 1982); the basic finding is that amphetamine accelerates feeding while decreasing meal duration and total food intake. The acceleration of feeding which can be seen with systemic doses of amphetamine can be produced with central amphetamine as well; injections into the nucleus accumbens produce this effect (Colle and Wise, 1986). It remains an open question as to whether subtle facilitation of feeding will be found when other stimulant drugs are tested in these paradigms.

5. REWARD PATHWAYS AND DRUG "CRAVING"

Clinicians attempting to help patients break compulsive drug self-administration habits are concerned with the subjective reports of "craving" which seem to predict relapse of detoxified individuals. Early theories of opiate addiction view opiate craving as a natural consequence of physical distress symptoms (Himmelsbach, 1943; Lindsmith, 1947), and methadone treatment programs were developed in the attempt to relieve opiate craving without producing opiate euphoria (Dole and Nyswander, 1965). More recently, clonidine and antidepressant therapies have been used in attempts to alleviate opiate craving in recently detoxified addicts (Gold and Kleber, 1981; Kleber *et al.*, 1983), and other drugs have been tried in attempts to alleviate craving for cocaine in recently detoxified compulsive users (Dackis and Gold, 1985b; Gawin and Kleber, 1984; Khantzian *et al.*, 1984). It is of some interest to attempt to relate the subjective symptoms of craving to the various effects of drugs and drug abstinence on the pathways of reward.

Attempts to understand craving for opiates in detoxified addicts have focused on the physical withdrawal symptoms (Gold *et al.*, 1978; Dole and Nyswander, 1965) which are alleviated by opiate effects in the negative reinforcement mechanisms and pathways of the periventricular system (Bozarth and Wise, 1984; Laschka *et al.*, 1976; Wei *et al.*, 1973b). Methadone and clonidine are each used to alleviate opiate withdrawal symptoms, substituting for heroin *as a negative reinforcer*.

The success of these therapies has served as a model for current attempts to find a pharmacological treatment for cocaine craving. The assumption is that the target for pharmacological intervention should be the distress syndrome associated with drug withdrawal, but in this case the distress syndrome is one of "psychological" dependence and not physical dependence. Since there is no evidence to suggest that stimulants interact with the periaqueductal gray pathways of opiate dependence, neither methadone nor clonidine is a viable candidate. Since there is no other negative reinforcement pathway associated with stimulant dependence, attention has focused on hypothesized changes in the primary reinforcement pathway; it has been suggested that cocaine craving is a correlate of dopamine depletion and receptor supersensitivity that can result from prolonged cocaine use (Dackis and Gold, 1985b; Gawin and Kleber, 1984).

The essence of this suggestion is that withdrawal distress marked by craving reflects a rebound condition resulting from prolonged and powerful activation of the positive reinforcement mechanism. Until it was clear that opiate positive reinforcement and opiate negative reinforcement involved anatomically—and thus functionally—distinct brain pathways (Bozarth and Wise, 1984), similar notions marked most discussions of possible mechanisms of opiate physical dependence; dependence was assumed to involve desensitization of the physiological mechanism of the drug's primary actions (Collier, 1968; Jaffe and Sharpless, 1968). The notion was that the mechanism of drug reinforcement was desensitized by exposure to drug, so that stronger and stronger doses were needed for a given psychological effect (tolerance) and so that some drug intake must be maintained to keep the system functioning even at normal levels. Such a model is viable logically, but it must be noted that it explains negative reinforcement, not positive reinforcement. In the case of the opiates, on which the model is based, it is now clear that the negative reinforcement mechanism does not involve rebound desensitization of the positive reinforcement mechanism (Bozarth and Wise, 1984). In the case of the opiates, two independent mechanisms mediate the positive and the negative reinforcing effects of the drugs.

This is not to deny that negative reinforcement could result from desensitization of the positive reinforcement mechanism. It is possible that chronic use of cocaine desensitizes the positive reinforcement mechanism, and that hypoactivity of that system results from drug abstinence after periods of heavy drug use. If such hypoactivity were the correlate of cocaine cravings, however, then it is obvious that the most effective pharmacological treatment for craving would be the normal dose of the habitual drug. Any drug that is substituted for the abused drug, producing negative reinforcement by activating the depressed positive reinforcement system, would be a substance that had abuse liability in its own right. It would be remarkable to find a drug that would stimulate the positive reinforcement system only when this system was depressed during cocaine abstinence. It would be even more remarkable to find a drug that could stimulate the system only to its normal level of activity. Bromocriptine, which has been used to treat cocaine craving in humans, is a selective dopamine receptor agonist, and this compound (Bozarth and Wise, unpublished observations; Woolverton *et al.*, 1984) like other dopamine agonists (Baxter *et al.*, 1974; Davis and Smith, 1977; Risner and Jones, 1976; Woolverton *et al.*, 1984; Yokel and Wise, 1978) is self-administered by rats and monkeys. If it proves to be the case that chronic activation of the positive reinforcement mechanism desensitizes that mechanism and causes dysphoria which can be alleviated by more drug, then this dysphoria will be difficult to treat with pharmacological approaches. Any drug which activates the positive reinforcement mechanism should be expected to have abuse liability.

Methadone and bromocriptine may alleviate heroin and cocaine cravings because they alleviate withdrawal distress by acting as negative reinforcers. Alternatively, they may alleviate heroin and cocaine cravings because, like heroin and cocaine, they activate the pathways of positive reinforcement. If they substitute in the positive reinforcement pathways, why do they not have addiction liability which is comparable in strength to that of heroin and cocaine? Bromocriptine has aversive side-effects, which may limit its attractiveness. Both bromocriptine and methadone are long-acting and slowly absorbed, and this may make them weaker reinforcers than cocaine and heroin. Morphine is a less potent positive reinforcer than heroin, and the difference is attributed to its slower entry into the brain (Oldendorf *et al.*, 1972). This fact takes on major significance when the importance of delay of reinforcement is appreciated. Operant psychologists attempt to make reinforcement follow the desired response as rapidly as possible when rapid learning is desired, and a delay of a single second greatly impairs acquisition of a lever-pressing habit rewarded by hypothalamic brain stimulation (Black *et al.*, 1985). If "craving" represents a condition of abnormal depression of the positive reinforcement mechanism and if the normalization of this depression constitutes a case of negative reinforcement involving the positive reinforcement pathways, then drugs like methadone and bromocriptine, which would alleviate depression of the mechanism for a long duration (thus reducing the number of reinforced responses in a given period) and which would alleviate this depression rather slowly, might be the best approach to pharmacological treatment. While positive reinforcement is greatly diminished by delays of a second or two, the ability to alleviate symptoms of craving should survive such delays.

If there is no depression of the reward pathways when chronic use of cocaine or heroin is terminated, what other explanation is there for feelings of drug craving and instances of drug relapse? One possibility is simply that the subject remembers the last reinforcement, and the reactivation of this memory by associated environmental stimuli is sufficient to activate feelings of craving. Rats clearly remember their last few rewarding brain stimulations, adjusting their speed of running for access to more brain stimulation in proportion to the amount of stimulation received on the last trial. The running speed is the same whether the last trial was five minutes earlier or five days earlier; the rat simply remembers what it has been receiving for lever-pressing (Gallistel *et al.*, 1974). If the rat remembers strong reinforcement, it runs quickly; this has nothing, apparently, to do with the state of its dopamine receptors, since five days should make a difference in any changes in receptor supersensitivity which were caused by the last reinforcement experiment. Craving for cocaine or heroin may, like craving for nicotine in a smoker who has been nicotine free for many years, simply be triggered by memories of past experience. Like a cat that has tasted fish, a human that has tasted cocaine may be unwilling to give up the hope of repeating the experience. If this view, suggested by the behavior of rats activating the reward pathways by medial forebrain bundle electrical stimulation, is correct, then it may be more appropriate to look for the biological correlate of craving in the neurobiology of memory, and not in the neurobiology of positive reinforcement.

6. SUMMARY AND CONCLUSIONS

In commenting on the discovery of "opiate" receptors, Goldstein (1976) said: "It seemed unlikely, a priori, that such highly stereospecific receptors should have been developed by nature to interact with alkaloids from the opium poppy" (p. 1081). Endogenous opioid peptides and opioid receptor systems have now been identified in invertebrates that are unlikely to have had ancestors exposed to opium poppies (Kavaliers *et al.*, 1983; Kream *et al.*, 1980; Leung and Stefano, 1984; Stefano *et al.*, 1980). Moreover, endogenous opioids play a role in stress-induced feeding in the slug (Kavaliers and Hirst, 1986) just as they play a role in stress-induced feeding in rodents (Lowy *et al.*, 1980; Morley and Levine, 1980). If we are to understand the actions of opiates and other drugs of abuse we must understand them in terms of their abilities to interact with neural systems that evolved in the service of primitive biological functions, long before any serious incidence of addiction itself.

The most primitive axes of the biological substrates of behavior are the axes of approach and withdrawal. Addictive drugs appear to be able to activate the mechanisms of approach, which is termed "positive reinforcement" and to inhibit the mechanisms of withdrawal, which is termed "negative reinforcement." anatomically distinct sets of pathways have evolved to serve these two forms of reward.

Activation of the medial forebrain bundle and associated structures serves positive reinforcement and induces forward locomotion. Approach and forward locomotion are the unconditioned responses to positive reinforcing stimuli such as food and sex partners, and approach to environmental objects and positive reinforcement is induced by electrical stimulation of this structure. The locomotor stimulating effects and the positive reinforcing effects of opiates and psychomotor stimulants result from their activation of this mechanism; stimulants activate the mechanism at the level of dopaminergic synapses of the nucleus accumbens, frontal cortex, and perhaps other forebrain structures, while opiates activate the system at two points: at the level of the dopaminergic synapse and at the level of the afferents to the dopaminergic cell bodies. Ethanol, nicotine, caffeine and phencyclidine stimulate both locomotor activity and dopamine turnover, but their sites of interaction with reward pathways have not yet been identified. Benzodiazepines and barbiturates stimulate locomotor activity without stimulating dopamine turnover; they may interact with reward pathways at a synapse efferent to the dopaminergic link in the pathways. On the basis of present evidence, it is not unreasonable to expect that there is a "final common path" for the positive reinforcement produced by natural rewards like food and water, laboratory rewards like medial forebrain bundle electrical stimulation, and drug rewards associated with all addictive substances.

The negative reinforcing properties of drugs involve a distinct mechanism from those of positive reinforcement and are unlikely to have any final common path. The mechanisms of opiate negative reinforcement are understood in some detail in relation to physical pain. Opiates activate pathways of the periaqueductal gray and spinal cord that can attenuate incoming pain signals. Opiates appear to alleviate the distress of their own withdrawal syndrome through actions in multiple brain and peripheral regions; their most dramatic effects on opiate withdrawal distress are mediated at or near sites where opiates activate brain pathways of analgesia. The negative reinforcing properties of other addictive substances are not known, but it is likely that a variety of pathways are involved and that there is a good deal of specificity associated with the negative reinforcement mechanisms associated with different classes of dependence-producing drugs. Considerable overlap is expected in the mechanisms mediating the negative reinforcing properties of ethanol, barbiturates, and benzodiazepines, since there is considerable cross-dependence between these agents. To the degree that physical dependence syndromes and negative reinforcement can be linked to the psychomotor stimulants, very different pathways are expected to play a role. Where psychomotor stimulants and various dependent classes may activate common pathways of positive reinforcement, they must either affect different pathways of negative reinforcement, or, if the same pathways are involved, they must affect them in opposite directions. There are no data from animal models to suggest that negative reinforcement plays a significant role in stimulant reinforcement.

REFERENCES

Abel, E. L. (1971) Effects of marihuana on the solution of anagrams, memory and appetite. *Nature* **231**: 260–261.

Abood, L. G., Lowry, K., Tometsko, A. and Booth, H. (1978) Electrophysiological, behavioral, and chemical evidence for a noncholinergic, stereo-specific site for nicotine in rat brain. *J. Neurosci. Res.* **3**: 327–333.

Adams, W. J., Lorens, S. A. and Mitchell, C. L. (1972) Morphine enhances lateral hypothalamic self-stimulation in the rat. *Proc. Soc. Exp. Biol.* **140**: 770–771.

Ahlenius, S. (1979) An analysis of behavioral effects produced by drug-induced changes of dopaminergic neurotransmission in the brain. *Scand. J. Psychol.* **20**: 59–64.

Akil, H., Mayer, D. J. and Liebeskind, J. C. (1976) Antagonism of stimulation-produced analgesia by naloxone, a narcotic antagonist. *Science* **191**: 961–962.

Alexander, B. K. (1984) When experimental psychology is not empirical enough: The case of the "exposure orientation." *Can. Psychol.* **25**: 84–95.

Alexander, B. K. and Hadaway, P. F. (1982) Opiate addiction: The case for an adaptive orientation. *Psychol. Bull.* **92**: 367–381.

Alexander, B. K., Coambs, R. B. and Hadaway, P. F. (1978) The effect of housing and gender on morphine self-administration in rats. *Psychopharmacology* **58**: 175–179.

ALEXANDER, B. K., BEYERSTEIN, B. L., HADAWAY, P. F. and COAMBS, R. B. (1981) The effect of early and later colony housing on oral ingestion of morphine in rats. *Pharmac. Biochem. Behav.* **15**: 571–576.

AMARAL, D. G. and ROUTTENBERG, A. (1975) Locus coeruleus and intracranial self-stimulation: a cautionary note. *Behav. Biol.* **13**: 331–338.

AMIR, S., BROWN, Z. W. and AMIT, Z. (1980) The role of endorphins in stress: Evidence and speculations. *Neurosci. Biobehav. Rev.* **4**: 77–86.

ARQUEROS, L., NAQUIRA, D. and ZUNINO, E. (1978) Nicotine-induced release of catecholamines from rat hippocampus and striatum. *Biochem. Pharmac.* **27**: 2667–2674.

ATWEH, S. F. and KUHAR, M. J. (1977) Autoradiographic localization of opiate receptors in rat brain. III. The telencephalon. *Brain Res.* **134**: 393–405.

AXELROD, J. (1970) Amphetamine: Metabolism, physiological disposition, and its effects on catecholamine storage. In: *Amphetamines and Related Compounds*, pp. 207–216, COSTA, E. and GARATTINI, S. (eds) Raven Press, New York.

AYHAN, I. H. and RANDRUP, A. (1973) Behavioural and pharmacological studies on morphine-induced excitation of rats. Possible relation to brain catecholamines. *Psychopharmacologia* **29**: 317–328.

BABBINI, M. and DAVIS, W. M. (1972) Time-dose relationships for locomotor activity effects of morphine after acute or repeated treatment. *Br. J. Pharmac.* **46**: 213–224.

BAILEY, C. S., HSIAO, S. and KING, J. E. (1985) Reward summation functions separate pimozide's motor and hedonic effects in rats lever-pressing for sucrose. *Soc. Neurosci. Abstr.* **11**: 720.

BARBEAU, A. (1974) Drugs affecting movement disorders. *Annu. Rev. Pharmac.* **14**: 91–113.

BARCHAS, J. D., AKIL, H., ELLIOTT, G. R., HOLMAN, R. B. and WATSON, S. J. (1978) Behavioral neurochemistry: Neuroregulators and behavioral states. *Science* **200**: 964–973.

BASBAUM, A. I. and FIELDS, H. L (1978) Endogenous pain control mechanisms: Review and hypothesis. *Ann. Neurol.* **4**: 451–462.

BAXTER, B. L., GLUCKMAN, M. I., STEIN, L. and SCERNI, R. A. (1974) Self-injection of apomorphine in the rat: Positive reinforcement by a dopamine receptor stimulant. *Pharmac. Biochem. Behav.* **2**: 387–391.

BECKMAN, A. L., LLADOS-ECKMAN, C., STANTON, T. L. and ADLER, M. W. (1982) Seasonal variation of morphine physical dependence. *Life Sci.* **30**: 147–153.

BEECHER, H. K. (1959) *Measurement of Subjective Responses: Quantitative Effects of Drugs*, Oxford University Press, Oxford.

BELLUZZI, J. D. and STEIN, L. (1977) Enkephalin may mediate euphoria and drive-reduction reward. *Nature* **266**: 556–558.

BENINGER, R. J. (1982) The behavioral function of dopamine. *Behav. Brain Sci.* **5**: 55–56.

BENINGER, R. J., BELLISLE, F. and MILNER, P. (1977) Schedule control of behavior reinforced by electrical stimulation of the brain. *Science* **196**: 547–549.

BIELAJEW, C. and SHIZGAL, P. (1982) Behaviorally derived measures of conduction velocity in the substrate for rewarding medial forebrain bundle stimulation. *Brain Res.* **237**: 107–119.

BIELAJEW, C. and SHIZGAL, P. (1986) Evidence implicating descending fibers in self-stimulation of the medial forebrain bundle. *J. Neurosci.* **6**(4): 919–929.

BISHOP, M. P., ELDER, S. T. and HEATH, R. G. (1963) Intracranial self-stimulation in man. *Science* **140**: 394–396.

BLACK, J., BELLUZZI, J. D. and STEIN, L. (1985) Reinforcement delay of one second severely impairs acquisition of brain self-stimulaton. *Brain Res.* **359**: 113–119.

BLOOM, F. E., BATTENBERG, E., ROSSIER, J., LING, N. and GUILLEMIN, R. (1978) Neurons containing β-endorphin in rat brain exist separately from those containing enkephalin: Immunocytochemical studies. *Proc. Natl. Acad. Sci. U.S.A.* **75**: 1591–1595.

BLUNDELL, J. E. and LATHAM, C. J. (1978) Pharmacological manipulation of feeding: possible influences of serotonin and dopamine on food intake. In: *Central Mechanisms of Anorectic Drugs*, pp. 83–109, SAMANIN, R. and GARATTINI, S. (eds) Raven Press, New York.

BLUNDELL, J. E. and LATHAM, C. J. (1982) Behavioural pharmacology of feeding. In: *Drugs and Appetite*, pp. 41–80, SILVERSTONE, T. (ed) Academic Press, London.

BOREN, J. L. and CONSROE, P. F. (1981) Behavioral effects of phencyclidine (PCP) in the dog: A possible animal model of PCP toxicity in humans. *Life Sci.* **28**: 1245–1251.

BOZARTH, M. A. and WISE, R. A. (1981a) Heroin reward is dependent on a dopaminergic substrate. *Life Sci.* **29**: 1881–1886.

BOZARTH, M. A. and WISE, R. A. (1981b) Intracranial self-administration of morphine into the ventral tegmental area of rats. *Life Sci.* **28**: 551–555.

BOZARTH, M. A. and WISE R. A. (1982) Localization of the reward-relevant opiate receptors. In: *Problems of Drug Dependence, 1981*, (National Institute on Drug Abuse Research Monograph 41), pp. 158–164, HARRIS, L. S. (ed.) U.S. Government Printing Office, Washington, D.C.

BOZARTH, M. A. and WISE, R. A. (1983) Dissociation of the rewarding and physical dependence-producing properties of morphine. In: *Problems of Drug Dependence, 1982* (National Institute on Drug Abuse Research Monograph 43), pp. 171–177, HARRIS, L. S. (ed.) U.S. Government Printing Office, Washington, D.C.

BOZARTH, M. A. and WISE, R. A. (1984) Anatomically distinct opiate receptor fields mediate reward and physical dependence. *Science* **224**: 516–517.

BOZARTH, M. A. and WISE, R. A. (1986) Involvement of the ventral tegmental dopamine system in opioid and psychomotor stimulant reinforcement. In: *Problems of Drug Dependence, 1985*, (National Institute on Drug Abuse Reseach Monograph 67), pp. 190–196, HARRIS, L. S. (ed.) U.S. Government Printing Office, Washington, D.C.

BRITT, M.D. and WISE, R. A. (1983) Ventral tegmental site of opiate reward: Antagonism by a hydrophilic opiate receptor blocker. *Brain Res.* **258**: 105–108.

BRITTON, D. R. and BRITTON, K. T. (1981) A sensitive open field measure of anxiolytic drug activity. *Pharmac. Biochem. Behav.* **15**: 577–582.

Broekkamp, C. L. E. (1975) The modulation of rewarding systems in the animal brain by amphetamine, morphine and apomorphine. Unpublished thesis, University of Nijmegen.

Broekkamp, C. L. E., Pijnenburg, A. J. J., Cools, A. R. and Van Rossum, J. M. (1975) The effect of microinjections of amphetamine into the neostriatum and the nucleus accumbens on self-stimulation behavior. *Psychopharmacologia* **42**: 179–183.

Broekkamp, C. L. E., Van den Bogard, J. H., Heijnen, H. J., Rops, R. H., Cools, A. R. and Van Rossum, J. M. (1976) Separation of inhibiting and stimulating effects of morphine on self-stimulation behavior by intracerebral microinjections. *Eur. J. Pharmac.* **36**: 443–446.

Broekkamp, C. L. E., Phillips, A. G. and Cools, A. R. (1979) Facilitation of self-stimulation behavior following intracerebral microinjections of opioids into the ventral tegmental area. *Pharmac. Biochem. Behav.* **11**: 289–295.

Brown, Z. W., Gill, K., Abitbol, M. and Amit, Z. (1982) Lack of effect of dopamine receptor blockade on voluntary ethanol comsumption in rats. *Behav. Neural Biol.* **36**: 291–294.

Browne, R. G. and Segal, D. S. (1980) Behavioral activating effects of opiates and opioid peptides, *Biol. Psychiatry* **15**: 77–86.

Bush, H. D., Bush, M. A., Miller, M. A. and Reid, L. D. (1976) Addictive agents and intracranial self-stimulation: Daily morphine and lateral hypothalamic self-stimulation. *Physiol. Psychol.* **4**: 79–85.

Carlsson, A. (1970) Amphetamine and brain catecholamines. In: *Amphetamines and Related Compounds*, pp. 289–300, Costa, E. and Garattini, S. (eds) Raven Press, New York.

Carr, K. D. and Simon, E. J. (1983) Effects of naloxone and its quarternary analogue on stimulation-induced feeding. *Neuropharmacology* **22**: 127–130.

Castellani, S. and Adams, P. M. (1981) Effects of dopaminergic drugs on phencyclidine-induced behavior in the rat. *Neuropharmacology* **20**: 371–374.

Chein, I., Gerard, D. L., Lee, R. S. and Rosenfeld, E. (1964) *The Road to H: Narcotics, Delinquency, and Social Policy*, Basic Books, New York.

Cheramy, A., Nieoullon, A. and Glowinski, J. (1977) Blockade of the picrotoxin-induced *in vivo* release of dopamine in the cat caudate nucleus by diazepam. *Life Sci.* **20**: 811–816.

Chin, J. H. and Goldstein, D. B. (1977) Drug tolerance in biomembranes. A spin label study of the effect of ethanol. *Science* **196**: 684–685.

Clarke, P. B. S. and Kumar, R. (1984) Effects of nicotine and *d*-amphetamine on intracranial self-stimulation in a shuttle box test in rats. *Psychopharmacology* **84**: 109–114.

Clarke, P. B. S. and Pert, A. (1985) Autoradiographic evidence for nicotine receptors on nigrostriatal and mesolimbic dopaminergic neurons. *Brain Res.* **348**: 355–358.

Clarke, P. B. S. Pert, C. B. and Pert, A. (1984) Autoradiographic distribution of nicotine receptors in rat brain. *Brain Res.* **323**: 390–395.

Clarke, P. B. S., Hommer, D. W., Pert, A. and Skirboll, L. R. (1985) Electrophysiological actions of nicotine on substantia nigra single units. *Br. J. Pharmac.* **85**: 827–835.

Clavier, R. M. and Routtenberg, A. (1974) Ascending monoamine-containing fiber pathways related to intracranial self-stimulation: histochemical fluorescence study. *Brain Res.* **72**: 25–40.

Cohen, G. and Collins, M. (1970) Alkaloids from catecholamines in adrenal tissue: Possible role in alcoholism. *Science* **167**: 1749–1751.

Cohen, S. R. and Melzack, R. (1985) Morphine injected into the habenula and dorsal posteromedial thalamus produces analgesia in the formalin test. *Brain Res.* **359**: 131–139.

Cole, S. O. (1967) Experimental effects of amphetamine: A review. *Psychol. Bull.* **68**: 81–90.

Cole, S. O. (1970) Experimental effects of amphetamine: Supplementary report. *Percept. Mot. Skills* **31**: 223–232.

Colle, L. M. and Wise, R. A. (1986) Facilitation of lateral hypothalamic self-stimulation by amphetamine microinjections into nucleus accumbens. *Soc. Neurosci. Abst.* **12**: 930.

Collier, H. O. J. (1968) Supersensitivity and dependence. *Nature* **220**: 228–231.

Collier, T. J. and Routtenberg, A. (1984) Electrical self-stimulation of dentate gyrus granule cells. *Behav. Neural Biol.* **42**: 85–90.

Cooper, S. J. (1980) Benzodiazepines as appetite-enhancing compounds. *Appetite* **1**: 7–19.

Corbett, D. and Wise, R. A. (1979) Intracranial self-stimulation in relation to the ascending noradrenergic fiber systems of the pontine tegmentum and caudal midbrain: A moveable electrode mapping study. *Brain Res.* **177**: 423–436.

Corbett, D. and Wise, R. A. (1980) Intracranial self-stimulation in relation to the ascending dopaminergic systems of the midbrain: A moveable electrode mapping study. *Brain Res.* **185**: 1–15.

Corrodi, H., Fuxe, K. and Hokfelt, T. (1966) The effects of barbiturates on the activity of the catecholamine neurons in the rat brain. *J. Pharm. Pharmac* **18**: 556–558.

Cox, B. M., Goldstein, A. and Nelson, W. T. (1984) Nicotine self-administration in rats. *Br. J. Pharmac.* **83**: 49–55.

Crow, T. J. (1970) Enhancement by cocaine of intra-cranial self-stimulation in the rat. *Life Sci* **9**: 375–381.

Crow, T. J. (1972) A map of the rat mesencephalon for electrical self-stimulation. *Brain Res.* **36**: 265–273.

Crow, T. J. (1973) Catecholamine-containing neurones and electrical self-stimulation: 2. Theoretical interpretation and some psychiatric interpretations. *Psychol. Med.* **3**: 66–73.

Csontos, K., Rust, M., Höllt, V., Mahr, W., Kromer, W. and Teschemacher, H. J. (1979) Elevated plasma beta-endorphin levels in pregnant women and their neonates. *Life Sci.* **25**: 835–844.

Dackis, C. A. and Gold, M. S. (1985a) Bromocriptine as treatment of cocaine abuse. *Lancet* **1**: 1151–1152.

Dackis, C. A. and Gold, M. S. (1985b) New concepts in cocaine addiction: The dopamine depletion hypothesis. *Neurosci. Biobehav. Rev.* **9**: 469–477.

Davis, V. E. and Walsh, M. J. (1970) Alcohol, amines and alkaloids: A possible biochemical basis for alcohol addiction. *Science* **167**: 1005–1006.

DAVIS, W. M. and SMITH, S. G. (1975) Effect of haloperidol on (+)-amphetamine self-administration. *J. Pharm. Pharmac.* **27**: 540–542.

DAVIS, W. M. and SMITH, S. G. (1977) Catecholaminergic mechanisms of reinforcement: Direct assessment by drug self-administration. *Life Sci.* **20**: 483–492.

DENEAU, G., YANAGITA, T. and SEEVERS, M. H. (1969) Self-administration of psychoactive substances by the monkey: A measure of pyschological dependence. *Psychopharmacologia* **16**: 30–48.

DEWEY, W. L. SNYDER, J. W., HARRIS, L. S. and HOWES, J. F. (1969) The effects of narcotics and narcotic antagonists on the tail-flick response in spinal mice. *J. Pharm. Pharmac.* **21**: 548–550.

DE WIT, H. and WISE, R. A. (1977) Blockade of cocaine reinforcement in rats with the dopamine receptor blocker pimozide but not with the noradrenergic blockers phentolamine or phenoxybenzamine. *Can. J. Psychol*, **31**: 195–203.

DE WITTE, P. and BADA, M. F. (1983) Self-stimulation and alcohol administered orally or intraperitoneally, *Exp. Neurol.* **82**: 675–682.

DINGEMANSE, J. and BREIMER, D. D. (1984) Benzodiazepine receptors. *Pharm. Int.* **5**: 33–36.

DOLE, V. P. and NYSWANDER, M. (1965) A medical treatment for diacetylmorphine (heroin) addiction. *J. Am. Med. Assoc.* **193**: 646–650.

DOLE, V. P. and NYSWANDER, M. (1967) Heroin addiction—A metabolic disease. *Arch. Intern. Med.* **120**: 19–24.

DOMINO, E. F. (1962) Sites of action of some central nervous system depressants. *Ann. Rev. Pharmac.* **2**: 215–268.

DOMINO, E. F., VASKO, M. R. and WILSON, A. E. (1976) Mixed depressant and stimulant actions of morphine and their relationship to brain acetylcholine. *Life Sci.* **18**: 361–376.

DOUGHERTY, J. D., MILLER, D., TODD, G. and KOSTENBAUDER, H. B. (1981) Reinforcing and other effects of nicotine. *Neurosci. Biobehav. Rev.* **5**: 487–495.

DREWNOWSKI, A. and GRINKER, J. A. (1978) Temporal effects of delta-9-tetrahydrocannabinol on feeding patterns and activity of obese and lean Zucker rats. *Behav. Biol.* **23**: 112–117.

DUNNETT, S. B., BJORKLUND, A., STENEVI, U. and IVERSEN, S. D. (1981) Behavioural recovery following transplantation of substantia nigra in rats subjected to 6-OHDA lesions of the nigrostriatal pathway. I. Unilateral lesions. *Brain Res.* **215**: 147–161.

DUNNETT, S. B., BJORKLUND, A., SCHMIDT, A., STENEVI, U. and IVERSEN, S. D. (1983) Intracerebral grafting of neuronal cell suspensions. IV. Behavioural recovery in rats with unilateral implants of nigral cell suspensions in different forebrain sites. *Acta Physiol. Scand. Suppl.* **522**: 29–37.

DUNNETT, S. B., BUNCH, S. T., GAGE, F. H. and BJORKLUND, A. (1984) Dopamine-rich transplants in rats with 6-OHDA lesions of the ventral tegmental area. I. Effects on spontaneous and drug-induced locomotor activity. *Behav. Brain Res.* **13**: 71–82.

EDMONDS, D. E. (1976) The effect of alpha-methyl-*p*-tyrosine methyl ester on temporal summation in the neural substrate for the reinforcement effect in self-stimulation. In: *Brain Stimulation Reward*, pp. 261–263, WAUQUIER, A. and ROLLS, E. T. (eds) Elsevier, Amsterdam.

EDMONDS, D. E. and GALLISTEL, C. R. (1974) Parametric analysis of brain stimulation reward in the rat: III. Effect of performance variables on the reward summation function. *J. Comp. Physiol. Psychol.* **87**: 876–883.

EIKELBOOM, R. and STEWART, J. (1979) Conditioned temperature effects using morphine as the unconditioned stimulus. *Psychopharmacology* **61**: 31–38.

ESPOSITO, R. U., FAULKNER, W. and KORNETSKY, C. (1979) Specific modulation of brain stimulation reward by haloperidol. *Pharmac. Biochem. Behav.* **10**: 937–940.

ESPOSITO, R. U. and KORNETSKY, C. (1978) Opioids and rewarding brain stimulation. *Neurosci. Biobehav. Rev.* **2**: 115–122.

ESPOSITO, R. U., PERRY, W. and KORNETSKY, C. (1980) EFFECTS OF *d*-amphetamine and naloxone on brain stimulation reward. *Psychopharmacology* **69**: 187–191.

ESSIG, C. F., JONES, B. E. and LAM, R. C. (1969) The effect of pentobarbital on alcohol withdrawal in dogs, *Arch. Neurol.* **20**: 554–558.

ESTLER, C. -J. (1979) Influence of pimozide on the locomotor hyperactivity produced by caffeine. *J. Pharm. Pharmac.* **31**: 126–127.

ETTENBERG, A. (1982) Behavioral effects of neuroleptics: Performance deficits, reward deficits or both? *Behav. Brain Sci.* **5**: 56–57.

ETTENBERG, A. and CAMP, C. H. (1986a) Haloperidol induces a partial reinforcement extinction effect in rats: Implications for a dopamine involvement in food reward. *Pharmac. Biochem. Behav.* **25**: 813–821.

ETTENBERG, A. and CAMP, C. H. (1986b) A partial reinforcement extinction effect in water-reinforced rats intermittently treated with haloperidol. *Pharmac. Biochem. Behav.* **25**: 1231–1235.

ETTENBERG, A., CINSAVICH, S. A. and WHITE, N. (1979) Performance effects with repeated-response measures during pimozide-produced dopamine receptor blockade. *Pharmac. Biochem. Behav.* **11**: 557–561.

ETTENBERG, A., KOOB, G. F. and BLOOM, F. E. (1981) Response artifact in the measurement of neuroleptic-induced anhedonia. *Science* **213**: 357–359.

ETTENBERG, A., PETTIT, H. O., BLOOM, F. E. and KOOB, G. F. (1982) Heroin and cocaine intravenous self-administration in rats: Mediation by separate neural systems. *Psychopharmacology* **78**: 204–209.

FENTON, H. M. and LIEBMAN, J. M. (1982) Self-stimulation response decrement patterns differentiate clonidine, baclofen and dopamine antagonists from drugs causing performance deficit. *Pharmac. Biochem. Behav.* **17**: 1207–1212.

FIBIGER, H. C. (1978) Drugs and reinforcement mechanisms: A critical review of the catecholamine theory. *Annu. Rev. Pharmac. Toxicol.* **18**: 37–56.

FIBIGER, H. C., CARTER, D. A. and PHILLIPS, A. G. (1976) Decreased intracranial self-stimulaton after neuroleptics or 6-hydroxydopamine: Evidence for mediation by motor deficits rather than by reduced reward. *Psychopharmacology* **47**: 21–27.

FOURIEZOS, G. and WISE, R. A. (1976) Pimozide-induced extinction of intracranial self-stimulation: Response patterns rule out motor or performance deficits. *Brain Res.* **103**: 377–380.

Fouriezos, G., Hansson, P. and Wise, R. A. (1978) Neuroleptic-induced attenuation of brain stimulation reward in rats. *J. Comp. Physiol. Psychol.* **92**: 661–671.

Franklin, K. B. J. (1978) Catecholamines and self-stimulation: Reward and performance effects dissociated. *Pharmac. Biochem. Behav.* **9**: 813–820.

Franklin, K. B. J. and McCoy, S. N. (1979) Pimozide-induced extinction in rats: Stimulus control of responding rules out motor deficit. *Pharmac. Biochem. Behav.* **11**: 71–75.

Fraser, H. F., Wikler, A. Isbell, H. and Johnson, N. K. (1957) Partial equivalence of chronic alcohol and barbiturate intoxications. *Q. J. Stud. Alcohol* **18**: 541–551.

Freed, W. J. and Mendelson, J. (1974) Airlicking: Thirsty rats prefer a warm dry airstream to a warm humid airstream. *Physiol. Behav.* **12**: 557–561.

Friedman, H. J., Carpenter, J. A., Lester, D. and Randall, C. L. (1980) Effect of alpha-methyl-*p*-tyrosine on dose-dependent mouse strain differences in locomotor activity after ethanol. *J. Stud. Alcohol* **41**: 1–7.

Frye, G. D. and Breese, G. R. (1981) An evaluation of the locomotor stimulating action of ethanol in rats and mice. *Psychopharmacology* **75**: 372–379.

Gallistel, C. R. and Davis, A. J. (1983) Affinity for the dopamine D_2 receptor predicts neuroleptic potency in blocking the reinforcing effect of MFB stimulation. *Pharmac. Biochem. Behav.* **19**: 867–872.

Gallistel, C. R. and Karras, D. (1984) Pimozide and amphetamine have opposing effects on the reward summation function. *Pharmac. Biochem. Behav.* **20**: 73–77.

Gallistel, C. R., Stellar, J. R. and Bubis, E. (1974) Parametric analysis of brain stimulation in the rat: I. The transient process and the memory-containing process. *J. Comp. Physiol. Psychol.* **87**: 848–859.

Gallistel, C. R. Shizgal, P. and Yeomans, J. (1981) A portrait of the substrate for self-stimulation. *Psychol. Rev.* **88**: 228–273.

Gallistel, C. R., Boytim, M., Gomita, Y. and Klebanoff, L. (1982) Does pimozide block the reinforcing effect of brain stimulation? *Pharmac. Biochem. Behav.* **17**: 769–781.

Gawin, F. H. and Kleber, H. D. (1984) Cocaine abuse treatment. *Gen. Psychiatry* **41**: 903–909.

Gerber, G. J., Bozarth, M. A. and Wise, R. A. (1981a) Small-dose intravenous heroin facilitates hypothalamic self-stimulation without response suppression in rats. *Life Sci.* **28**: 557–562.

Gerber, G. J., Sing, J. and Wise, R. A. (1981b) Pimozide attenuates lever pressing for water reinforcement in rats. *Pharmac. Biochem. Behav.* **14**: 201–205.

Gerhardt, G. and Rose, G. (1985) Presynaptic action of phencyclidine (PCP) in the rat striatum defined using *in vivo* electrochemical methods. *Soc. Neurosci. Abstr.* **11**: 1205.

German, D. C. and Bowden, D. M. (1974) Catecholamine systems as the neural substrate for intracranial self-stimulation: A hypothesis. *Brain Res.* **73**: 381–419.

Gessa, G. L., Muntoni, F., Collu, M., Vargiu, L. and Mereu, G. (1985) Low doses of ethanol activate dopaminergic neurons in the ventral tegmental area. *Brain Res.* **348**: 201–204.

Gilbert, R. M. (1976) Caffeine as a drug of abuse. In: *Research Advances in Alcohol and Drug Problems*, Vol. 3, pp. 49–176, Gibbons, R. J., Israel, Y., Kalant, H., Popham, R. E., Schmidt, W. and Smart, R. G. (eds) John Wiley, New York.

Giorguieff-Chesselet, M. F., Kemel, M. L., Wandscheer, D. and Glowinski, J. (1979) Regulation of dopamine release by presynaptic nicotinic receptors in rat striatal slices: effect of nicotine in low concentration. *Life Sci.* **25**: 1257–1262.

Glick, S. D. and Milloy, S. (1972) Increased and decreased eating following THC administration. *Psychon. Sci.* **29**: 6.

Glickman, S. E. and Schiff, B. B. (1967) A biological theory of reinforcement. *Psychol. Rev.* **74**: 81–109.

Glimcher, P. W., Giovino, A. A., Margolin, D. H. and Hoebel, B. G. (1984) Endogenous opiate reward induced by an enkephalinase inhibitor. *Behav. Neurosci.* **98**: 262–268.

Goeders, N. E. and Smith, J. E. (1983) Cortical dopaminergic involvement in cocaine reinforcement. *Science* **221**: 773–775.

Goeders, N. E., Lane, J. D. and Smith, J. E. (1984) Self-administration of methionine enkephalin into the nucleus accumbens. *Pharmac. Biochem. Behav.* **20**: 451–455.

Gold, M. S., and Kleber, H. D. (1981) Clinical utility of clonidine in opiate withdrawal: A study of 100 patients. In: *Pharmacology of Clonidine*, pp. 299–306, Harbans, L. and Fielding, S. (eds) Alan Liss, New York.

Gold, M. S., Redmond, D. E. and Kleber, H. D. (1978) Clonidine in opiate withdrawal. *Lancet* **1**: 599–601.

Goldberg, S. R., Woods, J. H. and Schuster, C. R. (1971) Nalorphine-induced changes in morphine self-administration in rhesus monkeys. *J. Pharmac. Exp. Ther.* **176**: 464–471.

Goldstein, A. (1976) Opioid peptides (endorphins) in pituitary and brain. *Science* **193**: 1081–1086.

Goldstein, D. B. and Goldstein, A. (1961) Possible role of enzyme inhibition and repression in drug tolerance and addiction. *Biochem. Pharmac.* **8**: 48.

Goldstein, A. and Judson, B. A. (1971) Alcohol dependence and opiate dependence: Lack of relationship in mice. *Science* **172**: 290–292.

Goldstein, A., Lowney, L. I. and Pal, B. K. (1971) Stereospecific and nonspecific interactions of the morphine congener levorphanol in subcellular fractions of mouse brain. *Proc. Natl. Acad. Sci. U.S.A.* **68**: 1742–1747.

Govoni, S., Petkov, V. V., Montefusco, O., Missale, C., Battaini, F., Spano, P. F. and Trabucchi, M. (1984) Differential effects of caffeine on dihydroxyphenylacetic concentrations in various rat brain regions. *J. Pharm. Pharmac.* **36**: 458–460.

Gramling, S. E., Fowler, S. C. and Collins, K. R. (1984) Some effects of pimozide on nondeprived rats licking sucrose solutions in an anhedonia paradigm. *Pharmac. Biochem. Behav.* **21**: 617–624.

Gratton, A. and Wise, R. A. (1983) Brain stimulation reward in the lateral hypothalamic medial forebrain bundle: mapping of boundaries and homogeneity. *Brain Res.* **274**: 25–30.

Gratton, A. and Wise, R. A. (1985) Hypothalamic reward mechanism: Two first-stage fiber populations with a cholinergic component. *Science* **227**: 545–548.

GROSSMAN, S. P. (1966) The VMH: A center for affective reactions, satiety, or both? *Physiol. Behav.* **1**: 1–9.

GUERIN, G. F., GOEDERS, N. E., DWORKIN, S. I. and SMITH, J. E. (1984) Intracranial self-administration of dopamine into the nucleus accumbens. *Soc. Neurosci. Abstr.* **10**: 1072.

GUILLEMIN, R., VARGO, T. M., ROSSIER, J., MINICK, S., LING, N., RIVIER, C., VALE, W. and BLOOM, F. E. (1977) β-endorphin and adrenocorticotropin are secreted concomitantly by the pituitary gland. *Science* **197**: 1367–1369.

GUNNE, L. M., ANGGARD, E. and JONSSON, L. E. (1972) Clinical trials with amphetamine-blocking drugs. *Psychiatr. Neurol. Neurochir.* **75**: 225–226.

HAEFELY, G. W. (1984) Benzodiazepine interactions with GABA receptors. *Neurosci. Lett.* **47**: 201–206.

HAUGER, R. L., HULIHAN-GIBLIN, R., SKOLNICK, P. and PAUL, S. M. (1984) Characteristics of [^{3}H](+)-amphetamine binding sites in the rat central nervous system. *Life Sci.* **34**: 771–782.

HEBB, D. O. (1949) *The Organization of Behavior*, Wiley, New York.

HEIKKILA, R. E., ORLANSKY, H. and COHEN, G. (1975) Studies on the distinction between uptake inhibition and release of [^{3}H]dopamine in rat brain tissue slices. *Biochem. Pharmac.* **24**: 847–852.

HENNINGFIELD, J. E. and GOLDBERG, S. R. (1983) Nicotine as a reinforcer in human subjects and laboratory animals. *Pharmac. Biochem. Behav.* **19**: 989–992.

HENNINGFIELD, J. E. and JASINSKI, D. R. (1983) Human pharmacology of nicotine. *Psychopharmac. Bull.* **19**: 413–415.

HERMAN, B. H. and PANKSEPP, J. (1978) Effects of morphine and naloxone on separation distress and approach attachment: Evidence for opiate mediation of social affect. *Pharmac. Biochem. Behav.* **9**: 213–220.

HERMAN, B. H. and PANKSEPP, J. (1981) Ascending endorphin inhibition of distress vocalization. *Science* **211**: 1060–1062.

HERZ, A., ALBUS, K., METYS, J., SCHUBERT, P. and TESCHEMACHER, H. (1970) On the central sites for the antinociceptive action of morphine and fentanyl. *Neuropharmacology* **9**: 539–551.

HEYMAN, G. M., KINZIE, D. L. and SEIDEN, L. S. (1986) Chlorpromazine and pimozide alter reinforcement efficacy and motor performance. *Psychopharmacology* **88**: 346–353.

HIMMELSBACH, C. K. (1943) Morphine, with reference to physical dependence. *Fed. Proc.* **2**: 201–203.

HOEBEL, B. G., MONACO, A., HERNANDEZ, L., AULISI, E., STANLEY, B. G. and LENARD, L. (1983) Self-injection of amphetamine directly into the brain. *Psychopharmacology* **81**: 158–163.

HOLLISTER, L. E. (1971) Hunger and appetite after single doses of marijuana, alcohol and dextroamphetamine. *Pharmac. Ther.* **12**: 44–49.

HOLMES, L. J. and WISE, R. A. (1985) Contralateral circling induced by tegmental morphine: Anatomical localization, pharmacological specificity, and phenomenology. *Brain Res.* **326**: 19–26.

HOLMES, L. J., BOZARTH, M. A. and WISE, R. A. (1983) Circling from intracranial morphine applied to the ventral tegmental area in rats. *Brain Res. Bull.* **11**: 295–298.

HOLTZMAN, S. G. (1974) Behavioral effects of separate and combined administrations of naloxone and *d*-amphetamine *J. Pharmac. Exp. Ther.* **189**: 51–60.

HOLTZMAN, S. G. (1975) Effects of narcotic antagonists on fluid intake in the rat. *Life Sci.* **16**: 1465–1470.

HORNYKIEWICZ, O. (1975) Parkinsonism induced by dopaminergic antagonists. In: *Advances in Neurology*, Vol. 9, pp. 155–164, KALNE, D. B., CHASE, T. N. and BARBEAU, A. (eds) Raven Press, New York.

HU, X.-T. and WANG, R. Y. (1984) Comparison of morphine-induced effects on dopamine and non-dopamine neurons in the rat ventral tegmental area. *Soc. Neurosci. Abstr.* **10**: 66.

HUSTON, J. P. (1982) Searching for the neural mechanism of reinforcement (of "stamping-in"). In: *The Neural Basis of Feeding and Reward*, pp. 75–83, HOEBEL, B. G. and NOVIN, D. G. (eds) Haer Institute, Brunswick, Maine.

IRWIN, S., HOUDE, R. W., BENNETT, D. R., HENDERSHOT, L. C. and SEEVERS, M. H. (1951) The effects of morphine, methadone and meperidine on some reflex responses of spinal animals to nociceptive stimulation. *J. Pharmac. Exp. Ther.* **101**: 132–143.

IWAMOTO, E. T. (1981) Locomotor activity and antinociception after putative mu, kappa and sigma opioid receptor agonists in the rat: Influence of dopaminergic agonists and antagonists. *J. Pharmac. Exp. Ther.* **217**: 451–460.

IWAMOTO, E. T. (1984) An assessment of the spontaneous activity of rats administered morphine, phencyclidine, or nicotine using automated and observational methods. *Psychopharmacology* **84**: 374–382.

JACOBS, B. L. and FAREL, P. B. (1971) Motivated behaviors produced by increased arousal in the presence of goal objects. *Physiol. Behav.* **6**: 473–476.

JACOBS, H. L. (1967) Taste and the role of experience in the regulation of food intake. In: *The Chemical Senses and the Nutritive Process*, pp. 187–200, KARE, M. and MALLER, O. (eds) Johns Hopkins Press, Baltimore, Maryland.

JACOBS, H. L. and SHARMA, K. N. (1969) Taste versus calories: Sensory and metabolic signals in the control of food intake. *Ann. N.Y. Acad. Sci.* **157**: 1084–1125.

JAFFE J. H. (1980) Drug addiction and drug abuse. In: *The Pharmacological Basis of Therapeutics*, pp. 535–584, GILMAN, A. G., GOODMAN, L. S. and GILMAN, A. (eds) Macmillan, New York.

JAFFE, J. H. and SHARPLESS, S. K. (1968) Pharmacological denervation super-sensitivity in the central nervous system: A theory of physical dependence. In: *The Addictive States*, pp. 226–246, WIKLER, A. H. (ed.) Williams and Wilkins, Baltimore, Maryland.

JALOWIEC, J. E., PANKSEPP, J., ZOLOVICK, A. J., NAJAM, N. and HERMAN, B. H. (1981) Opioid modulation of ingestive behavior. *Pharmac. Biochem. Behav.* **15**: 477–484.

JENCK, F., GRATTON, A. and WISE, R. A. (1986a) Effects of pimozide and naloxone on latency for hypothalamically induced eating. *Brain Res.* **375**: 329–337.

JENCK, F., GRATTON, A. and WISE, R. A. (1986b) Opposite effects of ventral tegmental and periaqueductal gray morphine injections on lateral hypothalamic stimulation-induced feeding. *Brain Res.* **399**: 24–32.

JONES, R. T. (1980) Human effects: An overveiw. In: *Marijuana Research Findings: 1980 Cocaine*, pp. 54–80, PETERSON, R. C. (ed.) National Institute on Drug Abuse Research Monograph 31, Washington, D.C.

JONES, R. T. (1984) The pharmacology of cocaine. In: *Cocaine: Pharmacology, Effects, and Treatment of Abuse*, pp. 34–53, GRABOWSKI, J. (ed.) National Institute on Drug Abuse Research Monograph 50, Washington, D.C.

JONSSON, L., ANGGARD, E. and GUNNE, L. (1971) Blockade of intravenous amphetamine euphoria in man. *Clin. Pharmac. Ther.* **12**: 889–896.

JOYCE, E. M. and IVERSEN, S. D. (1979) The effect of morphine applied locally to mesencephalic dopamine cell bodies on spontaneous motor activity in the rat. *Neurosci. Lett. 14*: 207–212.

JOYCE, E. M., KOOB, G. F., STRECKER, R., IVERSEN, S. D. and BLOOM, F. E. (1981) The behavioral effects of enkephalin analogues injected into the ventral tegmental area and globus pallidus. *Brain Res.* **221**: 359–370.

KALANT, H. (1977) Comparative aspects of tolerance to, and dependence on, alcohol, barbiturates, and opiates. In: *Alcohol Intoxication and Withdrawal III*, pp. 169–186, GROSS, M. M. (ed.) Plenum, New York.

KALIVAS, P. W. and BRONSON, M. (1985) Mesolimbic dopamine lesions produce an augmented behavioral response to enkephalin. *Neuropharmacology* **24**: 931–936.

KALIVAS, P. W., WIDERLOV, E., STANLEY, D., BREESE, G. and PRANGE, A. J. (1983) Enkephalin action on the mesolimbic system: A dopamine-dependent and a dopamine-independent increase in locomotor activity. *J. Pharmac. Exp. Ther.* **227**: 229–237.

KAVALIERS, M. and HIRST, M. (1986) Naloxone-reversible stress-induced feeding and analgesia in the slug Limax Maximus. *Life Sci.* **38**: 203–209.

KAVALIERS, M., HIRST, M. and TESKEY, G. C. (1983) A functional role for an opiate system in snail thermal behavior. *Science* **220**: 99–101.

KELLY, P. H., SEVIOUR, P. W. and IVERSEN, S. D. (1975) Amphetamine and apomorphine responses in the rat following 6-OHDA lesions of the nucleus accumbens septi and corpus striatum *Brain Res.* **94**: 507–522.

KENNEDY, L. T. and HANBAUER, I. (1983) Sodium-sensitive cocaine binding to rat striatal membrane: Possible relationship to dopamine uptake sites. *J. Neurochem.* **41**: 172–178.

KHANTZIAN, E. J. (1974) Opiate addiction: A critique of theory and some implications for treatment. *Am. J. Psychother.* **28**: 59–70.

KHANTZIAN, E. J., GAWIN, F. H., KLEBER, H. D. and RIORDAN, C. E. (1984) Methylphenidate (Ritalin) treatment of cocaine dependence: A preliminary report. *J. Subst. Abuse Treat.* **1**(2): 107–112.

KLEBER, H. D., WEISSMAN, M. M., ROUNSAVILLE, B. J., WILBUR, C. H., PRUSOFF, B. A. and RIORDAN, C. E. (1983) Imipramine as treatment for depression in addicts. *Arch. Gen. Psychiatry* **40**: 649–653.

KOOB, G. F. (1982) The dopamine anhedonia hypothesis: A pharmacological phrenology. *Behav. Brain Sci* **5**: 63–64.

KORNETSKY, C. and ESPOSITO, R. U. (1979) Euphorigenic drugs: Effects on the reward pathways of the brain. *Fed. Proc.* **38**: 2473–2476.

KORNETSKY, C., ESPOSITO, R. U., MCLEAN, S. and JACOBSON, J. O. (1979) Intracranial self-stimulation thresholds: A model for the hedonic effects of drugs of abuse. *Arch. Gen. Psychiatry* **36**: 289–292.

KREAM, R. M., ZUKIN, R. S. and STEFANO, G. B. (1980) Demonstration of two classes of opiate binding sites in the nervous tissue of the marine mollusc *Mytilus edulis. J. Biol. Chem.* **225**: 9218–9224.

KUSCHINSKY, K. and HORNYKIEWICZ, O. (1974) Effects of morphine on striatal dopamine metabolism: Possible mechanism of its opposite effects on locomotor activity in rats and mice. *Eur. J. Pharmac.* **26**: 44–50.

LASCHKA, E., TESCHEMACHER, H., MAHRAEIN, P. and HERZ, A. (1976) Sites of action of morphine involved in the development of physical dependence of rats: II. Morphine withdrawal precipitated by application of morphine antagonists into restricted parts of the ventricular system and by microinfusion into various brain areas. *Psychopharmacologia* **46**: 141–147.

LÊ, A. D., KHANNA, J. M., KALANT, H. and GROSSI, F. (1986) Tolerance to and cross-tolerance among ethanol, pentobarbital and chlordiazepoxide. *Pharmac. Biochem. Behav.* **24**: 93–98.

LESTER, D. (1966) Self-selection of alcohol by animals, human variation and the etiology of alcoholism: A critical review. *Q. J. Stud. Alcohol* **27**: 395–438.

LESTER, D. and FREED, E. X. (1973) Criteria for an animal model of alcoholism. *Pharmac. Biochem. Behav.* **1**: 103–108.

LEUNG, M. K. and STEFANO, G. B. (1984) Isolation and identification of enkephalins in pedal ganglia of *Mytilus edulisa* (Mollusca). *Proc. Natl. Acad. Sci. U.S.A.* **81**: 955–958.

LEVINE, J. D., LANE, S. R., GORDON, N. C. and FIELDS, H. L. (1982) A spinal opioid synapse mediates the interaction of spinal and brainstem sites in morphine analgesia. *Brain Res.* **236**: 85–91.

LEVITT, R. A., BALTZER, J. H., EVERS, T. M., STILWELL, D. J. and FURBY, J. E. (1977) Morphine and shuttle-box self-stimulation in the rat: a model for euphoria. *Psychopharmacologia* **54**: 307–311.

LEWIS, M. J., ANDRADE, J. R., MEBANE, C. and PHELPS, R. (1984) Differential effects of ethanol and opiates on BSR threshold. *Soc. Neurosci. Abst.* **10**: 960.

LICHTENSTEIGER, W., FELIX, D., LIENHART, R. and HEFTI, F. (1976) A quantitative correlation between single unit activity and fluorescence intensity of dopamine neurons in zona compacta of substantia nigra, as demonstrated under the influence of nicotine and physostigmine. *Brain Res.* **117**: 85–103.

LICHTENSTEIGER, W., HEFTI, F., FELIX, D., HUWYLER, T., MELAMED, E. and SCHLUMPF, M. (1982) Stimulation of nigrostriatal dopamine neurones by nicotine. *Neuropharmacology* **21**: 963–968.

LIEBMAN, J. M. (1983) Discriminating between reward and performance: A critical review of intracranial self-stimulation methodology. *Neurosci. Biobehav. Rev.* **7**: 45–72.

LINDSMITH, A. R. (1947) *Opiate Addiction*, Principia Press, Bloomington, Indiana.

LIPPA, A. S., ANTELMAN, S. M., FISHER, A. E. and CANFIELD, D. R. (1973) Neurochemical mediation of reward: A significant role for dopamine? *Pharmac. Biochem. Behav.* **1**: 23–28.

LJUNGBERG, T. and UNGERSTEDT, U. (1976) Reinstatement of eating by dopamine agonists in aphagic dopamine denervated rats. *Physiol. Behav.* **16**: 277–283.

LOH, H. H., TSENG, L. F., WEI, E. and LI, C. H. (1976) β-endorphin is a potent analgesic agent. *Proc. Natl. Acad. Sci. U.S.A.* **73**: 2895–2898.

LORENS, S. A. and MITCHELL, C. L. (1973) Influence of morphine on lateral hypothalamic self-stimulation in the rat. *Psychopharmacologia* **32**: 271–277.

LORENS, S. A. and SAINATI, S. M. (1978) Naloxone blocks the excitatory effect of ethanol and chlordiazepoxide on lateral hypothalamic self-stimulation in the rat. *Life Sci.* **23**: 1359–1364.

LOWY, M. T., MAICKEL, R. P. and YIM, G. K. W. (1980) Naloxone reduction of stress-related feeding. *Life Sci.* **26**: 2113–2118.

LYNCH, M. R. and WISE, R. A. (1985) Relative effectiveness of pimozide, haloperidol and trifluoperazine on self-stimulation rate-intensity functions. *Pharmac. Biochem. Behav.* **23**: 777–780.

LYNESS, W. H., FRIEDLE, N. M. and MOORE, K. E. (1979) Destruction of dopaminergic nerve terminals in nucleus accumbens: effect on d-amphetamine self-administration. *Pharmac. Biochem. Behav.* **11**: 553–556.

MAIKEL,, R. P., BRAUDE, M. C. and ZABIK, J. E. (1977) The effects of various narcotic agonists and antagonists on deprivation-induced fluid consumption. *Neuropharmacology* **16**: 863–866.

MALMO, R. B. (1975) *On Emotions, Needs, and Our Archaic Brain*, Holt, Rinehart and Winston, New York.

MARGULES, D. L. and STEIN, L. (1968) Increase of "antianxiety" activity and tolerance of behavioral depression during chronic administration of oxazepam. *Psychopharmacologia* **13**: 74–80.

MARTIN, B. R. and ACETO, M. (1981) Nicotine binding sites and their localization in the central nervous system. *Neurosci. Biobehav. Rev.* **5**: 473–478.

MARTIN, W. R. (1967) Opioid antagonists. *Pharmac. Rev.* **19**: 464–521.

MARTIN, W. R. (1968) A homeostatic and redundancy theory of tolerance and dependence to narcotic analgesics. *Res. Publ.—Assoc. Res. Nerv. Ment. Dis.* **46**: 206–225.

MASON, S. T., BENINGER, R. J., FIBIGER, H. C. and PHILLIPS, A. G. (1980) Pimozide-induced suppression of responding: Evidence against a block of food reward. *Pharmac. Biochem. Behav.* **12**: 917–923.

MATTHEWS, R. T. and GERMAN, D. C.(1984) Electrophysiological evidence for excitation of rat ventral tegmental area dopaminergic neurons by morphine. *Neuroscience* **11**: 617–626.

MAYER, D. J. and HAYES, R. (1975) Stimulation-produced analgesia: Development of tolerance and cross-tolerance to morphine. *Science* **188**: 941–943.

MAYER, D. J. and MURPHIN, R. (1976) Stimulation-produced analgesia (SPA) and morphine analgesia (MA): Cross-tolerance from application at the same brain site. *Fed. Proc.* **35**: 385.

MAYER, D. J. and PRICE, D. D. (1976) Central nervous system mechanisms of analgesia. *Pain* **2**: 379–404.

MAYER, D. J., WOLFE, T. L., AKIL, H., DARDER, B. and LIEBESKIND, J. C. (1971) Analgesia from electrical stimulation in the brainstem of the rat. *Science* **174**: 1351–1354.

MEISCH, R. A. and BEARDSLEY, P. (1975) Ethanol as a reinforcer for rats: Effects of concurrent access to water and alternate positions of water and ethanol. *Psychopharmacology* **43**: 19–23.

MELLO, N. K. (1973) A review of methods to induce alcohol addiction in animals. *Pharmac. Biochem. Behav.* **1**: 89–101.

MELLO, N. K., MENDELSON, J. H. and BREE, M. P. (1981) Naltrexone effects on morphine and food self-administration in morphine-dependent rhesus monkeys. *J. Pharmac. Exp. Ther.* **218**: 550–557.

MELZACK, R. (1970) Pain perception. *Percept. Disorders* **48**: 272–285.

MELZACK, R. and PERRY, C. (1975) Self-regulation of pain: The use of alpha-feedback and hypnotic training for the control of chronic pain. *Exp. Neurol.* **46**: 452–469.

MELZACK, R. and WALL, P. D. (1965) Pain mechanism: A new theory. *Science* **150**: 971–979.

MELZACK, R., STILLWELL, D. M. and FOX, E. J. (1977) Trigger points and acupuncture points for pain: correlations and implications. *Pain* **3**: 3–23.

MENDELSON, J. and CHILLAG, D. (1970) Tongue cooling: A new reward for thirsty rodents. *Science* **170**: 1418–1419.

MILIARESSIS, E., MALETTE, J. and COULOMBE, D. (1986) The effects of pimozide on the reinforcing efficacy of central grey stimulation in the rat. *Behav. Brain Res.* **21**: 95–100.

MILNER, P. M. (1970) *Physiological Psychology*, Holt, Rinehart and Winston, New York.

MOGENSON, G. J. (1964) Effects of sodium pentobarbital on brain self-stimulation. *J. Comp. Physiol. Psychol.* **58**: 461–462.

MOGENSON, G. J. and NIELSON, M. A. (1983) Evidence than an accumbens to subpallidal GABAergic projection contributes to locomotor activity. *Brain Res. Bull.* **11**: 309–314.

MOHLER, H. and OKADA, T. (1977) Benzodiazepine receptor: Demonstration in the central nervous system. *Science* **198**: 849–851.

MORLEY, J. E. and LEVINE, A. S. (1980) Stress-induced eating is mediated through endogenous opiates. *Science* **209**: 1259–1261.

MORLEY, J. E. and LEVINE, A. S. (1981) Dynorphin-(1-13) induces spontaneous feeding in rats. *Life Sci.* **29**: 1901–1903.

MORLEY, J. E., LEVINE, A. S., GOSNELL, B. A., KNEIP, J. and GRACE, M. (1983) The kappa opioid receptor, ingestive behaviors and the obese mouse (ob/ob). *Physiol. Behav.* **31**: 603–606.

MORLEY, J. E., LEVINE, A. S., GRACE, M. and KNEIP, J. (1982) Dynorphin-(1-13), dopamine and feeding in rats. *Pharmac. Biochem. Behav.* **16**:701–705.

MORRISON, C. F. and STEPHENSON, J. A. (1973) Effects of stimulants on observed behavior of rats on six operant schedules. *Neuropharmacology* **12**: 297–310.

MURRAY, T. F. and HORITA, A. (1979) Phencyclidine-induced stereotyped behavior in rats: Dose response effects and antagonism by neuroleptics. *Life Sci.* **24**: 2217–2226.

NAKAJIMA, S. and MCKENZIE, G. M. (1986) Reduction of the rewarding effect of brain stimulation by blockade of dopamine D1 receptor with SCH 23390. *Pharmac. Biochem. Behav* **24**: 919–923.

NIEHOFF, D. L. and KUHAR, M. J. (1983) Benzodiazepine receptors: Localization in rat amygdala. *J. Neurosci.* **3**: 2091–2097.

NORTON, P. R. E. (1970) The effects of drugs on barbiturate withdrawal convulsions in the rat. *J. Pharm. Pharmac.* **22**: 763–766.

OLDENDORF, W. H., HYMAN, S., BRAUN, L. and OLDENDORF, S. Z. (1972) Blood-brain barrier: Penetration of morphine, codeine, heroin, and methadone after carotid injection. *Science* **178**: 984–986.

Olds, J. (1956) Pleasure centers in the brain. *Sci. Am.* **195**: 105–116.

Olds, J. (1958) Effects of hunger and male sex hormones on self-stimulation of the brain. *J. Comp. Physiol. Psychol.* **51**: 320–324.

Olds, J. (1966) Facilitatory action of diazepam and chlordiazepoxide on hypothalamic reward behavior. *J. Comp. Physiol. Psychol.* **62**: 136–140.

Olds, J. (1972) Postscript. In: *Current Status of Physiological Psychology Readings*, pp. 152–153, Singh, D. and Morgan, C. T. (eds) Brooks/Cole, Monterey, California.

Olds, J. (1976) Reward and drive neurons. In: *Brain Stimulation Reward*, pp. 1–27, Wauquier, A. and Rolls, E. T. (eds) Elsevier, Amsterdam.

Olds, J. and Milner, P. M. (1954) Positive reinforcement produced by electrical stimulation of septal area and other regions of rat brain. *J. Comp. Physiol. Psychol.* **47**: 419–427.

Olds, J. and Olds, M. E. (1965) Drives, rewards, and the brain. In: *New Directions in Psychology*, Vol. II, pp. 327–410, Holt, Rinehart and Winston, New York.

Olds, J. and Travis, R. P. (1960) Effects of chlorpromazine, meprobamate, pentobarbital and morphine on self-stimulation. *J. Pharmac. Exp. Ther.* **128**: 397–404.

Olds, M. E. and Olds, J. (1963) Approach-avoidance analysis of rat diencephalon. *J. Comp. Neurol.* **120**: 259–295.

Olsen, R. W. (1982) Drug interactions at the GABA receptor ionophore complex. *Annu. Rev. Pharmac. Toxicol.* **22**: 245–277.

Ostrowski, N. L., Hatfield, C. B. and Caggiula, A. R. (1982) The effects of low doses of morphine on the activity of dopamine containing cells and on behavior. *Life Sci.* **31**: 2347–2350.

Panksepp, J. and Bishop, P. (1981) An autoradiographic map of (^{3}H)diprenorphine binding in rat brain: Effects of social interaction. *Brain Res. Bull.* **7**: 405–410.

Panksepp, J., Gandelman, R. and Trowill, J. (1970) Modulation of hypothalamic self-stimulation and escape behavior by chlordiazepoxide. *Physiol. Behav.* **5**: 965–969.

Panksepp, J., Herman, B. H., Conner, R., Bishop, P. and Scott, J. P. (1978a) The biology of social attachments: Opiates alleviate separation distress. *Biol. Psychiatry* **13**: 607–618.

Panksepp, J., Vilberg, T., Bean, N. J., Coy, D. H. and Kastin, A. H. (1978b) Reduction of distress vocalization in chicks by opiate-like peptide. *Brain Res. Bull.* **3**: 663–667.

Panksepp, J., Bean, N. J., Bishop, P., Vilberg, T. and Sahley, T. L. (1980a) Opioid blockade and social comfort in chicks. *Pharmac. Biochem. Behav.* **13**: 673–683.

Panksepp, J., Herman, B. H., Vilberg, T., Bishop, P. and DeEskinazi, F. G. (1980b) Endogenous opioids and social behavior. *Neurosci. Biobehav. Rev.* **4**: 473–487.

Pavlov, I. P. (1927) *Conditioned Reflexes*, Oxford University Press, Oxford.

Peele, S. and Brodsky, A. (1975) *Love and Addiction*, New American Library of Canada, Scarborough.

Pert, A. and Chiueh, C. C. (1986) Effects of intracerebral nicotinic agonists on locomotor activity: Involvement of mesolimbic dopamine. *Soc. Neurosci. Abstr.* **12**: 917.

Pert, A. and Sivit, C. (1977) Neuroanatomical focus for morphine and enkephalin-induced hypermotility. *Nature*, **265**: 645–647.

Pert C. B. and Snyder, S. H. (1973) Opiate receptor: Demonstration in nervous tissue. *Science* **179**: 1011–1014.

Pettit, H. O., Ettenberg, A., Bloom, F. E. and Koob, G. F. (1984) Destruction of dopamine in the nucleus accumbens selectively attenuates cocaine but not heroin self-administration in rats. *Psychopharmacology* **84**: 167–173.

Phillips, A. G. (1984) Brain reward circuitry: A case for separate systems. *Brain Res. Bull.* **12**: 195–201.

Phillips, A. G. and LePiane, F. G. (1980) Reinforcing effects of morphine microinjection into the ventral tegmental area. *Pharmac. Biochem. Behav.* **12**: 965–968.

Phillips, A. G. and LePiane, F. G. (1982) Reward produced by microinjection of (D-Ala^2)-Met^5 enkephalinamide into the ventral tegmental area. *Behav. Brain Res.* **5**: 225-229.

Phillips, A. G., Mora, F. and Rolls, E. T. (1981) Intracerebral self-administration of amphetamine by rhesus monkeys, *Neurosci. Lett.* **24**: 81–86.

Phillips, A. G., Broekkamp, C. L. E. and Fibiger, H. C. (1983) Strategies for studying the neurochemical substrates of drug reinforcement in rodents. *Prog. Neuro-Psychopharmac. Biol. Psychiat.* **7**: 585–590.

Pickens, R. and Harris, W. C. (1968) Self-administration of d-amphetamine by rats. *Psychopharmacologia* **12**: 158–163.

Pimoule, C., Schoemaker, H., Javoy-Agid, F., Scatton, B., Agid, Y. and Langer, S. Z. (1983) Decrease in [^{3}H]cocaine binding to the dopamine transporter in Parkinson's disease. *Eur. J. Pharmac.* **95**: 145–146.

Poschel, B. P. H. (1971) A simple and specific screen for benzodiazepine-like drugs. *Psychopharmacologia* **19**: 193–198.

Pradhan, S. N. (1970) Effects of nicotine on several schedules of behavior in rats. *Arch. Int. Pharmacodyn. Thér.* **183**: 127–138.

Prado-Alcala, R. and Wise, R. A. (1984) Brain stimulation reward and dopamine terminal fields. I. Caudate-putamen, nucleus accumbens and amygdala. *Brain Res.* **297**: 265–273.

Prado-Alcala, R., Streather, A. and Wise, R. A. (1984) Brain stimulation reward and dopamine terminal fields. II. Septal and cortical projections. *Brain Res.* **301**: 209–219.

Quirion, R., Hammer, R. P., Herkenham, M. and Pert, C. (1981) Phencyclidine (angel dust)/sigma "opiate" receptor: Visualization by tritium-sensitive film. *Proc. Natl. Acad. Sci. U.S.A.* **78**: 5881–5885.

Randall, L. O., Schallek, W., Heise, G. A., Keith, E. F. and Bagdon, R. E. (1960) The psychosedative properties of methaminodiazepoxide. *J. Pharmac. Exp. Ther.* **129**: 163–171.

Randrup, A. and Munkvad, I. (1966) Role of catecholamines in the amphetamine excitatory response. *Nature* **211**: 540.

Randrup, A. and Munkvad, I. (1970) Biochemical, anatomical and psychological investigations of stereotyped behaviour induced by amphetamines. In: *Amphetamines and Related Compounds*, pp. 695–713, Costa, E. and Garattini, S. (eds) Raven Press, New York.

RANGARAJ, N. and KALANT, H. (1980) Acute and chronic catecholamine-ethanol interactions on rat brain (Na^+ + K^+)-ATPase. *Pharmac. Biochem. Behav.* **13**: (Suppl. 1): 183–189.

REDGRAVE, P., DEAN, P., DONOHOE, T. P. and POPE, S. G. (1980) Superior colliculus lesions selectively attenuate apomorphine-induced oral stereotypy: A possible role for the nigrotectal pathway. *Brain Res.* **196**: 541–546.

REID, L. D., GIBSON, W. E., GLEDHILL, S. M. and PORTER, P. B. (1964) Anticonvulsant drugs and self-stimulation behavior. *J. Comp. Physiol. Psychol.* **7**: 353–356.

REITH, M. E. A., SERSHEN, H. and LAJTHA, A. (1980) Saturable [^{3}H] cocaine binding in the central nervous system of mouse. *Life Sci.* **27**: 1055–1062.

REYNOLDS, D. V. (1969) Surgery in the rat during electrical analgesia induced by focal brain stimulation. *Science* **164**: 444–445.

RISNER, M. E. and JONES, B. E. (1976) Role of noradrenergic and dopaminergic processes in amphetamine self-administration. *Pharmac. Biochem. Behav.* **5**: 477–482.

RISNER, M. E. and JONES, B. E. (1980) Intravenous self-administration of cocaine and norcocaine by dogs. *Psychopharmacology* **71**: 83–89.

ROBBINS, D. (1971) Partial reinforcement: A selective review of the alleyway literature since 1960. *Psychol. Bull.* **76**: 415–431.

ROBERTS, D. C. S. and KOOB, G. (1982) Disruption of cocaine self-administration following 6-hydroxydopamine lesions of the ventral tegmental area in rats. *Pharmac. Biochem. Behav.* **17**: 901–904.

ROBERTS, D. C. S. and ZITO, K. A. (1987) Interpretation of lesion effects on stimulant self-adminsitration. In: *Methods of Assessing the Reinforcing Properties of Abused Drugs*, p. 87–104, BOZARTH, M. A. (ed.) Springer-Verlag, New York.

ROBERTS, D. C. S., CORCORAN, M. E. and Fibiger, H. C. (1977) On the role of ascending catecholaminergic systems in intravenous self-administration of cocaine. *Pharmac. Biochem. Behav.* **6**: 615–620.

ROBERTS, D. C. S., KOOB, G. F., KLONOFF, P. and FIBIGER, H. C. (1980) Extinction and recovery of cocaine self-administration following 6-OHDA lesions of the nucleus accumbens. *Pharmac. Biochem. Behav.* **12**: 781–787.

ROSSIER, J., FRENCH, E. D., RIVIER, C., LING, N., GUILLEMIN, R. and BLOOM, F. E. (1977) Foot-shock induced stress increases β-endorphin levels in blood but not brain. *Nature* **270**: 618–620.

ROUTTENBERG, A. (1964) Self-starvation caused by "feeding-center" stimulation. *Am. Psychol.* **19**: 502–507.

SANGER, D. J. and MCCARTHY, P. S. (1980) Differential effects of morphine on food and water intake in food deprived and freely feeding rats. *Psychopharmacology* **72**: 103–106.

SANGER, D. J. and MCCARTHY, P. S. (1981) Increased food and water intake produced in rats by opiate receptor agonists. *Psychopharmacology* **74**: 217–220.

SANGER, D. J. and MCCARTHY, P. S. (1982) A comparison of the effects of opiate antagonists on operant and ingestive behavior. *Pharmac. Biochem. Behav.* **16**: 1013–1015.

SCHAEFER, G. J. and MICHAEL, R. P. (1980) Acute effects of neuroleptics on brain self-stimulation thresholds in rats. *Psychopharmacology* **67**: 9–15.

SCHAEFER, G. J. and MICHAEL, R. P. (1981) Threshold differences for naloxone and naltrexone in the hypothalamus and midbrain using fixed ratio brain self-stimulation in rats. *Psychopharmacology* **74**: 17–22.

SCHECHTER, M. D. (1981) Effect of fenfluramine and nicotine upon a stimulant-depressant continuum. *Pharmac. Biochem. Behav.* **15**: 371–375.

SCHLATTER, J. and BATTIG, K. (1979) Differential effects of nicotine and amphetamine on locomotor activity and maze exploration in two rat lines. *Psychopharamacology* **64**: 155–161.

SCHLEMMER, R. F., JACKSON, J. A., PRESTON, K. L., BEDERKA, J. P., GARVER, D. and DAVIS, J. M. (1978) Phencyclidine-induced stereotyped behavior in monkeys: Antagonism by pimozide. *Eur. J. Pharmac.* **52**: 379-384.

SCHNEIRLA, T. C. (1959) An evolutionary and developmental theory of biphasic processes underlying approach and withdrawal. In *Nebraska Symposium on Motivation*, pp. 1–42, JONES, M. R. (ed.) University of Nebraska Press, Lincoln, Nebraska.

SEEMAN, P. (1972) The membrane actions of anesthetics and tranquilizers. *Pharmac. Rev.* **24**: 583–655.

SHEFFIELD, F. D. and ROBY, T. B. (1950) Reward value of a non-nutritive sweet taste. *J. Comp. Physiol. Psychol.* **43**: 471–481.

SHIFFMAN, S. (1979) The tobacco withdrawal syndrome. In: Cigarette Smoking as a Dependence Process (National Institute on Drug Abuse Research Monograph), pp. 158–184, KRASNEGOR, N. A. (ed.) U.S. Government Printing Office, Washington, D.C.

SHIZGAL, P., BIELAJEW, C., CORBETT, D., SKELTON, R. and YEOMANS, J. (1980) Behavioral methods for inferring and anatomical linkage between rewarding brain stimulation sites. *J. Comp. Physiol. Psychol.* **94**: 227–237.

SIMON, E. J., HILLER, J. M. and EDELMAN, I. (1973) Stereospecific binding of the potent narcotic analgesic [^{3}H]etorphine to rat brain homogenate. *Proc. Natl. Acad. Sci. U.S.A.* **70**: 1947–1949.

SIMON, H., LEMOAL, M. and CARDO, B. (1975) Self-stimulation in the dorsal pontine tegmentum in the rat. *Behav. Biol.* **13**: 339–347.

SINCLAIR, J. D. (1974) Rats learning to work for alcohol. Nature **249**: 590–592.

SKINNER, B. F. (1935) Two types of conditioned reflex and a pseudotype. *J. Gen. Psychol.* **12**: 66–77.

SLOAN, J. W., BROOKS, J. W., EISENMAN, A. J. and MARTIN, W. R. (1962) Comparison of the effects of single doses of morphine and thebaine on body temperature, activity, and brain and heart levels of catecholamines and serotonin. *Psychopharmacologia* **3**: 291–301.

SOPER, W. Y. (1976) Effects of analgesic midbrain stimulation on reflex withdrawal and thermal escape in the rat. *J. Comp. Physiol. Psychol.* **90**: 91–101.

SPEALMAN, R. D. and GOLDBERG, S. R. (1982) Maintenance of schedule-controlled behavior by intravenous injections of nicotine in squirrel monkeys. *J. Pharmac. Exp. Ther.* **223**: 402–408.

SPYRAKI, C., FIBIGER, H. C. and PHILLIPS, A. G. (1982) Attenuation by haloperidol of place preference conditioning using food reinforcement. *Psychopharmacology* **77**: 379–382.

SPYRAKI, C., FIBIGER, H. C. and PHILLIPS, A. G. (1983) Attenuation of heroin reward in rats by disruption of the mesolimbic dopamine system. *Psychopharmacology* **79**: 278–283.

Squires, R. F. and Braestrup, C. (1977) Benzodiazepine receptors in rat brain. *Nature* **266**: 732–734.

Stapleton, J. M., Merriman, V. J., Coogle, C. L., Gelbard, S. D. and Reid, L. D. (1979) Naloxone reduces pressing for intracranial stimulation of sites in the periaqueductal gray area, accumbens nucleus, substantia nigra and lateral hypothalamus. *Physiol. Psychol.* **7**: 427–436.

Stark, P., Turk, J. A., Redman, C. E. and Henderson, J. K. (1969) Sensitivity and specificity of positive reinforcing areas to neuro-sedatives, antidepressants and stimulants. *J. Pharmac. Exp. Ther.* **166**: 163–169.

Stefano, G. B., Hall, B., Markham, M. H. and Dvorkin, B. (1980) Opioid inhibition of dopamine release from nervous tissue of *Mytilus edulis* and *Octopus bimaculatus. Science* **213**: 928–930.

Stein, L. (1968) Chemistry of reward and punishment. In: *Proceedings of the American College of Neuropsychopharmacology*, pp. 105–123, Efron, D. H. (ed.) U.S. Government Printing Office, Washington, D.C.

Stein, L. (1971) Neurochemistry of reward and punishment: Some implications for the etiology of schizophrenia. *J. Psychiat. Res.* **8**: 345-361.

Stein, L. and Ray, O. S. (1960) Brain stimulation reward "thresholds" self-determined in rat. *Psychopharmacology* **1**: 251-256.

Stein, L. and Wise, C. D. (1969) Release of norepinephrine from hypothalamus and amygdala by rewarding medial forebrain bundle stimulation and amphetamine. *J. Comp. Physiol. Psychol.* **67**: 189–198.

Stellar, J. R. and Neeley, S. P. (1982) Reward summation function measurements of lateral hypothalamic stimulation reward: Effects of anterior and posterior medial forebrain bundle lesions. In: *The Neural Basis of Feeding and Reward*, pp. 431–443, Hoebel, B. G. and Novin, D. G. (eds), Haer Institute, Brunswick, Maine.

Stellar, J. R., Kelley, A. E. and Corbett, D. (1983) Effects of peripheral and central dopamine blockade on lateral hypothalamic self-stimulation: Evidence for both reward and motor deficits. *Pharmac. Biochem. Behav.* **18**: 433-442.

Stinus, L., Koob, G. F., Ling, N., Bloom, F. E. and Le Moal, M. (1980) Locomotor activation induced by infusion of endorphins into the ventral tegmental area: Evidence for opiate-dopamine interactions. *Proc. Natl. Acad. Sci. U.S.A.* **77**: 2323-2327.

Stinus, L., Winnock, M. and Kelly, A. E. (1985) Chronic neuroleptic treatment and mesolimbic dopamine denervation induce behavioral supersensitivity to opiates. *Psychopharmacology* **85**: 323-328.

Stinus, L., Nadaud, D., Jauregui, J. and Kelley, A. E. (1986) Chronic treatment with five different neuroleptics elicits behavioral supersensitivity to opiate infusion into the nucleus accumbens. *Biol. Psychiat.* **21**: 34–48.

St Laurent, J. and Olds, J. (1967) Alcohol and brain centers of positive reinforcement. In: *Alcoholism Behavioral Research, Therapeutic Approaches*, pp. 85–106, Fox, R. (ed.) Springer, New York.

Stricker, E. M. and Zigmond, M. J. (1976) Recovery of function after damage to central catecholamine-containing neurons: A neurochemical model for the lateral hypothalamic syndrome. In: *Progress in Psychobiology and Physiological Psychology*, Vol. 6, pp. 121–188, Sprague, J. M. and Epstein, A. N. (eds) Academic Press, New York.

Strombon, U. H. and Liedman, B. (1982) Role of dopaminergic neurotransmission in locomotor stimulation by dexamphetamine and ethanol. *Psychopharmacology* **78**: 271-276.

Svensson, T. H., Grenhoff, J. and Aston-Jones, G. (1986) Midbrain dopamine neurons: Nicotinic control of firing pattern. *Soc. Neurosci. Abstr.* **12**: 1154.

Teasdale, J. A. P., Bozarth, M. A. and Stewart, J. (1981) Body temperature responses to microinjections of morphine in brain sites containing opiate receptors. *Soc. Neurosci. Abstr.* **7**: 799.

Terenius, L. (1973) Stereospecific interaction between narcotic analgesics and a synaptic plasma membrane fraction of rat cerebral cortex. *Acta Pharmac. Toxicol.* **32**: 317-320.

Terman, G. S., Shavit, Y., Lewis, J. W., Cannon, J. T. and Liebeskind, J. C. (1984) Intrinsic mechanisms of pain inhibition: Activation by stress. *Science* **226**: 1270–1277.

Ticku, M. K. (1983) Benzodiazepine-GABA receptor-ionophore complex. *Neuropharmacology* **22**: 1459–1470.

Ticku, M. K. and Davis, W. C. (1981) Evidence that ethanol and pentobarbital enhance [^{3}H]diazepam binding at the benzodiazepine-GABA receptor-ionophore complex indirectly. *Eur. J. Pharmac.* **71**: 521-522.

Tombaugh, T. N., Tombaugh, J. and Anisman, H. (1979) Effects of dopamine receptor blockade on alimentary behaviors: Home cage food consumption, magazine training, operant acquisition, and performance. *Psychopharmacology* **66**: 219–225.

Tombaugh, T. N., Anisman, H. and Tombaugh, J. (1980) Extinction and dopamine receptor blockade after intermittent reinforcement: Failure to observe functional equivalence. *Psychopharmacology* **70**: 19–28.

Trowill, J. A., Panksepp, J. and Gandelman, R. (1969) An incentive model of rewarding brain stimulation. *Psychol. Rev.* **76**: 264–281.

Trujillo, K. A., Belluzzi, J. D. and Stein, L. (1984) Naltrexone and self-stimulation: Extinction-like response pattern suggests selective reward deficit. *Soc. Neurosci. Abstr.* **10**: 308.

Tung, A. S. and Yaksh, T. L. (1982) *In vivo* evidence for multiple opiate receptors mediating analgesia in the rat spinal cord. *Brain Res.* **247**: 75–83.

Vaccarino, F. J., Bloom, F. E. and Koob, G. F. (1985) Blockade of nucleus accumbens opiate receptors attenuates intravenous heroin reward in the rat. *Psychopharmacology* **86**: 37–42.

Valenstein, E. S., Cox, V. C. and Kakolewski, J. W. (1970) Reexamination of the role of the hypothalamus in motivation. *Psychol. Rev.* **77**: 16–31.

van der Kooy, D., LePiane, F. G. and Phillips, A. G. (1977) Apparent independence of opiate reinforcement and electrical self-stimulation systems in the rat brain. *Life Sci. 20*: 981–986.

van Ree, J. M. and de Wied, D. (1980) Involvement of neurohypophyseal peptides in drug-mediated adaptive responses. *Pharmac. Biochem. Behav.* **13**(Suppl. 1): 257–263.

Vickroy, T. W. and Johnson, K. M. (1982) Similar dopamine-releasing effects of phencyclidine and nonamphetamine stimulants in striatal slices. *J. Pharmac. Exp. Ther.* **223**: 669–674.

Vincent, S. R., Hokfelt, T., Christensson, I. and Terenius, L. (1982) Dynorphin-immunoreactive neurons in the central nervous system of the rat. *Neurosci. Lett.* **33**: 185–190.

Waldeck, B. (1973) Modification of caffeine-induced locomotor stimulation by a cholinergic mechanism. *J. Neural Trans.* **34**: 61–72.

WATKINS, L. R. and MAYER, D. J. (1982) Organization of endogenous opiate and nonopiate pain control systems. *Science* **216**: 1185–1192.

WATSON, P. J. and COX, V. C. (1976) An analysis of barbiturate-induced eating and drinking in the rat. *Physiol. Psychol.* **4**: 325–332.

WATSON, S. J., KHACHATURIAN, H., AKIL, H., COY, D. H. and GOLDSTEIN, A. (1982a) Comparison of the distribution of dynorphin systems and enkephalin systems in brain. *Science* **218**: 1134–1136.

WATSON, S. J., KHACHATURIAN, H., COY, D., TAYLOR, L. and AKIL, H. (1982b) Dynorphin is located throughout the CNS and is often co-localized with alpha-neo-endorphin. *Life Sci.* **31**: 1773–1776.

WAUQUIER, A. and NIEMEGEERS, C. J. E. (1974) Intracranial self-stimulation in rats as a function of various stimulus parameters. V. Influence of cocaine on medial forebrain bundle stimulation with monopolar electrodes. *Psychopharmacologia* **38**: 201–210.

WAY, E. L. (1983) Some thoughts about opiopeptins, peptides with opiate-like activity. *Drug Alcohol Depend.* **11**: 23–31.

WEEKS, J. R. (1962) Experimental morphine addiction: Method for automatic intravenous injections in unrestrained rats. *Science 138*: 143–144.

WEI, E. (1981a) Pharmacological aspects of shaking behavior produced by AG-3-5, TRH and morphine withdrawal. *Fed. Proc.* **40**: 1491–1496.

WEI, E. T. (1981b) Enkephalin analogs and physical dependence. *J. Pharmac. Exp. Ther.* **216**: 12–18.

WEI, E. T. and LOH, H. H. (1976) Physical dependence on opiate-like peptides. *Science* **193**: 1262–1263.

WEI, E. T., LOH, H. H. and WAY, E. L. (1973a) Quantitative aspects of precipitated abstinence in morphine-dependent rats. *J. Pharmac. Exp. Ther.* **184**: 398–403.

WEI, E., LOH, H. H. and WAY, E. L. (1973b) Brain sites of precipitated abstinence in morphine-dependent rats. *J. Pharmac. Exp. Ther.* **185**: 108–115.

WEI, E., SIGEL, S. and WAY, E. L. (1975) Regional sensitivity of the rat brain to the inhibitory effects of morphine on wet shake behavior. *J. Pharmac. Exp. Ther.* **193**: 56–63.

WEI, E. T., TSENG, L. F., LOH, H. H. and LI, C. H. (1977) Comparison of the behavioral effects of β-endorphin and enkephalin analogs. *Life Sci.* **21**: 321–328.

WEINER, W. J., GOETZ, C., NAUSIEDA, P. A. and KLAWANS, H. L. (1977) Clonazepam and dopamine-related stereotyped behavior. *Life Sci.* **21**: 901–906.

WESNES, K. and WARBURTON, D. M. (1983) Effects of smoking on rapid visual information processing. *Neuropsychobiology* **9**: 223–229.

WESNES, K., WARBURTON, D. M. and MATZ, B. (1983) Effects of nicotine on stimulus sensitivity and response bias in a vigilance task. *Neuropsychobiology* **9**: 41–44.

WEST, C. K., SCHAEFER, G. J. and MICHAEL, R. P. (1983) Increasing the work requirements lowers the threshold of naloxone for reducing self-stimulaton in the midbrain of rats. *Pharmac. Biochem. Behav.* **18**: 705–710.

WEST, T. E. G. and WISE, R. A. (1986) Relative effects of naltrexone on nucleus accumbens, lateral hypothalamic, and ventral tegmental self-stimulation in the rat. *Soc. Neurosci. Abstr.* **12**: 931.

WIKLER, A. A. (1952) A psychodynamic study of a patient during self-regulated readdiction to morphine. *Psychiatr. Q.* **26**: 270–293.

WINTERS, W. D., MORI, K., SPENCER, C. E. and BAUER, R. O. (1967) The neurophysiology of anesthesia. *Anesthesiology* **28**: 65–80.

WISE, C. D. and STEIN, L. (1970) Amphetamine: Facilitation of behavior by augmented release of norepinephrine from the medial forebrain bundle. In: *Amphetamine and Related Compounds*, pp. 463–485, COSTA, E. and GARATTINI, S. (eds) Raven Press, New York.

WISE, R. A. (1978a) Neuroleptic attenuation of intracranial self-stimulation: Reward or performance deficits? *Life Sci.* **22**: 535–542.

WISE, R. A. (1978b) Catecholamine theories of reward: A critical review. *Brain Res.* **152**: 215–247.

WISE, R. A. (1980) Action of drugs of abuse on brain reward systems. *Pharmac. Biochem. Behav.* **13**(Suppl. 1): 213–223.

WISE, R. A. (1981) Intracranial self-stimulation: Mapping against the lateral boundaries of the dopaminergic cells of the substantia nigra. *Brain Res.* **213**: 190–194.

WISE, R. A. (1982) Neuroleptics and operant behavior: The anhedonia hypothesis. *Behav. Brain Sci.* **5**: 39–87.

WISE, R. A. (1985) The anhedonia hypothesis: Mark III. *Behav. Brain Sci.* **8**: 178–186.

WISE, R. A. and BOZARTH, M. A. (1984) Brain reward circuitry: Four circuit elements "wired" in apparent series. *Brain Res. Bull.* **12**: 203–208.

WISE, R. A. and BOZARTH, M. A. (1987) A psychomotor stimulant theory of addiction. *Psychol. Rev.* **94**: 469–492.

WISE, R. A. and DAWSON, V. (1974) Diazepam-induced eating and lever-pressing for food in sated rats. *J. Comp. Physiol. Psychol.* **86**: 930–941.

WISE, R. A., YOKEL, R. A. and DE WIT, H. (1976) Both positive reinforcement and conditioned taste aversion from amphetamine and from apomorphine in rats. *Science* **191**: 1273–1274.

WISE, R. A., SPINDLER, J., DE WIT, H. and GERBER, G. J. (1978a) Neuroleptic-induced "anhedonia" in rats: Pimozide blocks the reward quality of food. *Science* **201**: 262–264.

WISE, R. A., SPINDLER, J. and LEGAULT, L. (1978b) Major attenuation of food reward with performance sparing doses of pimozide in the rat. *Can. J. Psychol.* **32**: 77–85.

WISE, R. A., JENCK, F. and RAPTIS, L. (1986) Morphine potentiates feeding via the opiate reinforcement mechanism. In: *Problems of Drug Dependence*, 1985, (NIDA Research Monograph 67), pp. 228–234, HARRIS, L. S. (ed.) U.S. Government Printing Office, Washington, D.C.

WOLGIN, D. L., CYTAWA, J. and TEITELBAUM, P. (1976) The role of activation in the regulation of food intake. In: *Hunger: Basic Mechanisms and Clinical Implications*, pp. 179–191, NOVIN, D., WYRWICKA, W. and BRAY, G. (eds) Raven Press, New York.

WOOD, P. L. (1982) Actions of GABAergic agents on dopamine metabolism in the nigrostrial pathway of the rat. *J. Pharmac. Exp. Ther.* **222**: 674–679.

WOOLVERTON, W. L., GOLDBERG, L. I. and GINOS, J. (1984) Intravenous self-administration of dopamine receptor agonists by rhesus monkeys. *J. Pharmac. Exp. Ther.* **230**: 678–683.

Woolverton, W. L., Wessinger, W. D. and Balster, R. L. (1982) Reinforcing properties of clonidine in rhesus monkeys. *Psychopharmacology* **77**: 17–23.

Xenakis, S. and Sclafani, A. (1982) The dopaminergic mediation of a sweet reward in normal and VMH hyperphagic rats. *Pharmac. Biochem. Behav.* **16**: 293–302.

Yaksh, T. L. and Rudy, T. A. (1978) Narcotic analgetics: CNS sites and mechanisms of action as revealed by intracerebral injection techniques. *Pain* **4**: 299–359.

Yaksh, T. L. and Rudy, T. A. (1979) Studies on the direct spinal action of narcotics in the production of analgesia in the rat. *J. Pharmac. Exp. Ther.* **202**: 411–428.

Yaksh, T. L., Yeung, J. C. and Rudy, T. A. (1976) Systematic examination in the rat of brain sites sensitive to the direct application of morphine: Observation of differential effects within the periaqueductal gray. *Brain Res.* **114**: 83–103.

Yeomans, J. S. (1979) Absolute refractory periods of self-stimulation neurons. *Physiol. Behav.* **22**: 911–919.

Yeomans, J. S. (1982) The cells and axons mediating medial forebrain bundle reward. In: *The Neural Basis of Feeding and Reward*, pp. 405–417, Hoebel, B. G. and Novin, D. (eds) Haer Institute, Brunswick, Maine.

Yeung, J. C. and Rudy, T. A. (1980) Multiplicative interactions between narcotic agonisms expressed at spinal and supraspinal sites of antinociceptive action as revealed by concurrent intrathecal and intracerebroventricular injections of morphine. *J. Pharmac. Exp. Ther.* **215**: 633–642.

Yokel, R. A. and Pickens, R. (1974) Drug level of d- and l-amphetamine during intravenous self-administration. *Psychopharmacologia* **34**: 255–264.

Yokel, R. A. and Wise, R. A. (1975) Increased lever pressing for amphetamine after pimozide in rats: Implications for a dopamine theory of reward. *Science* **187**: 547–549.

Yokel, R. A. and Wise, R. A. (1976) Attenuation of intravenous amphetamine reinforcement by central dopamine blockade in rats. *Psychopharmacology* **48**: 311–318.

Yokel, R. A. and Wise, R. A. (1978) Amphetamine-type reinforcement by dopamine agonists in the rat. *Psychopharmacology* **58**: 289–296.

Yoon, K. -W. P., Gessa, G. L., Boi, V., Naes, L., Mereu, G. and Westfall, T. C. (1986) Electrophysiological effects of nicotine on dopamine mid-brain neurons. *Soc. Neurosci. Abstr.* **12**: 1515.

Young, W. S. and Kuhar, M. J. (1980) Radiohistochemical localization of benzodiazepine receptors in rat brain. *J. Pharmac. Exp. Ther.* **212**: 337–346.

Zamir, N., Palkovits, M., Weber, E., Mezey, E. and Brownstein, M. J. (1984) A dynorphinergic pathway of leu-enkephalin production in the rat substantia nigra. *Nature* **307**: 643–645.

Zarevics, P. and Setler, P. (1979) Simultaneous rate-independent and rate-dependent assessment of intracranial self-stimulation: Evidence for the direct involvement of dopamine in brain reinforcement mechanisms. *Brain Res.* **169**: 499–512.

CHAPTER 3

CLASSICAL CONDITIONING AND OPIATE TOLERANCE AND WITHDRAWAL

SHEPARD SIEGEL
Department of Psychology, McMaster University
Hamilton, Ontario, Canada

1. INTRODUCTION

Many of the effects of a variety of drugs, including opiates, decrease over the course of successive administrations. This phenomenon is termed *tolerance*. Also, in the drug-experienced (and drug-tolerant) organism, cessation of drug administration often results in a constellation of symptoms that are generally characterized as opposite in direction to the effects of the drug. These are termed *withdrawal symptoms*. With respect to opiates, it is generally assumed that common mechanisms account for both tolerance and withdrawal symptoms. For example, it has been hypothesized (e.g., Goldstein, 1976) that morphine initially supplements the activity of enkephalin. As morphine is repeatedly administered, feedback processes suppress the activity of enkephalin neurons. As a result of this suppression, the response to morphine decreases, or more morphine is needed to achieve the initial effect of the drug (i.e., tolerance develops). If morphine administration ceases, neither the exogenous opiate nor the endogenous ligand is present at the receptor. This lack of endophinergic activity results in withdrawal symptoms that persist until normal enkephalin activity is reestablished.

There is an increasing amount of data that attest to the importance of such neurochemical feedback processes in opiate tolerance and withdrawal effects. It is apparent, however, that such feedback processes are supplemented by feedforward processes. "Feedforward means anticipation. It means responding, not to disturbances, but to stimuli that have been associated with disturbances in the past" (Toates, 1979). That is, the effects of a drug are modulated not only by drug-elicited homeostatic responses, but also by responses made in the presence of drug-signaling environmental cues. As discussed by Houk (1980), an appreciation of feedforward regulation requires an appreciation of Pavlovian conditioning principles.

2. THE PAVLOVIAN CONDITIONING SITUATION

Living organisms respond not only reflexively to stimuli, but also in anticipation of stimuli. The analysis of such anticipatory responding uses procedures and terminology developed by Ivan Pavlov, and is called Pavlovian (or classical) conditioning (Pavlov, 1927).

In the Pavlovian conditioning situation, a contingency is arranged between two stimuli: typically, one stimulus reliably predicts the occurrence of the second stimulus. Using the usual terminology, the second of these paired stimuli is termed the *unconditional stimulus* (UCS). The UCS, as the name implies, is selected because it elicits relevant activities from the outset (i.e., unconditionally), prior to any pairings. Responses elicited by the UCS are termed unconditional responses (UCRs). The stimulus signaling the presentation of the UCS is "neutral," (i.e., it elicits little relevant activity prior to its pairing with the UCS), and is termed the *conditional stimulus* (CS). The CS, as the name implies, becomes capable of eliciting new responses as a function of (i.e., conditional upon) its pairing with the unconditional stimulus.

In Pavlov's well-known conditioning research, the CS was a conveniently manipulated exteroceptive stimulus (bell, light, etc.), and the UCS was either food or orally-injected dilute acid (both of which elicited a conveniently monitored salivary UCR). After a number of CS-UCS pairings, it was noted that the subject salivated not only in response to the UCS, but also in anticipation of the UCS (i.e., in response to the CS). The subject is then said to display a conditional response (CR).

2.1. Drugs As Unconditional Stimuli

A wide range of exteroceptive and interoceptive stimuli have been used in Pavlovian conditioning experiments (Razran, 1961). Drugs constitute a particularly interesting class of UCSs. After some number of drug administrations, each administration reliably signaled by a CS, pharmacological CRs can be observed in response to the CS. It was Pavlov who first demonstrated such pharmacological conditioning. He paired a tone with administration of apomorphine. The drug induced restlessness, salivation, and a "disposition to vomit." After several tone–apomorphine pairings, the tone alone "sufficed to produce all the active symptoms of the drug, only in a lesser degree" (Pavlov, 1927).

Additional research by Krylov (reported by Pavlov, 1927) indicated that even if there is not an explicit CS (such as an auditory cue), naturally occurring predrug cues (opening the box containing the hypodermic syringe, cropping the fur, etc.) could serve as CSs. In Krylov's experiments, a dog was repeatedly injected with morphine, each injection eliciting a number of responses including copious salivation. After five or six such injections, it was observed that "the preliminaries of injection" (Pavlov, 1927) elicited many morphine-like responses, including salivation.

2.2. The Pharmacological Conditional Response

Most pharmacological conditioning research has been greatly influenced by Pavlov's theory of CR formation. According to this theory, the CR is a replica of the UCR, and, indeed, much drug conditioning work has demonstrated CRs that mimick the drug effect (Siegel, 1985; Stewart and Eikelboom, 1987). In contrast, in 1937 Subkov and Zilov reported that dogs with a history of epinephrine administration (each injection eliciting a tachycardiac response), displayed a conditional *brady*cardiac response. Subkov and Zilov cautioned against "the widely accepted view that the external modifications of the conditional reflex must always be identical with the response of the organism to the unconditional stimulus" (Subkov and Zilov, 1937). Subsequent research has suggested that the characteristics of the pharmacological CR depend very much on the nature and mechanism of the drug effect (See Eikelboom and Stewart, 1982; Paletta and Wagner, 1986; Siegel, 1989). For many effects of many drugs, the CR is an anticipatory compensation for the drug effect. For example, the subject with a history of morphine administration (and its analgesic consequence) often displays a CR of hyperalgesia (Krank, 1987; Krank *et al.*, 1981; Siegel, 1975). Similar compensatory CRs have been reported with respect to the thermic (Siegel, 1978), locomotor (Mucha *et al.*, 1981; Paletta and Wagner, 1986), behaviorally sedating (Hinson and Siegel, 1983), and gastrointestinal (Raffa and Porreca, 1986) effects of morphine. The CR seen with many non-opiate drugs is similarly opposite to the drug effect, e.g., atropine (Mulinos and Lieb, 1929), chlorpromazine (Pihl and Altman, 1971), amphetamine (Obál, 1966), methyl dopa (Korol and McLaughlin, 1976), lithium chloride (Domjan and Gillan, 1977), haloperidol (King *et al.*, 1978), ethanol (Lê *et al.*, 1979), and caffeine (Rozin *et al.*, 1984).

2.3. Pavlovian Conditioning and Drug Tolerance

Drug-compensatory CRs would be expected to be a feature of normal drug administration procedures. In those cases in which the same drug is repeatedly administered with discrete environmental stimuli signaling each drug administration, drug-compensatory CRs should function to increasingly attenuate the drug effect. A decreasing response to a drug, over the course of successive administrations, defines tolerance. Thus, it is likely that pharmacological conditioning contributes to tolerance.

3. ENVIRONMENTAL SPECIFICITY OF OPIATE TOLERANCE

On the basis of the conditioning analysis, tolerance should *not* invariably result from repeated drug administrations. Rather, tolerance should be displayed only when the drug is administered in the context of the usual drug-predictive cues because it is these cues that elicit the drug-compensatory CRs that mediate tolerance. In fact, results of many studies have demonstrated that tolerance is more pronounced when the drug is administered in the presence of the usual predrug cues than if the drug is administered in the presence of alternative cues.

Early demonstrations of the contribution of predrug cues to tolerance were conducted by Mitchell and colleagues (e.g., Adams *et al.*, 1969). In these experiments, rats responded in the expected analgesia-tolerant manner to the last of a series of morphine injections only if this final injection occurred in the same environment as the prior injections of morphine. Much subsequent research has extended these demonstrations of the importance of predrug cues in tolerance to the analgesic effect of morphine (see Siegel and MacRae, 1984).

The details of the designs of experiments demonstrating the environmental specificity of morphine analgesic tolerance differed, but all incorporated two groups of rats, both receiving the drug a sufficient number of times for tolerance to develop during the initial, tolerance-development phase of the experiment. The analgesic effect of the drug was evaluated in a subsequent tolerance test phase. For one of the two groups, this test was conducted following the same cues that signaled the drug during the tolerance development phase (Same-Tested). For the second group, the tolerance test was conducted following different cues than those that signaled the drug during the tolerance development phase (Different-Tested). In addition, the design of the experiments enabled evaluation of the magnitude of the analgesic response in rats receiving the drug for the very first time (Control). Results obtained during the tolerance test in a number of experiments using this procedure are summarized in Fig. 1.

Figure 1A summarizes results of an experiment in which analgesia in rats was assessed following a tenth morphine injection (5 mg/kg), this tenth injection being paired with an audiovisual cue (Siegel *et al.*, 1978). Pain sensitivity was measured by noting the rat's latency to lick a paw when placed on a 54°C surface (the "hot plate" procedure). For Same-Tested rats, the nine pretest injections were signaled by the same cue that signaled the test injection. Different-Tested rats, in contrast, received their nine prior drug injections and cue presentations in an unpaired manner. As can be seen by comparing Control rats with Same-Tested rats, tolerance to the analgesic effect of morphine was obtained: Control rats, which received the drug for the first time on the tolerance test session, were significantly less sensitive to the thermal stimulation (i.e., were more analgesic) than Same-Tested rats, which received the drug for the tenth time on the test session. However, results obtained from Different-Tested rats demonstrate that analgesic tolerance is not the inevitable consequence of repeated morphine administration. Different-Tested rats had the same pharmacological history as Same-Tested rats (i.e., they received the same dose of morphine, equally often, and at the same intervals), but Different-Tested rats were as profoundly analgesic as Control animals.

Other studies, using different drug doses and/or analgesia assessment procedures, have similarly demonstrated that Same-Tested rats are more tolerant than Different-Tested rats, although such environmental specificity of tolerance is not always complete; that is, both groups of drug-experienced animals may be more tolerant than drug-naive Control animals. Figure 1B illustrates results of an experiment in which pain sensitivity was assessed with a paw-pressure analgesiometer; the rat was free to withdraw its paw from a source of gradually and constantly increasing pressure, with the amount of pressure applied before the withdrawal response occurs (i.e., the paw-withdrawal threshold), providing a measure of pain sensitivity (Siegel, 1976). As can be seen in Fig. 1B, Same-Tested rats, with a pretest history of eight, 5 mg/kg morphine injections, evidenced greater sensitivity to the paw pressure (i.e., more analgesic tolerance) than the equally drug-experienced Different-Tested rats. Thus, again, equivalent opiate exposure does not lead to equivalent levels of toler-

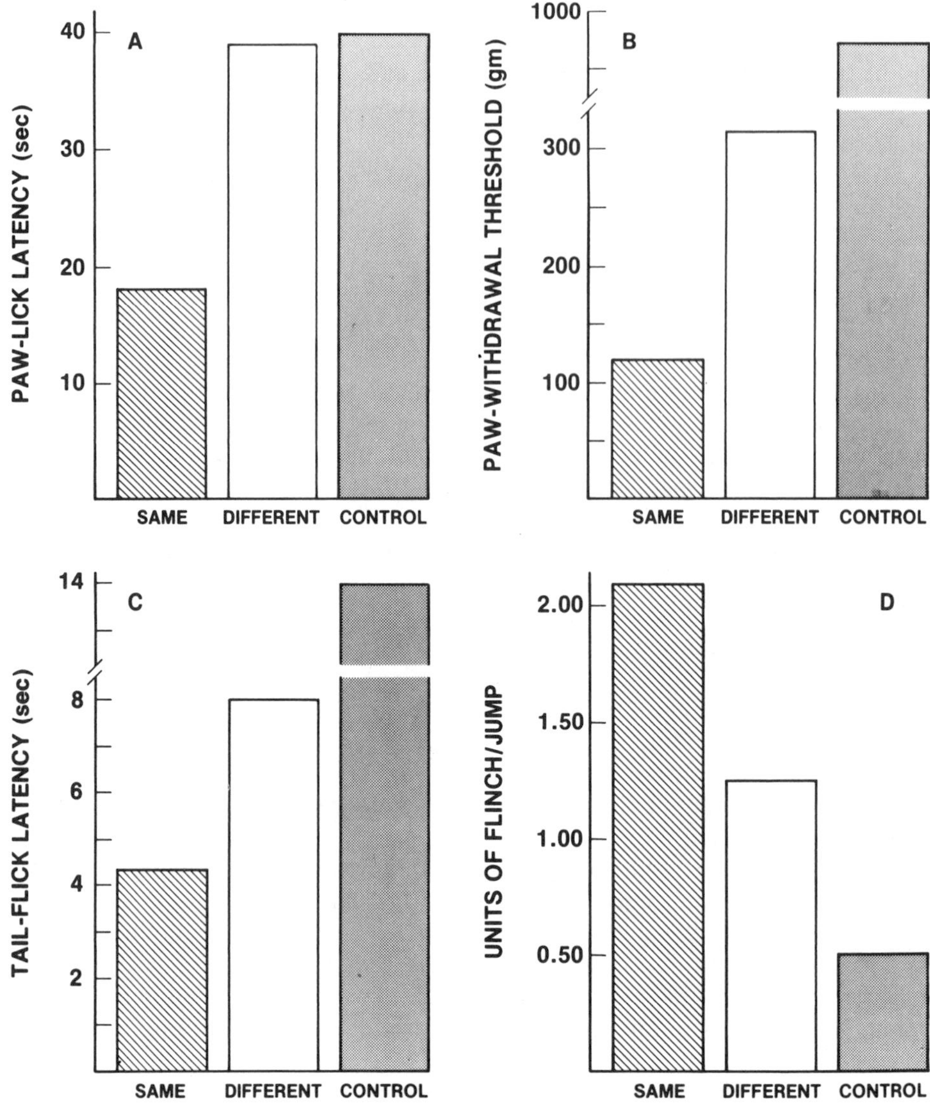

FIG. 1. Environmental specificity of tolerance to the analgesic effect of morphine demonstrated with the hot-plate (A), paw-pressure (B), tail-flick (C), and flinch/jump (D) analgesia assessment techniques. These results are based on Siegel *et al.* (1978), Siegel (1976), Advokat (1980), and Tiffany and Baker (1981), respectively.

ance. As is apparent in Fig. 1B, both Same- and Different-Tested rats displayed more tolerance than Control rats, perhaps indicating a nonenvironmental component of tolerance as well.

A similar pattern of results may be seen in a study of analgesic tolerance, as assessed by tail-flick latency following eight injections of morphine (7.5 mg/kg) (Advokat, 1980). As depicted in Fig. 1C, Control rats are profoundly analgesic. Although both drug-experienced groups display shorter tail-flick latencies than the Control level, they differed significantly: Same-Tested animals were more tolerant than Different-Tested animals. This pattern of results was confirmed in a different experiment (Tiffany and Baker, 1981), using a different number of pretest sessions (five), a different dose of morphine (20 mg/kg), and a different analgesia-assessment procedure (digitalized flinch/jump magnitude to electric shocks, with smaller numbers indicating less sensitivity to shock, i.e., greater analgesia). The results of this experiment are presented in Fig. 1D. Again, Same-Tested animals were more tolerant than Different-Tested animals, although neither were as analgesic as Control animals.

The environmental-specificity of tolerance to the analgesic effect of morphine is rather general, having recently been demonstrated in the terrestrial gastropod snail, *Cepaea nemoralis* (Kavaliers and Hirst, 1986), suggesting that such specificity "may be a general phenomenon having an early evolutionary development and broad phylogenetic continuity" (Kavaliers and Hirst, 1986).

The finding that opioid tolerance is more pronounced in the drug administration environment than an alternative environment has been demonstrated with respect to effects of the drug other than analgesia. It has been reported that rats tested in the context of the usual predrug cues are more tolerant to the thermic (Siegel, 1978), locomotor (Mucha *et al.*, 1981), and behaviorally sedating (Hinson and Siegel, 1983) effects of morphine than equally drug-experienced rats tested in the context of alternative cues.

3.1. Environmental Cues and Opiate Overdose

An especially dramatic demonstration of the contribution of environmental cues to tolerance is the finding that tolerance to the lethal effect of diacetylmorphine hydrochloride (heroin) is affected by such cues (Siegel *et al.*, 1982). The design of the experiment is summarized in Fig. 2.

During the initial tolerance-development phase of the experiment, three groups of rats with chronically implanted jugular cannula received 15 intravenous infusions in each of two different environments: a distinctive room and their colony (where they were continuously housed). For two groups, half the infusions consisted of heroin and half of dextrose (the vehicle), with the groups differing with respect to the location associated with each injected substance. One group was administered heroin in the room environment and dextrose in the colony environment. For the second group, the relationship between the administration location and the substance administered was reversed. The dose of heroin was systematically increased over the course of the 15 infusions from 1 mg/kg to 8 mg/kg. For a third group, all 30 infusions (half in each environment) consisted of dextrose. Finally, all 107

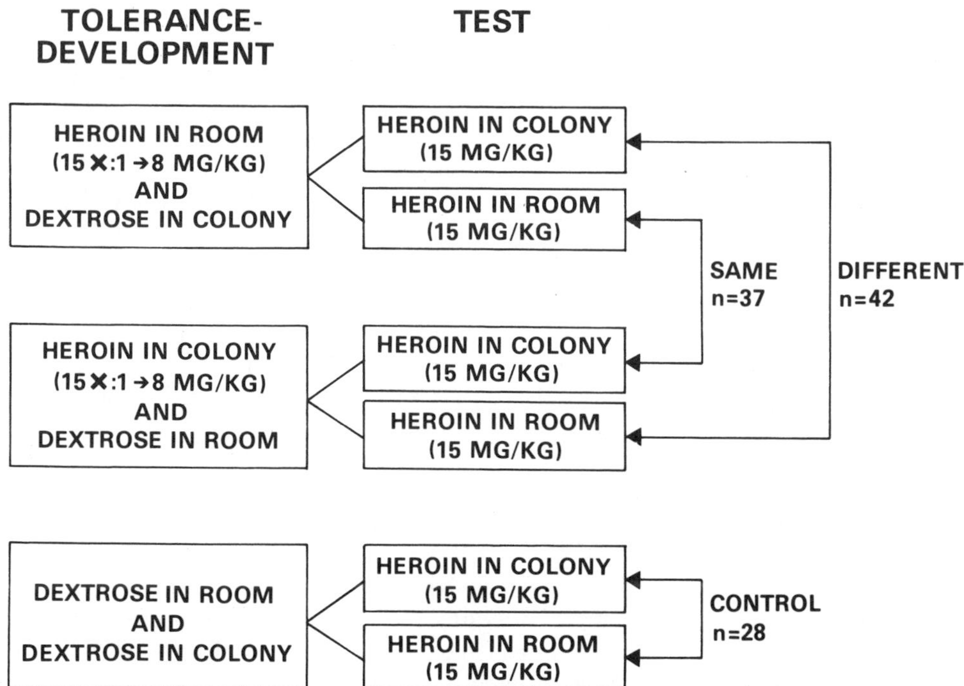

Fig. 2. Design of Siegel *et al.* (1982) experiment demonstrating environmental specificity of tolerance to the lethal effect of heroin.

subjects in the experiment received a final test session, in which they were administered 15 mg/kg heroin. Approximately half the subjects administered each of the three pretest treatments received their test infusion in the colony environment, and half in the room environment. As indicated in Fig. 2, then, some rats were administered the high dose of heroin in the same environment where they received lower doses (designated Same-Tested), and some rats received the high drug dose in an environment different from that associated with lower doses (Different-Tested). Control rats received heroin for the first time on the test session. Prior to the final test session, all groups were equated with respect to their exposure to both injection environments.

Test session mortality differed significantly between groups: Control = 96.4%, Different-Tested = 64.3%, and Same-Tested = 32.4%. Both groups with pretest experience with sublethal doses of heroin were more likely to survive the highest dose than control animals, suggesting that tolerance resulted from the pretest heroin injections independently of the environment associated with these injections. However, mortality was significantly higher in Different-Tested than Same-Tested Rats. This experiment demonstrated that groups of rats with the same history of heroin administration can differ in mortality following administration of a high dose of the drug: Same-Tested animals, which received the potentially lethal dose of opiate in the context of cues previously associated with sublethal doses, were more likely to survive than Different-Tested animals, which received the potentially lethal dose in the context of cues not previously associated with the drug.

The contribution of Pavlovian conditioning to heroin overdose has further been supported by retrospective reports provided by human overdose survivors (Siegel, 1984). These victims frequently report that the overdose occurred when the drug was administered in atypical circumstances. [Although contrary data have been reported by Neumann and Ellis (1986).] Pavlovian conditioning may not only contribute to death in illicit opiate users, but may also be relevant to some instances of death from overdose of licitly used opiates. A recent case report describes an instance of death from apparent morphine overdose in a patient receiving the drug for relief of pancreatic cancer (Siegel and Ellsworth, 1986). The circumstances of this death from medically prescribed morphine are readily interpretable by the Pavlovian conditioning account of tolerance.

3.2. Environmental Cues and Tolerance to Nonopiate Drugs

Although this chapter is concerned primarily with opiates, it should be noted that environmental specificity of tolerance has been demonstrated with respect to tolerance to many effects of a variety of non-opiate drugs, as well as opiates: ethanol (see review by Siegel, 1987), pentobarbital (Cappell *et al.*, 1981; Hinson *et al.*, 1982), scopolamine (Poulos and Hinson, 1984), haloperidol (Poulos and Hinson, 1982), chlordiazepoxide (Greeley and Cappell, 1985), and polyinosinic:polycytidylic acid (poly I:C, an immunostimulatory drug; Dyck *et al.*, 1987).

As already discussed, an especially dramatic demonstration of the contribution of environmental cues to tolerance concerns tolerance to the lethal effects of heroin. Heroin-experienced rats are especially likely to die following heroin administration in the presence of cues not previously associated with the drug (Siegel *et al.*, 1982). Similar environmental specificity of tolerance to the lethal effects of ethanol (Melchior and Tabakoff, 1982) and pentobarbital (Vila, 1989) has also been reported.

3.3. Summary of Environmental Cues and Tolerance

Results of many studies have demonstrated environmental specificity of tolerance. That is, speaking casually, tolerance is more pronounced when the drug is expected than when it is not expected. It should be noted that such environmental specificity is often not absolute (i.e., some tolerance is noted in Different-Tested subjects, compared to Control subjects receiving the drug for the first time). Furthermore, there are contradictory data concerning environmental specificity of tolerance with some drugs. For example, with respect to midazolam (a short-acting benzodiazepine), King *et al.* (1987) have reported clear environmental specificity of tolerance to the drug's sedative effect, while Griffiths and Goudie (1986) reported no environmental specificity of tolerance to the drug's hypothermic effect. However, the general finding, obtained with many drugs, dosages, species, and procedural variations, is that tolerance is more pronounced when the drug is administered in the context of the usual predrug cues than when it is administered in the context of alternative cues.

4. EVIDENCE FOR THE CONTRIBUTION OF CONDITIONING TO TOLERANCE

The observation that there often is pronounced environmental specificity to the display of tolerance is readily interpretable by an analysis of tolerance that incorporates Pavlovian conditioning principles. If the repeatedly drugged organism is administered the drug in the context of normal predrug cues, the compensatory CR partially cancels the drug effect, thus tolerance is apparent. However, if this organism is administered the drug in the context of cues not previously associated with the drug, there would be no CR attenuating the drug effect, and tolerance attributable to such a CR would not be observed. In addition, there are a variety of other findings that implicate conditioning in tolerance.

4.1. Retardation of Tolerance

If tolerance is a manifestation of a conditioning process, it would be expected that manipulations of the putative CS (i.e., environmental cues present at the time of drug administration) known to be effective in retarding the acquisition of CRs would similarly retard the acquisition of tolerance. Two such manipulations have been assessed: partial reinforcement and CS preexposure.

4.1.1. *Partial Reinforcement of Tolerance*

It has frequently been reported that if CS-alone presentations are interspersed among paired CS-UCS presentations, the acquisition of CRs is substantially attenuated (Mackintosh, 1974). This procedure of following only a portion of the CSs with the UCS is termed *partial reinforcement*.

The implication of the partial reinforcement literature for the conditioning theory of tolerance is clear: a group in which only a portion of the presentations of the drug administration cues are actually followed by the drug (i.e., a partial reinforcement group) should be slower to acquire tolerance than a group which never has exposure to environmental cues signaling the drug without actually receiving the drug (i.e., a continuous reinforcement group), even when the two groups are equated with respect to all pharmacological parameters. Such findings have been reported with respect to tolerance to several effects of morphine: analgesic (Krank *et al.*, 1984; Siegel, 1977), thermic (Siegel, 1978), and anorexigenic (Krank *et al.*, 1984).

4.1.2. *CS Preexposure Effect*

Another procedure that, like partial reinforcement, has a deleterious effect on CR formation is preconditioning exposure to the CS. It has been reported that in many conditioning preparations, with both human and a variety of infrahuman subjects, presentations of the CS prior to the start of acquisition serve to decrease the effectiveness of that stimulus when it is subsequently paired with a UCS during conditioning. The deleterious effect of CS preexposure has been termed the *CS preexposure effect*. If tolerance results (in part) from an association between the predrug environmental CS and the pharmacological UCS, the course of tolerance acquisition should be affected by the relative novelty of environmental cues present at the time of drug administration. Thus, organisms with extensive experience with the administration procedure prior to its actual pairing with a drug should be relatively retarded in the acquisition of tolerance, compared with organisms with minimal prior experience with these environmental cues, despite the fact that both groups suffer the systemic effects of the same dose of drug, given the same number of times, at the same intervals.

Both Siegel (1977) and Tiffany and Baker (1981) have demonstrated the detrimental effects of CS preexposure on the development of tolerance to the analgesic effect of morphine. Similar findings have been reported with respect to tolerance to the immunostimulatory synthetic polynucleotide, poly I:C.

4.2. Disruption of Established Tolerance

Findings that nonpharmacological manipulations that retard CR acquisition similarly retard tolerance suggest that conditioning contributes to tolerance. Other nonpharmacological manipulations are known to decrease the strength of well-established CRs; thus, it would be expected that these procedures should similarly decrease the magnitude of tolerance.

4.2.1. *Extinction of Tolerance*

Following a number of CS–UCS pairings sufficient for CR acquisition, presentation of the CS without the UCS causes diminution of CR strength. The phenomenon is termed "extinction." If drug tolerance is, in part, attributable to conditioning, tolerance should be subject to extinction. In other words, it would be expected that placebo sessions would attenuate established tolerance. Although there are numerous procedural differences among the experiments demonstrating such extinction of tolerance, all incorporate two groups, both of which receive a series of morphine injections sufficient to induce pronounced tolerance. Typically, for each injection the rat is removed from its home cage in the colony room, transported to a distinctly different room, and injected with morphine. These sessions constitute the tolerance development phase of the experiment. Some days later all animals receive at least one further injection of morphine in the distinctive room. This final drug injection constitutes the tolerance-test phase of the experiment. The two groups differ only with respect to their treatment during the interval between the tolerance-development phase and the tolerance-test phase. One group receives daily placebo sessions. They are treated in the same manner as on morphine sessions, except that physiological saline, rather than the drug, is injected. The response of this Extinction group to the drug during the tolerance test indicates the effects of repeated presentations of the morphine administration procedure, in the absence of the drug, on tolerance acquired during the tolerance development phase. Rats in the second group are simply left undisturbed in their home cages during the period between tolerance development and tolerance testing. The response of subjects in this Rest group during the tolerance test provides a measure of any alteration in tolerance attributable simply to the interval between the phases of the experiment. In addition, data from a Control group indicates the response to morphine in rats with no pretest experience with the drug.

Tolerance-test results of two morphine tolerance–extinction experiments are shown in Fig. 3. Figure 3A summarizes Siegel's (1975) original demonstration of the extinction of analgesic tolerance. The analgesic effect of morphine was assessed with the hot-plate procedure described previously, and Fig. 3A depicts mean (± 1 SEM) paw-lick latencies. As can be seen in Fig. 3A, Rest group rats displayed faster latencies (they were more tolerant to the analgesic of morphine) than Extinction group rats, despite the identical pretest history of morphine administration for the two groups. Indeed, the extinction procedure was so effective in attenuating tolerance that the morphine-experienced, Extinction group animals responded with the long response latency seen in rats receiving the drug for the first time. Subsequent research has confirmed the extinguishability of morphine analgesic tolerance (Siegel, 1977; Siegel *et al.*, 1980). Such extinction can be observed with a vari-

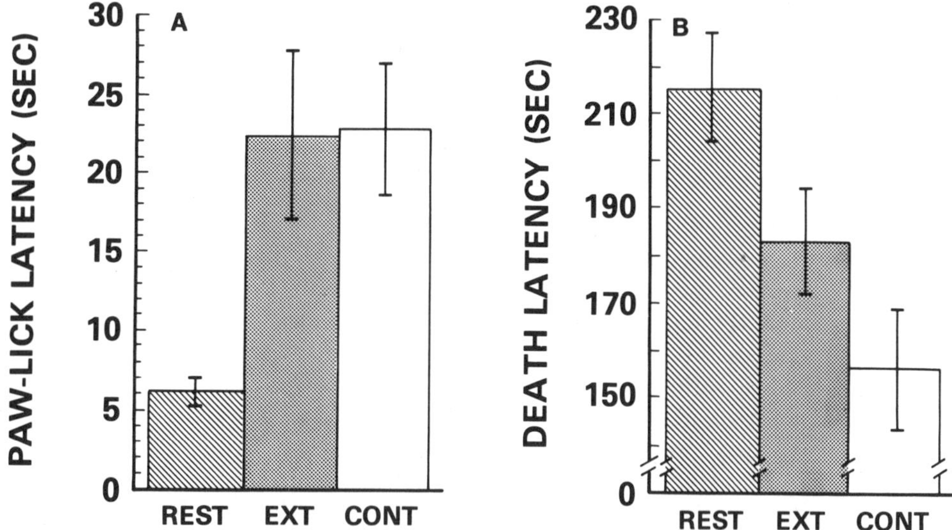

FIG. 3. Summary of results of experiments demonstrating extinction of tolerance to the analgesic (A) and lethal (B) effect of morphine, based on Siegel (1975) and Siegel *et al.* (1979), respectively.

ety of routes of drug administration, including administration directly into the ventricles of the brain (MacRae and Siegel, 1987).

Figure 3B summarizes results obtained in a study concerned with extinction of tolerance to the lethal effect of morphine (Siegel *et al.*, 1979). In this study of tolerance to the lethal effect of morphine, in contrast to the previously described study of tolerance to the lethal effect of heroin (Siegel *et al.*, 1982), the opiate dose used on the final test session was sufficient to kill almost all the rats (thus mortality did not differ between groups). The measure of the drug's effect in this Siegel *et al.* (1979) morphine-lethality extinction experiment was the time from the start of opiate infusion until death (as determined by lack of heartbeat). Experimental rats were initially given an ascending series of sublethal intravenous morphine infusions. On the test session, following intravenous infusion of a lethal dose of morphine, rats in both groups with pretest experience with the drug survived longer than rats in the Control group, which suggests that extinction was incomplete or that some tolerance occurred that was not attributable to associative mechanisms. However, some extinction of tolerance did occur, as extinction group rats were less tolerant to the lethal effect of morphine (their death latencies were significantly shorter) than Rest group rats.

Extinction of tolerance to the thermic (Siegel, 1978) and locomotor (Fanselow and German, 1982) effects of morphine has also been reported. Furthermore, extinction of tolerance has also been demonstrated with respect to many effects of general other drugs: ethanol (see Siegel, 1987), amphetamine (Poulos *et al.*, 1981), poly I:C (Dyck *et al.*, 1986), and midazolam (a short-acting benzodiazepine; King *et al.*, 1987).

4.2.2. *Explicitly Unpaired Presentations of CS and UCS and Loss of Tolerance*

In addition to extinction, another procedure for decreasing the strength of established CRs is to continue to present *both* the CS and UCS, but in an unpaired manner (see Mackintosh, 1974). That is, the subject receives both conditioning stimuli, but the CS does not signal the UCS; rather the UCS is presented only during intervals between CS presentations. With this procedure (in contrast with the CS–UCS pairings used to establish CRs), the CS signals a period of UCS absence. Fanselow and German (1982) demonstrated that this procedure can be used to attenuate tolerance to the behaviorally sedating effect of morphine in rats. Morphine was administered on a number of occasions in the presence of a distinctive environmental cue. When tolerance was established, continued presentation of the drug and cue, but in an explicitly unpaired manner, eliminated the tolerance. That is (as expected on the basis of a conditioning analysis of tolerance), despite the fact that morphine-tolerant rats continue to receive morphine, tolerance is reversed if the continued morphine administrations are unpaired with a cue that was initially paired with the drug.

4.3. Associative Inhibition of Tolerance

In most Pavlovian conditioning research, the CS is paired with the UCS. However, organisms can learn not only that a CS predicts the presence of the UCS, but also that a CS predicts the *absence* of the UCS. Such associations are termed *inhibitory* to distinguish them from the more commonly studied excitatory associations. An example of an inhibitory training procedure is one in which the CS signals a long period free of the UCS (Rescorla, 1969). The association between the CS and UCS *absence* is not readily detectable because it does not result in overt CRs. However, the inhibitory association resulting from this "explicitly unpaired" procedure may be seen by subsequently arranging the CS to predict the presence of the UCS (i.e., the CS and UCS are paired). The prior inhibitory training will retard the acquisition of the excitatory association; that is, CRs will be slow to develop. This is a "retardation of acquisition" demonstration of conditional inhibition (Rescorla, 1969).

If morphine tolerance is, in part, attributable to a drug-compensatory CR, it should be subject to inhibitory learning. Such inhibitory learning would be an especially dramatic and counterintuitive demonstration of the contribution of learning to tolerance, as tolerance would be retarded by a procedure involving administration of the drug.

Consider the situation in which the analgesic effect of morphine is tested, in drug-experienced subjects, in the context of a distinctive environmental cue. Subjects that receive pretest cue presentations and morphine administrations in an explicitly unpaired manner (i.e., the cue always signals a long, drug-free period) should be retarded in the acquisition of tolerance when subsequently administered morphine in the presence of the cue. It has, in fact, been reported that such an explicitly unpaired technique of cue and drug presentation *does* result in an inhibitory association between the environmental and pharmacological stimuli, as evidenced by the retarded development of tolerance to the analgesic (Siegel *et al.*, 1981) and behaviorally sedating (Fanselow and German, 1982) effects of morphine. Similar findings have been reported with respect to tolerance to the thermic effects of pentobarbital (Hinson and Siegel, 1986). The finding that tolerance acquisition may be retarded by a treatment involving drug administration is not readily interpretable by theories of tolerance that do not acknowledge a role for learning in the development of tolerance.

4.4 Morphine Tolerance and Compound Predrug Cues

Although pairing of a CS and UCS will generally promote an association between them (as evidenced by the development of CRs), it is possible to pair the two events without an association developing between them. This situation is seen in "compound conditioning," i.e., conditioning preparations in which at least two CSs simultaneously signal the UCS. It is well established that the effectiveness of any one of the CSs in becoming associated with the UCS depends on the characteristics of the stimuli with which this CS is compounded. Such compound conditioning effects may be seen in phenomena termed *blocking* and *overshadowing*. On the basis of the conditioning account, drug tolerance, like other CRs, should be subject to blocking and overshadowing.

4.4.1. *Blocking of Tolerance*

If a CS has initially been presented such that it is a good predictor of the UCS, it will prevent a second, simultaneously presented CS from becoming associated with the UCS (see Kamin, 1969). For example, if a particular CS (say, CS_A) has been associated with a

UCS, and CS_A is subsequently compounded with a second CS (say, CS_B), with this CS_A + CS_B compound still being paired with the UCS, little is learned about CS_B. That is, prior training with one component of a compound stimulus will block the subsequent conditioning of a second component; in this example, CS_A blocks CS_B (CS_A is the blocking stimulus, and CS_B is the blocked stimulus). If tolerance is attributable to conditioning, it should be subject to blocking. Consider the case of a subject repeatedly administered a drug in the context of a compound environmental cue, and which displays tolerance in the presence of this compound CS. This subject may or may not display tolerance in the presence of each of the components of the compound CS, depending on the conditioning history of the alternative component. That is, tolerance should be displayed in the presence of the blocking CS, but not in the presence of the blocked CS. This finding has been reported with respect to tolerance to the analgesic effect of morphine (Dafters *et al.*, 1983).

4.4.2. *Overshadowing of Tolerance*

In the case of blocking, one CS (the blocking CS) is pretrained prior to being compounded with a second CS (the blocked CS). With this procedure, subjects learn little about the added CS. Sometimes, even if there is no prior training of an element of a compound CS, subjects will still learn about only one of the elements. This occurs if one element is more salient than the other. Other things being equal, a group trained with a more salient CS will learn more rapidly than a group trained with a less salient CS. For example, if CS_A and CS_B are both effective CSs, but subjects learn a CS_A–UCS association faster than a CS_B–UCS association, CS_A is said to be more salient than CS_B. In this case, the effect of pairing a UCS with a CS_A + CS_B compound will be to strongly associate CS_A with the UCS. Little associative strength will develop between CS_B and the UCS; CS_A (the more salient CS) overshadows CS_B (the less salient CS). The overshadowing phenomenon was originally described by Pavlov (1927), and has been extensively investigated by Kamin (1969).

If tolerance is mediated by conditioning, it would be expected that overshadowing should be a feature of tolerance. That is, if subjects become tolerant to a drug consistently administered in the presence of a compound CS, these subjects should display more tolerance in the presence of the more salient component of the CS than they do in the presence of the less salient component. Indeed, these subjects should display less tolerance in the presence of the less salient component than they would if this less salient CS alone had signaled the drug (rather as a part of a compound CS constructed of components differing in salience). This result, demonstrating the applicability of a compound conditioning phenomenon to tolerance to the analgesic effect of morphine, was reported by Walter and Riccio (1983).

4.5. Compound Predrug Cues Normally Signaling a Drug

The study of compound conditioning effects with respect to drug tolerance provides further evidence in support of the conditioning analysis of tolerance. Moreover, it is possible that drug effects are typically signaled by compound stimuli, thus these compound conditioning effects may be especially important for understanding tolerance.

It is not difficult to specify the multiple CSs that conceivably could accompany drug administration. Although the drug may be made contingent on a single nominal CS [e.g., the tone used in Pavlov's (1927) original demonstration of pharmacological conditioning], there are typically other cues present uniquely at the time of drug administration. For example, handling an animal in conjunction with drug administration and piercing the skin with a hypodermic needle would appear to provide readily detectable signals of an impending drug effect. In fact, it is well established that such injection-ritual cues may become CSs for drugs in the absence of other, explicit CSs (see Siegel, 1985). When there is an explicit CS, these injection-ritual cues become components of a compound CS.

4.5.1. *Injection-ritual Cues and the Conditioning Model of Tolerance*

Evidence summarized thus far provide substantial evidence that Pavlovian conditioning contributes to tolerance. There are, however, ostensibly contrary data. For example, in contrast to previously described results indicating environmental specificity of tolerance, some investigators have reported that tolerance acquired as a result of consistent drug administration in one environment is sometimes fully displayed in a very different environment (e.g., Jørgensen and Hole, 1984; Kesner and Cook, 1983). These investigators suggested that the existence of cross-situational tolerance indicates that some tolerance is not associative. This, of course, is quite possible (Siegel, 1983); however, it is also possible that a failure to demonstrate environmentally specific tolerance may result from overshadowing. That is, both drug-administration environment and injection-ritual cues are paired with the drug. Under some circumstances, the latter cues might be much more salient than the former cues, thus the injection-ritual cues will overshadow other, simultaneously present environmental cues. Recently, Dafters and Bach (1985) have argued that such circumstances have prevailed in studies that have failed to demonstrate environmental specificity of morphine tolerance. If the injection-ritual cues have overshadowed other cues, it would be expected that subjects made tolerant to morphine in one environment would display this tolerance in a different environment because, despite the environmental alteration, the *effective* signal for the drug is unaltered. This effective signal is comprised of injection-ritual cues (i.e., picking up the rat and injecting it) which are similar in the test environment and in the environment in which tolerance has been acquired.

In an experiment designed to evaluate this overshadowing interpretation of instances of apparent environment-independent tolerance, Dafters and Bach (1985) reduced the salience of the injection-ritual cues. They used a CS preexposure procedure to decrease the effectiveness of this putative CS, (i.e., they repeatedly injected rats with an inert substance prior to administration of morphine). This would be expected to reduce the ability of injection-ritual cues to overshadow other environmental cues present at the time of drug administration. Dafters and Bach (1985) found that predrug exposure to the injection procedure enhanced the environmental specificity of tolerance to the analgesic effect of morphine; indeed, in conditions in which no attempt was made to decrease the salience of the injection-ritual cues, no evidence of tolerance environmental specificity was obtained. Although previously such transsituational tolerance has been interpreted as evidence contrary to an associative account of tolerance (e.g., Kesner and Cook, 1983), it is likely that it is attributable to overshadowing.

4.5.2. *Interoceptive Drug Cues and the Conditioning Model of Tolerance*

A second source of potential unauthorized CSs for a drug is provided by the interoceptive effects of the drug itself. That is, the early effect of a drug inevitably signals a later effect; thus, the maximal effects of a drug are announced by a compound CS consisting of interoceptive components, as well as exteroceptive components.

It has, in fact, recently been demonstrated that a drug can serve as a cue for itself, and this association may contribute to tolerance (Greeley *et al.*, 1984). The drug used in this experiment was ethanol. Although there are no reports of a similarly designed experiment with morphine, the results of this Greeley *et al.* (1984) experiment have important implications for understanding drug tolerance in general. In this study, rats in one group (Paired) consistently received a low dose of ethanol (0.8 g/kg) 60 minutes prior to a high dose (2.5 g/kg). Another group of rats (Unpaired) received the low and high doses on an unpaired basis. When tested for the tolerance to the hypothermic effect of ethanol, Paired subjects, but not Unpaired subjects, displayed tolerance. Moreover, if the high dose of ethanol was *not* preceded by the low dose, Paired rats failed to display their usual tolerance. This tolerance, dependent on an ethanol–ethanol pairing, was apparently mediated by an ethanol-compensatory thermic CR; Paired rats, but not Unpaired rats, evidenced a hyperthermic CR (opposite to the hypothermic effect of the drug) in response to the low dose of ethanol. Moreover, the tolerance seen in Paired rats, in common with tolerance resulting from environment–drug pairings, was subject to extinction; repeated presentation of the low dose *not* followed by the high dose led to diminution of tolerance established in Paired rats.

Results of this Greeley *et al.* (1984) study provide convincing evidence that a small dose of a drug can serve as a signal for a larger dose of that same drug. Because a gradual increase in systemic concentration is an inevitable consequence of most drug administration procedures, such drug–drug associations may play a hitherto unappreciated role in the effects of repeated drug administrations. For example, Walter and Riccio (1983) suggested that interoceptive stimuli produced by a drug may sometimes be more salient than external drug signals, and thus may overshadow environmental cues present at the time of drug administration. Therefore, transsituational tolerance, rather than having a fundamentally different mechanism than tolerance attributable to conditioning (e.g., Goudie and Griffiths, 1984; Kesner and Cook, 1983), may be due to the relatively greater effectiveness of the interoceptive–pharmacological component of the predrug compound CS. Such differential effectiveness may arise because of procedural features of the drug administration procedure that promote overshadowing or blocking:

> Tolerance controlled by internal, morphine-produced stimuli, unlike that mediated by environmental stimuli, would be expected to be relatively transsituational or "pharmacological" in nature, even though the same underlying conditioning mechanisms would be involved. The question then becomes one of establishing the extent to which tolerance, in any given case, is controlled by one or the other of these two general classes of stimuli, rather than one of making a distinction between two different "kinds" of tolerance. (Walter and Riccio, 1983, p. 661)

5. CUES FOR DRUGS

Most of the research summarized thus far has indicated the importance of drug-predictive environmental cues in the display of tolerance. However, the findings of Greeley *et al.* (1984), already summarized, indicate that a drug may serve as a cue for itself, and thus pharmacological cues, as well as environmental cues, may contribute to tolerance. Other experiments also indicate that non-environmental cues may become associated with morphine and contribute to the expression of morphine tolerance.

5.1. Pharmacological Cues and State-Dependent Learning of Morphine Tolerance

In addition to the findings of Greeley *et al.* (1984), there is a considerable amount of other evidence that the effects of a variety of drugs can serve as CSs. That is, if a given drug (D1) is repeatedly administered before a second drug (D2), a pharmacological CR is elicited by D1. Such drug–drug associations may importantly contribute to tolerance (Krank and Bennett, 1987; Lett, 1983, Taukulis, 1982, 1986a, 1986b). Results of recent research concerning the effects of pentobarbital on morphine tolerance are readily interpretable as a result of an association between a pharmacological signal (generated by the interoceptive effects of the barbiturate) and morphine.

Terman and colleagues (Terman *et al.*, 1983; Terman *et al.*, 1985) reported that rats with a history of morphine administration who were administered pentobarbital prior to a final injection of morphine do not display the analgesic tolerance seen in nonanesthetized rats. That is, the barbiturate apparently blocks morphine tolerance. Some interpretations of pentobarbital blockage of morphine tolerance have postulated direct pharmacodynamic interaction between the barbiturate and the opiate (Pontani *et al.*, 1985). Results of a recent experiment, however, indicate that "state-dependent learning," rather than pharmacodynamic interaction, best accounts for such barbiturate–opiate effects (Siegel, 1988).

There is a considerable amount of evidence that drug states in general, and the state generated by barbiturates in particular, can serve as salient stimuli (see Järbe, 1986; Overton, 1984). That is, learned responses acquired when the subject is *not* under the influence of a centrally acting drug, such as pentobarbital, may fail to be displayed when the subject is subsequently tested while under the influence of this drug. To the extent that tolerance to morphine's analgesic effect is mediated by learning, it might be expected that tolerance will display such drug state dependency—pharmacological cues, such as those generated by pentobarbital, may function very much like environmental cues in affecting the display of tolerance. In other words, just as there is environmental specificity of morphine tolerance (because of associations between morphine-signaling environmental cues and the opiate), there might also be state-specificity of morphine tolerance (because of associations between morphine-signaling pharmacological cues and the opiate).

Siegel (1988) confirmed the finding that pentobarbital interferes with the expression of morphine tolerance in rats that had not previously received barbiturate–opiate pairings. Additionally, the results supported the state-dependency interpretation of this interference.

This Siegel (1988) experiment consisted of six, daily sessions: five tolerance training sessions followed by a tolerance test session. During each session, rats received two injections, with a 15-min interval between injections. The CS drug was administered during the first of the two injections, and the UCS drug was administered during the second. Depending on the subject's group assignment and phase of the experiment, the CS drug was either pentobarbital or physiological saline, and the UCS drug was either morphine or saline. Subjects were assigned to one of the eight cells of a 2 × 2 × 2 factorial design. The groups differed with respect to the CS drug used during the training sessions (pentobarbital or saline), the UCS drug used during training sessions (morphine or saline), and the CS drug used for the test session (pentobarbital or saline). For all rats, the UCS drug used for the test session was morphine. Following the test-session morphine administration, the level of analgesia was assessed in all subjects.

Group abbreviations indicate the CS and UCS drugs used during training and testing. For example, subjects in Group Pent-MOR/Pent-MOR received pentobarbital prior to each morphine injection during training, and were also tested for the analgesic effect of morphine subsequent to pentobarbital administration. Similarly, subjects in Group Sal-SAL/Pent-MOR received physiological saline as both CS and UCS drugs during training, and received pentobarbital prior to their first morphine administration on the test session. Thirty minutes following the morphine administration on the test session, analgesia level was assessed in all subjects. Their tail was immersed in a 50°C water bath, and the latency to flick their tails out of the water was measured.

The results of the experiment are shown in Fig. 4. The mean response latencies (± SEM) are displayed separately for groups tested with pentobarbital as the CS drug (left panel) and saline as the CS drug (right panel). Figure 4 depicts the findings obtained when the dose of pentobarbital was 20 mg/kg [the same pattern of results was obtained with a 55 mg/kg dose of the barbiturate (see Siegel, 1988)]. As can be seen in the left panel of Fig. 4, there was no evidence of tolerance in the morphine-experienced group that received pentobarbital prior to the final morphine administration if pretest administrations were not signaled by the barbiturate (i.e., subjects in Groups Sal-MOR/Pent-MOR did not display shorter response latencies than subjects in Group Sal-SAL/Pent-MOR, despite the fact that subjects in this latter group received morphine for the first time on the test session). However, as can further be seen in the left panel of Fig. 4, signaling the test administration of morphine with pentobarbital does not inevitably interfere with morphine tolerance. Morphine-experienced subjects tested *and* trained with pentobarbital as the CS drug (Group Pent-MOR/Pent-MOR) displayed analgesic tolerance following the test administration of the opiate, i.e., they evidenced shorter response latencies than did subjects with the same exposure to the barbiturate that received morphine for the first time on the test session (Group Pent-SAL/Pent-MOR).

These results depicted in the left panel of Fig. 4 confirm and extend the findings of Terman *et al.* (1983, 1985). That is, rats with a history of morphine administration do not display the expected tolerance to a test injection of the opiate if it is preceded, for the first time, by pentobarbital. Results obtained from additional groups suggest that the effect of pentobarbital on morphine tolerance is a result of state-dependent learning. As would be expected from a state-dependency analysis, rats that had pretest administrations of morphine, as well as the test administration, signaled by pentobarbital displayed substantial tolerance to the analgesic effect of morphine (i.e., subjects in Group Pent-MOR/Pent-MOR evidenced shorter response latencies than subjects in Group Pent-SAL/Pent-MOR). Although this finding is readily explicable by the state-dependency interpretation, there is an alternative explanation. It is possible that the relevant effect of pretest exposure to pentobarbital in Group Pent-MOR/Pent-MOR was to establish tolerance to pentobarbital, rather than to associate pentobarbital with morphine. Such barbiturate tolerance, rather than state-dependent learning, could conceivably account for the ineffectiveness of pentobarbital in interfering with morphine tolerance. This alternative, nonassociative interpretation is unlikely, however, considering the results obtained with subjects tested with physiological saline as the CS (see right panel of Fig. 4).

Examination of the right panel of Fig. 4 indicates that saline-tested subjects, like pentobarbital-tested subjects, displayed an interaction between the magnitude of tolerance and the similarity of the training CS and test CS. Greater tolerance is displayed by subjects trained with saline (Group SAL-MOR/Sal-MOR compared to Group Sal-SAL/Sal-MOR) than by subjects trained with pentobarbital (Group Pent-MOR/Sal-MOR compared to Group Pent-SAL/Sal-MOR). That is, for saline-tested subjects trained with pentobarbital as the CS drug, the *omission* of the barbiturate cue on the test session attenuated the expression of morphine tolerance.

These results further indicate that pharmacological cues, as well as environmental cues, may come to control tolerance. Furthermore, not only may a drug serve as a cue for itself and control tolerance (as demonstrated by Greeley *et al.*, 1984), but also one type of drug (e.g., a barbiturate) may serve as a cue for another type of drug (e.g., an opiate) and similarly control tolerance. Such findings suggest that some cross-drug effects may represent instances of state-dependent learning, rather than pharmacodynamic interactions (see Siegel, 1988).

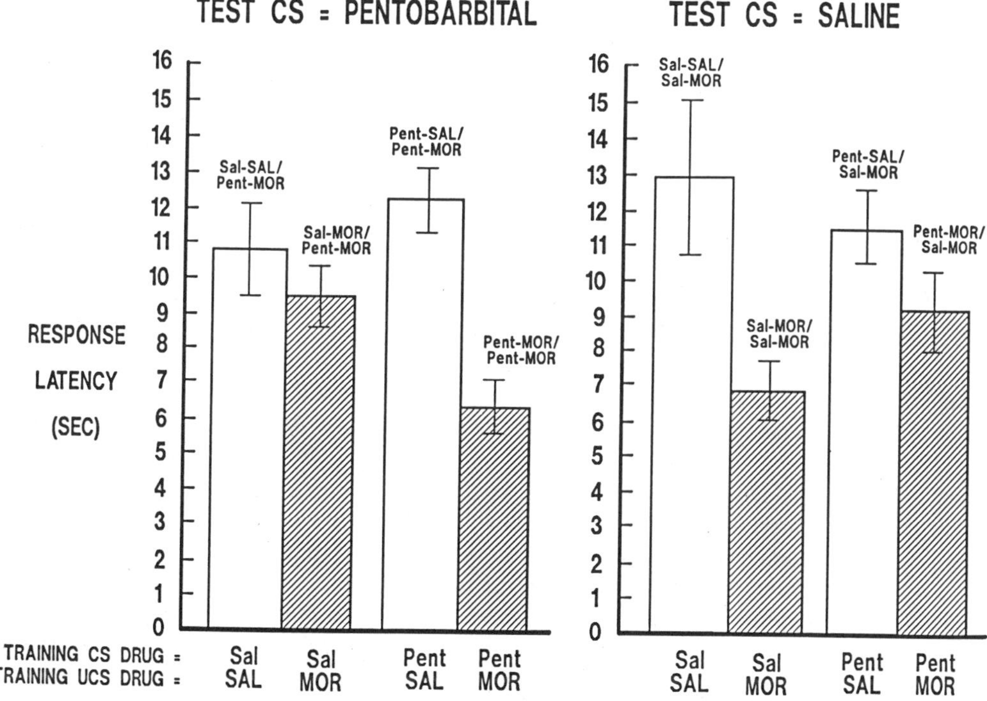

FIG. 4. Mean tail-flick latencies (± 1 SEM) following morphine administration on the tolerance tests session in the experiment of Siegel (1988). Rats received 20 mg/kg pentobarbital (left panel) or physiological saline (right panel) as a CS drug prior to the test session administration of morphine, and received the indicated combinations of CS and UCS drugs during pretest training sessions. (From Siegel, S. State-dependent learning of morphine tolerance. *Behavioral Neuroscience*, 1988. Copyright 1988 by the American Psychological Association. Reprinted by permission).

5.2. Pharmacological Cues and External Inhibition of Morphine Tolerance

Conditional responses, once established, can be disrupted by the presentation of a novel, extraneous stimulus. The phenomenon was termed "external inhibition" by Pavlov (1927), who described its operation in the salivary conditioning situation:

> The dog and the experimenter would be isolated in the experimental room, all the conditions remaining for a while constant. Suddenly some disturbing factor would arise—a sound would penetrate the room; some quick change in illumination would occur, the sun going behind a cloud; or a draught would get in underneath the door, and maybe bring some odour with it. If any of these extra stimuli happened to be introduced just at the time of application of the conditioned stimulus, it would inevitably bring about a more or less pronounced weakening or even a complete disappearance of the reflex response depending on the strength of the extra stimulus (Pavlov 1927, p. 44).

On the basis of the conditioning analysis of tolerance, it would be expected that the display of tolerance should be disrupted merely by presentation of a novel stimulus. Results of a recent experiment (Siegel and Sdao-Jarvie, 1986) supported this prediction with respect to tolerance to the hypothermic effect of ethanol. In this experiment, the display of hypothermic tolerance was disrupted by the presentation of novel environmental stimulus (a flashing light). Recently, Poulos *et al.* (1988) demonstrated disruption of morphine tolerance by a pharmacological stimulus.

During the tolerance acquisition phase of the Poulos *et al.* (1988) experiment, two groups of rats were repeatedly injected with morphine (5 mg/kg), and became tolerant to the drug's analgesic effect. One of these groups was additionally injected with ethanol (1.2 g/kg) 15 min after each morphine injection. Following tolerance acquisition, all rats were tested for morphine analgesic tolerance with a novel state being introduced following morphine administration, i.e., they experienced either the novel introduction, or the novel omission, of the alcohol cue. Both novel states attenuated tolerance.

It would appear that just as there is external inhibition of ethanol tolerance by a novel environmental cue (Siegel and Sdao-Jarvie, 1986), there is also external inhibition of morphine tolerance by a novel pharmacological state.

5.3. Magnetic Fields and the Conditioning Analysis of Tolerance

Results of experiments summarized thus far indicate that both environmental and pharmacological stimuli can become cues for morphine, and importantly contribute to tolerance. Results of an experiment by Kavaliers and Ossenkopp (1985) indicate that yet another category of stimuli may similarly be associated with morphine—magnetic fields. In the Kavaliers and Ossenkopp (1985) experiment, groups of mice received 10 daily injections of morphine, either in the presence or absence of rotating magnetic fields (2–35 gauses). Analgesia was assessed following each of these pretest drug administrations. Subjects were then tested for analgesic tolerance both in the presence and absence of magnetic stimuli.

The results of this experiment indicated that magnetic fields *per se* affect the development of tolerance. During the pretest phase of the experiment, mice repeatedly administered morphine in conjunction with magnetic field exposure were relatively retarded in the acquisition of tolerance to the analgesic effect of morphine. In addition, the field also functioned as an effective cue for the drug. On the test session, tolerance was more pronounced following drug administration in the presence of the same magnetic stimuli (either presence or absence of field) that prevailed during the pretest drug administrations than following drug administration in the presence of the alternative magnetic stimuli.

As discussed by Kavaliers and Ossenkopp (1985), the results extend the conditioning analysis of tolerance. The finding that magnetic field exposure during pretest sessions attenuated the acquisition of tolerance is congenial with suggestions that such exposure detrementally affects the acquisition of learned responses (see Kavaliers and Ossenkopp, 1985). The further finding that magnetic fields can become associated with morphine and influence the display of tolerance suggests that subtle stimuli may play a heretofore unappreciated role in the development of tolerance. The authors also suggest that their results may be relevant to reported circadian differences in morphine effects in mice.

6. RELATIONSHIP BETWEEN CONDITIONING AND NONASSOCIATIVE INTERPRETATIONS OF TOLERANCE

It is important to emphasize that the conditioning analysis of tolerance is not an alternative to traditional interpretations. Rather, the conditioning analysis is complementary to views of tolerance that do not acknowledge a role for learning. Many such nonassociative analyses of tolerance emphasize the role of drug-elicited homeostatic corrections that restore pharmacologically induced physiological disturbances to normal levels. Several investigators have indicated the potential adaptive advantage if these homeostatic corrections actually antedate the pharmacological insult (e.g., Wikler, 1973). Pavlov was certainly aware of the importance of such anticipatory responding: "Under natural conditions the normal animal must respond not only to stimuli which themselves bring immediate benefit or harm, but also to other physical or chemical agencies—waves of light and the like—which in themselves only signal the approach of these stimuli" (Pavlov, 1927, p. 14). On the basis of a conditioning model, the systemic alterations that mediate tolerance occur not only in response to the pharmacological stimulation, but may also occur in response to reliable environmental signals of this stimulation. That is, tolerance is controlled by feedforward mechanisms as well as feedback mechanisms.

It should be apparent that conditioning is irrelevant to some preparations that have been valuable in the study of tolerance. For example, tolerance studied in isolated tissue samples, or tolerance studied by continuous administration procedures (e.g., inhalation or liquid diet) is not amenable to alteration by environmental manipulations (see Melchoir and Tabakoff, 1984). On the other hand, conditioning processes likely contribute to tolerance under the usual conditions of drug administration (regular administrations, at widely spaced intervals, with discrete environmental cues uniquely present at the time of each administration). These are the conditions that favor the development of an association between predrug cues and the systemic effects of the drug.

7. ALTERNATIVE INTERPRETATIONS

A considerable amount of data has been summarized suggesting that an appreciation of Pavlovian conditioning principles is important for understanding morphine tolerance. The particular Pavlovian analysis of tolerance emphasized here ascribes an important role for drug-compensatory CRs in the development of tolerance. There are other theories that recognize the importance of learning in the development of morphine tolerance. These alternative theories differ somewhat in emphases and theoretical foundations.

7.1. Tolerance and Conditional "Autoanalgesia"

Demonstrations of environmental specificity of morphine analgesic tolerance, and hyperalgesia in response to predrug cues, have been interpreted as support for the compensatory-CR analysis of morphine tolerance, i.e., compensatory CRs evidenced in anticipation of morphine attenuate the effect of the drug administered in the context of the usual predrug cues. Recently, Rochford and Stewart (1987) suggested that these phenomena may be better understood as the result of responses made in anticipation of the pain sensitivity assessment, rather than CRs made in anticipation of the drug.

7.1.1. *Autoanalgesia and Conditioned Autoanalgesia*

Several investigators (e.g., Ross and Randich, 1985; Sherman *et al.*, 1984) have reported that presentations of nociceptive stimuli can activate endogenous pain-suppression mechanisms, causing an animal to become analgesic. Such pain-elicited analgesia has been termed *autoanalgesia*. In addition, these investigators report that if the animal is repeatedly exposed to the nociceptive stimuli in the presence of distinctive cues, these cues come to elicit a conditional analgesic response (i.e., conditioned autoanalgesia). According to Rochford and Stewart (1987), the results of at least some experiments, usually interpreted as support for the compensatory-CR account of morphine analgesic tolerance, are better interpreted as demonstrations of conditioned autoanalgesia. The usual design of these experiments may be expected to promote the development of such an analgesic CR:

> The typical demonstration of situation-specific tolerance to the analgesic effect of morphine comes from experiments in which two groups of animals are compared for pain reactivity over a series of days. The experimental group is transported to a distinctive environment, administered morphine and then given a test for analgesia sometime after injection. The control group is administered saline in the distinctive environment prior to the pain test and is administered morphine elsewhere . . . Provided that the intensity of the nociceptive stimulation produced by analgesic testing is strong enough to recruit endogenous pain-suppression mechanisms, it is likely that the environment in which testing is conducted will become capable of eliciting conditioned autoanalgesia (Rochford and Stewart [1987], p. 690).

7.1.2. *Conditioned Autoanalgesia, Tolerance, Environmental Specificity, and Compensatory Conditioning*

Although both experimental and control groups might be expected to develop conditioned autoanalgesia, it would be expected that such conditioning would be more pronounced in experimental subjects. These subjects receive morphine in conjunction with each analgesia assessment, thus the nociceptive stimulation would be expected to be functionally less intense for these subjects: "As a result, when both groups are tested under saline, the experimental group will appear hyperalgesic relative to the control because morphine attenuated the development of conditioned autoanalgesia" (Rochford and Stewart, 1987, pp. 690–691).

Differences in conditional autoanalgesia account not only for findings of apparent hyperalgesia, but also findings of tolerance environmental specificity: "because it has been shown that conditioned autoanalgesia is synergistic with morphine-induced analgesia (Sherman *et al.*, 1984), when both groups are administered analgesia tests following morphine administration in the distinctive environment, the experimental group should show greater tolerance to the analgesic effect of morphine than the control group because the experimental group would have lower levels of conditioned autoanalgesia with which to synergize with morphine analgesia" (Rochford and Stewart, 1987, p. 691).

7.1.3. *Compensatory Conditioning and Conditioned Autoanalgesia*

Rochford and Stewart (1987) present evidence that some data used in support of the compensatory CR analysis of tolerance to the analgesic effect of morphine are also congenial with their conditioned autoanalgesia account. There are, however, data that are not readily interpretable by conditioned autoanalgesia (e.g., MacRae and Siegel, 1987). Also, phenomena such as tolerance environmental specificity and compensatory pharmacological CRs are very general. As previously discussed, evidence for the compensatory-CR interpretation has been obtained with respect to tolerance to a variety of effects of many drugs, and not just tolerance to the analgesic effect of morphine.

7.2. Tolerance as Habituation

The term *tolerance* is used to describe the decreasing response to a drug over the course of successive administrations of that drug. The term *habituation* is used to describe the decreasing response to a peripheral stimulus over the course of successive presentations of that stimulus. Despite the obvious similarities in operations and outcomes, these two phenomena have typically been subject to quite different theoretical treatments.

An influential model of habituation has been developed by Wagner (1976, 1978). Following suggestions of Siegel (1977, 1982), Baker and Tiffany (1985) elaborated the application of Wagner's model to tolerance. A detailed discussion of the similarities and differences between the compensatory-CR and habituation analyses of tolerance is beyond the scope of this chapter. Briefly, the two accounts make many similar predictions (concerning, for example, environmental specificity of tolerance and extinction of tolerance), but there are some theoretical distinctions (see Baker and Tiffany, 1985; Mackintosh, 1987; Paletta and Wagner, 1986; Siegel, 1989).

Of the several analyses of tolerance that emphasize Pavlovian conditioning, the compensatory CR account is unique inasmuch as it addresses the appearance of withdrawal symptoms (following termination of drug use), as well as tolerance (when the drug is repeatedly administered).

8. PAVLOVIAN CONDITIONING AND "WITHDRAWAL SYMPTOMS"

According to most current views, tolerance and withdrawal symptoms are both manifestations of homeostatic mechanisms that correct for pharmacological disturbances—the feedback mechanisms that mediate tolerance (when the drug is administered) are expressed as withdrawal symptoms (when the drug is not administered) (see Siegel *et al.*, 1987). It has become increasingly apparent that just as feedforward or anticipation (as well as feedback) contributes to tolerance, it also contributes to withdrawal symptoms. Thus, some withdrawal symptoms are due not to alterations in feedback mechanisms induced by past drug administrations, but rather to the anticipation of the next drug administration. That is, some drug withdrawal symptoms are, more accurately, drug preparation symptoms; they result from drug-compensatory CRs.

In discussing the role of compensatory CRs in so-called withdrawal symptoms, it is important to make a distinction between the acute withdrawal reaction seen shortly after the initiation of abstinence (which typically lasts for days or, at most, weeks) and the apparently similar symptoms often noted after detoxification is presumably complete (see Hinson and Siegel, 1982). In the latter case it is likely that it is the anticipation of the drug, rather than the drug itself, that is responsible for the symptoms.

> Consider the situation in which the addict expects a drug, but does not receive it; that is, no drug is available, but the addict is in an environment where he or she has frequently used drugs in the past, or it is the time of day when the drug is typically administered, or any of a variety of drug-associated stimuli occur. Research with animals demonstrates that presentation of cues previously associated with drug administration, but now not followed by the drug, results in the occurrence of drug-compensatory CRs . . . In the situation in which the drug addict expects but does not receive the drug, it would be expected that drug-compensatory CRs would also occur. These CRs normally counter the pharmacological disruption of functioning which occurs when the anticipated drug is administered. However, since the expected drug is not forthcoming, the CRs may achieve expression as overt physiological reactions, e.g., yawning, running nose, watery eyes, sweating . . . or form the basis for the subjective experience of withdrawal sickness and craving (Hinson and Siegel, 1982, p. 499).

Actually, the role of environmental cues in the display of withdrawal symptoms and relapse has been known for a long time. The following observation is from *The Anatomy of Drunkenness*, written in 1859:

> Man is very much the creature of habit. By drinking regularly at certain times he feels the longing for liquor at the stated return of these periods—as after dinner, or immediately before going to bed, or whatever the period may be. He even finds it in certain companies, or in a particular tavern at which he is in the habit of taking his libations (Macnish, 1859, p. 151).

More recently, many other investigators have noted that environmental cues affect the display of the symptoms of withdrawal from a variety of drugs.

8.1. Environmental Elicitation of Withdrawal Distress

One way to evaluate the role of environmental cues in withdrawal distress is simply to ask addicts to recall the circumstances in which they suffer such distress. Several investigators have done just this, and have noted that both opiate addicts and alcoholics report that such distress is especially pronounced in the presence of drug-associated cues (see reviews by Siegel, 1983, 1987). Several clinicians have reported that opiate withdrawal symptoms are displayed when, during behavior therapy (even with long-detoxified former addicts), drugs are discussed (O'Brien, 1976; Wikler, 1977) or the paraphernalia of addiction (syringe and tourniquet) are viewed (Teasdale, 1973). The appearance of such symptoms in these circumstances can be enigmatic to an observer not acquainted with the phenomenon of pharmacological conditioning, as one of Wikler's (1977) recollections demonstrates:

> On two separate occasions, psychiatrists at the U.S. Public Health Service Hospital told me that in group therapy with long detoxified postaddicts, the patients would suddenly blow their noses, wipe their eyes, and yawn incessantly when the subject under discussion turned to dope. The psychiatrists, unaware of this theory of relapse, were puzzled by the reappearance of opioid abstinence phenomena 3 to 6 months after detoxification (Wikler, 1977, p. 35).

One's own personal experience may provide similar evidence of the importance of drug-associated cues in withdrawal distress and craving—environmental cues associated with smoking (or seeing others smoking, or talking about smoking) often elicit craving for a cigarette in individuals addicted to nicotine.

In the case of orally ingested drugs, such as alcohol and tobacco, an especially effective cue for the drug's systemic effects should be the flavor of the drug. It has been reported that cigarette smokers will display nicotine-withdrawal symptoms if they experience the taste of the cigarette without the usual accompanying nicotine administration, i.e., they puff on a cigarette containing much less than the usual amount of nicotine (Schachter, 1977). It is well known that alcoholics find the taste of alcohol a potent elicitor of craving (e.g., Ludwig and Stark, 1974) and have difficulty in refraining from drinking if they sample an alcoholic beverage (Hodgson and Rankin, 1976). This loss of control is apparently elicited by the taste cue, since if the taste of the alcoholic beverage is masked, a sip does not elicit such craving (Merry, 1966).

Drug-associated olfactory cues can apparently also elicit withdrawal sickness and craving. Teasdale (1973) noted that several heroin addicts who had usually injected themselves in public lavatories reported that a lavatory smell elicited craving. Many other anectodal reports of environmentally elicited withdrawal symptoms and craving are reported by Biernacki (1986) in his study of recovery from heroin addiction:

> Those in the study who were able to isolate the source of their cravings to use drugs again usually pointed to some olfactory or visual cue that they associated in their past experience with obtaining the drug and/or using it. Being in an area where they once had obtained the drug, seeing old addict associates, or (especially) witnessing another person using drugs were the most frequent reported events that engendered craving to use opiates. One man, who had been addicted for five years prior to his being interviewed, recalled how drug cravings were prompted when he saw a group of actors seem to inject heroin in a movie that he was watching on television (Biernacki, 1986, pp. 107–108).

Another of Biernacki's respondents displayed remarkable insight. He "likened himself to one of Pavlov's dogs when he felt the nausea accompanying a craving. He explained: 'I had the objectivity to even see my own behavior for what it was and that was like getting nauseous whenever I'd even think about fixing. Like one of Pavlov's dogs'" (Biernacki, 1986, p. 115).

Animals, experimentally addicted to morphine, also display environmentally elicited withdrawal symptoms. Consider Ternes' (1977) description of the behavior of monkeys that were repeatedly injected with morphine in the presence of an arbitrary auditory cue—tape-recorded music. This music became capable of eliciting withdrawal symptoms and relapse in these monkeys after a considerable period of abstinence:

> After the animal had been weaned from the drug and maintained drug-free for several months, the experimenter again played the tape-recorded music and the animal showed the following signs: he became restless, had piloerection, yawned, became diuretic, showed rhinorrhea, and again sought out the drug injection (Ternes, 1977, pp. 167–168).

There are several laboratory demonstrations of the ability of drug-associated cues to elicit withdrawal distress. For example, it has been noted that former addicts display physiological signs of narcotic withdrawal when they performed the "cooking up" ritual while being monitored by a polygraph (O'Brien *et al.*, 1976). Teasdale (1973) showed addicts slides of both opiate-related material (e.g., inserting a syringe into a vein) and non-opiate-related material (e.g., a hand holding a cup of coffee). On the basis of a variety of psychometric measures, Teasdale (1973) concluded that the opiate-related slides induced more emotional responding and evidence of withdrawal distress than the nondrug related slides. Sideroff and Jarvik (1980) also reported that drug-associated cues elicit symptoms of withdrawal. They presented a videotape depicting scenes of heroin preparation and administration to groups of both heroin addict–patients and nonaddicts. They found that the videotape elicited evidence of withdrawal (changes in heart rate and galvanic skin response, and subjective ratings of anxiety and craving) in only the addict group.

Similar findings have been reported with respect to alcohol. Ludwig and colleagues (Ludwig *et al.*, 1974, 1977) have reported that alcoholics, in the presence of laboratory-reconstructed alcohol-associated cues (e.g., a mock barroom, or the odor of bourbon), display withdrawal sickness, subjective reports of alcohol craving, and (if liquor is available) relapse to drinking (see also Siegel, 1987).

8.2. Environmental Cues, Relapse, and Abstinence

As indicated above, withdrawal symptoms are especially pronounced in the presence of drug-associated stimuli. According to the Pavlovian conditioning analysis, these stimuli have come to elicit CRs that are compensatory to the drug effect, and these CRs are often interpreted as symptoms of withdrawal. It follows that such withdrawal distress should be much less pronounced if the drug-experienced organism is not exposed to drug-associated stimuli. Such findings have been reported both in epidemiological studies with humans, and experimental studies with animals.

8.2.1. *Epidemiological Studies*

Not only is relapse related to the presence of drug-associated cues, but successful abstinence is related to the *absence* of these cues. Evidence in support of the salutatory effect of protection from drug-associated cues is provided by follow-up studies of returning Vietnam veterans who were addicted to heroin while in Vietnam:

> During the summer and fall of 1971, drug use by United States servicemen in Vietnam had, by all estimates, reached epidemic proportions (Robins, 1973, p. 1). The high rates of narcotic use and addiction there were truly unlike anything prior in the American experience (Robins *et al.*, 1975, p. 960).

A study of a sample of enlisted men departing Vietnam in September, 1971 indicated that approximately 20% of them were addicted to heroin while in Vietnam (Robins *et al.*, 1974). Although known heroin users were treated before release, a substantial social problem was anticipated. Since there is a very high relapse rate following all known forms of treatment, it was expected that a new, large population of relapsing heroin addicts would substantially add to the indigenous civilian addict population:

> This will obviously lead to crime and other problems with law enforcement when he (the returning Vietnam heroin user) brings his addiction home. . . . They will be unable to cut off this drug use (Senate Testimony, 1972, p. 481).

Unlike most civilian addicts, following treatment these Vietnam addicts returned to an environment very different than that in which they used drugs. They also evidenced much less relapse than civilian addicts. In one report, United States narcotic use by returned veterans addicted in Vietnam was compared to that seen in addicts of comparable age treated at the large federal facilities in Lexington, Kentucky, and Fort Worth, Texas (Robins *et al.*, 1975). Those addicted in Vietnam (and returned to a very different environment) were much less likely to relapse than those addicted in the environment to which they subsequently returned—indeed, the veterans evidenced "rates of remission unheard of among narcotics addicts treated in the United States" (Robins *et al.*, 1975, p. 958). Many of Robins' conclusions have been substantially confirmed in a more recent follow-up study of a different population of returned soldiers who were addicted in Vietnam (O'Brien *et al.*, 1980).

In addition to the Vietnam veteran findings, other data suggest that alteration in the addict's environment promotes long-lasting abstinence. Ross (1973) studied 109 opiate addicts in Detroit, and noted that physical relocation was significantly associated with abstinence from illicit drugs:

> It appears that for a large group of a treatment population (almost 40%) cessation of illegal drug use meant moving away physically from an area of high drug use (p. 561).

Frykholm (1979) evaluated 58 intravenous drug users in Sweden who had been abstinent for three years or more. Residence relocation was considered a prime factor in achieving this abstinence:

> When asked what they had done to change their lives in order to give up drugs, a majority of the respondents answered that they had felt it necessary to change residence (p. 376).

More recently, Maddux and Desmond (1982) studied patterns of abstinence in heroin addicts in San Antonio. They found that frequency of one-year abstinence was three times higher in relocated respondents than in respondents staying in San Antonio. These and many other reports [see review by Maddux and Desmond, (1982)] all indicate that environmental alteration favors long-term drug abstinence.

8.2.2. *Experimental Studies with Animals*

An early demonstration that environmental cues play an important role in relapse was provided by Thompson and Ostlund (1965). In the first phase of their experiment (addiction phase), rats were orally addicted to morphine by having it as their only available fluid for 60 days. They were then withdrawn from morphine by replacing the opiate solution with water for 30 days. Finally, during the readdiction phase of the experiment, the rats were again permitted to drink the morphine solution. For half the rats, readdiction occurred in the same environment as that used during the addiction phase. For the remaining rats, readdiction took place in a very different environment. During readdiction, rats displayed greater avidity for morphine solution when it was presented in the environment where original addiction had occurred than when readdiction occurred in an alternative environment.

More recently, Hinson *et al.*, (1986) confirmed and extended the results of Thompson and Ostlund (1965). In this Hinson *et al.* (1986) experiment, rats received a series of morphine injections in one environment (the DR, or "distinctive room" environment), and also a series of saline injections in another environment (the HR, or "home room" environment). When subsequently given the opportunity to consume morphine solution in both environments, the rats drank significantly more morphine solution in the morphine-associated DR environment than in the saline-associated HR environment.

9. ROLE OF SELF-ADMINISTRATION

The Pavlovian conditioning analysis emphasizes the contribution of predrug cues to drug tolerance and dependence. In the discussion thus far, these cues have been conceptualized as environmental (i.e., the physical location of drug administration), pharmacological (i.e., one drug signaling another, or the early effect of a drug signaling the later effect), or other detectible stimuli (magnetic fields). Often, of course, drugs are self-administered. It might be expected that interoceptive cues accompanying self-administration (e.g., cognitive–volitional or proprioceptive signals for the systemic effect of the drug) similarly contribute to the effects of repeated pharmacological stimulation.

Self-administration cues have been evaluated in experiments that compare the effects of drugs in animals that self-administer the drug with effects in animals yoked to these self-administering animals. Typically, the self-administering subject is prepared with a chronic jugular cannula, allowing for repeated intraveneous injection. They can inject themselves with an opiate by pressing a lever in an experimental chamber. Yoked animals are similarly cannulated, and placed in a similar chamber, but lever presses have no consequence. Rather, the yoked subject receives the drug at the same time as the self-administering subject. Thus, yoked animals have no control over drug delivery, but rather receive the same doses of the drug, equally often, and at the same intervals as the self-administering animals.

There is evidence that the physiological effects of opiates are different in self-administering and yoked rats (Smith *et al.*, 1982, 1984a, 1984b). It has also recently been demonstrated that the severity of withdrawal symptoms is different in self-administering and yoked rats, despite their identical pharmacological histories (MacRae and Siegel, unpublished data).

In this experiment demonstrating the different effects of self-administered and passively received morphine (MacRae and Siegel, unpublished data), rats participated in squads of three. For each experimental session, members of a simultaneously run trio (each preexperimentally implanted with chronic intraveneous cannulae) were individually confined in one of three identical experimental chambers. Each subject's cannula was attached to an automatic syringe pump. For one member of a trio (assigned to the Self-infused group), each operation of a lever in the chamber operated all three syringe pumps. The pumps delivered 0.69 mg of morphine sulfate to both the Self-infused rat and a rat in another chamber (Yoked-morphine). The third member of the trio (Yoked-ringer's) received an infusion of an equivalent volume of the vehicle, Ringer's solution, whenever the Self-infused and Yoked-morphine rats received morphine infusions. The experiment was conducted in repeated seven-day cycles. For the first six days of each cycle, the drugs were administered in accordance with the above procedure. For the seventh day, no drugs were administered to any subject; rather, their withdrawal behaviour was systematically observed and scored in accordance with standard procedures (Gianutsos *et al.*, 1975).

The various withdrawal behaviours observed in the three groups are depicted in Fig. 5. As can be seen, there was much more pronounced withdrawal distress in Self-infused subjects than in the equally morphine-experienced Yoked-morphine subjects. It would appear that interoceptive signals of a drug, incidental to voluntary self-administration, can importantly influence the magnitude of withdrawal symptoms.

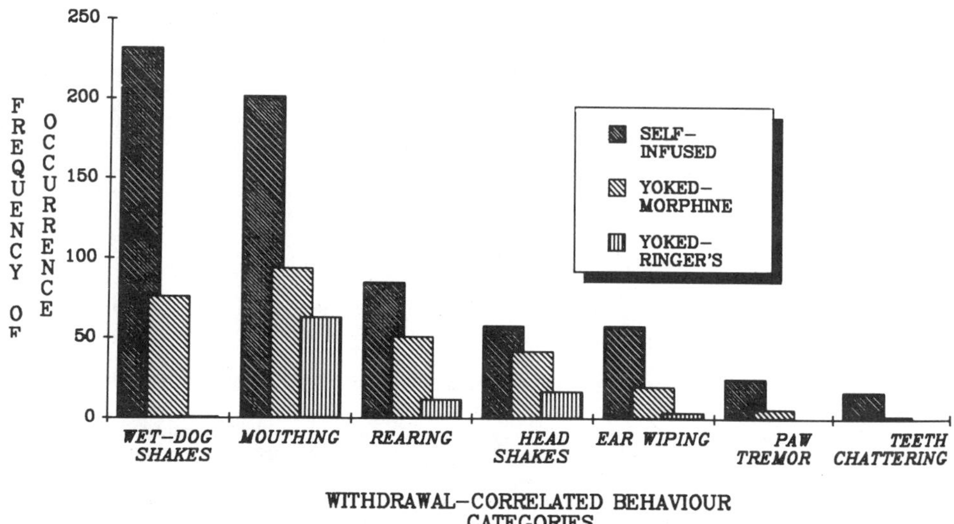

FIG. 5. Withdrawal behaviors in groups of rats that had self-administered morphine (Self-infused), or had been yoked to these self-administrators and passively received either morphine (Yoked-morphine) or Ringer's solution (Yoked-ringers).

10. CONCLUSIONS

It is well established that morphine tolerance is influenced by experience with drug-paired cues, as well as the drug. An interpretation of this influence emphasizes the interaction between learning and pharmacology; the organism learns, via Pavlovian conditioning, an association between predrug cues and the systemic effects of the drug. It has frequently been noted that conditional drug responses (elicited by presenting predrug signals without the drug) are opposite to the drug effect. According to the conditioning analysis, these conditional drug-compensatory responses contribute to tolerance by attenuating the drug effect when the drug is administered following the usual predrug cues. Results of many experiments support the conditioning analysis of tolerance by demonstrating that nonpharmacological manipulations of drug-predictive stimuli affect the acquisition of tolerance in much the same way as they effect the acquisition of Pavlovian conditional responses.

When the usual predrug signals are not followed by the usual pharmacological consequences, drug-compensatory conditional responses may sometimes be manifest as withdrawal symptoms. There is a substantial amount of experimental, clinical, and epidemiological data that attest to the role of such conditional responses in so-called withdrawal symptoms.

The cues that become associated with morphine may be environmental (e.g., the location of drug administration), pharmacological (e.g., the early effect of a drug signaling a later effect) or internal states that accompany volitional self-administration. There is evidence that other subtle cues, such as magnetic fields, can become associated with morphine. Thus, in addition to an understanding of pharmacodynamic and pharmacokinetic principles, a complete account of drug tolerance and withdrawal requires an appreciation of the many potential signals for the systemic effect of a drug.

REFERENCES

ADAMS, W. J., YEH, S. Y., WOODS, L. A. and MITCHELL C. L. (1969) Drug–test interaction as a factor in the development of tolerance to the analgesic effect of morphine. *J. Pharmacol. Exp. Ther.* **168**: 251–257.

ADVOKAT, C. (1980) Evidence for conditioned tolerance of the tail flick reflex. *Behav. Neural Biol.* **29**: 385–389.

BAKER, T. B. and TIFFANY, S. T. (1985) Morphine tolerance as habituation. *Psychol. Rev.* **92**: 78–108.

BIERNACKI, P. (1986) *Pathways from Heroin Addiction: Recovery Without Treatment*. Temple University Press, Philadelphia.

CAPPELL, H., ROACH, C. and POULOS, C. X. (1981) Pavlovian control of cross-tolerance between pentobarbital and ethanol. *Psychopharmacol.* **74**: 54–57.

DAFTERS, R. and BACH, L. (1985) Absence of environment specificity in morphine tolerance acquired in nondistinctive environments: Habituation or stimulus overshadowing? *Psychopharmacol.* **87**: 101–106.

DAFTERS, R., HETHERIGTON, M. and MCCARTNEY, H. (1983) Blocking and sensory preconditioning effects in morphine analgesic tolerance: Support for a Pavlovian conditioning model of drug tolerance. *Quart. J. Exp. Psychol.* **35B**: 1–11.

DOMJAN, M. and GILLAN, D. J. (1977) After-effects of lithium-conditioned stimuli on consummatory behavior. *J. Exp. Psychol: Animal Behav. Proc.* **3**: 322–334.

DYCK, D. G., DRIEDGER, S. M., NEMETH, R., OSACHUK, T. A. G. and GREENBERG, A. H. (1987) Conditioned tolerance to drug-induced (poly I:C) natural killer cell activation: Effects of drug-dosage and context specificity parameters. *Brain, Behavior, and Immunity* **1**: 251–266.

DYCK, D. G., GREENBERG, A. H. and OSACHUK, T. A. G. (1986) Tolerance to drug-induced (poly I:C) natural killer (NK) cell activation: Congruence with a Pavlovian conditioning model. *J. Exp. Psychol.: Animal Behav. Proc.* **12**: 25–31.

EIKELBOOM, R. and STEWART, J. (1982) Conditioning of drug-induced physiological responses. *Psychol. Rev.* **89**: 507–528.

FANSELOW, M.S. and GERMAN, C. (1982) Explicitly unpaired delivery of morphine and the test situation: Extinction and retardation of tolerance to the suppressing effects of morphine on locomotor activity. *Behav. Neural Biol.* **35**: 231–241.

FRYKHOLM, B. (1979) Termination of the drug career: An interview study of 58 ex-addicts. *Acta Psychiat. Scand.* **59**: 370–380.

GIANUTSOS, G., DRAWBAUGH, R., HYNES, M. and LAL, H. (1975) The narcotic withdrawal syndrome in the rat. In: *Methods in Narcotics Research*, pp. 293–309, EHRENPREIS, S. and NEIDLE, A. (eds) Marcel Dekker, New York.

GOLDSTEIN, A. (1976) Opioid peptides (endorphins) in pituitary and brain. *Science* **193**: 1081–1086.

GOUDIE, A. J. and GRIFFITHS, J. W. (1984) Environmental specificity of tolerance. *Tr. NeuroSci.* **7**: 310–311.

GREELEY, J. and CAPPELL, H. (1985) Associative control of tolerance to the sedative and hypothermic effects of chlordiazepoxide. *Psychopharmacol.* **86**: 487–493.

GREELEY, J., LÊ, D. A., POULOS, C. X. and CAPPELL, H. (1984) Alcohol is an effective cue in the conditional control of tolerance to alcohol. *Psychopharmacol.* **83**: 159–162.

GRIFFITHS, J. W. and GOUDIE, A. J. (1986) Analysis of the role of drug-predictive environmental stimuli in tolerance to the hypothermic effects of the benzodiazepine midazolam. *Psychopharmacol.* **90**: 513–521.
HINSON, R. E. and SIEGEL, S. (1982) Nonpharmacological bases of drug tolerance and dependence. *J. Psychosom. Res.* **26**: 495–503.
HINSON, R. E. and SIEGEL, S. (1983) Anticipatory hyperexcitability and tolerance to the narcotizing effect of morphine in the rat. *Behav. Neurosci.* **97**: 759–767.
HINSON, R. E. and SIEGEL, S. (1986) Pavlovian inhibitory conditioning and tolerance to pentobarbital-induced hypothermia in rats. *J. Exp. Psychol.: Animal Behav. Proc.* **12**: 363–370.
HINSON, R. E., POULOS, C. X. and CAPPELL, H. (1982) Effects of pentobarbital and cocaine in rats expecting pentobarbital. *Pharmacol. Biochem. Behav.* **16**: 661–666.
HINSON, R. E., POULOS, C. X., THOMAS, W. and CAPPELL, H. (1986) Pavlovian conditioning and addictive behavior: Relapse to oral self-administration of morphine. *Behav. Neurosci.* **100**: 368–375.
HODGSON, R. J. and RANKIN, H. J. (1976) Modification of excessive drinking by cue exposure. *Behav. Res. Ther.* **14**: 305–307.
HOUK, J. C. (1980) Homeostasis and control principles. In: *Medical Physiology, Volume 1*, pp. 246–267, MOUNTCASTLE, V. (ed) Mosby, St. Louis.
JÄRBE, T. U. C. (1986) State-dependent learning and drug discriminative control of behaviour: An overview. *Acta Neurol. Scand.* **74** (Supplement 109): 37–59.
JØRGENSEN, H. A. and HOLE, K. (1984) Learned tolerance to ethanol in the spinal cord. *Pharmacol. Biochem. Behav.* **20**: 789–792.
KAMIN, L. J. (1969) Predictability, surprise, attention, and conditioning. In: *Punishment and Aversive Behavior*, pp. 279–296, CAMPBELL, B. A. and CHURCH, R. M. (eds) Appleton-Century-Crofts, New York.
KAVALIERS, M. and HIRST, M. (1986) Environmental specificity of tolerance to morphine-induced analgesia in a terrestrial snail: Generalization of the behavioral model of tolerance. *Pharmacol. Biochem. Behav.* **25**: 1201–1206.
KAVALIERS, M. and OSSENKOPP, K.-P. (1985) Tolerance to morphine-induced analgesia in mice: Magnetic fields function as environmental specific cues and reduce tolerance development. *Life Sci.* **37**: 1125–1135.
KESNER, R. P. and COOK, D. G. (1983) Role of habituation and classical conditioning in the development of morphine tolerance. *Behav. Neurosci.* **97**: 4–12.
KING, D. A., BOUTON, M. E. and MUSTY, R. E. (1987) Associative control of tolerance to the sedative effect of a short-acting benzodiazepine. *Behav. Neurosci.* **101**: 104–114.
KING, J. J., SCHIFF, S. R. and BRIDGER, W. H. (1978) Haloperidol classical conditioning—Paradoxical results. *Soc. Neurosci. Abstr.* **4**: 495.
KOROL, B. and MCLAUGHLIN, L. J. (1976) A homeostatic adaptive response to alpha-methyl-dopa in conscious dogs. *Pavlovian J. Biol. Sci.* **11**: 67–75.
KRANK, M. D. (1987) Conditioned hyperalgesia depends on the pain sensitivity measure. *Behav. Neurosci.* **101**: 854–857.
KRANK, M. D. and BENNETT, D. (1987) Conditioned activity and the interaction of amphetamine experience with morphine's activity effects. *Behav. Neural Biol.* **48**: 422–433.
KRANK, M. D., HINSON, R. E. and SIEGEL, S. (1981) Conditional hyperalgesia is elicited by environmental signals of morphine. *Behav. Neural Biol.* **32**: 148–157.
KRANK, M. D., HINSON, R. E. and SIEGEL, S. (1984) The effect of partial reinforcement on tolerance to morphine-induced analgesia and weight loss in the rat. *Behav. Neurosci.* **98**: 79–85.
LÊ, A. D., POULOS, C. X. and CAPPELL, H. (1979) Conditioned tolerance to the hypothermia effect of ethyl alcohol. *Science* **206**: 1109–1110.
LETT, B. T. (1983) Pavlovian drug-sickness pairings result in the conditioning of an antisickness response. *Behav. Neurosci.* **97**: 779–784.
LUDWIG, A. M. and STARK, L. H. (1974) Alcohol craving: Subjective and situational aspects. *Quart. J. Stud. Alc.* **35**: 899–905.
LUDWIG, A. M., CAIN, R. B., WILER, A., TAYLOR, R. M. and BENDFELDT, F. (1977) Physiologic and situational determinants of drinking behavior. In: *Alcohol Intoxication and Withdrawal—IIIb: Studies in Alcohol Dependence,* pp. 589–600, GROSS, M. M. (ed) Plenum Press, New York.
LUDWIG, A. M., WIKLER, A. and STARK, L. H. (1974) The first drink: Psychobiological aspects of craving. *Arch. Gen. Psychiat.* **30**: 539–547.
MACKINTOSH, N. J. (1974) *The Psychology of Animal Learning.* Academic Press, London.
MACKINTOSH, N. J. (1987) Neurobiology, psychology and habituation. *Behav. Res. Ther.* **25**: 81–97.
MACNISH, R. (1859) *The Anatomy of Drunkeness.* W. R. McPuhn, Glascow.
MACRAE, J. R. and SIEGEL, S. (1987) Extinction of tolerance to the analgesic effect of morphine: Intracerebroventricular administration and effects of stress. *Behav. Neurosci.* **101**: 790–796.
MACRAE, J. R. and SIEGEL, S. (unpublished data) Differential effects of morphine in self-administering and yoked-control rats.
MADDUX, J. F. and DESMOND, D. P. (1982) Residence relocation inhibits opioid dependence. *Arch. Gen. Psychiat.* **39**: 1313–1317.
MELCHIOR, C. L. and TABAKOFF, B. (1982) Environment-dependent tolerance to the lethal effects of ethanol. *Alc.: Clin. Exp. Res.* **6**: 306.
MELCHIOR, C. L. and TABAKOFF, B. (1984) A conditioning model of alcohol tolerance. In: *Recent Developments in Alcoholism, Volume 2*, pp. 5–16, GALANTER, M. (ed) Plenum, New York.
MERRY, J. (1966) The "loss of control" myth. *Lancet* **1**: 1257–1258.
MUCHA, R. F., VOLKOVSIKS, C. and KALANT, H. (1981) Conditioned increases in locomotor activity produced with morphine as an unconditioned stimulus, and the relation of conditioning to acute morphine effect and tolerance. *J. Comp. Physiol. Psychol.* **95**: 351–362.
MULINOS, M. G. and LIEB, C. C. (1929) Pharmacology of learning. *Am. J. Physiol.* **90**: 456–457.
NEUMANN, J. K. and ELLIS, A. R. (1986) Some contradictory data concerning a behavioral conceptualization of drug overdose. *Bulletin of the Society of Psychologists in Addictive Behaviors* **5**: 87–90.

OBÁL, F. (1966) The fundamentals of the central nervous control of vegetative homeostatis. *Acta Physiol. Acad. Sci. Hung.* **30**: 15–29.
O'BRIEN, C. P. (1976) Experimental analysis of conditioning factors in human narcotic addiction. *Pharmacol. Rev.* **27**: 533–543.
O'BRIEN, C. P., NACE, E. P., MINTZ, J., MEYERS, A. L. and REAM, N. (1980) Follow-up of Vietnam veterans. 1. Relapse to drug use after Vietnam service. *Drug Alc. Dep.* **5**: 333–340.
O'BRIEN, C. P., TESTA, T., O'BRIEN, T. J. and GREENSTEIN, R. (1976) Conditioning in human opiate addicts. *Pavlovian J. Biol. Sci.* **4**: 195–202.
OVERTON, D. A. (1984) State dependent learning and drug discriminations. In: *Handbook of Psychopharmacology*, Volume 18, pp. 59–127, IVERSEN, L. L., IVERSEN, S. D. and SNYDER, S. H. (eds) Plenum, New York.
PALETTA, M. S. and WAGNER, A. R. (1986) Development of context-specific tolerance to morphine: Support for a dual-process interpretation. *Behav. Neurosci.* **100**: 611–623.
PAVLOV, I. P. (1927) *Conditioned Reflexes* (G. V. ANREP, trans.), Oxford University Press, London.
PIHL, R. O. and ALTMAN, J. (1971) An experimental analysis of the placebo effect. *J. Clin. Pharmacol.* **11**: 91–95.
PONTANI, R. B., VADLAMANI, N. L. and MISRA, A. L. (1985) Potentiation of morphine analgesia by subanecthetic doses of pentobarbital. *Pharmacol. Biochem. Behav.* **22**: 395–398.
POULOS, C. X. and HINSON, R. E. (1982) Pavlovian conditional tolerance to haloperidal catelepsy: Evidence of dynamic adaptations in the dopaminergic system. *Science* **218**: 491–492.
POULOS, C. X. and HINSON, R. E. (1984) A homeostatic model of Pavlovian conditioning: Tolerance to sopoloamine-induced adipisa. *J. Exp. Psychol.: Animal Behav. Proc.* **10**: 75–89.
POULOS, C. X. WILKINSON, D. A. and CAPPELL, H. (1981) Homeostatic regulation and Pavlovian conditioning in tolerance to amphetamine-induced anorexia. *J. Comp. Physiol. Psychol.* **95**: 735–746.
POULOS, C. X., HUNT, T. and CAPPELL, H. (1988) Tolerance to morphine analgesia is reduced by the novel addition or omission of an alcohol cue. *Psychopharmacol.* **94**: 412–416.
RAFFA, R. B. and PORRECA, F. (1986) Evidence for a role of conditioning in the development of tolerance to morphine-induced inhibition of gastrointestinal transit in rats. *Neurosci. Let.* **67**: 229–232.
RAZRAN, G. (1961) The observable unconscious and the inferable conscious in current soviet psychophysiology: Interoceptive conditioning, semantic conditioning and the orienting reflex. *Psychol. Rev.* **68**: 81–147.
RESCORLA, R. A. (1969) Pavlovian conditioned inhibition. *Psychol. Bull.* **72**: 77–94.
ROBINS, L. N. (1973) *The Vietnam Drug User Returns.* (Executive Office of the President, Special Action Office for Drug Abuse Prevention, Special Action Office Monograph, Series A, Number 2). U. S. Government Printing Office, Washington DC.
ROBINS, L. N., DAVIS, D. H. and GOODWIN, D. W. (1974) Drug use by U. S. Army enlisted men in Vietnam: A follow-up on their return home. *Am. J. Epidemiol.* **99**: 235–249.
ROBINS, L. N., HELZER, J. E. and DAVIS, D. H. (1975) Narcotic use in southeast Asia and afterwards. *Arch. Gen. Psychiat.* **32**: 955–961.
ROCHFORD, J. and STEWART, J. (1987) Morphine attenuation of conditioned autoanalgesia: Implications for theories of situation-specific tolerance. *Behav. Neurosci.* **101**: 690–700.
ROSS, S. (1973) A study of living and residence patterns of former heroin addicts as a result of their participation in a methadone treatment program. In: *Proceedings of the Fifth National Conference on Methadone Treatment*, pp. 554–561, National Association for the Prevention of Addiction to Narcotics, New York.
ROSS, R. T. and RANDICH, A. R. (1985) Associative aspects of conditioned analgesia evoked by a discrete CS. *Anim. Learn. Behav.* **13**: 419–431.
ROZIN, P., REFF, D., MARK, M. and SCHULL, J. (1984) Conditioned responses in human tolerance to caffeine. *Bull. Psychon. Soc.* **22**: 117–120.
SCHACHTER, S. (1977) Studies of the interaction of psychological and pharmacological determinants of smoking: 1. Nicotine regulation in heavy and light smokers. *J. Exp. Psychol.: General* **106**: 5–12.
SENATE TESTIMONY (1972) *Hearing Before the Subcommittee to Investigate Juvenile Delinquency of the Committee of the Judiciary United States Senate, Ninety-Second Congress.* Superintendent of Documents, U. S. Government Printing Office, Washington, DC.
SHERMAN, J. E., STRUB, H. and LEWIS, J. W. (1984) Morphine analgesia: Enhancement by shock-associated cues. *Behav. Neurosci.* **98**: 293–309.
SIDEROFF, S. I. and JARVIK, M. E. (1980) Conditioned responses to a video tape showing heroin related stimuli. *Int. J. Addict.* **15**: 529–536.
SIEGEL, S. (1975) Evidence from rats that morphine tolerance is a learned response. *J. Comp. Physiol. Psychol.* **89**: 498–506.
SIEGEL, S. (1976) Morphine analgesic tolerance: Its situation specificity supports a Pavlovian conditioning model. *Science* **193**: 323–325.
SIEGEL, S. (1977) Morphine tolerance acquisition as an associative process. *J. Exp. Psychol.: Animal Behav. Proc.* **3**: 1–13.
SIEGEL, S. (1978) Tolerance to the hyperthermic effect of morphine in the rat is a learned response. *J. Comp. Physiol. Psychol.* **92**: 1137–1149.
SIEGEL, S. (1982) Pharmacological habituation and learning. In: *Quantitative Analyses of Behavior: Volume III (Acquisition)*, pp. 195–217, COMMONS, M. L., HERRNSTEIN, R. and WAGNER, A. R. (eds) Ballinger, Cambridge.
SIEGEL, S. (1983) Classical conditioning, drug tolerance, and drug dependence. In: *Research Advances in Alcohol and Drug Problems, Volume 7*, pp. 207–246, ISRAEL, Y., GLASER, F. B., KALANT, H., POPHAM, R. E., SCHMIDT, W. and SMART, R. G. (eds) Plenum, New York.
SIEGEL, S. (1984) Pavlovian conditioning and heroin overdose: Reports by overdose victims. *Bull. Psychon. Soc.* **22**: 428–430.
SIEGEL, S. (1985) Drug anticipatory responses in animals. In: *Placebo: Theory, Research, and Mechanisms*, pp. 288–305, WHITE, L., TURSKY, B. and SCHWARTZ, G. (eds) Guilford Press, New York.
SIEGEL, S. (1987) Pavlovian conditioning and ethanol tolerance. In: *Advances in Biomedical Alcohol Research*, pp. 25–36, LINDROS, K. O., YLIKAHRI, R. and KIIANMAA, K. (eds) Pergamon Press, Oxford (Published as Supplement No. 1, *Alcohol and Alcoholism*, 1987).

SIEGEL, S. (1988) State-dependent learning of morphine tolerance. *Behav. Neurosci.* **102**: 228–232.
SIEGEL, S. (1989) Pharmacological conditioning and drug effects. In: *Psychoactive Drugs: Tolerance and Sensitization*, p. 115–180, GOUDIE, A. J. and EMMETT-OGLESBY M. W. (eds), Humana Press, Clifton, NJ.
SIEGEL, S. and ELLSWORTH, D. (1986) Pavlovian conditioning and death from apparent overdose of medically prescribed morphine: A case report. *Bull. Psychon. Soc.* **24**: 278–280.
SIEGEL, S. AND MACRAE, J. (1984) Environmental specificity of tolerance. *Tr. NeuroSci.* **7**: 140–142.
SIEGEL, S. and SDAO-JARVIE, K. (1986) Reversal of ethanol tolerance by a novel stimulus. *Psychopharmacol.* **88**: 258–261.
SIEGEL, S., HINSON, R. E. and KRANK, M. D. (1978) The role of predrug signals in morphine analgesic tolerance: Support for a Pavlovian conditioning model of tolerance. *J. Exp. Psychol.: Animal Behav. Proc.* **4**: 188–196.
SIEGEL, S., HINSON, R. E. and KRANK, M. D. (1979) Modulation of tolerance to the lethal effect of morphine by extinction. *Behav. Neural Biol.* **25**: 257–262.
SIEGEL, S., HINSON, R. E. and KRANK, M. D. (1981) Morphine-induced attenuation of morphine tolerance. *Science* **212**: 1533–1534.
SIEGEL, S., HINSON, R. E. and KRANK, M. D. (1987) Anticipation of pharmacological and nonpharmacological events: Classical conditioning and addictive behavior. *J. Drug Issues* **17**: 83–110.
SIEGEL, S., HINSON, R. E., KRANK, M. D. and MCCULLY, J. (1982) Heroin "overdose" death: The contribution of drug-associated environmental cues. *Science* **216**: 436–437.
SIEGEL, S., SHERMAN, J. E. and MITCHELL, D. (1980) Extinction of morphine analgesic tolerance. *Learn. Motiv.*, **11**: 289–301.
SMITH, J. E., CO, C., FREEMAN, M. E. and LANE, J. D. (1982) Brain neurotransmitter turnover correlated with morphine-seeking behavior of rats. *Pharmacol. Biochem. Behav.* **16**: 509–519.
SMITH, J. E., CO, C. and LANE, J. D. (1984a) Limbic acetylcholine turnover rates correlated with rat morphine-seeking behaviors. *Pharmacol. Biochem. Behav.* **20**: 429–442.
SMITH, J. E., CO, C. and Lane, J. D. (1984b) Limbic muscarinic cholinergic and bezodiazepine receptor changes with chronic morphine self-administration. *Pharmacol. Biochem. Behav.* **20**: 443–450.
STEWART, J. and EIKELBOOM, R. (1987) Conditioned drug effects. In: *Handbook of Psychopharmacology, Volume 19*, pp. 1–57, IVERSEN, L. L., IVERSEN, S. D. and SNYDER, S. H. (eds) Plenum, New York.
SUBKOV, A. A. and ZILOV, G. N. (1937) The role of conditioned reflex adaptation in the origin of hyperergic reactions. *Bulletin de Biologie et de Médecine Experimentale* **4**: 294–296.
TAUKULIS, H. K. (1982) Attenuation of lithium-elicited hypothermia in rats with a history of pentobarbital-LiCl pairings. *Pharmacol. Biochem. Behav.* **17**: 695–697.
TAUKULIS, H. K. (1986a) Conditional hyperthermia in response to atropine associated with a hypothermic drug. *Psychopharmacol.* **90**: 327–331.
TAUKULIS, H. K. (1986b) Conditional shifts in thermic responses to sequentially paired drugs and the "conditional hyperactivity" hypothesis. *Pharmacol. Biochem. Behav.* **25**: 83–87.
TEASDALE, J. D. (1973) Conditioned abstinence in narcotic addicts. *Int. J. Addict.* **8**: 273–292.
TERMAN, G. W., LEWIS, J. W. and LIEBSKIND, J. C. (1983) Sodium pentobarbital blocks morphine tolerance and potentiation in the rat. *Physiologist* **26**: A-111.
TERMAN, G. W., PECHNICK, R. N. and LIEBSKIND, J. C. (1985) Blockade of tolerance to morphine analgesia by pentobarbital. *Proc. West. Pharmacol. Soc.* **28**: 157–160.
TERNES, J. W. (1977) An opponent process theory of habitual behavior with special reference to smoking. In: *Research on Smoking Behavior* (National Institute on Drug Abuse Research Monograph 17), pp. 157–182, JARVIK, M. E., CULLEN, J. W., GRITZ, E. R., VOGT, T. M. and WEST, L. J. (eds) Superintendent of Documents, U.S. Government Printing Office, Washington, DC.
THOMPSON, T. and OSTLUND, W. JR. (1965) Susceptibility to readdiction as a function of the addiction and withdrawal environments. *J. Comp. Physiol. Psychol.* **60**: 388–392.
TIFFANY, S. T. and BAKER, T. B. (1981) Morphine tolerance in the rat: Congruence with a Pavlovian paradigm. *J. Comp. Physiol. Psychol.* **95**: 747–762.
TOATES, F. M. (1979) Homeostasis and drinking. *Behav. Brain Sci.* **2**: 95–139.
VILA, C. J. (1989) Death by pentobarbital overdose mediated by Pavlovian conditioning. *Pharmacol. Biochem. Behav.* **32**: 365–366.
WAGNER, A. R. (1976) Priming in STM: An information processing mechanism for self-generated or retrieval-generated depression in performance. In: *Habituation: Perspectives for Child Development, Animal Behavior, and Neurophysiology*, pp. 95–128, TIGHE, T. J. and LEATON, R. N. (eds) Erlbaum, Hillsdale, NJ.
WAGNER, A. R. (1978) Expectancies and the priming of STM. In: *Cognitive Processes in Animal Behavior*, pp. 179–209, HULSE, S. H., FOWLER, H., and HONIG, W. K. (eds) Hillsdale, NJ: Lawrence Erlbaum.
WALTER, T. A. and Riccio, D. C. (1983) Overshadowing effects in the stimulus control of morphine analgesic tolerance. *Behav. Neurosci.* **97**: 658–662.
WIKLER, A. (1973) Conditioning of successive adaptive responses to the initial effects of drugs. *Condit. Reflex* **8**: 193–210.
WIKLER, A. (1977) The search for the psyche in drug dependence: A 35-year retrospective survey. *J. Nerv. Mental Dis.* **165**: 29–40.

CHAPTER 4

TREATMENT PERSPECTIVES IN DRUG MISUSE: THE OPIATE PARADIGM

B. B. JOHNSTON

Drug Dependence Service, Tayside Health Board and Department of Psychiatry, University Medical School, Dundee, Scotland

1. INTRODUCTION

Man has been using psychoactive or psychotropic substances since time immemorial. It would appear that there is an almost innate need for some sort of anodyne to assuage the hardship of life, to dull the hardness of unpleasant reality, to soothe "The heartache and the thousand natural shocks that flesh is heir to . . ." *Hamlet*, Act III, scene 1.

In a historical context, alcohol is thought to have been first used by man in prehistoric times (Hofmann, 1983). It would seem that serendipity was at work with mild alcoholic beverages resulting from the accidental fermentation of grain or fruit. Stronger drinks (spirits) were available only after the discovery of the distillation process more than 1100 years ago around A.D. 800. The hypnotic properties of the opium poppy were known to the Sumerians 6000 years ago while Greek and Roman writers and physicians such as Homer, Aristotle and Galen were aware of opium as a thymoleptic and its use in the form of a medicinal wine (Stimson and Oppenheimer, 1982). In the Incan civilization dignitaries indulged themselves by chewing coca leaves, but with the advent of the Spanish Conquistadors the habit became widespread in the population, encouraged by the latter as a political move to quell discontent (Hofmann, 1983).

Later came tobacco and caffeine (tea and coffee) and as the use of these substances became widespread and popular throughout Europe, voices were also raised in condemnation of devotees. Attitudes to the use or misuse of psychoactive substances vary within a society or culture and also change over time. In the mid-nineteenth century the discovery of the anesthetic properties of nitrous oxide (laughing gas), ether and chloroform were hailed as major advances in the control of pain and allowed surgery on a scale that could never before have been contemplated. Yet Horace Wells, who first noticed the anesthetic effects of nitrous oxide on a participant who injured himself at a public spectacle and exhibition of laughing gas, became perhaps one of the first victims of the chronic effects of solvent inhalation. His constant use of chloroform and absinthe affected his personality and behaviour to the extent that he committed suicide in prison. Ether parties were apparently popular in certain Middle European countries after the First World War—glue-sniffing is not such a modern addiction! Although there were vogues for both opium and cocaine, which caused serious problems in the late nineteenth century through into the early twentieth century in both Britain and the United States, this review will concern itself primarily with treatment approaches to opiate abuse problems over the last 25 years or so, drawing mainly on the British experience.

Published statistics on the misuse of drugs in the United Kingdom by the Home Office in London indicate that in 1985 there were 30,500 seizures of controlled drugs, a 6.6% increase on the 1984 figure of 28,600 and almost three times that of 1975. Three thousand two hundred of the seizures were of heroin (200 more than 1984) totalling 365 kg. Although seizures of cocaine (another class A drug like the opiates) fell somewhat during 1985, the total amount of the drug found increased by 20 kg to 85 kg. The number of seizures of class B drugs (including cannabis and amphetamines) was 26,900 showing an increase of 7% on 1984, the tenth successive year of an upward trend. The biggest increase here was in the seizure of amphetamines. Also in 1985, a record number of 26,000 people were found guilty of, or cautioned for, controlled drug offences, an increase of 6% over the previous year. Of these, 5800 received a custodial sentence, an increase of 21%.

What are the reasons behind this comparatively worldwide proliferation of illicit drugs? What are the forces creating the market for them? Why do people use them? What can be done about it? It is surely no accident that countries cultivating and producing heroin, cocaine and cannabis are underdeveloped or in political turmoil or revolution, as well as having the appropriate terrain and climate. Local, if not national economies, depend on the cultivation and export of a particular crop and heroin, for example, is regarded as "our mineral wealth" in the Northwest Frontier Province (Lewis, 1985). Elaborate networks of distribution for heroin and cocaine have evolved to supply Western Europe and the United States, and the enormous profits to be made have attracted organized crime (Adler, 1985; Freemantle, 1985). Even so, at street level heroin is relatively cheap, comparing favorably with alcohol, and usually readily available. It may be significant that all of this has occurred during a period of worldwide economic recession and high levels of unemployment. Tackling these international social and political aspects of the drug abuse problem is important but clearly beyond the scope of this review. The answers to the last two of the above questions are not. However, it seems logical firstly to discuss some of the many general theories of causation, since there are no specific etiologies with related pathognomonic clinical presentations and radically different treatments which might distinguish dependency on one psychoactive substance from another. In other words, it is difficult to employ the systematic approach taken in medicine where an illness has a particular etiology, clinical course, pharmacological or surgical treatment, with a fairly predictable outcome and the patient cast in a largely passive role.

2. ETIOLOGICAL FACTORS: IMPLICATIONS FOR TREATMENT, PREVENTION AND CONTROL

In recent years there has been a tendency to refrain from the use of all-embracing and somewhat pejorative terms such as alcoholism and alcoholic, because they are 'all or nothing' phenomena and imply that an affected individual has a 'disease' or illness. The concept of alcohol dependence is preferred and there is a notion that someone who is dependent on alcohol or who drinks excessively, experiences problems (whether physical, psychological, social or legal) related to his or her drinking. Similarly there has been a trend among those dealing with drug misuse problems to shy away from nomenclature such as 'drug addiction' and 'addict'. These terms reflect a preoccupation with the physiological aspects of addiction, the physical symptoms of withdrawal, and the pharmacological properties of the substance involved. The WHO (1969) definition of drug dependence is as follows "A state, psychic, and sometimes also physical, resulting from the interaction between a living organism and a drug, characterised by behavioural and other responses that always includes a compulsion to take the drug on a continuous or periodic basis in order to experience its psychic effects, sometimes to avoid the discomfort of abstinence." Here psychological as well as physical manifestations of dependence are stressed with special emphasis given to obsessive-compulsive and behavioural aspects. The shift to a problem-oriented approach is embodied in the Advisory Council on the Misuse of Drugs (1982) definition of the problem drug taker as "someone who experiences social, psychological, physical or legal problems related to intoxication and/or regular excessive consumption and/or dependence as a consequence of his own use of drugs or other chemical substances (excluding alcohol or tobacco)."

This philosophy eschews what is seen as the narrow, traditional, substance-based approach to addiction espousing, instead, a more diversified *modus operandi* to confront the wide range of problems presented by drug misusers. Preoccupation with the pharmacological properties of the drug, the development of tolerance, physical dependence and withdrawal together with lurid media portrayals has led to the popular conception of a 'junkie' stereotype. In fact, there is a spectrum of drug-taking behaviour ranging from initial use on an experimental basis through recreational, regular to heavy compulsive-dependent use. Whether an individual does or does not progress through these phases depends on a variety of factors, including his expectations of the drug and the pattern of use, which may be much more important than its pharmacological characteristics (Strang, 1985). There is not necessarily a causal link between any of these phases.

2.1. Models of Use and Misuse

Drugs may be used by an individual in a number of ways and for one or more of the following reasons, e.g. to change perception of self or the environment, to create new, exciting or pleasurable experiences (hedonism), to generate confidence, enhanced performance and a sense of accomplishment in work, social or sexual spheres or simply to alter mood. The pattern of drug use is governed by a number of exogenous and endogenous factors. Depending on the emotional needs and expectations of an individual and the anticipated effects of the substance, the nature of the drug experience can be intensely subjective (Hofmann, 1983). In addition to inter-personal variation in the drug experience, there may be intra-personal variation in that the same substance produces different effects at different times (e.g. LSD may result in good or bad trips in the same individual on different occasions). Other important factors bearing on the pattern of use are the peer group, which substances have a current vogue or are being used by celebrity or superstar, the availability of these substances, and their price and quality. Peer group pressure, price and availability are probably particularly relevant to initial or experimental use.

All of the above elements can be integrated in the 'epidemiological triangle' (see Fig. 1) which attempts to give a balanced view of their inter-relationship (de Haes, 1986). Behavior related to drug-taking is the result of the interaction between drug, personality and environment (Edwards, 1974). In explaining illicit drug use and in proposing a basis for controlled intoxicant use Zinberg (1984) uses a similar model embodying the relationship of drug, set and setting. Drug in this context is defined as the pharmacological action of the substance, set as the attitude of the person at the time of use, including personality structure, and setting, as the influence of the physical and social environment within which use occurs.

2.2. The Moral Model

Other models are, or have been, used to conceptualize drug addiction or misuse, and have at different times attained pre-eminence in determining society's attitude and response to treatment and prevention. The earliest of these was the Moral Model which held sway throughout most of the nineteenth century and first two decades of the twentieth and is to date by no means effete. Addiction, according to this theorem is a vice, a deviant form of self-indulgence deserving public censure and the full rigor of the law. Drug misuse is, therefore, seen as a criminal act and activities such as possession, use and supply of proscribed substances attracts prosecution and protracted custodial sentences on conviction. In the United States such moral principles were enthusiastically embraced by the legislators in relation to alcohol use and led to the disastrous social consequences of the prohibition era during the twenties when organized crime created a lucrative black-market. During World War I in the United Kingdom, there was a distinct emphasis on the moral model and drug use and addiction were viewed as social problems which might seriously

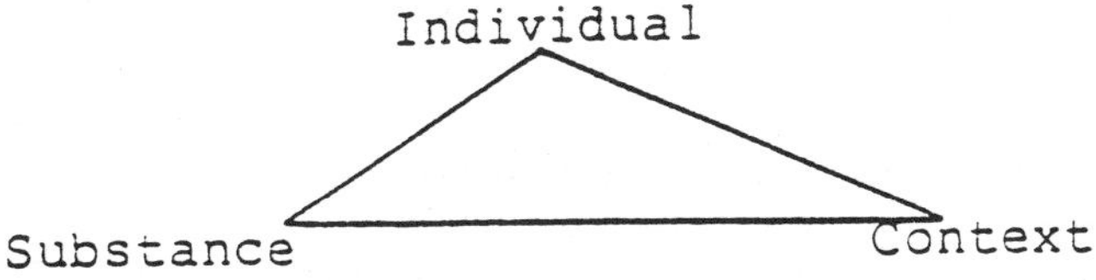

Fig. 1. Epidemiological triangle.

undermine the war effort and must therefore be prohibited. This resulted in the Defence of the Realm Act, 1917 in which controls on alcohol, opiates, cocaine and other psychoactive substances were introduced.

2.3. THE MEDICAL MODEL

Another paradigm used to view addiction is the Medical or Disease Model in which conditions such as alcohol or drug addiction are construed as illnesses or diseases in the face of which the individual becomes a helpless victim. This concept is central to the philosophy of bodies such as Alcoholics Anonymous, but has the singular disadvantage of allowing a dependent individual to retreat into illness, thus abdicating all responsibility for his current situation and condition, and to place the burden of redress on the therapist. The disease model is explained by the physiological and psychological mechanisms through which physical tolerance and psychological craving develop, often seen as withdrawal phenomena and uncontrolled use; while relapse, after a period of abstinence, is interpreted as a symptom of the re-emerging disease (Cummings *et al.*, 1980).

With the realization that earlier prohibitive legislation was in many ways an unsatisfactory response to drug misuse, there was a general feeling in government circles in the U.K. in the early twenties that a more humane approach should be taken but not without first consulting medical opinion. Consequently, the report of a committee on Morphine and Heroine Addiction under the Chairmanship of Sir Humphrey Rolleston, President of the Royal College of Physicians (The Rolleston Report) appeared in 1926. Among the main conclusions reached were that addiction was to be regarded as an illness, institutional treatment was favored for withdrawal from drugs and patients were to undergo gradual withdrawal since otherwise serious symptoms would result. Where withdrawal failed then the patient had to be maintained on a determined minimum dose, which was considered necessary to allow a relatively normal and useful life to be led. This report was the enshrinement of the Medical or Disease Model of Addiction and the foundation of the 'British System' which although modified was later reaffirmed in the second Brain Committee Report (1965), a government response to the alarming increase in the numbers of young people misusing drugs, especially heroin, known to the Home Office (Stimson and Oppenheimer, 1982; Yates, 1981). Because over-prescribing by a small number of doctors, mainly in the London area, was a significant factor in the rise in the number of addicts, one of the main recommendations of the second Brain Committee was the restriction of prescribing heroin and cocaine to doctors specially licensed by the Home Secretary. Heroin addicts were to be notified to the Chief Medical Officer at the Home Office and special treatment centres or clinics in National Health Service hospitals under Consultant Psychiatrists were to be established. Maintenance therapy was still regarded as an advantage by introducing an element of stability into the addict's life and hopefully would undercut the expansion of the illicit market.

2.4. THE SOCIAL LEARNING MODEL

In more recent years a Social Learning Model (Bandura, 1969) has been used to explain the etiology of addiction and relapse. Theoretical considerations are quite complex and in some areas still controversial (Cummings *et al.*, 1980) but both classical (Pavlovian) and instrumental (operant) learning or conditioning are applied to the development and maintenance of addictive behavior. Very simply drug-taking behavior can result from and be maintained by the association with tension-reducing and pleasurable experiences (operant learning). Eventually, with the development of tolerance and withdrawal phenomena, the latter, according to classical conditioning theory, become the conditioned stimuli evoking the conditioned response of craving, leading to drug-taking behavior. Drug addiction is, therefore, viewed as a learned behavioral response which, by suitable retraining and appropriate reinforcement, can be unlearned or modified. Consequently, a variety of behavioral therapies has been developed including aversion therapy (chemical, electrical, covert), desensitization, skills training and contingency management (Childress *et al.*, 1985). A behavioral approach known as the cue exposure response prevention method for treating compulsive disorders has been applied to alcohol abuse (Blakey and Baker, 1980; Rankin *et al.*, 1983) and other addictive problems including drug abuse. If, e.g. drinking or drug taking is the unconditioned stimulus and the resultant physiological changes, the unconditioned response, then in classical conditioning terms (which is only one explanation of the behavioral mechanisms involved), the sight and smell and other aspects of alcohol or drug use would be the conditioned stimuli. The conditioned response, e.g. the desire to drink, can then be extinguished by appropriate intervention and control techniques. From the principles of social learning, behavior modification and cognitive psychology there has evolved the concept of 'addictive behaviors,' which includes drug taking, problem drinking, smoking, obesity, gambling and compulsive sexual activity. It should be noted that there is no substance involved in the two latter. Orford (1985) has applied the concept of 'excessive appetites' to addictive behavior, recognizing the importance of personality and a range of environmental and social factors in the development and strengthening of a particular habit. Research into the common features of these addictive behaviors has indicated that initiation of behavior change (e.g. abstinence) is much easier than maintenance of that desired behavior over a period of time. This has led to the development of a behavior maintenance approach to relapse in the treatment of addictive behaviors (Marlatt and Gordon, 1980; Marlatt and George, 1984). In Marlatt's Relapse Prevention Model individuals are offered specific intervention strategies to help them cope more effectively with specifically defined high-risk situations, in addition to which global self-control strategies can be used where more general change in lifestyle seems appropriate.

2.5. Biological Factors: The Endogenous Opiates

Having highlighted the limitations of the disease or medical model used earlier to conceptualize addiction, research over the past 10–15 years has led to the discovery of endogenous opiate receptors (Kuhar *et al.*, 1973) and corresponding opiate-like substances within the CNS (Hughes, 1975; Terenius and Wahlstrom, 1975; Pasternak *et al.*, 1975) and compelled a reappraisal of the etiological significance of constitutional factors in addiction.

The first two endogenous opiates discovered were two short-chain pentapeptides (five amino acid chain) named leucine-enkephalin and methionine-enkephalin, since these peptides differed only at the fifth amino acid position of the chain. Further research has revealed much longer peptides, e.g. beta-endorphin, a 31 amino acid peptide, the first five amino acids of which are identical to methionine-enkephalin. There are now thought to be three major classes of endogenous opiate peptides, viz. the enkephalins, beta-endorphins and dynorphins (Bloom, 1983). Various studies have suggested that these endogenous ligands have effects similar to those of exogenous morphine at opiate receptors and may function as neurotransmitters which can control other neurotransmitter systems within the CNS, and by a process of inhibition, produce analgesia. This has led a number of workers, e.g. Kosterlitz and Hughes (Hughes, 1975) to explain narcotic addiction in terms of the interaction between endogenous and exogenous opiates. As a result of prolonged administration of an exogenous opiate (e.g. heroin) tolerance develops and the endogenous opiate system is suppressed, as in a biological feedback mechanism. Sudden cessation of administered heroin results in withdrawal symptoms because of overactivity in excitatory systems in the absence of the inhibitory influence of the endogenous opiates. Dynorphin, one of the groups of endogenous peptides mentioned above, has been shown to suppress heroin withdrawal symptoms (Wen and Ho, 1982).

In a more general context there are broad sociocultural and economic factors which seem important in the genesis of health and social problems including drug misuse. These factors include poverty, unemployment, educational disadvantage, inadequate housing and membership of a minority group (Advisory Council on Misuse of Drugs, 1984). In addition poorly developed leisure, sports and entertainment facilities result in young people from such deprived backgrounds adopting their own lifestyle, the ethos of which is derived from the drug subculture. Such a response has been described as 'anomie' or 'alienation' on the basis of sociological theory (Plant, 1980). This, of course, implies that society should change in the direction of redressing these imbalances, to eliminate these apparently inherent inequalities which place certain groups within it at serious disadvantage. (For more extensive and detailed review of the literature on etiology see Fazey, 1977 and Plant, 1981).

3. HISTORICAL ASPECTS OF OPIATE ABUSE AND THE DEVELOPMENT OF TREATMENT APPROACHES

British merchants and in particular the British East India Company were among the first to exploit opium commercially in the latter part of the eighteenth century by trading it illicitly for Chinese tea and silk. The deleterious effects on the Chinese economy and the general health of the population on the one hand and the British determination to continue the trade and safeguard their financial investments on the other eventually led to the First Opium War (1839–1842). Opium use was widespread in Britain during the nineteenth century and the drug was taken in a variety of patent medicines and other products freely available across the counter. Medicinally, it was a panacea, recreationally, it rivalled alcohol; in fact, at one time it was said to be cheaper than gin or beer (Stimson and Oppenheimer, 1982).

This easy availability of opiates was gradually curbed by a series of legislative enactments culminating in the Dangerous Drugs Act of 1920 and 1923, which restricted importation under penalty, and introduced regulations governing the manufacture, sale, distribution and possession of these drugs. There then followed the previously mentioned Rolleston Report of 1926 in which opiate addiction was regarded as an illness, but was comparatively rare and confined to professional groups having access to drugs. There was an awareness during the fifties of a significant increase in the recreational use of amphetamines and barbiturates, but it was the sudden upsurge in the numbers of young heroin addicts, mainly in the London area, in the early sixties which resulted in the Brain Committee (1965) making specific recommendations leading to the establishment of the special treatment centres or clinics mentioned earlier, the Dangerous Drugs Act (1967) and its associated Regulations (1968). Addicts, who were previously prescribed heroin and cocaine by general or private practitioners, must per force attend the new clinics where prescription of these drugs was strictly limited to specially licenced doctors. Thus the primary function of the clinics was to deal with individuals who were addicted to heroin and cocaine, and although there were a few exceptions, the majority of centres did not attempt to treat barbiturate or amphetamine addiction (Edwards, 1979).

Implicit in the philosophy of the clinics and embodied in the attendant legislation were certain preventive and treatment strategies, the conceptualization of which has been described in detail and critically reviewed by Edwards (1979, 1981). These included *inter alia* concepts such as competitive prescribing, control of the prescriber, drugs as the lure to treatment and maintenance treatment. The intention behind competitive prescribing was to undercut the black market but this stratagem in turn was undermined by an increase in illicitly imported heroin. By restricting the prescription of heroin and cocaine to specially licenced doctors, the identification of maverick practitioners who persisted in prescribing irresponsibly was made easier for the officers of the Home Office Drugs Inspectorate. The rationale behind the notion of drugs as the lure to treatment was that the offer of free opiates would prove irresistible to addicts, who would thus be tempted into a therapeutic situation in which, over time and in an almost imperceptibly subtle way, the associated emotional, social and legal problems could be broached.

The original intention of the clinics was to prescribe an opiate on a maintenance basis for a varying period of time to introduce a degree of stability into an individual's life before effecting a gradual withdrawal of the drug, so that ultimately a drug-free state would be achieved in the majority of attenders. It was recognized that there was likely to be a small percentage of addicts, usually older and with a long history of drug use, who would require long term maintenance on a non-progressive dosage regime, otherwise they would be unable to lead a relatively normal or useful life.

In practice there was considerable variation in prescribing habits around the country ranging from injectable forms of heroin and methadone to tablet forms and occasionally combinations of the two drugs taken orally. Some clinics provided 'fixing' rooms, sterile needles and syringes, swabs and distilled water to reduce the risk of infection (Stimson and Oppenheimer, 1982). Addicts were attracted in numbers but were often merely looking for a source of supply and many very quickly ceased attending when an opiate prescription was not immediately forthcoming. Therapeutic gains were limited and apparently the formula did not work well at a practical level. It was extremely difficult to facilitate withdrawal from opiates and the clinics were increasingly forced into long-term maintenance prescribing. This did not undercut the illicit market which, ironically, was sustained to a large extent by the quantities of drugs legitimately supplied to the clinic attenders. Staff came to view themselves as having a greatly diminished therapeutic role mainly because it became clear that the clinics could not fulfil the dual responsibilities of treatment and control expected of them. The problem of control of addiction now tended to be viewed, not as a medical matter, but the responsibility of government requiring appropriate legislative and enforcement measures. Results of a study comparing the effects of prescribing injectable heroin against oral methadone (Mitcheson and Hartnoll, 1978; Hartnoll *et al.*, 1980) were widely interpreted as showing the latter to be more therapeutic than the former, which was said to maintain the *status quo*, i.e. individuals maintained on heroin were less likely to change in terms of their opiate use. Although there was evidence that many of the clinics were already changing their prescribing policies before the appearance of these results (Ghodse, 1983), they did provide added impetus so that in time the majority of clinics changed to prescribing methadone in tablet or linctus form because it was believed that there was a greater likelihood of achieving abstinence and a decreased risk of infection and overdose. In terms of control it was felt that there was less likelihood of methadone, especially in linctus form, being used as currency within the drug subculture.

3.1. Methadone and Methadone Maintenance

Methadone is an opiate first synthesized in Germany towards the end of World War II as an analgesic substitute for morphine and heroin, the formula being seized by the United States following the cessation of hostilities (Peck and Beckett, 1976). It differs from heroin and morphine by possessing a longer duration of action and is much more effective than the other two drugs when taken orally, having an effect approximately equivalent to 45% of an intramuscular dose. It has been suggested that these differences combined with the phenomena of cross tolerance and physical dependence render methadone an extremely useful drug in short term detoxification (i.e. supervised withdrawal from heroin) and long-term maintenance (Hofmann, 1983; Blum, 1984a). However, being an opiate, it has significant inherent abuse potential and does present problems in its own right. For more detailed information on the pharmacology and clinical applications of methadone, particularly in the United States context, the reader should consult Blum (1984b) and Senay (1985).

Methadone maintenance as a successful treatment for heroin addiction was postulated by Dole and Nyswander (1965, 1968) and quickly attracted enthusiastic acclaim by many workers in the field of opiate addiction on both sides of the Atlantic, but particularly so in the United States. According to Dole and Nyswander (1967) there is a metabolic defect in susceptible individuals resulting in a biologically altered response to opiates. Narcotic addiction, on this model, is seen as a metabolic disorder which requires to be treated by methadone in a way analogous to the treatment of diabetes by parenteral insulin or other oral hypoglycaemic drugs. Methadone, in carefully titrated single doses, sometimes to a level of 80–120 mg per day, is thought to 'blockade' the abnormal response to heroin, prevent euphoria without inducing dysphoria, and eliminate withdrawal as a stimulus for drug-seeking behavior. It has been claimed that other attributes rendering the drug relatively safe and of value in the maintenance treatment setting are its low toxicity, few side effects (especially dysphoria) and long duration of action when taken orally.

In their review of methadone maintenance Peck and Beckett (1976) extol the virtues of the treatment in quotations from various sources, e.g.:

"The Dole-Nyswander hypothesis is that medical administration of methadone in quantities that can produce a high tolerance, in combination with other rehabilitative techniques, will lead to an end of abuse of illicit narcotic opiates . . ." (Dole and Nyswander, 1966).

"Patients on methadone feel no craving, are almost never subjected to withdrawal symptoms, are sensitive to pain, respond 'normally' to analgesics, eat, sleep and work normally, have normal reaction times, are alert and have normal sex lives," (Du Pont and Katon, 1971a).

"Mental and neuromuscular functions appear unaffected, and one cannot tell a methadone maintained person from someone not on methadone, except by urine analysis," (Reinert, 1965).

Other advantages of the treatment are that the act of taking drugs is decriminalized for the individual in a program. There is increased independence and self support, a decreased risk of infection, and a strong element of control over drug taking is introduced. Another goal of methadone maintenance therapy is to introduce the addict into a therapeutic relationship (Senay, 1985) with both counsellor and program, thereby facilitating provision of medical, psychological, social and legal support.

In the United States methadone, as used in maintenance therapy, is regarded as an experimental or investigative drug and its use in a treatment program must be licenced under Federal Law. In addition there are various criteria which must be met before entry into a typical program can be secured, e.g. the individual must be a volunteer, at least 18 years of age, have no major medical contra-indications, with 2 years or more history of heroin abuse, and have experienced several relapses after withdrawal and rehabilitation. In contrast to the British clinics which became involved in methadone prescribing on a maintenance basis in an almost arbitrary and unsystematic way, the American facilities provided very structured programs with considerable inherent control enabling greater organization of the individual attender's daily life. Nevertheless, in a survey of treatment available at London clinics 15 years on Ghodse (1983) noted that most were more actively engaged in offering some form of "treatment contract package" along the lines of contingency management procedures. Continuing methadone prescription would be contingent on abandoning illicit drug use, attending weekly, cooperating with other treatment approaches, and finding employment.

Dole *et al.* (1969) and Dole (1971) claimed that 80% remained in the program at least 2 years, 90% of those involved in criminal activity ceased while 75% of those retained in the program returned to productive lives. Senay (1985), in a review of methadone use, points out that success rates as highly favorable as those initially reported by Dole and Nyswander have not subsequently been maintained but goes on to describe several United States evaluation studies which have since produced very encouraging results. For example, the Drug Abuse Reporting Project (1979) is cited as having findings of more than 50% of clients retained in treatment for 1 year or more, rates of illicit opiate use and criminality decreased sharply, and employment rates increased from 39% pre-treatment to 62% in the year after leaving treatment.

In contra-distinction to the favorable results reported above, Gossop (1978) is severely critical of methadone maintenance as a treatment for narcotic addiction. The concept of narcotic addiction is viewed as untenable since it is not a unitary phenomenon in that there are major dissimilarities among individual addicts in areas such as personality and psychological characteristics, and attitudinal and behavioral responses. The analogy between heroin addiction and methadone maintenance on the one hand and diabetes and insulin on the other is unsupported by the facts, i.e. most drug users, including heroin users, do not become addicted and evidence from a study in which 40% of the sample had used heroin, but only 10% seemed ever to have been addicted, is quoted. Gossop is also highly critical of some of the studies cited as evidence in favor of methadone maintenance, on the basis that they were highly selective and discriminated between different sub-groups of addicts, e.g. individuals known to be multiple-drug abusers (commonest form of drug misuse) or to have alcohol problems were excluded. He also criticised them for inadequate control conditions and quoting inflated estimates of success rates by providing percentages based on individuals remaining in treatment rather than the original samples.

Ghodse (1983) reviewed some earlier British follow-up studies of opiate addicts attending London clinics and came to the conclusion that although many of the findings were interesting they shed little light on how effective these treatment centers were. In one study quoted there was a trend towards abstinence (9% at 1 year, 17% at 3 years, 23% at 6 years) but the role of the clinics in this trend was uncertain. He noted that about half of those who became abstinent did so within 18 months of notification, i.e. while they were still 'new' addicts, while in another study results again suggested that it was the less chronic group who were likely to become abstinent. Studies of heroin addicts in London over a 10 year period from 1969 to 1979 (Thorley *et al.*, 1977; Stimson and Oppenheimer, 1982) enabled the latter workers to come to certain conclusions. They found a decline in the number of individuals remaining addicted, and a majority no longer attended the clinics after 10 years. Thirty-eight percent who had stopped using heroin and other opiates had made significant changes in their lives and by and large had not inclined to alcohol or other drugs as substitutes. However, less optimistically, a majority of a further 38% who remained clinic attenders, had received prescriptions continuously for 10 years. Fifteen percent were dead and 9% lost to the study. A quite separate 10 year follow up study (1970–1980) of clinic attenders (Gordon, 1983) looking particularly at the relationship between drugs and delinquency, produced results showing that 18% of the sample had died, 75% of the survivors had been abstinent for 5 years while 25% were still addicted. Ninety-seven percent had been convicted by 1981 and 83% were convicted during follow-up. It was concluded that abstinence was not related to hospital treatment, receipt of a clinic prescription or imprisonment. Continued addiction and reconviction were associated with early parental loss, poor academic achievement, conviction before drug use, longer imprisonment and a high conviction rate. Gordon concluded "criminality emerges as the predominant and continuing expression of deviancy" in this group.

Methadone maintenance as a therapy for opiate dependence has its exponents and its critics, but even the former admit to certain inherent disadvantages of the treatment. The drug itself induces chronic dependence and some individuals seem to be maintained for indeterminate or indefinite periods of time. There are troublesome side-effects such as chronic constipation, decreased libido and amenorrhoea in the female. The dosages dispensed, frequently in linctus form (and in orange juice in some United States programs), can be lethal to non-tolerant individuals, especially children. There may be diversion of the drug on to the black market, and it may be used manipulatively by some individuals to maintain a degree of control over an escalating illicit heroin habit, particularly its financial aspects.

More seriously the treatment has been strongly criticized on moral, ethical, and sociological grounds (Gossop, 1978; Yates, 1981; Faigel, 1971; Jonas, 1969; Myerson, 1969). The disease model of addiction has already been referred to and has attracted severe criticism from all sides. The doctor may be seen as colluding with the user in maintaining dependence rather than helping the individual strive for a drug-free existence. He may also be viewed as prescribing a dangerous substance with which harm is already being done to the individual, in a way described by Szasz (1973) as like "treating addiction to scotch with bourbon." Injustice is inherent in a situation where society regards individuals maintained on methadone as law-abiding while users of other psychoactive substances are seen as criminals. The confusion engendered between treatment and social control frequently results in uncertainty among medical staff who perceive themselves as being in a nontherapeutic role, in charge of the state-licensed opiate dispensary. Control of illicit drug use is not a medical problem.

There therefore exists a broad spectrum of views and opinions in relation to methadone maintenance treatment ranging from uncritical acclaim and use in poorly controlled conditions to outright condemnation and rejection of it as a treatment under any circumstances. These kinds of reactions have parallels in the history of development of many previously new drugs or treatments which have survived the vacillations of medical opinion to find a useful niche in the therapeutic armamentarium. This may be the case with methadone prescribing *vis-à-vis* the major threats to public health posed by the spread of the Hepatitis B and AIDS viruses due to the sharing of equipment by intra-venous drug abusers. These circumstances have prompted some governmental bodies and other authorities (McLelland, 1986) to take the view that there is a greater danger to human life by the spread of HIV (Human Immuno-deficiency Virus) infection than through drug misuse, which may justify issuing sterile equipment to those who cannot or will not give up i.v. use, and prescribing a substitute, such as methadone, for those who may be persuaded to reduce or cease injecting.

In the United States levo-alpha-acetyl-methadol (LAAM), a long-acting methadone congener, is currently still undergoing clinical evaluation but is not routinely available as an alternative to methadone in the treatment of opiate dependence. Its usefulness in this respect was suggested in the early fifties by Fraser and Isbell (1952) who demonstrated LAAM's ability to prevent the onset of withdrawal symptoms for 72 hr or longer. The main advantages of LAAM's long duration of action is that it suppresses withdrawal on a thrice weekly dosage schedule (Zaks *et al.*, 1972) and causes minimal inconvenience and disruption in an individual's daily routine.

3.2. Methadone in the Management of Withdrawal Symptoms and Detoxification

Physical dependence results from the regular use of certain drugs such as opiates and central nervous system depressants (e.g. alcohol, barbiturates and benzodiazepines) and is characterized by the development of tolerance (i.e. a decrease in the intensity of effects with repeated administration of a given dose) and the onset of a withdrawal or abstinence syndrome within a variable period of cessation of the drug. Thus the onset of manifestations of heroin withdrawal are usually present 4–6 hr after the last dose, peak at around 36–72 hr and thereafter gradually subside over 5–10 days. The time scale of appearance and the severity of opiate withdrawal symptoms have been graded (0–4) by Blachly (1966) and range from early anxiety, yawning, lacrimation and rhinorrhea to peak symptoms such as vomiting, diarrhea, restlessness, myalgia, insomnia, with increased temperature, respiratory and cardiac rates. Psychotic symptoms or convulsions are not features of the opiate withdrawal syndrome and their presence in addition to the above should raise suspicions that there has been concomitant abuse of a central nervous system depressant such as a benzodiazepine or barbiturate.

In the absence of underlying serious physical illness, opiate withdrawal can be unpleasant and distressing but it is not life-threatening, although the individual concerned would often have the observer believe otherwise, in a manipulative attempt to secure attention and treatment, i.e. a further supply of opiates. Withdrawal is usually a common experience in a career of narcotic addiction and many misusers have had frequent 'cold turkey' episodes often associated with imprisonment when their supply may be cut-off. A psychogenic component of opiate withdrawal has long been recognized (Wikler, 1948; Kleber, 1981) and the role of conditioning, personality, mental set and setting at the time of withdrawal, have all been regarded as impinging on the severity of these phenomena to an extent as great as any pharmacological factors. Looking at the influence of psychological factors on opiate withdrawal Phillips *et al.* (1986) found that neuroticism and the degree of anticipated distress were related to subsequent severity and that since both these factors are anxiety-related, may intensify the symptoms of withdrawal. Such findings deserve serious consideration, especially in the clinical situation, and should be given equal weight along with pharmacological aspects, as determinants of the detoxification regime. Methadone regimes for the management of withdrawal symptoms vary (Preston and Bigelow, 1985; DHSS Guidelines, 1984; NIDA Treatment Manual, 1980) and may be carried out on an inpatient or outpatient basis, but they generally have in common certain principles such as basic supportive techniques, establishing a baseline dosage, and gradual reduction over a variable period of time.

3.3. Methadone and Pregnancy

Since opiates cross the placenta, it follows that the fetus of an opiate dependent mother will also be dependent, and attempts at detoxification may place the pregnancy at risk by endangering the fetus. Immaturity of the neonatal central nervous system and enzyme systems mean that the withdrawal syndrome is much more likely to be protracted and severe, and constitute a significant risk of death (Senay, 1985). Gradual withdrawal on a methadone regime may be accomplished during the early part of the pregnancy (14–28 weeks) by weekly 5 mg reduction, but should be avoided in the third trimester because of the danger of early labor and fetal withdrawal (NIDA Treatment Manual, 1980). Otherwise the opiate-dependent mother should be maintained through pregnancy on a low-dose methadone regime (less than 25 mg daily) after which neonatal withdrawal symptoms may be mild enough not to require further treatment. Of course, the many other emotional, social and physical complications which may occur, including HIV infection, must also be confronted and may require the expertise of a multi-professional team throughout the antenatal and post-natal periods (Dixon, 1987, Riley, 1987).

4. OTHER PHARMACOLOGICAL TREATMENTS

4.1. Narcotic Antagonists

Not long after the turn of the century a search began for specific antidotes or substances that could antagonize the various effects of opiates. This led to the development in the forties of nalorphine which, however, was found to have both agonist and antagonist properties which limited its usefulness in the treatment of overdose and in maintaining abstinence from opiates (Blum, 1984). Most compounds studied for use as antagonists have been found to possess varying degrees of agonist activity, but it has to be said that a few have proved useful in other ways, e.g. pentazocine possesses both agonist and antagonist properties but is a very effective analgesic. The same can be said of buprenorphine which has also been considered as promising in the treatment of opiate dependence (Preston and Bigelow, 1985). Eventually in the early sixties naloxone was developed as the first pure antagonist followed a few years later by naltrexone. Naloxone, since it is an antagonist with a shorter duration of action, has become the drug of choice in the treatment of opiate overdose.

The use of naloxone in the treatment of opiate dependence has been restricted by the need for a frequent dosage schedule because of its relatively short duration of action (Jasinski *et al.*, 1967). Naltrexone, on the other hand, is a long-acting antagonist with a half-life of about 10 hr (Preston and Bigelow, 1985) and at an appropriate dosage of 70 mg is said to completely block heroin-induced euphoria and the development of physical dependence for 48–72 hr (NIDA Treatment Manual, 1980). It has also been used in combination with clonidine to achieve rapid withdrawal from methadone (Charney *et al.*, 1986).

4.2. Clonidine

This drug has been used for many years now and has an established place in the treatment of hypertension and migraine. It is thought that clonidine exerts its anti-hypertensive effect by acting at central alpha-2-adrenoceptors in the medulla oblongata but interest in its use in the treatment of abstinence reactions has been stimulated by the discovery that its alpha-2-adrenoceptor agonist effect also inhibited ascending noradrenergic systems, particularly those in the locus coeruleus (Svensson, 1986).

The first report of the use of clonidine to reduce opiate withdrawal symptoms in laboratory rats was that of Tseng *et al.* (1975) which was followed by a series of clinical studies by Yale researchers (Gold *et al.*, 1978a,b, 1979, 1980). Subsequent American and

European studies have been reviewed in considerable detail by Agren (1986) giving numbers involved, dosage schedules, side effects and remarks on outcome. He opines "There is little evidence that a successful detoxification using clonidine should influence the long-term prognosis of opiate addiction in any other way than rapidly offering an opportunity for patient and therapist to plan ahead from a new vantage point."

4.3. Benzodiazepines

As a result of criticisms highlighting some of the limitations of methadone maintenance, an increasing number of treatment centers have moved in the direction of opiate-free or drug-free therapeutic approaches to problems associated with narcotic dependence (Drummond *et al.*, 1986; Preston and Bigelow, 1985; Sells and Simpson, 1979). Drummond *et al.* noted that, following a change from methadone to chlordiazepoxide prescribing at a Glasgow day center, the clientele, *inter alia*, were younger, more likely to be single and tended to come into treatment earlier in their drug career. They emphasize, however, that the study was not designed to evaluate the relative efficacy of an opiate-free policy compared with methadone prescribing.

Benzodiazepines such as diazepam and chlordiazepoxide have been widely used in alcohol withdrawal and their anxiolytic, hypnotic and muscle relaxant properties would indicate their utility in treating certain symptoms of opiate withdrawal such as anxiety, muscle cramps, tremor and insomnia, presumably as a result of their CNS depressant action. On the other hand benzodiazepine dependency itself can become a major problem, with abstinence symptoms following treatment of less than 2 months duration or presenting as an emergency situation with psychotic features and convulsions following abrupt withdrawal (Lader and Higgit, 1986; Murphy *et al.*, 1984; Tyrer and Sievewright, 1984). Benzodiazepines can also be used with a non-benzodiazepine hypnotic (e.g. chloral hydrate) and an anti-diarrheal (e.g. diphenoxylate plus atropine) in the symptomatic treatment of opiate withdrawal.

5. NON-PHARMACOLOGICAL TREATMENT APPROACHES

While there is always likely to be a place for pharmacological treatment in drug misuse, perhaps as much due to the inability of many dependent individuals to contemplate entering treatment without medication of some sort or another, it should not be allowed to obscure the fact that there are important psychological, behavioral and social factors which are of major therapeutic significance. Some of these treatment approaches have already been referred to in the earlier discussion of a social-learning model. Drug misuse is an extremely complex phenomenon and although abstinence may be the ideal goal or cure, it is probably an unrealistic one in many cases, since attaining and maintaining a drug-free state over a lengthy period of time is the exception rather than the rule. Success in treatment requires to be viewed more pragmatically and Conrad (1977) interprets this as reduced frequency of use, use under medical supervision, improved family and interpersonal relationships, return to employment, decreased criminality and overall improvement in social adjustment. It is also interesting to note that the latter regards the use of narcotic drugs as an epiphenomenon and that most misusers lives were chaotic and disordered "long before they stuck a needle in their arm."

It is perhaps therefore not altogether surprising that more formal psychological treatment approaches such as psycho-analysis and group psychotherapy, even in very structured and institutional settings, have not been singularly successful (Conrad, 1977), but then this applies to most other treatments. The fact that no particular treatment seems to be greatly superior to another should not result in a retreat into therapeutic nihilism, but rather a more serious attempt to meet the individual misuser's needs with appropriate treatment and supportive strategies of some practical merit. In recent years a spirit of electicism has become more prevalent and many now feel that alcohol and drugs-related problems can be tackled together (Raistrick and Davidson, 1985).

There has been a concomitant search for common features in treatment approaches, areas of commonality, which are useful in helping individuals change harmful habits and achieve new lifestyles, a concept familiar in health education (Ritson, 1986). It is not only internal psychological problems which have to be confronted but the individual's entire lifestyle may require major modification, frequently by significant environmental manipulation. The drug user is no longer seen as the passive recipient of treatment but is actively involved in modifying and changing his habits by the use of self-help manuals and self-monitoring diaries. Thus the desire for change may be fostered and enhanced by cognitive and behavioral techniques which facilitate the individual gradually assuming control of the necessary decision-making process over a period of time (Prochaska and Di Clemente, 1982).

In the late sixties and early seventies various alternatives to the hospital-based clinics began to appear in London and gradually throughout the rest of the country. These facilities ranged from day centres or drop-in street agencies, attempting to help drug users with an assortment of social and legal problems by providing advice and counselling at a practical level, to more structured residential rehabilitation establishments, often run as therapeutic communities. Particular examples of the former are the Lifeline Project in Manchester (Yates, 1981) and the Blenheim Project, and the Hungerford and the Community Drug Projects in London. According to Dorn and South (1985) these latter three "are best understood not as separate agencies but as complementary pieces in a wider jigsaw of response to drug-related problems. They operate primarily at two levels—locally and London-wide—and in two main ways—services to individual clients and families and friends, and to other agencies (statutory and non-statutory: drug-specialist, generic and specialising in fields other than drug problems)." Examples of the latter concept are Phoenix House (London and other areas of England), the Ley Community (Oxfordshire), Kilmahew House and Spectrum House (Scotland). The more structured residential facilities or communities largely in the voluntary sector, usually insist that the individual is drug-free before admission and the problem is approached from a socio-psychological angle, often with a strong confrontational element between staff and fellow residents, over periods ranging from 6 weeks to 6 months (Sessions, 1976). In recent years there has been a proliferation of agencies and projects, statutory and non-statutory, helped by government funding (Home Office, 1986) and resulting from the Advisory Council on the Misuse of Drugs 1982 Report. The Advisory Council recommended *inter alia*, that there should be much less pre-occupation with the physical aspects of abuse (less substance orientation) and more emphasis placed on a problem-solving approach within the context of a multiprofessional team which might include medical, social work, psychology and community nursing staff. Interaction and liaison between the various caring agencies was seen as desirable in the development of a network of care and support, in which the range of problems presented by drug misusers could be met with appropriate intervention. Other recommendations included the creation of local drug problem teams and drug advisory committees, to coordinate these services to suit local needs, and development of training and research. Important and useful organizations have been established such as the Institute for the Study of Drug Dependence (ISDD) and the Standing Conference on Drug Abuse (SCODA). The ISSD has a comprehensive reference library on the non-medical use of drugs and is an invaluable source of information and materials for health and social education, and for the training of professionals. SCODA is a national organization with responsibility for the coordination of non-statutory or voluntary agencies involved in drug misuse. It promotes the development of existing organizations, and gives advice and support in the establishment of additional facilities and research into problems associated with drug misuse (Home Office, 1986).

6. PREVENTION

Given the complex multifactorial nature of causation in drug misuse, preventive measures require to be extensive and wide-ranging. In the broadest sense there is a need for government to improve health, education and housing, to reduce unemployment and provide better leisure and recreational facilities through appropriate social and economic measures (Advisory Council, 1982, 1984). The need for health education has been seen as increasingly important, particularly in an effort to reach young people and prevent them being attracted to drug misuse. Bodies such as the Health Education Council and the Scottish Health Education Group have responsibilities for community aspects of health education including cigarette smoking and alcohol use as well as drugs.

The main legislative measures to control the availability of drugs in the United Kingdom are the Misuse of Drugs Act, 1971 and its associated regulations (The Misuse of Drugs Regulations, 1973, 1985) as well as the Medicine's Act (1968) and the Customs and Excise Act (1979). This body of legislation restricts the import, export, manufacture, sale, distribution, supply and possession of such drugs as opium, morphine, heroin, cocaine and cannabis, which are specified as controlled drugs and categorized as A (e.g. heroin, morphine and cocaine), B (e.g. amphetamines and cannabis) and C (e.g. certain amphetamine-related drugs). There are restrictions on prescribing and there is a requirement on the part of the doctor to notify patients who are suspected or confirmed as being addicted to Class A drugs, to the Chief Medical Officer at the Home Office. The Home Office Drugs Branch Inspectorate ensures that drugs are not diverted from legitimate sources and deals with irresponsible prescribing by some practitioners, while there are police powers to inspect controlled drugs registers at pharmacies. Penalties for some offences concerning controlled drugs have been increased by the Controlled Drugs (Penalties) Act (1985). The sentence that may now be meted out for the production, supply and possession with intent to supply a Class A drug has been raised from 14 years to life imprisonment, and penalties under the 1979 Customs Act have also been increased. The Drug Trafficking Offences Bill (1985) provides new powers for tracing and freezing the proceeds of drug trafficking and such assets are liable to be seized on conviction. This recent proliferation of legislation reflects a determination on the part of government to fight what is widely viewed as the menace to society of the spread of drug addiction. Efforts have been made to stem the supply of drugs from source countries by crop eradication and substitution, but these have had limited success for a variety of reasons, not least of which is the fact that growing such crops is an economic necessity. This has led Stimson (1985) to question whether a war on drugs can succeed and to suggest, among other things, the encouragement of a Third World pharmaceutical industry based on locally grown crops to promote economic development and legalize production under controlled conditions. The conclusion he comes to is that investment in law enforcement alone is unlikely to succeed and that it is necessary to have an equitable distribution of public expenditure on education, prevention and treatment.

REFERENCES

Adler, P. (1985) *Wheeling and Dealing. An Ethnography of an Upper-Level Drug Dealing and Smuggling Community*. Columbia University Press, New York.

Advisory Council on the Misuse of Drugs (1982) Report. *Treatment and Rehabilitation*. DHSS, London HMSO.

Advisory Council on the Misuse of Drugs (1984) Report. *Prevention*. Home Office, London. HMSO.

Agren, H. (1986) Clonidine treatment of the opiate withdrawal syndrome. A review of clinical trials of a theory *Acta Psychiat. Scand.* **73 (Suppl. 73):** 91–113.

Bandura, A. (1969) *Principles of Behaviour Modification*. Holt, Rinehart and Winston, New York.

Blachly, P. H. (1966) Management of the opiate abstinence syndrome. *Am. J. Psychiat.* **122**:742–744.

Blakey, R. and Baker, R. (1980) An exposure approach to alcohol abuse. *Behav. Res. Ther.* **18:** 319–325.

Bloom, F. E. (1983) The endorphins. A growing family of pharmacologically pertinent peptides. *Annu. Rev. Pharmacol. Toxicol.* **23:** 151–170.

Blum, K. (1984a) Methadone and other narcotic maintenance drugs. In: *Handbook of Abusable Drugs*, pp. 101–144. Gardner Press, New York.

Blum, K. (1984b) In: *Handbook of Abusable Drugs*, pp. 81–100. Gardner Press, New York.

Brain, R. (1985) *Interdepartmental Committee on Drug Addiction*, 2nd Report. London, HMSO.

Charney, D. S., Heninger, G. R. and Kleber, H. D. (1986) The combined use of clonidine and naltrexone as a rapid, safe effective treatment of abrupt withdrawal from methadone. *Am. J. Psychiat.* **143:** 831–837.

Childress, A. R., McLennan, A. T. and O'Brien, C. P. (1985) Behavioral therapies for substance abuse. *Int. J. Addict.* **20:** 947–969.

Conrad, H. T. (1977) Psychiatric treatment of narcotic addiction. In: *Drug Addiction I. Section II. Morphine Dependence*, pp. 259–276. Martin, W. R. (ed.) Springer, Berlin.

Cummings, C., Gordon, J. R. and Marlatt, G. A. (1980) Relapse: Prevention and prediction. In: *The Addictive Behaviors*, Miller, W. R. (ed.) Pergamon Press, Oxford.

DHSS Guidelines (1984) Report of the Medical Working Group on Drug Dependence. *Guidelines of Good Clinical Practice in the Treatment of Drug Misuse*, DHSS, London.

Dixon, A. (1987) The pregnant addict. *Druglink*, **2:** 6–8.

Dole, V. P. (1971) Methadone maintenance treatment for 25,000 heroin addicts. *J. Am. Med. Assoc.* **215:** 1131–1134.

Dole, V. P. and Nyswander, M. (1965) A medical treatment for diacetylmorphine (heroin) addiction. *J. Am. Med. Assoc.* **193:** 646–650.

Dole, V. P. and Nyswander, M. (1966) Narcotic blockade. *Arch. Intern. Med.* **118:** 303–309.

Dole, V. P. and Nyswander, M. (1967) Heroin addiction. A metabolic disease. *Arch. Intern. Med.* **120:** 19–24.

Dole, V. P. and Nyswander, M. (1968) The use of methadone for narcotic blockade. *Br. J. Addict.* **63:** 55–57.

Dole, V. P., Robinson, J. W., Orraca, J., Towns, E., Searcy, P. and Caine, E. (1969) Methadone treatment of randomly selected criminal addicts. *New Engl. J. Med.* **280**: 1372–1375.

Dorn, N. and South, N. (1985) *Helping Drug Users*. Gower, Aldershot, Hampshire. Brookfield, Vermont.

Drummond, D. C., Taylor, J. A. and Mullin, P. J. (1986) Replacement of a prescribing service by an opiate-free day programme in a Glasgow drug clinic. *Br. J. Addict.* **81:** 559–565.

Du Pont, R. and Katon, R. (1971a) Development of a heroin-addiction treatment program: effect on urban crime. *J. Am. Med. Assoc.* **216:** 1320–1324.

Du Pont, R. and Katon, R. (1971b) Physicians and the heroin epidemic. *Mod. Med.* June 28, 123–129.

Edwards, G. (1974) Drugs, drug dependence and the concept of plasticity. *Q. J. Stud. Alcohol.* **35:** 179–195.

Edwards, G. (1979) British policies on opiate addiction: ten years working of the revised response, and options for the future. *Br. J. Psychiat.* **134:** 1–13.

Edwards, G. (1981) The background. In: *Drug Problems in Britain: A Review of Ten Years*, pp. 5–23, Edwards, G. and Busch, C. (eds) Academic Press, London.

Faigel, H. (1971) Methadone maintenance treatment of addiction. *J. Am. Med. Assoc.* **215:** 299.

Fraser, H. F. and Isbell, H. (1952) Actions and addiction liabilities of alpha-acetylmethadols in man. *J. Pharmacol. Exp. Ther.* **105:** 458–465.

Freemantle, B. (1985) *The Fix.* Michael Joseph, London.

Ghodse, A. H. (1983) Treatment of drug addiction in London. *Lancet* **i:** 636–639.

Gold, M. S., Redmond, D. E. Jr and Kleber, H. D. (1978a) Clonidine in opiate withdrawal. *Lancet* **i:** 929–930.

Gold, M. S., Redmond, D. E. Jr and Kleber, H. D. (1978b) Clonidine blocks acute opiate-withdrawal symptoms. *Lancet* **ii:** 599–602.

Gold, M.S., Redmond, D. E. Jr and Kleber, H. D. (1979) Noradrenergic hyperactivity in opiate withdrawal supported by clonidine reversal of opiate withdrawal. *Am. J. Psychiat.* **136**: 100–102.

Gold, M. S., Pottash, A. L. C., Sweeny, D. R. and Kleber, H.D. (1980) Efficacy in opiate withdrawal. A study of thirty patients. *Drug Alcohol Depend.* **6:** 201–208.

Gordon, A. M. (1983) Drugs and delinquency: A ten year follow up of drug clinic patients. *Br. J. Psychiat.* **142:** 169–173.

Gossop, M. (1978) A review of the evidence for methadone maintenance as a treatment for narcotic addiction. *Lancet* **i:** 812–815.

de Haes, W. F. M. (1986) Drug education: Yes, but how? *Research Symposium on Addictive Behaviour*, March, 1986. University of Dundee, Scottish Health Education Group.

Hartnoll, R. L., Mitcheson, M. C., Battersby, A., Brown, G., Ellis, M., Fleming, P. and Hedley, N. (1980) Evaluation of heroin maintenance in controlled trial. *Arch. Gen. Psychiat.* **37:** 877–884.

Hofmann, F. G. (1983) *A Handbook on Drug and Alcohol Abuse. The Biomedical Aspects*, 2nd edn. Oxford University Press, New York.

Home Office (1986) *Tackling Drug Misuse: A Summary of the Governments Strategy*. 2nd edn. Home Office, London.

Hughes, J. (1975) Isolation of an endogenous compound from the brain with pharmacological properties similar to morphine. *Brain Res.* **88:** 295–306.

Hughes, J. (1976) Enkephalin and drug dependence. *Br. J. Addict.* **71:** 199–209.

Jasinski, D. R., Martin, W. R. and Hoeldtke, R. D. (1967) The human pharmacology and abuse potential of *N*-allylnoroxymorphine (naloxone). *J. Pharmacol. Exp. Ther.* **157:** 420–426.

Jonas, S. (1969) Methadone treatment of addicts. *New Engl. J. Med.* **281:** 391.

Kleber, H. D. (1981) Detoxification from Narcotics. In: *Substance Abuse*, Lowinson, J. and Ruiz, P. (eds) Williams & Wilkins, Baltimore.

Kuhar, M. J., Pert., C. B. and Snyder, S. H. (1973) Regional distribution of opiate receptor binding in monkey and human brain. *Nature* **245:** 447–450.

Lader, M. H. and Higgit, A. C. (1986) Management of benzodiazepine dependence—Update 1986. *Br. J. Addict.* **81:** 7–10.

Lewis, R. (1985) Serious Business—the global heroin economy. In: *Big Deal, The Politics of the Illicit Drug Business.* Henman, A., Lewis, R. and Maylon, T. (eds) Pluto Press, London.

Marlatt, G. A. and George, W. H. (1984) Relapse prevention: Introduction and overview of the model. *Br. J. Addict.* **79:** 261–273.

Marlatt, G. A. and Gordon, J. R. (1980) Determinants of relapse: Implications for the maintenance of behavior change. In: *Behavioural Medicine: Changing Health Lifestyles*, Davidson, P. O. and Davidson, S. M. (eds) Brunner/Mazel, New York.

McLelland, D. B. L. (1986) Report of Scottish Committee on HIV Infection and Intravenous Drug Misuse. *HIV Infection in Scotland*. Scottish Home and Health Department.

Mitcheson, M. C. and Hartnoll, R. L. (1978) Conflicts in deciding treatment with drug dependency clinics. In: *Problems of Drug Abuse in Britain*, West, D. J. (ed.) Institute of Criminology, Cambridge.

Murphy, S. M., Owen, R. T. and Tyrer, P. J. (1984) Withdrawal symptoms after 6 weeks treatment with diazepam. *Lancet* **ii:** 1389.

MYERSON, D. J. (1969) Methadone treatment of addicts. *New Engl. J. Med.* **281:** 390–391.
NIDA TREATMENT MANUAL (1980) *Detoxification Treatment Manual.* NIDA Treatment Program Monograph Series No. 6 U.S. Department of Health and Human Services.
ORFORD, J. (1985) *Excessive Appetites—A Psychological View of Addictions.* Wiley, London.
PASTERNAK, G. W., GOODMAN, R. and SNYDER, S. H. (1975) An endogenous morphine-like factor in mammalian brain. *Life Sci.* **16:** 1765–1769.
PECK, D. G. and BECKETT, W. (1976) Methadone maintenance: A review and critique. *Br. J. Addict.* **71:** 369–376.
PHILLIPS, G. T., GOSSOP, M. and BRADLEY, B. (1986) The influence of psychological factors on the opiate withdrawal syndrome. *Br. J. Psychiat.* **149:** 235–238.
PLANT, M. A. (1980) Drugtaking and prevention: The implications of research for social policy. *Br. J. Addict.* **75:** 245–254.
PLANT, M. A. (1981) What aetiologies? In: *Drug Problems in Britain: A Review of Ten Years.* pp. 245–280. EDWARDS, G. and BUSCH, C. (eds) Academic Press, London.
PRESTON, K. L. and BIGELOW, G. E. (1985) Pharmacological advances in addiction treatment. *Int. J. Addict.* **20:** 845–867.
PROCHASKA, J. O. and DI CLEMENTE, C. C. (1982) Transtheoretical therapy: Towards a more integrative model of change. *Psychother. Theory Res. Pract.* **19:** 276–288.
RAISTRICK, D. and DAVIDSON, R. (eds) (1985) *Alcoholism and Drug Addiction.* Churchill Livingstone.
RANKIN, H., HODGSON, R. and STOCKWELL, T. (1983) Cue exposure and response prevention with alcoholics: A controlled trial. *Behav. Res. Ther.* **21:** 435–446.
REINERT, J. (1965) Now—A drug that "cures" drug addicts. *Sci. Dig.* Nov. 38–41.
RILEY, D. (1987) The management of the pregnant addict. *Bull. Royal. Coll. Psychiat.* **11**: 362–365.
RITSON, B. (1986) Trends in the treatment response to substance abuse. *Research Symposium on Addictive Behaviour.* University of Dundee, March, 1986. Scottish Health Education Group.
ROLLESTON, H. (1926) *Departmental Committee on Morphine and Heroin Addiction*, Report. HMSO, London.
SELLS, S.B. and SIMPSON, D. D. (1979) On the effectiveness of treatment for drug abuse: Evidence from the DARP research program in the United States. *Bull. Narcot.* **31:** 1-11.
SENAY, E. C. (1985) Methadone maintenance treatment. *Int. J. Addict.* **20:** 803–821.
SESSIONS, K. B. (1976) Maintenance or suppression? A comparative look at the heroin addiction policies of Great Britain and the U.S. *Br. J. Addict.* **71:** 385–389.
STIMSON, G. V. (1985) Can a war on drugs succeed? *New Soc.* **74:** 275–278.
STIMSON, G. V. and OPPENHEIMER, E. (1982) *Heroin Addiction: Treatment and Control in Britain.* Tavistock, London.
STRANG, J. (1985) Breaking out of Procrustes' bed—services for problem drug takers. *Bull. Roy. Coll. Psychiat.* **9:** 150–152.
SVENSSON, T. H. (1986) Clonidine in abstinence reactions: Basic mechanisms. *Acta Psychiat. Scand.* **73:** (*Suppl. 327*) 19–42.
SZASZ, T. S. (1973) *The Second Sin*, p. 63, Routledge, London.
TERENIUS, L. and WAHLSTROM, A. (1975) Search for an endogenous ligand for the opiate receptor. *Acta Psychol. Scand.* **94:** 74–81.
THORLEY, A., OPPENHEIMER, E. and STIMSON, G. V. (1977) Clinic attendance and opiate prescription status of heroin addicts over a six year period. *Br. J. Psychiat.* **130:** 565–569.
TSENG, L.-F., LOH, H. H. and Wei, E. T. (1975) Effects of clonidine on morphine withdrawal signs in the rat. *Eur. J. Pharmacol.* **30:** 93–99.
TYRER, P. J. and SEIVEWRIGHT, N. (1984) Identification and management of benzodiazepine dependence. *Postgrad. Med. J.* **60** (*Suppl. 2*): 41–46.
WEN, H. L. and HO, W. K. K. (1982) Suppression of withdrawal symptoms by dynorphin in heroin addicts. *Eur. J. Pharmacol.* **82:** 183–186.
WHO (1969) *Expert Committee on Drug Dependence*, 16th Report. Technical Report Series 407. WHO Vienna.
WIKLER, A. (1948) Recent progress in research on the neurophysiologic basis of morphine addiction. *Am. J. Psychiat.* **105:** 329–338.
YATES, R. (1981) *Out From the Shadows.* Lifeline Project 10th Anniversary Report, NACRO, London.
ZAKS, A., FINK, M. and FREEDMAN, A. M. (1972) Levomethadyl in maintenance treatment of opiate dependence. *J. Am. Med. Assoc.* **220:** 811–813.
ZINBERG, N. E. (1984) *Drug, Set and Setting: The Basis for Controlled Intoxicant Use.* Yale University Press, New Haven.

CHAPTER 5

THE MOLECULAR PHARMACOLOGY OF THE MINOR TRANQUILIZERS

IAN L. MARTIN

MRC Molecular Neurobiology Unit, MRC Centre
Hills Road, Cambridge, UK

1. INTRODUCTION

Anxiety is a normal human emotion and forms an integral and necessary part of our daily lives. Should the anxiety become persistent or severe, a pathological anxiety syndrome may be diagnosed and treatment with a minor tranquilizer instituted. Since the introduction of the 1,4-benzodiazepines into clinical practice, they have become the drugs of choice for such indications.

The first in this series of compounds was synthesized in 1955 and the intriguing story of its discovery is recounted by Sternbach (1979). In 1957, the compound was subjected to pharmacological screening and was shown to have sedative, muscle relaxant, anticonvulsant, taming and appetite stimulating effects; it also exhibited low toxicity. The initial trials in human subjects were carried out in six hospitalized geriatric patients and the only effects noted were ataxia and sedation at doses of 50 to 150 mg/day; in a further series of ten patients with convulsive disorders it was again shown to be sedative but with no useful anticonvulsant effects. The enthusiasm of Lowell Randall for the novel pharmacological spectrum of this compound, however, remained unabated and later successful trials in anxious patients marked the dawn of a remarkable success story for the benzodiazepines in clinical medicine (see Randall, 1982). This compound, chlordiazepoxide (Fig. 1), was introduced in 1960 under the trade name Librium. Three years later the structural analog diazepam (Fig. 2) was marketed as Valium.

Since that time the compounds of this chemical class have become the most frequently prescribed of all psychotropic drugs being used not only as anxiolytics, but anticonvulsants, muscle relaxants, sedative/hypnotics and pre-anaesthetics. In 1977 the population of the U.S.A. was conservatively estimated to have ingested 8000 tons of these medicines (Tall-

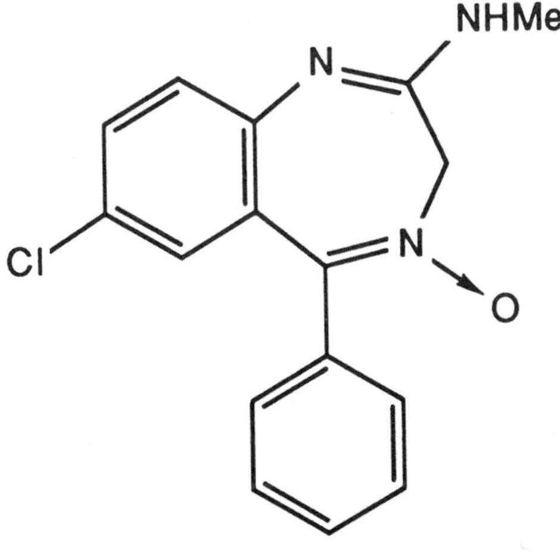

FIG. 1. Structure of chlordiazepoxide.

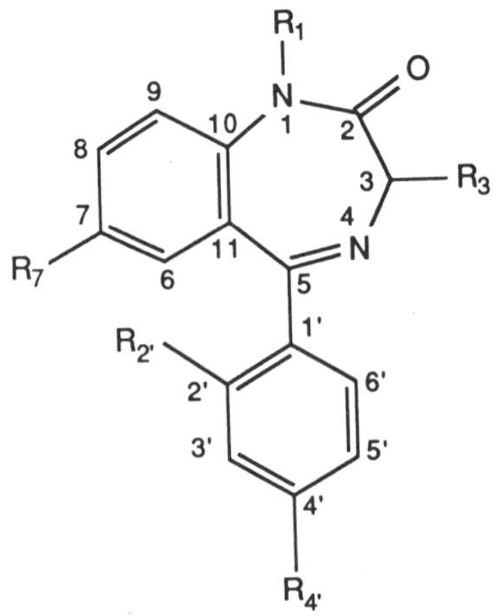

	R_1	R_3	R_7	$R_{2'}$	$R_{4'}$
Diazepam	Me	H	Cl	H	H
Flunitrazepam	Me	H	NO_2	F	H
Clonazepam	H	H	NO_2	Cl	H
Lorazepam	H	OH	Cl	Cl	H
Flurazepam	alkyl	H	Cl	F	H
Ro 5-4864	Me	H	Cl	H	Cl

where alkyl = $-(CH_2)_2NEt_2$

FIG. 2. Structures of 1,4-benzodiazepines.

man *et al.*, 1980). There are now over 40 analogues available to the clinician in various countries throughout the world. The details of their overt effects in both animals and man are the subject of other chapters in this volume and will not be addressed further here.

It is clear that the impact of these medicines has been enormous. Equally remarkable has been the progress made in the elucidation of the mechanisms by which they produce their effects. It is now widely accepted that the pharmacology of the benzodiazepines is intimately connected with the actions of the major inhibitory neurotransmitter gamma-aminobutyric acid (GABA).

2. GAMMA-AMINOBUTYRIC ACID: BIOCHEMISTRY AND RECEPTOR PHARMACOLOGY

2.1. INTRODUCTION

GABA was first isolated from the mammalian CNS, using simple chromatographic techniques, in 1949. Interest in this substance originally centered around its possible role in cerebral glucose metabolism, but, for the past 20 years, few have doubted its importance as a major inhibitory neurotransmitter in the mammalian CNS (Roberts, 1984).

2.2. DISTRIBUTION

GABA exhibits a ubiquitous occurrence in the mammalian brain where it has a differential topographical distribution. All brain regions contain GABA, although it is particularly abundant in the substantia nigra, globus pallidus and hypothalamus (Iversen and

Bloom, 1972; Ottersen and Storm-Mathison, 1984). It is localized in nerve terminals (Neal and Iversen, 1969) from which it can be released by depolarizing stimuli in a calcium-dependent manner (Bradford, 1970). High affinity uptake systems for GABA have been identified in neurons; this system is thought to be responsible for its removal from the synaptic cleft subsequent to release (Iversen and Neal, 1968). There is also evidence that it can be taken up into glial cells (Iversen and Kelly, 1975), from which it may be released by potassium depolarization (Minchin and Iversen, 1974).

It is thought to mediate inhibition, largely through hyperpolarization, at many synapses in the CNS (Kelly and Beart, 1975). The majority of these sites involve release from interneurons, though there are some long projection pathways which use this transmitter, such as the cerebellar output neuron, the Purkinje cell (ten Brugencatte and Engberg, 1969), the striatonigral pathway (Precht and Yoshida, 1971; Nagy *et al.*, 1978) and the nigrotectal pathway (Garcia-Munoz *et al.*, 1977).

2.3. Synthesis and Catabolism

This amino acid is synthesized almost exclusively from glutamic acid through decarboxylation by the enzyme glutamic acid decarboxylase (GAD; EC 4.1.1.15). GAD is localized exclusively in neurons and the product, GABA, follows the distribution of the enzyme. These conclusions have been possible from histochemical studies with antibodies, raised against the purified protein (Saito, 1976) at both the light (Barber and Saito, 1976; Mugnaini and Oertel, 1985) and electron microscope level (Wood *et al.*, 1976). Detailed biochemical characterization of the purified enzyme has been carried out (Wu *et al.*, 1973; Wu, 1976). Recently the primary amino acid sequence of a protein exhibiting the enzymatic properties of GAD has become available from the cloning techniques of molecular biology (Kaufman *et al.*, 1986; Kobayashi *et al.*, 1987). This has allowed the localization of mRNA encoding the synthesis of the enzyme using in situ hybridisation (Wuenschell *et al.*, 1986; Julien *et al.*, 1987). There is evidence for multiple forms of the enzyme in rat brain (Legay *et al.*, 1987).

GABA is degraded by transamination. The enzyme responsible, 4-amino butyrate:2-oxo glutarate aminotransferase has also been purified and characterized (Schousboe *et al.*, 1974; Wu, 1976). Again, antibodies were raised against the purified protein and the immunocytochemical distribution of the material has been studied at the light microscope level (Barber and Saito, 1976; Nagai *et al.*, 1984). It is clear that this immunoreactive material has a much wider distribution than that of GABA.

There have been many attempts to study the consequences of the pharmacological manipulation of the GABA system. GAD is the rate limiting step in the synthesis of this neurotransmitter and it can be effectively inhibited by a number of sulphydryl reagents, such as p-chloromercuribenzoate (Wu and Roberts, 1974), several thiol compounds e.g., 3-mercaptopropionic acid (Karlsson *et al.*, 1974) and a variety of carbonyl trapping agents, of which semicarbazide, thiosemicarbazide and isonicotinic acid hydrazide have been the most popular for experimental purposes (Wu & Roberts, 1974; Tapia, 1975). Inhibition of GAD leads to a decrease in the concentration of CNS GABA and there appears to be threshold level of GAD activity below which convulsions occur (Tapia *et al.*, 1975).

Inhibition of the degradative enzyme GABA-T results in an increase in the levels of brain GABA with a concomitant increase in seizure threshold. Aminooxyacetic acid is a potent inhibitor of GABA-T at low doses, though at higher concentrations GAD is also inhibited (Schousboe *et al.*, 1974). This compound has a multitude of other effects that should be taken into account in the interpretation of experimental data accumulated with this compound (Johnston, 1978). Several agents have been developed for the irreversible inhibition of GABA-T, ethanolamine-O-sulphate (Fowler and John, 1972), gamma-acetylenic GABA (Jung and Metcalf, 1975), gamma-vinyl GABA (Jung *et al.*, 1977) and gabaculine (Kobayashi *et al.*, 1976). All of these compounds exhibit anticonvulsant activity.

2.4. Uptake

GABA is taken up into both neurons and glia via energy-dependent processes. There appears to be a different substrate specificity for these two cell types: diamino-butyric acid is preferentially taken up into neurons, while in the case of beta-alanine the uptake is largely into glia (Iversen and Kelly, 1975); both are competitive inhibitors of GABA uptake. The structural requirements of GABA analogues required to further specify this differentiation have been investigated (Breckenridge *et al.*, 1981). Nipecotic acid is also a potent inhibitor of GABA uptake into neurons (Johnston *et al.*, 1976) and various analogs in this series have also been studied (Krogsgaard-Larsen and Johnston, 1975). There are a number of other compounds, of diverse chemical structure, which are potent inhibitors of the uptake of this neurotransmitter (Johnston, 1978).

2.5. GABA Receptors

Three subtypes of receptor for GABA have so far been delineated in terms of their ligand specificity. However, a precise pharmacological definition has so far been hindered by the lack of sufficient compounds with the appropriate specificity. The GABA-A and GABA-B subtypes are readily differentiated, bicuculline being a potent antagonist at the GABA-A receptor but without effect at GABA-B receptors. The pharmacology of the third type, the autoreceptor, is very similar to the A subtype though delta-amino laevulinic acid is a weak agonist at the autoreceptor, but not at the GABA-A receptor.

Bicuculline sensitive actions of GABA are observed in the mammalian CNS and also in the periphery. The structure activity relationships for agonists at this receptor binding site have been studied in considerable detail (Krogsgaard-Larsen *et al.*, 1984; 1986). Experimentally, the most widely used agonists are GABA, muscimol, 3-aminopropane sulphonic acid (3-APS), piperidine-4-sulphonic acid (P4S), isoguvacine and 4,5,6,7-tetrahydroisoxazolo{5,4-c}pyridin-3-ol (THIP) (see Fig. 3 for structures). Many of these compounds are available labelled with tritium and there is a large amount of data concerning their interaction with the GABA-A recognition site. Under the appropriate conditions they all bind in a mutually exclusive and competitive manner. The binding isotherms for many of these compounds to brain membranes are nonlinear on Scatchard transformation (Falch and Krogsgaard-Larsen, 1982; Jordan *et al.*, 1982; Quast and Brenner, 1983). This is not sufficient evidence to suggest that there are multiple GABA-A receptors. In fact it has been shown that the rank order of potency for the displacement of radiolabelled GABA, THIP or P4S by a number of other agonist ligands is very similar, suggesting that a single binding site exists in multiple conformational states (Krogsgaard-Larsen *et al.*, 1981). The significance of this interpretation of the data is still a matter of considerable discussion.

There are a number of specific antagonists for GABA-A receptor mediated events. Bicuculline is thought to interact directly with the GABA receptor to produce competitive inhibition of the neurotransmitter (Johnston, 1976; Frere *et al.*, 1982; Nowak *et al.*, 1982) as do certain pyridazinyl derivatives of GABA such as SR95531 (Heaulme *et al.*, 1986; Wermuth and Biziere, 1986). The effects are stereospecific and the structure activity relationships of a number of related alkaloids have been studied (Kardos *et al.*, 1984). ^{3}H-bicuculline has been used in binding studies; it is suggested that the binding interaction takes place with a different conformational state of the GABA-A recognition site (Mohler and Okada, 1977a; Olsen and Snowman, 1983; Olsen, Snowhill, *et al.*, 1984). On the other hand, picrotoxin does not interact with the recognition site for the neurotransmitter but produces potent noncompetitive inhibition (Simmonds, 1980; Barker *et al.*, 1980). There are several other antagonists which act to inhibit GABA-A mediated transmission at sites distinct from the amino acid binding site; these include anisatin (Kudo *et al.*, 1981), a series of bicyclophosphates (Bowery *et al.*, 1976; 1977), tetramethylenedisulpotetramine (Bowery *et al.*, 1975), bemegride and pentylenetetrazole (Simmonds, 1978).

The early electrophysiological evidence suggested that the interaction of GABA with the

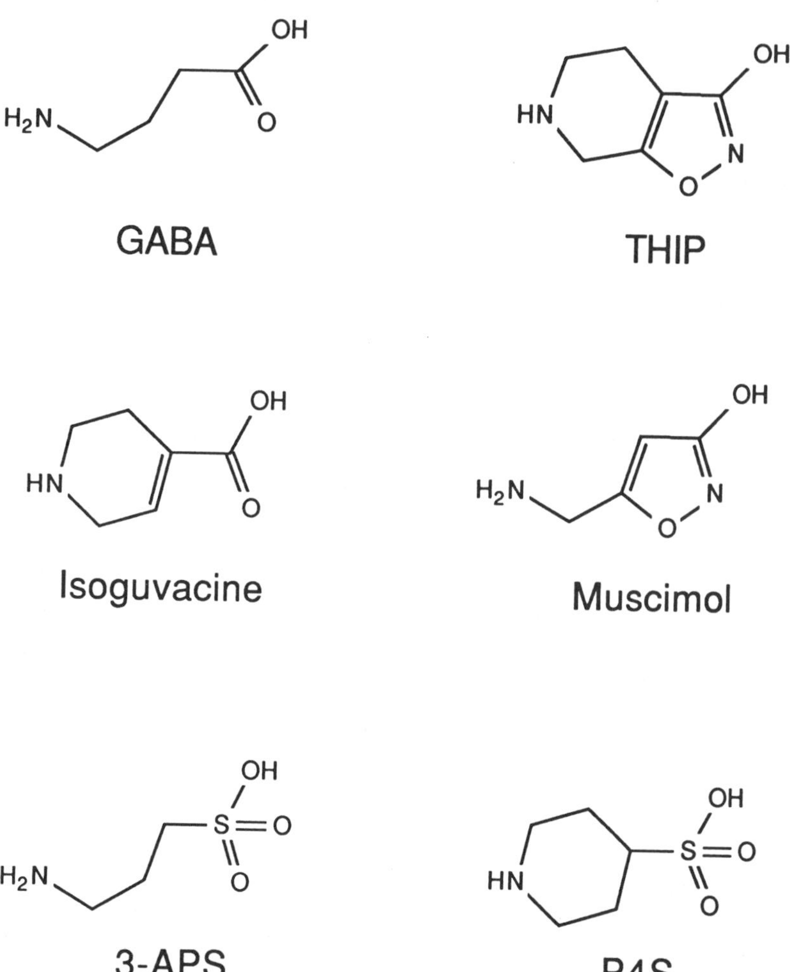

FIG. 3. Structures of $GABA_A$ receptor agonists.

A receptor subtype results in the hyperpolarization of the target cell, which is largely due to an increase in the chloride conductance of the postsynaptic membrane (Curtis *et al.*, 1968; Kelly *et al.*, 1969). The relative chloride concentration gradient across the membrane will clearly have a marked effect on the response, for when the ion channel is opened chloride will flow down its electrochemical gradient. There are examples where GABA causes a depolarization (Adams and Brown, 1975; Gallagher *et al.*, 1978) via the same ionic mechanism. The subject is lucidly discussed by Simmonds (1984). Two GABA molecules are required to bind to the GABA-A site in order to induce a channel opening event, as evidenced by Hill coefficients approaching 2 in dose response studies (Barker and Ransom, 1978; Nistri and Constanti, 1979). This is not apparent from the many radioligand binding studies carried out with a variety of agonists; however, recent evidence suggests that cooperativity can be observed in such experiments if they are carried out under more physiological conditions (Kardos *et al.*, 1985). Subsequent studies have analyzed the detail of the channel opening events in cultured cells using both fluctuation and patch clamp techniques (Barker *et al.*, 1982; Hamill *et al.*, 1983; McBurney, 1984; Bormann and Clapham, 1985; McBurney *et al.*, 1985; Bormann *et al.*, 1987). Current–voltage relationships obtained from whole cell measurements indicate that channel gating is voltage-sensitive with a reversal potential consistent with chloride-selective channels. Studies of anion selectivity of the channel indicate that the pore diameter is probably about 5.6 Å, as both phosphate and propionate are able to permeate the channel. The channels show multiple conductance states. In excised cell patches, bathed on both sides with 145 mM chloride solution, four conductance states are found, though the one with the greatest frequency (approximately 80%) exhibited a conductance of 30 pS (Bormann *et al.*, 1987).

The work that led to the discovery of the GABA-B receptor was carried out in the periphery. Bowery and his colleagues noted that GABA was able to depress the release of noradrenaline elicited from atrial muscle in a dose-dependent manner. The amino acid was effective whether the release was induced by either transmural stimulation or potassium ions. The effect of GABA was not blocked by either bicuculline or picrotoxin, both of which are able to completely block GABA-A responses, and the rank order of potency of a range of GABA agonists was completely different from that observed in GABA-A responses. The most outstanding finding was that (−) baclofen was equipotent with GABA while the (+) isomer was about 100 times weaker (Bowery and Hudson, 1979; Bowery *et al.*, 1981).

The demonstration that binding sites with these recognition characteristics were present in the mammalian brain suggested that indeed it was a true subtype of the GABA receptor and it was designated GABA-B (Hill and Bowery, 1981). These binding sites were further characterized when the binding of GABA was markedly increased in the presence of either calcium or magnesium ions; this calcium-dependent binding exhibited the ligand recognition characteristics of the GABA-B subtype (Bowery *et al.*, 1983). The distribution of the GABA-B receptor subtype has been studied in the mammalian CNS using either ^{3}H-GABA or ^{3}H-baclofen and shown to be markedly different from that of the A subtype (Bowery *et al.*, 1984; Bowery *et al.*, 1987). The GABA-B receptor is not linked to chloride channels; the affinity of agonist ligands for this receptor are decreased, however, by GTP. Although agonist ligands do not increase the basal level of cAMP, they are able to markedly enhance the ability of several other neurotransmitters to stimulate the production of this nucleotide (Karbon *et al.*, 1984; Karbon and Enna, 1985; Hill, 1985; Asano *et al.*, 1985; Watling and Bristow, 1986). The most potent GABA-B receptor antagonist so far identified is 3-amino-2-(p-chlorophenyl) propyl phosphonic acid (phaclofen; Kerr *et al.*, 1987), however, its relatively low potency and limited solubility have restricted its experimental use. Its antagonism is thought to be competitive.

The third type of GABA receptor that has been defined in the CNS is the autoreceptor. It appears that the function of this receptor is to control the release of GABA from its presynaptic terminals (Mitchell and Martin, 1978a; Snodgrass, 1978; Arbilla *et al.*, 1979). The pharmacological specificity of this receptor remains ill-defined. The recognition characteristics appear to be very similar to those of the GABA-A subtype, though delta-aminolaevulinic acid is a more potent agonist at the autoreceptor than at the A subtype (Brennan and Cantrill, 1979; Brennan *et al.*, 1981). The action of the agonists at the autoreceptor result in a decrease in the amount of GABA released from the presynaptic terminal; the antagonists, such as bicuculline, increase the release which occurs in response to a given stimulus. It has not so far been possible to design compounds which effectively differentiate between the autoreceptor and the GABA-A subtype.

While there is considerable neurochemical evidence to differentiate these GABA receptor subtypes, there remain some interesting questions with particular regard to their subclassification. Of particular concern to us here is the relationship between the benzodiazepines and the GABA-A receptor. While the distribution of these two receptor binding sites displays a good degree of similarity, there are areas within the CNS which exhibit marked differences. The granule cell layer of the cerebellum shows about five times the number of GABA binding sites than the molecular layer (Bowery *et al.*, 1987), while the benzodiazepine sites are approximately evenly distributed between the two regions (Young and Kuhar, 1980), though some interspecies variation has been noted. There is little evidence to support the contention that benzodiazepine responses are mediated by other than via GABA-A type receptors, but the reverse remains a possibility, i.e., some GABA-A receptors are not modulated by the benzodiazepines.

2.6. Summary

GABA is the major inhibitory transmitter of the mammalian central nervous system. It produces its effects through three quite distinct receptor systems. It has been argued that these may themselves be further subdivided, and evidence to define the precise mechanisms by which these receptors manipulate cellular excitability continues to appear in the literature. The benzodiazepines, however, appear to produce their effects through interactions with the GABA-A subtype of receptor; it is the evidence for this conclusion which will now be addressed.

3. THE MECHANISM OF ACTION OF THE BENZODIAZEPINES

3.1. Electrophysiological Studies

In retrospect, the first indications that the benzodiazepines produced their effects through modulation of GABA-mediated responses came from the work of Schmidt and co-workers in 1967. They showed that intravenous diazepam produced a dose-dependent increase in the amplitude of the dorsal root potential (DRP) elicited by cutaneous nerve stimulation in the spinalized cat (Schmidt *et al.*, 1967). It is now believed that the primary afferent depolarization (PAD), which underlies the DRP, is produced by the release of GABA from interneurons onto primary afferent nerve terminals; the so-called presynaptic inhibition (Curtis and Johnston, 1974; Levy, 1977). At the time when Schmidt performed his experiments, however, the concept of presynaptic inhibition was not universally accepted and the notion that GABA was the neurotransmitter involved had not yet been suggested. The implications of these findings were, therefore, not immediately apparent. Subsequently, however, the experiments were repeated and extended to show that the effect of the benzodiazepines, in this preparation, could be abolished by the prior treatment of the animals with thiosemicarbazide, a GABA synthesis inhibitor. Further, the effect of the benzodiazepines on the DRP could be inhibited, in a surmountable manner, with the GABA-A antagonist bicuculline (Polc *et al.*, 1974). The action of the benzodiazepines on the DRP had an absolute requirement for a functional GABAergic system.

While it was clear from these later studies that GABA-mediated presynaptic inhibition in the spinal cord was facilitated by the benzodiazepines, there was no evidence that the phenomenon generalized to postsynaptic inhibition. Postsynaptic inhibition in the spinal cord was thought to be mediated by glycine (Curtis and Johnston, 1974). However, in the dorsal column nuclei, the cuneothalamic relay cells are known to suffer both pre- and postsynaptic inhibition which is mediated by GABA (Curtis and Johnston, 1974). The demonstration that diazepam was able to increase both types of inhibition in this structure (Polc and Haefely, 1976) suggested that the facilitation of GABA-mediated transmission by the benzodiazepines may be a general phenomenon.

In the hippocampus, recurrent inhibition onto the main output cells of this structure, pyramidal cells and the dentate granule cells, is known to occur. This is thought to be GABA mediated. The benzodiazepines facilitate this inhibition (Adamec *et al.*, 1981; Lee *et al.*, 1979; Tsuchiya and Fukushima, 1978; Wolf and Haas, 1977).

In the cerebellum, four of the five types of identified neuron are inhibitory and are thought to use GABA as the transmitter. The neuronal circuitary in this structure is complex, but inhibition of the Purkinje cells, the only output neurons of the cerebellum, can be studied by surface stimulation. Single electrical stimuli applied to the surface of the cerebellar cortex result in activation of the parallel fibers, which are the axons of the excitatory granule cells. This results in the monosynaptic activation of the Purkinje cell. After a short latency, the firing rate of the Purkinje cell is depressed due to the recruitment of the inhibitory effects from GABAergic stellate and basket cells. Benzodiazepines, applied either locally or systemically, facilitate this inhibition (Curtis *et al.*, 1976; Geller *et al.*, 1978; Lippa *et al.*, 1979; Okamoto and Sakai, 1979; Pieri and Haefely, 1976; Sinclair *et al.*, 1982).

Similar examples can be found in many other brain areas including the cerebral cortex, the hypothalamus, the olfactory bulb and the late phase of recurrent Renshaw cell inhibition in the spinal cord (Polc and Haefely, 1982); this late phase is thought to be GABA-mediated (Cullheim and Kellerth, 1981). There is now, therefore, a considerable amount of electrophysiological evidence that all known GABA-mediated inhibition, whether postsynaptic or presynaptic, is facilitated by the agonist benzodiazepines and for a further detailed discussion of this subject the reader is referred to Haefely and Polc (1986).

3.2. Biochemical Studies

In parallel with electrophysiological investigations, evidence began to accumulate from the biochemical approach that GABA formed an important link in the actions of the benzodiazepines. In the early to mid-1970s there was much interest in attempts to define the importance of individual neurotransmitters by studies designed to investigate their rate of usage or the neurochemical consequences of the elevation of their levels in the CNS.

It was shown that the net activity of the cerebellar Purkinje cell was related to its content of cyclic GMP (Costa *et al.*, 1975; 1976). Activation of the Purkinje cell results in an increase in its cyclic GMP content and inhibition results in a decrease in the content of this second messenger (Biggio *et al.*, 1977). Both muscimol and diazepam caused a decrease in the content of cyclic GMP of the cerebellar cortex. Further, pretreatment of the animals with isoniazid, an inhibitor of GAD, caused an increase in the content of cyclic GMP, presumably due to a reduction of GABA-mediated inhibition. This effect of isoniazid could be completely reversed by muscimol. However, although diazepam could counteract the effect of isoniazid if the fall in levels of GABA in the cerebellum were limited to 30%, a depletion of the neurotransmitter content greater than this resulted in diazepam being unable to prevent the effects of isoniazid. The explanation accepted for this phenomenon was that the benzodiazepines required a functional GABA system to produce their effects on cyclic GMP levels in the cerebellum; it was unable to act as a GABA agonist (Costa *et al.*, 1978). There remained two possibilities: either the benzodiazepines increased the release of GABA in response to a given stimulus or these drugs amplified the signal transduction mechanism at some point beyond the postsynaptic GABA receptor.

To differentiate between these two alternatives, studies were conducted on the turnover of GABA in the CNS (Mao *et al.*, 1977). This group was able to demonstrate that while neither muscimol nor diazepam altered the steady state levels of GABA in the caudate nucleus, nucleus accumbens, or the globus pallidus, the turnover rate of the neurotransmitter was reduced in the former two regions. These results were inconsistent with the notion that diazepam increased the release of GABA.

Later direct studies showed that while some benzodiazepines were able to facilitate the potassium-stimulated release of GABA in certain brain regions at micromolar concentrations, not all the clinically active benzodiazepines exhibited this property. Only those compounds which possessed an alkyl substituent on the N-1 nitrogen produced this facilitation (Mitchell and Martin, 1978b and unpublished results).

In 1976, a substantial body of evidence had accrued to suggest that the benzodiazepines produced their effects by modulation of GABA-mediated transmission in the mammalian CNS. It was clear that they did not act directly as GABA agonists nor by the facilitation of the release of this transmitter, but the precise mechanism by which this occurred remained a matter of conjecture. However, a technical advance was about to occur which was to pervade the investigations with these compounds for the next decade.

4. THE BENZODIAZEPINE RECEPTOR

4.1. Initial Radioligand Binding Studies

The demonstration of saturable, specific, high-affinity binding of ^{3}H-diazepam to membrane fractions obtained from the rat CNS in 1977 was a watershed in the investigations into the mechanism of action of the benzodiazepines (Bosmann *et al.*, 1977; Mohler and Okada, 1977b, 1977c; Squires and Braestrup, 1977). These binding sites were found in the CNS of both animals (Braestrup and Squires, 1978b; Lippa *et al.*, 1978; Mackerer *et al.*, 1978; Squires and Braestrup, 1977; Muller *et al.*, 1978) and man (Braestrup and Squires, 1978a; Braestrup *et al.*, 1977; Mohler and Okada, 1978; Mohler *et al.*, 1978b).

Diazepam binding can be displaced from its binding sites on CNS membranes in a competitive manner by other benzodiazepines of similar structure. There is a very high correlation (0.99) between the affinity estimates made in these experiments from cerebral cortical membranes obtained from both rat and man. Attempts were therefore made to compare the apparent affinity constants of a series of benzodiazepine analogues, obtained from such competition experiments carried out in human cerebral cortex membranes, with their potency in a variety of pharmacological tests. The correlation coefficient with cat muscle relaxant activity was 0.92, while that for the antagonism of pentylenetetrazole-induced convulsions in mice was 0.90. There was, however, no significant correlation with the activity of these compounds in several other tests, including electric shock induced convulsions in mice, the taming effect in vicious monkeys and a series of conditioned avoidance tasks (Mohler and Okada, 1978; Braestrup *et al.*, 1977). Significant correlation coefficients were also obtained when the average therapeutic dose in man was used as the measure of pharmacological potency (Mohler and Okada, 1978; Braestrup *et al.*, 1977). This latter observation is surprising when one considers the trauma that a drug must undergo prior to arrival at its site of action, in this case, the CNS. In fact closer observation of their data indicates that those benzodiazepines which undergo metabolism, such as medazepam, are outlyers in the data set. Nevertheless, the outcome of these investigations gave confidence that the benzodiazepine binding site was, in fact, part of the pharmacological receptor through which these compounds produced their overt effects.

It was clear from the initial experiments that diazepam binding could not be demonstrated *in vitro* at physiological temperatures. The use of ^{3}H-flunitrazepam (Fig. 2) in such experiments, however, revealed specific high-affinity binding sites at these elevated temperatures. Flunitrazepam has an affinity for the binding site about four times that of diazepam, but the temperature dependence of the off rate of diazepam is nearly five times that of flunitrazepam at 30°C, while at 0°C the ratio of the off rates is eightfold. The result of this is that during the filtration procedure used to separate the free from the bound ligand, at the termination of the assay, some of the diazepam dissociates. At elevated temperatures the dissociation is so pronounced that little specific binding remains subsequent to filtration and washing.

Flunitrazepam appears to bind to the same population of receptors as diazepam at 0°C and the rank order of displacement of both ligands by a series of nine clinically active benzodiazepines was similar (Braestrup and Squires, 1978a). Since that time flunitrazepam has been the radioligand of choice to study the binding of these agonists.

4.2. Localization

4.2.1. *Peripheral Versus Central Type Sites*

High-affinity binding sites for both ^{3}H-diazepam and ^{3}H-flunitrazepam are found in the CNS, liver, kidney, lung, heart and peritoneal mast cells (Braestrup and Squires, 1977; Mohler and Okada, 1977c; Taniguchi *et al.*, 1980; Davies and Huston, 1981; Gallager *et al.*, 1981; Regan *et al.*, 1981). The binding sites in peripheral tissues, however, exhibit quite different recognition characteristics from those in the CNS. Clonazepam (Fig. 2), with a very high affinity for the central sites, exhibits a very low affinity for the peripheral type site, while the reverse is the case for Ro 5-4864 (Fig. 2). No function has yet been proposed for these peripheral type binding sites though they appear to be associated with the mitochondrial outer membrane (Anholt *et al.*, 1986). The peripheral type binding site is found in the central nervous system though it may easily be resolved in standard binding assay protocols by the use of clonazepam to define nonspecific binding. ^{3}H-Ro 5-4864 has been used to study the peripheral type of benzodiazepine binding site (Marangos *et al.*,

1982; Schoemaker *et al.*, 1983; Moingeon *et al.*, 1983; Beaumont *et al.*, 1984). The isoquinoline carboxamide derivative PK 11195 has also been used for the same purpose (Benavides *et al.*, 1983).

There is also a high capacity low affinity binding of the benzodiazepines to human serum albumin. The recognition properties of this site are also quite distinct from those of the CNS specific site (Sjodin *et al.*, 1976; Lucek and Coutinho, 1976; Mohler and Okada, 1977c; Albic-Kolbah *et al.*, 1979).

The remainder of this discussion will address only the central type of benzodiazepine binding site.

4.2.2. *Regional Distribution*

The benzodiazepine binding sites are unevenly distributed in the CNS of both animals (Squires and Braestrup, 1977; Mohler and Okada, 1977b; Muller *et al.*, 1978) and man (Braestrup *et al.*, 1977; Mohler and Okada, 1978; Speth *et al.*, 1978). The receptor capacity is highest in cortical regions (approximately 1 pmol/mg protein) and cerebellum (0.7 pmol/mg protein), with intermediate values in the thalamus, hypothalamus, and caudate nucleus; the lowest levels are in the pons, medulla and spinal cord (0.1 to 0.2 pmol/mg protein). It is almost absent from white matter. The apparent affinity of the site is almost uniform throughout the brain although minor differences do occur (Supavilai and Karobath, 1980b).

Within the major anatomical areas available to dissection methods, there are considerable variations of receptor density which are revealed by light microscopic autoradiographic techniques (Kuhar, 1978). These studies have mapped the distribution of benzodiazepine binding sites in some detail throughout the CNS (Richards *et al.*, 1983; Schlumpf *et al.*, 1983) and have revealed, in addition, subtle interspecies differences (Young and Kuhar, 1979; 1980; Biscoe *et al.*, 1984). The use of tritium sensitive film, together with computer-assisted densitometry, have allowed quantitative pharmacological characterization of these sites (Palacios *et al.*, 1981; Penney *et al.*, 1981; Unnerstall *et al.*, 1982). Central type binding sites have also been located in bovine adrenal chromaffin cells (Kataoka *et al.*, 1984) and in rat pituitary (Brown and Martin, 1984a).

4.2.3. *Cellular Localization*

Subcellular fractionation studies have demonstrated that the benzodiazepine binding site is associated largely with the synaptosomal fraction and, after osmotic shock, with the crude synaptic membranes (Braestrup and Squires, 1977; Mohler and Okada, 1978; Mackerer *et al.*, 1978). Attempts have also been made to locate specific neuronal populations which express the binding site. Two strategies have been used to achieve this: the first, the use of neurotoxic agents and the second, the investigation of mutant animal strains with a known anatomical deficit.

Kainic acid injected into the cerebellum, corpus striatum or the substantia nigra resulted in the loss of about 50% of the benzodiazepine binding sites (Braestrup and Squires, 1978a; Braestrup *et al.*, 1979; Chang *et al.*, 1980; Biggio *et al.*, 1980). In the hippocampus the similar use of ibotenic acid produced a decrease of only 30% (Fuxe *et al.*, 1981). Benzodiazepine binding assays carried out in the neurologically mutant mouse strains “staggerer” and “nervous” indicated that the sites were present on the Purkinje cells, but, due to the incomplete loss clearly other cell types were involved. There is a marked decrease in the number of benzodiazepine binding sites found in the putamen and caudate nucleus in Huntington’s disease (Mohler and Okada, 1978; Reisine *et al.*, 1980), a degenerative disorder characterized largely by a diffuse loss of neurons particularly from the striatum.

More direct evidence for the neuronal localization of the benzodiazepine binding site was obtained from autoradiography in combination with electron microscopy. This was carried out by the irreversible labelling of the benzodiazepine binding site using ^{3}H-flunitrazepam as a photoaffinity label (for a detailed discussion of this technique see later section). The radioligand was injected into rats *in vivo*; the brain was subsequently removed, tissue sections cut and the brain slices subsequently exposed to UV light. Silver grains were found located exclusively over regions of synaptic contact in the cerebral and cerebellar cortices and the hippocampus. There was no evidence for a generalized location of benzodiazepine binding sites over glial cells (Mohler *et al.*, 1980).

There is considerable evidence, therefore, that the benzodiazepine binding sites in the mammalian CNS are associated with neurons. This conclusion is supported by tissue culture studies of both neurons and glia which have yielded the observations expected from such a hypothesis (Braestrup *et al.*, 1978; Syapin and Skolnick, 1979; Baraldi *et al.*, 1979; Huang *et al.*, 1980; McCarthy and Harden, 1981; White *et al.*, 1981).

4.3. Phylogeny and Ontogeny

Phylogenetically, the benzodiazepine binding sites appear to have developed rather late. The recognition properties of the site in species lower than the bony fishes is atypical (Nielsen *et al.*, 1978; Fernholm *et al.*, 1979). This is quite distinct from the high affinity GABA binding sites which are present in cyclostomes and chondrichthyes (Mann and Enna, 1980); in these the benzodiazepine binding sites are absent. This is in general agreement with the electrophysiological studies in which responses to GABA can be found in invertebrates (Takeuchi and Takeuchi, 1975), though the effects of this neurotransmitter are not potentiated by chlordiazepoxide (Mathews and Wickelgren, 1979).

In the rat the ontogenesis of the benzodiazepine binding site is found early; specific ^{3}H-diazepam binding could be detected eight days before birth, while at birth the levels were already about 35% of the adult value, which was reached by four weeks (Braestrup and Nielsen, 1978). In a postnatal study these results were broadly confirmed, although differences were found in the rate of the development between the cerebral cortex and the cerebellum (Candy and Martin, 1979). The autoradiographic studies of Richards and coworkers have since provided much more detailed information. It is clear from these investigations that the development of the benzodiazepine binding sites in different brain regions parallels axonal growth and synaptogenesis, occurring much earlier in the spinal cord than in the cerebral cortex or cerebellum. In the latter structure the development of the benzodiazepine binding sites was closely associated with that of the Purkinje cell dendritic tree in the molecular layer (Richards *et al.*, 1983; Schlumpf *et al.*, 1983). This is in marked contrast to the development of high affinity binding sites for GABA in this structure, which followed that of the granule cells (Palacios and Kuhar, 1982). Although there appears to be a disparity in the rates of development here between GABA high affinity binding and that of the benzodiazepines, the modulation of ^{3}H-flunitrazepam binding by GABA *in vitro* seems to remain relatively constant throughout this period (Palacios *et al.*, 1979; Mallorga *et al.*, 1980; Regan *et al.*, 1980). It may be more rational, however, to compare the development of benzodiazepine binding sites with low affinity GABA sites which can be studied autoradiographically with ^{3}H-bicuculline methochloride (Olsen *et al.*, 1984). This has not yet been done.

5. CHARACTERIZATION OF THE BENZODIAZEPINE RECEPTOR

5.1. Neurochemical Characterization

The initial studies carried out with the benzodiazepine binding site suggested that it was indeed an integral part of the pharmacological receptor through which these compounds exerted their effects. These investigations suggested that only compounds with the benzodiazepine structure were able to displace ^{3}H-diazepam from its binding sites on brain membranes (Squires and Braestrup, 1977; Braestrup and Squires, 1978b; Mackerer *et al.*, 1978), and further that this interaction was stereospecific (Mohler and Okada, 1977c). The radioligand binding appeared to obey simple mass action kinetics, suggesting a homogeneous population of noninteracting sites. These conclusions retain their credence, but detailed investigations over the past several years have shown that the situation is a good deal more complicated.

5.2. Non-Benzodiazepine Ligands

The first non-benzodiazepine structure found to completely displace the benzodiazepines from their binding sites was the triazolopyridazine, CL 218872 (Fig. 4). This compound was found to have an apparent Ki value of about 70nM in competition experiments with either ^{3}H-diazepam of ^{3}H-flunitrazepam; the Hill coefficient, however, was significantly less than unity (Squires *et al.*, 1979). The hypothesis advanced to explain this observation was that the benzodiazepine receptor population was heterogeneous. The benzodiazepines were unable to differentiate between the two putative subtypes but CL 218872 bound to one population of sites with a Ki value about two orders of magnitude greater than to the other. The data aroused considerable interest when the same group reported that CL 218872 possessed anxiolytic and anticonvulsant activity but was devoid of sedative effects (Lippa *et al.*, 1979). This spectrum of activity was in marked contrast to the classical benzodiazepines, which are all sedative. The possibility that ligands for this receptor could be developed with a more restricted pharmacological profile was clearly an exciting idea, though subsequent investigations have suggested that the sedative properties of this triazolopyridazine are quite marked (Oakley *et al.*, 1984).

Later studies with the esters of beta-carboline-3-carboxylic acid (Fig. 5) were subsequently shown to exhibit very similar binding characteristics. In displacement experiments carried out with ^{3}H-flunitrazepam, the ethyl ester (beta-CCE), caused complete inhibition of the radioligand binding, although the potency was about four times greater in the cerebellum than in the hippocampus. The Hill coefficient in the hippocampus, 0.75, was again significantly less than unity but this was not the case in the cerebellum, where the displacement appeared to obey simple mass action kinetics (Nielsen and Braestrup, 1980). The data was again rationalized in terms of multiple benzodiazepine receptors. In the cerebellum, the beta-CCE was postulated to bind to the BZ1 subtype with high affinity; this anatomical region consisted almost entirely of this subtype. The hippocampus, however, contained an equal proportion of another receptor subtype, BZ2, which exhibited a lower affinity for the beta-carboline. The classical benzodiazepines were unable to differentiate between these two receptor subtypes, as their affinity at each was identical. Subsequently, beta-CCE, together with its methyl and n-propyl ester analogues, have become available labelled with tritium, and it has been confirmed that these ligands do appear to preferentially label a subpopulation of benzodiazepine receptors with high affinity (Braestrup and Nielsen, 1980; 1981a; Nielsen *et al.*, 1981). It is difficult to characterize the lower affinity site in any detail due to the rapid increase in nonspecific binding at the higher ligand concentrations in saturation experiments (Mitchell and Wilson, 1984); displacement analyses are consistent with such a hypothesis (Toll *et al.*, 1984). These types of data offer no conclusive proof of receptor heterogeneity and alternative explanations are equally viable (see later section and Martin *et al.*, 1983; Chiu and Rosenberg, 1983b).

The pyrazoloquinolinones (Fig. 6) also displace the benzodiazepines from their binding sites with very high affinity (Czernik *et al.*, 1982; Yokoyama, *et al.*, 1982). The first of this

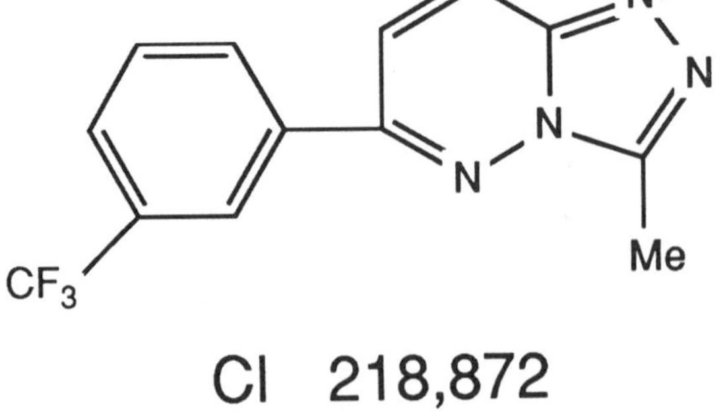

Cl 218,872

Fig. 4. Structure of the triazolopyridazine CL 218, 872.

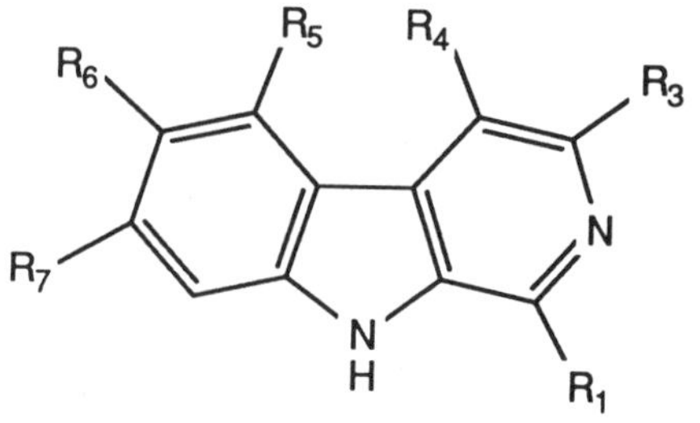

	R_1	R_3	R_4	R_5	R_6	R_7
Beta-CCM	H	COOMe	H	H	H	H
Beta-CCE	H	COOEt	H	H	H	H
Beta-CCPr	H	COOn-Pr	H	H	H	H
DMCM	H	COOMe	H	H	OMe	OMe
ZK93426	H	COOEt	Me	O-iPr	H	H
ZK91296	H	COOEt	alkyl	aryl	H	H
ZK93423	H	COOEt	alkyl	H	aryl	H

alkyl = $-CH_2OMe$; aryl = $-OCH_2$phenyl

FIG. 5. Structures of beta-carboline-3-carboxylic acid esters.

Zopiclone

Quazepam

PK 8165

Ro 15-1788

CGS 9896 R=Cl
CGS 9895 R=OMe
CGS 8216 R=H

Tracazolate R=HN-nC_4H_9

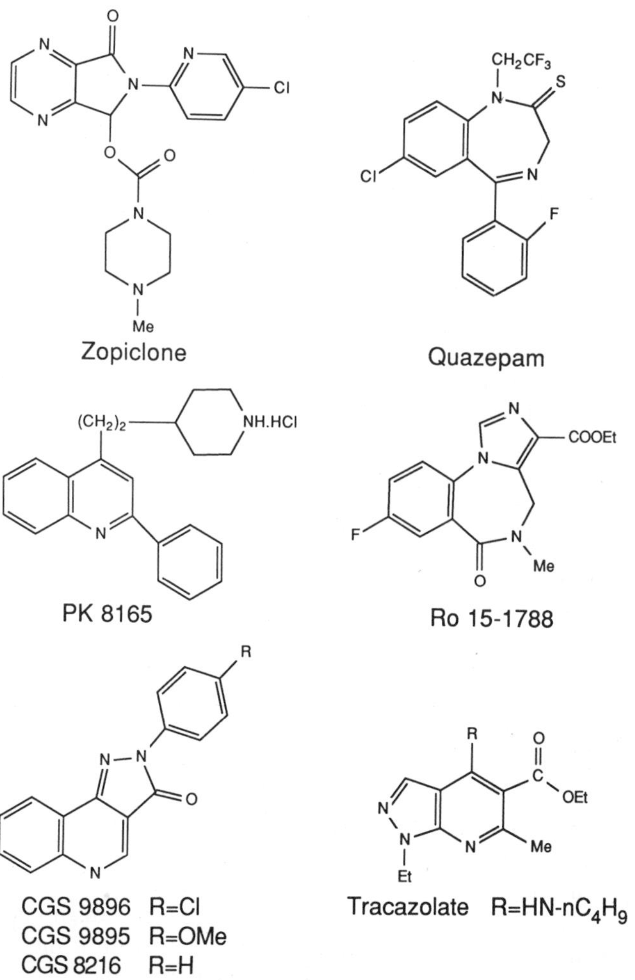

FIG. 6. Structures of some compounds which interact with the $GABA_A$-benzodiazepine receptor complex.

series to be described, ^{3}H-CGS 8216, was displaced by a number of benzodiazepines in the same rank order as that found in competition experiments with ^{3}H-flunitrazepam, suggesting that the two ligands bound to the same population of sites. In a series of saturation experiments, however, the Bmax values obtained with CGS 8216 were consistently below those found for flunitrazepam. The displacement of ^{3}H-flunitrazepam by CGS 8216 is not strictly competitive and the Hill coefficients obtained in membranes from both the cerebellum and hippocampus of the rat are significantly greater than unity (Baker and Martin, unpublished observations).

The imidazobenzodiazepine, Ro 15-1788 (Fig. 6), also displays a high potency in the displacement of ^{3}H-flunitrazepam binding. The interaction appears to be strictly competitive and studies with the tritium labelled compound indicate that the distribution of its binding sites are identical with those of the classical benzodiazepines (Hunkeler *et al.*, 1981).

Compounds of several other structural classes have also been found to displace the benzodiazepines from their binding sites. These include the sedative hypnotic zopiclone (Fig. 6; Blanchard *et al.*, 1979) and its analogue suriclone (Blanchard and Joulou, 1983), the isoquinoline derivatives PK 8165 and PK 9084 (Fig. 6; Lefur *et al.*, 1981) and the imidazopyridines EMD 39593 and EMD 41717 (Skolnick *et al.*, 1983).

5.3. Irreversible Labelling

Incubation of flunitrazepam with either CNS membrane preparations or brain slices, followed by irradiation of the material with UV light, results in the irreversible attachment of a fragment of flunitrazepam to the protein matrix in the vicinity of the recognition site (Battersby *et al.*, 1979; Mohler *et al.*, 1980). This procedure of photoaffinity labelling of the benzodiazepine receptor has proved extremely useful, not only for the autoradiographic localization of the benzodiazepine binding sites, but also to probe further the mechanisms by which the different ligand classes interact with the receptor complex.

The precise nature of the interaction remains uncertain. It is clear, however, that only those benzodiazepines with a nitro substituent in the 7 position can be used in the interaction (Johnson and Yamamura, 1979; Sieghart and Mohler, 1982). The amount of irreversible labelling is dependent on the concentration of the flunitrazepam in the reaction and there is an absolute requirement for the ligand to be bound to its recognition site before the irreversible labelling can occur; it can be completely blocked by the excess presence of other active benzodiazepines.

Subsequent to photoaffinity labelling and removal of the excess unused ligand, saturation analysis with either ^{3}H-diazepam or ^{3}H-flunitrazepam reveals that up to 90% of the high affinity binding sites have been lost, although it has not proved possible to reduce this capacity further. The stoichiometry of the reaction is difficult to ascertain. If the photoaffinity labelling is carried out with ^{3}H-flunitrazepam, a maximum 25% of the total number of sites available appear to be labelled (Thomas and Tallman, 1981); under certain conditions this figure may be increased to 40% (Herblin and Mechem, 1984). Even though the precise figure remains a matter of dispute, it is clear that the loss of the high affinity site, subsequent to photolabelling, is markedly greater than the number of sites labelled during the reaction. These observations are consistent with a cooperative interaction within the binding site population.

This irreversible labelling of the benzodiazepine receptor causes a drastic modification of the recognition properties of the binding site for the classical agonist benzodiazepines, with up to 90% of the high affinity sites apparently being lost. However, saturation analysis with ^{3}H-beta-CCE, the propyl ester or ^{3}H-Ro 15-1788, subsequent to photoaffinity labelling, suggest that the recognition site for these ligands is not so compromised. If the modified receptor population is labelled with one of these radioligands it is clear that the agonist benzodiazepines can still cause displacement, but with a much reduced affinity (Brown and Martin, 1982; Gee and Yamamura, 1982b; Hirsch, 1982; Karobath and Supavilai, 1982; Mohler, 1982). It has been suggested that the different types of ligand, agonist, antagonist and inverse agonist (see later section for explanation of these terms) can be differentiated by this procedure: after photoaffinity labelling the agonists show a reduced affinity, the antagonists exhibit no change while in the case of the inverse agonists an increase in affinity is apparent (Braestrup *et al.*, 1983). This has proved to be not generally correct. Within a series of pyrazoloquinolinones, compounds have been identified which exhibit agonist, antagonist or inverse agonist activity; they all suffer only a slight reduction in their affinity constants as a result of photoaffinity modification of the receptor population (Brown and Martin, 1983; 1984b).

This observation has led to some interesting speculations about the recognition site characteristics of the different ligand classes. The classical benzodiazepines function as agonists at their receptor; they cause a clear functional response. The interaction of an agonist with its receptor can be envisaged as an initial recognition process of the ligand, and then subsequently, or in some concerted fashion, a conformational change occurs in the protein as the first stage in the initiation of the effector sequence of events that leads to an overt response (Franklin, 1980). A marked loss in the affinity of the agonist benzodiazepines as a result of photoaffinity modification of the receptor population could be the result of changes in the recognition site process or the effector sequence. It has been proposed that the increase in the affinity of compounds for the benzodiazepine receptor, seen *in vitro* on the addition of GABA to the incubation medium, is indicative of an agonist profile (see later section). It has now been shown that the GABA facilitation of benzodiazepine binding remains unimpaired after photoaffinity labelling, suggesting that the modification which occurs is the result of the modification of the recognition site process and not its effector sequence (Brown and Martin, 1983; 1984b; Martin and Brown, 1983; Borea *et al.*, 1984). Such an explanation is also consistent with electrophysiological experiments in which photoaffinity labelling of cells in tissue culture showed markedly reduced responses to chlordiazepoxide compared to cells not so treated (Chan *et al.*, 1983).

In a series of very detailed experiments, carried out over several years, Sieghart and colleagues have shown that the polypeptide chains that constitute the benzodiazepine receptor are apparently different in several brain regions (Sieghart and Karobath, 1980; Sieghart and Drexler, 1983). The methods used here relied upon the photoaffinity labelling of membrane preparations with ^{3}H-flunitrazepam, solubilization of the affinity labelled material under denaturing conditions and the separation of these fragments using polyacrylamide gel electrophoresis. The cerebellum was found to consist almost entirely of a fragment with a weight of 51,000 daltons, while in the hippocampus an additional band of 55,000 daltons was found. The ontogenetic development of the labelled polypeptide chains in the cerebellum is interesting. While the adult rat cerebellum showed the single labelled polypeptide described above, in the 3-day-old animal several bands were seen in the same size range as those found in the adult rat hippocampus, for example (Sieghart, 1986). The significance of this development pattern has yet to be elucidated.

Later studies have also shown that Ro 15-4513 may be used as photoaffinity label. The characteristics of this molecule are quite different. More than 90% of the benzodiazepine binding sites can be labelled with this ligand, a property quite different from that of flunitrazepam. The pattern of polypeptide labelling found with this compound was essentially identical to that found for flunitrazepam in all brain areas except the cerebellum. In this latter region an additional band was labelled, with an apparent size of 57,000 daltons. However, this was not thought to be part of the benzodiazepine receptor complex as irreversible labelling of this peptide could not be prevented by excess diazepam (Mohler *et al.*, 1984).

The use of irreversible alkylating ligands for the benzodiazepine receptor have also been reported (Rice *et al.*, 1979; Williams *et al.*, 1980). This work suggests that certain populations of the benzodiazepine receptors interact reversibly with the alkylating ligand, kenazepine, while with others an irreversible reaction occurs.

5.4. Kinetics and Thermodynamics of the Binding Interaction

A detailed study of ligand interactions under nonequilibrium conditions can give information of the mechanism by which the interactions occur. In the case of the benzodiazepine ligands, this has been studied in detail with diazepam (Chiu and Rosenberg, 1982), flunitrazepam (Chiu *et al.*, 1982; Quast and Mahlmann, 1982) and Ro 15-1788 (Chiu and Rosenberg, 1983a, 1983b; Brown and Martin, 1984c).

Biphasic association kinetics have been observed with both diazepam and flunitrazepam (Chiu *et al.*, 1982; Quast and Mahlmann, 1982). The nuances of the interpretation of these data are beyond the scope of this review, but it is consistent with the idea that the agonists first bind to a recognition site complex, a reaction which takes place very rapidly; subsequent to this there is a slower isomerization step which may represent the first stage in the conformation change of the receptor protein, which presumably results from the interaction with these agonists.

In the case of the dissociation kinetics both monophasic (Quast and Mahlmann, 1982) and biphasic (Chiu *et al.*, 1982) dissociation of flunitrazepam have been reported. We have also observed biphasic dissociation kinetics of flunitrazepam from rat cerebellar membranes (Brown and Martin, unpublished). The reason for this discrepancy between the reports is not clear, although the experimental conditions were quite different. The data from such experiments really addresses the manner in which the ligand is removed from the binding site complex. Simplistically, we can imagine it dissociating from the initial recognition site complex or from the complex formed after the second slower isomerisation step. The data of Chiu *et al.* (1982) would suggest that the dissociation from these two ligand-receptor complexes takes place at different rates, but under different conditions the mechanism of dissociation may not be identical. Only further experimentation will allow us to define this more fully.

Similar experiments have been carried out with the putative antagonist ligand Ro 15-1788. Brown and Martin (1984c) have shown that the association of this compound with its binding site is strictly monophasic, as would be expected for an antagonist; presumably an antagonist does not induce a conformational change in the receptor protein. The dissociation kinetics in the cerebellum are again monophasic and consistent with the antagonist classification of Ro 15-1788. In membranes prepared from the rat hippocampus the dissociation kinetics are quite clearly biphasic. Biphasic dissociation kinetics of this ligand have also been observed in the cerebral cortex (Chiu and Rosenberg, 1983a). The conclusion is that the receptor complex in the cerebellum is distinct from that in the hippocampus. Do we then have to assume that Ro 15-1788 has some agonist activity in the hippocampus but not in the cerebellum? Such a conclusion would be very premature but there is evidence that this compound does have weak partial agonist activity (File and Pellow, 1987) and the receptor complex found in the cerebellum is distinct in a number of respects from that in the hippocampus (see next section).

While studies of the kinetics of the interaction of ligand with its receptor can give useful information about the mechanism by which this occurs, the study of the thermodynamics provides additional data concerning the energy barriers which control those mechanisms. Studies of this type with the beta-adrenergic receptor have led Weiland *et al.* (1979) to suggest that generality may exist in the thermodynamic parameters exhibited by agonist receptor interactions which can be differentiated from those of antagonists.

The equilibrium dissociation constant Kd is related to the free energy change (ΔG) on ligand receptor interaction by the equation:

$$\Delta G = RT \ln Kd$$

where R is the gas constant and T the absolute temperature. This free energy change can be resolved into an enthalpic (ΔH) and an entropic (ΔS) component by the Gibbs equation. Thus:

$$\Delta G = \Delta H - T\Delta S$$

hence,

$$\ln Kd = \frac{\Delta H}{RT} - \frac{\Delta S}{R}$$

By plotting ln *Kd* against $1/T$ (van't Hoff plot), estimates of both enthalpic and entropic components of the interaction can be obtained. Therefore, studies of the temperature dependence of the *Kd* values for various ligands will indicate the type of forces involved in their binding site interaction.

The majority of the benzodiazepine receptor ligands show a significant decrease in their affinity with increase in temperature (Speth *et al.*, 1979; Quast *et al.*, 1982; Doble, 1983), although the reverse is true for triazolam (Fig. 7; Kochman and Hirsch, 1982). The van't Hoff plots for flunitrazepam (Speth *et al.*, 1979; Quast *et al.*, 1982; Doble, 1983) and clonazepam (Mohler and Richards, 1981) show discontinuities. However, this is not a universal phenomenon, as it is not observed with diazepam and N-desmethyl diazepam (Quast *et al.*, 1982). Beta-CCE again shows this discontinuity (Doble, 1983), although Ro 15-1788 does not (Mohler and Richards, 1981). The explanation of these discontinuities remains unclear and no generalization about the phenomenon can be made at present.

At temperatures above the discontinuities (and throughout the temperature range for those ligands with linear van't Hoff plots), the binding interaction is largely enthalpically driven, though at lower temperatures a significant entropic component appears. The data is consistent with the idea that the interaction between ligand and its receptor does not rely completely on hydrophobic interaction.

The estimation of the enthalpic driving force of the reaction at 37°C for flunitrazepam, diazepam and its desmethyl analogue suggest values of between 40 and 50 kJ/mole (Quast *et al.*, 1982).

5.5. Multiple Receptors

In the final analysis, the singularity of a receptor population will be defined by the primary amino acid structure of the protein and, perhaps also, by the environment in which it resides. The primary structural information for the GABA-A-benzodiazepine receptor has recently become available (see section on molecular biology) but, as yet, analysis sufficiently detailed to address the question of receptor multiplicity has not been possible. In the absence of this type of data, a series of second-order criteria have been used to argue for the multiplicity of the benzodiazepine receptor system. These data have been derived from behavioral, electrophysiological and receptor binding studies, but have resulted in a

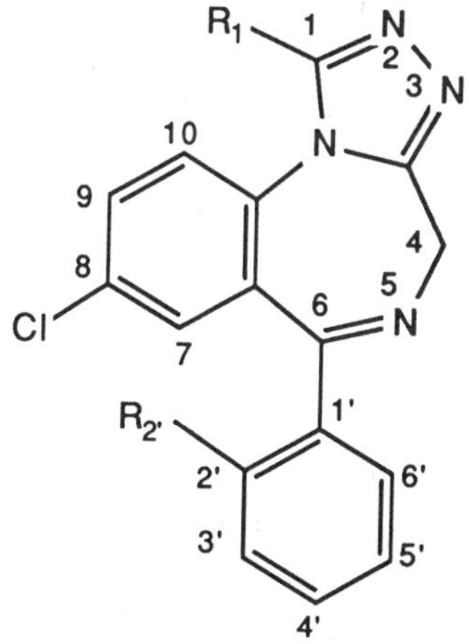

	R_1	$R_{2'}$
Triazolam	Me	Cl
Alprazolam	Me	H

Fig. 7. Structures of 1,2-annelated benzodiazepines.

considerable amount of confusion in the literature. The problem has been with the definition of receptor multiplicity. We can devise a set of functional criteria, from both the behavioral and electrophysiological studies, but we must not expect that data obtained from radioligand binding studies will explain functional observations. The interaction of a ligand with its recognition site is only the first stage in the sequence of events leading to an overt response from the system under observation. The affinity constants measured reflect only free energy changes that occur in this interaction of ligand with receptor. The neurochemical experiments which are used to define these constants are frequently carried out in membrane preparations obtained from broken cells and the secondary events which occur in the cell as part of the efficacy machinery may well be lost after such disruption. This, together with the nonphysiological conditions used, in terms of temperature and buffer, may well give a completely false impression of the reactions taking place. This is not to say that the binding assay is of no value; the data from such studies must be interpreted within a strict set of criteria which apply to this type of data. The conclusions reached may be used outside this defined environment but considerable caution must be exercised. This in mind we address the question of receptor multiplicity.

Behavioral and clinical data obtained with the classical agonist benzodiazepines is reviewed in some detail in other chapters of this book; suffice it to say here that all full agonists of this class appear to exhibit the same pharmacodynamic profile. It is possible that in the future partial agonists, with a more restricted spectrum of activity, will become available to the clinician, but at the present time these are only available for use in experimental animals.

Once we look at compounds from other chemical classes which appear to displace the benzodiazepines from their binding sites in brain membrane preparations, in the behavioral sense we find some remarkable differences. Beta-CCE has been shown to be proconvulsant and anxiogenic (Tenen and Hirsch, 1980; Cowan *et al.*, 1981; Dorow *et al.*, 1983), effects diametrically opposed to those found with the classical benzodiazepines. Within the beta-carboline series of compounds we now have the complete range of activity from full agonists, such as ZK 93423, partial agonists like ZK 91296, to the antagonist ZK 93426 and the full inverse agonists beta-CCM and DMCM (see Fig. 5 for structures). Electrophysiological data adds a further dimension to these behavioral observations. While the benzodiazepines appear to increase the rate of chloride channel opening in response to a given GABA stimulus, the inverse agonists decrease this rate (Barker *et al.*, 1983). The behavioral and electrophysiological data are within themselves consistent; however they need not lead us to the conclusion that we are dealing with a multiple receptor population.

Displacement of ^{3}H-flunitrazepam with CL 218872 or propyl beta-carboline-3-carboxylate at 0°C yield Hill coefficients significantly less than unity in rat hippocampal membranes, though in the cerebellum the Hill coefficient is unity; the potency of each compound is much greater in the cerebellum than in the hippocampus. This was the type of data that led to the suggestion of multiple benzodiazepine receptor subtypes, as discussed previously. If the experiments are carried out at 37°C, the Hill coefficient in each brain area is unity, though there remains a marked difference between the potency of the compounds in displacing ^{3}H-flunitrazepam in the two brain regions (Gee and Yamamura, 1982a). This suggests that the Hill coefficient is telling us something about a complexity in the binding interaction in the hippocampus, for example, which has nothing to do with the difference in potency of the ligands between this region and the cerebellum. Such a conclusion is supported by the observation that if ^{3}H-Ro 15-1788 is used in similar experiments, the Hill coefficient in the hippocampus remains significantly less than unity even if the experiments are carried out at physiological temperatures (Martin and Brown, 1983). The potency difference between the regions, however, remains. There does appear to be a difference between the benzodiazepine receptor populations in the hippocampus and the cerebellum. Such a conclusion is supported by the differences found in the dissociation characteristics of Ro 15-1788 between these two regions (Brown and Martin, 1984c) and the photoaffinity labelling pattern of the polypeptide chains in the same structures (Sieghart and Drexler, 1983).

Let us briefly examine the behavioral profile of those compounds which appear to differentiate between benzodiazepine receptor subtypes according to the binding assay classification. All the classical benzodiazepines are agonists and fail to distinguish between the receptor subtypes; also Ro 15-1788, with a largely antagonist profile, again does not differentiate between the subtypes in binding assays. There are some compounds of this benzodiazepine class, such as quazepam (Fig. 6) and some of its chemical analogues, which show a profile of action similar to the benzodiazepines (Kales *et al.*, 1980; Ongini *et al.*, 1982), but do display a preference for the putative BZ1 subtype of receptor (Sieghart, 1983). The inverse agonist beta-carboline analogues exhibit a preference for the BZ1 subtype but the partial agonist from the same series, ZK 91296 (Fig. 5) does not. CL 218872 also appears to be a partial agonist but displays the atypical binding characteristics which first led to the idea of benzodiazepine receptor subtypes. There appears to be no correlation between the behavioral profile of action and the ability of the compounds to differentiate in binding assays between the putative receptor subtypes.

In conclusion, we must accept that a considerable variety of biochemical evidence is consistent with the multiple receptor hypothesis; these differences may well be clarified as we learn more about the structural detail of the receptor complex. However, at the present time, there appears to be no relationship established between these biochemical observations and the pharmacodynamic profile of the compounds concerned.

6. BENZODIAZEPINE RECEPTOR FUNCTION

6.1. *In Vivo* Receptor Binding

An integral part of understanding the means by which a drug produces its overt effects on any particular system is a measure of the proportion of receptors which have to be occupied to achieve the desired response. *In vitro* binding assays clearly cannot address this problem. However, it has proved possible to carry out benzodiazepine binding studies *in vivo* using ^{3}H-diazepam (Tallman *et al.*, 1979), ^{3}H-flunitrazepam (Chang and Snyder, 1978; Duka *et al.*, 1979) and ^{3}H-beta-CCE (Hirsch and Lydigsen, 1981). The procedure is relatively simple and involves the injection of the radioligand, normally via the tail vein. The animal is subsequently killed at some determined time point after injection, the brain is removed, rapidly homogenized and filtered; the radioactivity remaining on the filter represents the amount of ligand bound at the time of death. The definition of non-specific binding can be carried out in two ways. The animal is given a high dose of a benzodiazepine at some time prior to the injection of the radiolabelled ligand, the dose being selected such that it is sufficient to occupy the total receptor population; any radioactivity remaining in the samples obtained from such animals is defined as non-specific binding. This is the method of choice and that used in the references above. The alternative is to remove and homogenize the brain as before, but an aliquot is taken and a high concentration of a benzodiazepine is added to the homogenate; this is subsequently allowed to come to some equilibrium and it is this value which is accepted as the non-specific binding. This procedure allows redistribution of binding to go on after the animal has been killed and is not strictly a measure of the receptors occupied at the time of death.

Recently this procedure of *in vivo* binding has been used to carry out saturation experiments with ^{3}H-flunitrazepam in the intact animal (Braestrup and Nielsen, 1986). These studies have shown that flunitrazepam appears to obey simple mass action kinetics *in vivo*, the Bmax value obtained was almost identical to that found *in vitro* while the affinity constant increased from 1.2 nM *in vitro* to 148 nM *in vivo*. The experimental procedure can thus be used to estimate the absolute occupancy of the receptor population if various assumptions are made about the interaction of the test drug with the radioligand *in vivo*.

The characteristics of this *in vivo* binding compare favourably with those expected from the *in vitro* studies in terms of both distribution and ligand specificity (Chang and Snyder, 1978; Blanchard *et al.*, 1979).

6.2. Receptor Occupancy and Pharmacological Effect

The benzodiazepines produce an array of pharmacological effects and, in experimental animals, a variety of behavioral paradigms have been devised in attempts to quantify their anticonvulsant, anxiolytic, sedative/hypnotic and muscle relaxant properties. It has been possible by combining the *in vivo* binding studies, mentioned above, with appropriate behavioral testing to define the receptor occupancy required to obtain a given response with the drug under investigation. In the case of full agonists at the benzodiazepine receptor, it has been found that inhibition of pentylenetetrazole-induced convulsions occurs at about 25% receptor occupancy (Duka *et al.*, 1979), while anticonflict activity is not seen until 60% of the receptors are occupied (Petersen and Buus-Lassen, 1981); ataxia occurs at a still higher occupancy.

It must be clear, however, that the occupancy required to obtain a given end point will vary, not only with the precise definition of that end point but also with the test paradigm used. A clear example of this is seen in the case of audiogenic seizures induced in DBA/2 mice; these convulsions are extremely sensitive to the benzodiazepines, less than 10% receptor occupancy being required to inhibit the convulsant activity (Jensen *et al.*, 1983). A figure markedly different from the 25% occupancy required for anticonvulsant activity against pentylenetetrazole-induced convulsions.

Clearly the ability to estimate the receptor occupancy required for a given effect allows the comparison of different ligands and the definition of compounds with high and low efficacy. The compound CGS 9896 appears to be an agonist with low efficacy. It is able to block convulsions produced in mice by an i.v. injection of pentylenetetrazole. However, greater receptor occupancy was required to achieve the same end point for CGS 9896 than for diazepam. This is consistent with the classification of the latter compound as a partial agonist, a conclusion supported by the observation that CGS 9896 is able to inhibit the anticonvulsant effect of the full agonist, diazepam (Brown *et al.*, 1984).

Partial agonists would therefore be expected to have a pharmacological profile restricted to those effects which are normally seen with full agonists at low receptor occupancy for, even at high occupancy, the partial agonist will not be able to provide the receptor stimulation required to produce the ataxic effects. Such a compound is the beta-carboline analogue, ZK 91296, which is an anticonvulsant but does not produce ataxia (Petersen *et al.*, 1984). It has therefore been possible to restrict the pharmacological profile of the classical benzodiazepines through the selection of partial agonists.

6.3. *In Vitro* Measurement of "Function"

The history of pharmacology is pervaded with attempts to estimate the efficacy of drugs *in vitro*. While in the periphery this has yielded a great deal with the isolated organ bath preparations, the problem in the CNS has proved much more difficult to address.

The activation of the GABA-A receptor with agonists is known to increase the frequency of chloride channel openings in the neuronal membrane, and successful attempts have been made to study the flux of chloride ions in rat hippocampal slices (Wong *et al.*, 1984) or CNS neurons in culture (Thampy and Barnes, 1984). These effects are clearly observable in whole cell preparations, but recently it has been possible to obtain preparations alternatively referred to as cell free (Harris and Allan, 1985) or "synaptoneurosomes" (Schwartz *et al.*, 1984) from homogenates of CNS tissue which exhibit GABA or GABA agonist stimulated ^{36}Cl influx. The characterization of these preparations need not be discussed here, but their proponents have argued that the uptake or influx of chloride seen takes place into essentially sealed fragments of postsynaptic membrane (see Paul *et al.*, 1986; Harris and Allan, 1986). These preparations have shown clearly GABA-activated, dose-dependent increases in chloride flux, which is modulated by the barbiturates, and inhibited by bicuculline and picrotoxin. Desensitization of the response results from the pretreatment of the preparations with high concentrations of agonists (Schwartz *et al.*, 1985; Allan and Harris, 1986; Schwartz *et al.*, 1987). The development of these techniques is an exciting addendum to the armoury with which we may address the problems of functionality *in vitro*. The time resolution is clearly much less than that obtainable with electrophysiological techniques, but holds much promise for studies on specific membrane preparations.

6.4. The Three State Model

We have previously alluded to a further complexity with the benzodiazepine receptor system, the existence of the inverse agonists. The classical benzodiazepines possess a clearly defined profile of action as anticonvulsants, sedative/hypnotics, anxiolytics and muscle relaxants. It is clear, however, that certain compounds, which appear to interact specifically with the benzodiazepine receptor, are able to produce diametrically opposed effects and yet others can antagonise both types of action (Mitchell and Martin, 1980; Tenen and Hirsch, 1980; Cowan *et al.*, 1981; Dorow *et al.*, 1983).

It is possible to rationalize this data by assuming that an endogenous ligand is present for the benzodiazepine receptor which imposes some tone upon the system. The benzodiazepines would presumably displace this endogenous ligand and increase the tone. The compounds with the opposite effects to the benzodiazepines would displace the endogenous material and release that tone which it imposed upon the system. This endogenous ligand would be classified as a partial agonist, the benzodiazepines as full agonists, and the compounds with the opposite effects to the benzodiazepines as antagonists. Compounds which had no effect on the system but were able to antagonise both of these effects would be classed as partial agonists like the endogenous ligand. Such an explanation is entirely satisfactory and able to rationalize all the data that is at the present time available. It has not received widespread acceptance.

An alternative has been proposed: the three state model (Nutt *et al.*, 1982; Polc *et al.*, 1982; Jensen *et al.*, 1983; Prado de Carvalho *et al.*, 1983). The benzodiazepine receptor is envisaged as existing in three energy states. Occupation of the first results in no effect being observed on the GABA activation of chloride channel opening: the antagonist state. The second, when occupied, allows the receptor complex to relax into such a conformation that results in an increased coupling between the GABA stimulus and its effector mechanism; this is the so-called agonist state and results in the overt actions produced by the classical benzodiazepines. The third state is obtained when the receptor is occupied by a compound such as methyl beta-carboline-3-carboxylate with behavioral actions opposite to those of the benzodiazepines; this compound produces overt convulsions. It induces a conformational change in the receptor which results in a decrease in the coupling between the GABA stimulus and its effector sequence; this is termed the inverse agonist state. The model is thermodynamically sound though its novelty has limited its universal acceptance.

Recently, Kemp *et al.* (1987) have carried out a detailed electrophysiological analysis of the actions of a series of agonists, antagonists and inverse agonists at the benzodiazepine receptor using isoguvacine as the GABA-A agonist in the rat hippocampal slice preparation. They conclude that their data are consistent with the model of positive and negative modulation of GABA-A responses by benzodiazepine agonists and inverse agonists, and further that within this spectrum of activity partial agonists can be defined, the action of which is closely paralleled by their receptor occupancy predicted from *in vitro* binding studies.

The benzodiazepine receptor then is envisaged as a true modulatory site in that it produces a fine tuning of the GABA stimulus effector coupling.

6.5. Interactions with the Benzodiazepine Receptor

6.5.1. *GABA*

There is compelling evidence that the benzodiazepines produce their effects by modulation of GABA-mediated transmission (e.g. Haefely, 1984). It has proved much more difficult to observe this interaction *in vitro* using neurochemical methods. However, it has proved possible to demonstrate a facilitation of GABA binding to a low affinity population of sites in CNS membrane preparations (Skerritt *et al.*, 1982). An allosteric modulation in the opposite direction, which consists of an increase in the affinity of the benzodiazepine binding site for agonist ligands when the *in vitro* experiments are carried out in the presence of GABA, was demonstrated much earlier (Martin and Candy, 1978; Tallman *et al.*, 1978). The modulation appears to occur via a low affinity GABA receptor as high concentrations of GABA are required to demonstrate the effect. This neurotransmitter appears to affect both the association and dissociation kinetics of the agonist benzodiazepine ligands, the net effect, however, is to increase the affinity. The effects of various GABA agonists have been studied in this type of experiment. It was initially thought that the GABA receptor responsible for the modulation of benzodiazepine receptor binding was atypical as certain GABA agonists appeared ineffective (Braestrup *et al.*, 1979a; Karobath and Lippitsch, 1979; Karobath *et al.*, 1979). The question has been resolved, however, as the atypical response of THIP and piperidine-4-sulphonic acid are not apparent if the experiments are carried out at more physiological temperatures (Supavilai and Karobath, 1980a).

The observation has proved of considerable practical value. It appears that the affinity of all agonist ligands is increased in the presence of GABA, while the affinity of the inverse agonists is decreased. The antagonists seem to suffer no change in affinity in the presence of GABA (Braestrup and Nielsen, 1981b; Braestrup *et al.*, 1982; Mohler and Richards, 1981; Doble *et al.*, 1982; Fujimoto *et al.*, 1982; Skolnick *et al.*, 1982).

It has been possible to demonstrate the phenomenon *in vivo*, since the use of pharmacological agents that increase the GABA content of the CNS produce significant increases in the binding of the appropriate ligands to the benzodiazepine receptor (Tallman *et al.*, 1979).

6.5.2. *Effects of Various Ions*

It was initially shown that chloride ions were able to produce a synergistic effect with GABA, increasing the affinity of the binding site for ^{3}H-diazepam (Martin and Candy, 1978). The effect was later shown to generalize to other ions, which were able to reverse the GABA-mediated inhibitory postsynaptic potentials electrophysiologically (Costa *et al.*, 1979; Martin and Candy, 1980). It has since been shown that certain distilbene derivatives can, at least partially, block the facilitation of agonist binding caused by chloride ions, although the effects are complex (Costa *et al.*, 1981).

Both nickel and cadmium ions have also been shown to increase the affinity of the benzodiazepine receptor for ^{3}H-diazepam (Mackerer *et al.*, 1978).

6.5.3. *Barbiturates*

The overt pharmacological effects of the sedative barbiturates is very similar to the agonist benzodiazepines, although their mechanism of action is different. The agonist benzodiazepines produce an increase in the frequency of chloride channel opening in response to a given GABA stimulus, while the major effect of the barbiturates is to increase channel open-time (Study and Barker, 1981). The barbiturates exhibit no direct interaction with the benzodiazepine receptor *in vitro*; their locus of action appears to be closely associated with the recognition site which is labelled with dihydropicrotoxin (Ticku and Olsen, 1978), although it is distinct from this (Trifiletti *et al.*, 1985). It is possible to demonstrate an allosteric interaction of the sedative barbiturates, however, as they show a chloride-dependent enhancement of agonist binding to the benzodiazepine site (Leeb-Lundberg *et al.*, 1980). The enhancement is due to an affinity increase at the receptor with no change in capacity. The effects appear to be complex, with the anticonvulsant phenobarbital producing no such facilitation, though able to block the effects of pentobarbital which does (Leeb-Lundberg *et al.*, 1981; Olsen, 1981).

In a similar manner to the effects of GABA, pentobarbital enhances the affinity of the benzodiazepine receptor for its agonist ligands and decreases the affinity for inverse agonist ligands (Braestrup *et al.*, 1983; Honore *et al.*, 1983). In the case of the modulatory effects of the barbiturates there appear to be a number of anomalies and the predictive reliability of the "barbiturate shift," as it has become known, is not as good as that for GABA (Honore *et al.*, 1984).

6.5.4. *Steroids*

It has been known for many years that a number of natural and synthetic steroids are effective anesthetics. It was suggested that such compounds produced their effects by a facilitation of inhibitory neurotransmission in the CNS (Scholfield, 1980). This report received experimental support from Harrison and Simmonds (1984) when they were able to show that alphaxalone (5-alpha-pregnane-3-alpha-ol,11,20, dione) was able to potentiate GABA-mediated responses recorded from the cuneate slice preparation *in vitro*. The effects were restricted to GABA-mediated responses and they were stereospecific, the 3-beta hydroxy analogue, betaxolone, was without effect. It would appear from the voltage clamp studies that alphaxolone potentiates chloride currents evoked by GABA both in the mammalian CNS (Barker *et al.*, 1986; Cottrell, Lambert and Mistry, 1987) and in cultured bovine adrenomedullary chromaffin cells (Cottrell, Lambert and Peters, 1987). Mechanistically the effects of the steroids appear to be similar to those of the anesthetic barbiturates in that their effects are on channel open lifetime rather than opening frequency (Barker *et al.*, 1986; Lambert *et al.*, 1987). However, more recent detailed analysis does reveal significant differences between the two classes of compound.

Neurochemical studies have also been carried out with these compounds. They are able to inhibit the binding of TBPS (see next section) and facilitate that of flunitazepam (Majewska *et al.*, 1986). It has been possible to demonstrate that certain of the steroids stimulate chloride uptake into synaptoneurosomes directly (Majewska *et al.*, 1986), an observation which has also been found electrophysiologically (Cottrell, Lambert and Peters, 1987). The full implications of the interaction of these steroids with the GABA-benzodiazepine receptor complex may well have some exciting clinical implications.

6.5.5. *Others*

Tert-butyl bicyclophosphorothionate (TBPS) produces convulsions by reducing GABA-mediated transmission at a site close to the chloride ionophore itself. It is a member of a series of potent cage convulsants and can be labelled with ^{35}S. This compound has proved useful in the investigation of ligands which are thought to allosterically modulate the GABA receptor complex (Squires *et al.*, 1983). Ligands for the benzodiazepine receptor increase or reduce ^{35}S-TBPS binding depending on whether they are classified as agonists or inverse agonists (Supavilai and Karobath, 1984). The effects rely on the ability of the compounds to modify the association and dissociation kinetics of the TBPS from its binding sites; the experiments are carried out prior to equilibrium being reached (Maksay and Simonyi, 1985).

There are several other classes of compound which have been reported to modulate binding at the benzodiazepine receptor, though the mechanisms by which they accomplish this have been less well characterized.

The pyrazolopyridines tracazolate, etazolate and cartazolate (Fig. 6) produce a chloride-dependent affinity change at the benzodiazepine receptor, with characteristics similar to those exhibited by the barbiturates (Beer *et al.*, 1978; Williams and Risley, 1979; Supavilai and Karobath, 1979, 1981; Meiners and Salama, 1982).

Avermectin Bla (Williams and Yarbrough, 1979) and ivermectin (Williams and Risley, 1982, 1984) appear to affect both the affinity and capacity of the benzodiazepine receptor. These compounds are macrolide anthelmintics which are reported to affect the chloride channel at the lobster neuromuscular junction (Fritz *et al.*, 1979). The adenosine analogues EMD 28422, EMD 35993 and EMD 41717 (Skolnick *et al.*, 1980; Skolnick *et al.*, 1983), as well as the diaryltriazine L 781067 (Wong *et al.*, 1983), the H2-receptor antagonist, cimetidine (Lakoski *et al.*, 1983) and the novel anxiolytic buspirone (Oakley and Jones, 1983) also modify benzodiazepine binding either *in vitro* or *in vivo*. The interpretation of some of these data is difficult, however, as enhancement of *in vivo* benzodiazepine binding may be due to the effect of the compounds on the normal pharmacokinetic distribution of the radiolabel.

6.6. Endogenous Ligands

The identification of the opioid peptides as natural ligands for the opiate receptors inevitably resulted in attempts to identify compounds which would serve the same function at the benzodiazepine receptor. A good deal of effort has been expended in this search over the past eight years, although it has been argued that it is not necessary to envisage the existence of such a molecule (Mohler, 1981). Three candidates still show much promise.

The first of these was isolated in impure form in 1978 (Guidotti *et al.*, 1978). It has subsequently been purified and partially characterized; it has a molecular weight of about 11,000 and contains 104 amino acid residues. Intraventricular injection of the material (DBI: diazepam binding inhibitor) indicates that the compound has inverse agonist activity (Guidotti *et al.*, 1983). Antibodies have been raised to DBI and its CNS distribution mapped (Alho *et al.*, 1985); material with similar immunological properties is found in the human brain (Ferrero, Costa, *et al.*, 1986). It appears to be stored in certain neuronal populations and released in response to veratridine or high potassium induced depolarisation (Ferrarese *et al.*, 1987). Tryptic digestion of the material from the rat yields an octadecaneuropeptide (ODN) which exhibits some of the biological properties of DBI (Ferrero, Santi, *et al.*, 1986); it appears to have higher affinity in the displacement of methyl beta-carboline-3-carboxylate than the parent DBI (Ferrero, Santi, *et al.*, 1986). cDNA clones have now been obtained for DBI from both human (Gray *et al.*, 1986) and rat (Mocchetti *et al.*, 1986).

n-Butyl-beta-carboline-3-carboxylate has recently been isolated from the bovine cerebral cortex and it is suggested that this molecule subserves the function of an endogenous ligand (Pena *et al.*, 1986). Previous attempts to isolate benzodiazepine displacing activity from human urine identified the active principle as ethyl beta-carboline-3-carboxylic acid, later studies showed that this was an extraction artefact (Braestrup *et al.*, 1980). In the more recent study considerable pains have been taken to obviate this possibility.

In the above two procedures, classical methods of extraction have been used to isolate active materials. Two further studies have adopted a rather different approach. De Blas and coworkers have linked 3-hemisuccinyloxy-clonazepam to bovine serum albumin and used this material to raise monoclonal antibodies in mice. The antibodies were subsequently selected for those recognizing the epitope associated with the benzodiazepine skeleton. These were then used to localize similar immunologically active material in rat brain. The antibodies were also used to prepare immuno affinity columns which allowed the purification of a low molecular weight material (approximately 1000 daltons) which was able to inhibit the binding of several benzodiazepine ligands to the receptor (De Blas *et al.*, 1985; Sangameswaran and De Blas, 1985). The properties of this antibody, in terms of its binding characteristics, are very similar to those of a polyclonal antibody against Ro 7-1986 linked to keyhole limpet haemocyanin, and raised in rabbits. Both antibodies recognized the classical benzodiazepines with high affinity but showed little recognition of the beta-carboline-3-carboxylate esters or Ro 15-1788 (Ayad *et al.*, 1986; Fry *et al.*, 1987).

Prior to these studies there have been many suggestions concerning putative endogenous ligands for the benzodiazepine binding site of this receptor complex; many have disappeared into antiquity and only time will allow rational comments to be made further on this subject.

6.7. The Neurochemical Consequences of Tolerance and Withdrawal

It is clear that tolerance to the pharmacological effects of the benzodiazepines develops on chronic treatment, though the rate of its development is dependent on the particular response monitored. Considerable efforts have been made to elucidate the underlying mechanisms but, to date, little definitive progress has been made.

Mohler *et al.* (1978) failed to observe any change in diazepam binding to the benzodiazepine site after 30 days treatment with diazepam at 3 mg/kg/day, though they did observe a decrease in the Bmax of GABA binding in the striatum. Using heroic doses of flurazepam Chiu and Rosenberg (1978) observed a small (15%) decrease in the binding capacity of diazepam in rat cerebral cortex. Similarly large doses of diazepam or lorazepam also failed to consistently modify the binding of diazepam in rat brain membranes following withdrawal from eight weeks of treatment with these drugs (Braestrup, Nielsen, and Squires, 1979c). It would therefore appear that the biochemical effects underlying tolerance and withdrawal must be associated with events removed from the benzodiazepine binding site.

Electrophysiologically, it has been shown quite clearly, however, that 21 days treatment of rats with 5 mg/kg/day diazepam results in a decreased sensitivity to the iontophoretically applied GABA in cells of the dorsal raphe nucleus; the decreased sensitivity was rapidly reversed by the systemic administration of the antagonist Ro 15-1788. The decreased response appeared to be reflected in a decreased coupling between GABA and benzodiazepine sites as the ability of GABA to facilitate flunitrazepam binding in cortical membranes from these animals was markedly reduced (Gallager *et al.*, 1984).

In an interesting series of experiments, Little *et al.* (1986) have shown that seven days of treatment with flurazepam (40 mg/kg/day) resulted in significant alterations in the sensitivity of the animals to a spectrum of compounds thought to act at the benzodiazepine receptor. All the drugs tested appeared to shift their classification towards the inverse agonist end of the spectrum: flurazepam became a less efficacious agonist, while the antagonists, Ro 15-1788 and ZK 93426 (Fig. 5), exhibited inverse agonist activity in the animals treated chronically with flurazepam; the inverse agonists appeared to increase their propensity to cause convulsions. However, it was not a generalized response in the sense that the convulsant bicuculline retained the same convulsant threshold in both control and drug-treated groups.

Two explanations can be advanced for such observations. First, it is possible that the ability of the benzodiazepines to modulate GABA-mediated transmission may become displaced on chronic treatment with the agonist benzodiazepines; that is the receptor system actually changes its characteristics in response to the chronic insult. Alternatively one could envisage the increased production of some endogenous ligand during the course of chronic treatment which on withdrawal of the agonist benzodiazepine sets a new tone on the GABA system. We would have to envisage this to be an inverse agonist to explain the data. The latter possibility gains some support from the recent observations of Miyata *et al.* (1987). Here, the mRNA encoding DBI has been shown to increase significantly as a result of protracted treatment with diazepam. The experiments to differentiate between these two possibilities do not appear to have been carried out.

The problem of tolerance to and withdrawal from these compounds retain many of their mysteries and the neurochemical hypotheses advanced so far require ratification.

7. STRUCTURE ACTIVITY RELATIONSHIPS AT THE BENZODIAZEPINE RECEPTOR

The initial structure activity studies with the benzodiazepines were elucidated by the medicinal chemists involved in the original synthetic program with these drugs (Sternbach *et al.*, 1968). In this work correlations were found between the various structural modifications carried out with the benzodiazepine skeleton and tests designed to quantify the several behavioral actions of these compounds. The studies led to a number of empirical rules. Activity was increased by the substitution of electron withdrawing groups at positions 7 and 2′; alkyl substituents larger than methyl at position 1 decreased activity. The replacement of the carbonyl function at position 2 with hydrogen, reduction of the N4-C5 double bond, or the introduction of halo-substituents at the 3′ or 4′ positions drastically reduced activity (see Fig. 2 for the numbering system used).

Subsequent studies, using anticonvulsant potency as the measure of biological activity have suggested correlations with the charge on the N4 (Sarrazin *et al.*, 1976), the charge on the C2 carbonyl oxygen together with the total molecular dipole moment (Blair and Webb, 1977), the difference between the energies of the lowest empty and the highest occupied molecular orbitals (Gilli *et al.*, 1977), or the electron density on the p_y orbital at C10 (Lucek *et al.*, 1979). These investigations, together with the application of the Free-Wilson and Hansch analysis with larger numbers of these compounds by Borea and his colleagues (Borea *et al.*, 1979; Borea, 1981), have rationalized and validated the original empirical rules found with this series of compounds.

The estimation of biological potency derived from *in vivo* data is fraught with danger. Before the compound in question arrives at its site of action, it must be absorbed and possibly suffer metabolic degradation or sequestration at various sites within the animal. Studies of this type, therefore, are of limited value, if information about recognition properties of the pharmacologically relevant binding site are being sought. Clearly they are of paramount importance in the total activity profile of the compounds. The discovery of the benzodiazepine binding site in the mammalian CNS gave new impetus to the investigation of structure activity relationships within the series as this particular measure of biological activity is dependent solely on binding site recognition; the structural modifications of metabolic importance can then be addressed separately.

It soon became clear that the receptor had a specific stereochemical requirement, those compounds with the R-conformation being preferentially recognized by the receptor (Sunjic *et al.*, 1979; Blount *et al.*, 1983). Although many studies have been carried out over the last few years which have defined the detail of the structural requirements for binding site recognition, little has been achieved of predictive value (Borea, 1983; Borea and Gilli, 1984; Butcher *et al.*, 1984; Loew *et al.*, 1984).

The situation is complex with the benzodiazepine receptor, as not only do we have to accommodate the agonists and antagonists into the binding site topography, but also the inverse agonists. The problem is compounded by the several different chemical classes which appear to interact at this site. The initial benzodiazepine structure has been modified with heterocyclic rings fused to the a face, such as triazolam and alprazolam (Fig. 7; Hester *et al.*, 1971; Gall *et al.*, 1976), and many others which have previously been reviewed in some detail (Hamor and Martin, 1983). An exhaustive structural classification of ligands which interact with the benzodiazepine receptor can be found in Haefely *et al.* (1985).

However, attempts have been made to address the recognition site problem. Crippen (1982), using the distance geometry approach, has attempted to design a recognition site which will account for the interactions of the different ligand classes which take place at this receptor. Recognition site modelling has also been carried out by experienced medicinal chemists and hypotheses have been developed which in turn have led to the synthesis of active compounds at this receptor (Fryer, 1983; Fryer *et al.*, 1984; Fryer *et al.*, 1986). Other attempts have also been made using eye matches to identify the manner in which these compounds bind to the recognition site (Codding and Muir, 1985; Borea *et al.*, 1987).

A degree of care must be taken in attempts to model the recognition site for these ligands; we have no proof at this time that all these ligands interact with the same site. Clearly the interaction of agonists, inverse agonists and antagonists must be different, but are these sites discrete and separate or do they overlap with each other in some complex manner? It would be of considerable advantage if this question could be addressed. It is not sufficient to note the apparent competitive displacement of the individual ligands by each other as such a competitive displacement can be simulated by a tight allosteric coupling between sites.

The question is very complex and cannot be tackled rigorously here but the principle of the approach will be outlined. The interaction of any ligand with its binding site is composed of a number of simple chemical bonds between the ligand points on the ligand and the complementary site points on the macromolecule. The distribution of these ligand points in three dimensional space provides the recognition fingerprint of the ligand. The bonding between individual ligand points and their complementary site points may be via hydrogen bonds, hydrophobic interactions or derive from the electrostatic potential.

Clearly, they must take place within a restricted area of space which is defined by the van der Waals surface of the two reactants, ligand and receptor. With this set of criteria we can ask whether or not two ligands, from distinct chemical classes, and with the same efficacy at the receptor, are sufficiently similar that we can envisage them binding to the same discrete site.

The imidazobenzodiazepine, Ro 15-1788, and the beta-carboline-3-carboxylic acid analogue, ZK 93426, can both be classified as antagonists at the benzodiazepine receptor; they are essentially devoid of pharmacological activity but are able to block the overt effects of either the agonists or the inverse agonists which bind to this receptor *in vitro*. In collaboration with P.A. Borea, from the Department of Pharmacology at the University of Ferrara in Italy, and P.M. Dean and D.J. Danziger at the Department of Pharmacology in Cambridge, we have searched for structural similarities between these two molecules using a combinatorial optimization procedure developed by Danziger and Dean (1985). This involves the allocation of certain properties to atoms, or groups of atoms within the two molecules; these are then defined as the ligand points. Using the X-ray crystal structure of Ro 15-1788 (Codding and Muir, 1985) and similar structural data for ZK 93426 from the crystal structure data of methyl beta-carboline-3-carboxylate (Bertolasi *et al.*, 1984), the location of all these ligand point positions in three dimensional space can be determined. The method of Danziger and Dean uses an efficient algorithm to obtain the best match between the ligand points of the two molecules. In this particular case a very good ligand point match between the two compounds was obtained.

This procedure, however, clearly only addresses the atom positions themselves and, as was suggested above, the ligands, when bound to their recognition site, must fit into a physical space. The flesh can be put onto these atom positions in terms of the accessible surface which can be calculated; further molecular orbital computations allow one to superimpose the molecular electrostatic potential on this surface. It is difficult to convey this information without the use of colour and the interested reader is referred to Martin (1987), where a more detailed explanation is available which is supplemented with colour photographs. The information is numerical and can therefore be subjected to the normal statistical analysis. These data, both concerning the surface and the potential can be compared directly, for the two molecules, using a Spearman rank correlation (Namasivayam and Dean, 1986). The correlation coefficients Rrank of the pattern match are 0.957 for the surface and 0.847 for the potential.

These results indicate that the two molecules, ZK 93426 and Ro 15-1788, show a remarkable similarity in their structure—an observation which lends weight to the hypothesis that they both share the same binding site on this receptor complex. There is one further point that should be made concerning such an approach. The corollary of similarity is that of complementarity, that is the relationship between the cast and its mold; we can glean something about the geometry and molecular properties of the recognition site in a semi-quantitative manner using this approach.

Further studies of this nature with other ligands for this receptor may allow us, therefore, to generate a structural map of the recognition site. This will facilitate not only a greater understanding of the molecular details of the interaction, but may also suggest the synthesis of novel ligands; a development which has produced, in the past, considerable advances in our understanding of this receptor complex.

8. BIOCHEMICAL STUDIES WITH THE BENZODIAZEPINE RECEPTOR

The pharmacological and neurochemical characterization of this receptor was carried out in ignorance of the physical and structural properties of the complex itself; indeed this information was superfluous to the interpretation of such data. However, if we are to understand the details of the molecular events which take place in response to receptor activation, they must be interpreted in structural terms. The question has been tackled before with the nicotinic acetylcholine receptor and the obvious similarity between this and the GABA-benzodiazepine receptor, both producing their effects by the gating of ion channels, naturally inspired a similar approach.

The approach adopted in the case of the GABA-benzodiazepine receptor has been to purify the protein from an appropriate source which would allow not only experiments to be conducted on the isolated receptor appropriately reconstituted, but also allow the considerable powers of the molecular biologist to be unleashed on the problem with the ultimate goal of obtaining the primary structural information of the receptor protein itself. There are many stages in such an effort.

8.1. Solubilization of the Receptor

The first step in such a procedure is the removal of the receptor from the membrane by solubilization. Various detergents have been used to accomplish this and many groups have been involved in the effort: lysolecithin (Gavish *et al.*, 1979; Chude, 1979); sodium deoxycholate (Greenlee and Olsen, 1979; Sherman-Gold and Dudai, 1980; Asano and Ogasawara, 1981); Lubrol PX (Yousufi *et al.*, 1979); Triton X-100 (Lang *et al.*, 1979; Lo *et al.*, 1982); CHAPS (Stephenson and Olsen, 1982; Mernoff *et al.*, 1983); octylglucoside (Hammond and Martin, 1986); and n-octyl pentaoxy ethylene (Bristow and Martin, 1987a). Each of the detergents has its own particular advantages and disadvantages, though one of the most important criteria of suitability must be the ability to remove the protein from its native membrane environment with as little damage as possible. This is currently assessed by the ability to demonstrate the same accessory binding site interactions that are observed in the membrane (reviewed by Stephenson and Barnard, 1986). It is generally believed that the most appropriate conditions involve the use of CHAPS with the addition of a cocktail of protease inhibitors and lipid, though it has recently become clear that there are marked variations in the stability of these accessory binding sites depending on the species used for the solubilization, the region of the CNS used and the precise lipid composition adopted (Bristow and Martin, 1987b; unpublished observations).

Subsequent to the solubilization, the receptor protein can be purified using affinity column chromatography. Suitable affinity columns have been prepared by the immobilization of a variety of benzodiazepine ligands on appropriate matrices (Gavish and Snyder, 1981; Martini *et al.*, 1981; Martini *et al.*, 1982; Sigel *et al.*, 1983; Taguchi and Kuriyama, 1984; Stauber *et al.*, 1987). The principle is simple: the soluble receptor is allowed to percolate through a column upon which is immobilized the benzodiazepine ligand. The benzodiazepine recognition site on the protein binds to the immobilized ligand and is retained on the column. Other proteins may then be washed off, and subsequently the desired receptor protein is removed using biospecific elution with a water-soluble benzodiazepine, such as clorazepate or flurazepam. The purification factor achieved can be over one-thousand-fold, though the yield is poor (less than 10% of the benzodiazepine binding sites applied to the column in soluble form are recovered after the affinity column purification). Subsequently, the eluting benzodiazepine may be removed from the soluble receptor preparation by ion exchange (Sigel *et al.*, 1983; Martini *et al.*, 1981), gel filtration (Olsen, Wong, *et al.*, 1984b; Schoch *et al.*, 1984) or diafiltration (Tallman, 1984).

The protein appears to be a multi-subunit complex consisting of two alpha and two beta subunits, according to SDS gel electrophoresis and total molecular weight determinations. The alpha subunit has a molecular weight of about 53,000, while that of the beta subunit is around 57,000 (Chang and Barnard, 1982; Sigel *et al.*, 1983; Olsen, Wong *et al.*, 1984; Barnard *et al.*, 1984; Schoch *et al.*, 1984). Glycosylation of the subunits appears to be brain-region dependent, at least for the alpha subunit (Sweetnam and Tallman, 1986), which is thought to exhibit the binding site for the benzodiazepines. Although the current dogma suggests that the total molecular weight of the receptor complex is about 220 KD, there is some evidence, from radiation inactivation studies, which suggest that it may be considerably higher (Nielsen and Braestrup, 1983); this dichotomy has not yet been resolved.

The protein has been successfully inserted into liposomes either in an impure (Hammond and Martin, 1986) or purified form (Sigel *et al.*, 1985; Schoch *et al.*, 1984), as assessed from binding studies. These also indicate that essentially all the protein is oriented correctly with the binding sites facing outwards. There have been no reports of successful functional reconstitution.

The successful purification of receptor protein, albeit it in small quantities, allowed two further important advances to be made.

8.2. Antibodies to the Receptor

The first antibodies to be produced were a collection of monoclonals raised from the spleen cells of mice which had previously been injected with the GABA-benzodiazepine receptor purified from bovine cerebral cortex, as the antigen (Haring *et al.*, 1985). In the initial screen, 28 hybridoma cultures were identified that showed binding to receptor preparations, of which 16 were selected for further analysis. These were subsequently divided into four groups: Group 1 recognized the beta subunit in human, bovine and rat while Group 2 and Group 4 were specific for the alpha subunit; the difference between the two groups resides in the species specificity of the recognition. The recognition specificity of Group 3 could not be determined by immunoblotting, perhaps because of the conformational dependence of the epitopes recognized by this particular group. The authors were able to show that the binding sites for the benzodiazepines and the high- and low-affinity GABA binding sites could be quantitatively immunoprecipitated with monoclonal antibodies specific to either the alpha or the beta subunit, indicating that both of the subunits occur in each individual receptor complex. It could also be demonstrated that both the alpha and beta subunits were present in all brain regions tested, indicating that there is a uniform subunit composition of the receptor complex throughout the brain; a conclusion which is further supported by the immunohistochemical and cytochemical studies carried out by Richards *et al.* (1987). None of the antibodies were able to compete with either benzodiazepine or GABA binding, indicating that they were not directed at either of these recognition sites.

Polyclonal antibodies to this receptor were raised by the injection of protein, again purified from the bovine cerebral cortex, into New Zealand white rabbits (Stephenson *et al.*, 1986). None of the antibodies were directed against the recognition site for either GABA or the benzodiazepines, and it recognized only the alpha subunit of the complex, as shown by Western blot. Clearly a proportion of the antibody preparation was not conformationally dependent. It was possible using this material to precipitate the binding sites for GABA, the benzodiazepines, TBPS and propyl beta-carboline-3-carboxylate from a soluble preparation of bovine brain, indicating that all these recognition properties were associated in oligomeric complexes with at least one alpha subunit.

8.3. Amino Acid Sequence of the GABA-Benzodiazepine Receptor

The availability of purified receptor protein also paved the way to the cloning of the two peptide subunits, thought, as a result of the purification studies previously discussed, to constitute this receptor complex in the mammalian brain (Schofield *et al.*, 1987). The material obtained from bovine cerebral cortex, after purification, was cleaved with cyanogen bromide and the resultant peptides separated by HPLC. A number of these yielded partial amino acid sequences, obviously derived from the original protein. In addition it proved possible to isolate one of the subunits, alpha, in a pure state from an SDS gel and, after tryptic digestion, this also yielded partial sequence data. Synthetic oligonucleotide probes were prepared from these sequences and were used to screen bovine brain and calf cortex complementary DNA libraries. The hybridising clones found were analyzed by DNA sequencing and found to be of two types. One contained the amino acid sequence found in the enzymically cleaved protein from the alpha subunit and was therefore designated as encoding the alpha subunit, while the other did not contain this sequence and presumably encoded the beta subunit. The nucleotide and deduced amino acid sequences of the two subunits are shown in the publication cited above.

It is possible to inject total mRNA obtained from chick or rat brain into the Xenopus oocyte and allow it to translate the message and insert the protein into its membrane. This it appears to accomplish successfully for the GABA-benzodiazepine receptor, and using voltage clamp techniques, it can be demonstrated that the receptor inserted into the membrane exhibits all the functional characteristics that are seen in the neurone (Miledi *et al.*, 1982; Smart *et al.*, 1983; Houamed *et al.*, 1984). To confirm the authenticity of the cDNAs for the alpha and beta subunits they were transcribed *in vitro* and the resultant mRNA injected into the oocyte in a similar manner. It was found that after injection of only one of the mRNAs obtained from the cDNA encoding, either the alpha or the beta subunit alone, no response was obtained in the oocyte as a result of GABA application. However, if both mRNAs were injected Schofield *et al.* (1987) reported that not only were responses seen to the application of GABA, but the response to this neurotransmitter could be modulated by the barbiturate, pentobarbitone, and the benzodiazepine, clorazepate. This indicated that the two mRNAs were all that was required to provide for translation of the receptor in the oocyte. The cDNAs from which they were transcribed must therefore encode all the information required to form not only the recognition sites for GABA, the benzodiazepines and the other ligands but also the ion channel, which must be an integral part of the complex.

Since the publication of this initial molecular cloning work it has become clear that the situation is a good deal more complicated. It has proved extremely difficult to obtain consistent facilitation of the GABA response by the agonist benzodiazepines in the oocyte preparation with the two cloned subunits (now called alpha-1 and beta-1) mentioned in that study (see Levitan *et al.*, 1988a). Alpha and beta subunits, highly homologous to those previously identified in the bovine brain, have recently been cloned from the human brain (again referred to as alpha-1 and beta-1 because of the degree of homology with the bovine sequences previously obtained). In addition, a further subunit, so-called gamma-2, has been obtained; it is distinctly different from the alpha-1 and beta-1 subunits but shows greater homology to the alpha. Further, it has been shown that when human embryonic kidney cells are transfected with the cDNAs encoding all three of these subunits (human: alpha-1 + beta-1 + gamma-2) electrophysiological responses to the benzodiazepines are found consistently. It proved impossible to obtain the benzodiazepine facilitation of GABA responses in these cells when either alpha-1 + gamma-2 or beta-1 + gamma-2 or gamma-2 alone were used (Pritchett *et al.*, 1989). However, the expressed receptor still appears to lack the positive cooperativity in the GABA response found in oocytes injected with total mRNA extracted from chick brain, suggesting that it still remains incorrectly assembled (Sigel and Baur, 1988). Radioligand binding experiments have been carried out on the transfected cells. Only in the case where the cells were transfected with the cDNAs from all three subunits did the cells express significant levels of benzodiazepine binding sites, though binding sites for muscimol and tert-butyl bicyclophosphorothionate were present in cells transfected with the cDNAs from alpha-1 + beta-1 subunits (Pritchett *et al.*, 1988; Pritchett *et al.*, 1989). Why was the gamma subunit not seen on the gels from the original protein purification? The size of the mature protein, prior to glycosylation, is very similar to that of the alpha subunit and it is possible, that, after posttranslational modification, the alpha-1 and gamma-2 subunits cannot be separated on the SDS gels.

Additional molecular cloning studies have shown that there are several homologous but distinct alpha subunits present in the bovine CNS. These subunits, designated alpha-1, alpha-2, and alpha-3, have been individually coexpressed in oocytes together with the beta-1 subunit from the bovine brain, and shown to display significantly different dose response curves to GABA (Levitan *et al.*, 1988a). Their biophysical properties are very similar to native GABA-A receptors with regard to ion selectivity, multiple single-channel conductance states, voltage dependent gating, and rectification and desensitisation kinetics (Levitan *et al.*, 1988b). Further electrophysiological studies have also shown that GABA-activated responses can be obtained from oocytes which have been injected with mRNA for alpha or beta subunits alone. The responses are augmented by pentobarbital and blocked by picrotoxin, suggesting that the recognition sites for GABA, and these other agents, are present on both the alpha and beta subunits and should thus be coded by homologous segments of the sequences (Blair *et al.*, 1988).

In situ hybridisation techniques have been used to study the distribution of the mRNAs coding for these subunits in both the rat (Sequier *et al.*, 1988) and bovine brain (Wisden *et al.*, 1988). In the latter case it is clear that the mRNAs which code for the different alpha subunits are differentially expressed in specific regions of the bovine brain. Similar studies have not yet been published with beta subunits; until recently only the beta-1 subunit sequence from human (Pritchett *et al.*, 1989) and bovine (Schofield *et al.*, 1987) were available and these are very homologous, though a beta sequence from rat has now been published which shows only 80% sequence identity with those previously published sequences (Lolait *et al.*, 1989). Viewed in conjunction with the electrophysiological data, it thus seems distinctly possible that we may find subtle differences in the pharmacology of the mature receptors between brain areas; indeed it is possible that the multiplicity of the GABA-benzodiazepine receptor suggested from the ligand binding experiments previously may be a good deal more complex than thought.

Inspection of the amino acid sequences suggests that there are multiple concensus glycosylation sites in all subunits, while the beta and gamma subunits also contain putative phosphorylation sites. In each subunit sequence there are four hydrophobic segments which are thought to represent membrane spanning alpha-helices, the first occurring approximately 200 amino acids from the N-terminus of the mature protein. This N-terminal portion is thought to be extracellular and each subunit contains a relatively conserved cysteine-cysteine loop. The first membrane spanning region is followed almost immediately by the second and third membrane spanning segments; there is then a relatively large intracellular loop, prior to the fourth membrane spanning segment, which is found almost at the carboxy-terminus. It is the intracellular loop which is the least conserved region between the subunits and contains the concensus phosphorylation sites. There is little evidence yet available to indicate at which points recognition occurs with the multiplicity of ligands known to interact with this complex. There is no structural data available for this receptor complex, the above inferences are purely predictive (Schofield *et al.*, 1987; Barnard *et al.*, 1987). However, they appear to be very similar to those made for the single sequence so far cloned for the glycine receptor from rat spinal cord (Grenningloh *et al.*, 1987) and the many sequences available from similar experiments with the nicotinic acetylcholine receptor complex from various sources, suggest that all these ligand-gated ion channels form a single superfamily of receptors.

The nicotinic acetylcholine receptor is thus a useful template on which to model our ideas of the GABA-benzodiazepine receptor, as the structural information available with this receptor complex is at a much more advanced stage, the most recent observations being available to a resolution of about 1.7 nm in the electric ray, Torpedo marmorata (Toyoshima and Unwin, 1988). The receptor complex adopts a pseudosymmetric pentameric array, when viewed from above the plane of the membrane, each segment of the pentamer representing a single subunit. It would also appear that the post-synaptic glycine receptor is pentameric (Langosch *et al.*, 1988), although the experimental evidence here is from subunit cross-linking experiments. No evidence is available concerning the GABA-benzodiazepine receptor, although it is tempting to speculate that it also is pentameric. The nicotinic acetylcholine receptor operates a cationic channel while the GABA receptor gates chloride ions. In 1986, Imoto *et al.* were able to show that the second membrane spanning region of the delta subunit of the nicotinic acetylcholine receptor was intimately involved in the control of ion transport through the channel. Recent work from the same group, using site directed mutagenesis (Imoto *et al.*, 1988), has indicated that specific acidic amino acids, located in the vicinity of this second membrane spanning region, are responsible for the control. In the case of the GABA-benzodiazepine receptor comparable positions.

The analysis of this structural data may appear a considerable distance from the tenets of pharmacology, however, this information marks a major step forward. It will be our ability to relate this structural information to the mechanisms by which ligands recognize binding sites, and the means by which channel gating is controlled, that will limit the advances which we are able to make in the future.

9. CONCLUSIONS AND FUTURE PROSPECTS

Since the introduction of the benzodiazepines to the clinician in 1960, remarkable progress has been made in attempts to understand the mechanisms by which these agents produce their effects. We have also learned a good deal about the normal physiological processes which can be manipulated by these medicines. Despite this advance in our knowledge, many intriguing questions remain to be solved. The advent of the molecular biological techniques have heralded a new phase. Just as the development of radioligand binding methods over 15 years ago allowed the pharmacologist to ask a completely new series of questions, so the revelation of the amino acid sequence of this receptor protein will open up new avenues of investigation. The subtleties of structure which define ligand recognition are almost within grasp; clues to the underlying mechanisms of receptor desensitisation are within sight. It is these subtleties at the molecular level which seem far removed from the desire to produce more specific and efficacious medicines; but, in the final analysis it is the understanding of these very subtleties which will allow us to reach that goal.

REFERENCES

Adamec, R. E., McNaughton, B., Racine, R. and Livingstone, K. E. (1981) Effect of diazepam on hippocampal excitability in the rat: action in the dentate area. *Epilepsia* **22**: 205–215.

Adams, P. R. and Brown, D. A. (1975) Actions of gamma-aminobutyric acid on sympathetic ganglion cells. *J. Physiol. (Lond).* **250**: 85–120.

Albic-Kolbah, T., Kajfez, F., Rendic, S., Sunjic, V., Konowal, A. and Snatzke, G. (1979) Circular dichroism and gel filtration study of binding of prochiral and chiral 1,4-benzodiazepin-2-ones to human serum albumin. *Biochem. Pharmacol.* **28**: 2457–2464.

Alho, H., Costa, E., Ferrero, P., Fujimoto, M., Cosenza-Murphy, D. and Guidotti, A. (1985) Diazepam binding inhibitor: A neuropeptide located in selected neuronal populations of rat brain. *Science* **229**: 179–182.

Allan, A. M. and Harris, R. A. (1986) Gamma-aminobutyric acid agonists and antagonists alter chloride flux across brain membranes. *Mol. Pharmacol.* **29**: 497–505.

Anholt, R. R. H., Pedersen, P. L., de Souza, E. B. and Snyder, S. H. (1986) The peripheral type benzodiazepine receptor: localisation to the mitochondrial outer membrane. *J. Biol. Chem.* **261**: 576–583.

Arbilla, S., Kamal, L. and Langer, S. Z. (1979) Presynaptic GABA autoreceptors on GABAergic nerve endings of the rat substantia nigra. *Eur. J. Pharmac.* **57**: 211–217.

Asano, T. and Ogasawara, N. (1981) Soluble gamma-amino butyric acid and benzodiazepine receptors from rat cerebral cortex. *Life Sci.* **29**: 193–200.

Asano, T., Ui, M. and Ogasawara, N. (1985) Prevention of agonist binding to gamma-aminobutyric acid B receptors by guanine nucleotides and islet-activating protein, Pertussis toxin, in bovine cerebral cortex. *J. Biol. Chem.* **260**: 12653–12658.

Ayad, V. J., Fry, J. P., Martin, I. L. and Rickets, C. (1986) Immunochemical evidence for an endogenous benzodiazepine receptor ligand in the brain of the mouse. *J. Physiol. (Lond).* 377: 32P.

Baraldi, M., Guidotti, A., Schwartz, J. P. and Costa, E. (1979) GABA receptors in clonal cells lines: A model for study of benzodiazepine action at molecular level. *Science* **205**: 821–823.

Barber, R. and Saito, K. (1976) Light microscopic visualisation of GAD and GABA-T in immunocytochemical preparations of rodent CNS. In: *GABA in Nervous System Function*, pp. 113–132, Roberts, E., Chase, T. N. and Tower, D. B. (eds) Raven Press, New York.

Barker, J. L. and Ransom, B. R. (1978) Amino acid pharmacology of mammalian central neurons grown in tissue culture. *J. Physiol. (Lond).* **280**: 331–354.

Barker, J. L., McBurney, R. N., Mathers, D. A. and Vaughan, W. (1980) The actions of convulsant agents or ion-channels activated by inhibitory amino acids on mouse neurons in cell culture. *J. Physiol. (Lond).* **308**: 18P.

Barker, J. L., McBurney, R. and MacDonald, J. F. (1982) Fluctuation analysis of neutral amino acid responses in cultured mouse spinal neurons. *J. Physiol. (Lond).* **322**: 365–387.

Barker, J. L., Gratz, E., Owen, D. G. and Study, R. E. (1983) Pharmacological effects of clinically important drugs on the excitability of cultured mouse spinal neurons. In: *Actions and Interactions of GABA and benzodiazepines*, Bowery, N. G. (ed) Raven Press, New York.

Barker, J. L., Harrison, N. L., Lange, G. D., Majewska, M. D. and Owen, G. D. (1986) Voltage clamp studies of the potentiation of GABA-activated chloride conductance by the steroidal anaesthetic alphaxalone and a reduced metabolite of progesterone. *J. Physiol. (Lond).* **377**:38P.

Barnard, E. A., Darlison, M. G. and Seeberg, P. H. (1987) Molecular biology of the $GABA_A$ receptor: The receptor/channel superfamily. *Trends in Neurosciences* **10**: 502–509.

Barnard, E. A., Stephenson, F. A., Sigel, E., Mamalaki, C., Bilbe, G., Constanti, A., Smart, T. E. and Brown, D. A. (1984) Structure and properties of the brain GABA/benzodiazepine receptor complex. In: *Neurotransmitter receptors: Mechanisms of Action and Regulation*, pp. 235–254, Kito, S., Segawa, T., Kuriyama, K., Yamamura, H. I. and Olsen, R. W. (eds) Plenum Press, New York.

Battersby, M. K., Richards, J. G. and Mohler, H. (1979) Benzodiazepine receptor: photoaffinity labelling and localisation. *Eur. J. Pharmacol.* **57**: 277–278.

Beaumont, K., Moberly, J. B. and Fanestil, D. D. (1984) Peripheral type benzodiazepine binding sites in a renal epithalial cell line (MDCK). *Eur. J. Pharmacol.* **103**: 185–188.

Beer, B., Klepner, C. A., Lippa, A. S. and Squires, R. F. (1978) Enhancement of ^{3}H-diazepam binding by SQ65396: a novel antianxiety agent. *Pharmacol. Biochem. Behav.* **9**: 849–851.

Benavides, J., Quarteronet, D., Imbault, F., Malgouris, C., Uzan, A., Renault, C., Dubroeucq, M. C., Gueremy, C. and LeFur, G. (1983) Labelling of "peripheral type" benzodiazepine binding sites in rat brain by using [3H]PK11195, an isoquinoline carboxamide derivative: kinetic studies and autoradiographic localisation. *J. Neurochem.* **41**: 1744–1750.

Bertolasi, V., Ferretti, V., Gilli, G. and Borea, P. A. (1984) Structure of methyl beta-carboline-3-carboxylate. *Acta Cryst.* **C40**: 1981–1983.

Biggio, B., Brodie, B. B., Costa, E. and Guidotti, A. (1977) Mechanism by which diazepam, muscimol and other drugs change the content of cGMP in the cerebellar cortex. *Proc. Natl. Acad. Sci. USA* **74**: 3592–3596.

Biggio, G., Corda, M. G., de Montis, G. and Gessa, G. L. (1980) Differential effects of kainic acid on benzodiazepine receptors GABA receptors and GABA-modulin in the cerebellar cortex. In: *Receptors for Neurotransmitters and Peptide Hormones*, pp. 265–270, Pepeu, G., Kuhar, M. J. and Enna, S. J. (eds). Raven Press, New York.

Biscoe, T. J., Fry, J. P. and Rickets, C. (1984) Autoradiography of benzodiazepine receptor binding in the central nervous system of the normal C57BL6J mouse. *J. Physiol. (Lond).* **352**: 495–508.

Blair, L. A. C., Levitan, E. S., Marshall, J., Dionne, V. E. and Barnard, E. A. (1988) Single subunits of the $GABA_A$ receptor form ion channels with properties of the native receptor. *Science* **242**: 577–579.

Blair, T. and Webb, G. A. (1977) Electronic factors in the structure–activity relationship of some 1,4-benzodiazepine-2-ones. *J. Med. Chem.* **20**: 1206–1210.

Blanchard, J.-C. and Joulou, L. (1983) Suriclone: a new cyclopyrrolone derivative recognising receptors labelled by benzodiazepines in rat hippocampus and cerebellum. *J. Neurochem.* **40**: 601–607.

Blanchard, J. C., Boireau, A., Garret, C. and Joulou, L. (1979) In vitro and in vivo inhibition by zopiclone of benzodiazepine binding to rodent brain receptors. *Life Sci.* **24**: 2417–2420.

Blount, J. F., Fryer, R. I., Gilman, N. W. and Todaro, L. J. (1983) Quinazolines and 1,4-benzodiazepines: 92 conformational recognition of the receptor for 1,4-benzodiazepines. *Mol. Pharmacol.* **24**: 425–428.

Borea, P. A. (1981) Structure activity relationships in 1,4-benzodiazepines. *Boll. Soc. Ital. Biol. Sper.* **57**: 628–632.

Borea, P. A. (1983) De novo analysis of receptor binding affinity data of benzodiazepines. *Arzneim. Forsch.* **33**: 1086–1088.

Borea, P. A. and Gilli, G. (1984) The nature of 1,4-benzodiazepines–receptor interactions. *Arzneim. Forsch.* **34**: 649–652.

Borea, P. A., Gilli, G. and Bertolasi, V. (1979) Application of the Free-Wilson model to the analysis of three different pharmacological activity tests in benzodiazepines. *Farmaro. Ed. Sci.* **34**: 1073–1082.

Borea, P. A., Supavilai, P. and Karobath, M. (1984) Effect of GABA and photoaffinity labelling on the affinity of drugs for benzodiazepine receptors in membranes of the cerebral cortex of five-day-old rats. *Biochem. Pharmacol.* **33**: 165–168.

Borea, P. A., Gilli, G., Bertolasi, V. and Ferretti, V. (1987) Stereochemical features controlling binding and intrinsic activity properties of benzodiazepine receptor ligands. *Mol. Pharmcol.* **31**: 334–344.

Bormann, J. and Clapham, D. E. (1985) Gamma-aminobutyric acid receptor channels in adrenal chromaffin cells: a patch clamp study. *Proc. Nat. Acad. Sci. USA* **82**: 2168–2172.

Bormann, J., Hamill, O. P. and Sakmann, B. (1987) Mechanism of anion permeation through channels gated by glycine and gamma-aminobutyric acid in mouse cultured spinal neurones. *J. Physiol. (Lond).* **385**: 243–286.

Bosmann, H. B., Case, K. R. and Distefano, P. (1977) Diazepam receptor characterisation: specific binding of a benzodiazepine to macromolecules in various areas of rat brain. *FEBS Lett.* **82**: 368–372.

Bowery, N. G. and Hudson, A. L. (1979) Gamma-aminobutyric acid reduces the evoked release of [^{3}H]-noradrenaline from synapathetic nerve terminals. *Brit. J. Pharmacol.* **66**: 108P.

Bowery, N. G., Brown, D. A. and Collins, J. F. (1975) Tetramethylenedisulphotetramine: an inhibitor of gamma-aminobutyric acid induced depolarisation of the isolated superior cervical ganglion of the rat. *Brit. J. Pharmacol.* **53**: 422–424.

Bowery, N. G., Collins, J. F., Hill, R. G. and Pearson, S. (1976) GABA antagonism as a possible basis for the convulsant action of a series of bicyclic phosphorus esters. *Brit. J. Pharmacol.* **57**: 435P–436P.

Bowery, N. G., Collins, J. F., Hill, R. G. and Pearson, S. (1977) t-Butyl bicyclophosphate: a convulsant and GABA antagonist more potent than bicuculline. *Brit. J. Pharmacol.* **60**: 275P–276P.

Bowery, N. G., Doble, A., Hill, D. R., Hudson, A. L., Shaw, J. S., Turnbull, M. J. and Warrington, R. (1981) Bicuculline insensitive GABA receptors on peripheral autonomic nerve terminals. *Eur. J. Pharmac.* **71**: 53–70.

Bowery, N. G., Hill, D. R. and Hudson, A. L. (1983) Characteristics of GABA-B receptor binding sites on rat whole brain synaptic membranes. *Brit. J. Pharmacol.* **78**: 191–206.

Bowery, N. G., Hill, D. R., Hudson, A. L., Price, G. W., Turnbull, M. J. and Wilkin, G. P. (1984) Heterogeneity of mammalian GABA receptors. In: *Actions and Interactions of GABA and Benzodiazepines*, pp. 81–108, BOWERY, N. G. (ed) Raven Press, New York.

BOWERY, N. G., HUDSON, A. L. and PRICE, G. W. (1987) GABA-A and GABA-B receptor site distribution in the rat central nervous system. *Neuroscience* **20**: 365–383.

BRADFORD, H. F. (1970) Metabolic response of synaptosomes to electrical stimulation: release of amino acids. *Brain Res.* **19**: 239–247.

BRAESTRUP, C. and NIELSEN, M. (1978) Ontogenetic development of benzodiazepine receptors in the rat brain. *Brain Res.* **147**: 170–173.

BRAESTRUP, C. and NIELSEN, M. (1980) Multiple benzodiazepine receptors. *Trends Neurosci.* **3**: 301–303.

BRAESTRUP, C. and NIELSEN, M. (1981a) ^{3}H-propyl beta-carboline-3-carboxylate as a selective radioligand for the Bz1 benzodiazepine receptor subclass. *J. Neurochem.* **37**: 333–341.

BRAESTRUP, C. and NIELSEN, M. (1981b) GABA reduces binding of ^{3}H-methyl-beta-carboline-3-carboxylate to brain benzodiazepine receptors. *Nature* **294**: 472–474.

BRAESTRUP, C. and NIELSEN, M. (1986) Benzodiazepine receptor binding in vivo and efficacy. In: *Benzodiazepine/GABA Receptors and Chloride Channels: Structural and Functional Properties*, pp. 167–184, Alan R. Liss, New York.

BRAESTRUP, C. and SQUIRES, R. F. (1977) Specific benzodiazepine receptors in rat brain characterised by high affinity [3H]-diazepam binding. *Proc. Natl. Acad. Sci. USA* **74**: 3805–3809.

BRAESTRUP, C. and SQUIRES, R. F. (1978a) Brain specific benzodiazepine receptors. *Brit. J. Psychiat.* **133**: 249–260.

BRAESTRUP, C. and SQUIRES, R. F. (1978b) Pharmacological characterisation of benzodiazepine receptors in the brain. *Eur. J. Pharmacol.* **78**: 263–270.

BRAESTRUP, C., ALBRECHTSEN, R. and SQUIRES, R. F. (1977) High densities of benzodiazepine receptors in human cortical areas. *Nature* **269**: 702–704.

BRAESTRUP, C., NIELSEN, M. and HONORE, T. (1983) Binding of ^{3}H-DMCM, a convulsive benzodiazepine ligand, to rat brain membranes: preliminary studies. *J. Neurochem.* **41**: 454–465.

BRAESTRUP, C., NIELSEN, M., KROGSGAARD-LARSEN, P. and FALCH, E. (1979a) Partial agonists for brain GABA/benzodiazepine receptor complex. *Nature* **280**: 331–333.

BRAESTRUP, C., NIELSEN, M., BIGGIO, G. and SQUIRES, R. F. (1979b) Neuronal localisation of benzodiazepine receptors in cerebellum. *Neurosci. Lett.* **13**: 219–224.

BRAESTRUP, C., NIELSEN, M. and SQUIRES, R. F. (1979c) No changes in rat brain benzodiazepine receptors after withdrawal from continuous treatment with lorazepam or diazepam. *Life Sci.* **24**: 347–350.

BRAESTRUP, C., NIELSEN, M. and OLSEN, C. E. (1980) Urinary and brain beta-carboline-3-carboxylates as potent inhibitors of brain benzodiazepine receptors. *Proc. Natl. Acad. Sci. USA* **77**: 2288–2292.

BRAESTRUP, C., NISSEN, C., SQUIRES, R. F. and SCHOUSBOE, A. (1978) Lack of brain specific benzodiazepine receptors on mouse primary astroglial cultures. *Neurosci. Lett.* **9**: 5–49.

BRAESTRUP, C., SCHMIECHEM, R., NEFF, G., NIELSEN, M. and PETERSEN, E. N. (1982) Interaction of convulsive ligands with benzodiazepine receptors. *Science* **216**: 1241–1243.

BRECKENRIDGE, R. J., NICHOLSON, S. H., NICOL, A. J., SUCKLING, C. J., LEIGH, B. and IVERSEN, L. L. (1981) Inhibition of neuronal GABA uptake and glial beta-alanine uptake by synthetic GABA analogues. *Biochem. Pharmacol.* **30**: 3045–3049.

BRENNAN, M. J. W. and CANTRILL, R. C. (1979) Delta-aminolaevulinic acid is a potent agonist for GABA autoreceptors. *Nature* **280**: 514–515.

BRENNAN, M. J. W., CANTRILL, R. C. and KROGSGAARD-LARSEN, P. (1981) GABA autoreceptors: structure activity relationships for agonists. *Advances in Biochemical Psychopharmacology* **26**: 157–167.

BRISTOW, D. R. and MARTIN, I. L. (1987a) Solubilisation of the benzodiazepine receptor from rat cerebellum by the detergent n-octylpentaoxyethylene. *J. Neurochem.* **48**: 1537–1540.

BRISTOW, D. R. and MARTIN, I. L. (1987b) Solubilisation of the gamma-aminobutyric acid/benzodiazepine receptor from rat cerebellum: optimal preservation of the modulatory responses by natural brain lipids. *J. Neurochem.* **49**: 1386–1393.

BROWN, C. L. and MARTIN, I. L. (1982) Photoaffinity labelling of the benzodiazepine receptor does not occlude the beta-CCE binding site. *Brit. J. Pharmacol.* **77**: 312P.

BROWN, C. L. and MARTIN, I. L. (1983) Photoaffinity labelling of the benzodiazepine receptor cannot be used to predict ligand efficacy. *Neurosci. Lett.* **35**: 37–40.

BROWN, C. L. and MARTIN, I. L. (1984a) Autoradiographic localisation of benzodiazepine receptors in the rat pituitary gland. *Eur. J. Pharmacol.* **102**: 563–564.

BROWN, C. L. and MARTIN, I. L. (1984b) Photoaffinity labelling of the benzodiazepine receptor compromises the recognition site but not its effector mechanism. *J. Neurochem.* **43**: 272–273.

BROWN, C. L. and MARTIN, I. L. (1984c) Kinetics of ^{3}H-Ro 15-1788 binding to membrane-bound rat brain benzodiazepine receptors. *J. Neurochem.* **43**: 918–923.

BROWN, C. L., MARTIN, I. L., JONES, B. and OAKLEY, N. (1984) In vivo determination of efficacy of pyrazoloquinolines at the benzodiazepine receptor. *Eur. J. Pharmacol.* **103**: 139–143.

BUTCHER, H. T., CHANANONT, P., HAMOR, T. A. and MARTIN, I. L. (1984) Structure activity relationships in a series of 5-phenyl-1,4-benzodiazepines. Proc. 8th International Symposium on Medical Chemistry, Uppsala.

CANDY, J. M. and MARTIN, I. L. (1979) The postnatal development of the benzodiazepine receptor in the cerebral cortex and cerebellum of the rat. *J. Neurochem.* **32**: 655–658.

CHAN, C. Y., GIBBS, T. T., BORDEN, L. A. and FARB, D. H. (1983) Multiple embryonic benzodiazepine binding sites: evidence for functionality. *Life Sci.* **33**: 2061–2069.

CHANG, L.-R. and BARNARD, E. A. (1982) The benzodiazepine/GABA receptor complex: molecular size in brain synaptic membranes and in solution. *J. Neurochem.* **39**: 1507–1518.

CHANG, R. S. L. and SNYDER, S. H. (1978) Benzodiazepine receptors: labelling in intact animals with ^{3}H-flunitrazepam. *Eur. J. Pharmacol.* **38**: 213–218.

CHANG, R. S. L., TRAN, V. T. and SNYDER, S. H. (1980) Neurotransmitter receptor localisation: brain lesions induced alterations in benzodiazepine, GABA, beta-adrenergic and histamine H1-receptor binding. *Brain Res.* **190**: 95–110.

Chiu, T. H. and Rosenberg, H. C. (1978) Reduced diazepam binding following chronic benzodiazepine treatment. *Life Sci.* **23**: 1153–1158.

Chiu, T. H. and Rosenberg, H. C. (1982) Comparison of the kinetics of ^{3}H-diazepam and ^{3}H-flunitrazepam binding to cortical synaptosomal membranes. *J. Neurochem.* **39**: 1716–1725.

Chiu, T. H. and Rosenberg, H. C. (1983a) Conformational changes in benzodiazepine receptors induced by the antagonist Ro 15-1788. *Mol. Pharmacol.* **23**: 289–294.

Chiu, T. H. and Rosenberg, H. C. (1983b) Multiple conformational states of benzodiazepine receptors. *Trends Pharmacol. Sci.*, **4**: 348–350.

Chiu, T. H., Dryden, D. M. and Rosenberg, H. C. (1982) Kinetics of ^{3}H-flunitrazepam binding to membrane bound benzodiazepine receptors. *Mol. Pharmacol.* **21**: 57–65.

Chude, O. (1979) Solubilisation and partial purification of the GABA receptor from mouse brain and a binding assay for the soluble receptor. *J. Neurochem.* **33**: 621–629.

Codding, P. W. and Muir, A. K. S. (1985) Molecular structure of Ro 15-1788 and a model for the binding of benzodiazepine receptor ligands. *Mol. Pharmacol.* **28**: 178–184.

Costa, E., Guidotti, A. and Mao, C. C. (1976) A GABA hypothesis for the action of benzodiazepines. In: *GABA in Nervous System Functions*, pp. 413–426, Roberts, E., Chase, T. N. and Tower, D. B. (eds), Raven Press, New York.

Costa, E., Guidotti, A., Mao, C. C. and Suria, A. (1975) New concepts on the mechanism of action of the benzodiazepines. *Life Sci.* **17**: 167–186.

Costa, E., Guidotti, A. and Toffano, G. (1978) Molecular mechanisms mediating the action of diazepam on GABA receptors. *Brit. J. Psychiat.* **133**: 239–248.

Costa, T., Rodbard, D. and Pert, C. (1979) Is the benzodiazepine receptor coupled to a chloride anion channel? *Nature* **277**: 315–317.

Costa, T., Russell, L., Pert, C. B. and Rodbard, D. (1981) Halide and gamma-aminobutyric acid-induced enhancement of diazepam receptors in rat brain. Reversal by disulfonic acid stilbene blockers of anion channels. *Mol. Pharmacol.* **20**: 470–476.

Cottrell, G. A., Lambert, J. J. and Mistry, D. K. (1987) Alphaxalone potentiates GABA and activates GABA-A of mouse spinal neurons in culture. *J. Physiol. (Lond).* **382**: 133P.

Cottrell, G. A., Lambert, J. J. and Peters, J. A. (1987) Modulation of GABA-A receptor activity by alphaxalone. *Brit. J. Pharmacol.* **90**: 491–500.

Cowan, P. J., Green, A. R., Nutt, D. J. and Martin, I. L. (1981) Ethyl beta-carboline carboxylate lowers seizure threshold and antagonises flurazepam induced sedation in rats. *Nature* **290**: 54–55.

Crippen, G. M. (1982) Distance geometry analysis of the benzodiazepine binding site. *Mol. Pharmacol.* **22**: 11–19.

Cullheim, S. and Kellerth, J.-O. (1981) Two kinds of recurrent inhibition of cat spinal alpha-motoneurones as differentiated pharmacologically. *J. Physiol. (Lond).* **312**: 209–224.

Curtis, D. R. and Johnston, G. A. R. (1974) Amino acid transmitters in the mammalian central nervous system. *Ergebn. Physiol.* **69**: 97–118.

Curtis, D. R., Hosli, L., Johnston, G. A. R. and Johnston, I. H. (1968) Pharmacological study of the depression of spinal neurones by glycine and related amino acids. *Exp. Brain Res.* **6**: 1–18.

Curtis, D. R., Lodge, D., Johnston, G. A. R. and Brand, S. J. (1976) Central actions of benzodiazepines. *Brain Res.* **118**: 344–347.

Czernik, A. J., Petrack, B., Kalinsky, H. J., Psychoyos, S., Cash, W. D., Tsai, C., Rinehart, R. K., Granat, F. R., Lovell, R. A., Brundish, D. E. and Wade, R. (1982) CGS 8216: receptor binding characteristics of a potent benzodiazepine antagonist. *Life Sci.* **30**: 363–372.

Danziger, D. J. and Dean, P. M. (1985) The search for functional correspondences in molecular structure between two dissimilar molecules. *J. Theoret. Biol.* **116**: 215–224.

Davies, L. R. and Huston, V. (1981) Peripheral benzodiazepine binding sites in heart and their interaction with dipyridamole. *Eur. J. Pharmacol.* **73**: 209–211.

De Blas, A. L., Sangameswaran, L., Haney, S. A., Park, D., Abraham Jr., C. J. and Rayner, C. A. (1985) Monoclonal antibodies to benzodiazepines. *J. Neurochem.* **45**: 1748–1753.

Doble, A. (1983) Comparative thermodynamics of benzodiazepine receptor ligand interactions in rat neuronal membranes. *J. Neurochem.* **40**: 1605–1612.

Doble, A., Martin, I. L. and Richards, D. A. (1982) GABA modulation predicts biological activity of ligands for the benzodiazepine receptor. *Brit. J. Pharmacol.* **76**: 238P.

Dorow, R., Horowski, R., Paschelke, G., Amin, M. and Braestrup, C. (1983) Severe anxiety induced by FG7142, a beta-carboline ligand for benzodiazepine receptors. *Lancet* ii: 98–99.

Duka, T., Hollt, V. and Herz, A. (1979) In vivo receptor occupation by benzodiazepine and correlation with pharmacological effect. *Brain Res.* **179**: 147–156.

Falch, E. and Krogsgaard-Larsen, P. (1982) The binding of the GABA agonist 3H-THIP to rat brain synaptic membranes. *J. Neurochem.* **38**: 1123–1129.

Fernholm, B., Nielsen, M. and Braestrup, C. (1979) Absence of brain specific benzodiazepine receptors in cyclostomes and elasmobranchs. *Comp. Biochem. Physiol.* **C62**: 209–211.

Ferrarese, C., Vaccarino, F., Alho, H., Mellstrom, B., Costa, E. and Guidotti, A. (1987) Subcellular location and neuronal release of diazepam binding inhibitor. *J. Neurochem.* **48**: 1093–1102.

Ferrero, P., Costa, E., Conti-Tronconi, B. and Guidotti, A. (1986) A diazepam binding inhibitor (DBI)-like neuropeptide is detected in human brain. *Brain Res.* **399**: 136–142.

Ferrero, P., Santi, M. R., Conti-Tronconi, B., Costa, E. and Guidotti, A. (1986) Study of an octadecaneuropeptide derived from diazepam binding inhibitor (DBI): biological activity and presence in rat brain. *Proc. Natl. Acad. Sci. USA* **83**: 827–831.

Fowler, J. L. and John, R. A. (1972) Active site directed irreversible inhibition of rat brain 4-aminobutyrate aminotransferase by ethanolamine-O-sulphate in vitro and in vivo. *Biochem. J.* **130**: 569–573.

Franklin, T. J. (1980) Binding energy and the activation of hormone receptors. *Biochem. Pharmacol.* **29**: 853–856.

Frere, R. C., MacDonald, R. L. and Young, A. B. (1982) GABA binding and bicuculline in spinal cord and cortical membranes from adult rat and mouse neurons in cell culture. *Brain Res.* **244**: 145–153.

Fritz, L. C., Wang, C. C. and Gorio, A. (1979) Avermectin Bla irreversibility blocks postsynaptic potential at the lobster neuromuscular junction by reducing muscle membrane resistance. *Proc. Natl. Acad. Sci. USA* **76**: 2062–2066.

Fry, J. P., Rickets, C. and Martin, I. L. (1987) Polyclonal antibodies to agonist benzodiazepines. *Biochem. Pharmacol.* **36**: 3763–3770.

Fryer, R. I. (1983) Benzodiazepine ligand-receptor interactions. In: *The Benzodiazepines: From Molecular Biology to Clinical Practice*, pp. 7–20, Costa, E. (ed) Raven Press, New York.

Fryer, R. I., Cook, Ch., Gilman, N. W. and Walser, A. (1986) Conformational shifts at the benzodiazepine receptor related to the binding of agonists antagonists and inverse agonists. *Life Sci.* **39**: 1947–1957.

Fryer, R. I., Gilman, N. W., Madison, V. and Walser, A. (1984) Conformational differences for agonists and antagonists at the benzodiazepine receptor. Proc. of 8th International Symposium on Medicinal Chemistry, Uppsala.

Fujimoto, M., Hirai, K. and Okabayashi, T. (1982) Comparison of the effects of GABA and chloride ion on the affinities of ligands for the benzodiazepine receptor. *Life Sci.* **30**: 51–57.

Fuxe, K., Koehler, C., Agnati, L. F., Andersson, K., Oegren, S.O., Eneroth, P., Perex de la Mora, M., Karobath, M. and Krogsgaard-Larsen, P. (1981) GABA and benzodiazepine receptors. Studies on their localisation in the hippocampus and their interaction with central dopamine neurones in the rat brain. In: *GABA and Benzodiazepine Receptors*, pp. 61–76, Costa, E., DiChiara, G. and Gessa, G. L. (eds) Raven Press, New York.

Gall, M., Hester, J. B., Rudzik, A. D. and Lahti, R. A. (1976) Synthesis and pharmacology of novel anxiolytic agents derived from 2-[(dialkylamino)methyl-4H-triazolo-4-yl]benzophenones and related heterocyclic benzophenones. *J. Med. Chem.* **19**: 1057–1064.

Gallager, D. W., Mallorga, P., Oertel, W., Henneberry, R. and Tallman, J. (1981) 3H-diazepam binding in mammalian central nervous system: a pharmacological characterisation. *J. Neurosci.* **1**: 218–225.

Gallager, D. W., Lakoski, J. M., Gonsalves, S. F. and Rauch, S. L. (1984) Chronic benzodiazepine treatment decreases postsynaptic GABA sensitivity. *Nature* **308**: 74–77.

Gallagher, J. P., Higashi, H. and Nishi, S. (1978) Characterisation and ionic basis of GABA-induced depolarisations recorded in vitro from cat primary afferent neurones. *J. Physiol. (Lond).* **275**: 263–282.

Garcia-Munoz, M., Nicolaou, M. M., Tulloch, I. F., Wright, A. K. and Arbuthnott, G. B. (1977) Feedback loop or output pathway in striatonigral fibres. *Nature* **265**: 363–365.

Gavish, M. and Snyder, S. H. (1981) Gamma-amino butyric acid and benzodiazepine receptors: Copurification and characterisation. *Proc. Natl. Acad. Sci. USA* **78**: 1939–1942.

Gavish, M., Chang, R. S. L. and Snyder, S. H. (1979) Solubilisation of histamine H-1, GABA and benzodiazepine receptors. *Life Sci.* **25**: 783–790.

Gee, K. W. and Yamamura, H. I. (1982a) Regional heterogeneity of benzodiazepine receptors at 37 degrees: an in vitro study in various regions of the rat brain. *Life Sci.* **31**: 1939–1945.

Gee, K. W. and Yamamura, H. I. (1982b) Differentiation of benzodiazepine receptor agonist and antagonist: sparing [^{3}H]-benzodiazepine antagonist binding following the photolabelling of benzodiazepine receptors. *Eur. J. Pharmacol.* **82**: 239–241.

Geller, H. M., Taylor, D. H. and Hoffer, B. J. (1978) Benzodiazepines and central inhibitory mechanisms. *Naunyn Schmiedebergs Arch. Pharmacol.* **304**: 81–88.

Gilli, G., Borea, P. A., Bertolasi, V. and Sacerdoti, M. (1977) Stereochemical and electronic properties of benzodiazepines. Correlation with their anti-convulsant activity, p. 38, Abstracts, 4th European Crystallography Meeting, Oxford.

Gray, P. W., Glaister, D., Seeburg, P. H., Guidotti, A. and Costa, E. (1986) Cloning and expression of cDNA for human diazepam binding inhibitor, a natural ligand for an allosteric regulatory site of the gamma-aminobutyric acid type A receptor. *Proc. Natl. Acad. Sci. USA* **83**: 7547–7551.

Greenlee, D. V. and Olsen, R. W. (1979) Solubilisation of gamma-aminobutyric acid receptor protein from mammalian brain. *Biochem. Biophys. Res. Comm.* **88**: 380–387.

Grenningloh, G., Rienitz, A., Schmitt, B., Methfessel, C., Zensen, M., Beyreuther, K., Gundelfinger, E. D. and Betz, H. (1987) The strychnine binding subunit of the glycine receptor shows homology with nicotinic acetylcholine receptors. *Nature* **328**: 215–220.

Guidotti, A., Forschetti, C. M., Corda, M. G., Kondel, D., Bennett, C. D. and Costa, E. (1983) Isolation, characterisation, and purification to homogeneity of an endogenous polypeptide with agonistic action on benzodiazepine receptors. *Proc. Natl. Acad. Sci. USA* **80**: 3531–3535.

Guidotti, A., Toffano, G. and Costa, E. (1978) An endogenous protein modulates the affinity of GABA and benzodiazepine receptors in rat brain. *Nature* **275**: 553–555.

Haefely, W. (1984) Actions and interactions of benzodiazepine agonists and antagonists at GABA-eric synapses. In: *Actions and Interactions of GABA and Benzodiazepines*, pp. 263–285, Bowery, N. G. (eds) Raven Press, New York.

Haefely, W. and Polc, P. (1986) Physiology of GABA enhancement by benzodiazepines and barbiturates. In: *Benzodiazepine/GABA Receptors and Chloride Channels: Structural and Functional Properties*, pp. 97–133, Alan R. Liss, New York.

Haefely, W., Kyburz, E., Gerecke, M. and Mohler, H. (1985) Recent advances in the molecular pharmacology of benzodiazepine receptors and in structure–activity relationships of their agonists and antagonists. *Adv. Drug Res.* **14**: 165–322.

Hamill, O. P., Borman, J. and Sakman, B. (1983) Activation of multiple conductance state chloride channels in spinal neurons by glycine and GABA. *Nature* **305**: 805–808.

Hammond, J. R. and Martin, I. L. (1986) Solubilisation of the benzodiazepine/gamma-aminobutyric acid receptor complex. Comparison of the detergents octylglucopyranoside and 3-[(cholamidopropyl)-dimethyl(ammonio)] 1-propanesulfonate (CHAPS). *J. Neurochem.* **47**: 1161–1171.

HAMOR, T. A. and MARTIN, I. L. (1983) The benzodiazepines. *Progress in Medicinal Chemistry* **20**: 157–223.

HARING, P., STAHLI, C., SCHOCH, P., TAKACS, B., STAEHELIN, T. and MOHLER, H. (1985) Monoclonal antibodies reveal structural homogeneity of gamma-aminobutyric acid/benzodiazepine receptors in different brain areas. *Proc. Natl. Acad. Sci. USA* **82**: 4837–4841.

HARRIS, R. A. and ALLAN, A. M. (1985) Functional coupling of gamma-aminobutyric acid receptors to chloride channels in brain membranes. *Science* **228**: 1108–1110.

HARRIS, R. A. and ALLAN, A. M. (1986) GABA receptor mediated chloride transport in a "cell-free" membrane preparation from brain. *Science* **233**: 229.

HARRISON, N. L. and SIMMONDS, M. A. (1984) Modulation of the GABA receptor complex by a steroid anaesthetic. *Brain Res.* **323**: 287–292.

HEAULME, M., CHAMBON, J. P., LEYRIS, R., WERMUTH, C. G. and BIZIERE, K. (1986) Specific binding of a phenyl-pyridazinium derivative endowed with GABA-A receptor antagonist activity. *Neuropharmacology* **25**: 1279–1283.

HERBLIN, W. F. and MECHEM, C. C. (1984) Short wave ultraviolet radiation increases photoaffinity labelling of benzodiazepine sites. *Life Sci.* **35**: 317–324.

HESTER, J. B., DUCHAMP, D. J. and CHIDESTER, C. G. (1971) A synthetic approach to new 1,4-benzodiazepine derivatives. *Tetrahedron Lett.* **20**: 1609–1612.

HILL, D. R. (1985) GABA-B receptor modulation of adenylate cyclase activity in rat brain slices. *Brit. J. Pharmac.* **84**: 249–257.

HILL, D. R. and BOWERY, N. G. (1981) ^{3}H-baclofen and ^{3}H-GABA bind to bicuculline-insensitive GABA-B sites in rat brain. *Nature* **290**: 149–152.

HIRSCH, J. D. (1982) Photolabelling of benzodiazepine receptors spares ^{3}H-propyl beta-carboline binding. *Pharmacol. Biochem. Behav.* **16**: 245–248.

HIRSCH, J. D. and LYDIGSEN, J. L. (1981) Binding of beta-carboline-3-carboxylic acid ethyl ester to mouse brain benzodiazepine receptors in vivo. *Eur. J. Pharmacol.* **72**: 357–360.

HONORE, T., NIELSEN, M. and BRAESTRUP, C. (1983) Binding of ^{3}H-DMCM to benzodiazepine receptors; chloride dependent allosteric mechanisms. *J. Neural. Trans.* **58**: 83–98.

HONORE, T., NIELSEN, M. and BRAESTRUP, C. (1984) Barbiturate shift as a tool for determination of efficacy of benzodiazepine receptor ligands. *Eur. J. Pharmacol.* **100**: 103–107.

HOUAMED, K. M., BILBE, G., SMART, T. G., CONSTANTI, A., BROWN, D. A., BARNARD, E. A. and RICHARDS, B. M. (1984) Expression of functional GABA, glycine and glutamate receptors in Xenopus oocytes injected with rat brain mRNA. *Nature* **310**: 318–321.

HUANG, A., BARKER, J. L., PAUL, S. M., MONCADA, V. and SKOLNICK, P. (1980) Characterisation of benzodiazepine receptors in primary cultures of fetal mouse brain and spinal cord neurons. *Brain Res.* **190**: 485–491.

HUNKELER, W., MOHLER, H., PIERI, L., POLC, P., BONETTI, E. P., CUMIN, R., SCHAFFNER, R. and HAEFELY, W. (1981) Selective antagonists of benzodiazepines. *Nature* **290**: 514–516.

IMOTO, K., BUSCH, C., SAKMANN, B., MISHINA, M., KONNO, T., NAKAI, J., BUJO, H., MORI, Y., FUKUDA, K. and NUMA, S. (1988) Rings of negatively charged amino acids determine the acetylcholine receptor channel conductance. *Nature* **335**: 645–648.

IMOTO, K., METHFESSEL, C., SAKMANN, B., MISHINA, M., MORI, Y., KONNO, T., FUKUDA, K., KURASAKI, M., BUJO, H., FUJITA, Y. and NUMA, S. (1986) Location of a delta-subunit region determining ion transport through the acetylcholine receptor channel. *Nature* **324**: 670–674.

IVERSEN, L. L. and BLOOM, F. E. (1972) Studies of the uptake of ^{3}H-GABA and ^{3}H-glycine in slices and homogenates of rat brain and spinal cord by electron microscopic autoradiography. *Brain Res.* **41**: 131–143.

IVERSEN, L. L. and KELLY, J. S. (1975) Uptake and metabolism of gamma-aminobutyric acid by neurones and glial cells. *Biochem. Pharmacol.* **24**: 933–938.

IVERSEN, L. L. and NEAL, M. J. (1968) The uptake of ^{3}H-GABA by slices of rat cerebral cortex. *J. Neurochem.* **15**: 1141–1149.

JENSEN, L. H., PETERSEN, E. N. and BRAESTRUP, C. (1983) Audiogenic seizures in DBA/2 mice discriminate sensitively between low efficacy benzodiazepine receptor agonists and inverse agonists. *Life Sci.* **33**: 393–399.

JOHNSON, R. W. and YAMAMURA, H. I. (1979) Photoaffinity labelling of the benzodiazepine receptor in bovine cerebral cortex. *Life Sci.* **25**: 1613–1620.

JOHNSTON, G. A. R. (1976) Physiologic pharmacology of GABA and its antagonists in vertebrate nervous system. In: *GABA in Nervous System Function*, pp. 395–411, ROBERTS, E., CHASE, T. N. and TOWER, D. B. (eds) Raven Press, New York.

JOHNSTON, G. A. R. (1978) Neuropharmacology of amino acid inhibitory transmitters. *Ann. Rev. Pharmacol. Toxicol.* **18**: 269–289.

JOHNSTON, G. A. R., KROGSGAARD-LARSEN, P., STEPHANSON, A. L. and TWITCHIN, B. (1976) Inhibition of the uptake of GABA and related amino acids in rat brain slices by the optical isomers of nipecotic acid. *J. Neurochem.* **26**: 1029–1032.

JORDAN, C. C., MUTUS, A. I., PIOTROWSKI, W. and WILKINSON, D. (1982) Binding of ^{3}H-gamma-amino butyric acid and ^{3}H-muscimol in purified rat brain synaptic plasma membranes and the effects of bicuculline. *J. Neurochem.* **39**: 52–58.

JULIEN, J.-F., LEGAY, F., DUMAS, S., TAPPAZ, M. and MALLET, J. (1987) Molecular cloning, expression and in situ hybridisation of rat brain glutamic acid decarboxylase messenger RNA. *Neurosci. Lett.* **73**: 173–180.

JUNG, M. J. and METCALF, B. W. (1975) Catalytic inhibition of gamma-aminobutyric acid-alpha-ketoglutarate transaminase of bacterial origin by 4-aminohex-5-ynoic acid, a substrate analogue. *Biochem. Biophys. Res. Commun.* **67**: 301–306.

JUNG, M. J., LIPPERT, B., METCALF, B. W., BOHLEA, P. and SCHECHTER, J. (1977) Gamma-vinyl GABA, a new selective irreversible inhibitor of GABA-T: effect on brain GABA metabolism in mice.

KALES, A., SCHARF, M. B., SOLDATOS, C. R., BIXLER, E. O., BIANCHI, S. B. and SCHWEITZER, P. K. J. (1980)

Quazepam, a new benzodiazepine hypnotic: intermediate term sleep laboratory evaluation. *J. Clin. Pharmacol.* **20**: 184–192.
KARBON, E. W., DUMAN, R. S. and ENNA, S. J. (1984) GABA-B receptors and norepinephrine stimulated cAMP production in rat brain cortex. *Brain Res.* **306**: 327–332.
KARBON, E. W. and ENNA, S. J. (1985) Characterisation of the relationship between gamma-amminobutyric acid B (GABA-B) agonists and transmitter coupled cyclic neucleotide generatory systems in rat brain. *Mol. Pharmacol.* **27**: 53–59.
KARDOS, J., GLASKO, G., KEREKES, P., KOVACS, I. and SIMONYI, M. (1984) Inhibition of ^{3}H-GABA binding to rat brain synaptic membranes by bicuculline related alkaloids. *Biochem. Pharmacol.* **33**: 3537–3545.
KARDOS, J., MADERSPACK, K. and SIMONYI, M. (1985) Towards a more physiological approach to GABA binding. *Neurochem. Intl.* **5**: 737–743.
KARLSSON, A., FONNUM, F., MALTHE-SORENSSEN, D. and STORM-MATHISEN, J. (1974) Effect of the convulsive agent 3-mercaptopropionic acid on the levels of GABA, other amino acids and glutamate decarboxylase in different regions of the rat brain. *Biochem. Pharmacol.* **23**: 3053–3061.
KAROBATH, M. and LIPPITSCH, M. (1979) THIP and isoguavacine are partial agonists of GABA stimulated benzodiazepine binding. *Eur. J. Pharmacol.* **58**: 485–488.
KAROBATH, M. and SUPAVILAI, P. (1982) Distinction of benzodiazepine agonists from antagonists by photoaffinity labelling of benzodiazepine receptors in vitro. *Neurosci. Lett.* **31**: 65–69.
KAROBATH, M., PLACHETA, P., LIPPITSCH, M. and KROGSGAARD-LARSEN, P. (1979) Is stimulation of benzodiazepine receptor binding mediated by a novel GABA receptor. *Nature* **278**: 748–749.
KATAOKA, Y., GUTMAN, Y., GUIDOTTI, A., PANULA, P., WROBLEWSKI, J., COSENZA-MURPHY, D., WU, J. Y. and COSTA, E. (1984) Intrinsic GABAergic system of adrenal chromaffin cells. *Proc. Natl. Acad. Sci. USA* **81**: 3218–3222.
KAUFMAN, D. L., MCGINNIS, J. F., KREIGER, N. R. and TOBIN, A. J. (1986) Brain glutamate decarboxylase cloned in lambda gt-11: fusion protein produces gamma-aminobutyric acid. *Science* **232**: 1138–1140.
KELLY, J. S. and BEART, P. M. (1975) Amino acid receptors in CNS. II GABA in supraspinal regions. In: *Handbook of Psychopharmacology 4*, pp. 129–209, IVERSEN, L. L., IVERSEN, S. D. and SNYDER, S. H. (eds) Plenum Press, New York.
KELLY, J. S., KRNJEVIC, K., MORRIS, M. E. and YIM, G. K. W. (1969) Anionic permeability of cortical neurones. *Exp. Brain Res.* **7**: 11–31.
KEMP, J. A., MARSHALL, G. R., WONG, E. H. F. and WOODRUFF, G. N. (1987) The affinities, potencies and efficacies of some benzodiazepine receptor agonists, antagonists and inverse agonists at rat hippocampal $GABA_A$ receptors. *Brit. J. Pharmacol.* **91**: 601–608.
KERR, D. I. B., ONG, J., PRAGER, R. H., GYNTHER, B. D. and CURTIS, D. R. (1987) Phaclofen: a peripheral and central baclofen antagonist. *Brain Res.* **405**: 150–154.
KOBAYASHI, Y., KAUFMAN, D. L. and TOBIN, A. J. (1987) Glutamic acid decarboxylase cDNA: nucleotide sequence encoding an enzymatically active fusion protein. *J. Neurosci.* **7**: 2768–2772.
KOBAYASHI, K., MIYANZAWA, S., TERAHARA, A., MISHIMI, H. and KURIHARA, H. (1976) Gabaculine: gamma-aminobutyrate aminotransferase inhibitor of microbial origin. *Tetrahedron Lett.* **7**: 537–540.
KOCHMAN, R. L. and HIRSCH, J. D. (1982) Thermodynamic changes associated with benzodiazepine and alkyl beta-carboline-3-carboxylate binding to rat brain homogenates. *Mol. Pharmacol.* **22**: 335–341.
KROGSGAARD-LARSEN, P. and JOHNSTON, G. A. R. (1975) Inhibition of GABA uptake in rat brain slices by nipecotic acid, various isoxazoles and related compounds. *J. Neurochem.* **25**: 797–802.
KROGSGAARD-LARSEN, P., FALCH, E. and JACOBSEN, P. (1984) GABA agonists: structural requirements for interaction with the GABA-benzodiazepine receptor complex. In: *Actions and Interactions of GABA and the Benzodiazepines*, pp. 109–132, BOWERY, N. G. (ed) Raven Press, New York.
KROGSGAARD-LARSEN, P., NIELSEN, L. and FALCH, E. (1986) The active site of the GABA receptor. In: *Benzodiazepine/GABA Receptors and Chloride Channels: Structural and Functional Properties*, pp. 73–95, OLSEN, R. W. and VENTER, J. C. (eds) Alan R. Liss, New York.
KROGSGAARD-LARSEN, P., SNOWMAN, A., LUMMIS, S. C. and OLSEN, R.W. (1981) Characterisation of the binding of ^{3}H-piperidine-4-sulfonic acid to bovine brain synaptic membranes. *J. Neurochem.* **37**: 401–409.
KUDO, Y., OKA, J. I. and YAMADA, K. (1981) Anisatin a potent GABA antagonist, isolated from Illicium anisatum. *Neurosci. Lett.* **25**: 83–88.
KUHAR, M. J. (1978) Histochemical localisation of neurotransmitter receptors. In: *Neurotransmitter Receptor Binding*, pp. 113–126, YAMAMURA, H.I., ENNA, S.J. and KUHAR, M.J. (eds) Raven Press, New York.
LAKOSKI, J. M., AGHAJANIAN, G. K. and GALLAGER, D. W. (1983) Interaction of histamine H_2-receptor antagonists with GABA and benzodiazepine binding sites in the CNS. *Eur. J. Pharmacol.* **88**: 241–245.
LAMBERT, J. J., PETERS, J. A. and COTTRELL, G. A. (1987) Actions of synthetic and endogenous steroids on the GABA-A receptor. *Trends Pharmacol. Sci.* **8**: 224–227.
LANG, B., BARNARD, E. A., CHANG, L.-R. and DOLLY, J. O. (1979) Putative benzodiazepine receptor: a protein solubilised from brain. *FEBS Lett.* **104**: 149–153.
LANGOSCH, D., THOMAS, L. and BETZ, H. (1988) Conserved quaternary structure of ligand-gated ion channels: The postsynaptic glycine receptor is a pentamer. *Proc. Natl. Acad. Sci. USA* **85**: 7394–7398.
LEE, H. K., DUNWIDDIE, T. V. and HOFFER, B. J. (1979) Interaction of diazepam with synaptic transmission in the in vitro hippocampus. *Naunyn Schmiedeberg's Arch. Pharmacol.* **309**: 131–136.
LEEB-LUNDBERG, F., SNOWMAN, A. and OLSEN, B. W. (1980) Barbiturate receptors are coupled in benzodiazepine receptors. *Proc. Natl. Acad. Sci. USA* **77**: 7468–7472.
LEEB-LUNDBERG, F., SNOWMAN, A. and OLSEN, R. W. (1981) Perturbation of benzodiazepine receptor binding by pyrazolophridines involves picrotoxinin/barbiturate receptor sites. *J. Neurosci.* **1**: 471–477.
LEFUR, G., MIZOULE, J., BERGEVIN, M., FERRIS, O., HEAULME, M., GAUTHIER, A., GUEREMY, C. and UZAN, A. (1981) Multiple benzodiazepine receptor evidence of dissociation between anticonflict and anticonvulsant properties by PK8165 and PK9084 (two quinoline derivative). *Life Sci.* **28**: 1439–1448.

LEGAY, F., HENRY, S. and TAPPAZ, M. (1987) Evidence for two distinct forms of native glutamic acid decarboxylase in rat brain soluble extract: an immunoblotting study. *J. Neurochem.* **48**: 1022–1026.

LEVITAN, E. S., SCHOFIELD, P. R., BURT, D. R., RHEE, L. M., WISDEN, W., KOHLER, M., FUJITA, N., RODRIGUEZ, H. F., STEPHENSON, A., DARLISON, M. G., BARNARD, E. A. and SEEBERG, P. H. (1988a) Structural and functional basis for $GABA_A$ receptor heterogeneity. *Nature* **335**: 76–79.

LEVITAN, E. S., BLAIR, L. A. C., DIONNE, V.E. and BARNARD, E. A. (1988b) Biophysical and pharmacological properties of cloned $GABA_A$ receptor subunits expressed in Xenopus oocytes. *Neuron* **1**: 773–781.

LEVY, R. A. (1977) The role of GABA in primary afferent depolarisation. *Progress in Neurobiology* **9**: 211–267.

LIPPA, A. S., CRITCHETT, D. J., SANO, M. C., KLEPNER, C. A., GREENBLATT, F. N., COUPET, J. and BEER, B. (1979) Benzodiazepine receptors: cellular and behavioural characteristics. *Pharmacol. Biochem. Behav.* **10**: 831–843.

LIPPA, A. S., KLEPNER, C. A., YUNGER, L., SANO, M. C., SMITH, W. V. and BEER, B. (1978) Relationship between benzodiazepine receptors and experimental anxiety in rats. *Pharmacol. Biochem. Behav.* **9**: 853–856.

LITTLE, H. J., NUTT, D. J. and TAYLOR, S. C. (1986) Does chronic benzodiazepine administration cause a "withdrawal-shift" across the whole benzodiazepine ligand spectrum? *Brit. J. Pharmacol.* **89**: 796P.

LO, M. M. S., STRITTMATTER, S. M. and SNYDER, S. H. (1982) Physical separation and characterisation of two types of benzodiazepine receptor. *Proc. Natl. Acad. Sci. USA* **79**: 680–684.

LOEW, G. H., NIENOW, J. R. and POULSEN, M. (1984) Theoretical structure-activity studies of benzodiazepine analogues. Requirements for receptor affinity and activity. *Mol. Pharmacol.* **26**: 19–34.

LOLAIT, S. J., O'CARROLL, A. M. KUSANO, K., MULLER, J. M. BROWNSTEIN, M. J. and MAHAN, L. C. (1989) Cloning and expression of a novel rat $GABA_A$ receptor. *FEBS Letters* **246**: 145–148.

LUCEK, R. W. and COUTINHO, C. B. (1976) The role of substituents in the hydrophobic binding of 1,4-benzodiazepines by human plasma proteins. *Mol. Pharmacol.* **12**: 612–619.

LUCEK, R. W., GARLAND, W. A. and DAIRMAN, W. (1979) CNDO/2 molecular orbital study of selected 1,3- dih dro-5-phenyl-1,4-benzodiazepin-2-ones. *Fed. proc.* **38**: 541.

MACKERER, C. R., KOCHMAN, R. L., BIERSCHENK, B. A. and BREMNER, S. S. (1978) The binding of ^{3}H-diazepam to rat brain homogenerates. *J. Pharmacol. Exp. Ther.* **206**: 405–413.

MAJEWSKA, M. D., HARRISON, N. L., SCHWARTZ, R. D., BARKER, J. L. and PAUL, S. M. (1986) Steroid hormone metabolites are barbiturate-like modulators of the GABA receptor. *Science* **232**: 1004–1007.

MAKSAY, G. and SIMONYI, M. (1985) Benzodiazepine anticonvulsants accelerate and beta-carboline convulsants decelerate the kinetics of ^{35}S-TBPS binding at the chloride ionophore. *Eur. J. Pharmacol.* **117**: 275–278.

MALLORGA, P., HAMBURG, M., TALLMAN, J. F. and GALLAGER, D.W. (1980) Ontogenetic changes in GABA modulation of brain benzodiazepine binding. *Neuropharmacology* **19**: 405–408.

MANN, E. and ENNA, S. J. (1980) Phylogenetic distribution of bicuculline sensitive gamma-aminobutyric acid (GABA) receptor binding. *Brain Res.* **184**: 367–373.

MAO, C. C., MARCO, E., REVUELTA, A., BERTILSSON, L. and COSTA, E. (1977) The turnover rate of gamma-aminobutyric acid in the nuclei of the telencephalon: implications in the pharmacology of antipsychotics and of a minor tranquilliser. *Biol. Psychiat.* **12**: 359–371.

MARANGOS, P. J., PATEL, J., BOULENGER, J.-P. and CLARK-ROSENBERG, R. (1982) Characterisation of peripheral-type benzodiazepine binding sites in brain using ^{3}H-Ro 5-4864. *Mol. Pharmacol.* **22**: 26–32.

MARTIN, I. L. (1987) The benzodiazepines and their receptors: 25 years of progress. *Neuropharmacology* **26**: 957–970.

MARTIN, I. L. and BROWN, C. L. (1983) Interactions of different ligand classes with the benzodiazepine receptor. In: *Benzodiazepine Recognition Site Ligands: Biochemistry and Pharmacology*, pp. 65–72, BIGGIO, G. and COSTA, E. (eds) Raven Press, New York.

MARTIN, I. L. and CANDY, J. M. (1978) Facilitation of benzodiazepine binding by sodium chloride and GABA. *Neuropharmacology* **17**: 993–998.

MARTIN, I. L. and CANDY, J. M. (1980) Facilitation of specific benzodiazepine binding in rat brain membrane fragments by a number of anions. *Neuropharmacology* **19**: 175–179.

MARTIN, I. L., BROWN, C. L. and DOBLE, A. (1983) Multiple benzodiazepine receptors: structures in the brain or structures in the mind? A critical review. *Life Sci.* **32**: 1925–1933.

MARTINI, C., LUCACCHINI, A. and RONCA, G. (1981) Specific absorbents for affinity chromatography of benzodiazepine binding proteins. *Preparative Biochem.* **11**: 487–499.

MARTINI, C., LUCACCHINI, A., RONCA, G., HRELIA, S. and ROSSI, C. A. (1982) Isolation of putative benzodiazepine receptors from rat brain membranes by affinity chromatography. *J. Neurochem.* **38**: 15–19.

MATHEWS, G. and WICKELGREN, W. O. (1979) Glycine, GABA and synaptic inhibition of reticulospinal neurones of lamprey. *J. Physiol. (Lond)* **293**: 393–415.

MCBURNEY, R. N. (1984) Membrane actions of GABA in cultured central neurones. In: *Actions and Interactions of GABA and Benzodiazepines*, pp. 43–58, BOWERY, N. (eds) Raven Press, New York.

MCBURNEY, R. N., SMITH, R. N. and ZOREC, R. (1985) Conductance states of gamma-aminobutyric acid (GABA) and glycine activated chloride channels in rat spinal neurones in cell culture. *J. Physiol. (Lond).* **365**: 87P.

MCCARTHY, G. D. and HARDEN, T. K. (1981) Identification of two benzodiazepine binding sites on cells cultured from rat cerebral cortex. *J. Pharmacol. Exp. Ther.* **216**: 183–191.

MEINERS, B. A. and SALAMA, A. J. (1982) Enhancement of benzodiazepine and GABA binding by the novel anxiolytic tracazolate. *Eur. J. Pharmacol.* **78**: 315–322.

MERNOFF, S. T., CHERWINSKI, H. M., BECKER, J. W. and DEBLAS, A. L. (1983) Solubilisation of brain benzodiazepine receptors with a zwitterionic detergent: Optimal preservation of their functional interaction with the GABA receptors. *J. Neurochem.* **41**: 752–758.

MILEDI, R., PARKER, I. and SUMIKAWA, K. (1982) Synthesis of chick brain GABA receptors by frog oocytes. Proc. Roy. Soc. Lond. B216: 509–515.

MINCHIN, M. C. W. and IVERSEN, L. L. (1974) Release of ^{3}H-gamma-aminobutyric acid from glial cells in dorsal root ganglia. *J. Neurochem.* **23**: 533–540.

Mitchell, P. R. and Martin, I. L. (1978a) Is GABA release modulated by pre-synaptic receptors? *Nature* **274**: 904–905.

Mitchell, P. R. and Martin, I. L. (1978b) The effects of benzodiazepines on K+-stimulated release of GABA. *Neuropharmacology* **17**: 317–320.

Mitchell, P. R. and Martin, I. L. (1980) Ethyl beta-carboline-3-carboxylate antagonises the effect of diazepam on a functional GABA receptor. *Eur. J. Pharmacol.* **68**: 513–514.

Mitchell, P. R. and Wilson, L. (1984) Investigation of the effects of muscimol on different components of ^{3}H-propyl beta-carboline-3-carboxylate binding to rat hippocampal and cerebella membranes. *Eur. J. Pharmacol.* **97**: 315–319.

Miyata, M., Mocchetti, I., Ferrarese, C., Guidotti, A. and Costa, E. (1987) Protracted treatment with diazepam increases the turnover of putative endogenous ligands for the benzodiazepine/beta-carboline recognition site. *Proc. Natl. Acad. Sci. USA* **84**: 1444–1448.

Mocchetti, I., Einstein, R. and Brosius, J. (1986) Putative diazepam binding inhibitor peptide: cDNA clones from rat. *Proc. Natl. Acad. Sci. USA* **83**: 7221–7225.

Mohler, H. (1981) Benzodiazepine receptors: are there endogenous ligands in the brain? *Trends Pharmacol. Sci.* **1**: 116–119.

Mohler, H. (1982) Benzodiazepine receptors: differential interaction of benzodiazepine agonists and antagonists after photoaffinity labelling with flunitrazepam. *Eur. J. Pharmacol.* **80**: 425–536.

Mohler, H. and Okada, T. (1977a) GABA receptor binding with ^{3}H-(+)-bicuculline-methiodide in rat CNS. *Nature* **267**: 56–67.

Mohler, H. and Okada, T. (1977b) Properties of ^{3}H-diazepam binding to benzodiazepine receptors in rat cerebral cortex. *Life Sci.* **20**: 2101–2110.

Mohler, H. and Okada, T. (1977c) Benzodiazepine receptor: demonstration in the central nervous system. *Science* **198**: 849–851.

Mohler, H. and Okada, T. (1978) The benzodiazepine receptor in normal and pathological human brain. *Brit. J. Psychiat.* **133**: 261–268.

Mohler, H. and Richards, J. G. (1981) Agonist and antagonist benzodiazepine receptor interactions in vitro. *Nature*. (Lond). **294**: 763–765.

Mohler, H., Battersby, M. K. and Richards, J. G. (1980) Benzodiazepine receptor protein identified and visualised in brain tissue by a photoaffinity label. *Proc. Natl. Acad. Sci. USA* **77**: 1666–1670.

Mohler, H., Okada, T. and Enna, S. J. (1978) Benzodiazepine and neurotransmitter receptor binding in rat brain after chronic administration of diazepam and phenobarbital. *Brain Res.* **156**: 391–395.

Mohler, H., Okada, T., Ulrich, J. and Heitz, P. H. (1978) Biochemical identification of the site of action of benzodiazepines in human brain by ^{3}H-diazepam binding. *Life Sci.* **22**: 985–996.

Mohler, H., Schoch, P., Richards, J. G., Haring, P., Takacs, B. and Stahli, C. (1986) Monoclonal antibodies: probes for structure and location of the GABA receptor/benzodiazepine receptor/chloride channel complex. In: *Benzodiazepine/GABA Receptors and Chloride Channels: Structural and Functional Properties*, pp. 285–297, Alan R. Liss, New York.

Mohler, H., Sieghart, W., Richards, J. G. and Hunkeler, W. (1984) Photoaffinity labelling of benzodiazepine receptors with a partial inverse agonist. *Eur. J. Pharmacol.* **102**: 191–192.

Moingeon, H., Bidart, J. M., Alberici, G. F. and Bohoun, C. (1983) Characterisation of a peripheral-type benzodiazepine binding site on human circulatory hymphocytes. *Eur. J. Pharmacol.* **92**: 147–149.

Mugnaini, E. and Oertel, W. H. (1985) An atlas of the distribution of GABAergic neurons and terminals in the rat CNS as revealed by GAD immunohistochemistry. In: *Handbook of Chemical Neuroanatomy, Volume 4*, pp. 436–608, Bjorklund, A. and Hokfelt, T. (eds) Elsevier, New York.

Muller, W. E., Schlafer, U. and Wollert, U. (1978) Benzodiazepine receptor binding in rat spinal cord membranes. *Neurosci. Lett.* **9**: 239–243.

Nagai, T., McGeer, P. L., Arak, M. and McGeer, E. G. (1984) GABA-T intensive neurons in the rat brain. In: *Handbook of Chemical Neuroanatomy, Volume 3*, pp. 247–272, Bjorklund, A., Hokfelt, T. and Kuhar, M. J. (eds) Elsevier, New York.

Nagy, J. I., Carter, D. A. and Fibiger, H. C. (1978) Anterior striatal projections to the globus pallidus, entopeduncular nucleus and substantia nigra in the rat: the GABA connection. *Brain Res.* **158**: 15–29.

Namasivayam, S. and Dean, P. M. (1986) Statistical method for surface pattern-matching between dissimilar molecules: electrostatic potentials and accessible surfaces. *J. Mol. Graphics* **4**: 46–50.

Neal, M. J. and Iversen, L. L. (1969) Subcellular distribution of endogenous ^{3}H-GABA in rat cerebral cortex. *J. Neurochem.* **16**: 1245–1252.

Nielsen, M. and Braestrup, C. (1980) Ethyl beta-carboline-3-carboxylate shows differential benzodiazepine receptor interaction. *Nature* **286**: 606–607.

Nielsen, M. and Braestrup, C. (1983) The molecular target size of brain TBPS binding sites. *Eur. J. Pharmacol.* **96**: 321–322.

Nielsen, M., Braestrup, C. and Squires, R. F. (1978) Evidence for a late evolutionary appearance of brain specific benzodiazepine receptors: an investigation of 18 vertebrate and 5 invertebrate species. *Brain Res.* **141**: 342–346.

Nielsen, M., Setton, H. and Braestrup, C. (1981) [^{3}H]-propyl-beta-carboline binds specifically to brain benzodiazepine receptors. *J. Neurochem.* **36**: 276–285.

Nistri, A. and Constanti, A. (1979) Pharmacological characterisation of different types of GABA and glutamate receptors in vertebrate and invertebrates. *Prog. Neurobiol.* **13**: 117–235.

Nowak, L. M., Young, A. B. and MacDonald, R. L. (1982) GABA and bicuculline actions on mouse spinal cord and cortical neurones in cell culture. *Brain Res.* **244**: 155–164.

Nutt, D. J., Cowen, P. J. and Little, H. J. (1982) Unusual interactions of benzodiazepine receptor antagonists. *Nature* **295**: 436–438.

Oakley, N. R. and Jones, B. J. (1983) Buspirone enhances ^{3}H-flunitrazepam binding in vivo. *Eur. J. Pharmacol.* **87**: 499–500.

OAKLEY, N. R., JONES, B. J. and STRAUGHAN, D. W. (1984) The benzodiazepine receptor ligand CL 218872 has both anxiolytic and sedative properties in rodents. *Neuropharmacology* **23**: 797–802.

OKAMOTO, K. and SAKAI, Y. (1979) Augmentation by chlordiazepoxide of the inhibitory effect of taurine, beta-alaine and GABA or spike discharges in guinea pig cerebellar slices. *Brit. J. Pharmacol.* **65**: 227–285.

OLSEN, R. W. (1981) GABA-benzodiazepine-barbiturate receptor interactions. *J. Neurochem.* **37**: 1–13.

OLSEN, R. W. and SNOWMAN, A. M. (1983) ^{3}H-bicuculline methochloride binding to low affinity gamma-aminobutyric acid receptor sites. *J. Neurochem.* **41**: 1653–1663.

OLSEN, R. W., SNOWHILL, E. W. and WAMSLEY, J. K. (1984) Autoradiographic localisation of low affinity GABA receptors with ^{3}H-bucuculline methochloride. *Eur. J. Pharmacol.* **99**: 247–248.

OLSEN, R. W., WONG, E. H. F., STAUBER, G. B., MURAKAMI, D., KING, R. G. and FISCHER, J. B. (1984) Biochemical properties of the GABA/barbiturate/benzodiazepine receptor-chloride ion channel complex. In: *Neurotransmitter Receptors: Mechanisms of Action and Regulation*, pp. 205–219, KITO, S., SEGAWA, T., KURIYAMA, K., YAMAMURA, H. I. and OLSEN, R. W. (eds) Plenum Press, New York.

ONGINI, E., PARRAVICINI, L., BAMONTE, F., GUZZON, V., IORIO, L. C. and BARNETT, A. (1982) Pharmacological studies with quazepam, a new benzodiazepine hypnotic. *Arzneim-Forsch* **32**: 1456–1462.

OTTERSEN, O. P. and STORM-MATHISON, J. (1984) Neurons containing or accumulating transmitter amino acids. In: *Handbook of Chemical Neuroanatomy, Volume 3*, pp. 141–246, BJORKLUND, A., HOKFELT, T. and KUHAR, M. J. (eds) Elsevier, New York.

PALACIOS, J. M. and KUHAR, M. J. (1982) Ontogeny of high affinity GABA and benzodiazepine receptors in rat cerebellum: an autoradiographic study. *Dev. Brain Res.* **2**: 531–539.

PALACIOS, J. M., NIEHOFF, D. L. and KUHAR, M. J. (1979) Ontogeny of GABA and benzodiazepine receptors: Effects of Triton X-100 and muscimol. *Brain Res.* **179**: 390–395.

PALACIOS, J. M., NIEHOFF, D. L. and KUHAR, M. J. (1981) Receptor autoradiography with tritium sensitive film: potential for computerised densitometry. *Neurosci. Lett.* **25**: 101–105.

PAUL, S. M., SCHWARTZ, R. D., CREVELING, C. R., HOLLINGSWORTH, E. B., DALY, J. W. and SKOLNICK, P. (1986) GABA receptor mediated chloride transport in a "cell-free" membrane preparation from brain. *Science* **233**: 228–229.

PENA, C., MEDINA, J. H., NOVAS, M. L., PALADINI, A. C. and DEROBERTIS, E. (1986) Isolation and identification in bovine cerebral cortex of n-butyl-beta-carboline-3-carboxylate, a potent benzodiazepine binding inhibitor. *Proc. Natl. Acad. Sci. USA* **83**: 4952–4956.

PENNEY, J. B., FREY, K. and YOUNG, A. B. (1981) Quantitative autoradiography of neurotransmitter receptors using tritium sensitive film. *Eur. J. Pharmacol.* **72**: 421–422.

PIERI, L. and HAEFELY, W. (1976) The effect of diphenylhydantoin, diazepam and clonazepam on the activity of Purkinje cells in the rat cerebellum. *Arch. Pharmacol.* **296**: 1–4.

PETERSEN, E. N. and BUUS-LASSEN, J. (1981) A water lick conflict paradigm using experienced rats. *Psychopharmacology* **75**: 236–239.

PETERSEN, E. N., JENSEN, L. H., HONORE, T., BRAESTRUP, C., KEHR, W., STEPHENS, D. N., WACHTEL, H. SEIDELMAN, D. and SCHMIECHEN, R. (1984) ZK91296, a partial agonist at benzodiazepine receptors. *Psychopharmacology* **83**: 240–248.

POLC, P. and HAEFELY, W. (1976) Effects of two benzodiazepines, phenobarbitone and baclofen on synaptic transmission in the cat cuneate nucleus. *Arch. Pharmacol.* **294**: 121–131.

POLC, P. and HAEFELY, W. (1982) Benzodiazepines enhance the bicuculline-sensitive part of recurrent Renshaw inhibition in the cat spinal cord. *Neurosci. Lett.* **28**: 193–197.

POLC, P., MOHLER, H. and HAEFELY, W. (1974) The effects of diazepam or spinal cord activities: possible sites and mechanisms of action. *Naunyn-Schmiedeberg's Arch. Pharmacol.* **284**: 319–337.

POLC, P., BONETTI, E. P., SCHAFFNER, R. and HAEFELY, W. (1982) A three state model of the benzodiazepine receptor explains the interactions between the benzodiazepine antagonist Ro 15-1788, benzodiazepine tranquilisers, beta-carbolines and phenobarbitone. *Naunyn-Schmiedeberg's Arch Pharmacol.* **321**: 260–264.

PRADO DE CARVALHO, L., GRECKSCH, G., CHAPOUTHIER, G. and ROSSIER, J. (1983) Anxiogenic and non-anxiogenic benzodiazepine antagonists. *Nature* **301**: 64–66.

PRECHT, W. and YOSHIDA, M. (1971) Blockage of caudate-evoked inhibitors of neurones in the substantia nigra by picrotoxin. *Brain Res.* **32**: 229–233.

PRITCHETT, D. B., SONTHEIMER, H., SHIVERS, B. D., YMER, S., KETTENMANN, H., SCHOFIELD, P. R. and SEEBERG, P. H. (1989) Importance of a novel GABA receptor subunit for benzodiazepine pharmacology. *Nature* **338**: 582–585.

PRITCHETT, D. B., SONTHEIMER, H., GORMAN, C. M., KETTENMANN, H., SEEBERG, P. H. and SCHOFIELD, P. R. (1988) Transient expression shows ligand gating and allosteric potentiation of $GABA_A$ receptor subunits. *Science* **242**: 1306–1308.

QUAST, U. and BRENNER, O. (1983) Modulation of ^{3}H-muscimol binding in rat cerebellar and cerebral cortical membrane by picrotoxin, pentobarbitone and etomidate. *J. Neurochem.* **41**: 418–425.

QUAST, U. and MAHLMANN, H. (1982) Interaction of ^{3}H-flunitrazepam with the benzodiazepine receptor: evidence for a ligand induced conformation change. *Biochem. Pharmacol.* **31**: 2761–2768.

QUAST, U., MAHLMANN, H. and VOLLMER, K.-O. (1982) Temperature dependence of the benzodiazepine-receptor interaction. *Mol. Pharmacol.* **22**: 20–25.

RANDALL, L. O. (1982) Discovery of benzodiazepines. In: *Pharmacology of Benzodiazepines*, pp. 15–22, USDIN, E., SKOLNICK, P., TALLMAN, J. F., GREENBLATT, D. and PAUL, S. M. (eds) MacMillan Press, New York.

REGAN, J. W., ROESKE, W. R. and YAMAMURA, H. I. (1980) The benzodiazepine receptor: its development and its modulation by gamma-aminobutyric acid. *J. Pharmacol. Exp. Ther.* **212**: 137–143.

REGAN, J. W., YAMAMURA, H. I., YAMADA, S. and ROESKE, W. R. (1981) High affinity renal ^{3}H-flunitrazepam binding: characterisation, localisation and alteration in hypertension. *Life Sci.* **28**: 991–998.

REISINE, T. D., OVERSTREET, D., GALE, K., ROSSOR, M., IVERSEN, L. L. and YAMAMURA, H. I. (1980) Benzodiazepine receptors: the effect of GABA on their characteristics in human brain and their alteration in Huntington's disease. *Brain Res.* **199**: 79–88.

RICE, K. C., BROSSI, A., TALLMAN, J., PAUL, S. M. and SKOLNICK, P. (1979) Irazepine, a non-competitive, irreversible inhibitor of ^{3}H-diazepam binding to benzodiazepine receptors. *Nature* **278**: 854–855.

RICHARDS, J. G., SCHOCH, P., HARING, P., TAKACS, B. and MOHLER, H. (1987) Resolving $GABA_A$/benzodiazepine receptors: cellular and subcellular localisation in the CNS with monoclonal antibodies. *J. Neurosci.* **7**: 1866–1886.

RICHARDS, J. G., SCHLUMPF, M., LICHTENSTEIGER, W. and MOHLER, H. (1983) Ontogeny of benzodiazepine binding sites in fetal rat brain: an in vitro autoradiographic study. *Monogr. Neural Sci.* **9**: 111–118.

ROBERTS, E. (1984) Gamma-aminobutyric acid (GABA): from discovery to visualisation of GABAergic neurons in the vertebrate nervous system. In: *Actions and Interactions of GABA and Benzodiazepines*, pp. 1–25, BOWERY, N. G. (eds) Raven Press, New York.

SAITO, K. (1976) Immunochemical studies of GAD and GABA-T. In: *GABA in Nervous System Function*, pp. 103–111, ROBERTS, E., CHASE, T. N. and TOWER, D. B. (eds) Raven Press, New York.

SANGAMESWARAN, L. and DEBLAS, A. (1985) Demonstration of benzodiazepine-like molecules in the mammalian brain with a monoclonal antibody to benzodiazepine. *Proc. Natl. Acad. Sci. USA* **82**: 5560–5564.

SARRAZIN, M., BOURDEAUX-POINTIER, M. and BRIAND, C. (1976) Etude de quelques relations structure-activité de benzodiazepines. *Ann. Phys. Biol. Med.* **9**: 211–220.

SCHLUMPF, M., RICHARDS, J. G., LICHTENSTEIGER, W. and MOHLER, H. (1983) An autoradiographic study of the pre-natal development of benzodiazepine-binding sites in rat brain. *J. Neurosci.* **3**: 1478–1487.

SCHMIDT, R. F., VOGEL, E. and ZIMMERMANN, M. (1967) Die Wirkung von Diazepam auf die pra-synaptische Hemmung und andere Ruckenmarks reflexe. *Naunyn-Schmiedeberg's Arch. Pharmacol.* **258**: 69–82.

SCHOCH, P., HARING, P., TAKACS, B., STAHLI, C. and MOHLER, H. (1984) The GABA/benzodiazepine receptor complex from bovine brain: purification, reconstitution and immunological characterisation. *J. Recept. Res.* **4**: 189–200.

SCHOEMAKER, H., BOLES, R. G., HORST, W. D. and YAMAMURA, H. I. (1983) Specific high affinity binding sites for [^{3}H]-Ro 5-4864 in rat brain and kidney. *J. Pharmacol. Exp. Ther.* **225**: 61–69.

SCHOFIELD, P. R., DARLISON, M. G., FUJITA, N., BURT, D. R., STEPHENSON, F. A., RODRIGUEZ, H., RHEE, L. M., RAMACHANDRAN, J., REALE, V., GLENCORSE, T. A., SEEBURG, P. H. and BARNARD, E. A. (1987) Sequence and functional expression of the $GABA_A$ receptor shows a ligand-gated receptor super-family. *Nature* **328**: 221–227.

SCHOLFIELD, C. N. (1980) Potentiation of inhibition by general anaesthetics in neurons of the olfactory cortex in vitro. *Pflugers Arch.* **383**: 249–255.

SCHOUSBOE, A., WU, J.-Y. and ROBERTS, E. (1974) Subunit structure and kinetic properties of 4-aminobutyrate-2-ketoglutarate transaminase purified from mouse brain. *J. Neurochem.* **23**: 1189–1195.

SCHWARTZ, R. D., JACKSON, J. A., WEIGERT, D., SKOLNICK, P. and PAUL, S. M. (1985) Characterisation of barbiturate-stimulated chloride efflux from rat brain synaptoneurosomes. *J. Neurosci.* **5**: 2963–2970.

SCHWARTZ, R. D., SKOLNICK, P., HOLINGSWORTH, E. B. and PAUL, S. M. (1984) Barbiturate and picrotoxin sensitive chloride efflux in rat cerebral cortical synaptoneurosomes. *FEBS Lett.* **175**: 193–196.

SCHWARTZ, R. D., SUZDAK, P. D. and PAUL, S. M. (1987) Gamma-aminobutyric acid (GABA) and barbiturate mediated $^{36}Cl^-$ uptake in rat brain synaptoneurosomes: evidence for rapid desensitisation of the GABA receptor coupled chloride ion channel. *Mol. Pharmacol.* **30**: 419–426.

SEQUIER, J. M., RICHARDS, J. G., MALHERBE, P., PRICE, G. W., MATHEWS, S. and MOHLER, H. (1988) Mapping of brain areas containing RNA homologous to cDNAs encoding alpha and beta subunits of the rat $GABA_A$ gamma-aminobutyrate receptor. *Proc. Natl. Acad. Sci. USA* **85**: 7815–7819.

SHERMAN-GOLD, R. and DUDAI, Y. (1980) Solubilisation and properties of a benzodiazepine receptor from calf cortex. *Brain Res.* **198**: 485–490.

SIEGHART, W. (1983) Several new benzodiazepine selectively interact with a benzodiazepine receptor-subtype. *Neurosci. Lett.* **38**: 73–78.

SIEGHART, W. (1986) Comparison of benzodiazepine receptors in cerebellum and inferior colliculus. *J. Neurochem.* **47**: 920–923.

SIEGHART, W. and DREXLER, G. (1983) Irreversible binding of ^{3}H-flunitrazepam to different proteins in various brain regions. *J. Neurochem.* **41**: 47–55.

SIEGHART, W. and KAROBATH, M. (1980) Molecular heterogeneity of benzodiazepine receptors. *Nature* **286**: 285–287.

SIEGHART, W. and MOHLER, H. (1982) 3H-clonazepam, like ^{3}H-flunitrazepam, is a photoaffinity label for the central type of benzodiazepine receptors. *Eur. J. Pharmacol.* **81**: 171–173.

SIGEL, E. and BAUR, R. (1988) Allosteric modulation by benzodiazepine receptor ligands of the $GABA_A$ receptor channel expressed in Xenopus oocytes. *J. Neurosci.* **8**: 289–295.

SIGEL, E., MAMALAKI, C. and BARNARD, E. A. (1985) Reconstitution of the isolated GABA/benzodiazepine receptors complex into phospholipid vesicles. *Neurosci. Lett.* **61**: 165–170.

SIGEL, E., STEPHENSON, F. A., MAMALAKI, C. and BARNARD, E. A. (1983) A gamma-aminobutyric acid/benzodiazepine receptor complex in bovine cerebral cortex. *J. Biol. Chem.* **258**: 6965–6971.

SIMMONDS, M. A. (1978) Presynaptic actions of gamma-aminobutyric acid in a slice preparation of cuneate nucleus. *Brit. J. Pharmacol.* **63**: 495–502.

SIMMONDS, M. A. (1980) Evidence that bicuculline and picrotoxin act at separate sites to antagonise gamma-aminobutyric acid in rat cuneate nucleus. *Neuropharmacology* **19**: 39–45.

SIMMONDS, M. A. (1984) Physiological and pharmacological characterisation of the actions of GABA. In: *Actions and Interactions of GABA and Benzodiazepines*, pp. 27–41, BOWERY, N. (eds) Raven Press, New York.

SINCLAIR, J. G., LO, G. F. and HARRIS, D. P. (1982) Flurazepam effects on rat cerebellar purkinje cells. *Gen. Pharmacol.* **13**: 453–456.

SJODIN, T., ROOSDORP, N. and SJOHOLM, I. (1976) Studies on the binding of benzodiazepines to human serum albumin by circular dichroism measurements. *Biochem. Pharmacol.* **25**: 2131–2140.

SKERRITT, J. H., WILLOW, M. and JOHNSTON, G. A. R. (1982) Diazepam enhancement of low affinity GABA binding to rat brain membranes. *Neurosci. Lett.* **29**: 63–66.

SKOLNICK, P., LOCK, K.-L., PAUGH, B., MARANGO, P., WINDSOR, R. and PAUL, S. (1980) Pharmacologic and behavioural effects of EMD 28422: a novel purine which enhances ^{3}H-diazepam binding to brain benzodiazepine receptors. *Pharmacol. Biochem. Behav.* **12**: 685–689.

SKOLNICK, P., PAUL, S., CRAWLEY, J., LEWIN, E., LIPPA, A., CLODY, IRMSCHER, K., SAIDO, O. and MINCK, K. (1983) Antagonism of the anxiolytic action of diazepam and chlordiazepoxide by the novel imidazopyridines EMD 39593 and EMD 41717. *Eur. J. Pharmacol.* **88**: 319–327.

SKOLNICK, P., SCHWERI, M. M., WILLIAMS, E. F., MONCADO, V. Y. and PAUL, S. M. (1982) An in vitro binding assay which differentiates benzodiazepine agonists and antagonists. *Eur. J. Pharmacol.* **78**: 133–136.

SMART, T. G., CONSTANTI, A., BILBE, G., BROWN, D. A. and BARNARD, E. A. (1983) Synthesis of functional chick brain GABA-benzodiazepine—barbiturate receptor complexes in mRNA injected Xenopus oocytes. *Neurosci. Lett.* **40**: 55–59.

SNODGRASS, S. R. (1978) Use of ^{3}H-muscimol for GABA receptor studies. *Nature* **273**: 392–394.

SPETH, R. C., WASTEK, G. J., JOHNSON, P. C. and YAMAMURA, H. I. (1978) Benzodiazepine binding in human brain: characterisation using ^{3}H-flunitrazepam. *Life Sci.* **22**: 859–866.

SPETH, R. C., WASTEK, G. J. and YAMAMURA, H. I. (1979) Benzodiazepine receptors: temperature dependence of ^{3}H-flunitrazepam binding. *Life Sci.* **24**: 351–358.

SQUIRES, R. F. and BRAESTRUP, C. (1977) Benzodiazepine receptors in rat brain. *Nature* **266**: 732–734.

SQUIRES, R. F., BENSON, D. I., BRAESTRUP, C., COUPET, J., KLEPNER, C. A., MYERS, V. and BEER, B. (1979) Some properties of brain specific benzodiazepine receptors: new evidence for multiple receptors. *Pharmacol. Biochem. Behav.* **10**: 825–830.

SQUIRES, R. F., CASIDA, J. E., RICHARDSON, N. M. and SAEDERUP, E. (1983) ^{35}S-t-butylbicyclophosphorothionate binds with high affinity to brain specific sites coupled to gamma-aminobutyric acid-A and ion recognition sites. *Mol. Pharmacol.* **23**: 326–336.

STAUBER, G. B., RANSOM, R. W., DILBER, A. I. and OLSEN, R. W. (1987) The gamma-aminobutyric acid/benzodiazepine receptor protein from rat brain: large scale purification and preparation of antibodies. *Eur. J. Biochem.* **167**: 125–133.

STEPHENSON, F. A. and BARNARD, E. A. (1986) Purification and characterisation of the brain GABA/benzodiazepine receptor. In: *Benzodiazepine/GABA Receptors and Chloride Channels: Structure and Functional Properties*, pp. 261–274, Alan R. Liss, New York.

STEPHENSON, F. A. and OLSEN, R. W. (1982) Solubilisation by CHAPS detergent of barbiturate-enhanced benzodiazepine-GABA receptor complex. *J. Neurochem.* **39**: 1579–1586.

STEPHENSON, F. A., CASALOTTI, S. O., MAMALAKI, C. and BARNARD, E. A. (1986) Antibodies recognising the $GABA_A$/benzodiazepine receptor including its regulatory sites. *J. Neurochem.* **46**: 854–861.

STERNBACH, L. H. (1979) The benzodiazepine story. *J. Med. Chem.* **22**: 1–7.

STERNBACH, L. H., RANDALL, L. O., BRAZIGER, R. and LEHR, H. (1968) Structure-activity relationships in the 1,4-benzodiazepine series. In: *Drugs Affecting the Central Nervous System, Volume 2*, pp. 237–264, BURGER, A. (eds) Marcel Dekker, New York.

STUDY, R. E. and BARKER, J. L. (1981) Diazepam and (−)-pentobarbital: fluctuation analysis reveals different mechanisms for potentiation of gamma-aminobutyric acid responses in cultured central neurons. *Proc. Natl. Acad. Sci. USA* **78**: 7180–7184.

SUNJIC, V., LISINI, A., SEGA, A., KOVAC, T., KAJFEZ, F. and RUSCIC, B. (1979) Conformation of 7-chloro-5-phenyl-d_5-3(S)-methyl-dihydro-1,4-benzodiazepin-2-one in solution. *J. Heterocyclic Chem.* **16**: 757–761.

SUPAVILAI, P. and KAROBATH, M. (1979) Stimulation of benzodiazepine receptor binding by SQ 20009 is chloride dependent and picrotoxin sensitive. *Eur. J. Pharmacol.* **60**: 111–113.

SUPAVILAI, P. and KAROBATH, M. (1980a) The effect of temperature and chloride ions on the stimulation of ^{3}H-flunitrazepam binding by the muscimol analogues THIP and piperidine-4-sulphonic acid. *Neurosci. Lett.* **19**: 337–341.

SUPAVILAI, P. and KAROBATH, M. (1980b) Heterogeneity of benzodiazepine receptors in rat cerebellum and hippocampus. *Eur. J. Pharmacol.* **64**: 91–93.

SUPAVILAI, P. and KAROBATH, M. (1981) Action of pyrazolpyridines as modulators of ^{3}H-fluntirazepam binding is the GABA/benzodiazepine receptor complex in the cerebellum. *Eur. J. Pharmacol.* **70**: 183–193.

SUPAVILAI, P. and KAROBATH, M. (1984) 35S-t-butylbicyclophosphorothionate binding sites are constituents of the gamma-aminobutyric acid benzodiazepine receptor complex. *J. Neurosci.* **4**: 1193–1200.

SWEETNAM, P. A. and TALLMAN, J. F. (1986) Regional difference in brain benzodiazepine receptor carbohydrates. *Mol. Pharmacol.* **29**: 299–306.

SYAPIN, P. J. and SKOLNICK, P. (1979) Characterisation of benzodiazepine binding sites in cultured cells of neural origin. *J. Neurochem.* **32**: 1047–1051.

TAGUCHI, J. and KURIYAMA, K. (1984) Purification of gamma-aminobutyric acid (GABA) receptor from rat brain by affinity column chromatography using a new benzodiazepine 1012-S, as an immobilised ligand. *Brain Res.* **323**: 219–226.

TAKEUCHI, A. and TAKEUCHI, N. (1975) The structure–activity relationship for GABA and related compounds in the crayfish muscle. *Neuropharmacology* **14**: 627–634.

TALLMAN, J. F. (1984) Properties of the purified GABA/benzodiazepine complex. *Clin. Neuropharmacol.* **7**: 558–559.

TALLMAN, J. F., PAUL, S. M., SKOLNICK, P. and GALLAGER, D. W. (1980) Receptors for the age of anxiety: pharmacology of the benzodiazepines. *Science* **207**: 274–281.

TALLMAN, J. F., THOMAS, J. W. and GALLAGER, D. W. (1978) GABAergic modulation of benzodiazepine binding site sensitivity. *Nature* **274**: 383–385.

TALLMAN, J. F., THOMAS, J. W. and GALLAGER, D. W. (1979) Identification of diazepam binding in intact animals. *Life Sci.* **24**: 873–880.

TANIGUCHI, T., WANG, J. K. T. and SPECTOR, S. (1980) Properties of ^{3}H-diazepam binding to rat peritoneal mast cells. *Life Sci.* **27**: 171–178.

TAPIA, R. (1975) Biochemical pharmacology of GABA in CNS. In: *Handbook of Psychopharmacology, Volume 4*, pp. 1–58, IVERSEN, L. L., IVERSEN, S. D. and SNYDER, S. H. (eds) Plenum Press, New York.

Tapia, R., Sandoval, M. E. and Contreras, P. (1975) Evidence for role of glutamate decarboxylase activity as a regulatory mechanism of cerebral excitability. *J. Neurochem.* **24**: 1283–1285.

ten Brugencatte, G. and Engberg, I. (1969) Effects of GABA and related amino acids on neurones in Deiters nucleus. *Brain Res.* **14**: 533–536.

Tenen, S. S. and Hirsch, J. D. (1980) Antagonism of diazepam activity by beta-carboline-3-carboxylic acid ethyl ester. *Nature* **288**: 609–610.

Thampy, K. G. and Barnes, E. M. (1984) Gamma-aminobutyric acid gated chloride channels in cultured cerebral neurons. *J. Biol. Chem.* **259**: 1753–1757.

Thomas, J. W. and Tallman, J. F. (1981) Characterisation of photoaffinity labelling of benzodiazepine binding sites. *J. Biol. Chem.* **256**: 9838–9842.

Ticku, M. K. and Olsen, R. W. (1978) Interaction of barbiturates with dihydropicrotoxinin binding sites related to the GABA receptor-ionipheres system. *Life Sci.* **22**: 1643–1652.

Toll, L., Keys, C., Spangler, D. and Loew, G. (1984) Computer-assisted determination of benzodiazepine receptor heterogeneity. *Eur. J. Pharmacol.* **99**: 203–209.

Toyoshima, C. and Unwin, N. (1988) Ion channel of acetylcholine receptor reconstructed from images of postsynaptic membranes. *Nature* **336**: 247–250.

Trifiletti, R. R., Snowman, A. M. and Snyder, S. H. (1985) Barbiturate recognition site on the GABA/benzodiazepine receptor complex is distinct from the pirotoxinin/TBPS recognition site. *Eur. J. Pharmacol.* **106**: 441–447.

Tsuchiya, T. and Fukushima, H. (1978) Effects of benzodiazepines and pentobarbitone on the GABAergic recurrent inhibition of hippocampal neurons. *Eur. J. Pharmacol.* **48**: 421–424.

Unnerstall, J. R., Niehoff, D. L. Kuhar, M. J. and Palacios, J. M. (1982) Quantitative receptor autoradiography using ^{3}H-ultrofilm: application to multiple benzodiazepine receptors. *J. Neurosci. Methods* **6**: 59–73.

Watling, K. J. and Bristow, D. J. (1986) GABA-B receptor mediated enhancement of vasoactive intestinal peptide-stimulated cyclic AMP production in slices of rat cerebral cortex. *J. Neurochem.* **46**: 1756–1762.

Weiland, G. A., Minneman, K. P. and Molinoff, P. B. (1979) Fundamental differences between the molecular interaction of agonists and antagonists with the beta-adrenergic receptor. *Nature* **281**: 114–117.

Wermuth, C. G. and Biziere, K. (1986) Pyridazinyl GABA derivatives a new class of synthetic GABA-A antagonists. *Trends Pharmacol. Sci.* **7**: 421–424.

White, W. J., Dichter, M. A. and Snodgrass, S. R. (1981) Benzodiazepine binding and interactions with the GABA receptor complex in living cultures of rat cerebral cortex. *Brain Res.* **215**: 162–176.

Williams, E. F., Rice, K. C., Paul, S. M. and Skolnick, P. (1980) Heterogeneity of benzodiazepine receptors in the central nervous system demonstrated with kenazepine, and alkylating benzodiazepine. *J. Neurochem.* **35**: 591–597.

Williams, M. and Risley, E. A. (1979) Enhancement of binding to rat brain membranes in vitro by SQ 20009, a novel anxiolytic agent, gamma-aminobutyric acid and muscimol. *Life Sci.* **24**: 833–841.

Williams, M. and Risley, E. A. (1982) Interactions of avermectins with ^{3}H-beta-carboline-3-carboxylate ethyl ester and ^{3}H-diazepam binding sites in rat brain cortical membranes. *Eur. J. Pharmacol.* **77**: 307–312.

Williams, M. and Risley, E. A. (1984) Ivermectin interactions with benzodiazepine receptors in rat cortex and cerebellum in vitro. *J. Neurochem.* **42**: 745–753.

Williams, M. and Yarbrough, G. G. (1979) Enhancement of in vitro binding and some of the pharmacological properties of diazepam by a novel anthelmintic agent avermectin B1a. *Eur. J. Pharmacol.* **56**: 273–276.

Wisden, W., Morris, B. J., Darlison, M. G., Hunt, S. P. and Barnard, E. A. (1988) Distinct $GABA_A$ receptor alpha subunit mRNAs show differential patterns of expression in bovine brain. *Neuron* **1**: 937–947.

Wolf, P. and Haas, H. L. (1977) Effects of diazepines and barbiturates on hippocampal recurrent inhibition. *Arch. Pharmacol.* **299**: 211–218.

Wong, D. T., Rathbun, R. C., Bymaster, F. P. and Lacefield, W. B. (1983) Enhanced binding of radioligands to receptors of gamma-aminobutyric acid and benzodiazepines by a new anti-convulsant agent, LY81067. *Life Sci.* **33**: 917–923.

Wong, E. H. F., Leeb-Lundberg, L. M., Teichberg, V. I. and Olsen, R. W. (1984) Gamma-aminobutyric acid activation of $^{36}Cl^{-}$ flux in rat hippocampal slices and its potentiation by barbiturates. *Brain Res.* **303**: 267–275.

Wood, J. G., McLaughlin, B. L. and Vaughn, J. E. (1976) Immunocytochemical localisation of GAD in electron microscope preparations of rodent CNS. In: *GABA in Nervous System Function*, p. 133, Roberts, E., Chase, T. N. and Tower, D. B. (eds) Raven Press, New York.

Wu, J.-Y. (1976) Purification, characterisation and kinetic studies of GAD and GABA-T from mouse brain. In: *GABA in Nervous System Function*, pp. 7–55, Roberts, E., Chase, T. N. and Tower, D. B. (eds) Raven Press, New York.

Wu, J.-Y. and Roberts, E. (1974) Properties of L-glutamate decarboxylase: inhibition studies. *J. Neurochem.* **23**: 759–767.

Wu, J.-Y., Matsuda, T. and Roberts, E. (1973) Purification and characterisation of glutamate decarboxylase from mouse brain. *J. Biol. Chem.* **248**: 3029–3034.

Wuenschell, C. W., Fisher, R. S., Kaufman, D. L. and Tobin, A. J. (1986) In situ hybridisation to localise mRNA encoding the neurotransmitter synthetic enzyme glutamate decarboxylase in mouse cerebellum. *Proc. Natl. Acad. Sci. USA* **83**: 6193–6197.

Yokoyama, N., Ritter, B., Neubert, A. D. (1982) Alpha-arylpyrazolo-[4,3-C]-quinolin-3-ones: novel agonist, partial agonist and antagonist of benzodiazepine. *J. Med. Chem.* **25**: 337–339.

Young, W. S. III. and Kuhar, M. J. (1979) Autoradiographic localisation of benzodiazepine receptors in the brains of humans and animals. *Nature* **280**: 393–395.

Young, W. S. and Kuhar, M. J. (1980) Radiohistochemical localisation of benzodiazepine receptors in rat brain. *J. Pharmacol. Exp. Ther.* **212**: 337–346.

Yousufi, M. A. K., Thomas, J. W. and Tallman, J. F. (1979) Solubilisation of benzodiazepine binding site from rat cortex. *Life Sci.* **25**: 463–470.

CHAPTER 6

BEHAVIORAL PHARMACOLOGY OF MINOR TRANQUILIZERS

S. E. FILE and S. PELLOW

Psychopharmacology Research Unit, UMDS Division of Pharmacology
University of London, Guy's Hospital, London SE1 9RT, U.K.

1. INTRODUCTION

The introduction into clinical practice of the benzodiazepines in 1967 saw a rapid replacement of barbiturates as the drugs of choice in a wide variety of disorders treated by minor tranquilizers. A concomitant advancement in the development of subtle and sensitive techniques in behavioral pharmacology has led to a wide and thorough investigation of the behavioral effects of benzodiazepines. A strong emphasis will be placed on animal studies, since they have contributed most to our current knowledge of the behavioral mechanisms underlying the therapeutic effects of the benzodiazepines.

Although the benzodiazepines have proved to be considerably more effective than the older classes of minor tranquilizers in the treatment of anxiety, it is accepted that there are certain undesirable side-effects: for example, sedative and amnesic effects; and there is a growing realization of their ability to induce dependence. The last few years have therefore seen the synthesis and pharmacological testing of a wide variety of nonbenzodiazepine compounds with extremely diverse chemical structures, that have been proposed as putative anxiolytic compounds. These compounds are listed in Table 1. Many of them have been claimed to provide significant advantages over the benzodiazepines, such as lower sedative potential. However, one thing that is clear is that certain of these compounds differ behaviorally from the benzodiazepines in a number of interesting ways. The behavioral effects of these compounds will also be discussed where information is available.

The review begins with a discussion of whether animals can detect the presence of benzodiazepines, and to what extent they consider their subjective effects to be similar to other drugs. We then continue with a discussion of the major effects of the benzodiazepines as related to their clinical uses. The emphasis is placed on the *behavioral* effects of the benzodiazepines, and so their effects on sleep mechanisms and muscle relaxation will not be discussed.

2. BENZODIAZEPINES AS DISCRIMINABLE STIMULI

A number of studies have been carried out on the ability of benzodiazepines both to serve as interoceptive discriminative stimuli (IDS) and to generalize to the IDS associated with other drugs. Colpaert *et al.* (1976) trained rats to discriminate chlordiazepoxide

TABLE 1. *Novel Putative Anxiolytic Compounds*

(A) *Acting at benzodiazepine receptor*	
CL 218,872	triazolopyridazine
CGS 9896	pyrazoloquinoline
PK 8165	phenylquinoline
PK 9084	phenylquinoline
ZK 91296	β-carboline
ZK 93423	β-carboline
Zopiclone	cyclopyrrolone
(B) *Non-benzodiazepine sites of action*	
Tracazolate	pyrazolopyridine
Buspirone	piperazinylpyrimidine
Tofisopam	3.4 benzodiazepine

(5 mg/kg) from saline on a fixed ratio schedule of food reinforcement. Several other benzodiazepines generalized to the IDS (bromazepam, diazepam, flurazepam, lorazepam, nitrazepam and oxazepam). The barbiturates pentobarbitone and phenobarbitone also generalized to the chlordiazepoxide IDS. Overton (1966) trained rats to escape shock by running in alternative directions in a T-maze after pentobarbitone or saline, and found that chlordiazepoxide (30 mg/kg) generalized to the barbiturate IDS. Similarly, in rats trained to discriminate ethyl alcohol (1200 mg/kg) from saline on a food-rewarded lever-pressing task, Kubena and Barry (1969) found that chlordiazepoxide (10 mg/kg) generalized to the alcohol IDS. However, although these studies have found cross-generalization between benzodiazepines and other minor tranquilizers, there are studies that have failed to do so (see Barry and Krimmer, 1978, for review). Studies have also shown that a wide variety of other compounds of different therapeutic classes do not generalize to the benzodiazepine IDS, and neither do benzodiazepines generalize to their IDS (see Barry and Krimmer, 1978).

A few studies have been carried out on the IDS properties of novel putative anxiolytics. McElroy and Feldman (1982) trained rats to discriminate 3 mg/kg chlordiazepoxide from saline in a milk-reinforced lever-pressing task. The novel putative anxiolytic CL 218,872 (0.5–10 mg/kg) dose-relatedly generalized to the benzodiazepine IDS. Shannon and Herling (1983) trained rats to discriminate between saline and diazepam (1 mg/kg) in a task using electric shock as a negative reinforcer. The pyrazoloquinoline CGS 9896 failed to generalize to the diazepam IDS. However, in rats trained to discriminate CGS 9896 from cornstarch (Bennett and Petrack, 1984) diazepam generalized to the IDS, as did the novel putative anxiolytics CL 218,872 and tracazolate. Rats trained to discriminate either oxazepam or pentobarbitone from vehicle identified buspirone as vehicle-like (Hendry *et al.*, 1983). Similarly, rats could only be poorly trained to discriminate buspirone from vehicle (Hendry *et al.*, 1983).

3. ANXIOLYTIC ACTIONS OF BENZODIAZEPINES

The anxiolytic actions of benzodiazepines in man are well-documented (see, for example, Greenblatt and Shader, 1974). However, although 1,4-benzodiazepines are effective in generalized anxiety states, they are believed to be less effective in the treatment of panic attacks (Klein, 1981). Although recent studies have shown high doses to be effective (Beaudry *et al.*, 1985; Rickels and Schweizer, 1986). In contrast, the triazolobenzodiazepines, such as alprazolam, are believed to be effective against both kinds of anxiety (Sheehan, 1982).

The actions of benzodiazepines have been studied in many animal tests that purport to model anxiety. The vast majority of early studies were carried out using conflict tests of anxiety. Geller and Seifter (1960) found that benzodiazepines increased responding for food on a punishment schedule of reinforcement combining food with delivery of footshock. There was no significant effect on unpunished responding for food. Cook and Davidson (1973) also reported such results in a modified Geller-Seifter procedure.

The above conflict tests are founded on responding that has been suppressed by the response-contingent delivery of punishment. However, in the conditioned emotional response model, responding is suppressed by punishment delivered independently of the animal's responses. Benzodiazepines have been reported to increase responding in conditioned emotional response situations, but there are also many reports of failure (e.g. Cook and Sepinwall, 1975; Millenson and Leslie, 1974). Huppert and Iversen (1975) showed that benzodiazepines are more effective in increasing behavior that is suppressed by contingent, rather than by non-contingent, shock.

Another model using responding suppressed by shock is the four-plate punished locomotor activity test of Boissier *et al.* (1968). Benzodiazepines release motor activity punished by shock. The Vogel punished drinking test is another widely used conflict procedure in which the drinking behavior of thirsty rats is suppressed by shock (Vogel *et al.*, 1971). Benzodiazepines also release suppressed responding in this test.

Benzodiazepine effects have also been considered in situations where punishment is not a major factor. Behavioral modifications induced by the omission of positive reinforcement habitually obtained after the emission of a response are interpreted as reactions to frustration (see Thiebot and Soubrie, 1983). Benzodiazepines have generally been found to attenuate behavioral inhibition introduced by the omission of reward; however, this is only true during the first periods of non-reward to which the animal is subjected (Dantzer, 1977). Benzodiazepines also attenuate the negative contrast that occurs when reinforcement is decreased (Flaherty *et al.*, 1980; Becker and Flaherty, 1983). However, the link between 'anxiety' and 'frustration' needs further investigation before these experiments can be taken as evidence of an anxiolytic action of benzodiazepines.

Several other tests have taken advantage of anxiety and/or fear induced by exposure to a novel environment to investigate benzodiazepine effects. The following procedures have been used: intensity of exploration in a novel environment such as a holeboard or Y-maze (Marriott and Spencer, 1965; Nolan and Parkes, 1973); however, tests based on exploration and locomotor activity have been heavily criticized in terms of validity (see File, 1985c; Pellow, 1986). The amount of food or water consumption in a novel enclosure has also been used as a measure of anxiety (Soubrie *et al.*, 1976b). One test that relies on the uncertainty generated by exposure to a novel environment, and on the unconditioned aversion that rats have to bright light, is the social interaction test of anxiety (File, 1980, 1985a). Benzodiazepines, after chronic administration, selectively increase social interaction between pairs of male rats only in anxiogenic test conditions, i.e. when lighting conditions are high or animals are unfamiliar with the environment. Another test, the elevated plus-maze test (Pellow *et al.*, 1985; Pellow, 1986) makes use of the unconditioned aversion that rats have for elevated and open places. In this test, rats choose to enter the two closed arms of an elevated plus-maze more frequently than they enter the two open arms. Benzodiazepines selectively increase the percentage of open arm entries, and the percentage of time spent on the open arms.

The effects of a number of novel putative anxiolytic compounds have also been widely investigated in these tests. The pyrazolopyridine tracazolate, that is believed to act at picrotoxinin sites on the GABA-benzodiazepine receptor complex, has anxiolytic activity in the Vogel punished drinking procedure but, interestingly, has no effect in the Geller-Seifter conflict test (Patel and Malick, 1982). Tracazolate also had an 'anxiolytic' action in a test using suppression of unconditioned motor activity as a measure (Patel and Malick, 1982), and has anxiolytic activity at low doses in the social interaction test (File and Pellow, 1985a) and the elevated plus-maze (Pellow and File, 1986a).

The pyrazoloquinoline CGS 9896, that is believed to act at benzodiazepine receptors, has anxiolytic activity in a Cook-Davidson conflict procedure (Yokoyama *et al.*, 1982); the Vogel punished drinking test (Patel *et al.*, 1983); the social interaction test (File and Pellow, 1986a) and the elevated plus-maze (File and Pellow, 1986a). The triazolopyridazine CL 218,872, believed to discriminate between two different subtypes of benzodiazepine receptor, has anxiolytic activity in a punished drinking test (Lippa *et al.*, 1979), the social interaction test (File, 1982a) and the elevated plus-maze (Pellow and File, 1986a).

An interesting compound that is claimed to possess anti-anxiety activity in man is buspirone. This compound is unusual in that it possesses no, or very little, activity in animal tests of anxiety (see File, 1985b, for review; McCloskey *et al.*, 1987). Another compound with a similar lack of activity in animal tests is the 3,4-benzodiazepine tofisopam, that is also claimed to be anxiolytic in man (see Pellow and File, 1986b, for review).

4. EFFECTS OF BENZODIAZEPINES ON STRESS

Benzodiazepines are able to attenuate several physiological, biochemical and pathological correlates of stress, including a decrease in the activation of the hypothalamic-pituitary-adrenocortical system (see below); a decrease in the reduced cerebral noradrenaline in response to footshock (Taylor and Laverty, 1969); a decrease in the elevation in frontal cortex DOPAC (Laveille *et al.*, 1979) and elevation of dopamine synthesis in frontal cortical slices (Kramarcy *et al.*, 1984); a decrease in the activity of noradrenergic neurones in the locus coeruleus (Chu and Bloom, 1974); reduced hypoglycaemia and hyperlactacidaemia (Satoh and Iwamato, 1966); hypertension (Benson *et al.*, 1970), and gastric ulceration (File and Pearce, 1981).

The most common measure of the anti-stress effects of benzodiazepines has been their effects on plasma corticosterone concentrations, which are elevated in response to stress. Benzodiazepines, both acutely and chronically, are able to prevent the increase in plasma corticosterone concentrations induced by stress (Lahti and Barsuhn, 1974, 1975; Keim and Sigg, 1977; LeFur *et al.*, 1979; File 1982b: File and Peet, 1980). At high doses of benzodiazepines, however, an increase in plasma corticosterone levels is observed in nonstressed animals. It has been hypothesized that this is due to the stress produced by high doses of benzodiazepines (Lahti and Barsuhn, 1975), particularly since rapid tolerance to this action is observed, as is observed to the depressant effects of benzodiazepines.

The ability of benzodiazepines to block the stress-induced elevation in plasma corticosterone levels is fairly specific, since this elevation in plasma corticosterone is not blocked by neuroleptics, psychostimulants, antidepressants, anticholinergics, α- and β-blockers, 5-HT antagonists or analgesics (LeFur *et al.*, 1979; Lahti and Barsuhn, 1974).

It is believed that the ability of benzodiazepines to prevent the corticosterone response to stress does not represent a direct stimulation of the adrenal cortex but is of central origin, because (a) benzodiazepines do not prevent the increase in plasma corticosterone concentrations produced by ACTH (LeFur *et al.*, 1979); (b) the effect of benzodiazepines could be suppressed by hypophysectomy or betamethasone treatment (LeFur *et al.*, 1979); (c) the *in vitro* reactivity of the adrenal glands in benzodiazepine-treated rats is no different from controls (Keim and Sigg, 1977). It is therefore possible that benzodiazepines centrally block the release of the ACTH at the hypothalamic or pituitary level. Consistent with this are observations that benzodiazepines decrease plasma ACTH concentrations (Bruni *et al.*, 1980).

The mechanism underlying the effects of high doses of benzodiazepines to increase corticosterone concentrations is not clear. Chabot *et al.* (1981) suggested that this was also not due to a direct stimulation of the adrenal cortex, since it could be prevented by blocking pituitary ACTH release. Lahti and Barsuhn (1975) suggested that the sedation and muscle relaxation produced by high doses of benzodiazepines is itself stressful, thus accounting for the rise in corticosterone concentrations.

File and Pellow (1985b) investigated the effects of the novel putative anxiolytic, tracazolate, on both basal corticosterone concentrations as measured in the home cage, and on the corticosterone response to novelty-stress. Tracazolate, at both anxiolytic and sedative doses (5 and 25 mg/kg) had no significant effect on corticosterone concentrations; however, in contrast, the phenylquinolines PK 8165 and PK 9084 that do not possess anxiolytic activity in animal tests, had benzodiazepine-like effects on corticosterone: they elevated basal corticosterone levels, and they attenuated the corticosterone response to stress. McElroy and Meyer (1983) found that the anxiolytic compound CL 218,872 did not inhibit the plasma corticosterone elevation in response to noise stress. The novel anxiolytic, buspirone, increases ACTH (Gilbert, *et al.*, 1987) and corticosterone concentrations (Urban *et al.*, 1986). These results suggest that drug effects on anxiety and stress are separable.

We do not believe that the elevations in basal corticosterone, as suggested by Lahti and Barsuhn, are due to the sedative effects of the compounds in question. Tracazolate did not elevate basal concentrations at sedative doses, and PK 8165 and 9084 elevated them at non-sedative doses. However, Stephens *et al.* (1986) have suggested that any novel drug effect that is strong enough may be the cause of elevated basal levels.

5. BENZODIAZEPINES AND CONVULSIONS

Benzodiazepines are effective against several types of epilepsy in man, and in particular they are used in the treatment of petit mal epilepsy and to reverse status epilepticus. They are potent at preventing a wide range of experimental convulsions in animals. The two methods that are most widely used for screening potential anticonvulsants are activity against pentylenetetrazol(PTZ)-induced seizures and activity against seizures induced by electroshock.

Chweh *et al.* (1983) found a high correlation between the potencies of several benzodiazepines at counteracting PTZ-induced seizures and their affinities for the ^{3}H-flunitrazepam binding sites. There were similar correlations between their anticonvulsant actions against seizures induced by bicuculline and picrotoxin, but no correlation between their potencies against electroshock or strychnine-induced seizures and their affinity for the benzodiazepine receptor. This suggests that these latter two anticonvulsant actions of the benzodiazepines may not be mediated by the high affinity benzodiazepine receptors. However, the correlation between receptor occupancy and diazepam's anti-PTZ effects (Paul *et al.*, 1979; File et al., 1989) is further evidence that this anticonvulsant activity is mediated by the benzodiazepine receptors. Benzodiazepines are also able to antagonize convulsions induced by bemegride, ouabain, local anesthetics, penicillin, nicotine, kainic acid, tetanus toxin and caffeine. This wide range of anticonvulsant action shows that this action is not restricted to any one neuronal system (Haefely *et al.*, 1981).

Benzodiazepines are also effective in rodent models of sensory epilepsy. They are effective against audiogenic seizures in mice (Lehmann, 1964; Robichaud *et al.*, 1970), against seizures induced by intermittent photic stimulation in photosensitive baboons (Killam *et al.*, 1973; Meldrum and Croucher, 1982) and against seizures produced by repeated electrical stimulation of discrete brain areas (Racine *et al.*, 1975; Albertson *et al.*, 1982).

Although the main action of benzodiazepines is an anticonvulsant one, it is possible to see the opposite effect. Even though the benzodiazepines have an anti-PTZ effect in neonates that is, if anything, more marked than in adult rats (Mares and Seidl, 1982), several benzodiazepines have been found to cause myoclonic jerks in newborn rats, possibly indicative of seizure-like activity (Barr and Lithgow, 1983; File and Wilks, 1986). These effects were not dose-related and disappeared after day 13. It has therefore been suggested that they might reflect activity at the type 2 benzodiazepine receptor subtype, since the type 1 receptors (which predominate in the adult) only start rapid proliferation after day 7. The lack of a dose-related effect suggests that the seizure activity was not just a reflection of the high brain concentrations that would be achieved in the neonate. Even in the adult rat it is possible at high doses to see benzodiazepine-induced seizures, particularly with flurazepam (Riegel and Bourn, 1983; Rosenberg, 1980). It has been suggested that the seizures may be mediated by benzodiazepine action at the picrotoxin site (see Olsen, 1982).

It is interesting to compare the anticonvulsant efficacy of the novel putative anxiolytics with those of the benzodiazepines. One group of compounds that has received considerable attention is the pyrazolopyridine class, e.g. tracazolate, cartazolate and etazolate. These compounds displace ligands that bind to sites on the chloride ionophore (Olsen, 1982) and enhance the binding of benzodiazepines to their receptors (Beer *et al.*, 1978; Meiners and Salama, 1982; Supavilai and Karobath, 1979). Tracazolate protects against seizures induced by PTZ and bicuculline (Patel and Malick, 1982), but is less potent than chlordiazepoxide. Etazolate, however, only weakly protected against PTZ-induced convulsions, and totally failed to counteract convulsions induced by strychnine or maximal electroshock (Beer *et al.*, 1978).

CGS 9896 is a pyrazoloquinoline that potently displaces benzodiazepines from their binding sites (Yokoyama *et al.*, 1982). There have been somewhat conflicting reports of its anticonvulsant activity. In rats it has been found to protect against seizures induced by bicuculline or PTZ (Gee and Yamamura, 1983; Yokoyama *et al.*, 1982), with a potency greater than that of diazepam. It is also potent at protecting mice against seizures induced by picrotoxin, which is thought to act at the same site as PTZ. Using a different strain of mice, Brown *et al.* (1984) failed to find an anti-PTZ action of CGS 9896 at the higher dose range of 30–100 mg/kg, and in this range CGS 9896 reduced by 50% the anti-convulsant action of diazepam. This suggests that the compound may be a partial, rather than a full, agonist at benzodiazepine receptors. Perhaps consistent with this is its inability to antagonize maximal electroshock seizures (Barbaz, cited in Bennett and Petrack, 1984).

Some of the other new compounds have mixed anti- and pro-convulsant actons. CL 218,872 is a triazolopyridazine that selectively displaces benzodiazepines from type 1 receptors, with a potency comparable to that of diazepam. In low doses, CL 218,872 is proconvulsant when combined with subconvulsant doses of β-CCM, bicuculline and picrotoxin, but interestingly not when combined with pentylenetetrazol; in higher doses it is anticonvulsant against PTZ-induced seizures, but not against picrotoxin-induced seizures (Melchior *et al.*, 1983, 1985; File and Wilks, 1985).

Tofisopam is a 3,4-benzodiazepine that does not displace benzodiazepines from their receptors, but that enhances their affinity for these receptors *in vivo* (Saano, 1982; Saano and Urtti, 1982) and that in high concentrations also displaces ligands binding to sites on the chloride ionophore (Ramanjaneyulu and Ticku, 1984). Although tofisopam is not effective in any animal test, it has been claimed to be clinically effective (for review, see Pellow and File, 1986b). On its own, tofisopam has no anticonvulsant action against seizures induced by electroshock, PTZ, nicotine and strychnine (Petocz and Kosoczky, 1975); however, it does enhance the anticonvulsant efficacy of diazepam against seizures induced by PTZ, picrotoxin, isoniazid and maximal electroshock, but not those induced by bicuculline, nicotine or strychnine (Briley *et al.*, 1984). In contrast to this action, tofisopam has been reported to *lower* the threshold for chemical seizures (Saano, 1982; Petocz and Kosoczky, 1975) and to be weakly proconvulsant in combination with PTZ and picrotoxin (Pellow and File, 1986c).

Buspirone is another new compound with a poor anxiolytic profile in animal tests (see File, 1985b, for review) but which has been claimed to be clinically effective. It has no anticonvulsant effects up to 400 mg/kg and in rats it *lowers* the convulsant threshold to picrotoxin (Eison and Eison, 1984), and causes convulsions when it is combined with antidepressant drugs (File, 1988).

6. BENZODIAZEPINES AND AGGRESSIVE BEHAVIOR

In assessing the effects of benzodiazepines on aggressive behavior it is important to distinguish between changes that are specific to aggression and those that reflect non-specific stimulant or sedative actions of the drug. Many of the early studies reporting antiaggressive actions of the benzodiazepines were simply providing further examples of the non-specific sedative effects of high doses of benzodiazepines. This review will concentrate on studies where the changes in aggression are likely to be specific. It is also important to realise that there are many different types of aggressive behavior and that the effects of benzodiazepines may vary according to the nature of the aggression. Their effects will therefore be considered separately for defensive behavior (self-defensive or maternal defense of the litter) and for offensive behavior.

6.1. DEFENSIVE BEHAVIORS

Chlordiazepoxide, in doses lower than those causing sedation, had a taming effect (reduced aggression towards a human experimenter) in monkeys, baboons, a variety of zoo animals, and cats (Randall, 1960; Heise and Boff, 1961; Scheckel and Boff, 1966; Heuschele 1961; Lister *et al.*, 1971; Hoffmeister and Wuttke, 1969). However, chlordiazepoxide only reduced aggression towards the experimenter shown by male mink in doses that caused ataxia (Bauen and Possanza, 1970). It is generally considered that aggression towards humans is a form of self-defensive behavior.

When rodents are exposed to inescapable foot-shock the aggressive behaviors that ensue are generally considered to be defensive in nature. Low doses of chlordiazepoxide reduce shock-elicited defense (Christmas and Maxwell, 1970; Hoffmeister and Wuttke, 1969; Irwin *et al.*, 1971; Robichaud and Goldberg, 1974; Sofia, 1969; Stille *et al.*, 1963; Tedeschi *et al.*, 1969). In contrast, Traversa *et al.* (1985) found that chlordesmethyldiazepam increased shock-elicited defense; this may represent an important difference among the various benzodiazepines. Kostowski *et al.* (1981) found that chlordesmethyldiazepam also increased shock-elicited defense in rats, but lorazepam (a metabolite of chlordesmethyldiazepam) was without effect below sedative doses.

Lactating female rats will vigorously defend their litters against male intruders and this form of aggression was increased by a low dose of chlordiazepoxide (Olivier *et al.*, 1986). This raises the possibility of the effects of chlordiazepoxide being in opposite directions for self-defensive and maternal defensive behaviors.

6.2. Offensive Behaviours

The most common way of assessing offensive behavior in rodents is to confront a resident rat or mouse with an intruder in its home-cage. Typically, mice are singly housed for 28 days to increase their level of aggression and they are then confronted with an intruder, who has usually been grouped-housed to reduce offensive behavior. Chlordiazepoxide, diazepam and midazolam all reduce attacks made by the resident mouse (Skolnick *et al.*, 1985; Rodgers and Waters, 1985; Yoshimura and Ogawa, 1984; Poshivalov, 1981; Miczek and O'Donell, 1980; Malick, 1978). Krsiak *et al.* (1981) found that diazepam and chlordiazepoxide reduced defensive and escape behavior of timid resident mice in lower doses than those reducing attack in aggressive residents. This suggests that changes in defensive and offensive behaviors are independent. This is confirmed by results with other benzodiazepines. Krsiak *et al.* (1984) found that nitrazepam and oxazepam reduced defensive and escape behavior, but were without effects on attack behavior. Other benzodiazepines, e.g. triazolam, clonazepam and flunitrazepam had no effect on aggressive behavior at doses below those causing sedation (Krsiak *et al.*, 1984).

In rats trained to run for food reward, the omission of food leads to fighting. Administration of low doses of chlordiazepoxide increased the number of attacks, bites and lateral threat postures. These behaviors were reduced by 20 mg/kg, which is a sedative dose (Miczek, 1974). In pairs of rats meeting in a neutral arena, chlordiazepoxide, oxazepam, loprazolam, nitrazepam, flurazepam and flunitrazepam all reduced aggressive behaviors (Gardner and Guy, 1984; Guy and Gardner, 1985). When chlordiazepoxide was given to the dominant monkey in a colony he dropped in status and received more aggression (Apfelbach and Delgado, 1974); there were no effects on the behavior of the subordinate monkey when he was given chlordiazepoxide, but this may be because it was not possible for him to display less aggression.

Similar effects on dominance were found in rats after chronic (5 days) administration of a low dose of chlordiazepoxide. In a chocolate competition test, File (1986a) found that chlordiazepoxide reduced the success of dominant and middle-ranking rats, and left unchanged the behavior of subordinate rats.

However, some change in subordinate behavior may occur in other situations. In one of the few studies to use chronic benzodiazepine administration, rats were treated for 5 days with a low dose of chlordiazepoxide and then placed as a single intruder in a colony of twelve resident rats; they received significantly less attacks than did the vehicle-injected control rats (File, 1982c). It was thought that this was because they emitted fewer escape responses, which would be in keeping with acutely administered chlordiazepoxide. The effects of lorazepam (0.025 mg/kg) has been studied in isolated mice; aggression was increased in the resident mice after acute administration and after 1,2 or 3 weeks of treatment (Wilks and File, 1986). Group-housed mice fed a diet of 0.03% chlordiazepoxide showed an increased incidence of aggression and deaths (Fox *et al.*, 1970). Although there are too few studies to draw firm conclusions, it is possible that with chronic treatment the effects of benzodiazepines are in the direction of *increasing* offensive behaviors.

In considering whether benzodiazepine-induced changes in aggression are specific changes, it is important to consider whether any decreases are secondary to drug-induced sedation or ataxia. It is also possible that changes in aggression are secondary to the anxiolytic action of the drugs. This is harder to assess and is not helped by the paucity of studies using chronic treatment. It has been argued (Rodgers and Waters, 1985) that the reduction in self-defensive behaviors reflects the anxiolytic action of the drugs, presumably by decreasing the effective threat of the human handler or the foot-shock. This may well be the case, but as well as modifying the impact of threatening stimuli, anxiety may independently change the threshold for attack. One could argue that this might explain the enhanced offensive behavior seen with chronic treatment. This issue cannot be resolved with our existing knowledge and more detailed studies of the neural bases of anxiety and of aggression are needed. An alternative strategy would be to identify particular benzodiazepines that produce atypical profiles in aggression and to determine whether they are also atypical in their profiles in anxiolytic tests.

7. BENZODIAZEPINES AND EXPLORATION

Benzodiazepines have been found to have significant effects in a number of tests that purport to measure exploration. This has resulted in a tendency to use tests of exploratory behavior to screen for benzodiazepine-like compounds. It is important to assess the value of using such tests to study the actions of benzodiazepines and related compounds. In low doses, benzodiazepines enhance exploration-related behaviors, whilst in high doses they reduce them. Is it possible to distinguish these actions from non-specific stimulant and depressant effects and can they be related to any of the clinical effects of benzodiazepines?

The definition of exploratory behavior and how to measure it have long been problems for psychologists (see Berlyne, 1960). Since exploration is behavior at its most spontaneous, by definition the experimenter has little control over it and thus it is important to measure the frequency, duration and temporal patterning of as many behaviors as possible. There are two major problems in the search for a model of exploratory behavior in rodents: (1) the problem of novelty and thus fear; and (2) the problem of separating locomotor activity from exploration. A problem with any test of exploration is that an animal will walk round an arena to explore it, or to escape from it, or both (Denenberg, 1969) and there is no way to separate out these factors. Clearly, then, the fear level of the animal (determined by the novelty of the situation, light level, past history of the animal) will be a strong determinant of his response to any test in which exploration is measured, and may be a confounding factor.

Where motor activity alone is the measure, it is also impossible to disentangle changes in exploration from changes in basal locomotor activity. Thus, tests such as the open field procedure are uninterpretable, as are situations measuring the number of entries into the arms of a T- or Y-maze, and the staircase test of Boissier *et al.* (1976). However, there have been attempts to separate out exploration and locomotor activity. The frequency and duration of approaches to a novel object can be measured (Berlyne, 1955; Delini-Stula, 1984; File, 1973a,b) either in the home cage or in a novel environment. Exploration has also been measured by the frequency and duration of exploratory head-dipping or nose-poking into holes in the floor or the wall of the apparatus, with independent measures of locomotor activity also taken (e.g. Boissier and Simon, 1962; File and Wardill, 1975).

Under certain conditions, benzodiazepines may enhance exploration. In general, it is easier to see enhanced exploratory activity with benzodiazepines in the mouse than in the rat (Crawley and Goodwin, 1980; File, 1985c). Increases have been found in open field and Y-maze activity, in tunnel entries and in head dipping and locomotor activity (Christmas and Maxwell, 1970; Itoh and Takaori, 1968; Iwahara and Sakama, 1972; Marriott and Smith, 1972; Marriott and Spencer, 1965; Sansone, 1979; File and Pellow, 1985c). The increased head-dipping in rats and mice is restricted to the first few minutes of the first trial (Nolan and Parkes, 1973). These stimulant effects, whether they are reflected in increased head-dipping or motor activity, are also seen in animals that have been chronically treated with benzodiazepines (Sansone, 1979; Gardner and Piper, 1982; File and Pellow, 1985c), in contrast to the rapid tolerance that develops to the sedative effects of benzodiazepines (see Section 12).

Is the increase in exploration secondary to non-specific stimulant effects of low doses of the benzodiazepines? This is not necessarily the case, as File and Pellow (1985c) found an elevation in exploratory head-dipping in mice without a concomitant elevation in locomotor activity. In rats, enhanced exploration can occur independently from motor stimulation: and Delini-Stula (1984) found increased object exploration with no change in motor activity. However, it is important to note that factors other than increased exploratory tendencies can account for elevated head-dipping and object exploration: a reduced capacity for information processing, for example, would also lead to longer responses to novelty—either because of sedation, or a more specific learning impairment such as has been found in other situations (see Section 8).

Few studies have investigated the possible effects of novel putative anxiolytics to elevate exploration. However, in the holeboard test in mice, we have shown (Pellow and File, 1986d) that the triazolopyridazine CL 218,872 (1 mg/kg), the pyrazolopyridine tracazolate (2.5 mg/kg) and the 3,4-benzodiazepine tofisopam (2.5 mg/kg) all elevate exploratory head-dipping. As with the benzodiazepines, tolerance to these effects was not observed in 10 days.

Although it seems that enhanced exploratory responses can be dissociated from locomotor activity, reductions in both behaviors tend to occur in parallel. File (1983a) calculated correlations for the four different behaviors measured in the holeboard after treatment with a dose of chlordiazepoxide (10 mg/kg) that reduced all measures. The reductions in number of head-dips and time spent head-dipping were highly correlated ($r = 0.8$); the correlations between these measures and motor activity and rearing were between 0.4 and 0.5, and there was a very high correlation ($r = 0.94$) between the latter two measures. Are the reductions in exploration and locomotor activity a reflection of the general CNS depressant effects of higher doses of benzodiazepines? The term 'sedation' has various usages in the literature. In many pharmacological papers it is used to describe the muscle relaxant and ataxic effects of the drugs. In other papers 'sedation' is used to mean drowsy or sleepy. In the AMA drug evaluation manual the term is used to define a dimension starting from the reduction in spontaneous behaviors and ending with the induction of sleep. The reduction of spontaneous behaviors in the holeboard would certainly fall into this latter definition. Although the benzodiazepines do also cause muscle relaxation and ataxia, there is no evidence that these effects fall on the same dimension as that of reduced alertness. The interchangeable use of these terms is therefore strongly discouraged.

A wide variety of benzodiazepines have now been found to have depressant effects on exploratory and locomotor activity in the holeboard, either in rats (e.g. triazolam, lorazepam, chlordiazepoxide; see File, 1985c) or in mice (chlordiazepoxide and diazepam, see File and Pellow, 1985c). The triazolobenzodiazepines alprazolam (0.2–2.0 mg/kg), adinazolam (0.5–5.0 mg/kg) and U-43, 465 (8–32 mg/kg) also caused dose-related reductions in spontaneous behavior in the holeboard in rats (File and Pellow, 1985d). Similarly the 3,4-benzodiazepine tofisopam caused reductions in spontaneous behavior in both rats (50 mg/kg, Pellow and File, 1986c) and mice (50 mg/kg, Pellow and File, 1986d). The sedative effects of chlordiazepoxide in the holeboard in mice were reversed by the benzodiazepine receptor antagonist, Ro 15-1788 (File *et al.*, 1985).

Since the decrease in spontaneous behavior is the most sensitive measure of the sedative effects of a drug, it is sensible to use tests such as the holeboard as an initial screen. This is a particularly important issue since there is a clear clinical requirement for a non-sedative anxiolytic. However, both the presence of an anxiolytic effect and the absence of a sedative one should be subject to rigorous testing.

The triazolopyridazine CL 218,872 was claimed to be non-sedative in doses up to 250 mg/kg (Lippa *et al.*, 1979). However, other experimenters have found it to be clearly sedative as measured by a decrease in spontaneous locomotor and/or exploratory behavior in both rats and mice (Oakley *et al.*, 1984; File *et al.*, 1985; McElroy *et al.*, 1985). The reductions in the holeboard in mice were antagonized by the benzodiazepine receptor antagonist, Ro 15-1788 (File *et al.*, 1985). Thus, although it has been shown to have anxiolytic properties in many animal tests, there is little to justify the claim that it is nonsedative. The original claim that the phenylquinolines PK 8165 and PK 9084 were nonsedative anxiolytics was based on the results from a punished drinking test in rats and measures of motor activity in mice. The claims for anxiolytic activity have not been substantiated (see File and

Lister, 1983a; Keane *et al.*, 1984; Pellow, 1985) and both compounds significantly reduce locomotor activity, rearing and head-dipping in the holeboard from doses of 10 mg/kg (File, 1983b; File and Pellow, 1984). Chlordiazepoxide reversed the reductions in head-dipping, but not in locomotor activity, caused by PK 8165. None of the reductions were antagonized by the benzodiazepine antagonist Ro 15-1788 (File and Pellow, 1984). The original evidence for no sedation came from results in mice where the ED50 for a decrease in spontaneous locomotor activity was 50 mg/kg (ten times higher than that required for an anticonflict effect in rats). However, the ED50 for the PK compounds was only twice the ED50 for chlordiazepoxide in these mice. This is exactly the ratio of dose effects found for rats in the holeboard (File, 1983b) and serves to highlight two important points. One is the danger of comparing doses across species; the other is the danger of selecting an animal or a test that is relatively insensitive to the behavioral effect of interest.

Other novel putative anxiolytics that have been observed to reduce spontaneous behavior in the holeboard are the pyrazoloquinolines, CGS 9896, that reduced exploratory head-dipping and motor activity in the rat at 10 mg/kg (File and Pellow, 1986a). The pyrazolopyridine tracazolate has been found to reduce exploratory and locomotor activity in the holeboard from 25 mg/kg in rats (File and Pellow, 1985a) and from 30 mg/kg in mice (Pellow and File, 1986d).

In conclusion, it is clearly premature to interpret the benzodiazepine enhancement of exploratory activity in terms of their anxiolytic activity, particularly given the interpretative problems inherent in the nature of most tests of exploration. The use of tests of exploratory behavior to screen for new potential benzodiazepine-like agents is therefore somewhat hazardous, unless accompanied by other tests and carefully interpreted. Although, in some circumstances, benzodiazepines may increase exploration, this effect is also characteristic of benzodiazepine receptor antagonists (see File and Pellow, 1986b,c). For a full discussion of tests of 'anxiety' that are based on measures of exploration, see Pellow (1986). On the other hand, it is quite likely that the reductions in exploratory behavior may reflect the sedative actions of the benzodiazepines. However, from tests such as the holeboard alone it is not usually possible to distinguish reductions in behavior resulting from sedation, from those resulting from, say, hypothermia or sickness. In these cases it would be necessary to obtain information from other tests.

8. EFFECTS OF BENZODIAZEPINES ON LEARNING AND MEMORY

In clinically effective doses, administration of benzodiazepines either to normal volunteers or to patients induces a wide range of cognitive impairments. One of the major impairments is that in learning and memory. Whilst this effect can be advantageous when combined with anesthesia in a surgical setting, it is extremely disadvantageous in a clinical setting. An impaired ability to acquire new visual and verbal material is the major effect of the benzodiazepines. Retrieval of already-learned information is not affected, i.e. the amnesia is anterograde. The effect is less on short-term than on long-term memory, and the deficit is episodic in nature (see Lister, 1985, and Taylor and Tinklenberg, 1986, for reviews).

In animals, the nature of the deficit to be found in learning and memory tests has not been well characterized. One of the tests that has been most used in the investigation of drug effects on learning and memory is the passive avoidance task: Jensen *et al.* (1979) found that diazepam (19 mg/kg) and lorazepam (20 mg/kg) given before training significantly impaired the acquisition of a passive avoidance task in mice as measured by the latency to enter the black compartment three days later. However, it must be noted that this is a huge dose of lorazepam compared with the effective sedative doses of this drug and the animals would have been comatose throughout the training period.

However, flurazepam (1 mg/kg) given immediately after training produced retrograde amnesia. Patel *et al.* (1979) showed that diazepam (0.6–0.5 mg/kg) and halazepam (10–40 mg/kg), administered before the training session, caused a dose-related decrease in passive avoidance responding in mice as measured by a reduced response latency 24 hr later. When benzodiazepines were administered both prior to training and prior to testing, there was significantly less amnesia. This suggested to the authors that state-dependent learning was a major factor in the amnesic effects of benzodiazepines. However, this has not been found in other studies (see Thiebot, 1985). Ongini *et al.* (1984) showed that a large variety of benzodiazepines, administered before training, could block the acquisition of a passive avoidance response in mice, when latencies to enter the dark compartment were compared with controls 24 hr later. The benzodiazepines and their ED50s were: triazolam (0.05 mg/kg), flunitrazepam (0.05 mg/kg), lormetazepam (0.1 mg/kg), lorazepam (0.2 mg/kg), diazepam (0.6 mg/kg), temazepam (0.9 mg/kg), nitrazepam (1 mg/kg), midazolam (1.4 mg/kg), flurazepam (1.7 mg/kg), halazepam (3.2 mg/kg), clobazam (3.7 mg/kg) and chlordiazepoxide (5.7 mg/kg). The effects of these drugs were reversed by the benzodiazepine antagonist, flumazenil (30 mg/kg).

In a more sophisticated avoidance learning situation, Kuribara and Tado (1984) investigated the effects of diazepam on two already-acquired conditioned lever-press procedures in mice: continuous avoidance and discrete avoidance. Diazepam (0.5–4 mg/kg) impaired avoidance behavior in both procedures.

Other investigators have used non-avoidance procedures involving punishment. For example, Soubrie *et al.* (1976b) placed rats in a novel enclosure, and administered electric footshock. The rats were returned 4 days later without shock and their locomotor activity measured. Rats treated with diazepam (2.5–20 mg/kg), lorazepam (0.6–5 mg/kg) or chlordiazepoxide (5–40 mg/kg) before training did not show such inhibition.

Procedures that have not used electric shock have also been utilized: for example, habituation to novel surroundings. An intersession decrease in exploration of an enclosure may indicate that an animal remembers having been there before. Conflicting results with chlordiazepoxide have been reported (File, 1976; Nolan and Parkes, 1973). Platel and Porsolt (1982) found that retention of information about the environment (taken as a decrease in locomotor activity on a second test) was impaired by chlordiazepoxide (5–20 mg/kg), when the drug was administered immediately after training and animals were tested after a three day delay. Hungry rats eat very little of an unknown but highly palatable food when faced with it for the first time. At a second presentation of this food, an increase in the amount eaten is observed in control rats, but not in rats given benzodiazepines before the first presentation, in spite of a benzodiazepine-induced increase in the initial consumption (Soubrie *et al.*, 1976a).

Discrimination learning procedures have been very popular in the investigation of drug effects on learning and memory. Schallek *et al.* (1972) showed that, in cats, chlordiazepoxide (10 mg/kg) increased non-rewarded responses in a discrimination procedure, but had no effect on rewarded responses. Nicholson and Wright (1974) showed that nitrazepam, diazepam and flurazepam impaired response accuracy on a delayed matching test. The impairment consisted mostly of an increase in no-go responding. Vachon *et al.* (1982) treated cats daily with chlordiazepoxide (0.4 mg/kg) during training on a go/no-go successive discrimination task. This treatment impaired the acquisition of the task. However, there was no effect of the benzodiazepine when the discrimination had already been learned. Cole (1982, 1983) also found an impairment with chlordiazepoxide (5 mg/kg) in acquisition of a discrimination task in rats.

Grimm and Hershkowitz (1981) investigated the effects of chronic diazepam treatment on performance of a previously-learned discrimination task in unavoidably shocked, or not, animals. The effect of diazepam depended on the previous experience of the rats: there was a significant improvement in the performance of shocked animals, but an impairment in the performance of non-shocked animals. Hughes *et al.* (1984) investigated the effects of chronic treatment with diazepam on the acquisition of appetitive discrimination learning in pigeons. Diazepam (2 mg/kg) throughout training led to an impairment in retention 30 days later when animals were tested drug-free. There was also a disruption in performance of an already-learned task; however, in the latter task this was likely to be due to sedation, because as tolerance developed to the sedative effects of the drug throughout the chronic treatment, performance was restored to baseline.

Hodges *et al.* (1986) trained rats to discriminate between different operant schedules of reinforcement. One group was trained to make a continuous reinforcement-time out discrimination (CRF-TO); the other group to make a variable interval-time out discrimination (VI-TO). Chlordiazepoxide (10 mg/kg) disrupted the acquisition of the CRF-TO discrimination only temporarily, whereas acquisition of the VI-TO discrimination was more severely impaired and the performance of pre-trained animals was disrupted. The chlordiazepoxide-induced disruption in performance was thus related to task difficulty. Hodges and Green (1986) tested discrimination learning in a radial-arm maze. Four out of eight arms were baited, under two cue conditions: random-cue, in which the location of the cues was changed before each trial, and constant-cue, in which the same arms were consistently cued and rewarded. Chlordiazepoxide (2.5–10 mg/kg) administered after rats had been trained to a 60–70% criterion, led to a decrease in efficiency in the random condition, in which both working memory (increased entries into arms already entered) and reference memory (entries into non-baited arms) errors occurred. In the constant condition, the reduced efficiency was less marked and consisted of working memory errors. In both situations, the high incidence of errors suggested a general disruption of information processing rather than of working memory, and the possibility of response perseveration.

Sahgal and Iversen have used tests of recognition memory. They found (Sahgal and Iversen, 1978) that chlordiazepoxide (8 mg/kg) impaired delayed comparison performance in pigeons. However, the same authors (1980) found few impairments on a Konorski pair comparison task, with or without delay in monkeys, even at very high doses (80 mg/kg).

In conclusion, on non-discrimination tasks, the vast majority of investigators have found that the benzodiazepines impair the acquisition, rather than the retention, of learning tasks. An interesting exception is a study by Cassone and Molinengo (1981), who found that a decay in rats' performance in a staircase maze ('forgetting') could be produced by an interruption of daily training for 13 days. Diazepam (0.07–0.35 mg/kg) daily during this period increased 'forgetting'. The vast majority of discrimination learning studies, on the other hand, have also shown impairments in performance of an already-learned task. However, it has been suggested by several authors that this disruption in performance is caused by a disinhibitory effect of benzodiazepines on no-go responding, rather than a specific deficit in memory processing.

9. BENZODIAZEPINES AND INTAKE OF FOOD OR WATER

Benzodiazepines are known to increase the intake of food (Cooper, 1980), and to increase drinking (Cooper, 1983). Since the above cited papers provide exhaustive reviews of this subject, we will not go into details here. The evidence is consistent with a direct effect to enhance appetite, at least at lower doses. However, at higher doses the benzodiazepines also show signs of reducing food neophobia (Cooper, 1980).

Triazolobenzodiazepines such as triazolam also increase food consumption, as do the β-carboline derivatives ZK 91296 and ZK 93423 (Cooper, 1986), which are a full and a partial agonist, respectively, at benzodiazepine receptors. Zopiclone and CL 218,872 elevated food intake (Cooper and Moores, 1985). The pyrazoloquinoline CGS 9896, in contrast, did not elevate food consumption (Cooper and Gilbert, 1985), and the pyrazolopyridine tracazolate actually reduced feeding (Cooper and Moores, 1985).

10. BENZODIAZEPINE DEPENDENCE AND WITHDRAWAL

When the benzodiazepines were introduced into clinical practice, it was believed for many years that their dependence potential was low (e.g. Marks, 1978). However, it is now widely appreciated that, in fact, the risk of dependence with the benzodiazepines is fairly high (e.g. Marks, 1983). Recently, Lader and File (1987) have proposed that the same withdrawal syndrome occurs on termination of high and low doses of benzodiazepines, regardless of whether they have been taken long- or short-term, and that a similar syndrome can even occur after a single administration.

The severity of the withdrawal syndrome following discontinuation of high-dose benzodiazepine use has been well documented (Petursson and Lader, 1984). Fits and delirium tremens-like syndromes are associated with abrupt withdrawal, but even gradual withdrawal may be followed by a specific syndrome, whether previous dosage was high or low (Hallstrom and Lader, 1981). The syndrome consists of psychological symptoms of anxiety, bodily symptoms of anxiety, and perceptual disturbances (Ladewig, 1984). The withdrawal syndrome may last for a few days or even weeks.

The appearance of dependence and withdrawal may be related to the particular benzodiazepine in use. It has been supposed that benzodiazepines with a short elimination half-life are most likely to invoke severe withdrawal reactions, whereas those with longer half-lives are likely to produce a mild but longer withdrawal syndrome (Hollister, 1983). However, although the elimination half-life may govern the delay to onset of withdrawal effects, and even its severity, it has been suggested (Lader and File, 1987) that the underlying mechanism of dependence is the same.

Benzodiazepine dependence in animals is assessed either from the withdrawal responses when chronic treatment is terminated abruptly, or by giving a benzodiazepine antagonist to precipitate withdrawal. Most of the studies on spontaneous benzodiazepine withdrawal in animals have used huge doses that are well above the equivalent of the human therapeutic range. In a sense, then, any observable changes could be considered as a manifestation of toxicity, but if the underlying mechanism of dependence is independent of dose these studies are pertinent.

After 24 days of administration of doses of diazepam 100–1000 times the anxiolytic dose, rats showed hyperactivity and a lowered threshold for audiogenic seizures (Kiianmaa and Boguslawsky, 1981). Hyperactivity, increased autonomic responses and enhanced polysynaptic activity in spinal neurones were found in rats withdrawn after 5 weeks of chlordiazepoxide in doses 100–200 times the anxiolytic dose (Ryan and Boisse, 1984). Using doses of diazepam and lorazepam about 100 times the anxiolytic dose, hyperactivity, seizures, explosive awakenings, wet dog shakes, hostility and decreased food and water intake have been found in dogs (McNicholas *et al.*, 1983). Using doses around 10 times the anxiolytic dose, hyperactivity and increased anxiety have been found in rats withdrawing from diazepam or chlordiazepoxide (McMillan and Leander, 1978; Emmett-Oglesby *et al.*, 1983a). It has also been possible to demonstrate increased anxiety on withdrawal from 21 days of treatment with an anxiolytic dose of chlordiazepoxide (File *et al.*, 1987) or diazepam (File, 1989). Whilst these studies provide description of the withdrawal syndrome in animals and suggest that the syndrome may not be qualitatively different following high or low doses, they provide no information as to the underlying mechanism. However, there is evidence that the enhanced anxiety seen in withdrawal after 3 weeks of chlordiazepoxide is due to the action of an anxiogenic endogenous ligand (File and Baldwin, 1987) because the increased anxiety was reversed by the benzodiazepine receptor antagonist flumazenil. Similarly, after 3 weeks of diazepam treatment both the increased anxiety and the decreased bicuculine seizure threshold 24 hr later were reversed by the benzodiazepine receptor antagonist flumazenil (Hitchott *et al.*, 1989) and by the inverse agonist FG 7142. Three further studies suggest that an endogenous ligand is not responsible for withdrawal responses after a single dose of lorazepam. Both mice and rats showed a withdrawal response several hours after lorazepam, indicated by a reduction in seizure threshold, hyperactivity and changes in exploratory head-dipping; none of these behaviors was modified by the administration of Ro 15-1788 (Lister and File, 1986; Lister and Nutt, 1986; Wilks and File, 1988).

The studies using precipitated withdrawal have also, in general, used very high doses of benzodiazepines. In the most extreme study, rats were given over 200 times the anxiolytic dose of diazepam for 6 months. When withdrawal was precipitated with the benzodiazepine antagonist, flumazenil, there was increased motor activity, poker tail, wet dog shakes, head and body tremor, occasional clonus and digging (McNicholas and Martin, 1982). Surprisingly, this precipitated withdrawal was found to be *less* intense than was spontaneous withdrawal. Using about 10–100 times the anxiolytic dose, mice and rats withdrawn from diazepam showed hyperactivity and mice showed an increased incidence of seizures, particularly after the higher doses (Cumin *et al.*, 1982). In contrast to the mild withdrawal seen in rats, it is easier to see withdrawal in cats, which are in any case very sensitive to benzodiazepines. After 35 days of about 10 times the anxiolytic dose of flurazepam, cats showed precipitated withdrawal responses of increased muscle tone, tremor, piloerection, pupil dilation and excess salivation (Rosenberg and Chiu, 1982). Similar changes were found after 16 days of 10 times the anxiolytic dose of lorazepam (Cumin *et al.*, 1982). Marked changes have been found in monkeys treated for 15 days with 10 times the anxiolytic dose of diazepam (Cumin *et al.*, 1982). In baboons, precipitated withdrawal can be seen even after doses of diazepam as low as 0.25 mg/kg for 7 days. This consisted of abnormal body postures, nose rubbing, retching and limb tremor. Head and body tremor and convulsions were seen only after 35 days of treatment at higher doses (Lukas and Griffiths, 1984). In this study, precipitated withdrawal had a more rapid onset, was *more* severe and of shorter duration than spontaneous withdrawal. In rats, enhanced anxiety has been found after treatment for 5–6 days with about 100 times the anxiolytic dose of diazepam (Emmett-Oglesby *et al.*, 1983b) or after 5 days of treatment with 4 times the anxiolytic dose of chlordiazepoxide (File and Pellow, 1985e). In the latter study, withdrawal was precipitated using the benzodiazepine receptor inverse agonist, CGS 8216. Ongini *et al.* (1985), in contrast, found that an abstinence syndrome in cats could not be precipitated by the β-carboline FG 7142, also an inverse agonist.

Thus there are at least two studies, one in rats and one in baboons, that suggest that it is possible to see precipitated withdrawal in animals following relatively short-term treatment with doses of benzodiazepines that fall within the therapeutic dose range. This, again, supports the proposal that a common mechanism of dependence is involved. The interpretation of benzodiazepine-precipitated withdrawal should be made with some care. Whilst it is true that at low doses flumazenil can reverse the behavioral effects of the benzodiazepines, at higher doses it has intrinsic behavioral effects, that include anxiogenic and proconvulsant actions (File and Pellow, 1986b,c). It has recently been argued that the apparent intrinsic effects of flumazenil may reflect antagonism of endogenous ligands, and that it is likely that both an anxiolytic and an anxiogenic ligand exist (File and Pellow, 1986b,c). Until such ligands have been firmly identified this must remain speculative, but clearly chronic benzodiazepine treatment may modify their release. The behavioral changes seen when withdrawal is precipitated with flumazenil will then be a complex effect of antagonism of benzodiazepines and of endogenous ligands. An interesting study by Lamb and Griffiths (1985) showed that with repeated applications of flumazenil there were significantly fewer signs of withdrawal in baboons that had received diazepam or triazolam for one month. This study will be discussed further in Section 12.

There is some evidence from animal studies that the development of dependence is not a necessary consequence of all anxiolytic drugs acting at the benzodiazepine binding site. It has not proved possible to produce a precipitated withdrawal response after chronic treatment with the novel putative anxiolytic CGS 9896, a pyrazoloquinoline, in either mice (Boast *et al.*, 1985) or baboons (Griffiths, 1984), and the behavioral changes of abstinence withdrawal in baboons were very mild. It has been suggested that a possible reason for this difference in dependence-liability between benzodiazepines and CGS 9896 is that the former, but not the latter, reduces the firing rate of zona reticulata neurones in the substantia nigra (Fallon and Sinton, 1985). Such regional differences could prove crucial, but the reason for them is unknown and cannot lie in differences in affinity for the benzodiazepine receptor.

11. REWARDING PROPERTIES OF MINOR TRANQUILIZERS

Griffiths and his colleagues, using human volunteer subjects with documented histories of drug abuse, have carried out an extensive series of investigations into the rewarding properties of minor tranquilizers. Griffiths *et al.* (1976) established that sodium pentobarbitone, diazepam and alcohol could all serve as reinforcers: Griffiths *et al.* (1979) showed that pentobarbitone (30 or 90 mg) and diazepam (10 or 20 mg) maintained self-administration. The higher doses were more effective than the lower doses.

Later studies from this group have assessed drug preferences. In these studies large single doses were given, rather than repeated moderate ones, which may account for some of the different results obtained. Pentobarbitone (200–900 mg) was liked by abuser subjects, whereas diazepam (50–400 mg) was not. Similarly, Roache and Griffiths (1985), comparing pentobarbitone (100–600 mg) with triazolam (0.5–3 mg), found that the latter was rated lowest on subjects' liking and estimate of street value. These data suggest that benzodiazepines have a lower abuse liability than barbiturates. Griffiths *et al.* (1984) have also compared different benzodiazepines: diazepam (40, 80 and 160 mg) was better liked and produced more euphoria than oxazepam (480 mg). In normal (non-abuser) subjects, dose and drug effects are more difficult to discern (de Wit *et al.*, 1984).

There are at least three ways of measuring the extent to which drugs are rewarding to animals: self-administration of the drug; conditioned place preference; and, possibly, by effects on electrical self-stimulation of the brain.

Rhesus monkeys and baboons will self-administer benzodiazepines, but at markedly lower rates than they will self-administer barbiturates and alcohol (Yanagita and Takahashi, 1973; Woods, 1982). It is also clear that not all benzodiazepines generate equal rates of self-administration and that procedural differences may be crucial in determining the drug preferences.

Some of the crucial determining factors have been highlighted by Singer (1985). Using a combination of self-injection and a schedule of food delivery to hungry rats, drugs were classified into various groups. Group 1 drugs (alcohol and heroin) were self-injected without the food delivery schedule, but injections were increased by the schedule and by reduced body weight. Group 2 drugs (amphetamine and cocaine) were greatly enhanced by reduced body weight. Self-injection of group 3 drugs (benzodiazepines, barbiturates, nicotine, Δ^9-THC and methadone) occurred only in the presence of a schedule and reduced body weight, i.e. some level of physiological stress.

Using the technique of conditioned place preference, lorazepam, diazepam and the triazolobenzodiazepines all produced significant preferences in doses that fall in the anxiolytic range. Chlordiazepoxide, and the non-benzodiazepine anxiolytic, buspirone, did not produce a significant preference (File, 1986b).

Electrical stimulation of the brain in certain sites, such as the lateral hypothalamus and ventral tegmentum, is rewarding and can be markedly enhanced by stimulants, opiates and barbiturates. In low doses, chlordiazepoxide, diazepam and clonazepam have all been reported to produce modest increases in self-stimulation, as have the non-benzodiazepine anxiolytics CL 218,872 and CGS 9896 (see Liebman, 1985, for review). There are two possible explanations for this effect. One is that the increased self-stimulation reflects the relatively mild rewarding aspects of the benzodiazepines, i.e. the minor tranquilizers enhance the rewarding properties of the stimulation. The other is that the benzodiazepines enhance self-stimulation by reducing concomitant aversive features of the stimulation where the latter play a major role (Herberg and Williams, 1983). Using a shuttle box in which the rat can both initiate and terminate stimulation, it is possible independently to assess rewarding and aversive properties. It is assumed that stimulation is terminated because aversive properties build up with continuous stimulation, possibly because of current spread into adjacent negatively reinforcing areas. Drugs that enhance dopaminergic function and have high reward value decrease the latency to initiate stimulation and do not affect the latency to terminate stimulation. Benzodiazepines have a nonsignificant tendency to shorten the initiation latency, but do significantly increase the latency to stop the stimulation. It would therefore seem that their effects of self-stimulation may be independent of their effects on reward mechanisms.

12. TOLERANCE TO THE BEHAVIORAL EFFECTS OF MINOR TRANQUILIZERS

Tolerance is said to have developed to the behavioral action of a drug when a given dose has significantly less effect as a result of previous administration. The term is used to describe the reduced behavioral efficacy and does not carry implications for the underlying mechanism(s).

In clinical practice, the benzodiazepines are extremely effective anxiolytics in the short term. However, both the U.K. Committee on Review of Medicines (1980) and the White House Office of Drug Policy (1979) concluded that they have not been shown to be effective over long periods. More specifically, the CRM concluded that "there was little convincing evidence that benzodiazepines were efficacious in the treatment of anxiety after four months' continuous treatment."

Studies in human volunteer subjects have shown that tolerance occurs to many of the behavioral effects of benzodiazepines. Lader *et al.* (1980) observed tolerance, after 15 days' administration of clorazepate, to the electroencephalographic and perceptual effects of the drug. File and Lister (1983b) found that tolerance developed in normal volunteers to some of the effects of lorazepam (2.5 mg), even when the interval between successive drug administrations was 7 days. After 3 doses, tolerance developed to the decrease in finger-tapping and to the self-ratings of dizziness observed with the drug. No tolerance was observed to the drug-induced impairments in a nonsense-syllable paired-associate learning task, or to self-ratings of sedation, or to drug effects on heart rate. Even more rapid development of tolerance can be seen after benzodiazepine overdose. In this case, the behavioral effects of benzodiazepines rapidly disappear, despite persisting high plasma concentrations (Greenblatt and Shader, 1978). This suggests that it is possible to demonstrate tolerance after both acute and chronic treatment even when there is still some drug at the receptor.

Tolerance has been demonstrated to most of the behavioral effects of benzodiazepines in animals. As was found for patients and for human volunteers, tolerance develops at very different rates for the various behavioral actions. It develops very rapidly to the sedative and anticonvulsant effects (from 3–5 days), but takes 10–15 days to develop to the anxiolytic effects, as measured in animal tests, and may not develop at all to the locomotor stimulant effects of low doses, (at least up to 20 days) (see File, 1985d, for review). There is no cross-tolerance between the sedative and stimulant effects of the benzodiazepines in mice (File and Pellow, 1985c), and in rats, as tolerance develops to sedative effects, EEG signs of stimulation emerge and persist (Mele *et al.*, 1984). Whilst the mechanism(s) of tolerance remains unknown, we can at least exclude certain possibilities. There is no evidence for any pharmacokinetic contribution to the tolerance seen to low and moderate doses (for review, see File, 1985d). Similarly, there is no evidence that a few days of treatment with these doses induces any change in benzodiazepine binding (see File, 1985d, for review). There is also evidence that tolerance does not involve a change in endogenous ligands, since the effects of the receptor antagonist Ro 15-1788 are unchanged after chronic treatment in rats (File *et al.*, 1986) or baboons (Lamb and Griffiths, 1985). There is recent evidence for a decrease in sensitivity of GABA receptors (Gonsalves and Gallager, 1985), but for this to account for the behavioral data additional assumptions have to be made. First, it has to be assumed that GABA receptors in different anatomical areas are crucially concerned with the different behaviors, and then one has to assume that any change in these receptors, such as phosphorylation, occurs at significantly different rates in different regions. These are not unreasonable assumptions, but as yet there is no supporting evidence. An alternative pharmacodynamic explanation of behavioral tolerance is that changes occur in the sensitivity of transmitter systems downstream from the GABA-benzodiazepine receptor complex. Since different neurotransmitters and different neuroanatomical pathways may mediate different behaviors, any differential changes in these pathways could easily result in different rates of tolerance to the various behaviors. An early report suggested that a reduction in noradrenaline turnover mediated the sedative effects of benzodiazepines, whereas a reduction in serotonin turnover mediated the anxiolytic effects. It was claimed that there was rapid tolerance to the changes in noradrenaline turnover, but not to those in serotonin (Wise *et al.*, 1972). Unfortunately, the data available do not support this suggestion, and, if anything, there may be a link between sedation and reduced serotonin function (see File, 1985d).

Whilst any change in the GABA-benzodiazepine receptor complex would be the direct result of repeated presence of benzodiazepines at their binding sites, any changes downstream from this complex might be less specific to the benzodiazepines, and the crucial factors may not be the physico-chemical features of the drug. It is possible that the circumstances in which the drug is administered might make a significant contribution to the rate at which tolerance develops. Three types of learned adaptation (habituation, classical conditioning and instrumental conditioning) have been shown to contribute to the development of tolerance to the behavioral actions of other drugs (Goudie and Demellweek, 1986). Some or all of these may play a role in benzodiazepine tolerance. So far, the evidence for any one of these is not strong and a possible reason for this could be the impairment that benzodiazepines produce in learning. In particular the benzodiazepines produce an anterograde episodic amnesia (see Section 8), and what little evidence there is suggests tolerance does not develop to this effect.

In recent years several non-benzodiazepine anxiolytics have been developed that also act at the benzodiazepine binding site. Tolerance seems to develop significantly more slowly to the behavioral effects of one of these, the triazolopyridazine CL 218,872. Tolerance does not develop to its sedative effects after 6 days of dosing (McElroy *et al.*, 1985) but is significantly present after 10 days (Pellow and File. 1986d) (as compared with marked tolerance to the sedative effects of benzodiazepines after 3 days); and it takes 15–20 days for tolerance to develop to its anticonvulsant actions (File and Wilks, 1985), compared with 5 days for the benzodiazepines. As with the benzodiazepines, tolerance was not observed to the stimulant effects of low doses (1 mg/kg) of CL 218,872 in the holeboard in mice (Pellow and File, 1986d). Tolerance was observed to the sedative, but not to the stimulant, effects of tracazolate, that acts at the picrotoxinin site, and similarly for the 3,4-benzodiazepine tofisopam (Pellow and File, 1986d). Tolerance to the anticonvulsant effects of the pyrazoloquinoline, CGS 9896, does not develop after 4 weeks of treatment (Gerhardt *et al.*, 1985). It is interesting to note that this compound also shows less evidence of inducing dependence (Boast *et al.*, 1985; Griffiths, 1984).

13. BENZODIAZEPINE EFFECTS IN THE DEVELOPING RAT

Behavioral teratology is the term used to describe long-term behavioral changes resulting from exposing the developing organism to drugs. These changes are usually assessed several weeks or months after the original treatment, and the animals can either be tested undrugged or given probe injections to determine whether their response to drugs has changed. Clearly the timing of early treatment is likely to be crucial for determining lasting effects. The CNS must be in a sufficiently advanced state to be able to respond to the drug, but still retain enough plasticity so that lasting changes are possible. In the rat, benzodiazepine binding sites start to proliferate rapidly from gestational day 14 and they reach adult levels at postnatal day 28. There are two sub-types of benzodiazepine receptors, although their functional relevance remains unclear. Type 2 receptors form first and reach adult levels at postnatal day 7; the type 1 receptors, which predominate in the adult, start rapid proliferation from around day 7 and continue increasing to day 28 (Lippa *et al.*, 1981; Braestrup and Nielsen, 1978). Thus either or both pre-and post-natal exposure to benzodiazepines in the rat is likely to affect the developing nervous system. This whole period would roughly correspond to the last trimester of human pregnancy and therefore maternal consumption of benzodiazepines could affect the developing fetus. There are only a few reports of physical malformations in rats following prenatal benzodiazepine exposure, but in mice, cleft palate has been reported (see Tucker, 1985, for review).

One of the main difficulties in reviewing this area is the lack of good experimental design applied to developmental studies. Before lasting behavioral changes can be unequivocally attributed to drug treatment, other sources of variability must be excluded. In particular, rats and mice show very marked differences between litters, and hence if only a small number of litters is used for each treatment it is impossible to distinguish between behavioral differences due to litter effects and those caused by drug treatment. Of the 15 studies reviewed by Tucker (1985) only two used the cross-fostering technique and three others made some attempt to re-assign litters after birth.

Prenatal administration of diazepam (2.5–10 mg/kg/day) reduced the normal peak of motor activity displayed by pups on day 16 if they are separated from the nest (Kellogg *et al.*, 1980; Lyubinov *et al.*, 1975), but in older animals no changes were found in activity in the open field, photocell cages or holeboard (Butcher and Vorhees, 1979; Shore *et al.*, 1983; Peruzzi *et al.*, 1983; Adams, 1982; Gai and Grimm, 1982). There have been few well-conducted studies in which learning has been assessed, but one study found that rats exposed prenatally (gestation days 14–20) to diazepam (up to 10 mg/kg) were impaired in a successive discrimination task (Frieder *et al.*, 1984).

When rats are exposed neonatally to drugs they should be randomly fostered to remove any genetic effects and pups within each new litter should be randomly allocated among all the groups to remove any effects due to differences in maternal care. Unfortunately, several studies failed to do this. In contrast to the effects of prenatal treatment, when diazepam is given postnatally to male rats, whether they are tested as adolescents or adults, they show an increase in open field activity and in locomotor activity in the holeboard (Fonseca *et al.*, 1976; Frieder *et al.*, 1984; File, 1986c). However, if the period of neonatal diazepam treatment is restricted to days 1–7, before the type 1 receptors start to proliferate rapidly, then the lasting effects in the holeboard were *reduced* levels of motor activity and rearing (File, 1987). In contrast to diazepam, after neonatal treatment with lorazepam (0.25–2.5 mg/kg/day from days 1–21) motor activity was unchanged in adult rats (File, 1986c) and after neonatal treatment with clonazepam (0.1–1 mg/kg/day 1–21) both motor activity and exploratory head-dipping were reduced in adult rats (File, 1986d). Thus it seems that both the timing of the treatment and the particular benzodiazepine are relevant factors in determining the direction of lasting effects on motor activity.

Treatment with diazepam throughout the preweaning period (days 1–21) led to increased social interaction in a neutral arena when the rats were tested undrugged as adults, but when they were challenged with yohimbine the rats that had been exposed to diazepam as neonates showed less reduction in social interaction (File, 1986c). Both these changes might be indicative of lasting effects in the direction of reduced anxiety. These two studies also demonstrate that the age of the rat when it is tested might determine the ease with which changes are detected, or even their nature. Neonatal treatment with diazepam increased offensive behaviors shown by a resident rat when confronted with a rat intruding into its home-cage; this effect was found whether the rats were tested as adolescents or as adults (File, 1986c,e). However, when the diazepam treatment was restricted to the first postnatal week there were no lasting effects on aggression (File, 1987). Neonatal (days 1–21) treatment with clonazepam (0.1 mg/kg) enhanced offensive behaviors of resident rats, but increased submissiveness in intruders. However, higher doses (0.5 and 1 mg/kg) enhanced dominance behaviors of intruder rats (File, 1986c). Neonatal treatment with lorazepam led to increased submissiveness of both resident and intruder rats (File and Tucker, 1983). Thus the detailed effects on aggression seem to depend on the time of treatment, the dose and on the particular benzodiazepine in question.

There was no change in the acquisition or retention of a passive avoidance task after neonatal (days 1–21) treatment with diazepam, lorazepam or clonazepam (File, 1986d). However, longer treatment with diazepam (days 5-45, 5-10 mg/kg/day) did result in impaired acquisition of a Lashley 111 Maze (Fonseca *et al.*, 1976). Acquisition of an active avoidance response was unimpaired in adolescent pups whose dams had received 1 mg/kg chlordiazepoxide in the drinking water from parturition until weaning (Adams, 1982). However, impaired acquisition was found in adulthood in pups whose dams had received chlordiazepoxide in the drinking water (Coen *et al.*, 1983; Peruzzi *et al.*, 1983). Following 10 mg/kg to dams during lactation, female pups were subsequently impaired as adults in both the acquisition and retention of a complex brightness discrimination; male pups were impaired only in the retention of this task (Frieder *et al.*, 1984).

Neonatal administration of lorazepam and diazepam did not change the PTZ-seizure threshold of adolescent rats (File, 1986e), but the incidence of myoclonic jerks elicited by a challenge dose of PTZ was reduced in adult rats exposed neonatally (days 1–21) to lorazepam and diazepam (File, 1986c).

In conclusion, perhaps the most marked changes found after treatment with benzodiazepines early in development are in aggressive behavior. The changes do not provide any clear indication of the neural compensations that might have occurred. The direction of change depends on the timing of treatment, the particular benzodiazepine, the dose and possibly also the age at testing. Clearly, global conclusions are not justified, but the possible clinical relevance of changes in aggression cannot be ignored.

14. CONCLUSIONS

It is apparent from the above discussion that benzodiazepines have a wide range of effects on a number of different behaviors. Since the major therapeutic use of benzodiazepines has been in the treatment of anxiety disorders, there has been a tendency for certain authors to consider all of the behavioral effects of the benzodiazepines as a reflection of, and as secondary to, their anti-anxiety effects. For example, it has frequently been assumed that animals given benzodiazepines explore more because they are less anxious, or that their anti-stress effects represent an aspect of their anxiolytic effects. However, this is an extremely naive approach that does not take into account other lines of evidence (behavioral or otherwise) for or against an association of anxiety and stress or of anxiety and exploration. A number of reviews have recently addressed such questions.

Pellow and File (1985) concluded that the effects of putative anxiolytic and anxiogenic agents on the rat corticosterone response to stress did not parallel their effects in tests of anxiety. Pellow (1985) concluded that an anticonvulsant effect is not necessarily concomitant with an anxiolytic effect. File (1985c) discussed the effects of benzodiazepines on exploration and concluded that they were quite separate from their anxiolytic effects.

REFERENCES

Adams, P. M. (1982). Effects of perinatal chlordiazepoxide exposure on rat preweaning and postweaning behavior. *Neurobehav. Toxicol. Teratol.* **4**: 279–282.

Albertson, T. E., Bowyer, J. F. and Paule, M. G. (1982) Modification of the anticonvulsant efficacy of diazepam by Ro15-1788 in the kindled amygdaloid seizure model. *Life Sci.* **31**: 1597–1601.

Apfelbach, R. and Delgado, J. M. R. (1974) Social hierarchy in monkeys (Macaca mulatta) modified by chlordiazepoxide hydrochloride. *Neuropharmacology* **13**: 47–63.

Barr, G. A. and Lithgow, T. (1983) Effect of age on benzodiazepine-induced behavioural convulsions in rats. *Nature* **302**: 431–432.

Barry, H. and Krimmer, E. C. (1978) Similarities and differences in discriminative stimulus effects of chlordiazepoxide, pentobarbitol, ethanol and other sedatives. In: *Stimulus Properties of Drugs: Ten Years of Progress*, pp. 31–51, Colpaert, F. C. and Rosecrans, J. A. (eds) Elsevier, Amsterdam.

Bauen, A. and Possanza, G. J. (1970) The mink as a psychopharmacological model. *Arch. Int. Pharmacodyn.* **186**: 133–136.

Beaudry, P., Fontaine, R., Chouinard, G. and Annable, L. (1985) An open trial of clonazepam in the treatment of patients with recurrent panic attacks. *Prog. Neuro-Psycho Pharmacol. Biol. Psychiatry* **9**: 589–592.

Becker, H. C. and Flaherty, C. F. (1983) Chlordiazepoxide and ethanol additively reduce gustatory negative contrast. *Psychopharmacology* **80**: 35–37.

Beer, B., Klepner, C. A., Lippa, A. S. and Squires, R. F. (1978) Enhancement of ^{3}H-diazepam binding by SQ 65,396: A novel anti-anxiety agent. *Pharmacol. Biochem. Behav.* **9**: 849–851.

Bennett, D. A. and Petrack, B. (1984) CGS 9896: A non-benzodiazepine, non-sedating potential anxiolytic. *Drug. Dev. Res.* **4**: 75–82.

Benson, H., Herd, J. A., Morse, W. H. and Kelleher, R. T. (1970) Hypotensive effects of chlordiazepoxide, amobarbital and chlorpromazine on behaviourally-induced elevated arterial blood pressure in the squirrel monkey. *J. Pharmacol. Exp. Ther.* **173**: 399–406.

Berlyne, D. E. (1955) The arousal and satiation of perceptual curiosity in the rat. *J. Comp. Physiol. Psychol.* **48**: 238–246.

Berlyne, D. E. (1960) *Conflict, Arousal and Curiosity*. McGraw-Hill, New York.

Boast, C. A., Gerhardt, S. C., Gajamy, Z. L. and Brown, W. N. (1985) Lack of withdrawal effects in mice after chronic administration of the non-sedating anxiolytic CGS 9896. *Soc. Neurosci. Abst.*

Boissier, J. R. and Simon, P. (1962) La réaction d'exploration chez la souris. *Therapie* **17**: 1225–1232.

Boissier, J. R., Simon, P. and Aron, C. (1968) A new method for rapid screening of minor tranquilisers in mice. *Eur. J. Pharmacol.* **4**: 145–151.

Boissier, J. R., Simon, P. and Soubrie, P. (1976) New approaches to the study of anxiety and anxiolytic drugs in animals. *Proc. 6th Int. Cong. Pharmacol.* **3**: 214–222.

Braestrup, C. and Nielsen, M. (1978) Ontogenetic development of benzodiazepine receptors in the rat brain. *Brain Res.* **147**: 170–173.

Briley, M., Charveron, M., Couret, E. and Stenger, A. (1984) Tofisopam enhances the anticonvulsant activity of diazepam against some, but not all, convulsive agents. *Br. J. Pharmacol.* Suppl. 82: 300P.

Brown, C. L., Jones, B. L., Martin, I. L. and Oakley, N. R. (1984) Efficacy at the benzodiazepine receptor: *In vivo* studies with pyrazoloquinolines. *Br. J. Pharmacol.* **82**: 236P.

BRUNI, G., DAL PRA, P., DOTTI, M. T. and SEGRE, G. (1980) Plasma ACTH and cortisol levels in benzodiazepine treated rats. *Pharmacol. Res. Comm.* **12**: 163–175.

BUTCHER, R. E. and VORHEES, C. V. (1979) A preliminary test battery for the investigation of the behavioral teratology of selected psychotropic drugs. *Neurobehav. Toxicol.* **1**: 207–212.

CASSONE, M. C. and MOLINENGO, L. (1981) Action of thyroid hormones, diazepam, caffeine and amitriptyline on memory decay (forgetting). *Life Sci.* **29**: 1983–1988.

CHABOT, G., BRESSETTE, Y. and GASCON, A. L. (1981) Relationship between plasma corticosterone and adrenal epinephrine after diazepam treatment in rats. *Can. J. Physiol. Pharmacol.* **60**: 589–596.

CHRISTMAS, A. J. and MAXWELL, D. R. (1970) A comparison of the effects of some benzodiazepines and other drugs on aggressive and exploratory behavior in rats and mice. *Neuropharmacology* 9: 17–29.

CHU, N.-S. and BLOOM, F. E. (1974) Activity patterns of catecholamine-containing neurons in the dorso-lateral tegmentum of unrestrained cats. *J. Neurobiol.* **5**: 527–544.

CHWEH, A. X., SWINYARD, E. A., WOLF, H. H. and KUPFERBERG, H. J. (1983) Correlation among minimal neurotoxicity, anticonvulsant activity, and displacing potencies in ^{3}H flunitrazepam binding of neurodiazepines. *Epilepsia* **24**: 668.

COEN, E. ABBRACHIO, M. P., BALDUINI, W., CAGIANO, R., CUOMO, V., LOMBARDELLI, G., PERUZZI, G. REGUSA, M. C. and CATTABENI, F. (1983) Early postnatal chlordiazepoxide administration: permanent behavioural effects in the mature rat and possible involvement of the GABA-benzodiazepine system. *Psychopharmacology* **81**: 261–266.

COLE, S. O. (1982) Effects of chlordiazepoxide on discrimination performance. *Psychopharmacology* **76**: 92–93.

COLE, S. O. (1983) Chlordiazepoxide-induced discrimination impairment. *Behav. Neural Biol.* **37**: 344–349.

COLPAERT, F. C., DESMEDELT, L. K. C. and JANSSEN, P. A. J. (1976) Discriminative stimulus properties of benzodiazepines, barbiturates, and pharmacologically related drugs: Relation to some intrinsic and anticonvulsant effects. *Eur. J. Pharmacol.* **37**: 113–123.

COOK, L. and DAVIDSON, A. B. (1973) Effects of behaviorally active drugs in a conflict-punishment procedure in rats. In: *The Benzodiazepines*, pp. 327–345, GARATTINI, S., MUSSINI, E. and RANDALL, L. O. (eds) Raven Press, New York.

COOK, L. and SEPINWALL, J. (1975) Behavioural analysis of the effects and mechanisms of actions of benzodiazepines. In: *Mechanism of Action of Benzodiazepines*, pp. 1–28, COSTA, E. and GREENGARD, P. (eds) Raven Press, New York.

COOPER, S. J. (1980) Benzodiazepines as appetite-enhancing compounds. *Appetite* **1**: 7–19.

COOPER, S. J. (1983) Benzodiazepines, barbiturates and drinking. In: *Theory in Psychopharmacology*, Vol. 2, pp. 115–148, COOPER, S. J. (ed.) Academic Press, London.

COOPER, S. J. (1986) Hyperphagic and anorectic effects of β-carbolines in a palatable food consumption test: Comparison with triazolam and quazepam. *E. J. Pharmacol.* **120**: 257–265.

COOPER, S. J. and GILBERT, D. B. (1985) Clonazepam-induced hyperphagia in nondeprived rats: Tests of pharmacological specificity with Ro5-4864, Ro5-3663, Ro5-1788 and CGS 9896. *Pharmacol. Biochem. Behav.* **22**: 753–760.

COOPER, S. J. and MOORES, W. R. (1985) Benzodiazepine-induced hyperphagia in nondeprived rat: comparisons with CL 218,872, zopiclone, tracazolate and phenobarbitone. *Pharmac. Biochem. Behav.* **28**: 169–172.

CRAWLEY, J. and GOODWIN, F. K. (1980) Preliminary report of a simple animal behavior model for the anxiolytic effects of benzodiazepines. *Pharmacol. Biochem. Behav.* **13**: 167–170.

CUMIN, R., BONETTI, E. P., SCHERSCHLICHT, R. and HAEFELY, W.E. (1982) Use of the specific benzodiazepine antagonist, Ro15-1788, in studies of physiological dependence on benzodiazepines. *Experimentia* **38**: 833–834.

DANTZER, R. (1977) Behavioural effects of benzodiazepines. A review. *Biobehav. Res.* **1**: 71–76.

DELINI-STULA, A. (1984) A change in novelty oriented responses as measures of the influence of drugs on behavioural habituation in the rat. Paper read at "Le medicament analyseur des comportements." Paris.

DENENBERG, V. H. (1969) Open-field behavior in the rat: What does it mean? *Ann. N. Y. Acad. Sci.* **159**: 852–859.

DE WIT, H., UHLENHUTH, E. H. and JOHANSON, C. E. (1984) Lack of preference for flurazepam in normal volunteers. *Pharmacol. Biochem. Behav.* **21**: 865–869.

EISON, M. S. and EISON, A. S. (1984) Buspirone as a midbrain modulator. Anxiolysis unrelated to traditional benzodiazepine mechanisms. *Drug. Dev. Res.* **4**: 109–119.

EMMETT-OGLESBY, M., SPENCER, JR., D., LEWIS, M. W., ELMESALLAMY, F. and LAL, H. (1983a) Anxiogenic aspects of diazepam withdrawal can be detected in animals. *Eur. J. Pharmacol.* **92**: 127–130.

EMMETT-OGLESBY, M., SPENCER, JR., D. G., ELMESALLAMY, F. and LAL, H. (1983b) The pentylenetetrazol model of anxiety detects withdrawal from diazepam in rats. *Life Sci.* **33**: 161–168.

FALLON, S. L. and SINTON, C. M. (1985) Evidence that CGS 9896 and diazepam differ in their actions on GABA transmission. *Abstr. Soc. Neurosci.* **11**: 425.

FILE, S. E. (1973a) Interaction between prior experience and effects of chlorpromazine on exploration in the rat. *Psychopharmacologia* **32**: 193–200.

FILE, S. E. (1973b) Potentiation of the effects of chlorpromazine on exploration in the rat by prior experience of the drug. *Psychopharmacologia* **29**: 357–363.

FILE, S. E. (1976) A comparison of the effects of ethanol and chlordiazepoxide on exploration and on its habituation. *Physiol. Psychol.* **4**: 529–532.

FILE, S. E. (1980) The use of social interaction as a method for detecting anxiolytic activity of chlordiazepoxide-like drugs. *J. Neurosci. Meth.* **2**: 219–238.

FILE, S. E. (1982a) Chlordiazepoxide-induced ataxia, muscle relaxation and sedation in the rat: Effects of muscimol, picrotoxin and nalaxone. *Pharmacol. Biochem. Behav.* **17**: 1165–1170.

FILE, S. E. (1982b) The rat corticosterone response: Habituation and modification by chlordiazepoxide. *Physiol. Behav.* **29**: 91–95.

FILE, S. E. (1982c) Colony aggression: Effects of benzodiazepines on intruder behavior. *Physiol. Psychol.* **10**: 413–416.

FILE, S. E. (1983a) Variability in behavioural responses to benzodiazepines in the rat. *Pharmac. Biochem. Behav.* **18**: 303–306.

FILE, S. E. (1983b) Sedative effects of PK 9084 and PK 8165, alone and in combination with chlordiazepoxide. *Br. J. Pharmacol.* **79**: 219–223.

FILE, S. E. (1985a) Animal models for predicting clinical efficacy of anxiolytic drugs: Social behaviour. *Neuropsychobiology* **13**: 55–62.

FILE, S. E. (1985b) Models of anxiety. *Br. J. Clin. Practice* **39**: 15–19.

FILE, S. E. (1985c) What can be learned from the effects of benzodiazepines on exploratory behavior? *Neurosci. Biobehav. Rev.* **9**: 45–54.

FILE, S. E. (1985d) Tolerance to the behavioral actions of benzodiazepines. *Neurosci. Biobehav. Rev.* **9**: 113–122.

FILE, S. E. (1986a) Effects of chlordiazepoxide on competition for a preferred food in the rat. *Behav. Brain Res.* **21**: 195–202.

FILE, S. E. (1986b) Aversive and appetitive properties of anxiogenic and anxiolytic agents. *Behav. Brain Res.* **21**: 189–194.

FILE, S. E. (1986c) Behavioral changes persisting into adulthood after neonatal benzodiazepine administration in the rat. *Neurobehav. Toxicol. Teratol.* **8**: 453–461.

FILE, S. E. (1986d) The effects of neonatal administration of clonazepam on passive avoidance and on social, aggressive and exploratory behavior of adolescent male rats. *Neurobehav. Toxicol. Teratol.* **8**: 447–452.

FILE, S. E. (1986e) Effects of neonatal administration of diazepam and lorazepam on performance of adolescent rats in tests of anxiety, aggression, learning and convulsions. *Neurobehav. Toxicol. Teratol.* **8**: 301–306.

FILE, S. E. (1988) Convulsant actions of the anxiolytic buspirone, in combination with antidepressants. *Human Psychopharm* **3**: 145–148.

FILE, S. E. (1989) Chronic diazepam treatment: Effect of dose on development of tolerance and incidence of withdrawal in an animal test of anxiety, *Human Psychopharm* **4**: 59–63.

FILE, S. E. and BALDWIN, H. A. (1987) Flumazenil: a possible treatment for benzodiazepine withdrawal anxiety. *Lancet* **II**: 106–107.

FILE, S. E. (1987) Diazepam and caffeine administration during the first week of life: Changes in neonatal and adolescent behavior. *Neurobehav. Toxicol. Teratol.* **9**: 9–16.

FILE, S. E. and LISTER, RR. E. (1983a) Quinolines and anxiety: Anxiogenic effects of CGS 8216 and partial anxiolytic profile of PK 9084. *Pharmacol. Biochem. Behav.* **18**: 185–188.

FILE, S. E. and LISTER, R. G. (1983b) Does tolerance to lorazepam develop with once weekly dosing? *Br. J. Clin. Pharmacol.* **16**: 645–650.

FILE, S. E. and PEARCE, J. B. (1981) Benzodiazepines reduce ulcers induced in rats by stress. *Br. J. Pharmacol.* **74**: 593–599.

FILE, S. E. and PEET, L. A. (1980) The sensitivity of the rat corticosterone response to environmental manipulations and to chronic chlordiazepoxide treatment. *Physiol. Behav.* **25**: 753–758.

FILE, S. E. and PELLOW, S. (1984) Behavioural effects of PK 8165 that are not mediated by benzodiazepine binding sites. *Neurosci. Lett.* **50**: 197–201.

FILE, S. E. and PELLOW, S. (1985a) The anxiolytic, but not the sedative, properties of tracazolate are reversed by the benzodiazepine receptor antagonist, RO 15-1788. *Neuropsychobiology* **14**: 193–197.

FILE, S. E. and PELLOW, S. (1985b) The effects of putative anxiolytic compounds (PK 8165, PK 9084 and tracazolate) on the rat corticosterone response. *Physiol. Behav.* **35**: 583–586.

FILE, S. E. and PELLOW, S. (1985c) No cross-tolerance between the stimulatory and depressant actions of benzodiazepines in mice. *Behav. Brain Res.* **17**: 1–7.

FILE, S. E. and PELLOW, S. (1985d) The effects of triazolobenzodiazepines in two animal tests of anxiety and the holeboard. *Br. J. Pharmacol.* **86**: 729–736.

FILE, S. E. and PELLOW, S. (1985e) Chlordiazepoxide enhances the anxiogenic actions of CGS 8216 in the social interaction test: Evidence for benzodiazepine withdrawal? *Pharmacol. Biochem. Behav.* **23**: 33–36.

FILE, S. E. and PELLOW, S. (1986a) The behavioral pharmacology of the pyrazoloquinoline CGS 9896, a novel putative anxiolytic. *Drug Dev. Res.* **7**: 245–253.

FILE, S. E. and PELLOW, S. (1986b) Intrinsic actions of the benzodiazepine receptor antagonist. RO 15-1788. *Psychopharmacology* **88**: 1–11.

FILE, S. E. and PELLOW, S. (1986c) Do the intrinsic actions of benzodiazepine receptor antagonists imply the existence of an endogenous ligand for benzodiazepine receptors. In: *Advances in Biochemical Pharmacology: Gabaergic Transmission and Anxiety*, pp. 187–202, BIGGIO, G. and COSTA E. (eds) Raven Press, New York.

FILE, S. E. and TUCKER, J. C. (1983) Lorazepam treatment in the neonatal rat alters submissive behavior in adulthood. *Neurobehav. Tox. Teratol.* **5**: 289–298.

FILE, S. E. and WARDILL, A. G. (1975) Validity of headdipping as a measure of exploration in a modified holeboard. *Psychopharmacologia* **44**: 53–59.

FILE, S. E. and WILKS, L. J. (1985) Effects of acute and chronic treatment on the pro- and anti-convulsant actions of CL 218,872, PK 8165 and PK 9084, putative ligands for the benzodiazepine receptor. *J. Pharm. Pharmacol.* **37**: 252–256.

FILE, S. E. and WILKS, L. J. (1986) The effects of benzodiazepines in new born rats suggest a function for type 2 receptors. *Pharmac. Biochem. Behav.* **25**: 1145–1148.

FILE, S. E., BALDWIN, H. A. and ARANKO, K. (1987) Anxiogenic effects in benzodiaepine withdrawal are linked to the development of tolerance. *Brain Res. Bull.* **19**: 607–610.

FILE, S. E., PELLOW, S., and WILKS, L. (1985) The sedative effects of CL218,872, like those of chlordiazepoxide, are reversed by benzodiazepine antagonists. *Psychopharmacology* **85**: 295–300.

FILE, S. E., WILKS, L. J. and MABBUTT, P.S. (1989) The role of the benzodiazepine receptor in mediating longlasting anticonvulsant effects and the late-appearing reductions in motor activity and exploration. *Psychopharm.* **97**: 349–354.

FILE, S. E., DINGEMANSE, J., FRIEDMAN, H. L. and GREENBLATT, D. J. (1986) Chronic treatment with RO 15-1788 distinguishes between its benzodiazepine antagonist, agonist and inverse agonist properties. *Psychopharmacology* **89**: 113–117.

FLAHERTY, C. F., LOMBARDI, B. R., WRIGHTSON, J. and DEPTULA, D. (1980) Conditions under which chlordiazepoxide influences gustatory contrast. *Psychopharmacology* **67**: 269–277.

Fonseca, N. M., Sell, A. B. and Carlini, E. A. (1976) Differential behavioral responses of male and female adult rats treated with 5 psychotropic drugs in the neonatal stage. *Psychopharmacology* **46**: 263–268.

Fox, K. A., Tuckosh, J. R. and Wilcox, A. H. (1970) Increased aggression among male mice fed chlordiazepoxide. *Eur. J. Pharmacol.* **11**: 119–121.

Frieder, B., Epstein, S. and Grimm, V. E. (1984) The effects of exposure to diazepam during various stages of gestation or during lactation on the development of behaviour of rat pups. *Psychopharmacology* **83**: 51–55.

Gai, N. and Grimm, V. E. (1982) The effect of prenatal exposure to diazepam on aspects of postnatal development and behavior in rats. *Psychopharmacology* **78**: 225–229.

Gardner, C. R. and Guy, A. P. (1984) A social interaction model of anxiety sensitive to acutely administered benzodiazepines. *Drug Dev. Res.* **4**: 207–216.

Gardner, C. R. and Piper, D. C. (1982) Effects of agents which enhance GABA-mediated neurotransmission on licking conflict in rats and exploration in mice. *Eur. J. Pharmacol.* **83**: 25–33.

Gee, K. W. and Yamamura, H. I. (1983) Selective anxiolytics: Are the actions related to partial 'agonist' activity or a preferential affinity for benzodiazepine receptor subtypes? In: *Benzodiazepine Recognition Site Ligands: Biochemistry and Pharmacology*, pp. 1–10, Biggio, G. and Costa, E. (eds) Raven Press, New York.

Geller, I. and Seifter, J. (1960) The effects of meprobamate, barbiturates, d-amphetamine and promazine on experimentally-induced conflict in the rat. *Psychopharmacology* **1**: 482–492.

Gerhardt, S. C., Gajamy, Z. L., Brown, W. N. and Boast, C. A. (1985) A non-sedating anxiolytic, CGS 9896, is differentiated from diazepam in behavioral tests of tolerance in mice. *Abst. Soc. Neurosci.* **11**: 425.

Gilbert, F., Dourish, C. T. and Stahl, S. M. (1987). Correlation between increases of food intake and plasma ACTH levels after administration of 5-HT_{1A} agonists in rats. *Neuroendocrin. Letters* **9**: 176.

Gonsalves, S. F. and Gallager, D. W. (1985) Spontaneous and Ro15-1788-induced reversal of subsensitivity to GABA following chronic benzodiazepines. *Eur. J. Pharmacol.* **110**: 163–170.

Goudie, A. J. and Demellweek, C. (1986) Conditioning factors in drug tolerance. In: *The Behavioural Basis of Drug Dependence*, pp. 225–285, Goldberg, S. R. and Stolerman, I. P. (eds) Academic Press, New York.

Greenblatt, D. J. and Shader, R. I. (1974) *Benzodiazepines in Clinical Practice*, Raven Press, New York.

Greenblatt, D. J. and Shader, R. I. (1978) Dependence, tolerance and addiction to benzodiazepines: Clinical and pharmacokinetic considerations. *Drug Metab.* **8**: 13–28.

Griffiths, R. R. (1984) Abuse liability of anxiolytic and sedative drugs. *Clin. Neuropharmacol.* **7**: S134.

Griffiths, R. R. Bigelow, G. E. and Liebson, I. (1976) Human sedative self-administration: Effects of interingestion interval and dose. *J. Pharmacol. Exp. Ther.* **197**: 488–494.

Griffiths, R. R., Bigelow, G. and Liebson, I. (1979) Human drug self-administration: Double-blind comparison of pentobarbital, diazepam, chlorpromazine and placebo. *J. Pharmacol. Exp. Ther.* **210**: 301–310.

Griffiths, R. R., McLeod, D. R., Bigelow, G. E., Liebson, I. A., Roache, J. D. and Nowowieski, P. (1984) Comparison of diazepam and oxazepam: Preference, liking and extent of abuse. *J. Pharmacol. Exp. Ther.* **229**: 501–508.

Grimm, V. E. and Hershkowitz, M. (1981) The effects of chronic diazepam treatment on discrimination performance and ^{3}H-flunitrazepam binding in brains of shocked and non-shocked rats. *Psychopharmacology* **74**: 132–136.

Guy, A. P. and Gardner, C. R. (1985) Pharmacological characterisation of a modified social interaction model of anxiety in the rat. *Neuropsychobiology* **13**: 194–200.

Haefely, W., Pieri, L., Polc, P. and Schaffner, R. (1981) General pharmacology and neuropharmacology of benzodiazepine derivatives. *Handb. Exp. Pharmacol.* **55**: 9–262.

Hallstrom, C. and Lader, M. (1981) Benzodiazepine withdrawal phenomena. *Int. Pharmacopsych.* **16**: 235–244.

Heise, G. A. and Boff, E. (1961) Taming action of chlordiazepoxide. *Fed. Proc.* **20**: 393.

Hendry, J. S., Balster, R. L. and Rosecrans, J. A. (1983) Discriminative stimulus properties of buspirone compared to central nervous system depressants in rats. *Pharmacol. Biochem. Behav.* **19**: 97–101.

Herberg, L. J. and Williams, S. F. (1983) Anticonflict and depressant effects of GABA agonists and antagonists, benzodiazepines and nonGABAergic anticonvulsants on self-stimulation and locomotor activity. *Pharmacol. Biochem. Behav.* **19**: 625–633.

Heuschele, W. P. (1961) Chlordiazepoxide for calming zoo animals. *J. Am. Vet. Med. Assoc.* **139**: 996.

Hitchcott, P. K., File, S. E., Little, H. J. and Nutt, D. A. (1989) Diazepam withdrawal: Decreased seizure threshold and increased anxiety reversed by FG 7142 and flumazenil. *Soc. Neurosci Abstr.* **15**: 414.

Hodges, H. and Green, S. (1986) Effects of chlordiazepoxide on cued radial maze performance in rats. *Psychopharmacology* **88**: 1–7.

Hodges, H., Baum, S., Taylor, P. and Green, S. (1986) Behavioural and pharmacological dissociation of chlordiazepoxide effects on discrimination and punished drinking. *Psychopharmacology* **89**: 155–161.

Hoffmeister, F. and Wuttke, W. (1969) On the action of psychotropic drugs on the attack and aggressive-defensive behaviour in mice and cats. In: *Aggressive Behaviour*, pp. 273–280. Garattini, S. and Sigg, E. B. (eds) Excerpta Medica Foundation, Amsterdam.

Hollister, L. E. (1983) *Clinical Pharmacology of Psychotherapeutic Drugs*, 2nd edn. Churchill Livingstone, New York.

Hughes, L. M., Wasserman, E. A. and Hinrichs, J. V. (1984) Chronic diazepam administration and appetitive discrimination learning: Acquisition versus steady-state performance in pigeons. *Psychopharmacology* **84**: 318–322.

Huppert, F. A. and Iversen, S. D. (1975) Response suppression in rats: A comparison of response-contingent and noncontingent punishment and the effect of the minor tranquilizer, chlordiazepoxide. *Psychopharmacology* **44**: 67–75.

Irwin, W., Kinohi, R., Van Sloten, M. and Workman, M. P. (1971) Drug effects on distress-evoked behaviour in mice: Methodology and drug class comparisons. *Psychopharmacologia* **20**: 172–185.

Itoh, H. and Takori, S. (1968) Effects of psychotropic agents on the exploratory behaviour of rats in a Y-shaped box. *Jpn. J. Pharmacol.* **18**: 344–352.

Iwahara, S. and Sakama, E. (1972) Effects of chlordiazepoxide upon habituation of open-field behavior in white rats. *Psychopharmacologia* **27**: 285–292.

JENSEN, R. A., MARTINEZ, J. L., VASQUEZ, B. J. and MCGAUGH, J. L. (1979) Benzodiazepines alter acquisition and retention of an inhibitory avoidance response in mice. *Psychopharmacology* **64**: 125–126.

KEANE, P. E. and SIMIAND, J., MOORE, M. (1984) The quinolines PK 8165 and PK 1084 possess benzodiazepine-like activity in vitro but not in vivo. *Neurosci. Lett.* **45**: 89–93.

KELLOGG, C., TERVO, D., ISON, J., PARISI, T. and MILLER, R. K. (1980) Prenatal exposure to diazepam alters behavioral development in rats. *Science* **207**: 205–206.

KEIM, K. L. and SIGG, E. B. (1977) Plasma corticosterone and brain catecholamines in stress: Effect of psychotropic drugs. *Pharmacol. Biochem. Behav.* **6**: 79–85.

KIIANMAA, K. and BOGUSLAWSKY, K. (1981) Behavioral effects following chronic treatment with chlormethiazole, pentobarbitol and diazepam in the rat. *Substance and Alcohol Actions/Misuse* **2**: 45–54.

KILLAM, E. K., MATSUZAKI, M. and KILLAM, K. F. (1973) Studies of anticonvulsant compounds in the papio papio model of epilepsy. In: *Chemical Modulations of Brain Functions*, pp. 161–171, SABELLI, H. C. (ed.) Raven Press, New York.

KLEIN, D. F. (1981) Anxiety reconceptualized. In: *Anxiety-New Research and Changing Concepts*, pp. 235–263, KLEIN, D. F. and RABKIN, J. G. (eds). Raven Press, New York.

KOSTOWSKI, W., PLAZNIK, A., PUCILOWSKI, O., TRZASKOWSKA, E. and LIPINSKA, T. Some behavioral effects of chloro-desmethyldiazepam and lorazepam. *Pol. J. Pharmacol. Pharm.* **33**: 597–602.

KRAMARCY, N. R., DELANOY, R. L. and DUNN, A. J. (1984) Footshock treatment activates catecholamine synthesis in slices of mouse brain regions. *Brain Res.* **290**: 311–319.

KRSIAK, M., SULCOVA, A., TOMASIKOVA, Z., DLOHOZKOVA, N., KOSAR, E. and MASEK, K. (1981) Drug effects on attack, defence, and escape in mice. *Pharmacol. Biochem. Behav.* **14**: 47–52.

KRSIAK, M., SULCOVA, A., DONAT, P., TOMASIKOVA, Z., DLOHOZKOVA, N., KOSAR, E. and MASEK, K. (1984) Can social and agonistic interactions be used to detect anxiolytic activity of drugs. In: *Ethopharmacological Aggression Research*, pp. 93–114, MICZEK, K. A., KRUK, M. R. and OLIVIER, B. (eds) Alan R. Liss, New York.

KUBENA, R. K. and BARRY, H. (1969) Generalization by rats of alcohol and atropine stimulus characteristics to other drugs. *Psychopharmacologia* **15**: 196–199.

KURIBARA, H. and TADOKORO, S. (1984) Conditioned lever-press avoidance in mice: Acquisition processes and effects of diazepam. *Psychopharmacology* **82**: 36–40.

LADER, M. H., CURRY, S. and BAKER, W. J. (1980) Physiological and psychological effects of chlorazepate in man. *Br. J. Clin. Pharmacol.* **9**: 83–90.

Lader, M. H. and FILE, S. E. (1987) The biological basis of benzodiazepine dependence. *Psychological Medicine* **17**: 539–547.

LADEWIG, D. (1984) Dependence liability of the benzodiazepines. *Drug Alcohol Depend.* **13**: 139–149.

LAHTI, R. A. and BARSUHN, C. (1974) The effect of minor tranquilizers on stress-induced increases in rat plasma corticosteroids. *Psychopharmacologia* **35**: 215–220.

LAHTI, R. A. and BARSUHN, C. (1975) The effects of various doses of minor tranquilizers on plasma corticosteroids in stressed rats. *Res. Commun. Chem. Path. Pharmacol.* **11**: 595–603.

LAMB, R. J. and GRIFFITHS, R. R. (1985) Effects of repeated Ro15-1788 administration in benzodiazepine-dependent baboons. *Eur. J. Pharmacol.* **110**: 257–261.

LAVEILLE, S., TASSIN, J.-P., THIERRY, A.-M., BLANC, G., HERVE, D., BARTHELEMY, C. and GLOWINSKI, J. (1979) Blockade by benzodiazepines of the selective high increase in dopamine turnover induced by stress in mesocortical dopaminergic neurons of the rat. *Brain Res.* **168**: 585–594.

LEFUR, G., GUILLOUX, F., MITRANI, N., MIZOULE J. and UZAN, A. (1979) Relationships between plasma corticosteroids and benzodiazepines in stress. *J. Pharmacol. Exp. Ther.* **211**: 305–308.

LEHMANN, A. (1964) Contribution a l'etude psychophysiologique et neuropharmacologique de l'epilepsie acoustique de la souris et du rat. *Agressologie* **5**: 311–351.

LIEBMAN, J. M. (1985) Anxiety, anxiolytics and brain stimulation reinforcement. *Neurosci. Biobehav. Rev.* **9**: 75–86.

LIPPA, A. S., BEER, B., SANO, M. C., VOGEL, R. A. and MEYERSON, L. R. (1981) Differential ontogeny of type I and type II benzodiazepine receptors. *Life Sci.* **28**: 2343–2347.

LIPPA, A. S., COUPET, J., GREENBLATT, E. N., KLEPNER, C. A. and BEER, B. (1979) A synthetic non-benzodiazepine ligand for benzodiazepine receptors: a probe for investigating neuronal substrates of anxiety. *Pharmacol. Biochem. Behav.* **11**: 99–106.

LISTER, R. G. (1985) The amnesic action of benzodiazepines in man. *Neurosci. Biobehav. Res.* **9**: 87–94.

LISTER, R. G. and FILE, S. E. (1986) A late-appearing benzodiazepine-induced hypoactivity that is not reversed by a receptor antagonist. *Psychopharmacology* **88**: 520–524.

LISTER, R. G. and NUTT, D. J. (1986) Mice and rats are sensitized to the proconvulsant action of a benzodiazepine receptor inverse agonist (FG 7142) following a single dose of lorazepam. *Brain Res.* **379**: 364–366.

LISTER, R. E., BEATTIE, I. A. and BERRY, P. A. (1971) Effects of drugs on the social behaviour of baboons. In: *Advances in Neuropsychopharmacology*, pp. 299–303, VINAR, O., VOTAVA, Z. and BRADLEY, P. B. (eds) North Holland, London.

LITTLE, H. J., NUTT, D. J. and TAYLOR, S. C. (1984) Acute and chronic effects of the benzodiazepine receptor ligand FG 7142: Proconvulsant properties and kindling. *Pharmacology* **83**: 951–958.

LUKAS, S. E. and GRIFFITHS, R. R. (1984) Precipitated diazepam withdrawal in baboons: effects of dose and duration of diazepam exposure. *Eur. J. Pharmacol.* **100**: 163–171.

LYUBINOV, B. I., SMOL'NIKOVA, N. M. and STREKALOVA, S. N. (1975) Effects of diazepam on development of the offspring. *Bull. Exp. Biol. Med.* **78**: 1156–1158.

MALICK, J. B. (1978) Selective antagonism of isolation-induced aggression in mice by diazepam following chronic administration. *Pharmacol. Biochem. Behav.* **8**: 497–499.

MARES, P. and SEIDL, J. (1982) Anti-metrazol effects of nitrazepam during ontogenesis in the rat. *Acta Biol. Med. Germ.* **41**: 251–253.

MARKS, J. (1978) *The Benzodiazepines. Use, Overuse, Misuse, Abuse.* MTP Press, Lancaster.

MARKS, J. (1983) The benzodiazepines—For good or evil. *Neuropsychobiology* **10**: 115–126.

MARRIOTT, A. S. and SMITH, E. F. (1972) An analysis of drug effects in mice exposed to a simple novel environment. *Psychopharmacologia* **24**: 397–406.
MARRIOTT, A. S. and SPENCER, P. S. J. (1965) Effects of centrally acting drugs on exploratory behaviour in rats. *Br. J. Pharmacol.* **25**: 432–441.
MCCLOSKEY, T. C., PAUL, B. K. and COMMISSARIS, R. L. (1987) Buspirone effects in an animal conflict procedure: Comparison with diazepam and phenobarbital. *Pharmac. Biochem. Behav.* **27**: 171–175.
MCELROY, J. F. and FELDMAN, R. S. (1982) Generalization between benzodiazepine and triazolopyridazine-elicited discriminative cues. *Pharmacol. Biochem. Behav.* **17**: 709–713.
MCELROY, J. F. and MEYER, J. S. (1983) Relationship between benzodiazepine receptors and the attenuation of stress-induced corticosterone elevations in rats. *Neurosci. Abs.* **9**: 413.
MCELROY, J. F., FLEMING, R. L. and FELDMAN, R. S. (1985) A comparison between chlordiazepoxide and CL 218,872—A synthetic nonbenzodiazepine ligand for benzodiazepine receptors on spontaneous locomotor activity in rats. *Psychopharmacology* **85**: 224–226.
MCMILLAN, D. E. and LEANDER, J. D. (1978) Chronic chlordiazepoxide and pentobarbital interactions on punished and unpunished behavior. *J. Pharmacol. Exp. Ther.* **207**: 515–520.
MCNICHOLAS, L. F. and MARTIN, W. R. (1982) The effect of a benzodiazepine antagonist, RO15-1788, in diazepam dependent rats. *Life Sci.* **31**: 731–737.
MCNICHOLAS, L. F., MARTIN, W. R. and CHERIAN, S. (1983) Physical dependence on diazepam and lorazepam in the dog. *J. Pharmacol. Exp. Ther.* **226**: 783–789.
MEINERS, B. A. and SALAMA, A. I. (1982) Enhancement of benzodiazepine GABA binding by the novel anxiolytic, tracazolate. *Eur. J. Pharmacol.* **78**: 315–322.
MELCHIOR, C. L., GARRETT, K. and TABAKOFF, B. (1983) Proconvulsant effects of the benzodiazepine agonist CL 218,872. *Soc. Neurosci. Abs.* **9**: 129.
MELCHIOR, C. L., GARRETT, K. and TABAKOFF, B. (1985) A benzodiazepine antagonist action of CL218,872. *Life Sci.* **34**: 2201–2206.
MELDRUM, B. S. and CROUCHER, M. J. (1982) Anticonvulsant action of clobazam and desmethylclobazam in reflex epilepsy in rodents and baboons. *Drug. Dev. Res.* (Suppl. 1) 33.
MELE, L., SAGRATELLA, S. and MASSOTTI, M. (1984) Chronic administration of diazepam to rats causes changes in EEG patterns and in coupling between GABA receptors and benzodiazepine binding sites in vitro. *Brain Res.* **323**: 93–102.
MICZEK, K. A. (1974) Intraspecies aggression in rats: Effects of d-amphetamine and chlordiazepoxide. *Psychopharmacologia* **39**: 275–301.
MICZEK, K. A. and O'DONNELL, J. M. (1980) Alcohol and chlordiazepoxide increases suppressed aggression in mice. *Psychopharmacology* **69**: 39–44.
MILLENSON, J. R. and LESLIE, J. (1974) The conditional emotional response (CER) as a baseline for the study of anti-anxiety drugs. *Neuropharmacology* **13**: 1–9.
NICHOLSON, A. N. and WRIGHT, C. M. (1974) Inhibitory and disinhibitory effects of nitrazepam, diazepam and flurazepam hydrochloride on delayed matching behaviour in monkeys (Macaca mulata). *Neuropharmacology* **13**: 919–926.
NOLAN, N. A. and PARKES, M. W. (1973) The effects of benzodiazepines on the behaviour of mice on a hole-board. *Psychopharmacologia* **29**: 277–288.
OAKLEY, N. R., JONES, B. J. and STRAUGHAN, D. W. (1984) The benzodiazepine receptor ligand CL 218,872 has both anxiolytic and sedative properties in rodents. *Neuropharmacology* **23**: 797–802.
OLIVIER, B., MOS, J. and VAN OORSCHOT, R. (1986) Maternal aggression in rats: Lack of interaction between chlordiazepoxide and fluprazine. *Psychopharmacology* **88**: 40–43.
OLSEN, R. W. (1982) Drug interactions at the GABA-receptor-ionophore complex. *Annu. Rev. Pharmacol. Toxicol.* **22**: 245–277.
ONGINI, E., BARZAGHI, C. and GUZZON, V. (1984) Comparative analysis of benzodiazepine-induced anterograde amnesia in mice. *Abstracts of 14th CINP Congress, Florence, Italy.*
ONGINI, E., MARZANATTI, M., BAMONTE, F., MONOPOLI, A. and GUZZON, V. (1985) A β-carboline antagonizes benzodiazepine actions but does not precipitate the abstinence syndrome in cats. *Psychopharmacology* **86**: 132–136.
OVERTON, D. A. (1966) State-dependent learning produced by depressant and atropine-like drugs. *Psychopharmacologia* **10**: 6–31.
PATEL, J. B. and MALICK, J. B. (1982) Pharmacological properties of tracazolate: A new non-benzodiazepine anxiolytic agent. *Eur. J. Pharmacol.* **78**: 323–333.
PATEL, J. B., CIOFALLO, V. B. and IORIO, L. C. (1979) Benzodiazepine blockade of passive avoidance task in mice: A state-dependent phenomenon. *Psychopharmacology* **61**: 25–28.
PATEL, J. B., MARTIN, C. and MALICK, J. B. (1983) Differential antagonism of the anticonflict effects of typical and atypical anxiolytics. *Eur. J. Pharmacol.* **86**: 295–298.
PAUL, S. M., SYAPIN, P. J., PAUGH, B. A., MONCADA, V. and SKOLNICK, P. (1979) Correlation between benzodiazepine receptor occupation and anticonvulsant effects of diazepam. *Nature* **281**: 688–689.
PELLOW, S. (1985) Can drug effects on anxiety and convulsions be separated? *Neurosci. Biobehav. Rev.* **9**: 55–74.
PELLOW, S. (1986) Anxiolytic and anxiogenic drug effects in a novel test of anxiety: Are exploratory models of anxiety in rodents valid? *Meth. Find. Exptl. Clin. Pharmacol.* **8**: 557–565.
PELLOW, S. and FILE, S. E. (1985) The effects of putative anxiogenic compounds (FG 7142, CGS 8216 and Ro 15-1788) on the rat corticosterone response. *Physiol. Behav.* **35**: 587–590.
PELLOW, S. and FILE, S. E. (1986a) Anxiolytic and anxiogenic drug effects in exploratory activity in an elevated plus-maze: A novel test of anxiety in the rat. *Pharmacol. Biochem. Behav.* **24**: 525–529.
PELLOW, S. and FILE, S. E. (1986b) Is tofisopam an atypical anxiolytic? *Neurosci. Biobehav. Rev.* **10**: 221–227.
PELLOW, S. and FILE, S. E. (1986c) The effects of tofisopam a 3,4-benzodiazepine, in animal models of anxiety, sedation and convulsions in rodents. *Drug. Dev. Res.* **7**: 61–73.
PELLOW, S. and FILE, S. E. (1987) Lack of cross-tolerance in mice between the stimulant and depressant actions of novel anxiolytics in the holeboard. *Behav. Brain Res.* **23**: 159–166.

PELLOW, S., CHOPIN, P., FILE, S. E. and BRILEY, M. (1985) Validation of open: closed arm entries in an elevated plus-maze as a measure of anxiety in the rat. *J. Neurosci. Meth.* **14**: 149–167.

PERUZZI, G., ABBRACHIO, M. P., CAGIANO, R., COEN, E., CUOMO, V., GALLI, C. L., LOMBARDELLI, G., MARINOVICH, M. and CATTABENI, F. (1983) Enduring behavioural and biochemical effects of perinatal treatment with caffeine and chlordiazepoxide. In: *Application of Behavioral Pharmacology and Toxicology*, Vol. 21, pp. 217–236. ZBINDEN, G., CUOMO, V., RACAGNI, G. and WEISS, B. (eds) Raven Press, New York.

PETOCZ, L. and KOSOCZKY, I. (1975) The main pharmacological characteristics of grandaxin (tofisopam,egyt-341). *Ther. Hung.* **23**: 134–138.

PETURSSON, H. and LADER, M. H. (1984) Dependence on tranquilizers. *Maudsley Monograph*, No. 28, Oxford University Press, Oxford.

PLATEL, A. and PORSOLT, R. D. (1982) Habituation of exploratory activity in mice: A screening test for memory enhancing drugs. *Psychopharmacology* **78**: 346–352.

POSHIVALOV, V. P. (1981) Pharmaco-ethological analysis of social behaviour of isolated mice. *Pharmacol. Biochem. Behav.* (Suppl. 1) **14**: 53–60.

RACINE, R., LIVINGSTONE, K. and JOAQUIN, A. (1975) Effects of procain HC1, diazepam and diphenylhydantoin on seizure development in cortical and subcortical structures in rats. *Electroencephalogr. Clin. Neurophysiol.* **38**: 355–365.

RAMANJANEYULU, R. and TICKU, M. K. (1984) Binding characteristics and interactions of depressant drugs with [35S] t-butylbicyclophosphorothionate, a ligand that binds to the picrotoxin site. *J. Neurochem.* **42**: 221–229.

RANDALL, L. O. (1960) Pharmacology of methaminodiazepoxide. *Dis. Nerv. Syst.*, Suppl. 21: 7–10.

RICKELS, K. and SCHWEIZER, E. E. (1986) Benzodiazepines for treatment of panic attacks: A new look. *Psychopharmaco. Bull.* **22**: 93–99.

RIEGEL, C. E. and BOURN, W. M. (1983) The effects of diazepam withdrawal on flurazepam, bicuculline and picrotoxin seizure threshold in diazepam-dependent rats. *Soc. Neurosci. Abst.* **9**: 155.

ROACHE, J. D. and GRIFFITHS, R. R. (1985) Comparison of triazolam and pentobarbital: Performance impairment, subjective effects abuse liability. *J. Pharmacol. Exper. Ther.* **234**: 120–133.

ROBICHAUD, R. C. and GOLDBERG, M. E. (1974) Pharmacological properties of two chlordiazepoxide metabolites following microsomal enzyme inhibition. *Arch. Int. Pharmacodyn. Ther.* **211**: 165–173.

ROBICHAUD, R. C., GYLYS, J. A., SLEDGE, K. L. and HILLYARD, I. W. (1970) The pharmacology of prazepam. A new benzodiazepine derivative. *Arch. Int. Pharmacodyn.* **185**: 231–237.

RODGERS, R. J. and WATERS, A. J. (1985) Benzodiazepines and their antagonists: A pharmacoethological analysis with particular reference to their actions on "aggression". *Neurosic. Biobehav. Rev.* **9**: 21–35.

ROSENBERG, H. C. (1980) Central excitatory actions of flurazepam. *Pharmacol. Biochem. Behav.* **13**: 415.

ROSENBERG, H. C. and CHIU, T. H. (1982) An antagonist-induced benzodiazepine abstinence syndrome. *Eur. J. Pharmacol.* **81**: 153–157.

RYAN, C. P. and BOISSE, N. R. (1984) Benzodiazepine tolerance, physical dependence and withdrawal: Electrophysiological study of spinal reflex function. *J. Pharmacol. Exp. Ther.* **231**: 464–471.

SAANO, V. (1982) Tofisopam selectively increases the affinity of benzodiazepam binding sites for 3H-flunitrazepam but not for 3H-B-carboxylic acid ethyl ester. *Pharmacol. Res. Commun.* **14**: 971–981.

SAANO, V. and URTTI, A. (1982) Tofisopam modulates the affinity of benzodiazepam receptors in the rat brain. *Pharmacol. Biochem. Behav.* **17**: 367–369.

SAHGAL, A. and IVERSEN, S. D. (1978) The effects of chlordiazepoxide on a delayed pair comparison task in pigeons. *Psychopharmacology* **59**: 57–64.

SAHGAL, A. and IVERSEN, S. D. (1980) Recognition memory, chlordiazepoxide and rhesus monkeys: Some problems and results. *Behav. Brain Res.* **1**: 227–243.

SANSONE, M. (1979) Effects of repeated administration of chlordiazepoxide on spontaneous locomotor activity in mice. *Psychopharmacology* **66**: 109–110.

SATOH, T. and IWAMOTO, T. (1966) Neurotropic drugs, electroshock and carbohydrate metabolism in the rat. *Biochem. Pharmacol.* **15**: 323–331.

SCHALLEK, W., KUEHN, A. and KOVACS, J. (1972) Effects of chlordiazepoxide hydrochloride on discrimination responses and sleep cycles in cats. *Neuropharmacology* **11**: 69–79.

SCHECKEL, L. L. and BOFF, E. (1966) Effects of drugs in aggressive behavior in monkeys. *Excerpta Medica Int.* **129**: 789–795.

SHANNON, H. E. and HERLING, S. (1983) Discriminative stimulus effects of diazepam in rats: evidence for a maximal effect. *J. Pharmacol. Exp. Ther.* **227**: 160–166.

SHEENAN, D. V. (1982) Current perspectives in the treatment of panic and phobic disorders. *J. Clin. Ther.* **12**: 179–193.

SHORE, C. O., VORHEES, C. V., BORNSCHEIN, R. L. and STEMMER, K. (1983) Behavioral consequences of prenatal diazepam exposure in rats. *Neurobehav. Toxicol. Teratol.* **5**: 565–570.

SINGER, G. (1985) Alcohol and drug abuse. *Fifty-first Beatie-Smith lecture.*

SKOLNICK, P., REED, G. F. and PAUL, S. M. (1985) Benzodiazepine-receptor mediated inhibition of isolation-induced aggression in mice. *Pharmacol. Biochem. Behav.* **23**: 17–20.

SOFIA, R. D. (1969) Effects of centrally-active drugs on four models of experimentally-induced aggression in rodents. *Life Sci.* **8**: 705–716.

SOUBRIE, P., DE ANGELIS, L., SIMON, P. and BOISSIER, J. R. (1976a) Effets des anxiolytques sur la prise de boisson en situation nouvelle et familiere. *Psychopharmacologia* **50**: 41–45.

SOUBRIE, P., SIMON, P. and BOISSIER, J. R. (1976b) An amnesic effect of benzodiazepines in rats? *Experientia* **32**: 359–360.

STEPHENS, D. N., KEHR, W. and DUKA, T. (1986) Anxiolytic and anxiogenic β-carbolines: Tools for the study of anxiety mechanisms. Gabergic transmission and anxiety, pp. 91–106, BIGGIO, G. and COSTA, E. (eds), Raven Press, New York.

STILLE, G., ACKERMAN, H., EICHENBERGER, E. and LAUENER, H. (1963) Vergleichende pharmakologische untersuchung eines neuen zentralen stimulans,1-p-tolyl-1-oxo-1-pyrrolidino-n-pentan-HC1. *Arzneim. Forsch.* **13**: 871–877.

SUPAVILAI, P. and KAROBATH, M. (1979) Stimulation of benzodiazepine receptor binding by SQ 20009 is chloride-dependent and picrotoxin-sensitive. *Eur. J. Pharmacol.* **60**: 111–113.

TAYLOR, K. M. and LAVERTY, R. (1969) The effects of chlordiazepoxide, diazepam and nitrazepam on catecholamine metabolism in regions of the rat brain. *Eur. J. Pharmacol.* **8**: 296–301.

TAYLOR, J. L. and TINKLENBERG, J. R. (1986) Cognative impairment and benzodiazepines in psychopharmacology. In: *The Third Generation of Progress: The Emergence of Molecular Biology and Biological Psychiatry*, MELTZER, H. Y. (ed.) Raven Press, New York (in press).

TEDESCHI, D. H., FOWLER, P. J., MILLER, R. B. and MACKO, E. (1969) Pharmacological analysis of footshock-induced fighting behaviour. In: *Aggressive Behavior*, pp. 245–252, GARATTINI, S. and SIGG, E. B. (eds) Excerpta Medica Foundation, Amsterdam.

THIEBOT, M.-H. (1985) Some evidence for amnesic-like effects of benzodiazepines in animals. *Neurosci. Biobehav. Rev.* **9**: 95–100.

THIEBOT, M.-H. and SOUBRIE, P. (1983) Biological pharmacology of the benzodiazepines. In: *The Benzodiazepines from Molecular Biology to Clinical Practice*, pp 67–92, E. COSTA (ed.) Raven Press, New York.

TRAVERSA, U., DE ANGELIS, L., DELLA LOGGIA, R., BERTOLISSI, M., NARDINI, G. and VERTUA, R. (1985) Effects of caffeine and chlordesmethyldiazepam on fighting behavior of mice with different reactivity baselines. *Pharmacol. Biochem. Behav.* **23**: 237–241.

TUCKER, J. C. (1985) Benzodiazepines and the developing rat: A critical review. *Neurosci. Biobehav. Rev.* **9**: 101–111.

U.K. COMMITTEE ON THE REVIEW OF MEDICINES (1980) Systematic review of the benzodiazepines. *Br. Med. J.* **1**: 910–912.

URBAN, J. H., VAN DER KAAR, L. D., LORENS, S. A. and BETHEA, C. L. (1986) Effect of the anxiolytic drug buspirone on prolactin and corticosterone secretion in stressed and unstressed rats. *Pharmac. Biochem. Behav.* **25**: 457–462.

VACHON, L., KITSIKIS, A. and ROBERGE, A. G. (1982) Effects of chlordiazepoxide on acquisition and performance of a go-no-go successive discrimination task, and on brain biogenic amines in cats. *Prog. Neuro-Psychopharmacol. Biol. Psychiat.* **6**: 463–466.

VOGEL, J. R., BEER, B. and CLODY, D. E. (1971) A simple and reliable conflict procedure for testing antianxiety agents. *Psychopharmacologia* **21**: 1–7.

WHITE HOUSE OFFICE OF DRUGS POLICY AND NATIONAL INSTITUTE ON DRUG ABUSE (1979) *F. D. A. Drug Bulletin 16.*

WILKS, L. J. and FILE, S. E. (1986) Withdrawal from three different anti-convulsant effects on aggression, exploration and seizure threshold. *Soc. Neurosci. Abs.* **12**: 906.

WILKS, L. J. and FILE, S. E. (1988) Behavioural activation detected after a single dose of lorazepam: evidence for a withdrawal response from a single dose of benzodiazepine. *Life Sci* (in press).

WISE, C. D., BERGER, B. D. and STEIN, L. (1972) Benzodiazepines: Anxiety-reducing activity by reduction of serotonin turnover in the brain. *Science* **177**: 180–183.

WOODS, J. H. (1982) Benzodiazepine dependence studies in animals. *Drug Dev. Res. Suppl.* **1**: 77–81.

YANAGITA, T. and TAKAHASHI, T. (1973) Dependence liability of several sedative-hypnotic agents evaluated in monkeys. *J. Pharmacol. Exp. Ther.* **185**: 307–316.

YOKOYAMA, N., RITTER, B. and NEUBERT, A. D. (1982) 2-arylpyrazolo 4,3-c quinolin-3-ones: Novel agonist, partial agonist and antagonist of benzodiazepines. *J. Med. Chem.* **25**: 337–339.

YOSHIMURA, H. and OGAWA, N. (1984) Pharmaco-ethological analysis of agnostic behavior between resident and intruder mice: effects of psychotropic drugs. *Folio Pharmacol. Jpn.* **84**: 221–228.

CHAPTER 7

DEPENDENCE AS A LIMITING FACTOR IN THE CLINICAL USE OF MINOR TRANQUILLIZERS

P. Tyrer
St. Charles Hospital, London, W10 6DZ, U.K.

1. INTRODUCTION

Thirty years ago there were few satisfactory drug treatments for anxiety and insomnia. The clinician had to rely on chloral and its derivatives, alcohol or barbiturates. All these were known to be toxic in overdosage and to produce an undue amount of sedation in doses needed to reduce anxiety. All these drugs also carried the serious risk of abuse and dependence and in the 1950's this was particularly well documented with the barbiturates (Isbell *et al.*, 1950). When Sternbach and his colleagues rediscovered the group of drugs with the benzodiazepine nucleus in 1961, they quickly noted that these drugs had anti-anxiety effects. Enthusiastic reports of their efficacy and safety of anti-anxiety drugs and hypnotics followed in quick succession (Harris, 1960; Randall *et al.*, 1961) and within a few years benzodiazepines had overtaken the barbiturates, and their immediate successors, the propanediols, in the prescription stakes. Indeed, by the early 1970's a new benzodiazepine was being introduced almost annually for no adequate clinical reason (Tyrer, 1974) and the level of prescription rose at such a rate that considerable alarm was expressed about its implications (Trethowan, 1975).

From the very beginning benzodiazepines were seen to be superior to barbiturates as anti-anxiety drugs and this was confirmed in clinical trials (Lader *et al.*, 1974). It was therefore reasonable to argue that one of the reasons for the escalation in prescriptions of benzodiazepines was that at long last we had an effective drug treatment for anxiety and, as anxiety was a ubiquitous problem, many people needed to be helped by these drugs.

An alternative explanation was that benzodiazepines were drugs of abuse and much of the increase in prescription could be explained by pharmacological dependence. This explanation deserves close examination.

2. EVIDENCE FOR DEPENDENCE ON MINOR TRANQUILLIZERS

2.1. Propanediols

For a few years before 1960 the propanediols were the most widely used anti-anxiety drugs in the USA and one of them, meprobamate, was the most frequently prescribed drug in that country. Although they are similar to the benzodiazepines in that they have sedative, hypnotic, muscle relaxant and anti-convulsant properties they are generally less effective, and this explains why benzodiazepines supplanted them so quickly. However, another reason was the demonstration that meprobamate was subject to abuse and associated with withdrawal symptoms when it was stopped suddenly (Hollister and Glazener, 1960; Swanson *et al.*, 1973). It was perhaps unfortunate that more attention was not paid to this evidence when the benzodiazepines were introduced because it was twenty years after the introduction of benzodiazepines that dependence was recognized to be a significant clinical problem.

2.2. Benzodiazepines

2.2.1. *High Dose Dependence*

It was recognized relatively early that benzodiazepines could be associated with withdrawal problems. Hollister *et al.* (1961) found that patients taking chlordiazepoxide in high dosage (above 100 mg daily) had major withdrawal symptoms when their drugs were stopped suddenly after periods of treatment ranging between one and seven months. Of eleven patients treated, two had epileptic seizures and all except one of the others developed new symptoms during the withdrawal phase. However, relatively little notice was taken of this report, perhaps because all the patients had schizophrenic psychoses rather than neurotic disorders, and also because in clinical practice it was found that patients did not tend to escalate dosage to this level. In fact, one of the satisfying consequences of the replacement of barbiturates with the benzodiazepines was a steady fall in the number of psychiatric admissions for abuse of minor tranquillizers (Allgulander, 1986). Although there continue to be isolated reports of high dose dependence (Gordon, 1967; Preskorn and Denner, 1977; De Bard, 1979) these suggested this problem was relatively small considering the vast scale of prescription of benzodiazepines. Marks (1978, 1980) examined the world literature and noted that most of the patients demonstrating dependence on high dosage of benzodiazepines were also taking other addictive drugs, particularly alcohol. Even though large doses of benzodiazepines were being taken it was difficult to be certain whether the withdrawal symptoms were due to the sudden cessation of benzodiazepines or reactions to stopping these other drugs. It was therefore understandable that Marks should conclude that the dependence risk with benzodiazepines was extremely small.

To some extent animal studies supported this conclusion. Self-administration experiments in rhesus monkeys showed that although some positive effects were demonstrated from receiving benzodiazepines in relatively high dosage so that the monkeys increased their drug consumption (Findley *et al.*, 1972; Yanagita and Takahashi, 1973) after several weeks of continuous treatment drug consumption actually fell (Yanagita, 1982). These results suggested that the pleasurable effects of benzodiazepines were much lower than those of barbiturates and the risk of dependence and drug abuse was correspondingly less. Although it is always unwise to generalize from animal experiments to clinical studies some support for this view has come from studies with opiates. These have demonstrated the close similarity between self-administration experiments in animals and subjective effects in man (Griffiths and Balster, 1979).

2.2.2. *Low Dose Dependence*

It has been mentioned already that one possible explanation for the rapid expansion in prescription of minor tranquillizers in the late 1960's onwards was an increased incidence of dependence. According to this hypothesis (Owen and Tyrer, 1983) a proportion of each group of new patients treated with benzodiazepines would develop dependence and go on taking the drugs in regular dosage. Even if this proportion was relatively small it would account for a significant number of prescriptions in an average year. If the number of new patients receiving benzodiazepines remained the same the total number of prescriptions would rise steadily because a 'ratchet effect' steadily increases the total number of prescriptions (Fig. 1). This argument has received some support from analysis of drug prescriptions and prescribing habits (Balter *et al.*, 1974; Williams, 1983; Mellinger *et al.*, 1985). These studies demonstrate that a significant proportion of all prescriptions is made up by a small group of chronic long term users that only now is beginning to be reduced.

In the past seven years it has become recognized that dependence can be a significant problem with benzodiazepines in therapeutic dosage. Indeed, from a position of complacency about their risks ten years ago the publicity given to reports of dependence have been such that the risks and dangers of addiction have been somewhat exaggerated. The earliest reports suggestive of dependence in therapeutic dosage all described epileptic seizures following abrupt withdrawal of benzodiazepines, mainly diazepam (Bant, 1975; Vyas and Carney, 1975; Rifkin *et al.*, 1976). An earlier controlled study had suggested that when diazepam was withdrawn after four months of regular use there was an increase in anxiety, tremor and other somatic symptoms of anxiety but this was interpreted more as symptom re-emergence than withdrawal symptoms (Covi *et al.*, 1973).

Two carefully monitored cases were reported in the literature soon afterwards (Pevnick *et al.*, 1978; Winokur *et al.*, 1980) which demonstrated that tremor, weight loss, tinnitus,

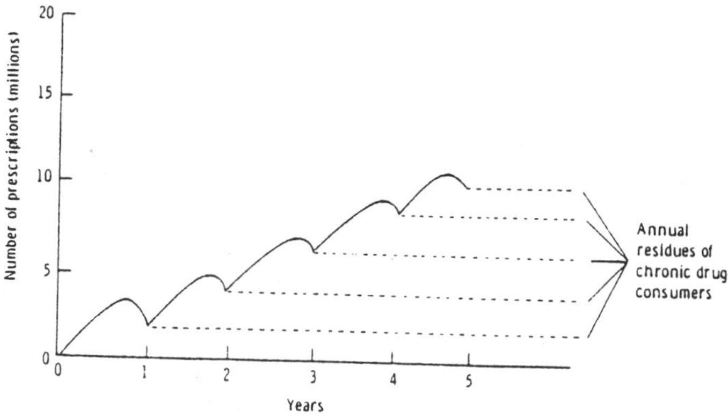

FIG. 1. Ratchet effect of drug dependence on prescribing practice. (Reproduced from *Drugs*, with permission.)

palpitations, hypersensitivity to noise and headaches were all associated with sudden withdrawal of diazepam in therapeutic dosage. However, these were still isolated reports and it is only since 1980 that there have been formal studies of groups of patients that have demonstrated unequivocally that withdrawal symptoms are a major problem after stopping benzodiazepines in therapeutic dosage and a cause of continued drug consumption (Tyrer, 1980a,b; Petursson and Lader, 1981; Tyrer *et al.*, 1983a; Ashton, 1984; Busto *et al.*, 1986). These studies have all demonstrated that pharmacological dependence is demonstrated primarily through the exhibition of a withdrawal syndrome rather than through increased tolerance, escalation of dosage, drug-seeking behavior and illegal use of the drugs. This probably explains why it has taken a relatively long time for the risks of dependence to be shown with benzodiazepines in normal dosage (Murphy and Tyrer, 1987).

Another reason for the delay in detection of withdrawal symptoms after stopping benzodiazepines is the degree of overlap between symptoms of withdrawal and symptoms found in anxiety. This is illustrated in Table 1; it is the combination of symptoms that suggests the presence of a withdrawal syndrome rather than individual complaints, none of which can be regarded as pathognomonic. Indeed, most of the symptoms reported after withdrawal from benzodiazepines can be detected in apparently normal people at times of stress (Rodrigo and Williams, 1986).

The only way of establishing the distinction between a true withdrawal syndrome and re-emergence of former anxiety symptoms after stopping treatment is to plot the time course of the symptoms. Withdrawal symptoms begin within two days of stopping a benzodiazepine of short elimination half life and within six days of stopping one with a long elimination half life. The symptoms last for a period ranging between three and 20 days and then resolve. If the symptoms merely represent a return to the anxiety that existed before treatment then onset is similar but the symptoms are less intense and rise gradually to the level which preceded the start of treatment. The most important difference is that there is no resolution of the symptoms after the withdrawal period is over.

Because definitions of withdrawal symptoms have differed and because the populations in clinical studies have suffered from various degrees of selection, it is difficult to give an exact figure of the incidence of withdrawal symptoms in patients taking benzodiazepines. Some investigators have found no examples of withdrawal syndromes (e.g. Bowden and Fisher, 1980) whereas others have demonstrated withdrawal problems in all patient studies (e.g. Petursson and Lader, 1981). In our own studies we have found, with a relatively unselected population referred to outpatient and general practice psychiatric clinics, that between 33% and 44% of all patients on long term benzodiazepines (regular therapy for longer than four months) have withdrawal symptoms after stopping treatment (Tyrer *et al.*, 1981, 1983a).

TABLE 1. *Hierarchy of Symptoms Between Anxiety and Withdrawal Reactions*

Symptom	Significance
Insomnia	Anxiety ↑
Fear	
Irritability	
Restlessness	
Dizziness	
Palpitations	
Tremor	
Muscle tension	
Mental tension	
Impaired concentration	
Sweating	
Depression	
Anorexia	
Weight loss	
Headaches	
Hyperacusis	
Hyperasthesiae	
Parasthesiae	
Depersonalization	
Derealization	
Ataxia	
Muscle twitching	
Tinnitus	
Formication	
Confusion	
Delirium	
Auditory hallucinations	
Other hallucinations	
Paranoid psychoses	
Myoclonic jerks	
Epileptic seizures	↓ Withdrawal phenomena

3. FACTORS PREDISPOSING TO BENZODIAZEPINE DEPENDENCE

Although benzodiazepines are the main drugs used for the relief of anxiety and for sedation to clinical practice there are other compounds that also need to be considered. Barbiturates now have no place in treatment because of their risks and should never be used for this purpose. However, there is a miscellaneous group of non-barbiturate sedative drugs that have a common property of facilitating GABA transmission and can be grouped together. This includes the propanediols, chlormethiazole and chloral derivatives. There are also some new anti-anxiety drugs that have been developed partly because of concern over the dependence potential of the benzodiazepines. These include buspirone and suriclone and the information about their risk of dependence to date is limited. Nevertheless, they need to be considered, not least because they are likely to be promoted because of lower dependence risks. The main factors affecting risk of dependence with each of these drugs are listed in Table 2.

Most of the larger studies of benzodiazepine dependence in therapeutic dosage have been carried out in patients who have taken the drugs for many months or years (Petursson and Lader, 1981; Tyrer *et al.*, 1981, 1983a; Busto *et al.*, 1986). Clinicians are therefore reminded to continue treatment with these drugs for as short a time as possible and preferably for only a few weeks (Committee on the Review of Medicines, 1980). The implication of this advice is that patients have no difficulty in stopping treatment after this has lasted for a few weeks only. However, in clinical practice it is common for patients to implore the doctor to go on prescribing a sedative drug after this period because of its apparent benefit. There is now reasonable evidence that withdrawal symptoms can take place after as little as four or six weeks treatment with benzodiazepines in regular dosage if they are suddenly withdrawn (Fontaine *et al.*, 1984; Murphy *et al.*, 1984). Although it could be

TABLE 2. *Factors Influencing Risk of Dependence with Minor Tranquilizers*

	Benzodiazepines	Other non-barbiturate sedative drugs (propanediols, chlormethiazole and chloral derivatives)	Newer non-benzodiazepine compounds (buspirone, suriclone)
Overall risk of dependence	Moderate	Moderate	Low (on evidence to date)
Duration of treatment	Increased risk after regular treatment for 4 weeks or longer	Not known, but probably similar to benzodiazepines	Not known. Little risk after 6 weeks treatment in regular dosage
Dosage	Greater risk of significant abuse in high dosage	As for benzodiazepines	No evidence that dosage is important
Personality characteristics	Greater risk in dependent personalities and in those who have abused drugs previously	Not known	Not known
Individual differences between drugs	Greater risk with potent benzodiazepines of short elimination half-life	Meprobamate of greater risk than tybamate. (chlormethiazole carries similar risks to benzodiazepines)	None known

argued that the apparent withdrawal symptoms represent the re-emergence of anxiety symptoms present before treatment this has not been borne out by continued assessment of these patients. The symptoms show the typical time course for a withdrawal reaction and it is significant that similar patients treated with the non-benzodiazepine drug, buspirone, do not show withdrawal symptoms after stopping regular treatment taken for the same period (Murphy *et al.*, 1984). If symptom re-emergence was the explanation for the return of symptoms it would apply equally no matter what drug was being prescribed. It is therefore reasonable to conclude that regular treatment for several weeks should be followed by gradual reduction if withdrawal symptoms are to be avoided.

In general, the higher the dose of a tranquillizing drug the greater the risk of dependence. This is a difficult subject to evaluate in controlled studies as maintenance dosage is determined by the level of symptoms and by the positive effects of a drug. It is well established that those who abuse drugs are more likely to take higher dosage and to take other drugs of abuse also (Allgulander, 1986). The classical picture of pharmacological dependence, with marked tolerance, escalation of dosage and drug-seeking behavior, is only found with high dosages of minor tranquillizers and has been described with all the established sedative drugs. Nevertheless, it would be wrong to assume that very low dosages of tranquillizers are safe from the risk of dependence. Although the amount of tolerance that develops with low dosages is generally low, there can be significant withdrawal symptoms from, for example, dosages of diazepam as low as 4 mg daily (Tyrer *et al.*, 1983a; Ashton, 1984). Often withdrawal symptoms develop only when patients have reduced to what many clinicians would regard as sub-therapeutic dosage, and the difficulty that patients have in withdrawing from this dosage cannot be explained entirely by psychological dependence.

It has also been found that there is an excess of abnormally dependent personalities in patients who are prone to dependence (Tyrer *et al.*, 1983a). It is always difficult to be certain whether dependence is secondary to the consumption of an addictive drug, but in our study personality assessment was made in all patients who had been taking diazepam long term *before* withdrawal and the personality assessment was made using an interview schedule that records premorbid personality before the onset of any psychiatric disorder (Tyrer and Alexander, 1979). The results demonstrated that the dependent personality characteristics of those who had withdrawal symptoms are significantly greater than those without such symptoms. By contrast, some personality features such as obsessional ones were more marked in those who did not have withdrawal symptoms. Studies of the patients most likely to be treated with benzodiazepines (neurotic disorder with anxiety, depressive and phobic features) have demonstrated that approximately 40% have some degree of personality disorder (Tyrer *et al.*, 1983b; Tyrer *et al.*, 1986). Taken together these figures suggest that between 15% and 20% of patients liable to be prescribed benzodiazepines have dependent personalities as opposed to only 2% in the normal population (Casey and Tyrer, 1986).

There is considerable variation in the apparent dependence potential of different minor tranquillizers although the subject is difficult to research and no common explanation for the differences has been put forward. In general, benzodiazepines with short elimination half lives are more likely to lead to pharmacological dependence, as measured by a higher incidence of withdrawal reactions, than those of long elimination half lives. However, an equally good case could be made out for benzodiazepines of high potency being significantly more likely to produce dependence than those of low potency. This is because the evidence available suggests that both potency and half life are significant factors in producing dependence potential (Table 3).

Unfortunately very few of the studies have compared withdrawal phenomena with different benzodiazepines and conclusions based on comparisons with other studies are prone to error. Both hypotheses to explain the difference in dependence potential between different benzodiazepines receive support from the data. The pharmacokinetic hypothesis that short-acting benzodiazepines are more likely to lead to dependence is also supported by evidence that patients who develop withdrawal symptoms after stopping diazepam have a more rapid fall in circulating blood levels than those who do not have withdrawal symptoms (Tyrer *et al.*, 1981) (Fig. 2).

It is, however, necessary to explain why a drug such as oxazepam has relatively little dependence potential compared with lorazepam, which has a very similar half life. The potency hypothesis receives support here although it is important not to equate potency with affinity to benzodiazepine receptors. Nevertheless, there is a rough correlation and it is reasonable to postulate that the key event in the withdrawal reaction is the affinity of a benzodiazepine for its receptor (Wesson and Smith, 1982).

The frequency of reports of dependence with an individual drug is an unsatisfactory way of measuring its dependence potential. For example, chlormethiazole, which also facilitates GABA transmission and has many similarities with the benzodiazepines, has frequently been reported as causing pharmacological dependence (e.g. Lundquist, 1966; Hession *et al.*, 1979) but as the drug was marketed early in its clinical history for the treatment of alco-

TABLE 3. *Differences in Dependence Potential of Benzodiazepines*

Benzodiazepine	Elimination half life (hr)	Daily dose (mg)	Potential for withdrawal reactions	References
Midazolam	2.5	10–30	high	Kales *et al.*, 1983
Triazolam	4	0.125–0.25	high	Kales *et al.*, 1976a; Morgan and Oswald, 1982
Temazepam	8	10–20	moderate	Ratna, 1981
Lormetazepam	10	1–2	moderate	Kales *et al.*, 1982
Lorazepam	15	2–5	high	Tyrer *et al.*, 1981; Schopf, 1983
Oxazepam	12	15–45	low	Pecknold *et al.*, 1982
Nitrazepam	28	5–15	low	Schopf, 1983
Flurazepam	90	15–30	low	Kales *et al.*, 1976b
Diazepam* after regular dosage	100	5–20	moderate	Lapierre, 1980; Tyrer *et al.*, 1981; Schopf, 1983; Fontaine *et al.*, 1984

*All of the benzodiazepines that are metabolised to nordiazepam (desmethyldiazepam) can also be included here. These include prazepam, clorazepate, ketazolam, medazepam, and chlordiazepoxide.

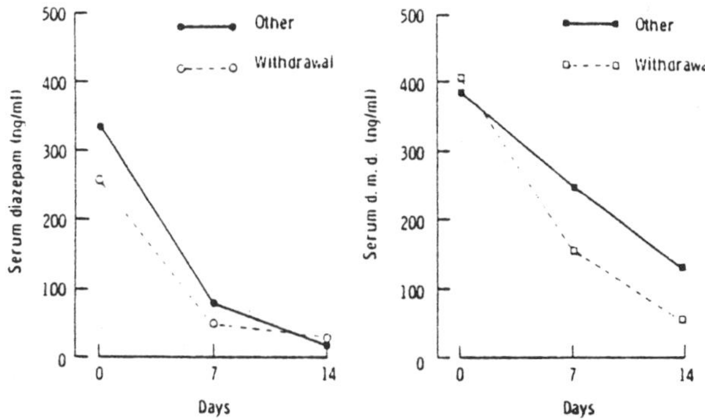

FIG. 2. Mean levels of diazepam and desmethyldiazepam (d.m.d.) in patients with withdrawal symptoms ($n = 7$) and others ($n = 13$) after stopping diazepam after long-term treatment. There is a significantly greater fall in desmethyldiazepam levels in those having withdrawal symptoms ($p < 0.01$). (Reproduced by permission of *The Lancet*.)

holism (Glatt *et al.*, 1965) it has been used widely in a population that is prone to addiction. The other major use of chlormethiazole, as a hypnotic in the elderly, has been associated with virtually no reports of dependence.

4. INFLUENCE OF DEPENDENCE ON PRESCRIBING PRACTICE

The demonstration that all minor tranquillizers known to be effective in relieving anxiety and insomnia also carry some risk of dependence is a sobering thought. The late recognition that benzodiazepines were similar to other compounds in this respect has caused particular concern. The clinical response to this has varied from a recommendation that benzodiazepines should be banned from further prescription (Snaith, 1984) through to the suggestion that as benzodiazepine hypnotics are safer than alcohol they should be freely available for purchase by the public at outlets such as off licences (Oswald, 1986). With this disparity of views it is not possible to reach a common synthesis. My personal view is that benzodiazepines and other minor tranquillizers still have a significant place in clinical practice but, because of dependence, this is reducing. Wherever possible, regular drug consumption should be avoided but as yet there is no alternative drug of equivalent efficacy and safety suitable for the short-term treatment of anxiety and insomnia (Tyrer, 1984). It is possible to chronicle the changes in prescribing habits that have occurred since dependence on minor tranquillizers was recognized as a universal phenomenon at the beginning of the 1980's and these give useful clues as to the impact of dependence on prescribing. In addition to the frequency of prescription and the type of drug prescribed, there have been changes in the duration of treatment and in the indications for their use.

4.1. FREQUENCY OF PRESCRIPTION

There has been a significant drop in the prescription of minor tranquillizers in the past few years. In the United States, the peak of prescription was reached in 1975 and has been associated with a steady fall since, accelerated since 1979. A similar trend has been found in the United Kingdom but the peak of prescription was delayed until 1977. The extent of the change has been quite dramatic for some groups of drugs. For example, 42 million prescriptions for hypnotic drugs were filed in drug stores in the United States in 1971 but this had fallen to 21 million by 1982 (Mellinger *et al.*, 1985). The prevalence of hypnotic drug use fell 3.5% of the population in 1970 to 2.4% in 1979 and all the evidence suggests it is now a great deal lower. In large measure this reduction can be attributed to greater care in prescription by clinicians but also greater awareness of the dangers of tranquillizers in potential patients (Clinthorne *et al.*, 1986). Although doctors like to think that they are the prime movers in any shift of prescribing policy, in the case of tranquillizers the social attitudes of the patients is probably much more important (Gabe and Williams, 1986). The change in prescribing habits includes fewer people taking minor tranquillizers and a smaller proportion of those that do take them becoming long-term users. Both these statistics are going to reduce the numbers of dependent patients in the future.

5. NATURE OF DRUG PRESCRIBED

5.1. Drug Group

In the 1960's there was a major change in the prescription of minor tranquillizers. Barbiturates were replaced gradually by benzodiazepines and overtaken by them in prescription volume in 1965. Subsequently, prescriptions for benzodiazepines continued to climb and barbiturates decreased virtually to zero. Although the improved efficacy of the benzodiazepines was one factor in this change, the lessened risk of dependence with benzodiazepines was at least equally important. The clinician now is in a dilemma. There is no class of drugs that is superior to the benzodiazepines for relieving anxiety and promoting sleep and almost all the well-established minor tranquillizers that are not benzodiazepines carry a risk of dependence that is equivalent to, if not considerably greater than, the benzodiazepines. We are therefore seeing a fall in the prescription of benzodiazepines that is not accompanied by a significant increase in the prescriptions of any other drug, unlike the replacement of the barbiturates by the benzodiazepines in the 1960's. This suggests that non-pharmacological ways of relieving anxiety and insommnia are being used more frequently. Certainly, by far the largest proportion of patients with significant sleep disturbance never take a hypnotic drug (Mellinger *et al.*, 1965). The picture of a society 'hooked on the happy pills' often promoted by the media is far off target.

The commercial rewards of a successor to the benzodiazepines that does not carry any risk of dependence are extremely great, so it is not surprising that the pharmaceutical industry is devoting considerable resources into developing new anti-anxiety agents. It is reasonable to adopt a considerable degree of pessimism about the likely success of these ventures in view of past experience with anti-anxiety drugs (Tyrer, 1985b) but it is reasonable to make the attempt. Newer drugs could include different classes of benzodiazepines. The development of benzodiazepine antagonists and inverse agonists has illustrated that some of the effects of benzodiazepines can be separated from each other, and it is possible that the potential to produce dependence can be separated from their anti-anxiety effects. However, it could be postulated that the dependence potential is so closely linked to the anti-anxiety effects of the compounds that it would be impossible to separate the two, and to date none of the new compounds has successfully produced this separation.

The fear of dependence could also lead to increased prescription of anti-psychotic drugs in low dosage as these carry no risk of dependence. However, the concern about tardive dyskinesia and other unwanted effects of these compounds is such that a significant shift in prescribing is unlikely and to date there is no evidence that it is taking place. Nevertheless, there is reasonably good evidence that anti-psychotic drugs such as flupenthixol are effective in reducing anxiety (Young *et al.*, 1976) and if further development of these drugs results in the introduction of compounds with a low risk of extrapyramidal side effects and subsequent dangers of developing tardive dyskinesia these may become attractive as anti-anxiety compounds. Currently there is a considerable amount of interest in the selective D2 receptor blocking drug, sulpiride, but its anti-anxiety effects in low dosage have not been evaluated. Even newer agents, such as GR38032F (Glaxo Laboratories), are alleged to be extremely effective in reducing anxiety without a significant risk of dependence and to have anti-schizophrenic effects as well.

There is also good evidence that some patients with anxiety respond well to beta-blocking drugs. These drugs carry no risk of dependence and it seems likely that most of their therapeutic effects are mediated through peripheral beta receptors (Bonn *et al.*, 1972). Patients who usually respond well have a high incidence of somatic complaints, particularly tremor, cardiac and respiratory symptoms (Tyrer and Lader, 1974; Kathol *et al.*, 1980). Patients who primarily complain of somatic symptoms are most likely to be seen by non-psychiatrists. Indeed, diagnostic labels such as hyperventialation syndrome, neurocirculatory asthenia, hyperdynamic circulatory adrenergic state, and irritable bowel syndrome could all be regarded as somatic presentations of anxiety states (Tyrer, 1976).

For this group of patients beta-blocking drugs may be extremely valuable and they may also have a role in combination with benzodiazepines in other anxiety states. There is evidence that combined treatment with a benzodiazepine and a beta-blocking drug is more effective than either alone and may allow reduction in the dosage of the benzodiazepine (Hallstrom *et al.*, 1981). Beta-blocking drugs may also be helpful in patients withdrawing from benzodiazepines (Tyrer *et al.*, 1981).

5.2. Choice of Benzodiazepine

It might be expected that the evidence suggesting that benzodiazepines of short elimination half life have greater dependence risks would lead to a reduction in their use. At the same time, however, the advantages of shorter duration of action have been promoted so heavily by the pharmaceutical industry that most new benzodiazepines have short half lives. Benzodiazepine hypnotic drugs with short half lives have a lower incidence of hangover (Bond and Lader, 1972) and so have some advantages over benzodiazepines of longer half life for induction of sleep. It is often desirable to have a short duration of action for a benzodiazepine given during the day (e.g. for the treatment of panic and phobias). In clinical practice there is therefore a demand for a short-acting drug that seems to outweigh the concern over dependence.

Diazepam, the most well known benzodiazepine, accounts for a significant proportion of the reduction in total prescriptions for benzodiazepines (Fig. 3). In regular treatment diazepam is a long acting benzodiazepine because of the accumulation of its active metabolite, desmethyldiazepam (nordiazepam), which has an elimination half life of some 90 hr. After regular dosage, blood levels of desmethyldiazepam exceed those of diazepam, and at steady state this drug is more important than the parent one in determining clinical effects (Kaplan *et al.*, 1973).

As diazepam was the most commonly prescribed benzodiazepine for many years it is not surprising that in the public consciousness the equation 'Benzodiazepines=Valium' rules. In my clinical practice I am constantly coming across patients who have persuaded their general practitioners to prescribe a different benzodiazepine to diazepam and believe that

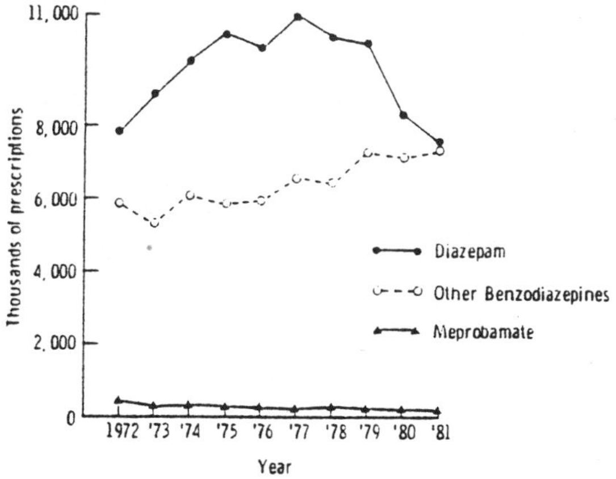

Fig. 3. Recent trends in the prescription of diazepam, other benzodiazepines and meprobamate in England and Wales. (Information about prescription provided by the Association of the British Pharmaceutical Industry).

as a consequence they are no longer addicted. It is therefore predictable that prescriptions for diazepam have shown a dramatic fall over the last few years, but more disturbing that those for other benzodiazepines have increased (Fig. 3).

The only other benzodiazepine to have encountered a similar level of opprobrium is triazolam, which for some years was banned in Holland because of concern expressed about its unwanted effects rather than its risks of dependence (van der Kroef, 1979). The debate for and against continued use of this drug was notable more for intemperate language than constructive comment and was criticized heavily by Lasagna (1980) for its 'trial by media'. It is quite possible that some of the alleged effects of triazolam in this debate were those of withdrawal. The very short elimination half life and potency of triazolam makes it the most dependence-prone of the benzodiazepines if either the 'potency' or 'pharmacokinetic' hypotheses of dependence described above are substantially correct. In an exhaustive survey of animal and human studies with triazolam Griffiths and his colleagues (1985) conclude that 'there is substantial speculation among clinical investigators and some limited data suggesting that the abuse liability of triazolam is greater than that of a variety of other benzodiazepines, and virtually no credible data or speculation that it is less'.

Prescription of other benzodiazepines still shows a trend in favor of compounds with a short elimination half life. This is reflected in the nature of the nine benzodiazepines on the NHS limited list. Four are short acting and relatively new (triazolam, temazepam, loprazolam, lormetazepam), two are intermediate elimination half lives (lorazepam, oxazepam) and three have a long elimination half life (in regular dosage) and may only retain their position because they were the first marketed benzodiazepines (diazepam, chlordiazepoxide and nitrazepam). Most of the compounds excluded from the limited list have long elimination half lives. It therefore seems likely that the proportion of short acting benzodiazepines prescribed will continue to increase.

6. DURATION OF TREATMENT

The recognition of dependence has had a major effect on the recommended duration of treatment with benzodiazepines. In the early 1970's it was recognized that up to one in five of patients prescribed a benzodiazepine took it regularly for greater than a year (Parish, 1971; Balter *et al.*, 1974). This fact did not arouse undue concern because of additional evidence that most doctors were prescribing these drugs responsibly (Mellinger *et al.*, 1978) and the diagnostic notion of 'chronic anxiety' was popular. It was therefore not surprising that some patients might require long-term treatment because they had a long-term affective disorder. However, clinical evidence that many of these patients were taking these drugs unnecessarily and for no good clinical reason (Tyrer, 1978) suggested that pharmacological dependence might indeed be one of the main reasons for continued prescription. When evidence of dependence in therapeutic dosage became established the recommended duration of treatment diminished rapidly. The Committee on the Review of Medicines (1980) recommended that 'prescriptions [of benzodiazepines] be limited to short-term use'. However, 'short-term use' was not defined further and could be interpreted as any period from several days to many months. Furthermore, the Committee also concluded that 'the true addiction potential of benzodiazepines was low' as at that time there had been few reports of withdrawal problems on therapeutic dosage. However, the more recent evidence that dependence may be a problem even after short courses of regular treatment lasting only a few weeks has led to an even shorter recommended duration of treatment. In the British National Formulary (1987) it is now recommended that a hypnotic 'may be useful but should not be given for more than three weeks and preferably only one' and that benzodiazepines prescribed as anti-anxiety drugs 'should be limited to the lowest possible dose for the shortest possible time'.

Unfortunately, it is still not known if there is a 'safe period' of regular treatment before dependence becomes a significant risk, but it seems likely that once steady state levels are reached there are likely to be withdrawal problems if the drug is stopped suddenly. Recommendations for short-term treatment of several weeks, such as those proposed by the Committee on the Review of Medicines, might be followed assiduously by the prescriber but if a proportion of patients become dependent after the end of this time, they will ask for further treatment. As they will present withdrawal symptoms, at the time, it is difficult to deny them further prescriptions despite the original plan to discontinue treatment after several weeks. Although there is still no satisfactory pharmacological explanation for benzodiazepine dependence, it seems likely that the pharmacological activity of an endogenous ligand is altered by persistent occupation of benzodiazepine receptors by a benzodiazepine drug and the consequent imbalance that becomes manifest when the drug is withdrawn leads to withdrawal symptoms. One way of avoiding this is to give benzodiazepines (and other minor tranquillizers) intermittently when required to avoid regular dosage. This makes sound clinical sense as the symptoms of anxiety and insomnia are extremely variable, and this policy of prescribing leads to a significantly reduced drug consumption (Winstead *et al.*, 1974). Now that patients are also more cautious about taking all minor tranquillizers it is possible to operate a policy of intermittent flexible dosage in which an agreed maximum dosage per day (or week) is agreed upon and dosage titrated against symptoms within the agreed dosage range. This is likely to become the pattern for the future and, if so, will lead to much more appropriate use of these drugs. This pattern of consumption also prevents the development of tolerance so the lower dosages are more effective.

7. SPECIFIC INDICATIONS FOR TREATMENT

7.1. Anxiety and Insomnia

Most minor tranquillizers are used for the treatment of anxiety and insomnia and this seems likely to continue. However, in addition to more careful prescription and greater use of psychological treatments for these disorders, there is much less 'open-ended' prescribing with consumption being determined by the patient and received relatively painlessly from the doctor through the medium of repeat prescriptions. We still have a cohort of dependent patients treated in the 1960's and 1970's who have tried and failed to stop taking their benzodiazepines but still continue on them reluctantly. This cohort will reduce steadily as there are many fewer new recruits. Epidemiological studies have shown that the old consume more benzodiazepines than the young and perhaps there is less concern about dependence in this group. In many instances psychological symptoms are associated with organic disease and so prescription of a minor tranquillizer can be justified more readily. It seems likely that the young–old differences in prescription will be maintained or even increased in succeeding years.

Another change in prescribing practice may follow from developments in diagnosis. The classification of anxiety disorders is in a state of flux and there is considerable argument over the extent to which they can be separated from those of other affective disorders such as depression. There is now abundant evidence that both tricyclic antidepressants and monoamine-oxidase inhibitors are effective in the treatment of anxiety. The improvement noted by patients is delayed and quite independent of the anticholinergic and sedative effects of antidepressant drugs (Klein, 1964). The delay in response is dependent on dose and is shorter when a higher dose is used (Tyrer *et al.*, 1980). There has been considerable argument over the status of panic as a separate diagnostic group. This is now fully accepted as a diagnosis in America, and one reason for this acceptance is the evidence that tricyclic antidepressants 'block panic attacks' (Klein, 1981).

In the American literature a consensus view is developing that panic and phobic disorder should be treated with antidepressants and the remaining group, termed Generalized Anxiety Disorder, is appropriate for treatment with benzodiazepines. However, it is equally possible to argue that these constitute one disorder (Tyrer, 1985a) and indeed there is evidence that in generalized anxiety there is a better response to antidepressants than to benzodiazepines (Johnstone *et al.*, 1980; Kahn *et al.*, 1986). There is therefore a strong argument for using antidepressants whenever the drug treatment of anxiety is expected to last for four weeks or longer. If treatment is predicted for less than this time there is little point in prescribing antidepressants because of their delay in response and high incidence of unwanted effects early in treatment.

The triazolobenzodiazepine, alprazolam, is not on the NHS limited list but is worth mentioning because it has been promoted strongly for the treatment of panic disorder. Although there is undoubted evidence that it is effective in the treatment of panic (Chouinard *et al.*, 1982; Alexander and Alexander, 1986) there is no evidence that it is superior to other benzodiazepines in this condition. As it is a potent benzodiazepine of relatively short half life it might be expected to be associated with significant withdrawal problems. This seems to be the case. Three cases of grand mal seizures have been reported after stopping alprazolam suddenly (Levy, 1984; Breier *et al.*, 1984), and of 17 patients withdrawn from alprazolam gradually after periods of treatment ranging between 12 and 47 weeks, 15 had further panic attacks and nine had significant new withdrawal symptoms (Fyer *et al.*, 1987). It therefore seems likely that the dependence risk with alprazolam will be a major factor in limiting its use.

7.2. Alcoholism

One important use of benzodiazepines is in the treatment of alcoholism. For many years chlordiazepoxide has been the most popular drug used for the treatment of alcohol withdrawal symptoms although diazepam is preferred in the United Kingdom. It is understandable that benzodiazepines have achieved such popularity as they are also anti-convulsant as well as sedative and therein lies superiority over other drug treatments (Kaim *et al.*, 1969). Because of the dependence risk with benzodiazepines it is understandable that concern should be expressed about using a drug of dependence to treat an addiction. However, there are few alternative treatments that are not themselves addictive. One currently under investigation is clonidine (Manhem *et al.*, 1985), but at present there is not sufficient information to recommend this as an alternative to the benzodiazepines.

Chlormethiazole has also been mentioned as a treatment for alcohol withdrawal symptoms. For some years the risk of dependence with this drug has led to clear recommendations that it only be used for a short period in the treatment of alcohol withdrawal with steadily reducing dosage over a five day period (British Medical Journal, 1981). This caution is now extending to the benzodiazepines and now diazepam is recommended in a dose of 40 mg daily reducing to 10 mg over a ten day period (Thorley, 1982).

7.3. Tardive Dyskinesia

At present there are no satisfactory treatments for the neuroleptic-induced dyskinesias, of which tardive dyskinesia is the most important. However, benzodiazepines have been suggested as possible treatments because of their facilitation of GABA receptors and they are at least as effective as the other treatments suggested for this condition (Mackay and Sheppard, 1979). If benzodiazepines proved to be of value in this and other movement disorders the dependence risk would be unlikely to limit prescription significantly.

7.4. Treatment for Medical Disorders

Benzodiazepines and propanediols are muscle relaxants and therefore have a place in the treatment of spasticity and other disorders in which there is increased muscle tone such as tetanus. Benzodiazepines are also anti-convulsants and have a place in the treatment of epilepsy, particularly when partial seizures and myoclonic jerks are common (Nanda *et al.*, 1977). Intravenous diazepam has for many years been the preferred treatment for status epilepticus because of its dramatic onset of action (Parsonage and Norris, 1967). It seems unlikely that any of these indications will be affected significantly by the knowledge that some patients might become dependent. It is also likely that fewer patients taking benzodiazepines for medical conditions will develop dependence because a smaller proportion have the dependent and other personality features associated with dependence risk (Tyrer *et al.*, 1983a). If a benzodiazepine, or rarely a propanediol, is superior to other drugs in the treatment of any of these conditions then it seems likely that this will take precedence and the drug prescribed even it if is given long term.

8. SUMMARY

The recognition that all minor tranquillizers carry the risk of dependence has had a significant impact in their prescription over the years. But it has only recently had the same impact on the prescribing of benzodiazepines because their dependence risks were not recognized until late. Approximately one third of all patients prescribed a benzodiazepine regularly for six weeks or longer will experience withdrawal symptoms if the drug is withdrawn suddenly after this time. Even if the drug is withdrawn gradually withdrawal symptoms may still lead to demands for further prescription. The major change in prescribing has been towards shorter and intermittent treatment so that tolerance is reduced and withdrawal symptoms avoided. This is appropriate for acute anxiety reactions but more difficult for longer term anxious and depressive neurotic disorders, which have a much longer natural history. Continuing evidence that other drugs not specifically marketed for the relief of anxiety, particularly the antidepressants, are effective in relieving this anxiety has led to increased prescription of antidepressants. Some patients may also be helped by treatment with beta-blocking drugs and new agents such as buspirone which have no significant dependence potential. There has also been a move away from drug treatment to psychological treatments for anxiety as a consequence of concern over dependence.

For some conditions, particularly medical ones such as spasticity and epilepsy, benzodiazepines may be considered for long-term treatment. They may also be regarded as necessary for more severe psychiatric disorders, usually as an adjunct to other therapy. In such instances the dependence risk is acknowledged but the benefits of treatment are considered to outweigh them. There may also be patients who are dependent on benzodiazepines but the alternative of withdrawing the drug may lead to dependence on a more dangerous drug such as alcohol. In such cases it is reasonable to regard continued prescription of the benzodiazepine as the least dangerous course of action.

It is important to maintain a perspective of dependence on minor tranquillizers, particularly as attitudes are in danger of being distorted by excessive media attention. To date there is no evidence that dependence on benzodiazepines leads to any dangerous long term sequelae although there is concern over their effects on higher cognitive function. Nevertheless, the dangers of barbiturates, alcohol and nicotine are so much greater that it would be unfortunate if public concern led to excessive restrictions on the use of benzodiazepines. Newer compounds that are as effective as the benzodiazepines and do not carry the same dependence risk are needed urgently but to date there are none that satisfy these requirements. It is salutary for clinicians to remind themselves that all drugs effective in the treatment of anxiety have proved to be major drugs of dependence and it seems unlikely that new compounds are going to escape the same fate.

REFERENCES

Alexander, P. E. and Alexander, D. D. (1986) Alprazolam treatment for panic disorders. *J. Clin. Psychiatry* **47**: 301–304.

Allgulander, C. (1986) History and current status of sedative–hypnotic drug use and abuse. *Acta Psychiat. Scand.* **73**: 465–478.

Ashton, H. (1984) Benzodiazepine withdrawal: An unfinished story. *Br. Med. J.* **288**: 1135–1140.

Balter, M. B., Levine, J. and Manheimer, D. I. (1974) Cross-national study of the extent of anti-anxiety/sedative drug use. *New Engl. J. Med.* **292**: 769–774.

Bant, W. (1975) Diazepam withdrawal symptoms. *Br. Med. J.* **4**: 285.

Bond, A. J. and Lader, M. H. (1972) Residual effects of hypnotics, *Psychopharmacologia* **25**: 117–132.

Bonn, J. A., Turner, P. and Hicks, D. C. (1972) Beta-andrenergic-receptor blockade with practolol in treatment of anxiety. *Lancet* **i**: 814–815.

Bowden, C. L. and Fisher, J. G. (1980) Safety and efficacy of long-term benzodiazepine therapy. *South. Med. J.* **73**: 1581–1584.

BREIER, A., CHARNEY, D. S. and NELSON, J. C. (1984) Seizures induced by abrupt discontinuation of alprazolam. *Am. J. Psychiatry* **141**: 1606–1607.

BRITISH MEDICAL JOURNAL (1981) Editorial–Management of alcohol withdrawal symptoms. *Br. Med. J.* **282**: 502.

BRITISH NATIONAL FORMULARY (1987) 13th edition. British Medical Association and the Pharmaceutical Society of Great Britain, London.

BUSTO, U., SELLERS, E. NARANJO, C. A., CAPPELL, H., SANCHEZ-CRAIG, M. and SYKORA K. (1986) Withdrawal reaction after long-term therapeutic use of benzodiazepines. *New Engl. J. Med.* **315**: 854–859.

CASEY, P. and TYRER, P. (1986) Personality, functioning and symptomatology. *J. Psychiat. Res.* **20**: 363–374.

CHOUINARD, G., ANNABLE, L., FONTAINE, R. *et al.* (1982) Alprazolam in the treatment of generalised anxiety and panic disorders: A double-blind placebo-controlled study. *Psychopharmacology* **77**: 229–233.

CLINTHORNE, J. K., CISIN, I. H., BALTER, M. H., MELLINGER, G. D. and UHLENHUTH, E. H. (1986) Changes in popular attitudes and beliefs about tranquillisers. *Arch. Gen. Psychiatry* **43**: 527–532.

COMMITTEE ON THE REVIEW OF MEDICINES (1980) Systematic review of the benzodiazepines. *Br. Med. J.* **280**: 910–912.

COVI, L., LIPMAN, R. S., PATTISON, J. A., DEROGATIS, L. R. and UHLENHUTH, E. H. (1973) Length of treatment with anxiolytic sedatives and response to their sudden withdrawal. *Acta Psychiatr. Scand.* **49**: 51–64.

DE BARD, M. L. (1979) Diazepam withdrawal syndrome: A case of psychosis, seizure and coma. *Am. J. Psychiatry* **136**: 105–106.

FINDLEY, J.D., ROBINSON, W. W. and PEREGRINO, L. (1972) Addiction to secobarbital and chlordiazepoxide in the rhesus monkey by means of a self-infusion preference procedure. *Psychopharmacologia* **26**: 93–114.

FONTAINE, R., CHOUINARD, G. and ANNABLE, L. (1984) Rebound anxiety in anxious patients after abrupt withdrawal of benzodiazepine treatment. *Am. J. Psychiatry* **141**: 848–852.

FYER, A. J., LIEBOWITZ, M. R., GORMAN, J. M. *et al.* (1987) Discontinuation of alprazolam treatment in panic patients. *Am. J. Psychiatry* **144**: 303–308.

GABE, J. and WILLIAMS, P. (eds) (1986) *Tranquillisers: Social, Psychological and Clinical Perspectives*, Tavistock, London.

GLATT, M. M., GEORGE, H. R. and FRISCH, E. P. (1965) Controlled trial of chlormethiazole in treatment of the alcoholic withdrawal phase. *Br. Med. J.* **2**: 401–404.

GORDON, E. B. (1967) Addiction to diazepam (Valium). *Br. Med. J.* **1**: 112.

GRIFFITHS, R. R. and BALSTER, R. L. (1979) Opioids: Similarity between evaluations of subjective effects and animal self-administration results. *Clin. Pharmacol. Therap.* **25**: 611–617.

GRIFFITHS, R. R., LAMB, R. J., ATOR, N. A., ROACHE, J. D. and BRADY, J. V. (1985) Relative abuse liability of triazolam: Experimental assessment in animals and humans. *Neurosci. Biobehav. Rev.* **9**: 133–151.

HALLSTROM, C., TREASADEN, I., EDWARDS, J. G. and LADER, M. (1981) Diazepam, propranolol and their combination in the management of chronic anxiety. *Br. J. Psychiatry* **139**: 417–421.

HARRIS, T. H. (1960) Methaminodiazepoxide. *J. Am. Med. Assoc.* **172**: 1162.

HESSION, M. A., VERMA, S. and MOHAN BHAKTA, K. G. (1979) Dependence on chlormethiazole and effects of its withdrawal. *Lancet* **i**: 953–954.

HOLLISTER, L. E. and GLAZENER, F. S. (1960) Withdrawal reactions from meprobamate, alone and combined with promazine: A controlled study. *Psychopharmacologia* **1**: 336–341.

HOLLISTER, L. E., MOTZENBECKER, F. P. and DEGAN, R.O. (1961) Withdrawal reaction from chlordiazepoxide (librium). *Psychopharmacologia* **2**: 63–68.

ISBELL, H., ALTSCHUL, S., KORNETSKY, C. H., EISENMAN, A. J., FLANARY, H.G. and FRASER, H. F. (1950) Chronic barbiturate intoxication. *Arch. Neurol. Psychiatry* **64**: 1–16.

JOHNSTONE, E. C., CUNNINGHAM OWENS, D. G., FRITH, C. D., MCPHERSON, K., DOWIE, C., RILEY, G. and GOLD, A. (1980) Neurotic illness and its response to anxiolytic and antidepressant treatment. *Psychol. Med.* **10**: 321–328.

KAHN, R. J., MCNAIR, D. M., LIPMAN, R. S., COVI, L., RICKELS, K., DOWNING, R., FISHER, S. and FRANKENTHALER, L. M. (1986) Imipramine and chlordiazepoxide in depressive and anxiety disorders: 2. Efficacy in anxious outpatients. *Arch. Gen. Psychiatry* **43**: 79–85.

KAIM, S. C., KLETT, C. J. and ROTHFELD, B. (1969) Treatment of the acute alcohol withdrawal state: A comparison of four drugs. *Am. J. Psychiatry* **125**: 1640–1646.

KALES, A., KALES, J. D., BIXLER, E. O., SCHARF, M. B. and RUSSEK, E. (1976a) Hypnotic efficacy of triazolam: Sleep laboratory evaluation of intermediate-term effectiveness. *J. Clin. Pharmacol.* **16**: 399–406.

KALES, A., BIXLER, E. O., SCHARF, M. and KALES, J. D. (1976b) Sleep laboratory studies of flurazepam: A model for evaluating hypnotic drugs. *Clin. Pharmacol. Ther.* **19**: 576–583.

KALES, A., BIXLER, E. O., SOLDATOS, C. R., MITSKY, D. J. and KALES, J. D. (1982) Dose-response studies of lormetazepam: Efficacy, side effects, and rebound insomnia. *J. Clin. Pharmacol.* **22**: 520–530.

KALES, A., SOLDATOS, C. R., BIXLER, E. O., GOFF, P. J. and VELA-BUENO, A. (1983) Midazolam: Dose-response studies of effectiveness and rebound insomnia. *Pharmacology* **26**: 138–149.

KAPLAN, S. A., JACK, M. L., ALEXANDER, K. and WEINFELD, R. W. (1973) Pharmacokinetic profile of diazepam in man following single intravenous and chronic oral administration. *J. Pharm. Sci.* **62**: 1789–1796.

KATHOL, R., NOYES, R. JR, SLYMEN, D. J. *et al.* (1980) Propranolol in chronic anxiety disorders: A controlled study. *Arch. Gen. Psychiatry* **37**: 1361–1367.

KLEIN, D. F. (1964) Delineation of two-drug-responsive anxiety syndromes. *Psychopharmacology* **5**: 397–408.

KLEIN, D. F. (1981) Anxiety reconceptualized. In: *Anxiety: New Research and Changing Concepts*, pp. 235–263, KLEIN, D.R. and RABKIN J. G. (eds) Raven Press, New York.

LADER, M. H., BOND, A. J. and JAMES, D. C. (1974) Clinical comparison of anxiolytic drug therapy. *Psychol. Med.* **4**: 381–387.

LAPIERRE, Y. D. (1980) Benzodiazepine withdrawal. *Can. J. Psychiatry* **26**: 93–95.

LASAGNA, L. (1980) The halcion story: Trial by media. *Lancet* **i**: 815–816.

LUNDQUIST, G. (1966) The clinical use of chlormethiazole. *Acta Psychiatr. Scand.* **42**(Suppl. 192): 113–114.

Mackay, A. V. P. and Sheppard, G. P. (1979) Pharmacotherapeutic trials in tardive dyskinesia. *Br. J. Psychiatry* **135**: 489–499.
Manhem, P., Nilsson, L. H., Moberg, A. L. *et al.* (1985) Alcohol withdrawal: Effects of clonidine treatment on sympathetic activity, the renin–aldosterone system, and clinical symptoms. *Alcoholism (N.Y.)* **9**: 238–243.
Marks, J. (1978) *The Benzodiazepines: Use. Overuse, Misuse, Abuse.* MTP Press, Lancaster.
Marks, J. (1980) The benzodiazepines: Use and abuse. *Arzneimittel-Forschung/Drug Research* **30**: 398–390.
Mellinger, G. D., Balter, M. B., Manheimer, D. I., Cisin, I. H. and Parry, H. J. (1978) Psychic distress, life crisis and the use of psychotherapeutic medications. *Arch. Gen. Psychiatry* **35**: 1045–1052.
Mellinger, G. D., Balter, M. B. and Uhlenhuth, E. H. (1985) Insomnia and its treatment: Prevalence and correlates. *Arch. Gen. Psychiatry* **42**: 225–232.
Morgan, K. and Oswald, I. (1982) Anxiety caused by a short-life hypnotic. *Br. Med. J.* **284**: 942.
Murphy, S. M. and Tyrer, P. (1987) The essence of benzodiazepine dependence. *Br. J. Addict.* (in press).
Murphy, S. M., Owen, R. T. and Tyrer, P. J. (1984) Withdrawal symptoms after six weeks treatment with diazepam. *Lancet* **ii**: 1389.
Nanda, R. N., Johnson, R. H., Keogh, H. J. *et al.* (1977) Treatment of epilepsy with clonazepam and its effects on other anticonvulsants. *J. Neurol. Neurosurg. Psychiatry* **40**: 538–543.
Oswald, I. (1986) Drugs for poor sleepers? *Br. Med. J.* **292**: 715.
Owen, R. T. and Tyrer, P. (1983) Benzodiazepine dependence: A review of the evidence. *Drugs* **25**: 385–398.
Parish, P. A. (1971) The prescribing of psychotropic drugs in general practice. *J. R. Coll. Gen. Pract.* **21** (Suppl. 14): 1–77.
Parsonage, M. J. and Norris, J. W. (1967) Use of diazepam in treatment of severe convulsive status epilepticus. *Br. Med. J.* **3**: 85–88.
Pecknold, J. C., McClure, D. J., Fleuri, D. and Chang, H. (1982) Benzodiazepine withdrawal effects. *Prog. Neuro-psychopharm. Biol. Psychiat.* **6**: 521–522.
Petursson, H. and Lader, M. H. (1981) Withdrawal from long-term benzodiazepine treatment. *Br. Med. J.* **283**: 643–645.
Pevnick, J. S., Jasinski, D. R. and Haertzen, C. A. (1978) Abrupt withdrawal from therapeutically administered diazepam. *Arch. Gen. Psychiatry* **35**: 995–998.
Preskorn, H. and Denner, J. (1977) Benzodiazepines and withdrawal psychosis: Report of three cases. *J. Am. Med. Assoc.* **237**: 36–38.
Randall, L. O., Heise, G. A., Schalleck, W., Bagdon, R. E., Banziger, R. F., Boris, A., Moe, R. A. and Abrams, W. B. (1961) Pharmacological and clinical studies on Valium, a new psychotherapeutic agent of the benzodiazepine class. *Curr. Ther. Res.* **3**: 465–469.
Ratna, L. (1981) Addiction to temazepam. *Br. Med. J.* **282**: 1837–1838.
Rifkin, A., Quitkin, F. and Klein, D. F. (1976) Withdrawal reaction to diazepam. *J. Am. Med. Assoc.* **236**: 2172–2173.
Rodrigo, E. K. and Williams, P. (1986) Frequency of self-reported 'anxiolytic withdrawal' symptoms in a group of female students experiencing anxiety. *Psychol. Med.* **16**: 467–472.
Schopf, J. (1983) Withdrawal phenomena after long-term administration of benzodiazepines: A review of recent investigations. *Pharmacopsychiatry* **16**: 1–8.
Snaith, R. P. (1984) Benzodiazepines on trial. *Br. Med. J.* **228**: 1379.
Swanson, D. W., Weddige, R. L., and Morse, R. M. (1973) Abuse of prescriptioned drugs. *Mayo Clinics Proc.* **48**: 359–367.
Thorley (1982) Alcohol. In: *Drugs in Psychiatric Practice*, p. 361, Tyrer, P. J. (ed.) Butterworths, London.
Trethowan, W. (1975) Pills for personal problems. *Br. Med. J.* **3**: 749–751.
Tyrer, P. (1974) The benzodiazepine bonanza. *Lancet* **ii**: 709–710.
Tyrer, P. (1976) *The Role of Bodily Feelings in Anxiety*. Oxford University Press, London.
Tyrer, P. (1978) Drug treatment of psychiatric patients in general practice. *Br. Med. J.* **2**: 1008–1010.
Tyrer, P. (1980a) Benzodiazepine dependence and propranolol. *Pharmaceutical J.* **225**: 158–160.
Tyrer, P. (1980b) Dependence on benzodiazepines. *Br. J. Psychiatry* **137**: 576–577.
Tyrer, P. (1984) Benzodiazepines on trial. *Br. Med. J.* **288**: 1101–1102.
Tyrer, P. (1985a) Neurosis divisible. *Lancet* **i**: 685–688.
Tyrer, P. (1985b) Prospects in treating anxiety. In: *Recent Advances in Psychopharmacology*, pp. 113–121, Iversen, S., (ed.) Oxford University Press, Oxford.
Tyrer, P. and Alexander, J. (1979) Classification of personality disorder. *Br. J. Psychiatry* **135**: 163–167.
Tyrer, P. J. and Lader, M. H. (1974) Response to propranolol and diazepam in somatic and psychic anxiety. *Br. Med. J.* **2**: 14–16.
Tyrer, P., Gardner, M., Lambourn, J. and Whitford, M. (1980) Clinical and pharmacokinetic factors affecting response to phenelzine. *Br. J. Psychiatry* **136**: 359–365.
Tyrer, P., Rutherford, D. and Huggett, T. (1981) Benzodiazepine withdrawal symptoms and propranolol. *Lancet* **i**: 520–522.
Tyrer, P., Owen, R. and Dawling, S. (1983a) Gradual withdrawal of diazepam after long-term therapy. *Lancet* **i**: 1402–1406.
Tyrer, P., Casey, P. and Gall, J. (1983b) Relationship between neurosis and personality disorder. *Br. J. Psychiatry* **142**: 404–408.
Tyrer, P., Casey, P. and Seivewright, N. (1986) Common personality features in neurotic disorder. *Br. J. Med. Psychol.* **59**: 289–294.
van der Kroef, C. (1979) Reactions to triazolam. *Lancet* **ii**: 526.
Vyas, I. and Carney, M. W. P. (1975) Diazepam withdrawal fits. *Br. Med. J.* **4**: 44.
Wesson, D. R. and Smith, D. E. (1982) Low dose benzodiazepine withdrawal syndrome—Receptor site mediated. *Calif. Soc. Treat. Alc. Drug. Depend. News* **9**: 1–5.
Williams, P. (1983) Patterns of psychotropic drug use. *Soc. Sci. Med.* **17**: 845–851.

Winokur, A., Rickles, K., Greenblatt, D. J., Snyder, P. J. and Schatz, N. J. (1980) Withdrawal reaction from long term low dosage administration of diazepam. *Arch. Gen. Psychiatry* **37**: 101–105.

Winstead, D. K., Anderson, A., Eilers, M. K. *et al.* (1974) Diazepam on demand. Drug-seeking behaviour in psychiatric inpatients. *Arch. Gen. Psychiatry* **30**: 349–351.

Yanagita, T. (1982) Dependence producing effects of anxiolytics. In: *Psychotropic Agents*, Part 2, pp. 395–406, Hoffmeister and Stille (eds) Springer Verlag, Berlin.

Yanagita, T. and Takahashi, S. (1973) Dependence liability of several sedative agents evaluated in monkeys. *J. Pharmacol. Exp. Ther.* **185**: 307–316.

Young, J. P. R., Hughes, W. C. and Lader, M. H. (1976) A controlled comparison of flupenthixol and amitriptyline in depressed outpatients. *Br. Med. J.* **1**: 1116–1118.

CHAPTER 8

PHARMACOLOGY OF ETHANOL

LARISSA A. POHORECKY AND JOHN BRICK
Rutgers—The State University, New Brunswick, New Jersey 08901, U.S.A.

1. INTRODUCTION

In this review we will focus on several aspects of ethanol pharmacology. We shall begin with a brief overview of ethanol pharmacokinetics. This is followed by a more detailed examination of the physiological changes in thermoregulation and cardiovascular functioning associated with ethanol administration. A survey then follows of the effects of acute and chronic ethanol use on brain neurochemistry and the endocrine system. Then, different types of tolerance are discussed, as well as pharmacological and non-pharmacological factors that contribute to ethanol tolerance. Finally, ethanol dependence and withdrawal in humans and animal models of alcoholism are examined.

1.1. ETHANOL

All alcohols have a similar structure, an hydroxyl group, OH, attached to a saturated carbon. There are many different types of alcohol but in this chapter, we will limit our discussion to ethyl alcohol or ethanol, the psychoactive agent in beverage alcohol. In this review, we will use the term ethanol to describe studies in which ethanol was administered, and alcohol to describe those studies in which ethanol was administered as beverage alcohol.

Ethanol is a relatively simple molecule, CH_3-CH_2-OH. Ethanol is formed during fermentation which occurs when certain yeasts combine with water and sugar. The yeast acts to recombine carbon, hydrogen, oxygen and water to form alcohol and carbon dioxide. The different types of alcoholic beverages are derived from the use of different fermenting ingredients. In the manufacture of wine, for example, fruits that are high in sugar such as grapes, apricots, berries, etc. provide the required oxygen in the fermentation process. When the concentration of ethanol reaches 15% (v/v)*, most yeasts die, terminating fermentation.

In the production of beer, starch may be substituted for sugar in the fermentation process so that cereal grains can be used instead of fruits. The starch must still be enzymatically converted to sugar, however, through a "malting" process. Malting involves sprouting cereal, such as barley, in water. The sprouts are then dried and mixed with water so that the enzymes formed during sprouting convert starch to sugar which allows fermentation to proceed. Most beers have an ethanol content of 4.5%–5.5% (v/v).

To obtain beverages with a higher ethanol content, a distillation process is used. The ethanol produced by fermentation is heated to its vaporization temperature and the vapor is condensed and collected. Distilled spirits (e.g., bourbon, gin, vodka, whiskey, etc.) are manufactured to very high ethanol levels usually 80–100 proof (40–50% v/v pure ethanol).

*The specific gravity of ethanol is 0.798 at 15°C. Therefore a 10% v/v solution is equivalent to a 7.98% w/v solution. In this review ethanol doses are expressed in millimolar (mM) or milligram/deciliter (mg/dl) concentrations; for comparison, 21.7 mM = 100 mg/dl.

1.2. ETHANOL PHARMACOKINETICS

1.2.1. *Routes of Administration*

In order for ethanol to exert either central nervous system or peripheral effects, it must get into the circulation. Ethanol may enter the circulatory system through a number of different routes which are discussed below.

1.2.1.1. *Pulmonary.* It has been known for over one hundred years that ethanol may enter the body through the pulmonary epithelium (Grehant and Quinquaud, 1883). Since alcohol is a volatile substance, it can be inhaled through the lungs, directly into the circulatory system. In humans, this is not a particularly efficient method of becoming intoxicated because only about 62% of the ethanol in inspired air is absorbed into the blood, regardless of the concentration of ethanol in the air (Lester and Greenberg, 1951). Since the rate of alcohol metabolism is similar to the rate of absorption through the lungs, it is difficult to produce any significant elevations in blood ethanol level using this method, although Lester *et al.* (1951) found that blood alcohol levels could reach 50 mg/dl. A second factor that limits the uptake of ethanol through the lungs is its concentration in air. High atmospheric ethanol concentrations, such as those above 20 mg/l, are so irritating (Lester *et al.*, 1951) that most people would find this route of administration aversive. If the discomfort of this route of administration can be tolerated (by accident or design), severe intoxication, even death, can result (Carpenter, 1929; Bowers *et al.*, 1942). In other species, inhaled ethanol can produce blood concentrations that can greatly exceed 100 mg/dl if animals are treated with pyrazole (Goldstein and Pal, 1971).

1.2.1.2. *Skin.* The simpler alcohol molecules (methyl to propyl) have very low oil-water partition coefficients, making it very difficult for them to diffuse through the keratin layer of the intact skin. Several early reports suggested that ethanol did pass through the skin of experimental animals, however, it is quite possible that in these studies the detection of ethanol in blood was due to inhalation through the pulmonary system rather than absorption through the skin. One of the most convincing studies of ethanol absorption through the skin (or lack thereof) was performed by Bowers *et al.*(1942). Human subjects had dressings soaked in 95% ethanol wrapped around their legs. The subjects' legs were then wrapped in a rubber sheet to minimize evaporation and maximize absorption. Blood ethanol measurements made every 3 h for 12 hr revealed no evidence of ethanol absorption through the skin (Bowers *et al.*, 1942). The use of ethanol-containing after shave lotions has been reported to produce a toxic reaction in patients treated with disulfiram (antabuse) but this reaction is more likely due to very low levels of ethanol that enter the circulation through the lungs.

1.2.1.3. *Injection, insertion.* In some cases, alcohol is taken parenterally, usually intravenously. This route of administration is not common and usually falls into the category of "recreational drug experimentation" rather than a regular route of administration. A more common technique is direct rectal administration or administration through the use of a douche containing alcohol. Alcoholics, suffering from gastrointestinal distress, usually caused by abusive drinking, have been known to take an alcohol enema.

1.2.1.4. *Oral.* The most common route of alcohol administration is through the mouth. Alcohol is swallowed, passing down the esophogus and into the stomach. Under laboratory conditions in which the pyloris has been ligated, 40–60% of a test dose of ethanol may be absorbed directly through the stomach (Karel and Fleisher, 1948; Haggard *et al.*, 1941; Kalant, 1971, for a review). Under natural drinking conditions, only a small percentage of alcohol, probably not more than 10% is absorbed directly from the stomach and the majority of ethanol passes from the stomach into the ileum or small intestine. Because the ethanol molecule is both lipid and water soluble, it easily passes through the walls of the small intestines into the dense network of capillary beds surrounding the intestines. From there, alcohol enters the hepatic portal vein to the liver whereafter it passes to the heart and is circulated to the brain and other parts of the body.

1.2.2. *Absorption*

1.2.2.1. *Rate of absorption.* The rate at which alcohol is absorbed from the gastrointestinal tract varies considerably. The range in time from the last drink to the peak level in blood is usually 30–90 min, with an average of 45–60 min. Several factors may alter the rate of absorption. For example, the time to reach a peak blood alcohol level may be shorter after a single drink or several drinks consumed over a short period of time (Dubowski, 1963). If alcoholic beverages are consumed over a period of many hours, the absorption of alcohol may also continue for several hours post drink (Dubowski, 1963). However, subjects that have been fasted overnight and then given alcohol reach a peak blood alcohol level in less than 30 min (Cocco *et al.*, 1986).

1.2.2.2. *Factors affecting absorption.* The amount and rate of alcohol that can be absorbed may also be affected by the concentration and type of alcoholic beverage. For example, in man the absorption of alcohol is most rapid when administered in a 15–30% solution and less rapidly when the concentration is below 10% or above 30%. Low concentrations of alcohol are probably absorbed more slowly due to the effect of volume on gastric emptying time (Hopkins, 1966) or, as Fick's Law would predict, the lower concentration gradient results in slower diffusion per unit area per unit time. Carbonated beverages, such as champagne, may also be absorbed faster than non-carbonated drinks (Edkins and Murray, 1924) although this finding is not undisputed (Haggard *et al.*, 1938). Higher concentrations may delay the absorption of alcohol due to the inhibition of gastric peristalsis and pylorospasm. The type of alcoholic beverage may also influence the rate of absorption. For example, beer is absorbed more slowly than whiskey or brandy (Mellanby, 1919; Haggard *et al.*, 1938). Interestingly, even if these beverages are diluted to the same ethanol concentration, differences in absorption rates between types of alcoholic beverage are still observed (Haggard *et al.*, 1938; Newman and Abramson, 1942; Dussault and Chappel, 1975), perhaps due to differences in carbohydrates or congeners. Genetic factors may also influence absorption (Kopun and Propping, 1977).

It is worth noting that in addition to variability in absorption, beverage type may produce differences in impairment at the same blood alcohol level. Newman and Abramson (1942) found more incoordination with dessert wines than with distilled liquors and Bjerver and Goldberg (1950) observed that driving ability was less impaired with beer than after equivalent amounts of distilled spirits.

The most significant factor influencing the absorption of alcohol from the gastrointestinal tract is the presence of food in the stomach (Mellanby, 1919; Miller *et al.*, 1966; Greenberg, 1968; Kalant, 1971; Santamaria, 1975). Alcohol is absorbed much more rapidly on an empty stomach than on a full one. The delay in absorption of ethanol from the gastrointestinal tract into the circulation is similar when food is consumed just before, during or just after alcohol. The presence of food in the stomach not only impairs absorption but will result in lower blood alcohol concentrations. Food type may also affect absorption. Haggard *et al.* (1938) found proteins and carbohydrates were more effective than fats in delaying ethanol absorption.

1.2.3. *Distribution*

Regardless of the route of administration, once ethanol enters the circulation, it is distributed throughout the water compartments of the body. Tissues with the greatest blood supply and capillarization receive alcohol more rapidly than tissues less vascularized. For example, it may take several hours for alcohol to be equilibrated in bone whereas brain, lung, kidney and liver tissues equilibrate very rapidly. Alcohol is infinitely soluble in water, so that at equilibrium, it is distributed equally throughout the body water.

1.2.4. *Elimination and Metabolism*

Alcohol elimination begins well before absorption is complete. Small amounts of unchanged alcohol are eliminated from the body through sweat, urine and expired air. The primary method through which alcohol is eliminated from the body is the metabolism of alcohol to carbon dioxide and water. In humans, the rate of alcohol elimination averages 15 mg/dl/hr although this rate can vary from 10–34 mg/dl/hr (Harger and Forney, 1963). Approximately 90% of all alcohol is eliminated from the body through enzymatic oxidation in the liver. Once absorption is complete, the elimination rate is quite linear along the descending limb of the blood alcohol curve, corresponding to a one compartment open model with zero order elimination. Under such circumstances, neither the dose or blood alcohol concentration affect the rate of elimination. There is evidence that in many subjects alcohol elimination follows a combination of zero order and first order kinetics. When the oxidizing enzyme is saturated, the elimination is constant; however, when there is an excess of enzyme, elimination proceeds at an exponential rate since a constant fraction of alcohol will be eliminated per unit time (Dubowski, 1985). In other words, under some circumstances the rate of elimination may be faster, the greater the initial consumption and subsequent BAC (Wagner *et al.*, 1976).

The interrelationship between the amount of ethanol consumed, body weight, elimination rate and the blood ethanol concentration was first formulated by Widmark (1932) and is authoritatively reviewed by Kalant (1971). Since then, Widmark's equation has been modified to take into account more recent advances in the estimation of total body water (Watson *et al.*, 1981).

Blood alcohol concentration is usually expressed in grams or milligrams of pure ethanol per 100 ml of whole blood although the results of clinical assays often express ethanol in milligrams of serum which yields a value approximately 17% higher than the equivalent amount of ethanol in whole blood. The prediction of blood ethanol concentration is made by dividing the amount of ethanol consumed by body weight and correcting for water dilution. Thus, the total grams of ethanol consumed are divided by the total body water weight in kilograms. Calculations for total body water weight vary, depending, in part, upon methodology but a value of 58% and 48% of total body weight, for men and women, respectively, yields accurate results (Watson *et al.*, 1981; Cocco *et al.*, 1986). The obtained quotient is then multiplied by the percentage of water in blood (80.65%). From this value must be subtracted the total amount of ethanol oxidized from the time of the first drink to a point in time after ethanol absorption is complete. Various slide rule devices (Center of Alcohol Studies, 1980) and computer software program (Cocco *et al.*, 1986) are available to facilitate this calculation.

1.2.4.1. *Alcohol dehydrogenase.* There are three metabolic pathways in the liver which can oxidize alcohol. Each of these pathways is shown below. Most alcohol is metabolized in the liver, by the cytoplasmic enzyme alcohol dehydrogenase. The cofactor nicotinamide adenine dinucleotide (NAD+) acts as a hydrogen acceptor in the oxidation of alcohol to acetaldehyde. In this process. NAD+ is reduced and converted to NADH. The affinity of alcohol for ethanol dehydrogenase is very high so that even at low alcohol levels the enzyme is saturated. In accord with the classic work of Widmark and many others, the disappearance of alcohol from the blood is almost completely linear until very low ethanol levels are reached. There is some evidence, however, that the rate of ethanol elimination is non-linear (Lundquist and Wolthers, 1958) and is concentration dependent (Von Wartburg, 1981). NADH oxidizing compounds such as pyruvate, D-glyceraldehyde, methylene blue, fructose and other compounds have been shown to increase the rate of ethanol metabolism and decrease acute alcohol intoxication (Lowenstein *et al.*, 1970; Thieden and Lundquist, 1967; Lieber and Pirola, 1982) but not consistently (Levy *et al.*, 1977). Sugar has been reported to antagonize some of ethanol's effects on behavior but not metabolism (Zacchio *et al.*, 1986). In this pathway, ethanol is metabolized to its primary metabolite acetaldehyde via ethanol dehydrogenase. Acetaldehyde is metabolized via mitochondrial aldehyde dehydrogenase to acetate which is then metabolized to water and carbon dioxide.

$$CH_3CH_2OH + NAD^+ \xrightarrow[ADH]{} CH_3CHO + NADH + H^+$$

1.2.4.2. *Microsomal ethanol oxidizing system (MEOS).* Up until about twenty years ago, it was believed that ethanol oxidation was catalyzed exclusively by alcohol dehydrogenase. However, Lieber and DeCarli (1986) have since characterized a second mechanism which they designated the microsomal ethanol-oxidizing system (MEOS). The MEOS requires oxygen and reduced nicotinamide adenine dinucleotide phosphate (NADPH) to oxidize long chain aliphatic alcohols. The repeated administration of ethanol increases the rate of ethanol metabolism (Hawkins *et al.*, 1966; Lieber and DeCarli, 1968; Tobon and Mezey, 1971). Chronic ethanol does increase MEOS and it has been suggested that MEOS can account for more than half of the observed increase in ethanol metabolism associated with chronic alcohol use (Lieber and DeCarli, 1972).

$$CH_3CH_2OH + NADPH + H^+ + O_2 \xrightarrow[MEOS]{} CH_3CHO + NADP^+ + 2H_2O$$

1.2.4.3. *Catalase.* The third pathway for ethanol metabolism is through catalase, an enzyme found primarily in liver peroxisomes. The primary role of catalase is to destroy toxic hydrogen peroxide which is naturally formed as a biproduct of several physiological reactions. The effect of catalase on ethanol metabolism is limited by the rate at which hydrogen peroxide is formed and not the amount of catalase present. In general, catalase probably contributes very little to ethanol metabolism in liver (Lieber and Pirola, 1982).

$$H_2O_2 + CH_3CH_2OH \xrightarrow[Catalase]{} 2H_2O + CH_3CHO$$

1.3. Factors Affecting Ethanol Pharmacokinetics

1.3.1. *Age*

Biological changes associated with aging can influence drug pharmacokinetics. Metabolism may be altered through reduced blood flow to the liver or reduced microsomal enzyme activity (Greenblatt *et al.*, 1982). Peak ethanol alcohol levels may also change as a function of alteration in body composition. This is particularly important in the elderly since there is a reduction of lean body mass and total body water with age. Greenblatt *et al.* (1982) found the body proportion of adipose increased with age. In men, body fat increased 18–36% and in women, increased 33–48% as a function of age. If total body weight remains constant, a shift in body mass from muscle to fat would decrease the total water compartments of the body decreasing the dilution of alcohol. These changes may account for the increased sensitivity to alcohol in elderly as compared to younger subjects (NIAAA, 1978, Jones and Jones, 1981; Gomberg, 1982; York, 1982; Vogel-Sprott and Barrett, 1984).

1.3.2. *Hormones*

Ethanol can produce a number of hormonal changes which may subsequently affect the activity of ethanol-metabolizing enzymes. As previously discussed, ethanol elimination depends upon the availability of alcohol dehydrogenase and the microsomal ethanol oxidizing system, but is also dependent upon coenzymes produced during ethanol oxidation. Since liver alcohol dehydrogenase can oxidize a number of physiological hormonal substrates (Li, 1977) ethanol can influence its own pharmacokinetics via its effect on hormones.

1.3.2.1. *Catecholamines.* Various stressors can activate endocrine systems, particularly the hypothalamine-hypophyseal-adrenocortical axis. Forbes and Duncan (1961) and others (Platonow and Coldwell, 1966; Videla *et al.*, 1975; Mezey and Potter, 1979) demonstrated that stress can alter ethanol metabolism. For example, repeated immobilization in rats increased the activity of liver ethanol dehydrogenase (Mezey *et al.*, 1979). After 2 weeks of immobilization (2.5 hr/day) Mezey *et al.* (1979) found an 83% increase in the activity of ADH enzyme and a doubling of alcohol elimination rate.

Stress-induced changes in catecholamines may be responsible, in part, for hormone induced changes in ethanol pharmacokinetics. Adrenalectomy prevents chronic ethanol-induced elevations in liver alcohol dehydrogenase activity (Sze, 1975) suggesting further that adrenal catecholamines may be responsible for stress or ethanol-induced changes in metabolism. Chronic administration of epinephrine increases the rate of ethanol elimination in male rats by increasing liver cell mitochondrial oxidation rate (Petermann *et al.*, 1979).

1.3.2.2. *Corticosteroids.* Although plasma corticoids are dramatically increased during stress, corticoid administration does not appear to alter liver ADH activity in rats (Mezey and Potter, 1979) or mice (Sze, 1975).

1.3.2.3. *Growth hormone.* Growth hormone causes a small increase in liver alcohol dehydrogenase activity (Mezey and Potter, 1979), as does stress.

1.3.2.4. *Androgens and estrogens.* In general, female rodents have higher levels of alcohol dehydrogenase activity and rates of ethanol elimination than their male counterparts (Erikkson and Malstrom, 1967; Collins *et al.*, 1975; Rachamin *et al.*, 1980). Testosterone administration has variable effects on alcohol dehydrogenase. Castration increases (Mezey and Potter, 1979; Cicero *et al.*, 1980) or decreases (Rachamin *et al.*, 1980) alcohol dehydrogenase activity depending upon the age of the animals. In castrated rats, increased alcohol dehydrogenase activity was associated with an increased rate of ethanol elimination (Mezey *et al.*, 1980).

In animals, estrogens do not appear to affect ethanol pharmacokinetics. Neither ovariectomy or the administration of estradiol alter alcohol dehydrogenase or the rate of ethanol elimination (Rachamin *et al.*, 1980; Mezey *et al.*, 1981).

In humans, the effect of endogenous gonadotrophic hormones on alcohol pharmacokinetics and behavior is controversial. In a number of studies, women were found to be more impaired than men on cognitive and behavioral tasks (Dubowski, 1976; Jones and Jones, 1976a,b). However, these effects may be due to differences in alcohol pharmacokinetics. In support of this, several studies have shown that given equal doses of alcohol, females achieved consistently higher blood alcohol levels than males (Jones and Jones, 1976a; Niaura *et al.*, in press).

Several studies reported nearly a decade ago suggested that menstrual cycle phase alters the absorption rate and peak alcohol level obtained for a given dose, as well as drinking pattern (Dubowski, 1976; Jones and Jones, 1976a,b). The same studies suggested that hormonal differences between men and women may be responsible for women reaching higher blood ethanol levels, and at a faster rate than men given the same dose (Dubowski, 1976; Jones and Jones, 1976a,b). These findings, though, may have resulted from the practice of dosing subjects by total body weight, rather than by body water weight. When doses were calculated based on total body water weight, no significant differences in blood alcohol levels between males and females are found (Marshall *et al.*, 1983; Sutker *et al.*, 1983; Goist and Sutker, 1985; Cocco *et al.*, 1986).

More recent studies have failed to confirm differences in alcohol pharmacokinetics as a function of menstrual phase (Hay *et al.*, 1984; Sutker *et al.*, 1986). These studies investigated the relationships among variations in blood ethanol level, blood alcohol discrimination and behavioral tolerance to alcohol in female social drinkers during each of the three phases of a full menstrual cycle. Contrary to some earlier reports (Jones and Jones, 1976a; Jones and Jones, 1984) no differences were found in indices of alcohol metabolism between women who were, and those who were not taking birth control pills (Hay *et al.*, 1984). Also, no differences in peak blood alcohol level were found as a function of menstrual cycle phase in humans (Hay *et al.*, 1984; Brick *et al.*, 1986) or monkeys (Mello *et al.*, 1984).

Of particular interest is the recent work of Sutker *et al.* (1986), who reported no difference in absorption or peak ethanol levels among females in the early follicular, ovulation or midluteal phases of the menstrual cycle. Women in the midluteal phase did, however, eliminate alcohol faster, as indicated by a reduction in the area under the total blood alcohol curve and alcohol disappearance rates, than the same subjects tested during early follicular and ovulatory phases. In a subsequent study these investigators found a significant interaction between dose and gender with regard to alcohol elimination. Men metabolized alcohol at a slower rate than women (11.3 mg/dl/hr vs. 14.4 mg/dl/hr) at high (approximately 110 mg/dl) but not moderate (approximately 76 mg/dl) blood alcohol levels. These complex interactions warrant further investigation with larger sample sizes and with a range of alcohol doses.

1.3.3. *Circadian Rhythms*

A number of studies have revealed variations in ethanol pharmacokinetics (Wilson *et al.*, 1956; Jones, 1974; Sturtevant *et al.*, 1976; Soliman and Walker, 1979) or nervous system sensitivity (Jones, 1974; Deimling and Schnell, 1980; Brick *et al.*, 1984) as a function of circadian rhythms. In rodents, greatest sensitivity to ethanol-induced hypothermia, toxicity, and ethanol clearance rate occur during the dark cycle, when these animals are normally quite active. Variations in behavioral and biological sensitivity may be regulated by light dark cycles but also type of test employed (Brick *et al.*, 1984) and feeding availability (Sturterant and Garber, 1980).

1.4. Alcohol Intoxication

Except as an antiseptic, there is no well-accepted medical use for ethanol. The primary use of this drug is related to its psychoactive properties. For the most part, alcohol is a central nervous system depressant, although it may have biphasic effects (Pohorecky, 1982). Low doses of alcohol often have stimulant-like properties, increasing sociability, gregariousness, etc. These effects are probably more due to the lessening of inhibitions than to an actual effect of alcohol.

The identification of alcohol intoxication is not a simple matter, even for skilled observers. Individual differences in response to alcohol may vary as a function of pharmacological tolerance, behavioral conditioned tolerance, genetic differences in sensitivity to alcohol and accepted cultural norms. With relative indifference to the above-mentioned factors, numerous correlational studies have been performed in which the relationship between blood alcohol concentration and resulting changes in behavior were examined (Jetter, 1938; Harger and Julpieu, 1956; Penner and Coldwell, 1958; Solarz, 1975; Penttila *et al.*, 1971; Zusman and Huber, 1979). In one of the more recent studies, Zusman and Huber (1979) found that skilled interviewers were unable to identify 74% of drivers with blood alcohol levels between 10–240 mg/dl. Accuracy of raters improved with higher blood alcohol levels. When blood alcohol levels were 50–90 mg/dl, raters correctly identified drinkers only 31% of the time, however, when blood alcohol levels were 150–240 mg/dl a staggering 30% of these subjects were not identified as intoxicated. Although there were relatively few subjects in this study, the results support, in part, the findings of an earlier study (e.g., Pentilla *et al.*, 1971). An examination of one of the most extensive studies performed (Penttila *et al.*, 1971) indicated that the raters, physicians with special training in the identification of alcohol intoxication, were successful in identifying intoxication in only 15–44% of the cases. Greatest accuracy was obtained when blood alcohol levels were in excess of 200 mg/dl. It is interesting to note that in most studies of this type, those persons making the diagnosis of alcohol intoxication were usually physicians or other professionals with prior specialized training in the identification of intoxication. In the non-alcoholic, typical effects of low alcohol levels (50 mg/dl) include talkativeness, relaxation, and tension reduction. Higher blood levels (above 100 mg/dl) significantly impair mental and cognitive ability, including judgement and there is depression of sensory-motor functioning. As blood ethanol levels exceed 200 mg/dl sensory and cognitive functioning is markedly impaired and intoxication is obvious. At 300 mg/dl most individuals would be stuporous. At higher concentrations (LD_{50} = 400 mg/dl), alcohol is lethal due to severe depression of respiratory function or other complications, such as aspiration of vomit.

The signs and symptoms of alcohol intoxication increase as a function of blood alcohol level and vary to some extent between individuals. Drinking history, and consequent degree of tolerance, also affect observable signs of intoxication. Maladaptive behavior such as fighting, impaired judgement, interference with social or occupational functioning as well as bio-behavioral signs such as slurred speech, uncoordination, unsteady gait, nystagmus or flushed face accompanied by euphoria are often taken as indicia of intoxication (APA, 1980). In addition, psychological changes in mood, irritability, loquacity, or impaired attention may also be indicative of alcohol intoxication (APA, 1980). The effects of acute ethanol intoxication have been extensively studied and excellent reviews are available (Mello and Mendelson, 1978; Barry, 1979).

Recently, Teplin and Lutz (1985) examined the frequency and reliability of various signs of intoxication and concluded that the most reliably detected indicia of alcohol intoxication included impairment of fine motor control (fumbling hand movements, etc), impaired gross motor control (stumbling or difficulty walking or balancing, slurred speech, change in speech volume, decreased alertness, excessive perspiration (not due to temperature or nervousness), slow or shallow respiration, sleepiness, changes in rate of speaking or bloodshot eyes. Unfortunately, the blood alcohol levels at which these indicia occur was not part of the study. These investigators found that the presence of 3–4 of the indicia noted above were necessary to make an identification of intoxication, when the blood levels were greater than 50 mg/dl; however, 4–5 of the above cited indicia were necessary to make an identification when the blood alcohol level was greater than 100 mg/dl.

In the post-intoxication phase, when blood alcohol levels have returned to zero, physical (fatigue, headache, thirst, nausea, malaise) and psychological (anxiety, depression, irritability, extreme sensitivity) changes associated with hangover are present (Badawy, 1986). Post-alcohol effects deserve continued exploration, particularly in light of a growing controversy over urine sampling of employees in the United States. Drug free urine may not be an indication of unimpairment. For example, in a recent study by Yesavage and Leirer (1986), 14 hr after consuming alcohol and well after blood alcohol levels returned to zero, pilots tested in a flight simulator showed impairment, compared with controls.

There are a number of ways in which the intoxicating effects of alcohol can be altered. Changes in the absorption, distribution or excretion of ethanol may increase or decrease the peak blood alcohol level and thus degree of intoxication (Goldberg, 1943). Rate of absorption alone, may also affect intoxication. Conners and Maisto (1979) found that the greater the rate of absorption, the greater the impairment and intoxication.

1.5. Conclusions

In summary, the two major pathways of ethanol metabolism within the liver are through alcohol dehydrogenase and the microsomal ethanol-oxidizing system. It is believed that at low ethanol concentrations, alcohol dehydrogenase oxidizes alcohol, but with higher concentrations or repeated ethanol administration, the MEOS system predominates. Hormones can influence the rate of ethanol elimination, although the effect of physiological levels of various hormones on ethanol metabolism is probably not very great. As a psychoactive drug, ethanol has biphasic effects; low doses have stimulant properties whereas higher doses depress cognitive, sensory and motor functioning in a dose-dependent fashion. In addition to dose and blood ethanol level, several additional factors, including rate of consumption, blood ethanol phase, and light–dark cycle may influence the degree of intoxication in non-alcoholic drinkers.

2. PHYSIOLOGICAL EFFECTS OF ETHANOL

2.1. Thermoregulation

2.1.1. *Human Subjects*

The effect of ethanol on thermoregulation in rodents has been extensively investigated. However the effect of ethanol on body temperature in man has generated less interest. The few studies at normal ambient temperature do not indicate a significant effect of ethanol in normal adults (Isbell *et al.*, 1955; Andersen *et al.*, 1963; Marbach and Schwertz, 1964; Martin and Cooper, 1978).

Many of the reports on the effects of ethanol in man have dealt with accidental hypothermia (Fernandez *et al.*, 1970; Henderson and Conn, 1974; Carter, 1976; Hirvonen, 1976; Paton, 1983). At low ambient temperature ethanol did not enhance hypothermia (Keatinger and Evans, 1960; Andersen *et al.*, 1963; Martin *et al.*, 1977; Fox *et al.*, 1979; Risbo *et al.*, 1981). In fact, subjects frequently felt warmer when they ingested ethanol (Keatinger and Evans, 1960; Martin *et al.*, 1977; Fox *et al.*, 1979). In support of this, ethanol has been shown to delay onset of shivering after a cold stress (Hobson and Collins, 1977; Martin *et al.*, 1977; Fox *et al.*, 1979; Risbo *et al.*, 1981). However, a significantly retarded fall in temperature (Gupta, 1960; Hobson and Collins, 1977; Graham and Baulk, 1980) has also been reported.

The feeling of warmth reported by human subjects after ingestion of ethanol most likely can be explained by changes in peripheral circulation. The increase in blood flow occurs primarily in the skin of the face and the extremities (Fewings *et al.*, 1966; Gillespie, 1967). Concurrently there is a decline in the blood supply to muscles. The net effect of these circulatory changes is a 72% increase in heat loss from the hands (Keating and Evans, 1960; Goldman *et al.*, 1973), as skin temperature rises (Risbo *et al.*, 1981). Peripheral vasodilation has been repeatedly demonstrated in man after ingestion of ethanol (Fewings *et al.*, 1966; Gillespie, 1967; Downey and Frewin, 1970; Allison *et al.*, 1971).

In conjunction with a physical stressor, such as exercise of variable severity, ethanol produced a relatively consistent hypothermia at low ambient temperatures (Haight and Keatinge, 1973; Graham and Dalton, 1980; Graham, 1981a, 1983; Simper *et al.*, 1983). Generally, the results seem to be influenced by the severity of exercise.

Except at low doses (Marbach and Schwartz, 1964), it is unlikely that changes in respiratory rate contribute to ethanol's hypothermia, since ethanol produces respiratory depression (Martin and Cooper, 1978). The hypothermia produced by ethanol is believed to be a consequence of either impaired thermoregulation (Garland *et al.*, 1960; Graham, 1981a; Risbo *et al.*, 1981), or hypoglycemia (Graham and Baulk, 1980; Huttenen *et al.*, 1980; Graham, 1981a; Oliveira Souza and Masur, 1982).

During withdrawal from ethanol, alcoholics showing severe symptoms also usually have hyperthermia (Isbell *et al.*, 1955; Gross *et al.*, 1975; Thompson *et al.*, 1975; Kramp *et al.*, 1979) which is accompanied by cutaneous vasodilation (Godfrey *et al.*, 1958) and sweating (Isbell *et al.*, 1955).

This evidence from human subjects indicates that ethanol impairs regulation of body temperature only under special circumstances. However, the evidence collected so far does not indicate the nature of the impairment (i.e., change in set point or impairment of thermoregulatory mechanism).

2.1.2. *Experimental Animals*

A large number of reports have documented the lowering of body temperature by ethanol in a variety of animal species. The effect of ethanol is dose-dependent and shows diurnal variation (Pohorecky and Jaffe, 1975; Kakihana and Moore, 1977; Demling and Schell, 1980; Brick and Horowitz, 1982). Peak hypothermia after ethanol treatment was noted when body temperature was at the lowest point of the circadian cycle (Brick *et al.*, 1984).

When ethanol treatment was combined with exposure to cold temperature, the resulting hypothermia was more severe (Lozinski *et al.*, 1969; Hirvonen and Huttunen, 1977; Meyers, 1981a; Malcolm and Alkana, 1981; Huttunen, 1982; Lomax and Lee, 1982). This decline in rectal temperature did not occur if animals were kept at a higher ambient temperature (30–38°C) (Tabakoff *et al.*, 1975; Vuorinen *et al.*, 1976; Ferko and Bobyock, 1978; Grieve and Littleton, 1979; George *et al.*, 1981; Myers, 1981a; Pohorecky and Rizeck, 1981). In fact, at 34–37°C, ethanol treatment can actually raise rectal temperature (Ritzmann and Tabakoff, 1976; Malcolm and Alkana, 1981; Myers, 1981a). These results indicate that ethanol produces poikilothermia rather than hypothermia (Myers, 1981a). That is, because of ethanol's effect on thermoregulation, the actual effect noted will depend on ambient temperature. At normal ambient temperature ethanol produces hypothermia, while there can be hyperthermia at high ambient temperatures. In fact at high ambient temperatures the toxicity of ethanol was reported to be increased (Thomas and Tremolieres, 1968; Freud, 1973; Dinh and Gailis, 1979; Grieve and Littleton, 1979b).

Ethanol could also alter body temperature by an effect on the set point regulating body temperature. An effect of ethanol on the thermoregulatory hypothalamic set point is indicated by one study. In this study ethanol (1.5 g/kg i.p.) decreased the latency to escape from radiant heat concurrently with a fall in rectal temperature (Lomax *et al.*, 1981).

With repeated exposures to ethanol there is significant development of tolerance to the hypothermic effect of ethanol (Ferko and Bobyock, 1978; Frankel *et al.*, 1978; Le *et al.*, 1979a; Rogers *et al.*, 1979; Rigter *et al.*, 1980; Mullin and Ferko, 1981; Brick and Horowitz, 1983; Pohorecky *et al.*, 1987). There is also a parallel shift in the dose-response curve to the right (Ritzmann and Tabakoff, 1976; Crabbe *et al.*, 1979; Rigter *et al.*, 1980a). The developed tolerance was proportional to the daily ethanol dose (i.e., the degree of hypothermia) and the duration of treatment (Ritzmann and Tabakoff, 1976a; Frankel *et al.*, 1978; Ferko and Bobyock, 1978; Crabbe *et al.*, 1981). This functional tolerance cannot be accounted for entirely by metabolic tolerance (Ferko and Bobyock, 1979). The rate of development of tolerance can be quite rapid. For instance tolerance can develop in mice that inhaled ethanol for 6 hr (Grieve and Littleton, 1979). Interestingly, as with other effects of ethanol, tolerance to the hypothermic effect of ethanol may involve a cognitive component, as reflected by effects of environmental cues in what is conceived as a Pavlovian conditioning paradigm (Le *et al.*, 1979b; Mansfield and Cunningham, 1980; Melchoir and Tabakoff, 1981; Crowell *et al.*, 1981).

In rodents there is little change in rectal temperature during withdrawal. Although mice show hypothermia during withdrawal (Ritzmann and Tabakoff, 1976a; Harris, 1979), no changes in temperature have been reported in rats (Brick and Pohorecky, 1977). Animals in the later study, however, showed preference for a warm ambient temperature when given a choice of environmental temperatures (2–30°C).

2.1.3. *Conclusions*

Ethanol generally lowers body temperature at normal ambient temperature. Because in man the thermoregulatory mechanism is more efficient, the hypothermia is generally negligible, except when the subject is concomitantly exposed to low ambient temperature. As succinctly discussed by Kalant and Le (1984) the currently available data suggests that ethanol impairs thermoregulatory mechanisms and also lowers the hypothalamic set point for body temperature control. It is likely that in rodents some of the observed biochemical and/or physiological effects of ethanol are secondary to the ethanol-induced hypothermia (Pohorecky and Rizek, 1981).

2.2. MYOCARDIAL EFFECTS

2.2.1. *Effect of Ethanol on Functional Activity of the Heart*

2.2.1.1. *Acute ethanol treatment.* To avoid the influence of central depressant effects of ethanol as well as other metabolic factors, the direct action of ethanol on the heart has been examined using isolated tissue preparations. The most commonly employed preparations for research on the myocardial effects of ethanol are the isolated heart-muscle preparation and the heart-lung preparation.

An effect of ethanol on the isolated heart preparation was originally reported in the early 1900s (Loeb, 1905; Dixon, 1907). Both studies indicated a biphasic effect of ethanol, with stimulation at concentrations below 300 mg/dl and depression at concentrations above 500 mg/dl. More recent research has shown a primarily depressant, dose-dependent effect of ethanol on contractility using atrial (Loomis, 1952; Gimeno *et al.*, 1962; Lake *et al.*, 1978; Kobayashi *et al.*, 1979) or ventricular preparations (Hirota *et al.*, 1976; Mason *et al.*, 1978). With the heart-lung preparations there was either no effect of ethanol (Webb *et al.*, 1967) or a small significant increase in left ventricular end diastolic pressure (LVEDP) at concentrations over 200 mg/dl ethanol (Mierzwiak *et al.*, 1972). At concentrations of ethanol below 300 mg/dl myocardial contractility and heart rate increased slightly; both parameters declined at higher concentrations (Nakano and Kessinger, 1972).

From early *in vivo* studies it became apparent that when the consequences of anoxia from respiratory depression are prevented by artificial respiration, the effects of ethanol on functional activity of the heart were negligible in up to nearly lethal concentrations (Haggard *et al.*, 1941; Loomis, 1952). At lethal concentrations of ethanol both the rate and force of contractility declined (Loomis, 1952). More recent *in vivo* studies show the myocardial depressant effects at much lower concentrations of ethanol. For example, LVEDP increased and stroke volume decreased during slow intravenous infusion of ethanol into pentobarbital anesthetized dogs (peak ethanol levels 200 mg/dl) without significant changes in heart rate or blood pressure. However, the effect of ethanol on LVEDP in chloralose anesthetized dogs was variable during the first half hour of a slow infusion (Wong, 1973). Thus the choice of anesthetic used in such studies is an important consideration. It is known that barbiturates depress compensatory cardiovascular reflexes and ventricular function while chloralose does not (Sawyer *et al.*, 1971; Pachinger *et al.*, 1973). It has also been reported that depression of cardiac output and the increase in LVEDP was greater, and occurred sooner, in chloralose anesthetized dogs with autonomic blockade (pretreatment with propranolol and atropine) (Wong, 1973). This suggested that the depressant effect of ethanol was partially masked through concomitant autonomic activation (Wong, 1973). However, in another study in which unanesthetized dogs were used the depressant effect of ethanol on ventricular function was not altered by β-noradrenergic blockade (Horowitz and Atkins, 1974).

The depressant effects of ethanol on the myocardium are accentuated if there is an additional stressor. For example very low levels of ethanol (16 mg/dl) combined with treadmill exercise in dogs, depressed heart rate and left ventricular peak systolic pressure, while it also increased coronary artery blood flow (Stratton *et al.*, 1981).

In non-alcoholic subjects an acute moderate dose of ethanol (approximately 5–6 oz of 90% proof whiskey – 120 mg/dl) increased cardiac output (Riff *et al.*, 1969; Juchems and Klobe, 1969; Blomqvist *et al.*, 1970). This increase in output was accounted for primarily by an increase in heart rate since stroke volume was not increased. At lower doses (2 oz of whiskey), the increase in cardiac output was accounted for by an increase in cardiac output while heart rate remained unchanged. Blood levels of 110 mg/dl had no effect on functional activity of the heart, however when combined with autonomic blockade (propranolol and atropine) ethanol decreased ventricular contractility (left ventricular preejection period/left ventricular ejection time ratio) (Child *et al.*, 1979). Similar to the study with dogs referred to earlier (Wong, 1973), the authors concluded that ethanol has a negative inotropic effect which is masked by ethanol-induced catecholamine release.

2.2.1.2. *Chronic ethanol treatment.* Most of the early studies involving long term treatment of dogs with ethanol, (by gavage or added to the drinking water for 3.2–22 months), reported minimal impairment of myocardial function (Pachinger *et al.*, 1973; Regan *et al.*, 1974). Even the longest duration of treatment with ethanol (3.2 g/kg/day for 22 months), representing 36% of total daily caloric intake, produced only a marginally significant increase in LVEDP and no change in heart rate, aortic pressure, and stroke volume (Regan *et al.*, 1974). However functional capacity of the myocardium was decreased (depressed left ventrical function during after load increments with angiotensin) in the chronic ethanol treated dogs compared to the control animals (Regan *et al.*, 1974). Similarly, after either 3.2 or 6 months of treatment, with 4.0 g/kg/day and 1.65 g/k/day respectively, there was no difference in cardiac output, stroke volume, heart rate, LVEDP, rate of rise of ventricular pressure or blood pressure compared with control animals (Goodkind *et al.*, 1975). In a more recent study on anesthetized dogs which had drunk up to a 40%* ethanol solution from 18 or 22 months, left ventricular contractility was decreased only in the 22 month group (Thomas *et al.*, 1980). However, end diastolic pressure was decreased about equally after both treatment durations.

In one study carried out in rats, animals ingested 25% ethanol in the drinking fluid for 7 months (Maines and Aldhinger, 1967). Isometric tension of ventricular muscle, measured at 5 week intervals, was increased in the control group but not in the ethanol-treated group. The difference between the 2 groups became significant after 4 months of treatment. However in another study with rats treated with ethanol for 17 weeks there was no change in isometric peak systolic pressure nor in myocardial contractility (Hastillo *et al.*, 1980).

In a recent study, rats were given an ethanol-containing liquid diet for up to 42 weeks (Posner *et al.*, 1985). When tested *in vitro*, atria from the ethanol-treated rats exhibited no change in maximum negative chronotropic responsivity to carbachol (a muscarinic agonist), but the maximum positive chronotropic response to isoproterenol (a β-adrenoceptor agonist) was lower compared with atria from control rats.

In an unusual animal model, turkeys were given a 5% ethanol solution as the only source of fluid for 28 to 56 days. Left ventricular diameter and left ventricular systolic time interval were decreased by the treatment with ethanol. However heart rate and systolic arterial blood pressure were not affected by the ethanol treatment (Noren *et al.*, 1983).

As with acute treatment, impairment in functional activity of the myocardium as a result of chronic ethanol ingestion may become evident only after an additional stressor. For example depression of the *in vitro* myocardial contractile function in guinea pigs ingesting 10% ethanol solution for 13–16 weeks, was unmasked by the additional stress of ischemia (Schreiber *et al.*, 1984). Spontaneously beating Langendorff perfused hearts from rats consuming a 20% solution of ethanol for 12 weeks did not differ from hearts from non-ethanol treated control rats. However, when the hearts were electrically paced, contractility of hearts from ethanol-treated animals deteriorated faster compared with hearts from control animals. The dose-response curve for isoproterenol was not altered unless Ca^{2+} was drastically decreased (Chan and Sutter, 1982).

Some of the above long-term studies have administered ethanol via the drinking fluid available to the subjects (dogs, rats, mice). Although technically this is the simplest method for long-term administration of ethanol, it may involve a serious pitfall, which has not been adequately evaluated. The problem centers around the dislike rodents have for concentrated solutions of ethanol. Forced to drink ethanol solutions (20% or more) rodents typically tend to limit their fluid intake and therefore also their food ingestion. For example, marked effects of chronic ethanol ingestion were reported as far as myocardial norepinephrine levels and histology (Ferreira *et al.*, 1975; Rossi *et al.*, 1976; Rossi and Oliviera, 1976). Subsequently, however, it was found that by pair watering the effects of ethanol on histology and on norepinephrine levels disappeared (Rossi, 1980). Similarly, functional myocardial effects (reduction in twitch tension) in myocardial tissues from mice ingesting 20% or more ethanol disappeared when the control group was pair-watered to the experimental group (Berk *et al.*, 1975). It is possible that the electrolyte imbalance as well as the changes in water in cellular compartments reported in some studies as a result of chronic ethanol ingestion reflect this problem (Thomas *et al.*, 1980; Polimeni *et al.*, 1983).

Chronic heavy ethanol consumption has been shown to be the cause of alcoholic cardiomyopathy which is known to be associated with the development of coronary heart disease. An association between heart disease and heavy alcohol consumption dates back to 1873 (Walshe, 1873). A few years later a connection between beer consumption and the

*Throughout this review the literature dealing with some of the experiments with experimental animals involved the administration of ethanol via the drinking fluid. The concentration of the employed ethanol solutions varied from low (5%) to rather high (40%). Since it was not always stated whether these solutions were w/v or v/v, this is omitted from the text and the provided numbers are given only as a relative index of the concentration of the employed solutions of ethanol.

incidence of heart dilation was reported (Bollinger, 1884). This review does not cover the cardiopathologic consequences of alcoholism. The reader is directed to other reviews on this and related topics (Klasky, 1982; Regan, 1984; Ashley, 1984; Dancy and Maxwell, 1986).

In alcoholic subjects, 6 oz of scotch had no effect on stroke volume or LVEDP (Wendt *et al.*, 1966; Regan *et al.*, 1969). Since however an increase in LVEDP and a small decline in stroke volume occurred after 12 oz (Wendt *et al.*, 1966), the dose difference probably reflects the tolerance to ethanol in these alcoholic subjects. Six ounces of whiskey significantly increased LVEDP but not stroke volume or cardiac output in long term alcoholics with heart failure (Regan, 1971). Thus such individuals appear to be more sensitive to ethanol either because of a loss of tolerance to ethanol or because of the already compromised myocardial function (Conway, 1968; Regan, 1971; Gould *et al.*, 1971).

2.2.2. *Electrophysiologic Effects of Ethanol*

A number of electrophysiological disturbances have been described as a result of both acute and chronic ethanol ingestion. Two ounces of whiskey delay conduction in atria, improve overall conduction (Gould *et al.*, 1978). In dogs ingestion of ethanol (30% of daily calories) for 3 years did not result in any impairment in atrial conduction, but depressed conduction through the A–V node and the bundle of His (Ettinger *et al.*, 1976). Direct intravenous application of ethanol in dogs dose-dependently depressed intracardiac conduction (through A–V node and bundle of His) (Goodkind *et al.*, 1975).

The basis of the functional myocardial depressant effects of ethanol may be a decrease in the duration of action potential in atrial and ventricular myocytes, and in cardiac Purkinje fibers (Fisher and Kavaler, 1973, Snoy *et al.*, 1980; Gimeno *et al.*, 1962). The shortening of the action potential by ethanol in combination with conduction defects may furthermore predispose the myocardium to arrhythmias and fibrillation.

Alcoholics show a number of conduction and rhythm disturbances (Evans, 1966; Alexander, 1968; Burch *et al.*, 1971). The most commonly reported conduction defects are: a tall peaked T-wave, slow slurred T-wave, prominent U-wave, increased or decreased P–R interval, right or left bundle branch block. Alterations of rhythm include: atrial and ventricular premature beats, ventricular prefibrillatory tachycardia, atrial and ventricular fibrillations. Heavy binge drinkers commonly show arrhythmias (atrial fibrillation, atrial flutter and atrial and ventrical tachycardia) after drinking (Ettinger *et al.*, 1978).

2.2.3. *Metabolic Effects of Ethanol*

2.2.3.1. *Mitochondrial function.* Considerable evidence indicates that the primary metabolic impairments in the myocardium are depression of mitochondrial function and lipid metabolism. In studies with dogs ingesting ethanol for periods up to 14 weeks, and rats ingesting ethanol, impairment of mitochondrial function was evident before there was functional impairment of the myocardium (Pachinger *et al.*, 1973; Bing *et al.*, 1974, Sarma *et al.*, 1975; Sarma *et al.*, 1976; Weishaar *et al.*, 1978; Segel *et al.*, 1979). Mitochondria had decreased respiratory function, (QO_2 and respiratory control index), after 4 weeks of liquid diet ingestion (35% of total calories) (Weishaar *et al.*, 1978) or after 6 months of ingestion of a 25% solution of ethanol (Sardesai and Provido, 1978). There was no change in the ADP/O ratio (Pachinger *et al.*, 1973). The mechanism for the defect in mitochondrial respiration has been suggested to be an impairment in pyruvate dehydrogenase or in the transport of pyruvate into mitochondria (Williams and Li, 1977). In addition, both glucose-6-phosphate dehydrogenase and glyceraldehyde phosphate dehydrogenase activities in the myocardium were increased after 6 months ingestion of a 25% solution of ethanol. Isocitrate dehydrogenase activity, on the other hand, was not altered by the treatment with ethanol (Weishaar *et al.*, 1978).

It is unclear whether ethanol affects high-energy phosphate in the myocardium. There was a slight decrease in myocardial ATP levels after dogs ingested a 25% solution of ethanol for either 14 weeks or 29 months (Pachinger *et al.*, 1973; Sarma *et al.*, 1976). However, others found no change in myocardial high energy phosphates (Whitman *et al.*, 1980).

Leakiness of both mitochondrial and cell membranes was indicated by an increase in creatine kinase and lactate dehydrogenase in plasma after chronic ethanol ingestion in both experimental animals and humans (Regan *et al.*, 1969). However myocardial enzyme levels (creatine kinase, lactic dehydrogenase, malate dehydrogenase) in plasma decreased in rats ingesting an ethanol solution (up to 40% of daily calories) for up to 12 weeks (Edes *et al.*, 1983). The possible contribution to the desired effects of impaired enzyme synthesis was not addressed in this study.

2.2.3.2. *Lipid metabolism.* An acute dose of ethanol increased cardiac triglyceralde content (Kikuchi and Kako, 1970; Regan *et al.*, 1977; Somer *et al.*, 1981). Oxidation of free fatty acids was depressed after both acute and chronic ethanol treatment in dogs (Regan *et al.*, 1979), or an acute dose of ethanol in rabbits (180 mg/dl) (Kikuchi and Kako, 1971). The elevated levels of triglycerides could possibly be accounted for by an increased uptake of plasma triglycerides (Regan *et al.*, 1977) and by the increased esterification of fatty acids (Lochner *et al.*, 1969; Kikuchi and Kako, 1970). It has been postulated that ethanol may alter the transfer of long-chain fatty acid acyl CoA into mitochondria as a result of direct damage to mitochondria (Kikuchi and Kako, 1970). Ingestion of ethanol as a 15% drinking solution for 18 months increased synthesis of lipids from labelled palmitate (Lochner *et al.*, 1969; Somer *et al.*, 1981) and, as mentioned above, decreased rate of fatty acid oxidation (Lochner *et al.*, 1969). Interestingly the fatty acid composition of the triglycerides that accumulate in the myocardium mirrors that of the fatty acids in plasma (Kako *et al.*, 1973). This finding suggests that the accumulated triglycerides are synthesized from precursors taken up from the circulation. The enzyme lipoprotein lipase is involved in making circulating lipids (high density lipoproteins and chylomicrons) available for myocardial metabolism. This enzyme is found in the endothelium of coronary vasculature as well as in the myocardial cells themselves. One would expect that if there is increased synthesis of myocardial triglycerides from lipid precursors taken up from the circulation then the activity of lipoprotein lipase would be increased. However, in one study in anesthetized rabbits 180 mg/dl ethanol increased cardiac triglyceride content but did not change lipoprotein lipase activity (Kikuchi and Kako, 1970). On the other hand, in rats a 3.0 g/kg dose of ethanol was found to depress cardiac neutral and lipoprotein lipase activities (Brick *et al.*, 1987).

An interesting recent finding concerns the demonstration of the production and accumulation of fatty acid ethyl esters in the myocardium after ethanol exposure (Lange *et al.*, 1981; Lange, 1983). Formation of these neutral lipids by esterification of free fatty acids was shown to be entirely due to ethanol and not to acetaldehyde. Furthermore, ethyloleate could decrease mitochondrial respiratory control index (loss of coupling or decrease in oxygen consumption). These compounds also bound preferentially to mitochondrial membranes (Lange and Sobel, 1983). Thus fatty acid ethyl esters formed as a consequence of ethanol exposure can have a direct toxic effect on mitochondria.

2.2.3.3. *Protein synthesis.* Generally, chronic ethanol does not produce significant impairment of total protein synthesis in the myocardium of adult animals (Schreiber *et al.*, 1972, 1974, 1984, 1986). A decline in protein synthesis has been reported (Weishaar *et al.*, 1978; Rawat, 1979). Of the relevant myocardial proteins, synthesis of actin, but not heavy or light chain myosin or tropomyosin, from (^{3}H)-labeled amino acid precursors was particularly impaired as a result of ethanol ingestion (Schreiber *et al.*, 1986). This impairment was suggested ultimately to lead to the observed myofibrillar disorganization and vacuolization seen in the myocardium with chronic exposure to ethanol.

An impairment in protein synthesis was, however, demonstrated in the presence of an additional stressor. A small decrease in protein synthesis *in vitro* was found in the loaded right ventricle but not in the unloaded left ventricle of the same heart from growing guinea pigs ingesting a 5.5% solution of ethanol for 8–11 weeks (Schreiber *et al.*, 1982). Impairment of protein synthesis was also found in hearts of growing guinea pigs ingesting 10% solution of ethanol (26% of total daily calories) for 13–16 weeks, and which were additionally stressed *in vitro* by reducing coronary flow (Schreiber *et al.*, 1984). In the absence of ischemia the experimental tissues did not show functional impairment, but were impaired in the presence of ischemia, indicating dissociation of protein synthesis and functional performance.

2.2.3.4. *Electrolyte balance.* Chronic ethanol also results in disturbances in myocardial electrolyte balance. A non-selective sarcolemmal "leakiness" and redistribution of myocardial electrolytes along their electrochemical gradient was found in rats that ingested a 25% solution of ethanol for up to 12 weeks (Polimeni *et al.*, 1983). Specifically water in the cellular compartment increased and decreased in the extracellular compartment. Concomitantly there was an increase in tissue Ca^{2+}, Na^+ and K^+ with no change in Mg^{2+}. This shift in myocardial electrolytes and tissue water requires prolonged ethanol exposure. An increase in cellular water and in Na^+ was not found in dogs that ingested ethanol (up to 40% solution) for 18 months, but was present after 52 months of ethanol ingestion (Thomas *et al.*, 1980). There were no changes in cellular K^+ or tissue Ca^{2+} in this study. Kinetics of Ca^{2+} in various subcellular organelles was also impaired by ethanol. Furthermore the uptake and binding of calcium in both microsomes (Swartz *et al.*, 1974; Noren *et al.*, 1983) and mitochondria (Bing *et al.*, 1974) of chronically ethanol treated animals was impaired. The release and uptake of Ca^{2+} by sarcoplasmic reticulum was also impaired by ethanol (Swartz *et al.*, 1974; Noren *et al.*, 1983). Another indicator of mitochondrial fragility was the altered distribution of the oligomycin sensitive Mg^{2+}-ATPase. This enzyme is bound to the inner mitochondrial membrane. The activity of this enzyme was decreased in mitochondria and increased in the tissue supernatant fraction prepared from hearts of guinea pigs ingesting a 15% solution of ethanol for 34 weeks (Schultheiss *et al.*, 1985).

Evidence for a role of calcium kinetics in the effects of ethanol on myocardial function comes from a recent study (Mantelli *et al.*, 1985). This study examined the effects of high concentrations of ethanol (323 mM) on the contractility of electrically-stimulated guinea-pig atria. It was found that the depressant effects of ethanol were decreased by increasing the extracellular calcium concentration. Similarly calcium also reduced the dose-dependent inhibition of contraction produced by field stimulation of adrenergic nerve terminals (Mantelli *et al.*, 1985). The authors concluded that the effect of ethanol was due to a possible decrease in calcium availability at the pre- and post-synaptic sites.

2.2.3.5. *ATPase activity.* Another mechanism by which ethanol may affect functional activity of the myocardium is by an effect on cell membrane Na^+/K^+ ATPase. The Ca^{2+}-stimulated myofibrillar ATPase enzyme was also depressed by ingestion of ethanol (5–25% ethanol) for 3–6 months (Segel *et al.*, 1975; Hastillo *et al.*, 1980). This biochemical impairment as well as the impaired mitochondrial function may be relevant to the functional and ultrastructural abnormalities noted in this study. By contrast, in another study (turkeys drinking 5% ethanol—25% of daily calories for up to 56 days) no change in the activity of Ca^{2+}-stimulated ATPase in myocardial sarcoplasmic reticulum was found (Noren *et al.*, 1983). However Na^+/K^+-ATPase was decreased after 56, but not 28 days of treatment (Noren *et al.*, 1983).

2.2.4. *Role of Ethanol Metabolites*

Alcohol dehydrogenase activity is very low in the heart (Forsyth, 1979). The lack of significant metabolism of ethanol in this organ is further confirmed by the lack of $^{14}CO_2$ formation after perfusion of (^{14}C)-ethanol through the heart (Lodmen *et al.*, 1969). Since under appropriate conditions blood levels of acetaldehyde can be elevated, it has been suggested that the myocardial effects of ethanol are due to the actions of its much more potent metabolite, acetaldehyde. As for the functional activity of the heart, and in contrast with other tissues, ethanol and acetaldehyde have opposite effects (Friedman *et al.*, 1979; Stratton *et al.*, 1981). In contrast to the depressant effects of ethanol in anesthetized closed-chest dogs, acetaldehyde had no effect on end-diastolic volume, LVEDP, it increased cardiac output and depressed systemic resistance (Friedman *et al.*, 1979). With respect to myocardial lipid metabolism, acetaldehyde (50 μM) did not alter significantly the uptake, oxidation or incorporation into lipids of oleate (Kiuiluoma and Hassinen, 1983). However, acetaldehyde is known to produce marked inhibition of cardiac protein synthesis (Schreiber *et al.*, 1974; Schreiber *et al.*, 1976). Interestingly, despite the inhibition of protein synthesis produced by acetaldehyde, it had positive inotropic and chronotropic effects (Schreiber *et al.*, 1974).

By contrast acetate (2 μM), the metabolite of acetaldehyde, had effects on lipid metabolism which were very similar to those of ethanol (inhibition of oleate oxidation, and increased its incorporation into tissue lipids) (Kiuiluoma and Hassinen, 1983). The depression in myocardial oxygen consumption and in oxidation of oleate, the increase in oleate incorporation into lipids, as well as the increase in coronary blood flow produced by ethanol, can all be reproduced by acetate in concentrations attainable *in vivo* (Peuhkurinen *et al.*, 1983). Therefore the possibility that acetate contributes to the impairment of myocardial lipid metabolism produced by ethanol needs to be further examined.

2.2.5. *Conclusions*

It can be concluded from the presented evidence that an acute dose of ethanol decreases cardiac output and increases LVEDP. The negative inotropic effect of ethanol may be masked by the autonomic activation produced by ethanol. Chronic ethanol treatment leads to some decrease in myocardial contractility. In alcoholics there is a significant increase in LVEDP and eventual development of cardiopathology.

Electrophysiologically, an acute dose of ethanol decreases the duration of the action potential in the myocardial conduction elements and myocytes, thus probably predisposing the heart to fibrillations and arrhythmias. Alcoholics exhibit a variety of rhythm disturbances.

At the biochemical level ethanol impairs myocardial function and possibly also decreases myocardial high-energy phosphates ATP—this impairment precedes development of functional disturbances. Chronic ethanol treatment may also impair myocardial protein synthesis, particularly that of actin. Lipid metabolism in the myocardium is also impaired by ethanol. Free fatty acid oxidation in the heart is decreased while triglyceride accumulation is increased by ethanol. In addition fatty acid ethyl esters may be formed in the myocardium as a result of metabolism of ethanol—these may have a direct toxic effect.

Electrolyte imbalance may develop in the myocardium as a result of increased permeability of some or all myocardial membranes. These changes in electrolytes may result, at least in part, from the impairment in ATPase activity produced by ethanol.

Lastly, it cannot be excluded, at this point, that some of the myocardial effects of ethanol are produced by ethanol metabolites, particularly acetate. One can also conclude that overall the depressant effects of ethanol on the myocardium become accentuated when the heart is subjected to an additional workload.

2.3. BLOOD CIRCULATION

Except as discussed earlier (Section 2.2.1) ethanol seems to have no significant effects on circulation until relatively high blood ethanol concentrations are reached. Furthermore there is significant regional specificity in the response of different vascular beds to ethanol.

An early study examined the effect of ethanol on cerebral blood flow using human subjects (Battey *et al.*, 1953). With the nitrous oxide technique no significant changes in cerebral blood flow oxygen extraction and consumption were found at blood ethanol concentrations ranging from 15 to 137 mg/dl. At higher concentrations oxygen uptake and cerebral blood flow were depressed. In rhesus monkey ethanol also decreased cerebral blood flow (McQueen, 1978).

In rats, using (^{14}C) antipyrine as a tracer, 0.48–4.8 g/kg ethanol decreased blood flow in the dorsal hippocampus at 2.5 g/kg and in the olfactory bulb, medulla and parietal cortex only at the highest dose of ethanol (Goldman *et al.*, 1973). A recent study examined regional blood flow in awake ethanol-treated dogs using the microsphere technique (Friedman *et al.*, 1984). At blood ethanol levels of 231 mg/dl, ethanol depressed blood flow in all brain areas examined, with the greatest effect in the cerebellum. In anesthetized animals the effects of ethanol were obscured because of the already depressed blood flow (Friedman *et al.*, 1984). Part of the mechanism by which blood flow might be decreased is the demonstration that ethanol produces spasms of the isolated canine middle cerebral and basilar arteries by a direct vascular action (Altura and Altura, 1984). Chronic ingestion of ethanol in man is associated with sharp decrease in cerebral blood flow. This is especially true in subjects over 50 years of age indicating that age is a significant contributing factor (Berglund and Invar, 1976). This topic will not be reviewed further here, but the interested reader is referred to an excellent review which focuses specifically on cerebral blood flow in long-term alcoholics (Berglund, 1981).

One of the earliest studies on the effect of ethanol on coronary blood flow used an anesthetized open-chest dog (Lasker *et al.*, 1955). Ethanol (375 mg/dl) administered intravenously produced an increase in coronary blood flow. In a conscious dog the intravenous administration of 1 g/kg dose of ethanol decreased coronary vascular resistance but not in anesthetized dogs (Pitt *et al.*, 1970). Using microspheres to assess regional distribution of flow in the myocardium, no regional differences were found up to 210 mg/dl ethanol despite an overall increase in coronary blood flow in isolated heart lung preparation (Abel, 1980). On the other hand, with a coincidence double counting system, an increase in coronary blood flow was found at blood concentration of 190 mg/dl ethanol and higher (Mendoza *et al.*, 1971). Similar effects of ethanol on coronary blood flow were obtained with human subjects. Employing the rubidium technique no changes in coronary blood flow were found after 65 mg/dl or 90 ml of whiskey (Mendoza *et al.*, 1971; Gould *et al.*, 1972). Only after ingestion of 12 oz of whiskey over a 2 hr period was there a small increase in coronary blood flow with the ^{85}Kr clearance technique (Regan *et al.*, 1969).

When dogs were subjected to an additional load such as exercise, the increase in coronary blood flow was less and developed only at higher blood ethanol levels (161 mg/dl) (Stratton *et al.*, 1981). When human subjects with angina pectoris and coronary artery disease underwent an exercise stress test, prior ingestion of 2 or 5 oz of whiskey decreased significantly the time necessary to precipitate an attack of angina (Orlando *et al.*, 1976). The results of this study point again to the limited margin of safety in myocardial tissues exposed to ethanol.

In the canine kidneys an acute high dose of ethanol (3 g/kg) had no effect on renal blood flow (using the method based on the extraction of *p*-aminohippurate). However, renal blood flow increased 10 hr after treatment (Sargent *et al.*, 1975). Animals that received chronic ethanol treatment had a small increase in renal blood flow (Sargent *et al.*, 1976).

Blood flow through muscles as affected by acute ethanol treatment was examined in a study using human subjects (Fewings *et al.*, 1966). Ethanol administered intraarterially in the forearm decreased blood flow through the skin and muscles. This appeared to be a direct effect of ethanol on the vasculature since the ethanol had no effect if subjects were pretreated with phenoxybenzamine (a noradrenergic receptor blocker). When given orally, ethanol dilated the blood vessels of the hand and forearm. The later effect was blocked by phenoxybenzamine and therefore most likely was mediated by the sympathetic nervous system.

In one study hepatic blood flow in baboons was estimated according to the Fick principle using sulfobromophthalein infusion. At elevated blood ethanol levels (about 275 mg/dl), hepatic blood flow increased (Shaw *et al.*, 1977). In the pancreas blood flow was decreased dose dependently by ethanol (0.5–1.5 g/kg) in dogs (Horwitz and Myers, 1980).

By quantatitively measuring splanchnic microvasculature with a high-resolution closed circuit television microscope, it was shown that ethanol dose-dependently dilates precapillary sphincters, arterioles and muscular vessels (Altura, 1978; Altura *et al.*, 1979; Altura, 1981; Altura and Altura, 1983). Furthermore ethanol (100 mM or more) non-specifically inhibited vascular constrictions produced by vasoactive substances such as catecholamines, serotonin, angiotensin, vasopression histamine, prostaglandins and Ca^{2+} (Altura *et al.*,

1979; Altura, 1981; Altura and Altura, 1983). But at low concentrations of ethanol, it potentiated the action of these vasoactive substances. Addition of ethanol to isolated venous or arterial smooth muscle preparations had a biphasic effect on their resting tension. At low concentrations ethanol (1–50 mM) lowered resting tension of arteries capable of developing a tone and inhibited spontaneous mechanical activity (Altura and Altura, 1976, 1978, 1981, 1983; Altura *et al.*, 1976, 1980). At high concentrations ethanol (over 100 mM) evoked dose-dependent contractions of blood vessels (Altura *et al.*, 1976; Edganian and Altura, 1976). There was, interestingly, a regional specificity in the effect of ethanol on isolated vascular preparations. Some vessels (coronary, cerebral, intrapulmonary, renal, femoral) did not exhibit a biphasic response to ethanol, but rather showed only vasoconstriction (Altura and Altura, 1983). On the basis of extensive pharmacologic manipulations, these investigators believe that the effects of ethanol on vascular responsiveness are due to changes in the availability of Ca^{2+} for the contractile mechanism (Altura and Altura, 1982).

Blood vessels from rats maintained on a liquid diet containing ethanol (6–8% v/v) for 6 weeks exhibited tolerance to *in vitro* effects of high concentrations of ethanol (170–430 mM) (Altura *et al.*, 1980). Furthermore, *in vivo* ethanol did not produce vasodilation in animals maintained on the ethanol-containing liquid diet for 6 weeks, and interestingly it potentiated the vasoconstrictor effect of locally administered catecholamines (Altura and Altura, 1980).

These effects of ethanol on the vasculature are apparently not mediated by acetaldehyde or acetate (Altura and Gebrowolt, 1981), which generally produce vasoconstriction.

2.3.1. *Conclusions*

The effect of ethanol on blood flow shows regional specificity. Blood flow in brain and pancreas is decreased by ethanol. Conversely, blood flow in liver, heart, skeletal muscles is increased, and blood flow through the kidneys is not influenced by ethanol.

Ethanol can have a direct effect on the vasculature. Its action on blood vessels is biphasic. At low concentrations ethanol potentiates the action of vasoactive substances, basal tone and the spontaneous activity of the vasculature. At higher concentrations (over 100 mM) ethanol decreases the action of vasoactive substances and increases spontaneous contractions of the vasculature. These actions of ethanol may be mediated by the availability of intracellular calcium. Also with chronic ethanol treatment, tolerance develops to its action on the vasculature.

2.4. BLOOD PRESSURE

Very few studies have examined the effect of ethanol on the regulation of blood pressure. In man, most of the evidence comes from epidemiologic studies which indicated in some cases a somewhat lower diastolic blood pressure in individuals drinking some alcohol than in the average population of abstainers (Kannel and Sorlil, 1974; Klatsky *et al.*, 1977; Gordon and Kannel, 1983; Welte and Greiserstein, 1985). However, the overwhelming evidence indicates a positive association between ethanol ingestion and blood pressure (Kondo and Ebihara, 1974; Gyntlberg and Meyer, 1974; Mathew, 1976; Barboriak *et al.*, 1982; Bellin and Pudley, 1984). This positive correlation, however, may be sex and age dependent since in women and young men, either there was no correlation between alcohol consumption and blood pressure or the association was negative for low to moderate levels of ethanol ingestion (Baghurst and Dwyer, 1981; Wallace *et al.*, 1981; Welte and Greiserstein, 1985). Epidemiologic studies also suggest that long-term alcoholics have a higher incidence of hypertension (D'Alonzo and Pell, 1968; Beevers, 1977; Klatsky *et al.*, 1977; Mathews, 1979; Saunders *et al.*, 1979; Harburgh *et al.*, 1980).

In rats although 0.5 g/kg of ethanol had no effect on baroreflex sensitivity, an acute dose of 3.0 g/kg significantly depressed it. Inhaling ethanol for 6 days produced a decrease in mean arterial blood pressure in rats with blood ethanol levels of more than 182 mg/dl

(Karanian *et al.*, 1986). This hypotension was associated with hypersensitivity to a thromboxane agonist, but not to norepinephrine. Longer exposure to ethanol (12 weeks of ingestion of 5–10% ethanol solution) by rats either had no effect (Khetapal and Volicer, 1979) or resulted in elevated blood pressure (5–20% solution) (Chan and Sutter, 1984). In a more extensive study using chronic ethanol treated (liquid diet for 30 days) rats, ethanol produced a differential effect on blood pressure control with respect to baroceptor function. Using anesthetized rats the baroreceptor system was found to be less sensitive to elevations in arterial pressure, but more sensitive in buffering decreases in arterial pressure in the ethanol compared with the control group (Adel-Rahman *et al.*, 1985). In unanesthetized rats systolic blood pressure was not altered by the chronic ethanol treatment, but there was a small decrease in heart rate. Since the depression of baroreflex sensitivity appeared to be smaller in the chronic ethanol group compared to the chronic sucrose control group, there was indication of development of tolerance to this effect of ethanol (Adel-Rahman *et al.*, 1985). The decrease in baroreflex sensitivity, in absence of alterations in systolic blood pressure, was suggested by the authors to possibly contribute to the development of ethanol-induced hypertension.

2.4.1. *Conclusions*

Ethanol affects baroreflex sensitivity which may, with chronic exposure to ethanol, lead to the development of hypertension.

3. NEUROCHEMICAL EFFECTS OF ETHANOL

As will become readily evident to the reader, the evidence on the overall neurochemical effects of ethanol is somewhat inconsistent. This variability of effects is frequently due not only to the multiplicity of effects of ethanol, but also to the proclivity of subject and treatment associated variables. Not only are the effects of ethanol biphasic with respect to dose and time after treatment, but are also significantly affected by the route of ethanol administration (oral, i.p., inhalation), the vehicle for its administration (e.g. liquid diet, dilute aqueous solution for fluid consumption), the stress involved in the treatment procedure, etc. (for reviews, see Pohorecky, 1981; Pohorecky, 1982). Additional considerations are organ as well as regional specificity in the brain.

Inconsistencies may also arise from the application of some techniques to ethanol research. A case in point was the use of monoamine oxidase inhibitors for assessment of the turnover of monoamines. As it turned out monomine oxidase inhibitors also affected the metabolism of ethanol, and thus affected blood ethanol levels (Dembiec *et al.*, 1976), confounding the interpretation of a number of published studies.

Neuronal membranes have been the focus of attention as a possible site of ethanol's action for the past decade. The simplicity of the ethanol molecule coupled with the lack of interaction *in vivo* with specific "receptors" has contributed to the hypothesis that ethanol acts more like a physical agent. This notion is based on the observed similarity of the effects of ethanol to that of other simple alcohols and anesthetics. According to the "Meyer–Overton" hypothesis (Meyer, 1937), the potency of various anesthetic drugs is directly proportional to their lipid solubility. Even better correlation existed if the molar concentration as well as the space the drug occupies in the membrane were considered (Mullins, 1954). Alcohols were also found to have the ability to expand membranes, either artificial ones or membranes prepared from erythrocytes (Seeman and Roth, 1972; Seeman, 1974).

In 1977 Chin and Goldstein reported that membrane fluidity of both red blood cells and synaptosomal membranes was increased in the presence of 20–40 mM ethanol. The effect was dose-dependent up to 350 mM. Using 5-doxylstearic acid, a spin-labeled electroparamagnetic probe they were able to demonstrate for the first time that ethanol dose-dependently reduces the order parameter in synaptosomal membranes from mouse brains. These data were interpreted to mean that ethanol disordered or fluidized neuronal membranes.

Since then extensive research has demonstrated that ethanol, as well as other aliphatic alcohols can alter fluidity of membranes. This property of alcohols correlates to their lipid solubility.

Since several recent excellent reviews/monograms exist on the pharmacology of the effects of ethanol on cellular membranes (Harris and Hitzemann, 1981; Hunt, 1985), the reader is referred to these for more detailed discussion on this topic. Instead we will discuss in more detail the effect of ethanol on two important cell membrane enzymes: Na^+/K^+ ATPase and the cyclic nucleotide cyclases.

3.1. Na^+/K^+ ATPase

Sodium- and potassium-activated adenosine triphosphatase (Na^+/K^+ ATPase) is a cell membrane enzyme vital to neuronal function. It is involved in maintaining the ionic gradients for both sodium and potassium across neuronal membranes. Evidence indicates that for every three sodium ions that are transported out of the neuron, two potassium ions are transported into the neuron. This function is essential for the maintenance of electrical excitability of neurons. The sequence of events involves at least two phosphorylated and two non-phosphorylated intermediates. During the process of phosphorylation of the enzyme by ATP, intracellular sodium is bound to the activated enzyme. The overall reaction, driven by conformational changes catalyzed by magnesium, leads to the transport of sodium through the cell membrane. Upon dephosphorylation of the enzyme by hydrolysis, extracellular K^+ is transported into the cell. The overall simplified reaction sequence with E_1 and E_2 representing different states of the enzyme, is the following (Fahn *et al.*, 1966):

$$E_1 + ATP \xrightarrow{Na^+} ADP + E_1P \rightarrow E_2P \xrightarrow[H_2O]{K^+} E_2 + Pi$$

3.1.1. *Acute Ethanol Treatment*

The effect of ethanol on Na^+/K^+ ATPase has been examined by a number of investigators. Probably the first study was that of Jarnfelt (1961) in which he demonstrated that ethanol inhibited Na^+/K^+ ATPase activity in microsomal preparations from rat brain homogenates. A number of subsequent studies using different tissue preparations obtained from different animal species (Israel *et al.*, 1965; Israel *et al.*, 1966; Sun and Samojarski, 1970; Tabakoff, 1974; Sun, 1974; Sun and Samojarski, 1975; Erwin *et al.*, 1975; Syapin *et al.*, 1976; Kalant *et al.*, 1978) have confirmed the inhibitory effect of ethanol on Na^+/K^+ ATPase activity. The effect of ethanol was dose-dependent (Israel *et al.*, 1965; Goldstein and Israel, 1972), and was competitive with respect to potassium ions (Israel *et al.*, 1965, 1966; Goldstein and Israel, 1972; Rangaraj and Kalant, 1978) and other alkali metals (rubidium, cesium) (Kalant *et al.*, 1978). Since the inhibitory effect of ethanol could be reversed by increasing the concentration of K^+ in the medium, it indicated that ethanol's inhibition resulted from an allosteric effect on the K^+ binding site (Kalant *et al.*, 1978).

Although the lipid composition and fluidity of membranes influence the activity of Na^+/K^+ ATPase, the enzyme activity is primarily affected by lipids immediately surrounding it (the boundary lipids) (Lin, 1980; Kimelberg and Papalidjopoulos, 1972). The transition temperature of enzymes as obtained from Arrhenius plots is believed to be an indication of the phase transition of lipids surrounding a given enzyme (Charnock and Bashford, 1975). Arrhenius analysis showed that 500 mM ethanol decreased the transition temperature for Na^+/K^+ ATPase (Levental and Tabakoff, 1980; Hoffman *et al.*, 1980; Rangaraj and Kalant, 1980). This means that the temperature at which the membrane changed from the gel to a liquid state was lower. These results, as well as other reports in the literature, confirm that Na^+/K^+ ATPase is sensitive to changes in membrane fluidity, and may therefore explain the temperature sensitivity of the enzyme (Sun and Seaman, 1980). As indicated earlier, membrane fluidity is considered one possible mechanism by which ethanol affects neuronal functioning. Ethanol affects the activation energy of the enzyme only above transition temperature, indicating that both the membrane matrix lipids as well as the membrane lipids adjacent to the enzyme (boundary lipids) were affected (Rangaraj and Kalant, 1980). It follows from the above discussion that the lipid composition of membranes may influence membrane fluidity as well as susceptibility of membrane Na^+/K^+ ATPase to ethanol. The effect of ethanol (500 mM) on enzyme activity from different membrane fractions (myelin, axolemma, synaptic membranes) varies with their lipid content (Levantal and Rakic, 1980). This might explain, at least in part, the observed regional differences in Na^+/K^+ ATPase activity (Rangaraj and Kalant, 1984).

Besides ethanol, acetaldehyde also inhibits Na^+/K^+ ATPase (Tabakoff, 1974; Gonzalez-Calvin, 1983). Other alcohols and depressant drugs also inhibit Na^+K^+ ATPase activity (Israel *et al.*, 1966; Rangaraj and Kalant, 1982). There is good positive correlation between anesthetic potency of various depressant drugs with their inhibitory potency on Na^+/K^+ ATPase activity (Israel and Salazar, 1967). Furthermore, endogenous and exogenous aldehydes also inhibit competitively Na^+/K^+ ATPase (Tabakoff, 1974; Erwin *et al.*, 1975), and have been found to be more potent inhibitors than ethanol (Erwin *et al.*, 1975).

Although Na^+/K^+ ATPase is just one of several ATPase enzymes present in tissues, most of the research with ethanol has focused on Na^+/K^+ ATPase because of its major physiological significance in neuronal function. Mg^{2+} ATPase has also been found to be reversibly inhibited by ethanol (Israel *et al.*, 1966; Israel and Salazar, 1967; Sun and Samojarski, 1970; Goldstein and Israel, 1972; Erwin *et al.*, 1975). Generally the Na^+/K^+ ATPase is more sensitive to ethanol than to the Mg^{2+}-stimulated enzyme (Sun and Samojarski, 1970; Goldstein and Israel, 1972; Erwin *et al.*, 1975), though the converse has also been reported (Israel and Salazar, 1967; Israel and Kuriyama, 1971). On the other hand, the Ca^{2+}-stimulated ATPase can be either inhibited (Sun and Seaman, 1980) or stimulated (Yamamoto and Harris, 1983) by ethanol.

The effect of ethanol on Na^+/K^+ ATPase activity is not restricted to the nervous system. A few studies examined ethanol's action on the enzyme in other tissues. Although *in vitro* ethanol (120 mM) inhibited Na^+/K^+ ATPase of hepatic plasma membranes by 20% (Gonzalez-Calvin *et al.*, 1983), *in vivo* treatment with ethanol (4.0 g/kg i.p., 3 hr post-treatment) elevated activity of hepatic microsomes (Israel and Kuriyama, 1971). *In vitro* ethanol (50–1000 mM) also inhibited the Na^+/K^+ ATPase in myocardial plasma membrane preparations (Williams *et al.*, 1975). On the other hand Ca^{2+}-stimulated ATPase activity in red blood cell membranes was stimulated by ethanol (50 mM) (Yamamoto and Harris, 1983). Lastly, in tissue cultures ethanol generally inhibited Na^+/K^+ ATPase, with the effect varying with the particular cell type under investigation (chick glia, glia tumor, etc.) (Ledig *et al.*, 1985), but no effect of ethanol was reported on Na^+/K^+ ATPase activity in astroblasts (Syapin *et al.*, 1976).

One approach used to examine the mechanism(s) by which ethanol affects Na^+/K^+ ATPase activity is to test the activity of K^+-*p*-nitrophenylphosphatase (pNNPase); pNNPase is believed to be part of the sodium/potassium transport system which is measured in the absence of sodium. By examining the activity of this enzyme the K^+ and Na^+ effects of Na^+/K^+ ATPase can be investigated independently and the effects of K^+ and ATP binding can be distinguished. pNNPase activity is believed to be a measure of the E_2 conformational state of the Na^+/K^+ ATPase enzyme (Swann, 1983). Li^+ activates the enzyme at the catalytic but not regulatory site; therefore, Li^+-stimulated phosphatase activity is independent of conformational changes of the enzyme and reflects only the catalytic activity of the enzyme in the E_2-conformation (Swann, 1983). Since ethanol at high concentrations (500 mM) inhibited pNNPase activity (Kalant *et al.*, 1978; Swann, 1983; Nhamburo *et al.*, 1986) direct inhibition of the enzyme protein by ethanol was suggested (Nhamburo *et al.*, 1986). This effect of ethanol involved decreased formation of the K^+-sensitive enzyme by cation binding and also stabilization of the K^+-sensitive enzyme in the presence of ATP (Swann, 1983). This was interpreted to indicate that ethanol acted by a combination of a membrane and solvent effect, since both cation binding and comformation of the enzyme were affected. After chronic ethanol treatment (ingestion of a liquid diet for 3 weeks) sensitivity of pNNPase to inhibition to *in vitro* added ethanol was significantly decreased (Swann, 1985). Interestingly, chronic noradrenergic stimulation *in vivo* by treatment with yohimbine, had effects opposite to those of ethanol on pNNPase activity (Swann, 1986).

Another approach to the understanding of the action of ethanol on Na^+/K^+ ATPase activity is to determine ouabain binding to cell membrane preparations (Israel *et al.*, 1965; Sharma *et al.*, 1977). The cardiac glycoside binds to the catalytic subunit of the enzyme, thus specifically inhibiting enzyme activity. *In vitro* ouabain binding was increased by ethanol in the presence of low Na^+, but inhibited at high Na^+ (Brody and Akera, 1976). Furthermore ethanol increased release of labeled ouabain already bound to Na^+/K^+ ATPase (Brody and Akera, 1976). This was interpreted by the authors as indicating that the action of ethanol on the enzyme is similar to that of sodium ions. In chronic ethanol treated cats (1.5–2.0 g/kg by intubation twice daily for 5 weeks) (^3H)-ouabain binding was also increased. Scatchard analysis indicated that the number of ouabain binding sites was increased by the ethanol treatment (Sharma *et al.*, 1977). To correctly assess the significance of these studies more research must be carried out since the catalytic subunit of brain ATPase exists in two forms (Sweander, 1979), which may be localized to specific cell types (Sweander, 1979), and may also vary with the age of the organism (Matsuda *et al.*, 1984; Specht, 1984).

Na^+/K^+ ATPase activity can be modulated by neurotransmitters (specifically biogenic amines) as well as some hormones (e.g., insulin). Na^+/K^+ ATPase activity is stimulated by biogenic amines (Yoshimura, 1973; Desaiah and Ho, 1976; Lee and Phillis, 1977). Furthermore stimulation of the enzyme can also be achieved by increasing noradrenergic activity *in vivo* (Swann *et al.*, 1981, Swann, 1984b). In the presence of low concentrations of norepinephrine Na^+/K^+ ATPase activity was more sensitive to the inhibition by ethanol (Rangaraj and Kalant, 1980; Kalant and Rangaraj, 1981). In fact concentrations of ethanol as low as 132.2 mM were found to be effective. Of further interest was that this facilitatory action of norepinephrine was receptor mediated. α-Noradrenergic antagonists blocked the effect of norepinephrine, while β-noradrenergic agonists were ineffective (Rangaraj and Kalant, 1978, 1980). This effect of norepinephrine was observed in all brain areas examined, except for the striatum. The sensitizing action of norepinephrine occurs at very low concentrations (10^{-12} M) (Rangaraj and Kalant, 1979), and is specific to l-norepinephrine (the d-form is ineffective) (Beauge *et al.*, 1983). Other catecholamines which are α-receptor agonists are also effective (Rangaraj and Kalant, 1979; Beauge *et al.*, 1983).

The mechanisms by which norepinephrine sensitizes Na^+/K^+ ATPase to inhibition by ethanol has been suggested to be a conformation change from the outwardly facing K^+-binding E_2P form to the inwardly facing Na^+-binding E_1P form (Kalant and Rangaraj, 1981). This effect of ethanol can occur at physiologically relevant K^+ concentrations (Kalant and Rangaraj, 1981). Arrhenius plots indicated that facilitation of ethanol inhibition by norepinephrine occurs by altering the activation energy only above the transition temperature (Rangaraj and Kalant, 1980). This suggested that norepinephrine acted by fluidizing membrane lipids thus facilitating the conformational change of Na^+/K^+ ATPase produced by ethanol (Rangaraj and Kalant, 1980). However, since there were discrepancies in the regional differences in enzyme susceptibility to ethanol, in the response to norepinephrine, in the development of tolerance and norepinephrine, and in Arrhenius plots from tissues from ethanol-tolerant animals, the authors indicated the unlikelihood that a simple mechanism (i.e. resistance to membrane "fluidization") is responsible for the development of tolerance (Rangaraj and Kalant, 1984).

A recent study failed to confirm the sensitizing effect of norepinephrine on the inhibition of Na^+/K^+ ATPase by ethanol (Nhamburo *et al.*, 1986). Based on the analysis of Arrhenius plots and of the correlation between inhibition of Na^+/K^+ ATPase and the membrane partition of various alcohols, these investigators suggest that partitioning of ethanol in membranes as well as an effect on the enzyme protein itself may be responsible for the inhibitory effect of ethanol (Nhamburo *et al.*, 1986).

The effect of ethanol on transition temperature of the Na^+/K^+ ATPase is specific to this enzyme. Ethanol did not affect the transition temperature of the Mg^{2+} ATPase, or of some other enzymes (5-nucleotidase, acetylcholinesterase) (Collins *et al.*, 1984).

The inhibitory effect of ethanol on Na^+/K^+ ATPase can be influenced by subject related variables. For example, the action of ethanol varies with age. Older mice are presumed to be more sensitive to ethanol's action on synaptosomal Na^+/K^+ ATPase (Sun and Samojarski, 1975). Also genetics play a role in susceptibility of the enzyme to ethanol. Ethanol's inhibitory effect on hepatic Na^+/K^+ ATPase activity is 65% higher in short sleep (SS) versus long sleep (LS) mice (Zysset *et al.*, 1983). These mice strains vary in their sensitivity to ethanol, the SS show a short-lasting loss of righting reflex, while the LS have a significantly longer depression to ethanol. Although the Na^+/K^+ ATPase activity in brain preparations and its sensitivity to ethanol did not differ in LS and SS mice (Marks *et al.*, 1984), the transition temperature of the high ouabain sensitive form of the enzyme was twice as sensitive to ethanol in LS versus SS mice (Collins *et al.*, 1984). Similarly Na^+/K^+ ATPase was higher in DBA mice compared with C57 mice (Zysset *et al.*, 1983). These mice differ in their preference for ethanol ingestion, the DBA prefer ethanol while C57 mice avoid it.

All of the preceding studies examined *in vitro* the effect of ethanol on Na^+/K^+ ATPase. The question remains what are the probable *in vivo* consequences of ethanol's action on this enzyme. When ethanol was injected as a solution in KCl rather than NaCl, its depressant effect was less (Israel *et al.*, 1965). The study suggested that ethanol's intoxication possibly involved depression of Na^+/K^+ ATPase, since *in vitro* K^+ had been shown to antagonize the effect of ethanol on Na^+/K^+ ATPase.

On the other hand, the intoxicating effects of ethanol could be potentiated by ions known to inhibit Na^+/K^+ ATPase (Kalant *et al.*, 1978). For example, lithium exhibits Na^+/K^+ ATPase (Kalant *et al.*, 1978). In goldfish, lithium and vanadate were found to increase the depression produced by ethanol (Guevri *et al.*, 1981), while cadmium increased sleep time and hypothermia produced by ethanol (Magour *et al.*, 1981, Yamamoto *et al.*, 1981). These results could not be explained by changes in blood ethanol levels (Magour *et al.*, 1981; Yamamoto *et al.*, 1981).

3.1.2. *Chronic Ethanol Treatment*

Studies on the effect of chronic ethanol treatment on Na^+/K^+ ATPase activity have not been entirely consistent. A number of studies indicate that Na^+/K^+ ATPase activity is increased in brain preparations from rats that received chronic ethanol treatment (Israel *et al.*, 1970; Knox *et al.*, 1972; Wallgren *et al.*, 1975; Guerri *et al.*, 1978; Cowan *et al.*, 1980; Guerri and Grisolia, 1983; Beauge *et al.*, 1983; Shiohara *et al.*, 1984; Ledig *et al.*, 1985). Other studies have not reported a change in the activity of this enzyme with chronic exposure to ethanol (Goldstein and Israel, 1972; Akera *et al.*, 1973; Levental and Tabakoff, 1980; Rangaraj and Kalant, 1984; Aloia *et al.*, 1985). During withdrawal from chronic ethanol treatment Na^+/K^+ ATPase activity was elevated (Roach *et al.*, 1973; Rangaraj and Kalant, 1978; Rangaraj and Kalant, 1980). Enzyme activity increased 12–48 hr after termination of ethanol treatment, with peak increase at 24 hr (Rangaraj and Kalant, 1982). Since a stressor (swimming), and enhanced release of norepinephrine (with amphetamine) also elevated Na^+/K^+ ATPase activity, it was postulated that the increase in enzyme activity observed during withdrawal resulted from its activation by the released norepinephrine.

It is interesting that the elevation in Na^+/K^+ ATPase activity with chronic treatment or withdrawal from ethanol shows regional specificity. The most sensitive brain area appears to be the cerebral cortex and hippocampus (Knox *et al.*, 1972; Rangaraj and Kalant, 1984) with no changes in enzyme activity in other areas such as the caudate, amygdala or reticular formation (Knox *et al.*, 1972). Interestingly, (^{3}H)-ouabain binding also increased in the cortex and hippocampus after 5 weeks of ethanol treatment (Sharma and Baney *et al.*, 1979). Furthermore, the effect of ethanol is primarily restricted to the Na^+/K^+ ATPase fractions associated with neurotransmission (Shiohara *et al.*, 1984). In this study 16 weeks of ethanol treatment increased Na^+/K^+ ATPase activity in synaptosomal plasma membrane preparations but not in microsomal preparations. This finding might explain some of the contradictory reports since in some cases (Goldstein and Israel, 1972; Nikander and Pekkanen, 1977) crude microsomal fractions rather than purified synaptosomal membrane preparations were used. For example, 4 weeks of ingestion of liquid diet containing ethanol did not alter Na^+/K^+ ATPase activity in whole homogenates (Rangaraj and Kalant, 1977), while 4 weeks of intragastric ethanol intubations resulted in up to an 18% increase in basal Na^+/K^+ ATPase activity in synaptosomal preparations (Beauge *et al.*, 1983) (differences in the method of ethanol treatment may have also contributed to these discrepancies).

There is general agreement on the apparent development of tolerance to effects of *in vitro* ethanol on enzyme preparations obtained from chronically ethanol-treated animals. That is, membrane preparations from rats chronically treated with ethanol show little if any inhibition of Na^+/K^+ ATPase activity in response to the *in vitro* addition of ethanol and to changes in transition temperature compared with preparations from control animals (Hoffman *et al.*, 1980; Beauge *et al.*, 1983; Guerri and Grisolia, 1983; Aloia *et al.*, 1985; Swann, 1985). In most of these studies presence of functional tolerance was demonstrated to either ethanol-induced motor impairment, motor impairment or to its hypothermic action.

Chronic treatment with ethanol results in a decrease in the effectiveness of norepinephrine in sensitizing Na^+/K^+ ATPase to ethanol (Rangaraj and Kalant, 1980; Rangaraj and Kalant, 1982; Rangaraj and Kalant, 1984; Rangaraj *et al.*, 1985). The tolerance to the inhibition of Na^+/K^+ ATPase by ethanol in brain preparations of ethanol-dependent animals could possibly be explained by a change in α-noradrenergic receptors. Ethanol tolerant rats showed a decrease in maximum number of binding sites (B_{max}) and the dissociation constant (K_D) of α_1-noradrenoceptors (Rangaraj *et al.*, 1985). A surprising additional finding was that tissue preparations from chronic sucrose treated animals also showed some sensitization to the stimulatory effect of norepinephrine on Na^+/K^+ ATPase activity (Rangaraj *et al.*, 1984).

Some of the above inconsistencies could be explained by differences in regional sensitivity of the enzyme, as referred to above. Thus, although the sensitizing effect of norepinephrine on Na^+/K^+ ATPase to ethanol was found in all brain areas except the striatum, tolerance developed to this effect only in some areas (cortex, hypothalamus, hippocampus) (Rangaraj and Kalant, 1984).

The effect of ethanol on Na^+/K^+ ATPase has also been examined in tissue cultures. Na^+/K^+ ATPase activity was increased in the presence of 43.4 mM ethanol in HeLa cells derived from human cervix but not in mouse fibroblasts (Lindsay, 1974). On the other hand an increase in both Mg^{2+} and Na^+/K^+ ATPase activity was seen in astroblasts but not in neuroblasts obtained from hamsters (Syapin *et al.*, 1976). In another study, neuronal cell lines were not sensitive to ethanol (Syapin *et al.*, 1976). Although after incubation in the presence of ethanol for 68 days one line of neuroblastoma showed increased Na^+/K^+ ATPase activity, other lines of neuroblastoma and astroblastoma were not affected by ethanol (Syapin *et al.*, 1976). Similar variability in response to ethanol by different cell types (chick glia, chick neurons, glia tumor, etc.) was reported in another study (Ledig *et al.*, 1985). One can conclude from these reports that the effect of ethanol on Na^+/K^+ ATPase varies with the type of tissue, possibly because of differences in cell membrane lipoprotein structure, or other yet unknown factors.

3.1.3. *Conclusions*

Ethanol inhibits the activity of Na^+/K^+ ATPase. This effect of ethanol is dependent on several subject related factors. Among these are the age and the genetic background of the subject. Presence of low concentrations of norepinephrine sensitizes Na^+/K^+ ATPase to inhibition by ethanol. With chronic exposure to ethanol, tolerance develops to its inhibitory effect. During withdrawal from ethanol Na^+/K^+ ATPase activity is elevated.

3.2. Cyclic Nucleotide System

3.2.1. *Adenyl Cyclase*

An important cellular regulatory mechanism is that of the cyclic nucleotides, cyclic adenosine 3′,5′-monophosphate (cAMP) and cyclic guanosine 3′,-5′-monophosphate (cGMP). These two cyclic nucleotides play the role as second messengers in the action of neurotransmitters and hormones. The synthesis of both nucleotides is catalyzed by the respective cyclases. Adenylate cyclase requires magnesium for its activity:

$$\text{ATP} \xrightarrow[\text{Adenylate cyclase}]{\text{Mg}^{2+}} \text{cAMP} + 5'\text{-AMP}$$

Adenyl cyclase is part of a cell membrane receptor-coupled system. This system consists of three major parts: a receptor, a regulatory protein and a catalytic unit. The function of the receptor unit is to interact with neurotransmitters; it is specific to a particular neurotransmitter. The regulatory protein is stimulated by guanosine nucleotide (GTP). Two forms of this protein exist, one stimulates and the other inhibits cyclase activity. The catalytic unit is stimulated by NaF which is located in the inner surface of the cell membrane where cAMP is synthesized. When an agonist interacts with the receptor a high-affinity ternary complex is formed which consists of agonist, the receptor unit and the guanine nucleotide binding regulatory protein. Formation of this complex results in the dissociation of the bound guanosine diphosphate from the regulatory protein. Upon rebinding GTP, the receptor reverts to a low affinity form with dissociation of the complex. Concomitantly the activated regulatory protein with bound GTP activates the catalytic unit of the adenyl cyclase leading to the formation of cAMP.

Cyclic AMP in turn produces its cellular effects by activating specific protein kinases which promote phosphorylation of protein or/and histones which affect changes in DNA/RNA transcription. Thus the immediate consequence of neurotransmitter receptor interaction is reflected by the stimulation of cAMP synthesis.

3.2.1.1. *Acute ethanol treatment.* The first attempts at examining the effects of ethanol on cyclic nucleotides focused on measuring brain levels of these compounds. The overall effect of the acute treatment with ethanol was a dose-dependent decrease in cAMP levels in brain (Volicer and Gold, 1973; Volicer *et al.*, 1976; Orenberg *et al.*, 1976; Volicer and Hunter, 1977) and in CSF of alcoholics (Orenberg *et al.*, 1976). In rats a single dose of ethanol (0.55–4.6 g/kg by intubation) decreased cAMP levels in CSF for up to 24 hr (Weitbrecht and Cramer, 1980). In the brain, largest decreases in cAMP levels were observed in cortex and cerebellum (Volicer *et al.*, 1976; Orenberg *et al.*, 1976; Volicer and Hunter, 1977). This observation was, however, not entirely reproducible since in an equal number of cases (Israel *et al.*, 1972; Redos *et al.*, 1976; Kuriyama, 1977) no changes in cAMP levels were found after ethanol treatment.

One confounding factor in some of the above mentioned post mortem studies is the possible increase in tissue cAMP levels that occur after death because of the different rates of inactivation of adenyl cyclase and phosphodiesterase (the enzyme that metabolizes cAMP) (Schmidt *et al.*, 1971). Studies which avoided this problem by using a focused high intensity microwave beam to kill animals showed no change in brain cAMP levels after ethanol treatment (Redos *et al.*, 1976; Breese *et al.*, 1979).

No change in adenyl cyclase activity with acute ethanol treatment has been reported (Israel *et al.*, 1972; Kuriyama, 1977). Analysis of Arrhenius plots further indicated, that in contrast to membrane Na^+/K^+ ATPase activity, adenyl cyclase (basal and dopamine or NaF stimulated) was not altered by ethanol. Recent work however indicates that ethanol added *in vitro* in the presence of GTP stimulates specific dopamine-sensitive adenyl cyclase from various brain areas (Rabin and Molinoff, 1981; Rabin and Molinoff, 1983; Luthin and Tabakoff, 1984). This stimulation occurred at pharmacologically relevant concentrations of ethanol (50 mM). The effect of ethanol was not due to the release of endogenous catecholamines since various antagonist drugs did not modify the effect of ethanol (Rabin and Molinoff, 1981). Ethanol's effect on dopamine-stimulated cyclase was also not mediated by a change in the affinity or number of dopaminergic receptors (Rabin and Molinoff, 1981). Enzyme activity in the presence of NaF was also stimulated by ethanol as was the V_{max} of the reaction. However, cholera toxin, which stimulates adenyl cyclase activity by blocking hydrolysis of GTP, did not modify the effect of ethanol on adenyl cyclase (Luthin and Tabakoff, 1984). Therefore, it is likely that ethanol acts on the guanine nucleotide regulatory protein, in some way favoring the formation of an active GTP protein-catalytic unit complex (Hoffman and Tabakoff, 1982).

The above findings receive support from a study carried out on S49 lymphoma cells. Several variants of this cell line differ in the components of the receptor–adenyl cyclase complex. Stimulation of adenyl cyclase by ethanol occurred in all variants of the cell line except in the one missing the regulatory subunit (Rabin and Molinoff, 1983).

In contrast with the effect of ethanol on Na^+/K^+ ATPase activity, discussed in the previous section, the effect of ethanol on adenyl cyclase apparently does not depend in the lipid microenvironment of adenyl cyclase. Thus ethanol had no effect on Arrhenius parameters of the basal or dopamine-stimulated adenyl cyclase (Hoffman and Tabakoff, 1982).

Opiates, via receptors, have been shown to inhibit striatal adenyl cyclase by interacting with the inhibitory form of the regulatory protein of adenyl cyclase. Ethanol had no effect on this inhibitory action of opiates (Hoffman and Tabakoff, 1986). However, ethanol increased prostaglandin E mediated cAMP formation in murine neuroblastoma cells (Stenstrom and Richelson, 1982).

3.2.1.2. *Chronic ethanol treatment*. Equally discrepant effects on adenyl cyclase are reported after chronic ethanol treatment. Four days of intragastric intubations with ethanol (Shen *et al.*, 1976) or long-term ingestion of a 20% ethanol solution decreased brain cAMP levels by 40–50% (Shen *et al.*, 1983). No changes in cAMP levels were noted in all other studies (Redos *et al.*, 1976; Volicer *et al.*, 1976; Volicer and Hunter, 1977), except for an increase in cAMP levels in one study (Kuriyama, 1977). During withdrawal from ethanol, brain levels of cAMP were elevated (Volicer *et al.*, 1976; Volicer and Hunter, 1977).

Chronic ethanol treatment has been reported to either increase (Israel *et al.*, 1972; Kuriyama, 1977) or have no effect on adenyl cyclase activity (Seeber and Kuschinsky, 1976 Hunt *et al.*, 1979). A small decrease in dopamine sensitive adenyl cyclase of the corpus striatum was seen in preparations from mice given an ethanol-containing liquid diet for 7 days and killed 24 hr after termination of treatment (Tabakoff and Hoffman, 1979). It was postulated that this decrease in sensitivity to dopamine reflects the continuous stimulation of the enzyme by the chronic exposure to ethanol. Addition of ethanol to the enzyme preparation reversed the small depression in adenyl cyclase activity. This finding, however, could not be replicated (Rabin *et al.*, 1980). The opiate mediated inhibition of striatal adenyl cyclase was not modified by chronic ethanol treatment (Hoffman and Tabakoff, 1986).

Receptor mediated accumulation of cAMP in brain slices has been examined by some investigators to assess the effect of ethanol on adenyl cyclase activity under controlled conditions. This method is based on the measurement of the accumulation of (^{3}H)-cAMP formed from (^{3}H)adenine in the presence of specific agonists. At least 4 days of gastric intubations with ethanol were necessary to elevate norepinephrine stimulated cAMP formation. An increase in cAMP accumulation could be observed after withdrawal from only 3 days of ethanol treatment (Smith *et al.*, 1981).

A change in sensitivity in the cAMP generating system was indicated by the 4.3-fold shift to the right for the norepinephrine dose-response curves obtained in tissues from rats consuming ethanol in their drinking fluid for 16 weeks (French *et al.*, 1974, 1975). The reverse, an increase in sensitivity to norepinephrine, was observed in tissues from animals in which ethanol treatment was discontinued (French *et al.*, 1975). Since the hypersensitivity of the adenyl cyclase system was also observed with other amines (histamine, 5HT), and α- and β-noradrenergic antagonists were only partially effective in reducing the increased adenyl cyclase activity, the authors suggested that during withdrawal from ethanol there is a non-specific postjunctional supersensitivity (French *et al.*, 1975).

The effect of ethanol on a related enzyme, protein kinase, was examined in one study. Two weeks of ethanol treatment via a liquid diet resulted in four-fold elevation of synaptosomal cAMP-dependent protein kinase (Kuriyama, 1977). A single large dose of ethanol (4.0 g/kg i.p.) had no effect on this enzyme (Kuriyama, 1977). On the other hand, phosphodiesterase activity was not affected by the chronic ethanol treatment.

3.2.2. *Effect of Ethanol on the Cyclic Guanyl Nucleotide System*

The guanylate cyclase system has been investigated less intensively than the adenyl cyclase system. Consequently, the effect of ethanol on the guanyl nucleotide system is less well defined. Like adenyl cyclase, guanyl cyclase can be stimulated by various putative neurotransmitters. The overall reaction for cGMP synthesis is:

$$\text{GTP} \xrightarrow[\text{Guanylate cyclase}]{\text{Mn}^{2+}} \text{cGMP} + 5'\text{-GMP}$$

3.2.2.1. *Acute ethanol treatment.* Acute treatment with ethanol consistently and dose-dependently depletes brain cGMP levels (Redos *et al.*, 1976; Volicer *et al.*, 1976; Thurman *et al.*, 1977; Hunt *et al.*, 1977; Mailman *et al.*, 1978; Breese *et al.*, 1979). cGMP levels in CSF are also decreased by ethanol (Weitbrecht and Cramer, 1980). Cerebellum is the brain area most sensitive to the depressant effects of ethanol (Volicer *et al.*, 1976; Hunt *et al.*, 1977; Mailman *et al.*, 1978). The largest depletion of cGMP occurs at the time of peak elevation in blood ethanol levels (Hunt *et al.*, 1977).

The significance of this consistent and large effect of ethanol on cGMP is uncertain. In studies in which the effects of motor activity, of changes in arterial carbon dioxide or of oxygen tension, all known to affect cerebellar cGMP levels, were controlled for, the ethanol-induced depression of cGMP levels were prevented (Breese *et al.*, 1979; Lundberg *et al.*, 1979). It is therefore possible that the depressant effect of ethanol reflects a secondary effect to other actions of ethanol.

3.2.2.2. *Chronic ethanol treatment.* Chronic ethanol treatment (26 days) resulted in development of little or no tolerance to the depressant effect of ethanol on cGMP levels (Volicer *et al.*, 1976; Volicer *et al.*, 1977a; Volicer *et al.*, 1977b). In fact a rebound increase in cGMP in the vestibular region was reported after ingestion of ethanol via a liquid diet for 14 days; the elevation was preceded by an increase in guanyl cyclase (Stenstrom and Richelson, 1982). After 8 weeks of treatment guanyl cyclase activity returned to control levels (Stenstrom and Richelson, 1982). During withdrawal from ethanol cGMP levels were elevated in cerebellum (Volicer *et al.*, 1976). Also a negative correlation was found between levels of cAMP and GABA levels in the cerebellum (Volicer *et al.*, 1977a; Volicer *et al.*, 1977b).

3.2.3. *Conclusions*

Acute ethanol treatment most likely decreases cAMP levels in brain and activates adenyl cyclase by an effect on the guanine nucleotide binding regulatory protein of the enzyme. With chronic ethanol treatment tolerance develops to these acute effects of ethanol. The effect of ethanol on the guanyl nucleotide system is not clear at the present.

3.3 Norepinephrine

The catecholamines dopamine and norepinephrine are synthesized from the precursor amino acid tyrosine. The rate limiting step in this synthesis is the first enzyme in the sequence, tyrosine hydroxylase. Metabolism of norepinephrine proceeds through three major pathways catalyzed by monoamine oxidase, by catechol *O*-methyl transferase (COMT) and by aldehyde reductase or aldehyde dehydrogenase. The abbreviated sequences for both syntheses of catabolism are shown in Fig. 1. Four types of noradrenergic receptors have been characterized. β-1 and β-2 receptors are differentiated on the basis of their affinities for norepinephrine as well as for specific inhibitors: β-1 receptors have equal affinity for norepinephrine and epinephrine, but β-2 receptors have greater affinity for epinephrine. Activation of both receptors results in stimulation of adenyl cyclase activity. α-1 and α-2 receptors are distinguished by the use of specific agonists and antagonists. Stimulation of these receptors results in the inhibition of adenyl cyclase activity.

3.3.1. *Acute Effect of Ethanol*

3.3.1.1. *Levels and turnover.* There is considerable inconsistency in the early reports on the effects of ethanol on noradrenergic neurons. For example, brain noreprinephine levels were reported to decrease (Corrodi *et al.*, 1966; Carlsson *et al.*, 1973; Aldegunde *et al.*, 1984), increase (Bradawy *et al.*, 1983), or to be unaffected (Haggendal and Lindqvist, 1961; Lundqvist, 1973; Rawat, 1974; Pohorecky, 1974; Erickson and Matchett, 1975) after a single dose of ethanol. Similarly, the turnover of norepinephrine, as estimated by a variety of methods, was reported to be decreased (Corrodi *et al.*, 1966; Hunt and Majchrowicz, 1974; Thadani *et al.*, 1976; Thadani and Truitt, 1977; Bacopoulos *et al.*, 1978; Carlsson and Lindqvist, 1973), increased (Svensson and Waldeck, 1973; Carlsson *et al.*, 1973; Hunt and Majchrowicz, 1974; Pohorecky and Jaffe, 1975; Bacopoulos *et al.*, 1978; Ahtee *et al.*, 1979) or unchanged (Haggendal and Lindqvist, 1961; Bacopoulos *et al.*, 1978).

It is clear that such discrepancies are due, at least in part, to regional specificity and the biphasic nature of ethanol's action. Low doses of ethanol increase norepinephrine turnover (Pohorecky and Jaffe, 1975; Bacopoulos *et al.*, 1978) and high doses decrease turnover (Carlsson and Lindqvist, 1973; Svensson and Waldeck, 1973; Carlsson *et al.*, 1973; Pohorecky, 1974; Bacopoulos *et al.*, 1978; Ahtee *et al.*, 1979; Aldegunde *et al.*, 1984; Engel and Rydberg, 1985). The effect of a given dose of ethanol also varies with time after injection. When blood ethanol levels were rising, the turnover of norepinephrine increased, but when ethanol levels were falling so did the turnover of norepinephrine (Hunt and Majchrowicz, 1974; Pohorecky and Jaffe, 1975; Smith *et al.*, 1985).

The regional non-uniformity of the effects of ethanol on noradrenergic neurons in the brain is evident from studies which examined norepinephrine turnover in several brain areas. A moderate dose of ethanol (2.0 g/kg i.p.) increased norepinephrine turnover in the

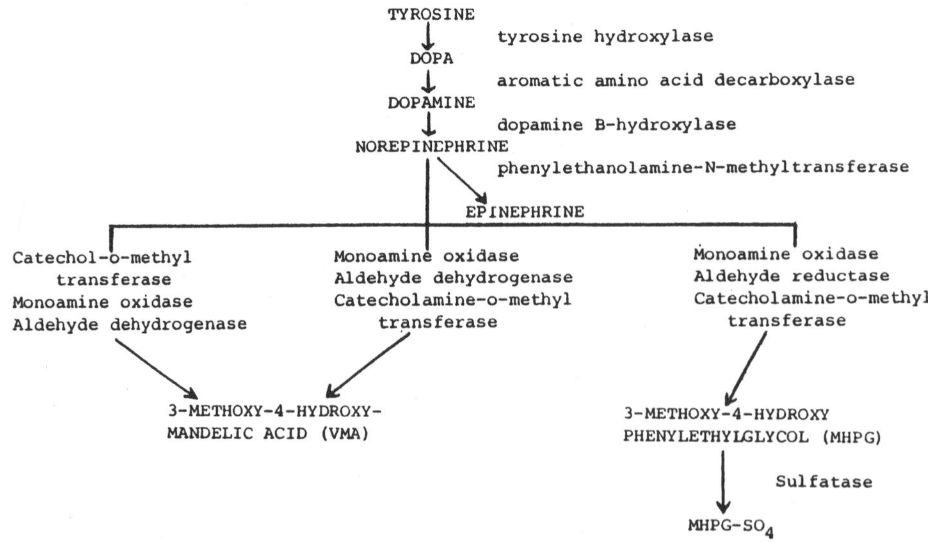

FIG. 1.

brain stem, decreased norepinephrine turnover in the hypothalamus and had no effect in the other areas that were examined (Bacopoulos *et al.*, 1978). This regional specificity could be interpreted as indicating that, in part, ethanol's action on these neurons is indirect. For example the direct effects of ethanol on norepinephrine metabolism in a given brain area could be modified by inputs from non-noradrenergic brain areas, by hormones, etc. However, regional differences in susceptibility to ethanol may also represent actual functional or biochemical differences between neuronal cell groups in the brain.

The effect of ethanol on levels of norepinephrine metabolites, primarily 3-methoxy-4-hydroxyphenylethylene glycol (MHPG) have also been examined. Accumulation of brain MHPG, or of its conjugated form (MHPG-sulfate) has been shown to be an index of central noradrenergic activity. Ethanol (6 g/kg by intubation) decreased MHPG sulfate in one study (Brown *et al.*, 1978) while an increase in unconjugated MHPG was found in another (5 g/kg by intubation) (Karoum *et al.*, 1976). In man ethanol (6 hr after ingestion of 0.9–1.2 g/kg) increased CSF levels of MHPG (Borg *et al.*, 1981, 1983). CSF levels of this metabolite have been employed as a possible index of norepinephrine turnover in brain. Therefore the results of this study indicated that ingestion of ethanol increased norepinephrine turnover in the brain.

Overall the peripheral sympathoadrenomedullary system is stimulated by ethanol in a dose-related fashion. Early studies with human subjects reported an increase in plasma levels and in urinary excretion of catecholamines and their metabolites, suggesting that ethanol stimulated the sympathoadrenomedullary system (Perman, 1961; Anton, 1965; Brohult *et al.*, 1970; Myrsten *et al.*, 1971). There was a change in the urinary pattern of catecholamine metabolites with a decrease in biogenic amine acid metabolites and an increase in biogenic amine aldehyde metabolites (Smith *et al.*, 1960; Perman, 1961; Davis *et al.*, 1967). It was postulated that there was a shift in the intraneuronal metabolism of catecholamines from an oxidative to a reductive pathway. However, subsequent research indicated that the shift in catecholamine metabolites represented primarily a shift in hepatic and not intraneuronal biogenic amine metabolism. Furthermore, no shift in catecholamine metabolism was found in the brain after an acute dose of ethanol (Karoum *et al.*, 1976; Thadani and Truitt, 1977). More recent studies using more sensitive techniques have shown an increase in catecholamines in plasma (Ireland *et al.*, 1984) and have confirmed the increase in the excretion of norepinephrine and epinephrine and their metabolites in urine (Brohult *et al.*, 1970; Myrsten *et al.*, 1971) after ingestion of ethanol in man. The excretion of catecholamines was larger in subjects showing flushing of the skin after ingestion of ethanol (Kijima, 1979). The excretion of epinephrine, but not that of norepinephrine remained high during hangover (Myrsten *et al.*, 1971) although in another study both catecholamines remained high in hangover (Brohult *et al.*, 1970). Small doses of ethanol produced primarily an increase in urinary norepinephrine excretion rather than that of epinephrine (Anton, 1965). On the other hand, after a 0.5 mg/kg dose of ethanol the rise in plasma epinephrine was very rapid, while the increase in plasma norepinephrine levels was delayed (Ireland *et al.*, 1984).

It is worthwhile noting that ethanol in small to moderate doses may actually alter activation of central and peripheral catecholamine systems in stressed subjects. For example, depletion of catecholamines in brain and adrenals produced in rats by immobilization at low temperature was decreased by pretreatment with ethanol (Kuriyama *et al.*, 1984). A larger dose (3.0 g/kg) was necessary for the protective effect to be also exerted on the adrenal medulla (Kuriyama *et al.*, 1984). Brain catecholamine levels were actually increased in guinea pigs subjected to cold and given a 2.0 g/kg injection of ethanol (Huttunen, 1982). Stress-induced decrease in brain catecholamines (DeTurck and Vogel, 1982) and the increase in plasma catecholamines (Hayashi *et al.*, 1978; DeTurck and Vogel, 1982) were lessened by ethanol. Ethanol may also have a "protective" effect in stressed human subjects. For example, individuals about to learn how to fly a glider showed an increased excretion of norepinephrine in urine. Small doses of ethanol blocked this stress-induced elevation of norepinephrine excretion (Goddard, 1958).

3.3.1.2. *In vitro effects of ethanol.* The effect of ethanol on noradrenergic function have also been examined in *in vitro* systems (brain slices, synaptosomes, peripheral tissues). The effect of ethanol on the uptake of radioactive norepinephrine was examined in a number of studies. Addition of ethanol to brain slices, synaptic vesicles (up to 600 mM) (Roach *et al.*, 1973; Majchrowicz, 1973) or perfused heart (up to 200 mM) did not affect (^{3}H)-norepinephrine uptake (Gothert *et al.*, 1976). At very high concentrations of ethanol (217 mM), uptake of (^{3}H)-norepinephrine in brain slices was decreased (Roach *et al.*, 1973; Israel *et al.*, 1973), the effect being larger at reduced potassium concentrations in the medium (Israel *et al.*, 1973). The potassium-stimulated release of (^{3}H)-norepinephrine from pre-labeled cortical brain slices was decreased by ethanol (Israel *et al.*, 1975; Howerton and Collins, 1984). However in another study employing cortical brain slices ethanol (100–250 mM) had no effect on potassium-stimulated release of norepinephrine (Holman and Snape, 1985; Murphy *et al.*, 1985; McBride *et al.*, 1986). On the other hand, although basal release of (^{3}H)-norepinephrine from superfused hypothalamic slices was not affected by a comparatively lower concentration of ethanol (69.6 mM) the potassium stimulated release of the amine was increased (Hyatt and Tyce, 1985).

Turning to peripheral noradrenergically innervated tissues, basal release of (^{3}H)-norepinephrine from pre-labeled vas deferens preparations was enhanced by ethanol at relatively low concentrations (65 mM) (Degani *et al.*, 1979; Howerton and Collins, 1984). Furthermore, when the intraneuronal metabolism of the amine was blocked by pretreated animals with an MAO inhibitor, the spontaneous efflux of norepinephrine in the presence of ethanol was increased even further. This effect of ethanol was dependent on the presence of calcium. All other alcohols tested had effects similar to those of ethanol. Because the rank order for the potentiation of spontaneous norepinephrine release from the vas deferens correlated with the antihemolytic potency of the tested alcohols, it was suggested that these represented non-specific actions of the alcohols on the presynaptic and vesicular membranes (Degani *et al.*, 1979). In the isolated perfused heart ethanol has been shown to depress stimulated release of norepinephrine (Gothert and Kennerknecht, 1975; Gothert *et al.*, 1976; Gothert and Thielecke, 1976). The inhibitory effect of ethanol was dependent on its concentration and on the method used for stimulating the release of norepinephrine. Basal release of norepinephrine was not affected by ethanol. Ethanol was most effective in inhibiting the release of norepinephrine induced by cholinergic stimulation. The concentrations of ethanol required to inhibit the release of norepinephrine by 50% (IC_{50}) were 1150 mM for electrical stimulation, 830 mM for potassium chloride, 148 mM for acetylcholine, and 129 mM for dimethylphenylpiperazine (a nicotinic agonist). The uptake of norepinephrine by the heart appeared to be less sensitive to ethanol (IC_{50} = 760 mM). It is noteworthy that the threshold concentration of ethanol for the dimethylphenylpiperazine-stimulated release of norepinephrine is compatible with moderate levels of intoxication *in vivo*. The extent of the selectivity of the effect of ethanol for the cholinergically induced release of norepinephrine is especially striking in view of a similar differential sensitivity of central cholinergic neurons to ethanol (Carmichael and Israel, 1975). Gothert and associates postulated that ethanol may uncouple the release of norepinephrine from its cholinergic activation (Gothert *et al.*, 1976). Tolerance to ethanol has also been demonstrated in another sympathetically innervated organ, the vas deferens of rats. In this tissue preparation ethanol dose-dependently decreases contractions induced by norepinephrine , KCl or by electrical transmural stimulation (DeTurck and Pohorecky, 1986). Chronic ethanol treatment for 2 weeks produced significant tolerance to this inhibitory action of ethanol.

Increasing the extracellular concentration of calcium decreased the in vitro inhibitory effectiveness of ethanol on contractions induced by NE, KCl or by electrical stimulation (DeTurck and Pohorecky, 1987a). Additional research using tissues from animals treated with ethanol, and incubated in vitro with the calcium blocker nifedipine, suggested that changes in calcium mobilization are involved in both the acute effects of ethanol on vas deferens contractions and in the development of tolerance to ethanol. Chronic treatment with ethanol also resulted in subsensitivity of the vas deferens to the in vitro effects of alpha-adrenoceptor agonist and antagonist drugs, as well as to adenosine and naloxone

(DeTurck and Pohorecky, 1987b). This was interpreted to indicate that both pre- and post-junctional mechanisms are involved in the modulation of neurotransmission in the rat vas deferens.

3.3.1.3. *Enzymes.* A number of studies examined the effect of ethanol on various enzymes involved in catecholamine synthesis. The activity of tyrosine hydroxylase, the first rate-limiting enzyme for catecholamine synthesis, was increased 25 min after an acute dose of ethanol in the striatum, locus coeruleus, and frontal cortex (Baizer *et al.*, 1981; French *et al.*, 1985) and in the adrenal medulla (French *et al.*, 1985). Also the oral administration of 4.0 g/kg of ethanol increased the activities of tyrosine hydroxylase, dopamine-β-hydroxylase (DBH), and phenylethanolamine-*N*-methyltransferase (PNMT) in the adrenals (Cohen *et al.*, 1980). The effect of ethanol was independent of adrenal innervation, which suggests that it acted directly on the adrenal medulla (enzyme activities rose probably in response to the enhanced release of catecholamines), or that it was a secondary response to its other peripheral and/or central effects (e.g. changes in blood glucose, hypothermia).

3.3.2. *Chronic Ethanol Treatment*

3.3.2.1. *Levels and turnover.* There is general agreement that chronic ethanol exposure increases the turnover of norepinephrine in both brain and peripheral tissues. Chronic ethanol treatment did not alter (Hunt and Majchrowicz, 1974; Pohorecky, 1974; Ahtee and Eriksson, 1975), increased (Post and Sun, 1973; Ortiz *et al.*, 1974; Rossi *et al.*, 1976; Chopde *et al.*, 1977), or decreased (Rawat, 1974) levels of norepinephrine in the brain. Turnover of norepinephrine on the other hand was increased in all the brain areas that have been examined (Hunt and Majchrowicz, 1974; Pohorecky, 1974; Ahtee and Svanstrom-Fraser, 1975; Pohorecky *et al.*, 1976; Karoum *et al.*, 1976; Thadani *et al.*, 1976). Turnover of norepinephrine was also increased during withdrawal from ethanol (Pohorecky, 1974; Ahtee and Svastrom-Fraser, 1975). There are no studies correlating changes in norepinephrine turnover with development of tolerance and/or physical dependence to ethanol. However, it is apparent from the literature that there is development of tolerance in the noradrenergic system since norepinephrine turnover was increased at blood ethanol levels which would depress norepinephrine turnover after an acute dose of the alcohol (Pohorecky, 1974; Pohorecky *et al.*, 1976).

In peripheral tissues chronic ethanol treatment also increased the turnover of catecholamines. Four days of severe intoxication (intubation with ethanol every 6 hr) decreased epinephrine/norepinephrine in adrenal medulla (Adams and Hirst, 1982b, 1984). However, a less severe but longer duration of ethanol treatment (liquid diet for up to 30 days) did not alter levels of catecholamines in the adrenals (Pohorecky, 1974; Pohorecky *et al.*, 1974; Guaza and Borrell, 1983). Chronic ethanol exposure did not alter endogenous norepinephrine levels in the heart (Pohorecky, 1974; Ahtee and Eriksson, 1975), nor did it alter the myocardial uptake of intravenously injected labeled norepinephrine (Pohorecky, 1974). Four days of ethanol intoxication (administered intragastrically every 6 hr) was shown to produce cardiomegaly in rats which correlated with the increase in plasma catecholamines. During the initial 2 days there was a decrease in cardiac catecholamines with a return to control levels by 4 days (Adams and Hirst, 1983, 1986).

The increase in norepinephrine turnover produced by chronic treatment with ethanol is supported by measures of postsynaptic sensitivity determined in tissue slices. For example, brain slices from rats kept on an ethanol-containing liquid diet showed decreased sensitivity to norepinephrine induced cAMP accumulation (French *et al.*, 1975). Similar changes in sensitivity to norepinephrine were observed in liver slices of similarly treated rats (French *et al.*, 1976).

In the perfused heart ethanol (150 mM) and other anesthetics had no effect on spontaneous release of norepinephrine nor on the uptake of exogenous norepinephrine, but the release of norepinephrine in response to activation of nicotinic receptors was decreased (Gothert *et al.*, 1976). This was interpreted as a hydrophobic interaction with the nicotinic receptors resulting in a conformational change leading to inhibition of stimulus formation.

The maximal firing rate of the sinus–atrial node in response to the β-agonist isoproterenol was decreased in tissues from rats ingesting ethanol for up to 40 weeks. These findings indicate that ethanol treatment resulted in decreased sensitivity of myocardial β-receptors (Posner *et al.*, 1985), which is what one would expect as a result of elevated turnover of norepinephrine.

3.3.2.2. *Receptors.* The effect of chronic ethanol treatment on norepinephrine receptors is dependent on the duration of treatment. Short term (4 days) continuous intoxication with ethanol had no effect on α- or β-receptor binding in brain (Hunt and Dalton, 1981). However, longer treatment durations with ethanol (7–60 days) did decrease β-receptors in brain without a consistent effect on α-receptors (Banerjee *et al.*, 1978; Muller *et al.*, 1980; Rabin *et al.*, 1980). The effect of ethanol was specific to the β-2 receptors (Rabin *et al.*, 1980). Acute treatment with ethanol decreased the affinity of the high affinity state of β-adrenoceptors for isoproterenol in the cerebral cortex (Hoffman *et al.*, 1987). Furthermore, ethanol also potentiated the action of guinine nucleotides on agonist binding. This suggested to the authors an action of ethanol at the level of the stimulatory guanine nucleotide-binding protein (Ns) which is one of the subunits of the β-adrenoceptor. Chronic treatment with ethanol resulted in the presence of only low affinity agonist binding sites, such as occurs after uncoupling of receptors (Hoffman *et al.*, 1987).

Although acute treatment with ethanol did not alter β-adrenergic receptor binding in the heart, chronic treatment did (Banerjee *et al.*, 1978). Specific binding of [^{3}H]-dihydroalprenolol (DHA) to heart particulate fractions was decreased by 43% in rats fed an ethanol-containing liquid diet for 60 days, compared with the control group. By contrast, in rats inhaling ethanol for 3 weeks neither α- nor β-adrenoceptors in the myocardium were affected (Sabourault *et al.*, 1981). In a more recent study, acute ethanol treatment increased the proportion of the low affinity binding site in the heart (Hoffman *et al.*, 1987). Mice consuming a liquid diet containing ethanol for 7 days showed a decrease in low affinity isoproterenol binding sites in the heart (Kwast *et al.*, 1987). Interestingly, a decrease in the high-affinity agonist binding sites was present in control animals treated with an equicaloric sucrose containing liquid diet.

A subsensitivity of peripheral sympathetic receptors with chronic ethanol treatment was indicated in another study. Animals treated with ethanol for 2 months showed a smaller increase in plasma cAMP after an isoproterenol challenge (Ihrig *et al.*, 1978). This was interpreted to reflect a subsensitivity of peripheral β-noradrenergic receptors. Long-term (250 days) exposure of rats to ethanol via drinking water did not alter β-receptor sensitivity evaluated *in vivo* (Liljequist *et al.*, 1978).

3.3.2.3. *Enzymes.* Chronic ethanol treatment elevates the activity of all the enzymes involved in catecholamine synthesis. However, short term treatment with ethanol (intubations every 8 hr for 48 hr) did not alter TOH activity in the adrenals or the brain (Masserano *et al.*, 1983). Longer ethanol treatment (ingestion of a liquid diet for up to 100 days) decreased TOH activity in the caudate and hypothalamus (Friedhoff and Miller, 1973). In the adrenals, TOH, DBH and PNMT were elevated in rats after chronic treatment with ethanol (liquid diet or a 5–25% solution for up to 12 weeks) (Pohorecky *et al.*, 1974; Cohen *et al.*, 1980; Rubio *et al.*, 1984). Catecholamine synthesis (Pohorecky *et al.*, 1974; Cohen *et al.*, 1980) and release from the adrenals was also increased (Cohen *et al.*, 1980). An intact adrenal innervation is essential for the ethanol-induced elevations of PNMT activity and catecholamine turnover, but not for elevations in the activities of tyrosine hydroxylase and DBH (Cohen *et al.*, 1980).

Sensitivity of noradrenergic neurons to ethanol may differ depending on the tissue. Treatment with a liquid diet containing ethanol for 2 weeks elevated DBH activity by 54% in the adrenals, but by only 16% in the superior cervical ganglion (Sze *et al.*, 1974). With 3 weeks of ethanol treatment, the activity of this enzyme in the adrenals was elevated by 303%, but decreased by 44% in the superior cervical ganglion. The mechanism for this organ specificity to ethanol is at present unknown, and these data need to be expanded to other peripheral tissues as well. It is known, however, that sympathetic nerves do differ in various tissues. For instance, sympathetic nerves that regulate blood pressure differ significantly from those that regulate heart rate (Simpson, 1980). Therefore caution should be exercised in generalizing the effects of ethanol from one tissue or organ to another.

Chronic immobilization stress results in a specific decline in α_2- but not α_1-receptors in the cortex of rats. Interestingly this stress-induced effect was decreased if the stressed animals were ingesting ethanol as part of a liquid diet (Lynch *et al.*, 1983).

Alcoholics have been shown to have altered MAO activity. MAO activity in postmortem brain samples from alcoholics who committed suicide was lower compared to samples from control subjects (Gothfries *et al.*, 1975; Oreland *et al.*, 1983). Also there was a significant decrease in MAO activity in platelets from abstinent alcoholics compared to nonalcoholic subjects (Takahashi *et al.*, 1976; Brown, 1977; Sullivan *et al.*, 1978a; Major and Murphy, 1978; Sullivan *et al.*, 1978b; Fowler *et al.*, 1981, Tsuji *et al.*, 1982). The depression persisted even after abstinence for one year (Sullivan *et al.*, 1978) but in one case platelet MAO activity recovered after 4 weeks of abstinence (Takahashi *et al.*, 1976). The depression in platelet MAO activity apparently did not correlate with chronicity or severity of alcohol drinking (Major and Murphy, 1978). Significance of these findings of depressed MAO activity in platelets of alcoholics is not clear. Besides questions concerning the assay procedure (e.g. type of substrate used), sample (how samples, especially postmortem brain samples, were obtained, handled and stored) and subject (psychological condition, use of medication by the subjects, etc.) related issues, there is the question of significance of platelet MAO activity in general—an issue that remains unresolved at the time of writing.

3.3.3. *Withdrawal*

Withdrawal from ethanol is generally characterized by an overall state of hyperexcitability (see Section 6.2). In alcoholics sympathoadrenal activation is indicated by such symptoms as tachycardia and other disturbances in cardiac function, and increases in blood pressure (Victor, 1966; Gross *et al.*, 1974). In experimental animals, time-related changes in turnover or norepinephrine have been described in the brain and the heart (Pohorecky, 1974; Pohorecky *et al.*, 1974; Ahtee and Svastrom-Fraser, 1975). After exposure to an ethanol-containing liquid diet, there was a 45% increase in the accumulation of newly synthesized norepinephrine in the brain and in the heart of animals 3–8 hr after the discontinuation of ethanol. (^{3}H)-Labeled metabolites of norepinephrine also showed a 40% increase during withdrawal. By 48 hr all parameters were normal. Ahtee and Svanstrom-Fraser found a 30% increase in norepinephrine turnover in hearts of rats withdrawn from ethanol after a 7 to 10 day exposure period (Ahtee and Svanstrom-Fraser, 1975). In the adrenals there were increases in the activities of tyrosine hydroxylase, DBH, and PNMT; in the release of catecholamines (Cohen *et al.*, 1980); and in catecholamine turnover (Pohorecky, 1974; Pohorecky *et al.*, 1974). Levels of catecholamines in the adrenals were unchanged during withdrawal from longer moderate treatment with ethanol (Pohorecky, 1974; Pohorecky *et al.*, 1974) but were decreased during withdrawal from short term severe intoxication (Adams and Hirst, 1982a, 1982b, 1984). Excretion of catecholamines in urine was increased during withdrawal (Pohorecky, 1974; Adams and Hirst, 1982b, 1984), while levels of epinephrine and norepinephrine in the adrenals decreased (Pohorecky, 1974; Adams and Hirst, 1982b). There does not appear to be a good correlation between the severity of the withdrawal syndrome and adrenomedullary activation (Adams and Hirst, 1982b). For instance, in rats pretreated with diazepam the withdrawal syndrome was significantly ameliorated, but the excretion of urinary catecholamines was not. However, propranolol decreased the excretion of catecholamines during withdrawal, but had only a small short term effect on the symptoms of withdrawal. Lastly, hexamethonium (a cholinergic antagonist) increased both the excretion of urinary catecholamines and aggravated the withdrawal syndrome.

During withdrawal tyrosine hydroxlase activity in brain and in the adrenals increased (Friedhoff and Miller, 1973; Masserano *et al.*, 1983). In the brain the increase in tyrosine hydroxlase was restricted to only the locus coeruleus (Masserano *et al.*, 1983). Furthermore by using immunotitration of the enzyme protein, it was demonstrated that the increase in tyrosine hydroxylase activity represents new enzyme synthesis (Masserano *et al.*, 1983).

CSF levels of MHPG were elevated in intoxicated alcoholics as well as during withdrawal from ethanol (Borg *et al.*, 1983a, 1983b). However, one to three weeks after withdrawal from ethanol MHPG levels in CSF were reported to be decreased (Borg *et al.*, 1983). In one study also levels of norepinephrine in CSF were increased during withdrawal from ethanol (Hawley *et al.*, 1981). During withdrawal from ethanol the urinary excretion of catecholamines in alcoholics was elevated (Ogata *et al.*, 1971; Sellers *et al.*, 1976; Borg *et al.*, 1983). A small increase in platelet MAO activity was observed during withdrawal from alcohol (Wiberg *et al.*, 1977).

Despite the increase in catecholamine turnover, β-receptor binding was elevated in brain and in the adrenals (Banerjee *et al.*, 1978; Kuriyama *et al.*, 1981). In the heart [^{3}H]-DHA binding increased 49% 48 hr after discontinuation of ethanol administration, and 136% by 72 hr. Further characterization indicated that the increased binding was due mainly to more binding sites (Banerjee *et al.*, 1978).

3.3.4. *Pharmacological Studies*

A number of investigators have used a pharmacological approach to delineate the role of brain catecholamines in ethanol's action in the organism. Agonists or antagonists of noradrenergic function were examined with respect to the effects of ethanol on motor activity, sedation, ethanol self-selection, and withdrawal severity in experimental animals. In man, various behavioral measures as well as withdrawal severity were evaluated.

The increase in motor activity produced by small to moderate doses of ethanol was blocked by pretreatment with α-methyl-*p*-tyrosine (AMPT), an inhibitor of catecholamine synthesis (Blum *et al.*, 1973a). On the other hand a decrease in catecholamines produced by pretreatment with 6-hydroxydopamine (6-OHDA), a neurotoxin for catecholaminergic neurons, had no effect on ethanol induced hyperactivity, but reversed the motor depressant effect of larger doses of ethanol (Masur *et al.*, 1979).

Ingestion of ethanol by rats in self-selection tests was increased by localized brain lesions that decrease norepinephrine levels (Kiianmaa *et al.*, 1975; Melchior and Myers, 1976). On the other hand a decrease in whole brain noradrenergic function has also been reported to decrease ethanol selection (Myers and Melchoir, 1975; Melchoir and Myers, 1976; Amit *et al.*, 1977; Brown *et al.*, 1977).

In experimental animals withdrawal severity (handling seizures) was increased by drugs that decrease noradrenergic function (reserpine, AMPT, phentolamine, propanolol) (Goldstein, 1973; Blum and Wallace, 1974). However, pretreatment with a noradrenergic neurotoxin 6-OHDA prior to induction of physical dependence did not alter the withdrawal syndrome (Ritzmann and Tabakoff, 1976; Frye *et al.*, 1977; Tabakoff and Ritzmann, 1977; Wood and Laverty, 1977). This was interpreted to mean that noradrenergic neurons are not necessary for the development of physical dependence (Ritzmann and Tabakoff, 1976; Tabakoff and Ritzmann, 1977).

The sedative action of ethanol was potentiated by AMPT and by the β-adrenergic blocking drug propanolol (Blum *et al.*, 1972; Erickson *et al.*, 1975; Munoz and Giuvernau, 1980), as well as by L-dopa (Blum *et al.*, 1973a, 1973b) which increases noradrenergic function. However in other studies ethanol induced sedation was decreased by pretreatment with L-dopa (Blum *et al.*, 1972) as well as by D-amphetamine (Erickson *et al.*, 1975). Potentiation of sedative action of ethanol by propranolol is, however, questionable due to its CNS depressant effect (Wimbish *et al.*, 1977) and because it decreases the metabolism of ethanol (Isselbacher and Carter, 1976).

Evidence for the involvement of catecholamines in the depressant effects of ethanol has been obtained from studies on LS and SS mice. These lines of mice have been selectively bred for their differential sensitivity to ethanol-induced loss of righting reflex (sleep time). The long sleep (LS) mice are more sensitive to the depressant effects of ethanol compared to the short sleep (SS) mice (McClearn and Kakihana, 1981), have 30% lower levels and turnover of NE only in the cerebellum (French and Weiner, 1984) and higher catecholamine content and tyrosine hydroxylase activity in the adrenal glands (French *et al.*, 1985). Treatment with ethanol decreased the turnover of catecholamines in some brain areas and the adrenal medulla of LS mice (French *et al.*, 1985) while it increased adrenals or had no effect (brain) on the turnover of catecholamines in SS mice (French and Weiner, 1984; French *et al.*, 1985). In reserpine pretreated mice ethanol decreased sleep time by 34% in LS mice (Masserano and Weiner, 1982).

A decrease in noradrenergic function produced by treatment with AMPT in man decreased the euphoria produced by an acute dose of ethanol (Ahlenius *et al.*, 1973). The β-adrenergic blocker propranolol also blocked the cognitive, perceptual and motor effects of ethanol, as well as the hypoglycemia, but not the elevation of blood fatty acids produced by ethanol (Mendelson *et al.*, 1974; Svedsen *et al.*, 1978). Other effects of ethanol, e.g. its psychomotor depression, were found to be potentiated by propranolol (Alkana *et al.*, 1976). Propranolol was reported to be more effective than diazepam in decreasing the tension in depressed alcoholics (Carlsson and Fusth, 1976). Also in alcoholics undergoing withdrawal, propranolol has been reported to decrease the withdrawal symptomology (Sellers *et al.*, 1977) but it had no effect on tremors occurring during withdrawal (Teravainen and Larsen, 1976). The α-adrenergic agonist clonidine was found to improve some of the symptoms occurring during withdrawal from ethanol (Bjokqvist, 1975).

3.3.5. *Conclusions*

Acute ethanol treatment results in a biphasic effect on noradrenergic neurons in brain. Turnover of norepinephrine increases with small doses of ethanol and while blood ethanol levels are rising, and decreases with large doses of ethanol and when blood ethanol levels fall. By contrast the release of catecholamines from the adrenal medulla is stimulated dose-dependently. Chronic ethanol treatment increases turnover of catecholamines in brain and peripheral tissues. Turnover of catecholamines is also increased during withdrawal. The increase in norepinephrine turnover in chronic ethanol-treated animals most likely results in the reported subsensitivity of β-receptors in brain and in the heart.

3.4. Dopamine

The synthesis of dopamine proceeds along the same pathway as that already described for norepinephrine, as shown in Section 3.3. The catabolism of dopamine involves the same enzyme systems already described for norepinephrine catabolism in Section 3.3; the schematic outline for dopamine is shown in Fig. 2.

Four different types of dopamine receptors may exist on the basis of their linkage with adenyl cyclase and their relative affinities for dopamine and dopamine antagonists. D-1 binding sites are linked to adenyl cyclase and differ from D-2 receptors on the basis of ligand affinity and in cellular localization. D-1 receptors are predominantly localized on non-

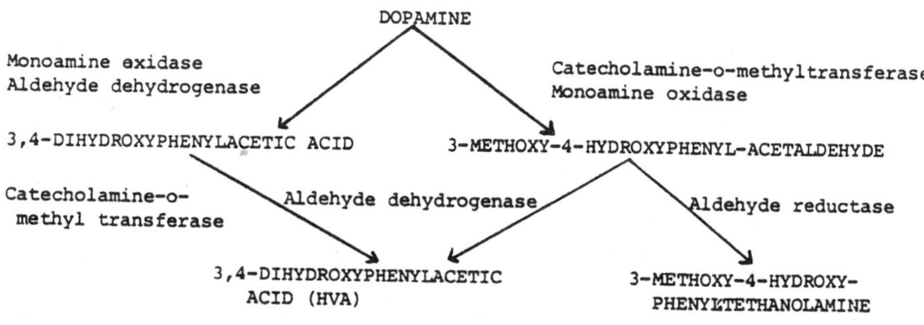

Fig. 2.

dopaminergic cell bodies, while D-2 receptors are predominantly localized on corticostriatal fibers. Very little is presently known about D-3 receptors, these receptors may be autoreceptors.

3.4.1. *Acute Effects of Ethanol*

3.4.1.1. *Levels and turnover.* Overall levels of dopamine are not affected by an acute dose of ethanol. Turnover of dopamine was increased by large acute doses of ethanol (Hunt and Majchrowicz, 1974; Karoum, *et al.*, 1976; Bustos and Roth, 1976; Wajda *et al.*, 1977; Bacopoulos *et al.*, 1978; Lai *et al.*, 1979; Reggiani *et al.*, 1980; Fadda *et al.*, 1980). Like with noradrenergic neurons, the effect of ethanol is dose, time, and region specific. Turnover of dopamine after 5 g/kg of ethanol was not affected during the first 3 hr and decreased thereafter (Hunt and Majchrowicz, 1974). As far as regional specificity, turnover of dopamine was increased in the olfactory tubercles, decreased in substantia nigra and caudate (Bacopoulos *et al.*, 1978) and was unchanged in the nucleus accumbens, amygdala and hypothalamus. After 3.2 g/kg of ethanol by intubation dopamine synthesis was increased in the caudate but not in substantia nigra or frontal cortex (Fadda *et al.*, 1980). In the rat doses below 4 g/kg ethanol had no effect on dopamine turnover, but in the monkey even 6.0 g/kg of ethanol by intubation had no effect on dopamine metabolism and release as examined using a push–pull cannula (Weiner *et al.*, 1980).

Recently the effect of ethanol on the metabolism of dopamine was examined in rats using transcerebral dialysis (Imperato and Di Chiara, 1986). Low doses of ethanol (0.25–0.5 g/kg i.p.) increased the release of dopamine from the nucleus accumbens. Doses from 1.0–2.5 g/kg of ethanol also increased the release of dopamine, as well as that of its metabolites dihydroxyphenylacetic acid (DOPAC) and homovanillic acid, from the nucleus accumbens and less so from the caudate. Finally, a very large dose of ethanol (5 g/kg i.p.) initially decreased and then increased dopamine release from both the accumbens and the caudate. These results were interpreted as indicating that ethanol preferentially increases dopaminergic neurotransmission in the mesolimbic system, possibly by activating the firing rate of these neurons. The latter hypothesis was based on the additional finding that a low dose of apomorphine completely reversed the stimulant effect of ethanol (0.5 g/kg) on dopamine release as well as on the motor stimulation. Furthermore γ-butyrolactone, which blocks the firing of dopaminergic neurons and the release of dopamine, also blocked the behavioral stimulation produced by the low dose of ethanol.

Interestingly, the effect of ethanol on dopamine metabolism is affected by genetic factors. C57BL mice, known to be relatively resistant to the behavioral and physiological effects of ethanol, were more resistant to the effect of ethanol on dopamine turnover, when compared to the more sensitive BALB and DBA mice (Kiianmaa and Tabakoff, 1983).

CSF levels of homovanillic acid, a major metabolite of dopamine, were not consistently altered by ethanol ingestion in man (Orenberg *et al.*, 1976; Major *et al.*, 1977).

3.4.1.2. In vitro *effects of ethanol.* The effect of ethanol on the potassium-stimulated release of (^{3}H)-dopamine was dependent on the dose and time after treatment (Darden and Hunt, 1978). Ethanol concentrations of 1–2 g/kg had no effect, 3–4 g/kg increased, and 6 g/kg first decreased and then 6–18 hr post ethanol treatment increased, (^{3}H)-dopamine release. In rats chronically treated with ethanol (4 days of daily intubations) (^{3}H)-dopamine release was higher but was reduced during withdrawal. Uptake returned to normal 7 days after termination of ethanol treatment (Darden and Hunt, 1978).

The potassium-stimulated synthesis of dopamine from (^{3}H)-tyrosine was examined in brain slices of olfactory tubercle in the presence of ethanol (43–174 mM) (Umezu *et al.*, 1980). Ethanol had no effect on dopamine synthesis at depolarizing concentrations of potassium. In striatal slices synthesis of dopamine was inhibited by ethanol at both low and high concentrations of potassium (Bustos *et al.*, 1976). Synthesis of (^{3}H)-dopamine was also inhibited in striatal synaptosomes obtained from rats injected with 2–4 g/kg ethanol (Pohorecky and Newman, 1977). This effect was time-related since 30 min post injection (^{3}H)-dopamine synthesis was actually increased.

3.4.1.3. *Receptor binding studies. In vitro* dopamine receptor binding (using ^{3}H-spiroperidol) was decreased in a dose-dependent manner. However, rather high concentrations of ethanol were needed (Hruska and Silbergeld, 1980; Rabin and Molinoff, 1981). Scatchard analysis indicated that ethanol decreased the affinity of (^{3}H)-spiroperidol for the receptor without affecting the number of binding sites (Hruska and Silberfeld, 1980). *In vivo* a 3 g/kg dose of ethanol (by intubation) had no effect on (^{3}H)-spiroperidol binding (Barbaccia *et al.*, 1980; Lal *et al.*, 1980).

3.4.1.4. *Pharmacological studies.* The effects of ethanol on body temperature may be mediated by dopaminergic mechanisms. Apomorphine (a dopamine agonist) potentiated the hypothermic effect of ethanol, while haloperidol (a dopamine antagonist) decreased it (Yamawaki *et al.*, 1984). In man, eight behavioral measures of intoxication in "moderate" male drinkers were enhanced by apomorphine, a dopamine agonist (Alkana *et al.*, 1982).

3.4.2. *Chronic Ethanol Treatment*

3.4.2.1. *Levels and turnover.* Although overall chronic treatment with ethanol does not alter dopamine levels, dopamine levels were increased in a few studies (Post and Sun, 1973; Littleton *et al.*, 1974; Wajda *et al.*, 1977; Mena and Herrera, 1980). Treatment with ethanol for 7 to 28 days depressed dopamine turnover in most studies (Hunt and Majchrowicz, 1974; Ahtee and Svarstrom-Fraser, 1975; Tabakoff and Hoffman, 1978); however, no effect on dopamine turnover has also been reported (Lucchi *et al.*, 1983). A decrease in dopamine turnover as a result of chronic ethanol treatment may indicate that tolerance develops to the initial effects of ethanol on this neuronal system. Ingestion of a 8–24% ethanol solution for 270 days reduced dopamine levels and increased its synthesis in the striatum—this was interpreted as indicating that dopamine turnover was increased during withdrawal (Liljequist and Engel, 1979).

3.4.2.2. In vitro *effects of ethanol.* Dopamine release was enhanced after rats treated with ethanol for 60 days were challenged with ethanol (3.2 g/kg) (Fadda *et al.*, 1980). Dopamine synthesis was not affected by ethanol treatment in this study. Similarly (^{3}H)-dopamine synthesis was also not altered in striatal synaptosomes prepared from rats ingesting a liquid diet containing ethanol (Pohorecky and Newman, 1977). A challenge dose of ethanol had no effect on striatal dopamine metabolism in animals tolerant to the behavioral effects of ethanol (Kiianmaa and Tabakoff, 1983). The potassium-stimulated release of dopamine from brain slices prepared from rats inhaling ethanol vapor for 24 hr was decreased (Mullin and Ferko, 1983). Dopamine synthesis in striated synaptosomes was depressed in animals undergoing withdrawal (Pohorecky and Newman, 1977).

3.4.2.3. *Receptor binding studies.* The effect of chronic ethanol on dopamine receptors was dependent on the duration of treatment. A short treatment with ethanol (4–7 days) had no effect on binding of (^{3}H)-spiroperidol or (^{3}H)-apomorphine in the caudate nucleus of mice (Tabakoff and Hoffman, 1979; Rabin *et al.*, 1980; Hunt and Dalton, 1981). In rats, chronic ethanol treatment (2 weeks of daily intubations or 3 weeks of liquid diet ingestion) increased striatal binding of (^{3}H)-spiroperidol or (^{3}H)-sulpiride (Lai *et al.*, 1980; Barbaccia *et al.*, 1982). By contrast, up to 15 days of intubations with ethanol resulted in a decline in (^{3}H)-haloperidol binding in mesolimbic areas and no change in the striatum (Muller *et al.*, 1980). Binding was reduced 4 weeks after withdrawal from 13 month long ethanol treatment (Pelham *et al.*, 1980). This long term treatment apparently decreased the apparent number of binding sites.

3.4.2.4. *Pharmacological studies.* Overall dopamine agonists and antagonist drugs injected into mice 24 hr after withdrawal from chronic ethanol treatment (using liquid diet) were found to be less effective in producing their respective biochemical, physiological or behavioral effects (Hoffman and Tabakoff, 1977; Tabakoff and Hoffman, 1978; Tabakoff *et al.*, 1978; Block *et al.*, 1980). By contrast, in one study 14 days of ethanol ingestion (6 g/kg/day) increased the sensitivity to apomorphine (general motor and stereotyped activity) tested 15 hr after the last dose of ethanol (Lai *et al.*, 1980). Dopaminergic supersensitivity (locomotor activity in response to injection of dopamine into the nucleus accumbens) was also enhanced during the latter part of withdrawal from ethanol in animals ingesting an ethanol-containing solution (8–24%) for at least 5 months (Engel and Liljequist, 1976; Liljequist, 1978).

3.4.3. *Withdrawal from Ethanol*

Levels of homovanillic acid in the CSF were lower during withdrawal in comparison to those in alcoholics not undergoing withdrawal (Major *et al.*, 1977). This was interpreted to indicate that dopamine turnover was decreased during withdrawal. In support of this is the reported improvement of certain withdrawal symptoms in alcoholics treated with dopamine agonists (Borg and Weinholdt, 1982).

3.4.4. *Conclusions*

Acute ethanol increases dopamine release and turnover primarily in mesolimbic neurons. There is also a decrease in the affinity for binding to dopamine receptors. Chronic ethanol treatment decreases dopamine turnover; however, the results on dopamine receptor binding are inconclusive suggesting both super- and subsensitivity of this neuronal system. Species differences or regional variability may account for these discrepancies. During late stages of withdrawal sensitivity of dopamine receptors is increased.

3.5. SEROTONIN

Serotonin is synthesized from the precursor amino acid tryptophan. The rate limiting enzyme in the synthesis is tryptophan hydroxylase. The abbreviated sequences of synthesis and catabolism of serotonin are outlined in Fig. 3.

Two types of serotonin receptors have been distinguished primarily on the basis of non-serotonergic drug binding. Serotonin-1 receptors are linked to adenylate cyclase activity, are regulated by guanine nucleotides and bind (^{3}H)-serotonin. Serotonin-2 receptors are not linked to adenylate cyclase or guanine nucleotides and have greater binding for (^{3}H)-spiroperidol, the dopamine receptor antagonist. Some evidence also indicates that activation of serotonin-1 receptors mediates the behavioral depressant effects of serotonin and that behavioral excitatory effects are mediated via serotonin-2 receptors.

3.5.1. *Acute Effects of Ethanol*

Acute treatment with ethanol has been found generally not to alter serotonin levels (Haggendal and Lindqvist, 1961; Feldstein, 1973; Tabakoff *et al.*, 1975; Pohorecky and Newman, 1978; Pohorecky *et al.*, 1978; Fukumori *et al.*, 1980), although small decreases (Gursey and Olson, 1960; Gothoni and Ahtee, 1980) or increases (Erikson and Matchett, 1975) have also been reported. In some cases where there was no change in serotonin levels; there was, however, a change in the serotonin levels of 5HIAA. Again, either a decrease (Feldstein, 1973), or an increase (Pohorecky and Newman, 1978; Fukumori *et al.*, 1980; Mena and Herrera, 1980; Gothoni and Ahtee, 1980) was also found. The elevated levels

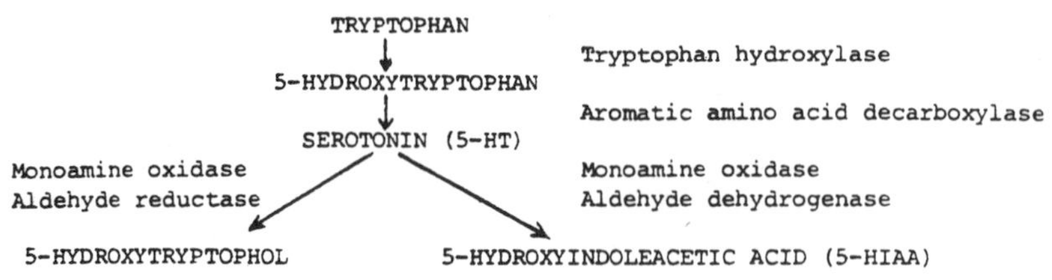

FIG. 3.

of 5HIAA after an acute dose of ethanol was absent in adrenalectomized rats (Pohorecky and Newman, 1978).

In man, levels of 5HIAA in CSF and in urine were decreased after ingestion of ethanol (Davis *et al.*, 1969; Orenberg *et al.*, 1976). In urine, there was a concomitant increase in 5-hydroxytryptophol (Davis *et al.*, 1969). As mentioned in the section on norepinephrine the pattern of urinary excretion of monoamine metabolites reflects the effect of ethanol on the metabolism of biogenic amines in the liver.

Turnover of serotonin was evaluated in several studies examining the effects of ethanol. Unfortunately these studies measured levels of serotonin after blockade of monoamine oxidase. An increase (Palaic *et al.*, 1971), a decrease (Tyce *et al.*, 1970) or no change (Kuriyama *et al.*, 1971) in serotonin turnover were found after ethanol treatment. Similarly the activity of tryptophan hydroxylase was either decreased (Rogawski *et al.*, 1974) or not affected by ethanol (Kuriyama *et al.*, 1971). Using (^{14}C)-serotonin no effect of ethanol was found on serotonin metabolism in the caudate nucleus (Tyce *et al.*, 1968) or in brain slices *in vitro* (Eccleston *et al.*, 1969).

In vitro addition of ethanol (over 43.4 mM) inhibited both (^{3}H)-serotonin and (^{3}H)-LSD binding in mouse brain membrane preparations (Hirsch, 1981). Scatchard analysis indicated an increase in the affinity for binding as well as a reduction in the apparent number of binding sites.

3.5.2. *Chronic Ethanol Treatment*

After chronic ethanol treatment levels of serotonin are generally unchanged (Wallgren, 1973; Rawat, 1974; Tabakoff and Bogan, 1974; Moscatelli *et al.*, 1975; Pohorecky *et al.*, 1978). An increase in serotonin levels were reported after 10 days of ethanol intubation (Littleton *et al.*, 1974) and in rats ingesting an ethanol-containing liquid diet (Pohorecky *et al.*, 1974). On the other hand 3 times daily intubation for 10 days decreased serotonin levels in most areas except the cortex (Gothoni and Ahtee, 1980). 5HIAA levels in brains of rats (Gothoni and Ahtee, 1980) were increased as a result of chronic exposure to ethanol.

Turnover of serotonin was higher in animals ingesting ethanol as part of their daily fluid or food supply for 14–21 days (Kuriyama *et al.*, 1971; Mena and Herrera, 1980). However, in other studies a decrease in serotonin turnover was found (Yamanaka and Kono, 1974; Tabakoff *et al.*, 1977). In one of these studies turnover was examined using (^{14}C)-serotonin rather than a monoamine oxidase inhibitor (Tabakoff *et al.*, 1977). No change in turnover of serotonin as a result of chronic ethanol treatment has also been reported (Frankel *et al.*, 1974). Levels of 5HIAA in brain were also elevated during withdrawal in mice (Tabakoff and Boggan, 1974). In intoxicated alcoholics 5HIAA levels in CSF were elevated (Zarcone *et al.*, 1975) but not in another study (Beck *et al.*, 1980). Levels in 5HIAA in CSF were decreased 28–63 days after withdrawal from ethanol (Ballenger *et al.*, 1979).

Tryptophan hydroxylase was elevated in animals ingesting ethanol as part of a liquid diet for 14 days (Kuriyama *et al.*, 1971; Sze and Neckers, 1974; Pohorecky *et al.*, 1974) as well as during withdrawal from ethanol (Pohorecky *et al.*, 1974).

Chronic treatment with ethanol (8 g/kg/day by intubation) for 15 days had no effect on (^{3}H)-serotonin binding in brain stem and the caudate nucleus, but decreased binding in hippocampus (Muller *et al.*, 1980). A shorter treatment with ethanol (4 days of inhalation) did not affect serotonin binding (Hunt and Dalton, 1981).

3.5.3. *Pharmacological Studies*

Pretreatment with the serotonergic antagonist methysergide prolonged the duration of anesthesia produced by an acute dose of ethanol (Blum *et al.*, 1974). The hypothermia produced by ethanol appears to involve serotonergic mechanisms. A decrease of serotonin release (after *p*-chloroamphetamine treatment) increased ethanol hypothermia, while blocking of serotonin reuptake at synapses with Lilly 110140 blocked the hypothermic effect of ethanol (Pohorecky *et al.*, 1976).

The blockade of serotonin metabolism with a monoamine oxidase inhibitor increased serotonin levels, increased gross motor activity and stereotyped behavior in ethanol-treated (2 g/kg) rats (Holman *et al.*, 1977). The stereotyped behavior could be blocked by *p*-chlorophenylalanine (PCPA) pretreatment (Holman *et al.*, 1977). The analgesic effect of ethanol is significantly decreased when brain serotonin levels are decreased with *p*-chloroamphetamine (PCA) (Brick *et al.*, 1976).

There has been considerable interest in the possibility that serotonergic mechanisms may be involved in mediating ingestion of ethanol. This research was stimulated by the observation that PCPA pretreatment decreases ethanol preference (Myers and Veale, 1968; Myers and Cicero, 1969; Veale and Myers, 1970). This research indicated that the decline in ethanol ingestion was a consequence of the decrease in brain serotonin levels. In fact, other manipulations of brain serotonin levels supported the hypothesis even though all the evidence was not consistent.

Adding tryptophan to the diet of rats (the precursor of serotonin) enhanced intake of ethanol (Myers and Melchior, 1975). Treatment with the MAO inhibitor pargyline decreased ethanol preference (Sanders *et al.*, 1976). However, decreasing brain levels of serotonin with the neurotoxin 5,6-dihydroxytryptamine increased ethanol intake (Myers and Melchior, 1975). While a decrease in brain serotonin produced by *p*-chloroamphetamine decreased ethanol preference (Stein *et al.*, 1977). Overall it is not clear how PCPA or *p*-chloroamphetamine decrease ethanol preference. The effect of PCPA appears to be due to its noxious effects (Nachman *et al.*, 1970) which result in general aversion, including decreased food and saccharin intakes (Parker and Radov, 1976; Stein *et al.*, 1977). PCPA has also been found to produce a learned aversion to ethanol (Walters, 1977). In contrast to tryptophan, the serotonin precursor 5-hydroxytryptophan decreased ethanol preference (Zabik *et al.*, 1978; Geller and Martenaun, 1981).

Decreasing serotonin levels with PCPA decreased the tolerance to the hypothermic effect of ethanol (Frankel *et al.*, 1975, 1978; Le *et al.*, 1979; Khanna *et al.*, 1980). Similarly, brain lesions that decrease serotonin levels (Le *et al.*, 1980, 1981) delayed development of tolerance to ethanol. There is regional specificity in the serotonergic pathways involved. Thus dorsal and magnus raphe lesions had no effect on development of tolerance to ethanol, lesions of only the median raphe nucleus were effective (Le *et al.*, 1981).

Other investigators examined whether drugs that modify serotonergic neuron activity modified the symptoms observed during withdrawal from chronic ethanol treatment. Although intracerebral methysergide, a serotonin antagonist, increased the number of handling-induced convulsions (Blum *et al.*, 1976), other investigators found no alteration of the withdrawal syndrome with these and other drugs affecting serotonin (Goldstein, 1973; Griffiths *et al.*, 1974). Head twitches occurring during withdrawal however were antagonized by serotonin antagonists (Collier *et al.*, 1976).

3.5.4. *Conclusions*

Although many studies have been carried out on the acute effects of ethanol on the serotonin neuronal system in brain, there is still no coherent picture. A variety of results have been reported, generally of small magnitude, which considering the sensitivity of the serotonergic system to stress, may reflect variability in the stress to which animals were subjected during treatment, rather than the effect of ethanol itself. Nevertheless, evidence is accumulating to implicate serotonin in the expression of preference for ingestion of ethanol.

3.6. ACETYLCHOLINE

The synthesis of acetylcholine (ACh) from the precursor amino acid choline is catalyzed by choline acetyltransferase. The outline of the pathway for ACh synthesis and metabolism is the following:

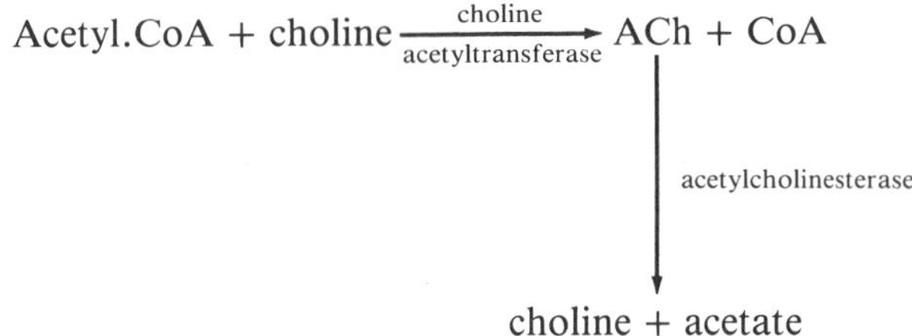

There are two general types of ACh receptors: nicotinic and muscarinic. The ligand for muscarinic receptors is (^{3}H)-quinuclidinyl benzylate (QNB). Muscarinic receptors predominate in brain. (^{3}H)-Nicotine is generally used as a ligand for studies on nicotine receptors.

3.6.1. *Acute Effects of Ethanol*

Acute ethanol treatment produces a dose-dependent increase in ACh levels in brain (Erickson and Graham, 1973; Hunt and Dalton, 1976). As with the catecholamines there are regional differences in the sensitivity of cholinergic neurons to ethanol with subcortical areas being more sensitive to ethanol than cortical areas (Erickson and Graham, 1973). Hunt and Dalton (1976) found an increase in ACh levels after ethanol treatment only in the caudate nucleus and in the brain stem.

In vitro ethanol did not alter the potassium-stimulated release of ACh from cortical brain slices (Kalant *et al.*, 1967). *In vivo* an acute dose of ethanol resulted in the decline in electrically-stimulated ACh release from cortical brain slices (Kalant *et al.*, 1967; Erickson and Graham, 1973; Carmichael and Israel, 1975; Hunt and Dalton, 1976; Sinclair and Lo, 1978). Spontaneous release of ACh *in vivo* was also decreased by an acute dose of ethanol (Kalant *et al.*, 1967; Erickson and Graham, 1973; Carmichael and Israel, 1975; Hunt and Dalton, 1976; Sinclair and Lo, 1978). There was very rapid (within 30 mins) development of tolerance to the depressant effects of ethanol on stimulated ACh release from cortical brain slices (Sinclair and Lo, 1978).

Since the rate of synthesis of ACh is directly dependent on the availability of its precursor choline, a number of investigators examined this particular aspect. Furthermore neuronal choline uptake is directly linked to the functional activity of cholinergic neurons. An acute dose of ethanol (2.0–4.5 g/kg by intubation) was found to inhibit choline uptake (Durkin *et al.*, 1982). The effect showed regional variability, with largest changes in the striatum and hippocampus (Durkin *et al.*, 1982; Howerton *et al.*, 1982). The effect of ethanol on high affinity choline uptake has a genetic component. Overall C57B1 mice were more sensitive than BALB/c mice to the depressant effect of ethanol on high affinity choline uptake (Durkin *et al.*, 1982; Furhmann *et al.*, 1986). *In vivo* ethanol (4.0–6.0 g/kg by intubation) increased choline uptake in the caudate nucleus, decreased it in the hippocampus, and had no effect in other brain areas of rats (Hunt *et al.*, 1979). A number of studies, however, did not show an effect of *in vitro* ethanol (up to 200 mM) on high affinity choline uptake (Durkin *et al.*, 1982; Howerton *et al.*, 1982). Therefore the changes in choline uptake observed *in vivo* were postulated to be indirect effects of ethanol (Durkin *et al.*, 1982).

Using the push–pull or the cortical cup perfusion techniques, an acute dose of ethanol (1.0–2.0 g/kg, intravenously) has been shown to decrease ACh release (Erickson and Graham, 1973) from several brain areas (Morgan and Phillis, 1975; Sinclair and Lo, 1978; Phillis *et al.*, 1980). The effects of ethanol on potassium or electrically-stimulated ACh release support these *in vivo* results. A depression of ACh release in the presence of ethanol (110–170 mM) was also found in cortical slices (110–170 mM) (Kalant and Grove, 1967; Carmichael and Israel, 1975; Sunahara and Kalant, 1980). There was no effect of ethanol on spontaneous release of ACh from cortical slices (Sunahara and Kalant, 1980) nor on stimulated release from slices of the midbrain (Richter and Werling, 1979).

3.6.2. *Chronic Ethanol Treatment*

After chronic ethanol treatment ACh release increased from cortical slices (Rawat, 1974; Hunt and Dalton, 1976). Furthermore tissues were tolerant to the *in vitro* inhibitory effect of ethanol in ACh release and choline uptake was normal (Clark *et al.*, 1977). Sodium dependent choline uptake in the hippocampus was decreased as a result of chronic ethanol treatment (Beracochea *et al.*, 1986). On the other hand, uptake of choline by neural cell cultures exposed to 100 mM ethanol for 20 days was increased (Massarelli *et al.*, 1976). Changes in the cholinergic system in response to ethanol appear to be rapid, possibly either because this neuronal system is more sensitive to ethanol, or because this system is inherently less able to cope with disturbance in its homeostasis. During withdrawal from chronic ethanol treatment ACh levels were lower in several brain areas, but within a few hours ACh levels as well as choline uptake were normal (Rawat, 1974; Hunt and Dalton, 1976; Hunt *et al.*, 1979). However, the elevated choline uptake in striatum did not disappear until 7 days after withdrawal from ethanol (Rawat, 1974).

Choline acetyltransferase and acetylcholinesterase, the enzymes involved in the synthesis and metabolism of ACh, respectively, were not affected by chronic ethanol treatment (Rawat, 1974). An exception was the elevated activity of choline acetyltransferase 1 hr after an acute dose of ethanol (Durkin *et al.*, 1972). After chronic ethanol treatment the activity of this enzyme increased in the striatum and decreased in the hippocampus (Ebel *et al.*, 1979). Postmortem brain samples from alcoholic subjects had slightly lower choline acetyltransferase activity compared to control samples (Nordberg *et al.*, 1983).

In vitro ACh receptor binding using (^{3}H)-QNB as a ligand was not affected by ethanol even at very high concentrations (920 mg/dl) (Hunt *et al.*, 1979). Chronic ethanol treatment (4 days inhalation or 11–15 days of intubation with 8 g/kg/day) had no effect on (^{3}H)-QNB binding (Muller *et al.*, 1980; Hunt and Dalton, 1981). However muscarinic receptor binding in the hippocampus and cerebral cortex was elevated in two other studies (ethanol-containing liquid diet intake for 7–8 days) (Tabakoff *et al.*, 1979; Rabin *et al.*, 1980) as indicated by Scatchard analysis. The effect on receptor binding was no longer apparent 24 hr after termination of the ethanol treatment (Muller *et al.*, 1980; Rabin *et al.*, 1980). Considerably longer treatment with ethanol (ingestion of an ethanol solution for up to 75 weeks) increased (^{3}H)-QNB binding in striatum but only if animals were withdrawn from ethanol at the time of testing (Nordberg and Wahlstrom, 1983). High affinity binding of (^{3}H)-nicotine to nicotinic receptors was decreased in the hippocampus and increased in hypothalamus and thalamus after 5 months of ethanol ingestion (8–12% solution) (Yoshida *et al.*, 1982). In postmortem brain samples of alcoholics there was a decline in the number of muscarinic, but no change in nicotinic receptors, compared to control samples (Noreberg *et al.*, 1983).

The functional significance and interpretation of these *in vitro* changes in receptor binding studies is not quite clear. For example, although there was an increase in (^{3}H)-QNB binding in synaptosomes prepared from brains of mice ingesting an ethanol-containing liquid diet for 7 days, there was no change in the muscarinic receptor-mediated incorporation of (^{32}P) into phosphotidylinositol (Smith, 1983).

The cholinergic system may mediate the effects of ethanol on motor activity in rodents. Cholinomimetic drugs (choline chloride and physostigmine) potentiated the decrease in motor activity produced by ethanol (Pohorecky *et al.*, 1979). Conversely, a decrease in cholinergic function produced by scopolamine antagonized the depressant effect of ethanol on motor activity (Pohorecky *et al.*, 1979).

3.6.3. *Conclusions*

There is rather good agreement in the literature to indicate that acute exposure to ethanol depresses the cholinergic neuronal system. Thus an acute dose of ethanol leads to a decrease in ACh release, elevates ACh levels and decreases choline uptake. Chronic treatment with ethanol activates the cholinergic system. Synthesis and release of ACh are increased, as is the number of muscarinic receptors as a result of chronic ethanol exposure.

3.7 GABA

γ-Aminobutyric acid (GABA) is synthesized from the precursor amino acid glutamic acid. The sequences of synthesis and catabolism of GABA are shown in Fig. 4.

The GABA receptor is part of a large GABA-benzodiazepine-chloride ionophore receptor complex present in some cellular membranes. Activation of the receptor results in the passage of chloride ions through the cell membrane channels. This complex consists of 3 distinct binding sites: GABA itself binds to one of the sites (identified by using (^{3}H)-GABA or (^{3}H)-muscimol as ligands), benzodiazepines bind to the second site (identified by labeled benzodiazepines), and picrotoxin binds to the third site (identified by the use of (^{3}H)-α-dihydropicrotoxin as ligand). The binding sites at the GABA and benzodiazepine receptors can either be of high and low affinity forms; for both forms there is an endogenous binding inhibitor present in tissue. Presence of such inhibitors requires that tissue samples be extensively washed before binding studies can be carried out.

3.7.1. *Acute Ethanol Treatment*

3.7.1.1. *Levels and turnover.* The effect of acute ethanol on the GABA neuronal system is controversial. Acute large doses of ethanol (4 g/kg and over, i.p.) increased GABA levels (Sutinsky *et al.*, 1975; Chan, 1976a; Hakkinen and Kulomen, 1981). In some cases, when regional levels were examined, the increase in GABA was localized to only some brain areas (Chan, 1976). A decrease in GABA levels was observed in other studies at similar or somewhat lower doses of ethanol (Volicer *et al.*, 1976; Chan, 1976; Volicer *et al.*, 1977; Volicer, 1980). The decrease in GABA levels usually was restricted to specific brain areas, with cerebellum being the most readily affected area (Volicer *et al.*, 1976, 1980; Chan, 1976; Wixon and Hunt, 1980; Hunt and Majchrowicz, 1983). In addition, a number of studies found no effect of 3–6 g/kg doses of ethanol (Hakkinen and Kulonen, 1961; Higgins, 1962; Gordon, 1967; Sutton and Simmonds, 1973; Hakkinen and Kulonen, 1976; Wixon and Hunt, 1980; Hunt and Majchrowicz, 1983). Turnover of GABA, generally measured by the accumulation of levels after inhibition of GABA metabolism, was either increased (1–4 g/kg ethanol) (Supavilal and Karobath, 1980), decreased (low doses of ethanol) in cerebellum and cortex (Wixon and Hunt, 1980; Hunt and Majchrowicz, 1983), or not altered (high doses of ethanol) (Wixon and Hunt, 1980; Hunt and Majchrowicz, 1983).

In vitro ethanol increased uptake of GABA, but only in the absence of glucose in the medium (Cerda and Israel, 1969). The synthesis and release of GABA were decreased by ethanol (Cerda and Israel, 1969; Strong and Wood, 1984). GABA release, from synaptosomes from chronic ethanol-treated animals, was inhibited in the presence of 500 mM ethanol (Strong and Wood, 1984).

Of the enzymes in GABA metabolism, GABA transaminase was not altered by acute ethanol treatment (Sutton and Simmonds, 1973; Sutinsky *et al.*, 1975), while glutamate decarboxylase activity (the enzyme that decarboxylates glutamate to GABA) was elevated in one study (Sutton and Simmonds, 1973).

3.7.1.2. *Receptor binding studies. In vitro* ethanol (230–460 mg/dl) decreased ^{3}H-α-dihydroxypicrotoxin binding to the GABA-benzodiazepine-chloride ionophore receptor complex in Lubrol solubilized tissue preparations (Davis and Ticku, 1981; Ticku and Davis, 1981). Ethanol (100 mM) had no effect on binding GABA to benzodiazepine receptor

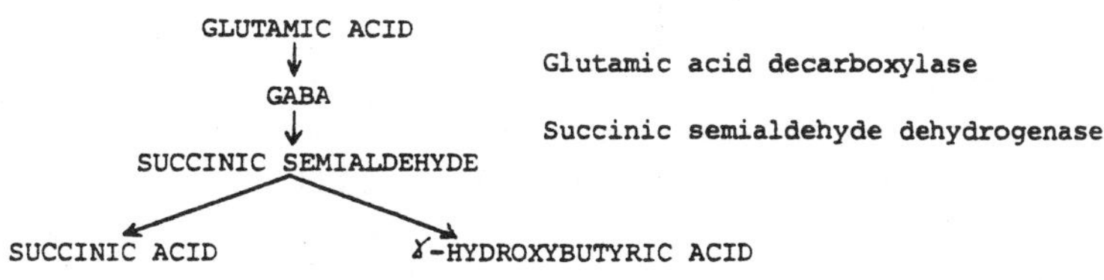

FIG. 4.

(Greenberg *et al.*, 1984). Binding of ^{35}S-T-butylbicyclophosphorothianate (^{35}S-TBPS) to membranes of cerebellum and cerebral cortex was dose-dependently decreased by ethanol (Liljequist *et al.*, 1986). The effect was due to decreased affinity of the ligand for its binding site.

An acute dose of ethanol (4 g/kg i.p.) has been shown to increase GABA binding (Ticku, 1980b; Ticku and Burch, 1980; Reggiani *et al.*, 1980a). Scatchard analysis indicated that there was an increase in the apparent number of low-affinity binding sites (Ticku and Burch, 1980) or in both low- and high-affinity binding sites (Reggiani *et al.*, 1980a). Somewhat lower blood ethanol levels (4 g/kg given orally) had no effect on GABA binding (Volicer and Biagioni, 1982b). Also no effect of an acute dose of ethanol on benzodiazepine binding was found in unwashed as well as in Triton X100 washed tissue preparations (Freund, 1980a; Volicer and Biagioni, 1982a). But a dose-dependent increase in benzodiazepine binding was found if tissues were solubilized with 1% Lubrol-Px (Davis and Ticku, 1981; Ticku and Davis, 1981).

Both the GABA and the benzodiazepine recognition binding sites of the postsynaptic GABA receptor complex are associated with the chloride-channel. The effect of ethanol on chloride-transport in synaptic vesicles has also been examined. 20–50 mM Ethanol stimulated ^{36}Cl-uptake, but uptake of the ion declined at higher concentrations of ethanol (Suzdak *et al.*, 1986). This effect of ethanol was decreased by GABA antagonists and was similar to that produced by pentobarbital. Depression of headpoke activity produced by ethanol was antagonized by R015-4513 (Lister, 1987). R015-4513 could increase the likelihood for the development of seizures during withdrawal from ethanol (Lister and Keranian, 1987), which would limit its potential clinical application. In primary spinal cord cultured neurons ethanol (50 mM) also potentiated the effect of GABA on ^{36}Cl-influx (Ticku *et al.*, 1986).

3.7.2. *Chronic Ethanol Treatment*

3.7.2.1. *Levels and turnover.* Chronic ethanol treatment ranging from 1 to 3 weeks elevated GABA levels in brain (Sutton and Simmonds, 1973; Volicer *et al.*, 1976; Wixon and Hunt, 1980). The effect of ethanol was region specific (ethanol given by intubation 3 times daily for 7 days), GABA was elevated in subcortical areas, but was unchanged in cerebellum (Volicer *et al.*, 1976). Several other studies found GABA levels unaltered by chronic ethanol treatment lasting from 14–30 days (Hagen, 1967; Patel and Lal, 1973; Wooles and DaVanzo, 1977; Cooper *et al.*, 1979; Supaviolai and Karobath, 1980). Turnover of GABA in animals ingesting an ethanol-containing liquid diet for 14 days was reported to be increased (Supavilai and Karobath, 1980) or decreased in cerebellum and pons medulla oblongata (Volicer, 1980). Chronic ingestion of ethanol via the drinking water by C57 mice decreased the turnover of GABA (as measured by GABA-induced accumulation of GABA) in a number of brain areas (striatum, cerebellum, amygdala, olfactory tubercle septum and hippocampus) and increased it in the posterior colliculus (Simler *et al.*, 1986).

During withdrawal from chronic ethanol treatment, GABA levels were generally decreased (Patel and Lal, 1973; Volicer *et al.*, 1976; Cooper *et al.*, 1979; Volicer, 1980; Wixon and Hung, 1980) in several brain areas (brain stem, medulla, cerebellum) as was its turnover. On the other hand, levels of GABA were found to be elevated during withdrawal from 3 days of exposure to ethanol by inhalation (Chopde *et al.*, 1977). Furthermore, levels of GABA in CSF of alcoholics undergoing withdrawal were elevated if the subjects experienced convulsions (Volicer, 1980; Goldman *et al.*, 1981). In another study, GABA levels in CSF were not changed (Hawley *et al.*, 1981).

3.7.2.2. *Receptor binding studies.* Available data on the effects of chronic ethanol treatment on GABA binding are very inconsistent. No changes in GABA binding was reported with 4 days in inhalation of ethanol (Hunt and Dalton, 1981), 7 days of daily multiple i.p. injections of ethanol (Volicer *et al.*, 1982b) and 21 days of ingestion of a 6% ethanol containing liquid diet (Ticku, 1980b). Intragastric intubation with ethanol for 5 days, and subsequent withdrawal from ethanol did not affect the benzodiazepine and picrotoxin binding sites in the brain (Rastogi *et al.*, 1986). In the last two reports, however, there was a decline in the affinity of the low affinity binding sites (Ticku, 1980b) or high affinity binding sites (Volicer *et al.*, 1982b). A decrease in the apparent number of binding sites was found during withdrawal from 4 days of ethanol inhalation (^{3}H-muscimol binding) (Linnoila *et al.*, 1981), after 14 days of consumption of a 10% solution of ethanol (Ticku and Burch, 1980) and consumption of a solution of ethanol increasing in concentration (Unwin and Tabemer, 1980).

Finally, an increase in apparent high- and low-affinity GABA binding in the striatum has been found after 21 days of ingestion of a 6% ethanol solution (Reggiani *et al.*, 1980). Elevated ^{3}H-muscimol binding was reported in postmortem specimens from alcoholics compared to control specimens (Tran *et al.*, 1981). A decrease in ^{35}S-TBPS binding was found in membranes of mice given ethanol for 7 days, similar to the response obtained in tissues from naive rats (Liljequist *et al.*, 1986). This indicates that there was no development of tolerance within 7 days of treatment.

Inhalation of ethanol for 14–19 days did not affect benzodiazepine binding to non-solubilized tissue preparations (Frye *et al.*, 1980; Karobath *et al.*, 1980). Shorter duration of ethanol treatment (4–5 days with 10 g/kg/day) decreased benzodiazepine binding in both non-solubilized (Kocheran *et al.*, 1981) and Triton X-100 solubilized tissue preparations (Volicer and Biagioni, 1982a). On the other hand 9 months treatment with ethanol resulted in a small decrease in the affinity as well as in the apparent number of binding sites of benzodiazepine receptors (Freund, 1980a).

As pointed out by Hunt (1986) one possible explanation for these discrepant findings is the preparation of the samples, which may or may not have removed the endogenous inhibitor of GABA and benzodiazepine binding. It is possible that ethanol affects not only GABA binding but it may also interact with these endogenous binding inhibitors.

3.7.2.3. *Pharmacological studies.* A number of pharmacological studies indicate that GABAergic mechanisms might mediate some of the effects of ethanol. Such studies indicate that GABA agonists increase, and GABA antagonists decrease, ethanol-induced depression (Frye and Breese, 1982; Liljequist and Engel, 1982; Martz *et al.*, 1983). Specifically the motor incoordinating and sedative effects of ethanol in both mice and rats could be potentiated by drugs that increase GABAergic function, and conversely could be antagonized by drugs that depress this neuronal system (McCabe *et al.*, 1971; Cott *et al.*, 1976; Hakkimen and Lukonen, 1976; Frye and Breese, 1982; Liljequist and Engel, 1982; Martz *et al.*, 1983; Dar and Wooles, 1985; Mendelson *et al.*, 1985). Also there is rather good evidence to indicate that drugs that elevate GABA levels protect against convulsions occurring during withdrawal from chronic ethanol treatment (Goldstein, 1973; Hillbom, 1975; Noble *et al.*, 1976; Cooper *et al.*, 1979; Goldstein, 1979; Frye *et al.*, 1983a,b). Forelimb tremors however were not affected by such drug treatment (Frye *et al.*, 1983b) nor was the overall withdrawal syndrome (LeBourhis and Aufrere, 1980). A benzodiazepine antagonist (R015-1788) had no effect on the severity of the withdrawal syndrome (Adinoff *et al.*, 1986). Diazepam however did decrease the severity of the ethanol withdrawal syndrome, and this was antagonized by R015-1788 (Adinoff *et al.*, 1986). Therefore, ethanol withdrawal syndrome may involve a central benzodiazepine recognition site. This evidence along with the data on GABA CSF levels in alcoholics, seems to indicate that impairment in GABAergic function is involved primarily with the convulsive component of the withdrawal syndrome. Furthermore, as indicated above, GABAergic neurons are probably involved in the CNS depressant effects produced by large doses of ethanol.

3.7.3. *Conclusions*

Chronic ethanol exposure may reduce GABA neurotransmission. Evidence on how ethanol affects the GABA neuronal system is rather inconsistent at the present time. For example, studies on the effect of ethanol on GABA receptor binding are difficult to compare and to interpret since tissue preparation and solubilization differed markedly amongst the studies. Nevertheless, the most recent data on chloride transport via the GABA receptor complex indicates enhanced GABA receptor function at concentrations of ethanol that are pharmacologically relevant.

3.8. Opiates

Significant evidence exists for at least three types of opiate receptors. These are the μ, δ- and κ-receptors. (^{3}H)-dihydromorphine is used to characterize μ-receptor binding; this binding is decreased by sodium. Opioid analgesia is believed to be mediated via μ-receptors. [(^{3}H)-D-Ala^2, D-Leu^5]enkephalin is used for binding to δ-receptors; the receptors may be linked to adenyl cyclase activity. Activation of the δ-receptor may mediate seizure activity as well as reward. Finally, dynorphin may be the endogenous substrate for κ-receptors.

3.8.1. *Levels and Turnover*

The effect of ethanol on brain opioid peptide has been carried out primarily on animals after chronic treatment. These studies were concerned primarily with measuring levels, synthesis, and receptors of opioid peptides.

The synthesis and release of β-endorphin-like opioid peptides in the neurointermediate lobe of the pituitary was increased by daily intubations of ethanol for 7 days (Gianoulakis *et al.*, 1981) or by ingestion of a liquid diet containing ethanol for 14 days (Gianoulakis *et al.*, 1983). In the later study β-endorphin levels were decreased in the anterior pituitary and increased in serum (Gianoulakis *et al.*, 1983). These findings indicate that in the anterior pituitary the turnover of the opioid was increased by chronic ethanol exposure. However, the processing of the precursor lipotropin to β-endorphin in the anterior pituitary was decreased (Schulz *et al.*, 1980; Seizinger *et al.*, 1983; Selinger *et al.*, 1984). There appear to be regional differences in the response of β-endorphin to ethanol. Thus although levels of β-endorphin in the anterior pituitary (Schultz *et al.*, 1980; Cheng and Tseng, 1982; Gianoulakis *et al.*, 1983; Wilkinson *et al.*, 1986) and in the intermediate pituitary (Wilkinson *et al.*, 1986) were decreased, levels were elevated in the hypothalamus (Cheng and Tseng, 1982). Duration of ethanol treatment is also important. Short term (3 day) exposure to ethanol did not affect β-endorphin levels in the pituitary (Gianoulakis *et al.*, 1983). Pyrazole-treated mice inhaling ethanol had lower β-endorphin levels in the anterior and neurointermediate lobes of the pituitary as well as in the hypothalamus and mid-brain—peak decline in β-endorphin occurred 24 hr after exposure to ethanol (Wilkinson *et al.*, 1986). In another study however, identical ethanol treatment resulted in an increase in whole brain β-endorphin levels, with peak elevation after 48 hr of exposure (Keith *et al.*, 1983). Levels of β-endorphin in the pituitary were not altered by chronic ethanol treatment in yet another study (Seizinger *et al.*, 1984).

Chronic treatment with ethanol also reduced brain levels of methionine enkephalin (Schulz *et al.*, 1980; Seizinger *et al.*, 1983, 1984). Acute or chronic ethanol treatment (5–7 days of liquid diet) had no effect on levels of enkephalin in several brain areas (Ryder *et al.*, 1981). Although leu-enkephalin levels in basal ganglia of mice ingesting ethanol in their drinking water for one year were decreased (Blum *et al.*, 1982), levels of methionine-enkephalin in the striatum were increased by ethanol (Schwarz *et al.*, 1980; Melchoir and Tabakoff, 1981).

Levels of β-endorphin and enkephalin in the CSF of alcoholics have been found to be reduced (Genazzani *et al.*, 1982; Borg *et al.*, 1982).

3.8.2. *Receptor Binding Studies*

In vitro the binding of (^{3}H)(L2-D-Ala-5-D-Leu)enkephalin to delta receptors (the high affinity receptors for enkephalin) was decreased selectively by ethanol in one study (200 mM) (Tabakoff *et al.*, 1981), but not in another (Jorgensen and Hole, 1986). The binding of (^{3}H)-dihydromorphine to μ-receptors (high affinity for morphine) was increased by ethanol, and the binding of (^{3}H)-naloxone (binds to both μ and δ receptors) was not affected (Hiller *et al.*, 1981). Very similar results were obtained in another study (Gianoulakis,

1983), except that in the study of Hiller *et al.*, the changes in binding produced by ethanol were explained by an alteration in the affinity of the receptor for ligand, and in the study by Gianoulakis by a change in receptor number. The effect of ethanol on (^{3}H)-dihydromorphine actually appears to be biphasic: 50 mM ethanol increased binding while 250–1000 mM inhibited binding in membrane preparations from caudate (Tabakoff and Hoffman, 1982). *In vitro* 460–4600 mg/dl ethanol decreased opiate receptor binding of whole brain or caudate nuclei preparations (Hiller *et al.*, 1981; Tabakoff and Hoffman, 1983; Hiller *et al.*, 1984). The decline in binding was found to be due to reduced affinity of the ligand for the receptors (Hiller *et al.*, 1981, 1984; Tabakoff and Hoffman, 1983), which in turn resulted from an increased rate of dissociation of the ligand from the receptor (Hiller *et al.*, 1983). Affinity of the receptor was also decreased by ethanol (Labella *et al.*, 1979; Tabakoff and Hoffman, 1983). There was no effect of ethanol κ-receptor binding (Hiller *et al.*, 1984). 50 mM ethanol increased binding to μ-receptor in caudate nucleus (Tabakoff and Hoffman, 1983). Scatchard analysis indicated an increase in affinity for these receptors. Also the apparent number of receptors was increased in another study (Levine *et al.*, 1983).

Chronic ethanol treatment did not modify binding of δ-receptor in mice, but decreased the affinity for binding in tissue preparations from rats given 9 g/kg orally for up to 60 days (Lucelin *et al.*, 1981). Similarly in mice the affinity of μ-receptors was reduced in the caudate nucleus 24 hr after withdrawal from chronic ingestion of an ethanol-containing liquid diet (Hoffman *et al.*, 1981). Twenty-one days of ingesting a 15% solution of ethanol increased affinity for δ-receptor but did not alter binding to μ-receptor (Pfeiffer *et al.*, 1981).

In addition to specific β-endorphin binding sites in brain, β-endorphin binding sites have also been reported recently in a variety of peripheral tissues (adrenals, kidney, spleen, testis, liver). Chronic ethanol treatment of rats (14 days of inhalation) decreased the number of β-endorphin binding sites in the liver and kidney (Dave *et al.*, 1986). Membranes from these peripheral tissues were tolerant to the enhancing effects of ethanol on β-endorphin binding seen in membrane preparations from control animals. This study also reported a significant decline in plasma β-endorphin levels.

3.8.3. *Pharmacological Studies*

Functional studies indicate that the intraventricular administration of β-endorphin increased both the sedative and hypothermic effects of ethanol (Luttinger *et al.*, 1981). On the other hand, a δ-receptor antagonist did not modify the analgesic, hypothermic or sedative effects of ethanol, nor its effect on sensorimotor performance (Jorgensen and Hole, 1986).

Naloxone, an opiate antagonist, decreased ethanol-induced coma, the duration of loss of righting reflex in mice (Kiianmaa *et al.*, 1983), ethanol-induced analgesia (Berkowitz *et al.*, 1976; Boada *et al.*, 1981), and the epileptiform-like activity produced by ethanol in monkeys (Berkowitz *et al.*, 1976; Triana *et al.*, 1980; Boada *et al.*, 1981; Seilicovich *et al.*, 1982; Pokras and Tabakoff, 1982). Naloxone also blocked the ethanol-induced decreases in brain catecholamines (Guaza and Borrell, 1985).

Naloxone attenuated morphine-induced hypothermia in mice selectively bred for differential sensitivity to ethanol (LS/SS lines) and attenuated ethanol-induced hypothermia in the SS mice (Brick and Horowitz, 1982).

3.8.4. *Conclusions*

Ethanol treatment decreases levels and increases synthesis and release of β-endorphin in the pituitary gland. There might be regional specificity in the effect of ethanol on β-endorphin levels since the response of β-endorphin in the hypothalamus was in the opposite direction from that of the pituitary gland. Methionine-enkephalin levels in both brain and CSF were decreased by ethanol. The three types of opiate receptors respond differently to *in vitro* ethanol: δ-receptor binding was decreased, μ-receptor binding was increased and

κ-receptor binding was unaltered. Chronic ethanol treatment decreased the affinity of opiate receptor binding. Pharmacological experiments also indicate involvement of opioid peptides in the action of ethanol in the brain. Specifically, the sedative and hypothermic effects of ethanol may involve opioid mechanisms.

4. ETHANOL AND THE ENDOCRINE SYSTEM

4.1. EFFECT OF ACUTE AND CHRONIC ETHANOL

4.1.1. *Vasopressin*

One of the most well known effects of acute ethanol on the endocrine system is diuresis (Murray 1932; Nicholson and Taylor 1938; Linkola 1974; Pohorecky 1985). That ethanol-induced diuresis was due to a central, rather than a peripheral effect of ethanol was suggested by Dyke and Ames (1951) who produced diuresis in dogs with minute amounts of ethanol. The dose was too small to have any direct effect on glomerular filtration or renal functioning but when injected into the carotid artery water loss was significantly increased, suggesting that ethanol acted centrally.

Linkola *et al.* (1978) found that ethanol induced diuresis was associated with increased plasma levels of vasopressin. This apparent paradox may be due to blood ethanol phase or age of subjects. For example, Helderman *et al.* (1978) reported that ethanol's inhibiting effect on vasopressin occurs only while blood ethanol levels are rising. In subjects older than age 50 ethanol increases vasopressin but in subjects below age 50, a sharp suppression of vasopressin is observed (Helderman *et al.*, 1978). More recently, a biphasic effect of ethanol has been observed on the ascending limb of the blood alcohol curve (Eisenhofer and Johnson, 1982). Plasma AVP levels fell after a 75 ml dose of ethanol was ingested, then rose while plasma ethanol levels were still rising (Eisenhofer and Johnson, 1982). Since the rise in plasma AVP coincided with a rise in plasma osmolarity, these researchers suggest that the "biphasic nature of the vasopressin response to ethanol is due to an increased osmolarity that overrides the inhibitory effects of ethanol." Thus, the effects of ethanol on vasopressin may involve a resetting of hypothalamic osmoreceptors (Eisenhofer and Johnson, 1982). In rats, the most consistent evidence suggests that central noradrenergic mechanisms play a key role in the diuretic action of ethanol (Pohorecky 1985; Pohorecky and Packard 1986).

In mice, vasopressin analogue, co-administered with ethanol during the onset of withdrawal increases the severity of withdrawal (Crabbe and Rigter 1980), although vasopressin alone has no effect on the withdrawal syndrome (Hoffman *et al.*, 1979). Plasma vasopressin is higher in alcoholics during withdrawal, than in alcoholics not showing withdrawal syndrome (Eisenhofer *et al.*, 1985).

4.1.2. *Cortisol/Corticosterone*

The earliest evidence of an effect of ethanol on corticosterone was a study reported by Smith (1951) who found that adrenal ascorbic acid, which is inversely proportional to adrenocorticotropin stimulating hormone (ACTH), was significantly reduced in rats given acute ethanol. In contrast, hypophysectomized rats showed no reduction in adrenal ascorbic acid (Ellis, 1966). These results suggest that adrenal stimulation by ethanol was at the level of either the anterior pituitary or hypothalamus. Similar results were reported using guinea pigs (Forbes and Duncan, 1951) thus indicating that the effect was not species specific. A few years later, Kalant *et al.* (1965) and others (Ellis, 1966; Pohorecky, 1974) confirmed these initial observations. Other studies (Noble, 1971) showed that the synthetic glucocorticoid, dexamethasone, inhibited the normal release of corticosterone after ethanol and decreased pituitary ACTH content (Noble, 1971; Nobel *et al.*, 1971). Part of the mechanism of ethanol's action on corticosterone release may involve central nervous system serotonin since metergoline, a serotonin antagonist, blocks the effect of ethanol on ACTH release (Rivier *et al.*, 1984). Experimental treatments that decrease brain serotonin also decreased the elevating effects of ethanol on corticosterone (Brick and Pohorecky, 1985).

Rivier *et al.* (1984) were the first to demonstrate that in nonanesthetized rats, ethanol caused a dose dependent increase in plasma ACTH that was dependent upon corticotropin releasing factor (CRF). Immunoneutralization of endogenous CRF abolished the effect of ethanol. These investigators suggest that the hypothalamus is a major site of ethanol's action on increasing ACTH and thus corticosterone secretion (1984). Redei *et al.* (1986) suggest that low doses of ethanol act directly on the pituitary to induce ACTH release and that high doses act primarily in the hypothalamus. Acute exposure of superfused rat pituitaries to 20–200 mg/dl of ethanol produced a dose-related increase in ACTH (Redei *et al.*, 1986).

Rivier and Vale (1988) examined the interaction between ethanol and stress on ACTH secretion and reported that the intraperitoneal infusion of ethanol (1 g/hr/kg body weight for three hours) attenuated the secretion of ACTH (and beta-endorphin) that was induced by a subsequent footshock. Conversely, three hours of mild footshock decreased the pituitary response to subsequent dose (1 g/kg) of ethanol. These findings suggest that there is a cross-tolerance between the pituitary effects of ethanol and stress with regard to the ACTH (and beta-endorphin). Since shock diminishes the pituitary response to CRF injections, an effect probably due to ACTH depletion and increased negative corticoid feedback (Rivier and Vale 1987), the finding of a cross tolerance between pituitary effects of ethanol and stress on the release of ACTH suggest that ethanol did not alter pituitary ACTH content. Since adrenalectomized rats exposed to ethanol also have an attenuated pituitary response to CRF, steroid feedback probably does not play a role in the diminished stimulatory action of CRF in rats infused to ethanol. Excessive use of alcohol is often associated with high circulating levels of cortisol and 'Pseudo-Cushings disease' (Van Thiel 1983; Van Thiel *et al.*, 1983).

In humans ACTH has been measured using sensitive radioimmunoassays, but ethanol's action of this hormone is controversial (Leppaluoto *et al.*, 1975; Jeffcoate *et al.*, 1980; Cobb and Van Thiel, 1982).

Stress may also play an important role in determining the way in which ethanol alters corticosterone. Various physical and psychological stressors also increase plasma corticosterone but pretreatment with low doses of ethanol 'protect' experimental animals from stress-induced elevations in this hormone (Pohorecky *et al.*, 1980; Brick and Pohorecky, 1982, 1983).

During ethanol withdrawal significant elevations in plasma ACTH, cortisol and corticosterone (Ellis, 1966; Mendelson *et al.*, 1971; Pohorecky, 1974; Tabakoff *et al.*, 1978; Valimaki *et al.*, 1984). Interestingly, cortisol levels return to normal if alcohol is administered during withdrawal (Merry and Marks, 1972). Plasma cortisol values often remain significantly elevated for several weeks after the last drink (Willingbring *et al.*, 1984). Several studies suggest that in chronic alcoholics going through withdrawal, the normal inhibition of cortisol produced by dexamethasone is inhibited. Although nonsuppression of cortisol in the dexamethasone suppression test has often been used as an index of alcohol withdrawal, methodological flaws, such as lack of control for liver disease, other illnesses and use of tobacco in alcoholic subjects may confound the interpretation of such results (Edelstein *et al.*, 1983; Swartz and Dunner, 1982; Rihmer and Arato, 1982; Wilkins *et al.*, 1982).

4.1.3. *Growth Hormone*

Several studies have suggested that ethanol inhibits growth hormone. Initially, it was believed that ethanol produced degenerative changes within the anterior pituitary gland, but more recent studies suggest that acute doses of ethanol decrease the spontaneous release of growth hormone (Redmond, 1980). In alcoholics with cirrhosis, the opposite effect is found. Alcoholics have elevated levels of growth hormone (Van Thiel *et al.*, 1978b).

Chronic alcohol consumption decreases growth hormone. In one study, growth hormone levels immediately returned to normal when alcohol was discontinued (Prinz *et al.*, 1980).

4.1.4. *Insulin*

The interrelationship between ethanol and insulin was first brought to attention by the observation that both alcoholics and fasted subjects exhibited significant hypoglycemia when exposed to ethanol. Most studies utilizing human subjects have reported only modest effects of ethanol on insulin (Raptis *et al.*, 1974). In chronic alcoholics, insulin has been reported to be increased (Trell *et al.*, 1981; Anderson *et al.*, 1983), normal (Nicholson and Paton, 1979; Iturriaga *et al.*, 1986) or decreased (Sereny and Endrenyi, 1978). In diabetic subjects, ethanol did not significantly alter basal immunoreactive insulin (Bagdade *et al.*, 1972). Holley *et al.* (1981) examined the effect of ethanol on glucose-stimulated insulin secretion and found insulin was initially unchanged but after 4 hr of ethanol infusion resulted in an enhancement of the glucose response. Similarly, Potter and Morris (1980) found that ethanol produced a dose-related suppression of insulin levels in rats. Ethanol induced hypoglycemia in both humans and animals is probably an inhibition of gluconeogenesis due to an increased ratio of NADH2 to NAD as a result of the hepatic oxidation of ethanol rather than a hormonal effect.

4.1.5. *Prolactin*

The effect of ethanol on prolactin, the hormone responsible for lactation, has not been extensively studied. Of the few animal and human studies performed, prolactin does not appear to be affected by acute ethanol administration (Ylikahri *et al.*, 1978, 1980). However, prolactin activity may be altered in the alcoholic. Loosen and Prange (1977) found that alcoholics had reduced prolactin levels although the number of prolactin secreting cells in the pituitary is greater in both male and female alcoholics who died from alcoholic liver disease (Jung and Russfield, 1972). On the other hand, prolactin values have been found to be elevated in nearly half of chronic alcoholics tested (Lindholm *et al.*, 1978). Alcoholics have an exaggerated prolactin response to thyrotropin releasing factor (Ylikahri *et al.*, 1976; Van Thiel *et al.*, 1978).

During alcohol withdrawal, prolactin is initially decreased, then returns to normal in about 4 weeks. Furthermore, the severity of alcohol withdrawal was found to be negatively correlated with prolactin levels (Majumdar, 1982).

4.1.6. *Gonadotropic Hormones*

4.1.6.1. *Hormonal changes in males.* Chronic ethanol produces testicular atrophy in male rats and ovarian dysfunction in female rats (Van Thiel, 1978, 1979). In humans, chronic ethanol use decreases production of androgens, and increases estrogens, changes that are associated with testicular atrophy, impotence gynocomastia and feminization (Rather, 1947; Van Thiel and Lester, 1976; Van Thiel, 1980, 1983). Mendelson and colleagues found that chronic administration of ethanol to alcoholic and nonalcoholic men resulted in a dose dependent decrease in testosterone levels (Mendelson *et al.*, 1977, 1978). The inhibitory effect of ethanol on testicular steroidogenesis has been observed *in vivo* and *in vitro* in rodents and human males but the exact mechanism of ethanol's action is not understood. Van Thiel and Lester (1976) suggested that the increased NADH:NAD ratio produced during ethanol oxidation may inhibit enzymes necessary for steroid metabolism. Ethanol may alter steroidogenesis indirectly, through its primary metabolite, acetaldehyde (Cobb *et al.*, 1978, 1980; Cicero *et al.*, 1980).

Cicero (1981) observed that pyrazole, an ethanol dehydrogenase inhibitor had no effect on ethanol-induced inhibition of testosterone. Since the administration of pyrazole and the corresponding elevation of blood ethanol had no effect on steroidogenesis, it suggests that ethanol alone is not the primary agent responsible for testosterone inhibition. Coupled with previous studies (Cobb *et al.*, 1978; Ellingboe and Varanelli, 1979; Gordon *et al.*, 1980) it appears that ethanol *per se* does not directly inhibit the biosynthesis of testosterone.

4.1.6.2. *Hormonal changes in females.* In female rats, ethanol administration disrupts menstrual cycle (Aron *et al.*, 1965; Kieffer and Ketchel, 1970; Eskay *et al.*, 1981; Bo *et al.*, 1982), decreased ovarian and uterine weights (Van Thiel *et al.*, 1977, 1978; Bo *et al.*, 1982;

Gavaler, 1983; Mello *et al.*, 1983), delayed vaginal opening (Boggan *et al.*, 1979), decreased estradiol and progesterone and increased estrone levels (Van Thiel *et al.*, 1977, 1978; Gavaler *et al.*, 1980), decreased lordosis (Merari *et al.*, 1973) and luteinizing hormone levels (Blake, 1978). In monkeys, self-administered low doses of ethanol do not affect estrus cycles or luteinizing hormone (Mello *et al.*, 1983). High doses of ethanol produce amenorrhea, decreased leuteinizing hormone levels, decreased ovarian mass and uterine atrophy (Mello *et al.*, 1983).

In women, chronic ethanol affects reproductive functioning in much the same way it does in animal models (Gavaler, 1985, for a review), namely by disrupting menstrual regularity and ovarian function (Ryback 1977; Jones-Saumty *et al.*, 1981; Valimaki, 1984). In a carefully controlled study, (Mendelson *et al.*, 1981) measured plasma prolactin, luteinizing hormone and estradiol in adult women on the same day of the menstrual cycle, over two consecutive cycles. Samples collected every 20 min for 6 hr before and after ethanol revealed no differences in luteinizing hormone or estradiol when compared to pre-ethanol baselines or with control beverages.

4.1.7. *Adrenal Catecholamines*

The effect of ethanol on peripheral catecholamines is discussed in section 3.3.1.1.

4.1.8. *Conclusions*

Acute administration of, and withdrawal from, ethanol alters a number of endocrine systems. Some of these effects may be due to a direct action of ethanol on endocrine glands or within the central nervous system whereas other effects may be due to indirect actions. The consequences of hormonal changes in response to acute or chronic ethanol or ethanol withdrawal are unknown, although some of these changes may be associated with mechanisms underlying tolerance and dependence.

5. ETHANOL TOLERANCE

There can be little doubt that alcohol abuse is a maladaptive behavior that is often associated with medical complications for the abuser as well as social problem for both the user and his or her social contacts (family, employer, society at large). In the United States, for example, each year ethanol related disabilities cost taxpayers millions of dollars in lost work, property damage, and hospital costs, not to mention over 50,000 ethanol related driving fatalities per year. Despite such consequences, alcohol continues to be abused in many societies. Little is known about the etiology of ethanol use/abuse, although considerable effort has gone into understanding factors that regulate the consumption of alcohol. For example, the possible positively and negatively reinforcing effects of alcohol has been the subject of considerable review (Cappell and Herman, 1972; Pohorecky, 1980; Cappell and LeBlanc, 1983; Wilson, 1987) and at least one major international symposium (Pohorecky and Brick, 1983). In an effort to gain insight into the etiology of this disease, researchers have focused on tolerance and physical dependence aspects of ethanol use. As an issue quite separate from that of physical dependence, the study of 'modulating' variables such as tolerance may be useful in understanding factors that differentiate alcohol use from alcohol abuse. For example, the interrelationships among an individual's ability to know when to stop drinking and tolerance may be relevant to pathological consequences of drinking (Lipscomb and Nathan, 1980; Lipscomb *et al.*, 1980; Cappell and LeBlanc, 1983).

Tolerance is a term used to describe behavioral and/or biological decreases in sensitivity with increased exposure to the drug. In other words, we say that tolerance has developed when there is a shift to the right in the dose–response curve, so that increasingly larger amounts of drug must be given to obtain the same pharmacological effect observed with the original dose. These changes are part of a general adaptive response in the organism. Although alcoholics may be able to consume up to twice the amount of alcohol as a teetotaler, in comparison to other drugs, such as morphine, tolerance to alcohol is rather modest (American Psychiatric Association, 1987). Recently, the APA has de-emphasized the importance of physiological symptoms such as tolerance and withdrawal in making a diagnosis of dependence. The presence of these symptoms are still diagnostic criteria, but dependence may exist in their absence. In part, this less restricted definition can be used to diagnose dependence on other drugs that have less pronounced tolerance and withdrawal associated with their use. This revised criteria can more easily include drinkers that show severe impairment of their control of alcohol but do not develop tolerance or withdrawal (e.g., binge drinkers).

5.1. Types of Tolerance

There are several different types of tolerance which are discussed below. It should be kept in mind that although various types of tolerance are known, the mechanisms involved in mediating these phenomena are not well understood. Furthermore, very little is known about the relationships that exist between these categories of tolerance. As discussed below, the development of tolerance not only varies with type of tolerance, but also with different responses to ethanol.

5.1.1. *Acute Tolerance*

Mellanby (1919) first proposed the concept of acute tolerance based upon his observation that in dogs, there was greater behavioral impairment while ethanol levels were rising compared to when they were falling at the same blood ethanol level. A similar effect in humans was described by Goldberg (1943). Acute tolerance, which is still referred to as the Mellanby effect, can therefore be defined as the difference in response at a given concentration of ethanol while its level in blood is rising compared to when it is falling. Unlike other forms of tolerance, acute tolerance develops very rapidly during the time course of a single ethanol administration (within-session tolerance) and is believed to represent an adaptive or compensatory change within the central nervous system that occurs in response to the drug (LeBlanc *et al.*, 1975). LeBlanc *et al.* (1976) demonstrated this effect using performance on a moving belt as a measure of tolerance. Rats were tested once, at three different times (9, 29 and 59 min) after the administration of ethanol. Immediately after each test, the rat was sacrificed and brain ethanol level was measured. Rats were less impaired at 60 min than at 10 min at the same brain ethanol level suggesting a rapid, acute tolerance (LeBlanc *et al.*, 1975).

Goldberg (1943) examined the time course of impairment following a single dose of ethanol and found that cognitive type tasks returned at higher blood ethanol levels than did motor-type tasks. It was suggested (Goldberg, 1943; Carpenter, 1963), and confirmed in later years, that ethanol impairment of cognitive function dissipates more rapidly for ethanol-induced motor impairment. Jones (1973) observed acute tolerance to ethanol-induced memory impairment in non-alcoholics. Vogel-Sprott (1976) found that the performance of social drinkers on a coding task was impaired on the rising portion of the blood ethanol curve but not on the descending limb. In a study of acute recovery and tolerance to low doses of ethanol, Vogel-Sprott (1979) found that cognitive performance on a divided attention coding task improved (acute tolerance) whereas performance on a pursuit rotor task did not (no acute tolerance). At least part of the acute tolerance detected in these studies may be due to task practice effects (Beirness and Vogel-Sprott, 1984; Vogel-Sprott *et al.*, 1984; Annear and Vogel-Sprott, 1985; Niaura *et al.*, 1986).

5.1.2. *Chronic Tolerance*

Chronic or repeated exposure to ethanol results in resistance to the intoxicating effects of the drug (Goldberg, 1943). Goldberg (1943) examined tolerance in three types of drinkers: heavy, light and abstainers. Impairment due to ethanol was measured using Goldberg's finger test (subject matches up forefingers). A plot of test accuracy vs blood ethanol level revealed parallel but different dose–response curves for the three groups of drinkers. Subjects with heavy drinking histories were less impaired than moderate drinkers or abstainers. Goldberg interpreted this finding as evidence of tolerance, although the results could have been due to innate differences. The clinical work of Jellinek (1960) suggested that ethanol tolerance required many years of heavy drinking, however experimental studies in humans and animals indicate tolerance can develop rapidly. After ten doses of ethanol (5 g/kg every other day), Wallgren and Lindbohm (1961) found rats to be less impaired on a tilting plane test. LeBlanc *et al.* (1969) studied tolerance to the effects of ethanol on a moving belt test. After two weeks of daily ethanol (3–6 g/kg/day) rats showed a parallel shift of the dose–response curve in which the ED_{50} had been increased by approximately 33%. More recent studies have shown that chronic ethanol administration results in tolerance to the effects of ethanol on several response measures, including hypothermia (Pohorecky, 1974; Crabbe *et al.*, 1982; Brick and Horowitz, 1983; Goldstein and Zaechelein, 1983; Kalant and Le, 1984; Pohorecky *et al.*, 1986), incoordination ataxia (Hunt and Overstreet, 1977; Crabbe *et al.*, 1982; Pohorecky *et al.*, 1986), startle response (Pohorecky *et al.*, 1976, 1986), analgesia (Pohorecky *et al.*, 1976, 1986), memory (Poulos *et al.*, 1981; Shapiro and Nathan, 1986), locomotor activity (Hunt and Overstreet, 1977) heart rate (Pohorecky *et al.*, 1986) and changes in electroencephalography (Zilm *et al.*, 1981, 1982). Generally, the development of tolerance to the effects of ethanol is rapid, particularly for responses such as hypothermia. For example, Brick and Horowitz (1983) found tolerance to ethanol induced hypothermia in only three days. However, the rate of tolerance development may be dependent on what response is being measured. For example, tolerance to the hypothermic effects of ethanol in rats is fully developed after 9 days of chronic ethanol treatment, but tolerance to loss of balance on a dowel test required 17 days and tolerance to a startle response required an even longer time to develop in the same subjects (Pohorecky *et al.*, 1986). Peris and Cunningham (1985) found the development of tolerance to the hypothermic, but not the cardioaccelerating effects of ethanol after 18 days of treatment.

5.1.3. *Dispositional and Metabolic Tolerance*

If there is less drug available to alter general cellular function, there will be less effect of the drug on whatever response is being measured. Dispositional tolerance could result from differences in ethanol absorption and distribution, however, the most important factor in altering drug availability to some target tissue is metabolism. With many drugs, their repeated administration results in enzyme induction so that more enzyme is available to metabolize the drug. Under such circumstances, the drug is metabolized more rapidly so it does not reach its full pharmacological effect due to metabolic tolerance. In human alcoholics, the magnitude of metabolic tolerance is unknown and is probably quite variable. In animals, chronic ethanol treatment may induce liver enzymes to increase ethanol metabolism by 30–50% (Lieber and DiCarli, 1972; Lieber, 1983).

5.1.4. *Cross Tolerance*

Cross tolerance between alcohol and other drugs may develop through several different mechanisms including the sharing of similar pathways of metabolism, or receptor systems. The most consistent evidence concerning mechanisms of cross-tolerance comes from research on metabolic tolerance in which two different drugs share the same metabolic pathways. Known pathways of ethanol metabolism, discussed in Section 1.2.4, include oxidative metabolism catalyzed by cytochrome P-450, reduced nicotinamine–adenine dinucleotide phosphate and MEOS. Drugs such as barbiturates and minor tranquillizers that utilize these systems may be removed from the body more slowly in the presence of ethanol. Thus the combination of ethanol with other drugs can be toxic because of unpredicted high drug concentrations (Chakraborty, 1980; Lieber and Pirola, 1982). Interactions between ethanol and environmental factors as well as other drugs may also contribute to cross-tolerance (Kalant and Khanna, 1980).

5.2. Theories of Tolerance

The most dramatic demonstration of drug tolerance involves cellular tolerance in which the physiological responses to various drugs decrease with repeated drug exposure. The precise mechanisms involved in cellular tolerance are not fully understood, but a number of theories and experiments have been generated in order to answer this question.

5.2.1. *Role of Neurotransmitters, Neuropeptides and Other Hormones*

Goldstein and Goldstein (1961) suggested that tolerance could develop as a result of changes in the neurotransmitters. They proposed that if a drug could inhibit the rate limiting enzyme in the formation of a neurotransmitter, the initial effect of the drug would be to lower the level and functional activity of that neurotransmitter. Thus, changes in the functional activity of various neurotransmitters produced the neuropsychopharmacological effects of the drug.

The expression of ethanol tolerance seems to depend upon an intact monoaminergic system (Frankel *et al.*, 1975, 1978a,b; Tabakoff *et al.*, 1977; Tabakoff and Ritzmann, 1977; LeBlanc *et al.*, 1978, Khanna *et al.*, 1979; Le *et al.*, 1981; Speisky and Kalant, 1985). For example, Le *et al.*, (1981) lesioned specific serotonin, norepinephrine and dopamine containing neurons and assessed the development of tolerance to ethanol-induced hypothermia and motor impairment. Lesion-induced depletion of serotonin retarded the development of tolerance but the combined depletion of norepinephrine and serotonin completely inhibited tolerance development. Similarly, dietary supplements of the serotonin precursor, L-tryptophan, increase the rate of tolerance acquisition to the effects of chronic ethanol on motor impairment and hypothermia (Le *et al.*, 1979, 1981; Khanna *et al.*, 1979). Tabakoff and Ritzmann (1977) examined the role of neurotransmitters and the relationship between tolerance and dependence. When mice were pretreated with 6-OHDA and treated with chronic ethanol they did not develop tolerance to the temperature lowering or hypnotic effects of ethanol. Even though pretreatment with 6-OHDA prevented the development of tolerance, it did not affect withdrawal. In other words, dopamine neurotoxin affected tolerance but not dependence, suggesting that these two phenomena are mediated by different neurochemical systems and are not simply points at opposite ends of a continuum.

From a biological survival perspective, adaptive responses must be learned and remembered in order to be useful to the organism when faced with a similar future environmental challenge. Therefore, neurochemical mechanisms believed to play a role in mediating learning and memory may also be involved in ethanol tolerance. Experimental manipulations that alter brain monoaminergic activity have been shown to impair the learning of new tasks (McGaugh *et al.*, 1975, 1980). In addition, brain neuropeptides such as the neurohypophyseal hormone 8-arginine vasopressin (AVP) has been shown to play a role in memory processing (deWeid, 1980) and, as discussed below, ethanol tolerance.

In mice, chronic ethanol administration results in an increase in basal levels of AVP although animals continued to show an inhibition of AVP in response to an acute ethanol challenge (Hoffman and Tabakoff, 1981). Furthermore, development of functional tolerance to the hypothermic and sedative effects of chronic ethanol treated animals is prolonged by AVP treatment (Hoffman and Tabakoff, 1979; Hoffman *et al.*, 1983; Hung *et al.*, 1984). The effect of AVP may be dependent upon brain noradrenergic neurons since the administration of 6-OHDA neurotoxin greatly reduced the tolerance prolonging effects of AVP (Hoffman and Tabakoff, 1983).

Glucocorticoid levels in plasma are elevated by acute and chronic ethanol (see Section 5). These hormones may also play a role in tolerance (Sze, 1983). Wood (1977) found that rats that were injected daily with dexamethasone and ethanol had a higher rate of tolerance development to the depressant effects of ethanol, compared to animals that received ethanol alone. Similarly, tolerance to the hypnotic effects of ethanol were antagonized by the co-administration of cortexolone, a glucocorticoid receptor blocker (Tabakoff and Yanai, 1979).

5.2.2. *Role of Biological Membranes*

Collier (1965) proposed that tolerance producing drugs reduce the level of activity at some postsynaptic site resulting in a compensatory increase in the number of postsynaptic receptors, presumably via the synthesis of new receptor protein. When the number of receptors has increased to sufficiently compensate for the decreased neurotransmitter level, it resulted in tolerance. In this disuse or supersensitivity theory, withdrawal hyperexcitability is also explained as a condition that develops with tolerance. Withdrawal results when the drug is withdrawn and receptors are then able to interact with the unrepressed neurotransmitter. Consistent with this theory, French (1975) found that chronic ethanol increased the sensitivity of adenylate cyclase to norepinephrine stimulated cAMP.

Research from several laboratories suggests that ethanol enters neuronal membrane and acts in some way to alter membrane fluidity (Hill and Bangham, 1975; Chin and Goldstein, 1977a,b). Ethanol is believed to cause an unfavorable shift in membrane dynamics, namely an increase in membrane fluidity caused by disordering of lipid-protein which disrupts the normal functioning of the cell. With chronic ethanol exposure, individual neurons respond to the increased fluidizing effects of ethanol by altering the lipid composition of the cell membrane so it is less fluid. In response to ethanol, rapid changes within neurons may include increased saturation of membrane phospholipids and increased cholesterol:phospholipid molar ratio (Chin *et al.*, 1978; Littleton *et al.*, 1979). These changes may underlie behavioral expressions of tolerance (Littleton, 1980). That is, larger amounts of ethanol are required to affect the compensated membrane and a state of tolerance exists. When the drug is withdrawn, the newly adapted membrane is now too rigid and the withdrawal syndrome occurs.

5.2.3. *Non-pharmacological Factors*

An area of considerable scientific interest is the role of non-pharmacological (i.e. environmental) factors in the development of tolerance. Although this is not a new concept, recent investigation of non-pharmacological factors in alcohol tolerance have added significantly to the field. One of the earliest learning-based theories of tolerance was the demonstration of state-dependent learning (Overton 1966, 1972). State dependency characterizes the observation that a task learned and practiced under a drug state is better performed in the same drug state. The demonstration of state dependent learning with ethanol suggested the possibility that tolerance and dependence can be explained in state dependent terms. Performance steadily improves in the drug state until tolerance develops. Abrupt removal of the drug shifts the organism to the non-drug state and performance deficits occur.

In an early study Chen (1968) injected rats with ethanol before a daily maze test session and found that initially, performance was markedly impaired. With repeated injections, however, performance improved until ethanol tolerance developed. If rats were given the same doses of ethanol after the test rather than before, subsequent testing after a single dose of ethanol revealed significant behavioral impairment. Since all rats received the same training and ethanol exposure, cellular tolerance should have been identical. Chen interpreted these findings as evidence of a purely psychological form of tolerance. In contrast, LeBlanc *et al.* (1975, 1976) suggested that intoxicated practice augmented the rate of tolerance acquisition. In the above cited studies, LeBlanc and colleagues found that if rats were exposed to ethanol, but not allowed to practice while intoxicated, they developed the same degree of tolerance as rats that practiced while intoxicated. Other investigators have not replicated these findings (Wenger *et al.*, 1981).

The work of Siegel and others has provided additional evidence that learning plays a significant role in the development of tolerance. Siegel's model (1978) of drug tolerance is by far the most influential and best supported model of its kind. Siegel suggests that environmental stimuli preceding drug intake elicit a conditioned compensatory response which attenuates the drug effect. In Siegel's classical Pavlovian conditioning paradigm, the conditioned stimuli (CS) consists of the various experimental procedures and environmental stimuli associated with the administration of the drug. The unconditioned stimuli (UCS) are the actual direct pharmacological effects of the drug. The conditioned response (CR), once formed by repeated administrations of the drug, may then be demonstrated with a placebo by presenting the usual drug administration cues (CS) in the absence of the pharmacological effects of the drug (UCS). Siegel initially proposed that in accord with a Pavlovian conditioning theory, the conditioned responses should then mimic the unconditioned response.

The conditioned response to certain drugs of abuse appears in many instances as preparation for, rather than a replica of the unconditioned response (Seward, 1970). In other words the conditioned responses to drug associated stimuli are often in the opposite direction to the pharmacological effects of the drug. These responses are presumably physiological changes made by the organism to negate the disruption in homeostasis produced by the pharmacological agent. For example, in a study by Crowell *et al.* (1981) two groups of rats were given alternating schedules of ethanol and saline injections and changes in body temperature were measured. For one group ethanol was administered in a distinctive environment and saline was administered in the animal colony room. In the second group the room in which ethanol or saline was administered was reversed from Group 1. After about 3 weeks of such pairings, all rats were subsequently injected with ethanol or saline in both the distinctive environment or the colony room. It was found that in rats previously receiving ethanol in the distinct environment, ethanol produced slight hypothermia but hypothermia was pronounced in rats previously injected in the colony room. When rats that were previously given saline in the distinctive environment were given saline there was little thermic response. If rats had previously received ethanol in this environment and were then given saline placebo, marked hyperthermia was observed (Crowell *et al.*, 1981). Conditioned tolerance has been demonstrated for many different drugs, including ethanol both in animals (Le *et al.*, 1979; Hinson and Siegel, 1980; Mansfield and Cunningham, 1980; Melchior and Tabakoff, 1981, 1985; Greeley *et al.*, 1984) and in humans (Dafters and Anderson, 1982; Newlin, 1985, 1986; Shapiro and Nathan, 1986; Tiffany and Baker, 1986).

According to Siegel (1978), the repeated pairing of stimuli associated with drug intake with the pharmacological effects of the drug leads to an increase in the magnitude of the conditioned compensatory response. Accordingly, when the drug is administered in conjunction with the usual pre-drug cues, the drug effect is reduced by these anticipatory conditioned compensatory responses. As these compensatory conditioned responses increase in magnitude, with continued drug intake, the effect of the drug continues to decrease. The decreasing effect of a drug as a function of repeated intake defines chronic tolerance.

Up until recently, most studies of conditioned tolerance have utilized animal subjects, but a preliminary exploration of the role of classical conditioning processes in human tolerance to ethanol was reported by Lightfoot and Vogel-Sprott (1981). These researchers tested tolerance to bead-stringing and coding vigilance measures of tolerance in male social drinkers before and after alcohol over the course of four sessions. Subjects in group 1 were given alcohol in the presence of a distinct set of environmental cues. Subjects in a second group were treated identically, except that they were not tested. Subjects in a third group received alcohol under a different set of environmental cues (and were tested before, rather than after, receiving alcohol). Subjects in a fourth group received a placebo during the phase of the study when tolerance developed. This phase of the study was followed by a tolerance test session in which all subjects received alcohol in the distinct environment and were then tested on the perceptual motor tasks. Subjects in the first and second groups were significantly less impaired, that is, more tolerant, on the coding vigilance task than those in group three, just as the classical conditioning model of tolerance would predict.

In two recent studies, Newlin and colleagues examined expectancy effects of alcohol. If subjects were told they were receiving alcohol, but actually received a placebo, subjects often showed physiological responses that were in the opposite direction to the acute effects of alcohol. Newlin (1985a,b) interpreted these findings as evidence of conditioned compensatory responses, further supporting a classical conditioning model of ethanol tolerance. Other investigators (Tiffany and Baker, 1986) have criticized such findings, pointing out inconsistent results both between and within physiological dependent variables used in such studies.

More recently, Shapiro and Nathan (1986) studied the role of Pavlovian conditioning in tolerance development in male subjects classified as light to moderate drinkers. Subjects were assigned to one of two groups and then participated in four experimental phases. Both groups received five administrations of alcohol and five administrations of an equal volume of tonic on an alternating schedule during a 10 session tolerance development phase. Group 1 received alcohol under environmental conditions designated the 'distinct environment' and received tonic in the 'home environment.' Group 2 was treated the same except the relationship between the environmental cues and the substance consumed was reversed. On the 11th session, both groups received alcohol in the distinct environment. On the 12th day both groups received tonic in the distinct environment.

Tolerance was assessed from cognitive, motor, physiological and affective responses. Subjects who received alcohol under cues previously associated with alcohol consumption (Group 1) were significantly less impaired (more tolerant) in Session 11 on the cognitive task than subjects who received alcohol under cues never before associated with alcohol (Group 2). Furthermore, in Session 12, Group 1 subjects evidenced compensatory responses opposite in direction to the unconditioned effect of the drug; that is, Group 1 subjects performed significantly better on the cognitive task than Group 2 subjects. Although all other measures were sensitive to the effects of alcohol, the presence or absence of cues predicting alcohol consumption did not impact significantly on these responses.

5.3. Effect of Stress on Tolerance

A recent study by Maier and Pohorecky (1986) provides evidence for an interaction between stress and ethanol tolerance. Footshock stress accelerated the development of tolerance to ethanol on several tasks, including hypothermia and motor impairment. However, a psychological stressor had the opposite effect; it retarded tolerance development.

5.4. Conclusions

Tolerance to ethanol is a multidimensional event. Tolerance may develop during the course of a single administration of ethanol (acute tolerance) but may also develop over the course of repeated ethanol administration (chronic or functional tolerance). Metabolic tolerance, cross-tolerance or stress may account for the decreased effect of the drug. Manipulations of central nervous system monoamines or peptide hormones alter the expression of tolerance. The precise mechanisms responsible for this are unknown but may involve perturbations of cell membranes to alter the functional activity of the nervous system.

6. ETHANOL DEPENDENCE AND WITHDRAWAL

Dependence can be defined as those adaptive biological changes induced by chronic drug exposure that are reflected in various behavioral and physiological responses expressed upon removal of the drug (i.e. withdrawal). Originally, it was believed that the development of tolerance and physical dependence shared similar biochemical mechanisms and that tolerance and withdrawal were part of the same continuum. The relationship between tolerance and dependence has been discussed in several reviews (Cicero, 1977; Goldstein, 1979; Tabakoff, 1980).

6.1. Alcoholism

In spite of the fact that alcohol abuse and alcoholism are major public health problems in most industrialized countries and have been around for centuries, it is difficult to define these concepts. An alcoholic diagnosis is complicated by inconsistent attitudes and definitions of what abusive drinking is (Mendelson and Mello, 1985). Cultural and social variables add further variability to defining alcoholism. The World Health Organization (WHO) Expert Committee (Edwards *et al.*, 1977) recommends replacing the term 'alcoholism' with 'ethanol-type drug dependence' and defines this disorder as follows:

> Drug dependence of the ethanol type may be said to exist when the consumption of ethanol by an individual exceeds the limits that are accepted by his culture, if he consumes ethanol at times that are deemed inappropriate within that culture, or his intake of ethanol becomes so great as to injure his health or impair his social relationships.

The ethanol dependence syndrome consists of clusters of phenomena including a 'narrowing in the repertoire of drinking behavior; salience of drink-seeking behavior; increased tolerance to ethanol; repeated withdrawal symptoms; repeated relief or avoidance of withdrawal symptoms by further drinking; subjective awareness of a compulsion to drink; reinstatement of the syndrome after abstinence (Edwards *et al.*, 1977). Psycho-social and medical sequellae are deliberately omitted from the WHO description of ethanol dependence.

In contrast, the American Psychiatric Association (APA) emphasizes impairment of personal health and social and occupational functioning. Drinking is considered a normal part of culture in many countries. Dependence is indicated when the culturally accepted drinking patterns are exceeded. Essential features of abusive drinking include a pattern of pathological use for at least a month that causes impairment in social or occupational functioning whereas alcohol dependence is reflected in a pathological pattern of alcohol use or impairment in social or occupational functioning due to alcohol, and either tolerance or withdrawal (APA, 1980). The APA diagnostic criteria for alcohol abuse include the need for daily use of alcohol for normal functioning, the inability to stop drinking, frequent attempts to stop drinking, binges (remaining intoxicated throughout the day for at least two days), blackouts and the occasional consumption of a fifth of spirits or its equivalent in other alcoholic beverages. Other behavioral criteria include social or occupational impairment such as violence, loss of job, legal difficulties due to drinking, and arguments with family or friends because of excessive ethanol use.

6.2. Ethanol Withdrawal Syndrome

The ethanol withdrawal syndrome has been known at least since the time of Hippocrates who noted, 'If the patient be in the prime of life and from drinking he has trembling hands, it may be well to announce beforehand either delerium or convulsion' (cited by Ballenger and Post, 1978). In more recent times, the relationship between abstinence in alcoholics and the withdrawal syndrome was described by Victor and Adams (1953). Later studies have helped establish the chronology of withdrawal, namely that the severity of withdrawal is positively correlated with the length of ethanol consumption prior to the period of abstinence (Isbell *et al.*, 1955; Mendelson, 1964).

Early or minor withdrawal and late or major withdrawal (Table 1) (delerium tremens or DTs) phases have been described in humans although there may be considerable overlap between these two phases. Symptoms of early withdrawal include insomnia, vivid dreaming and 'hangover' and are associated with decreases in blood ethanol concentration. Anxiety, tremor (the 'shakes'), agitation, hypertension and tachycardia may also develop shortly after the termination of drinking. In most cases these symptoms disappear within 48 hr (APA, 1980).

Major withdrawal symptoms include autonomic nervous system hyperactivity, disorientation, confusion and hallucinations may occur. Convulsions, identical to tonic-clonic seizures of grand mal epilepsy also occur. Autonomic overreactivity usually includes sweating, nausea, vomiting, diarrhea and fever. In both humans and animals acute or chronic administration of ethanol alters the functioning of the hypothalamic-hypophyseal-adrenocortical system, and produces a number of endocrine changes discussed below. The APA diagnosis for alcohol dependence is very similar to that of alcohol abuse adding the cri-

TABLE 1. *Qualitative and temporal differences between early and late alcohol withdrawal symptoms (adapted from Naranjo and Sellers, 1986)*

Clinical	Early/minor withdrawal	Late/major withdrawal
Symptoms	Mild agitation Anxiety Restlessness Tremor Anorexia Insomnia	Extreme psychomotor and autonomic activity Disorientation Confusion sensory-perceptual impairment
Time post-alcohol	0–48 hr	24–150 hr
Peak of withdrawal severity	24–36 hr Mild	72–96 hr potentially life threatening
Seizures	Yes, 6–48 hr post alcohol	Yes, 24–48 hr post alcohol

teria of tolerance (markedly increased amounts of alcohol to achieve the desired effect) and withdrawal (morning 'shakes,' and malaise relieved by drinking) after the cessation of, or reduction in, drinking (APA, 1980).

In animal models, symptoms associated with acute withdrawal are similar to those observed in humans and may include: tremors, anorexia, EEG manifestations, convulsions, temperature aberrations, hypersensitivity, piloerection and mydriasis (Tabakoff, 1977). Ethanol withdrawal in animals is discussed in detail in Section 6.4.5.

6.3. Medical–Physiological Consequences

During withdrawal from ethanol, both human and animal subjects show behavioral hyperexcitability. Some investigators have suggested that the acute and chronic effects of ethanol administration are on a 'biological continuum' (Cicero, 1978). Initial psychopharmacological effects of the drug are due to changes in the functional activity of biological systems, but with continued exposure to ethanol, the system adapts (tolerance). When ethanol is removed, a disruption of this adaptation results in the withdrawal syndrome. Thus, many investigators have postulated that tolerance and withdrawal are related (but see Section 6.2.1). It has been postulated that ethanol withdrawal may be a rebound or derepression of increased neurotransmitter activity (Goldstein and Goldstein, 1961) due to increased number of post-synaptic receptors (Collier, 1965), kindling (Post and Ballenger, 1981), and alterations in membrane fluidity (Hill and Bangham, 1975).

Ethanol abuse can result in a number of medical complications including: hepatic pathogenesis, fatty liver (Lieber, 1977, 1982); endocrine dysfunction, including changes in reproductive (Cicero, 1980) and pituitary-hypothalamic-adrenal functioning (Van Theil, 1983); impairment of cardiovascular functioning (Altura *et al.*, 1983; Ashley, 1982; Ettinger *et al.*, 1976; LaPorte *et al.*, 1980) and immunosuppression (Johnson, 1975; Strauss and Berenyi, 1973; Lundy *et al.*, 1975).

Specific neurochemical changes associated with ethanol withdrawal are discussed in Sections 3.3.3, 4.2.4, 5.3 and 7.2.1. Endocrine system changes during ethanol withdrawal are discussed in Section 4.2.

6.4. Animal Models of 'Alcoholism'

Animal models of alcoholism are essential for research aimed at unraveling the chronic effects of ethanol treatment on an organism, particularly its effects on the brain. A major difficulty, however, has been that experimental animals will not voluntarily ingest sufficient amounts of ethanol to result in physical dependence. The metabolic capacity of rats is approximately 9 g/kg/day of ethanol. Therefore, for significant levels of ethanol to accumulate in blood, daily ingestion of ethanol must approach and/or exceed the metabolic capacity of the organism. In order to achieve blood ethanol levels necessary to produce physical dependence, ethanol has been administered to experimental animals in a variety of ways. Since practically all of these methods are forceful, various degrees of stress are associated with them. None of the currently available methods is ideal, each has certain advantages and disadvantages. We shall outline briefly the currently available animal models. For in-depth discussion of this topic the reader is directed to several excellent reviews on this topic (Goldstein, 1978; Cicero, 1980; Freund, 1980; Pohorecky, 1981).

Criteria for an animal model of alcoholism were established in 1973 by Lester and Freed and have been subsequently modified (Pohorecky, 1981). Although most of these criteria have been met successfully by many of the existing animal models, one of these, the voluntary ingestion of pharmacologically relevant amounts of ethanol, has not been easy to meet. Recently, with the advent of pharmacogenetics, this criterion has now been adequately met (Waller *et al.*, 1984).

In experimental animals physical dependence is manifested by the withdrawal syndrome. Thus the only way the severity of the dependence can be evaluated is by quantitating the severity of the withdrawal syndrome. The withdrawal syndrome in rodents is dependent on the following variables:

(a) method of ethanol administration,

(b) duration and dose of ethanol treatment,

(c) age of subjects, and

(d) genetic factors.

Besides these variables, there is the problem of quantifying the withdrawal syndrome.

6.4.1. *Methods of Ethanol Administration*

Basically the methods of ethanol administration fall into three broad categories. These categories are based on the control exerted by the experimenter. Treatment of experimental animals with ethanol can be voluntary, semivoluntary or involuntary. The voluntary method of ethanol treatment has possibly the most relevance to alcohol ingestion in humans. It is the only method that allows investigation of the reinforcing properties of ethanol.

6.4.1.1. *Involuntary method.* With this method the exposure to ethanol is totally controlled by the experimenter. Exposure to ethanol can be continuous (inhalation, gastric infusion, sustained ethanol release tube) or discontinuous (gastric intubation).

(a) *Inhalation.* Goldstein and Pal (1971) developed this relatively simple and ingenious inhalation technique. As originally developed for mice, it was used in combination with daily injections of pyrazole to stabilize blood ethanol levels (Goldstein, 1972). Pyrazole retards ethanol elimination *in vivo* (Lester *et al.*, 1968; Goldberg and Rydberg, 1969) by inhibiting the metabolism of ethanol. Animals are first primed with a dose of ethanol necessary to achieve a specific level of ethanol in blood, which is then maintained through inhalation. There is good correlation between ethanol levels in the inspired air and in blood (Goldstein, 1974; Ferko and Bobyock, 1978). As metabolic tolerance develops, ethanol levels in the air must be increased (Goldstein, 1974). The inhalation method has also been adapted for rats. Roach *et al.* (1973) obtained stable blood ethanol levels of up to 300 mg/dl in rats exposed to ethanol for 7 days without the use of pyrazole. More recently Ferko and Bobyock (1978) and Rogers *et al.* (1979) have used this method to successfully maintain increasing levels of ethanol of up to 300 mg/dl for a period of over 10 days, without the use of pyrazole to stabilize ethanol levels in blood. The effects of rate and dose of ethanol on the severity of withdrawal produced by this procedure have been described (Le-Bourhis and Aufrere, 1983).

A modification of the inhalation model was recently described which incorporated voluntary selection of ethanol exposure (Rijk *et al.*, 1982). The procedure employed specially constructed chambers in which vaporized ethanol was, or was not, present. Mice could freely move from one chamber to the other. To facilitate initial selection of the chamber containing ethanol in the air, this chamber was darkened. This method produced significant blood ethanol levels (60 mg/dl) and resulted in the development of a withdrawal syndrome when exposure to ethanol vapor was terminated. However, when both the ethanol and non-ethanol containing chambers had equal illumination, preference for the chamber containing ethanol vapor waned after 3 days, suggesting factors other than ethanol were responsible for chamber selection.

(b) *Gastric intubation.* This is an extensively used method with a number of animal species (rats, dogs, cats, monkeys). The intubations can be done manually, or may be carried out with an infusion pump in animals with implanted gastric catheters. Majchrowicz (1975) and Majchrowicz and Hunt (1976) were the first to apply the intubation method to rats. Their procedure consisted of delivering aqueous solutions of ethanol via a stomach tube three to five times daily. Each dose, other than the initial one, was based on individual behavioral evaluation of the animals, with criteria differing during the early versus the latter part of the treatment. Cannon *et al.* (1974) developed a simplified version of this method. Animals received no food or water during the treatment period, and in contrast to other methods, the daily dose of ethanol decreased from 12 to 5 g/kg over the 2 day exposure period. Animals were treated every 8 hr with the dose adjusted to the state of each individual animal, which was evaluated according to selected behavioral criteria. Apparently animals did not become tolerant fast enough to adapt to exposure of high doses of ethanol.

An undesirable consequence of this method is weight loss, which among other things limits the total duration of treatment. To circumvent this side effect several investigators adopted a modified version (Hillbom, 1975; Mucha *et al.*, 1975; Noble *et al.*, 1976) in which a nutritionally complete liquid diet was intubated with ethanol (Mucha *et al.*, 1975), or was made available to the animals in their cages. Another problem with this method includes potential overdosing of the animals and perforation of the esophagus.

An automated oral infusion procedure was originally employed by Deutsch and Koopmans (1973) to study ethanol preference. This method has been adapted for producing ethanol dependence by French and his associates. An ethanol-containing liquid diet is infused at fixed intervals manually or by an infusion pump via an implanted gastric cannula (Pettit *et al.*, 1980; Tsukamoto *et al.*, 1985). High blood ethanol levels (250 to 300 mg/dl) can be easily maintained and animals do not have to be partially food-deprived prior to treatment. Tsukamoto (*et al.*, 1985) implanted animals with a double gastrostomy cannula, ethanol (8–12 g/kg/day) was infused through the lumen of one of the cannulas and a low fat liquid diet was infused through the other. This method resulted in blood ethanol levels as high as 300 mg/dl. It is noteworthy that besides primates this is the first animal model using rats that produced evidence of liver pathology. Thirty days of ethanol treatment resulted in focal necrosis with mononuclear cell infiltration in centrilobular areas of the liver. Also the accumulation of triglycerides in the liver was directly related to the levels of blood ethanol achieved.

A procedure whereby multiple-individually housed rats receive continuous or intermittent preprogrammed intragastric infusions of ethanol has also been described (Pohorecky *et al.*, 1987).

A programmed intravenous procedure for the administration of ethanol has also been described (Numan and Gilroy, 1978; Numan and Naparzewska, 1984). A total of 10–14 g/kg/day ethanol (30%) was infused in 4–12 fractions. After 7 days of treatment 63% of the rats developed audiogenic seizures during withdrawal.

6.4.1.2. *Semivoluntary methods.* With these methods ethanol is administered as part of the daily food or fluid ingested by the animals. Although these methods are probably the simplest, there is no control over the daily dose of ethanol since ingestion may vary both between and within days. However, there is less danger of overdosing the animals with this procedure because intoxication precludes further ingestion of ethanol.

(a) *Ethanol as part of fluid intake.* Ethanol exposure as part of fluid intake was originally described by Richter (1926) and consists of confining the animal's fluid intake to aqueous solutions of ethanol. Initially very dilute nonaversive solutions are offered (3 to 5%). As animals become adapted to the taste of the solution and develop metabolic tolerance, the ethanol content of the solutions is gradually raised. Animals are then maintained at the highest concentrations of ethanol they will ingest (15 to 30%).

A recently described modification of this procedure resulted in the consumption of rather high levels of ethanol with the consequent development of tolerance and physical dependence (Lindros *et al.*, 1984). The procedure consisted of starting animals on ethanol ingestion when they are young (5 weeks of age) and the concentration of the ethanol solution was increased gradually from 5% to 17.5% with peak consumption of 15–17 g/kg (35–40% of their liquid intake). If in addition 4-methylhydrazole is given daily, blood ethanol levels are more stable as is the development of tolerance and physical dependence.

(b) *Schedule induced polydipsia.* The model developed by Falk *et al.* (1972) is based on the observation that food-deprived rats will drink large amounts of fluid in a rather short period of time when food is presented in small portions every few minutes. The ingestion of ethanol in concentrations up to 6% during 1 hr sessions was maintained for periods of 4 to 6 months. Before training animals are reduced to 80% of their free-feeding weights, blood ethanol levels as high as 200 to 300 mg/dl were attained with this method. Others have been somewhat less successful in producing severe withdrawal reactions with this model (Heintzelman *et al.*, 1976; McMillan *et al.*, 1976).

(c) *Liquid diet.* One of the most successful and widely used animal methods is the liquid diet procedure. As originally developed for mice, by Freund (1969), it required that the animal's weight be reduced by about 30% prior to initiation of the treatment, to ensure high initial food intake while animals adapted to the adulterated diet. This procedure produces high blood ethanol levels (250 to 300 mg/dl) and, consequently, physical dependence is generated within a week. The liquid diet model was first employed with rats by Branchey *et al.* (1971), has also been used extensively with primates (Pieper and Skeen, 1972; Lieber and DeCarli, 1973). In rats, weight reduction is not necessary for adequate ingestion of the diet. For the control animals the ethanol-derived calories are replaced equicalorically with carbohydrate. Although sucrose has been used most frequently (Freund, 1969; Ritzmann and Tabakoff, 1976; Numan and Gilroy, 1978), other carbohydrates such as dextrose (Frye and Ellis, 1977) and a mixture of dextrin maltose (Lieber and DeCarli, 1973) have also been used. Since the control group is pair-fed with respect to the experimental groups, this method probably provides the best nutritional control.

Hunter *et al.*, 1975 have provided the most detailed parametric investigation of ethanol physical dependence with this method in rats. Freund (1970) and Goldstein and Arnold (1976) have extensively characterized this model using mice.

A new liquid diet incorporating nutrients specifically recommended for rodents was described by Miller *et al.* (1980). After 15 to 20 days of ingestion of this diet (32% of daily calories in the form of ethanol), blood ethanol levels of 300 mg/dl resulted. Tolerance to the depressant effects of ethanol was evident 7 days and physical dependence was produced in 10 days of treatment. Also an updated description of the Lieber and DeCarli liquid diet has been recently published (Lieber and DeCarli, 1986).

6.4.1.3. *Voluntary methods.* This category includes self administration of ethanol either intragastrically or intravenously. In general, the procedure consists of training animals to press a bar in order to receive an infusion of ethanol into the jugular vein or stomach. Of the animals that do respond to training, monkeys will infuse ethanol to the point where they become grossly intoxicated (up to 400 mg/dl). They will also show episodic periods of self abstinence during which withdrawal symptoms develop.

A procedure for self administration of ethanol intravenously in primates was developed (Altshuler and Fenimore, 1977). A variant of the self administration procedure method for primates was developed by Meisch and Thompson (1974). Initially, an operant response is paired with the delivery of food. After this association is learned, ethanol is substituted as the reinforcer. This method is also amenable to studying the reinforcing properties of ethanol, since ethanol is self-ingested orally. The model involved prior reduction in body weight; it has not yet been used for rodents. The advantage of this approach is that the administration of ethanol is oral rather than intravenous or intragastric.

Most recently, sufficiently high voluntary oral self ingestion of ethanol has been achieved using a genetic approach. By selective breeding an alcohol-preferring P line and a non-alcohol-preferring NP line of rats was developed from Wistar rats (Lumeng *et al.*, 1977; Li *et al.*, 1979; Waller *et al.*, 1982; Waller *et al.*, 1984). Rats of the P line consume over 5.0 g/kg/day of ethanol in the presence of ad libitum food and water and a 10% ethanol solution. In contrast, NP rats under the same conditions will consume only less than 1.0 g/kg/day of ethanol. Blood ethanol levels ranging from 92 to 415 mg/dl were achieved in P lines outfitted with transesophageal catheters for intragastric infusions of ethanol upon selection of a preferred flavored water solution (Waller *et al.*, 1984). Consumption of a 10% ethanol solution by partially food-deprived animals was greatly increased (7–14 g/kg/day for P rats and 1–12 g/kg/day of NP rats). After 8 weeks of consumption withdrawal developed in both lines of rats (Waller *et al.*, 1982).

6.4.2. *Duration and Dose of Ethanol Treatment*

In mice about 2 to 4 days, and in rats 3 to 9 days are required for development of dependence. The rate at which physical dependence develops depends mainly on the dose of ethanol, but other factors also play a significant role and account for the differences among the various methods. Some of these are: peak blood ethanol levels attained, maintenance of these ethanol levels, and use of auxiliary factors such as food deprivation. The effects of food ingestion on blood ethanol levels and on ethanol metabolism have been well documented (Baker *et al.*, 1977; Lumeng *et al.*, 1979). Withdrawal syndrome including audiogenic seizures were lower in animals that received the nutritional supplement during the chronic treatment with ethanol (Edmonds and Bellin, 1976; Edmonds *et al.*, 1983).

To summarize, physical dependence to ethanol develops fairly rapidly in rodents. Focusing on rats which are the most extensively investigated experimental animals, the gastric intubation procedure of Majchrowicz (1977) can produce physical dependence in 4 days of 9.0–15.9 g/kg/day (in up to 5 daily fractions) treatment with ethanol. Administration of liquid diet (35–40% of total calories as ethanol) results in the development of physical dependence within 10 days (Majchrowicz, 1975; Hunter *et al.*, 1976). Inhalation of ethanol results in physical dependence within 3 days of treatment (Goldstein, 1974). Similarly the gastric infusion procedure described by Tsukamoto *et al.* (1985) results in development of dependence with 3–4 days of treatment.

With the ingestion of ethanol via the drinking fluid, exposure time has to be relatively long, from a few weeks to several months. Some investigators have attempted to increase ethanol intake by making the solution of ethanol more palatable with sweetening agents, but without much success (Gilbert, 1974). This method of exposure to ethanol does not generally lead to the development of overt signs of withdrawal, however there is development of tolerance to ethanol. In a few cases, with prolonged exposure to ethanol, some dependence appears to develop. For instance, an increase in open field activity was noted in some rats on withdrawal from ethanol intake (7%) for 4 months (Cicero *et al.*, 1971). In another study, rats were maintained on aqueous solutions of ethanol (up to 34%) for a period of up to 270 days (Liljequist *et al.*, 1977). At this time rats ingested 11.2 g/kg/day of ethanol, and blood ethanol levels ranged from 80–200 mg/dl. When ethanol was discontinued, 45% of the animals showed audiogenic seizures and all exhibited other minor signs of withdrawal. With the inhalation procedure, exposure to ethanol for 2–4 days is sufficient to induce physical dependence (Goldstein, 1974).

Lastly, the withdrawal syndrome is more severe in animals that had experienced several cycles of intoxication and withdrawal (Baker and Cannon, 1979). Animals subjected to repeated withdrawal episodes (binge treatment with ethanol) showed accelerated development of tolerance to ethanol-induced motor impairment and hypothermia compared to animals receiving an equivalent treatment with ethanol but subjected to only one cycle of withdrawal (Maier and Pohorecky, 1987).

6.4.3. *Age of Subjects*

Age of the subjects affects not only the response to acute doses of ethanol but also the development of tolerance and physical dependence (Abel, 1978; Abel, 1979, Wood *et al.*, 1982; York, 1983; Ott *et al.*, 1985). Overall aging has been shown to be associated with an increased sensitivity to ethanol. It was found that even though blood ethanol levels were the same in young and middle aged (3 and 14 months) versus old (25 months) mice, the old mice were more intoxicated and had a more severe withdrawal syndrome (Wood *et al.*, 1982).

6.4.4. *Genetic Factors*

Although evidence for genetic factors in alcoholism has been known now for a long time, the application of genetics to the study of physical dependence in experimental animals is rather recent. Selective breeding of mice has resulted in the development of genetic lines which differ in their susceptibility for displaying seizures during withdrawal syndrome (Crabbe *et al.*, 1983; McSwigan *et al.*, 1984). These two lines of mice did not differ in susceptibility to other forms of induced convulsions (electrical, pentylene-tetrazole, strychnine, GABA, flurothyl) (McSwigan *et al.*, 1984; Harris *et al.*, 1984). The withdrawal seizure prone mice overall showed a more severe withdrawal syndrome (including tremors, greater reduction in exploratory activity) compared to the withdrawal seizure resistant line of mice (Kosobud and Crabbe, 1986), but did not differ in any other respect as far as their responsiveness to ethanol (blood ethanol levels, acute sensitivity to ethanol, tolerance to ethanol) (Crabbe and Kosobud, 1985). On the other hand the inbred C57BL/6J mice (ethanol preferring mice) show rapid development of tolerance, and had a brief and mild withdrawal syndrome while DBA2 mice (non-ethanol preferring mice) showed rapid development of tolerance and more severe and prolonged withdrawal syndrome after chronic treatment with ethanol (Grieve *et al.*, 1979). These results indicate that the adaptive capacity, whether to the presence or absence of ethanol in these mice, is genetically controlled.

6.4.5. *The Withdrawal Syndrome*

The withdrawal syndrome can be viewed as a hyperreactive state during which the CNS homeostasis is disturbed. The re-adaptation to homeostasis in the absence of ethanol underlies the withdrawal syndrome and the withdrawal symptoms can be thus viewed as the manifestation of the adaptive functions to the repeated presence of ethanol in the organism.

In rodents, symptoms of withdrawal include hyperreactivity, piloerection, wet dog shakes, tail stiffening and arching, teeth chattering, abnormal posture and a splayed, broad-sided gait, localized and general tremors, sprawling episodes, muscular fasiculations, bizarre behavior with stereotyped movements, sudden propulsions, spontaneous vocalizations, rigidity, spontaneous and sound- or handling-induced convulsions (Freund, 1980).

The beginning of the withdrawal syndrome is quite variable. It depends on how high were the blood ethanol levels after the last treatment dose of ethanol and on the rate at which blood ethanol levels fall. Generally symptoms begin to develop while there is still considerable ethanol in blood (about 100 mg/dl) (Majchrowicz, 1979) which can be anywhere from 2 to 12 hr after the last dose of ethanol. Generally most severe symptoms develop when blood ethanol levels reach zero (about 14–16 hr after the last dose of ethanol), and symptoms disappear by 24 hr (Majchrowicz, 1979).

One of the major problems in this field of research is the difficulty in quantitating the withdrawal syndrome. Determination of the severity of the withdrawal syndrome is difficult because: (1) the withdrawal symptoms generally are not sustained for long periods of time, but rather they tend to appear and disappear periodically, therefore continuous observation of the animals for long periods of time is necessary; (2) not all animals show all of the symptoms of withdrawal, the same severity, or time course despite equal treatment with ethanol; (3) most symptoms, although quite obvious when they occur, are difficult to quantitate, and therefore are graded subjectively (e.g., convulsions, tremors). Very few of the symptoms of withdrawal (e.g. startle response) are amenable to objective quantification. As a result, comparison of ethanol treatment conditions or the evaluation of pharmacological drugs to modify the withdrawal syndrome are subject to a high degree of variability and inconsistency. A few investigators have developed procedures to quantify particular parameters of the syndrome. These objective quantitative measures in most cases reflect the heightened neuroexcitability that is the hallmark of the withdrawal reaction. The simplest and most widely used procedures for mice are the convulsions elicited by handling (i.e. lifting the animal by the tail and gently rotating, if necessary) (Goldstein, 1972; Goldstein, 1974) and the hypothermia that develops during withdrawal (Tabakoff and Boggan, 1974). In rats, measures of CNS hyperexcitability such as the startle response to either sound (Pohorecky *et al.*, 1976) or electric shock (Hammond and Schneider, 1973) as well as indices of motor activity (Pohorecky, 1976) have been employed. Also, audiogenic seizures have been used in both mice (Freund and Walker, 1971) and rats (Hunter *et al.*, 1973; Samson and Falk, 1975; Baker *et al.*, 1977; Noble *et al.*, 1976; Frye and Ellis, 1977; Erickson *et al.*, 1978). Convulsions, whether audiogenic or induced with drugs or by handling, have generally been rated as an all-or-none response. However, it would be more meaningful to determine the threshold for inducing convulsions. This would allow for the grading of the severity of the response.

In a number of cases, the withdrawal syndrome has been successfully evaluated by scoring overt behavioral signs at various intervals over the first 1 or 2 (or more) days of withdrawal (Hunter *et al.*, 1975; Majchrowicz, 1975; Majchrowicz and Hunt, 1976; Pohorecky, 1976). Although such rating may be subjective and semiquantitative, this probably is the best approach currently available for the global assessment of the withdrawal syndrome.

Since physical dependence and the withdrawal syndrome are poorly understood, the relevance of particular signs during the withdrawal period is not known. For instance, is hypothermia, which develops during withdrawal in mice, an expression of primary changes in neurotransmission, or is it secondary to peripheral metabolic changes?

6.5. Conclusions

Alcoholism is not easy to define as its diagnosis may be confounded by cultural practices. Ethanol-type dependence is said to exist when drinking exceeds cultural norms or becomes so great that physical health and social relationships are jeopardized. Abstinence following long term heavy drinking results in withdrawal. Withdrawal symptoms vary in intensity from 'shakes' and tremors to frank hallucinations and, in some cases, death. Alcohol abuse is also associated with multiple medical disorders of the liver, heart, endocrine and immune system.

Animal models have been used to further study the development and etiology of dependence. A variety of methods for chronic treatment with ethanol have been described which result in the production of physical dependence as evaluated by the development of a withdrawal syndrome upon discontinuation of treatment. Each of the methods has its own particular problems. Overall, and irrespective of the method of ethanol administration, physical dependence with nearly maximum tolerable doses of ethanol develops in about 3–4 days. Doses above the daily metabolic rate of a given organism are necessary to induce physical dependence. Withdrawal severity is influenced by subject related variables such as nutritional status, age and genetic background. The withdrawal syndrome represents the transition stage during which the organism de-adapts from the chronic presence of ethanol. It consists of a sequence of symptoms which begin to appear as blood ethanol levels in the organism fall below 100 mg/dl. The withdrawal syndrome is evaluated using primarily subjective measures. Better measures for the evaluation of the withdrawal syndrome are needed.

REFERENCES

Abdel-Rahman, A.-R., Dar, M. S. and Wooles, W. R. (1985) Effect of chronic ethanol administration in arterial baroreceptor function and pressor and depressor responsiveness in rats. *J. Pharmacol. Exp. Ther.* **222**: 194–201.

Abel, E. (1978) Effects of ethanol and pentobarbital in mice of different ages. *Physiol. Psychol.* **6**: 366–368.

Abel, F. L. (1980) Direct effects of ethanol on myocardial performance and coronary resistance. *J. Pharmacol. Exp. Ther.* **212**: 28–33.

Abel E. and York, J. (1979) Age-related differences in response to ethanol in the rat. *Physiol. Psychol.* **7**: 391–395.

Adams, M. A. and Hirst, M. (1982) The ethanol withdrawal syndrome in the rat: Effects of drug treatment on adrenal gland and urinary catecholamines. *Subst. Alc. Actions Misuse* **3**: 287–298.

Adams, M. A. and Hirst, M. (1983) Myocardial hypertrophy, cardiac and urinary catecholamines during severe ethanol intoxication and withdrawal. *Life Sci.* **33**: 547–554.

Adams, M. A. and Hirst, M. (1984) Adrenal and urinary catecholamines during and after severe ethanol intoxication in rats: A profile of changes. *Pharmacol. Biochem. Behav.* **21**: 125–131.

Adinoff, B., Majchrowicz, E., Martin, P. R. and Linnoila, M. (1986) The benzodiazepine antagonists Ro 15–1788 does not antagonize the ethanol withdrawal syndrome. *Biol. Psychiat.* **21**: 643–649.

Ahlenius, S., Brown, R., Engel, J. and Lundborg, P. (1973) Learning deficits in 4 week old offspring of the nursing mothers treated with the neuroleptic drug penfluridol. *N.-S. Arch. Pharmacol.* **279**: 31–37.

Ahtee, L. and Eriksson, K. (1975) Dopamine and noradrenaline content in the brain of rat strains selected for their alcohol intake. *Acta Physiol. Scand.* **93**: 563–565.

Ahtee, L. and Svartstrom-Fraser, M. (1975) Effect of ethanol dependence and withdrawal on the catecholamines in rat brain and heart. *Acta Pharmacol. Toxicol.* **36**: 289–298.

Ahtee, L., Attila, L. M. J. and Kiianmaa, K. (1980) Brain catecholamines in rats selected for their alcohol behavior. In: *Animal Models in Alcohol Research*, pp. 55–55, Eriksson, K., Sinclair, J. D. and Kiianmaa, K. (eds) *Papers presented at the International Conference on Animal Models in Alcohol Research, Helsinki, Finland, 4–8 June, 1979.* Academic Press, New York.

Akera, T., Rech, R. H., Marquis, W. J., Tobin, T. and Brody, T. M. (1973) Lack of relationship between brain ($Na^+ + K^+$)-activated adenosine triphosphatase and the development of tolerance to ethanol in rats. *J. Pharmacol. Exp. Ther.* **185**: 594–601.

Aldegunde, M., Duran, R., Otero, P. F. and Marco, J. (1984) Effect of ethanol in preovulatory periods on brain monoamine levels. *Gen. Pharmacol.* **15**: 59–61.

Alexander, C. S. (1968) The concept of alcoholic cardiomyopathy. *Med. Clin. N. Am.* **52**: 1183–1192.

Alkana, R. L., Parker, E. S., Cohen, H. B., Birch, H. and Noble, E. P. (1976) Reversal of ethanol intoxication in humans: an assessment of the efficacy of propranolol. *Psychopharmacology.* **51**: 29–37.

Alkana, R. L., Parker, E. S., Malcolm, R. D., Cohen, H. B., Birch, H. and Noble, E. P. (1982) Interaction of apomorphine and amantadine with ethanol in men. *Alcoholism Clin. Exp. Res.* **6**: 403–411.

Allison, R. D., Kraner, J. C. and Rothe, G. M. (1971) Effects of alcohol and nitroglycerin on vascular responses in man. *Angiology* **22**: 211–222.

Aloi, R. C., Paxton, J., Daviau, J. S., van Gelb, O., Mlekusch, W., Truppe, W., Meyer, J. A. and Brauer, F. S. (1985) Effect of chronic alcohol consumption on rat brain microsome lipid composition, membrane fluidity and Na+-K+-ATPase activity. *Life Sci.* **36**: 1003–1017.

Altura, B. M. (1978) Pharmacology of venular smooth muscle: New insights. *Microvasc. Res.* **16**: 91–117.

Altura, B. M. (1981) Pharmacology of venules: Some current concepts and clinical potential. *J. Cardiovasc. Pharmacol.* **3**: 1413–1428.

Altura, B. M. and Altura, B. T. (1976) Vascular smooth muscle and prostaglandins. *Fed. Proc.* **35**: 2360–2366.

Altura, B. T. and Altura, B. M. (1978) Intravenous anesthetic agents and vascular smooth muscle function. Vanhoutte, P. M., Leusen, I. (eds) *Mechanisms of Vasodilation*, pp. 165–172, Karger, Basel.

Altura, B. M. and Altura, B. T. (1981) Alcohol induces cerebral arterial and arteriolar vasospasm by a direct action. *Circulation* **64**: Part II, 231–237.

Altura, B. M. and Altura, B. T. (1982) Microvascular and vascular smooth muscle actions of ethanol, acetaldehyde and acetate. *Fed. Proc.* **41**: 2447–2451.

Altura, B. M. and Altura, B. T. (1983) Peripheral vascular actions of ethanol and its interactions with neurohumoral substances. *Neurobehav. Toxicol Teratol.* **5**: 211–220.

Altura, B. M. and Gebrewold, A. (1981) Failure of acetaldehyde or acetate to mimic the splanchnic arteriolar venular dilator actions of ethanol: Direct in situ studies on the microcirculation. *Br. J. Pharmacol.* **73**: 580–582.

Altura, B. M., Edgarian, H. and Altura, B. T. (1976) Differential effects of ethanol and mannitol on contraction of arterial smooth muscle. *J. Pharmacol. Exp. Ther.* **197**: 352–361.

Altura, B. M., Altura, B. T. and Carella, A. (1983) Ethanol produced coronary vasospasm: Evidence for a direct action of ethanol on vascular muscle. *Br. J. Pharmacol.* **78**: 260–262.

Altura, B. M., Altura, B. T., Carella, A., Turlapaty, M. V. and Weinberg, J. (1980) Vascular smooth muscle and general anesthetics. *Fed. Proc.* **39**: 1584–1591.

American Psychiatric Association (1980) *Diagnostic and Statistical Manual of Mental Disorders*, 3rd Edn. APA, Washington, D.C.

American Psychiatric Association (1987) *Diagnostic and Statistical Manual of Mental Disorders (DSM III-R).* APA, Washington, D.C.

Amit, Z., Brown, A. W., Levitan, D. E. and Ogren, S.-O. (1977) Noradrenergic mediation of the positive reinforcing properties of ethanol. I. Suppression of ethanol consumption in laboratory rats following dopamine-beta-hydroxylase inhibition. *Arch. Int. Pharmacodyn.* **230**: 65–75.

Andersen, K. L., Hellstrom, B. and Lorentzen, F. V. (1963) Combined effect of cold and alcohol on heat balance in man. *J. Appl. Physiol.* **18**: 975–982.

ANNEAR, W. C. and VOGEL-SPROTT, M. (1985) Mental rehearsal and classical conditioning contribute to ethanol tolerance in humans. *Psychopharmacology* **87**: 90–93.

ANTON, A. H. (1965) Ethanol and urinary catecholamines. *Clin. Pharmacol. Ther.* **6**: 462–469.

ARON, E., FLANZY, M., COLMBESCOTT, C., PUISAIS, J., DEMARET, J., REYNOUARD-BRAULT, F. and IGERT, C. (1965) L'alcool est-il dans le vin l'element qui perturbe, chez la ratte, le cycle vaginal? *Bull. Acad. Natl. Med.* **149**: 112–120.

ASHLEY, J. M. (1982) Alcohol consumption, ischemic heart disease and cerebrovascular disease. *J. Stud. Alc.* **43**: 869–887.

ASHLEY, J. M. (1984) Alcohol consumption and ischemic heart disease. In: *Recent Advances in Alcohol and Drug Problems*, Vol. 8, pp. 99–147, SMART, R. G., CAPPELL, H. D., GLASER, F. B., ISRAEL, Y., KALANT, H., POPHAM, R. E., SCHMIDT, W. and SELLERS, E. M. (eds) Plenum, New York.

BACOPOULOS, N. G., BHATNAGAR, R. K. and VAN ORDEN, L. S. III. (1978) The effects of subhypnotic doses of ethanol on regional catecholamine turnover. *J. Pharmacol. Exp. Ther.* **204**: 1–10.

BADAWY, A. (1986) Alcohol intoxication and withdrawal. In: *Clinical Biochemistry of Alcoholism*, pp. 95–116, ROSALKI, E. B. (ed) Churchill Livingstone, New York.

BADAWY, A.A.-B., WILLIAMS, D. L. and EVANS, M. (1983) Role of tyrosine in the acute effects of ethanol on rat brain catecholamine synthesis. *Pharmacol. Biochem. Behav.* **18**: Suppl. 1, 389–396.

BAGHURST, K. I. and DWYER, T. (1981) Alcohol consumption and blood pressure in a group of young Australian males. *J. Hum. Nutr.* **35**: 257–264.

BAIZER, L., MASSERANO, J. M. and WEINER, N. (1981) Ethanol-induced changes in tyrosine hydroxylase activity in brains of mice selectively bred for differences in sensitivity to ethanol. *Pharmacol. Biochem. Behav.* **15**: 945–949.

BAKER, T. and CANNON, D. (1979) Potentiation of ethanol withdrawal by prior dependence. *Psychopharmacology.* **60**: 105–110.

BAKER, T. B., CANNON, D. S., BERMAN, R. F. and ATKINSON, C. A. (1977) The effect of diet on ethanol withdrawal symptomatology. *Addict. Behav.* **2**: 35–46.

BALLENGER, J. C. and POST, R. M. (1978) Kindling as a model for alcohol withdrawal syndrome. *Br. J. Psych.* **133**: 1–14.

BALLENGER, J. C., GOODWIN, F. K., MAJOR, L. F. and BROWN, G. L. (1979) Alcohol and central serotonin metabolism in man. *Arch. Gen. Psychiat.* **36**: 224–227.

BARBACCIA, M. L., REGGIANI, A., SPANO, P. F. and TRABUCCHI, M. (1980) Ethanol effects on dopaminergic function: Modulation by the endogenous opioid system. *Pharmacol. Biochem. Behav.* **13**: Suppl. 1, 303–306.

BARBACCIA, M. L., BOSIO, A., SPANO, P. F. and TRABUCCHI, M. (1982) Ethanol metabolism and striatal dopamine turnover. *J. Neural Trans.* **53**: 169–177.

BARBORIAK, J. J., ANDERSON, A. J. and HOFFMAN, R. G. (1982) Smoking, alcohol and coronary artery occlusion. *Atherosclerosis* **43**: 277–282.

BARRY, H. (1979) Behavioral manifestations of ethanol intoxication and physical dependence. In: *Biochemistry and Pharmacology of Ethanol*, Vol. 2, pp. 511–531, MAJCHROWICZ, E. and NOBLE, E. P. (eds) Plenum Press, New York.

BATTEY, L. L., HEYMAN A. and PATTERSON, J. L. (1953) Effects of ethyl alcohol on cerebral blood flow and metabolism. *JAMA* **152**: 6–10.

BEAUGE, F., STIBLER, H. and KALANT, H. (1983) Brain synaptosomal (Na^+ and K^+) ATPase activity as an index of tolerance to ethanol. *Pharmacol. Biochem. Behav.* **18**: Suppl. 1, 519–524.

BECK, O., BORG, S., HOLMSTEDT, B., KVANDE, H. and SKRODER, R. (1980) Concentration of serotonin metabolites in the cerebrospinal fluid from alcoholics before and during disulfiram therapy. *Acta Pharmacol. Toxicol.* **47**: 305–307.

BEEVERS, D. G. (1977) Alcohol and hypertension. *Lancet* **2**: 114–115.

BEILIN, L. J. and PUDDEY, I. B. (1984) Alcohol and essential hypertension. *Alc. Alcoholism* **19**: 191–195.

BEIRNESS, D. and VOGEL-SPROTT, M. (1984) Alcohol tolerance in social drinkers: Operant and classical conditioning effects. *Psychopharmacology* **84**: 393–397.

BELNAP, J. K. (1980) Genetic factors in the effects of alcohol: Neurosensitivity, functional tolerance and physical dependence. In: *Alcohol Tolerance and Dependence*, pp. 157–180, RIGTER, H. and CRABBE, J. C. (eds) Elsevier, Amsterdam.

BERACOCHEA, D., DURKIN, T. P. and JAFFARD, R. (1986) On the involvement of the central cholinergic system in memory deficits induced by long term ethanol consumption in mice. *Pharmacol. Biochem. Behav.* **24**: 519–524.

BERGLUND, M. (1981) Cerebral blood flow in chronic alcoholics. *Alcoholism Clin. Exp. Res.* **5**: 295–303.

BERGLUND, M. and INGVAR, D. H. (1976) Cerebral blood flow and its regional distribution in alcoholism and in Korsakoff's psychosis. *J. Stud. Alc.* **37**: 386–397.

BERK, S. L., BLOCK, P. J., TOSELLI, P. A. and ULLRICK, W. C. (1975) The effects of chronic alcohol ingestion in mice on contractile properties of cardiac and skeletal muscle: A comparison with normal and dehydrated-malnourished controls. *Experientia* **31**: 1302–1303.

BERKOWITZ, B. A., FINCK, A. D. and NGAI, S. H. (1976) Nitrous oxide analgesia: reversal by naloxone and development of tolerance. *J. Pharmacol. Exp. Ther.* **203**: 539–547.

BICHET, D., SZATALOWICZ, V., CHAIMOVITZ, C. and SCHRIER, R. W. (1982) Role of vasopressin in abnormal water excretion in cirrhotic patients. *Ann. Intern. Med.* **96**: 413–417.

BING, R. J., TILLMANNS, H., FAUVEL, J., SEELER, K. and MAO, J. (1974) Effect of prolonged alcohol administration on calcium transport in heart muscle of the dog. *Circ. Res.* **35**: 33–38.

BJEVERER, K. and GOLDBERG, L. (1950) Effect of alcohol ingestion on driving ability. Results of practical road tests and laboratory experiments. *Q. J. Stud. Alc.* **11**: 1–30.

BJORQVIST, S. E. (1975) Clonidine in alcohol withdrawal. *Acta Psychiat. Scand.* **52**: 256–263.

BLAKE, C. A. (1978) Paradoxical effects of drugs acting on the central nervous system on the preovulatory release of pituitary luteinizing hormone in pro-oestrous rats. *J. Endocrinol.* **79**: 319–326.

BLOOMQVIST, G., SALTIN, B. and MITCHELL, J. H. (1970) Acute effects of ethanol ingestion on the response to submaximal and maximal exercise in man. *Circulation* **42**: 463–470.

BLUM, K., MERRITT, J. H., WALLACE, J. E., OWEN, R., HAHN, J. W. and GELLER, I. (1972) Effect of catecholamine synthesis inhibition on ethanol narcosis in mice. *Curr. Ther. Res.* **14**: 324–329.

BLUM, K., CALHOUN, W., MERRITT, J. and WALLACE, J. E. (1973) 1-DOPA: Effect of ethanol narcosis and brain biogenic amines in mice. *Nature* **242**: 407–409.

BLUM, K., WALLACE, J. E., CALHOUN, W., TABOR, R. G. and EUBANKS, J. D. (1974) Ethanol narcosis in mice: Serotonergic involvement. *Experentia* **30**: 1053–1054.

BLUM, K., WALLACE, J. E., SCHWERTNER, H. A. and EUBANKS, J. D. (1976) Enhancement of ethanol-induced withdrawal convulsions by blockade of 5-hydroxytryptamine receptors. *J. Pharm. Pharmacol.* **28**: 832–835.

BLUM, K., BRIGGS, A. H., ELSTON, S. F. A., DELALLO, L., SHERIDAN, P. J. and SAR, M. (1982) Reduced leucine-enkephalin-like immunoreactive substance in hamster basal ganglia after long-term ethanol exposure. *Science* **216**: 1425–1426.

BO, W. J., KRUEGER, W. A., RUDEEN, P. K. and SYMMES, S. K. (1982) Ethanol-induced alterations in the morphology and function of the rat ovary. *Anat. Rec.* **202**: 255–260.

BOADA, J., FERIA, M., IBANEZ, T. and DARIAS, V. (1979) Action algesique de la serotoine administres par voie intra peritoneale chez la souris. *Interaction avec l'ethanol et la pentzocine Therapie* **34**: 111–115.

BOADA, J., FERIA, M. and SANZ, E. (1981) Inhibitory effect of naloxone on the ethanol-induced antinociception in mice. *Pharmacol. Res. Comm.* **13**: 673–678.

BOGGAN, W. O., RANDALL, C. L. and DODDS, H. M. (1979) Delayed sexual maturation in female C57Bl/6J mice prenatally exposed to alcohol. *Res. Commun. Chem. Pathol. Pharmacol.* **23**: 117–125.

BOLLINGER, O. (1884) Ueber der haufigkeit und ursachen der idiopathischen Herz hypertrophie in Munchen. *Drsch. Med. Wschr.* **10**: 180–181.

BORG, V. and WEINHOLDT, T. (1982) Bromocriptine in the treatment of the alcohol-withdrawal syndrome. *Acta Psychiat. Scand.* **65**: 101–111.

BORG, S., KVANDE, H. and SEDVALL, G. (1981) Central norepinephrine metabolism during alcohol intoxication in addicts and healthy volunteers. *Science* **213**: 1135–1137.

BORG, S., KVANDE, H., RYDBERG, U., TERENIUS, L. and WAHLSTROM, A. (1982) Endorphin levels in human cerebrospinal fluid during alcohol intoxication and withdrawal. *Psychopharmacology* **78**: 101–103.

BORG, S., CZARNECKA, A., KVANDE, H., MOSSBERG, D. and SEDVALL, G. (1983) Clinical conditions and concentrations of MOPEG in the cerebrospinal fluid and urine of male alcoholic patients during withdrawal. *Alcoholism. Clin. Exp. Res.* **7**: 411–415.

BORG, S., KVANDE, H., MOSSBERG, D., VALVERIUS, P. and SEDVALL, G. (1983) Central nervous system noradrenaline metabolism and alcohol consumption in man. *Pharmacol. Biochem. Behav.* **18**: 375–378.

BOWERS, R. V., BURLESON, W. D. and BLADES, J. F. (1942) Alcohol absorption from the skin in man. *Q. J. Stud. Alc.* **3**: 31–33.

BRANCHY, M., RAUSCHER, G. and KISSIN, B. (1971) Modification in the response to alcohol following the establishment of physical dependence. *Psychopharmacologia* **22**: 314–322.

BREESE, G. R., LUNDBERG, D. B. A., MAILMAN, R. B., FRYE, G. D. and MUELLER, R. A. (1979) Effect of ethanol on cyclic nucleotides in vivo: Consequences of controlling motor and respiratory changes. *Drug Alc. Depend.* **4**: 321–326.

BRICK, J. and HOROWITZ, G. P. (1982) Alcohol and morphine induced hypothermia in mice selected for sensitivity to ethanol. *Pharmacol. Biochem. Behav.* **16**: 473–479.

BRICK, J. and HOROWITZ, G. P. (1983) Tolerance and cross tolerance to morphine and ethanol in mice selectively bred for differential sensitivity to ethanol. *J. Stud. Alc.* **44**: 770–779.

BRICK, J. and POHORECKY, L. A. (1977) Ethanol withdrawal: Altered ambient temperature selection in rats. *Alcoholism. Clin. Exp. Res.* **1**: 207–211.

BRICK, J. and POHORECKY, L. A. (1982) Ethanol stress interactions: Biochemical findings. *Psychopharmacology* **77**: 81–84.

BRICK, J. and POHORECKY, L. A. (1983) The neuroendocrine response to stress and the effect of ethanol. In: *Stress and Alcohol Use*, pp. 389–402. POHORECKY, L. A. and BRICK, J. (eds) Elsevier Science, New York.

BRICK, J., SUN, J., DAVIS, L. and POHORECKY, L. A. (1976) Ethanol and the response to electric shock in rats. *Life Sci.* **18**: 1293–1298.

BRICK, J., POHORECKY, L. A., FAULKNER, W. and ADAMS, M. N. (1982) Circadian variations in behavioral and biological sensitivity to ethanol. *Alc. Clin. Exp. Res.* **8**: 204–211.

BRICK, J., NATHAN, P. E., WESTRICK, E., SHAPIRO, A. and FRANKENSTEIN, W. (1986) Effect of menstrual phase on behavioral and biological responses to alcohol. *J. Stud. Alc.* **47**: 472–477.

BRICK, J., POHORECKY, L. A. and DETURCK, K. (1987) Cardiac lipase: Effect of ethanol and stress. *Life Sci.* **40**: 1897–1901.

BRODY, T. M. and AKERA, T. (1976) Effects of ethanol on brain Na,K-ATPase and related reactions. *Pharmacology.* **18**: 189.

BROHULT, J., LEVI, L. and REICHARD, H. (1970) Urinary excretion of adrenal hormones in man; effects of ethanol ingestion, and their modification by chlormethiazole. *Acta Med. Scand.* **188**: 5–13.

BROWN, J. B. (1977) Platelet MAO and alcoholism. *Am. J. Psychiat.* **134**: 206–207.

BROWN, Z. W., AMIT, Z., LEVITAN, D. E., OGREN, S.-O. and SUTHERLAND, E. A. (1977) Noradrenergic mediation of the positive reinforcing properties of ethanol: II. Extinction of ethanol-drinking behavior in laboratory rats by inhibition of dopamine-beta-hydroxylase. Implications for treatment procedures in human alcoholics. *Arch. Int. Pharmacodyn.* **230**: 76–82.

BROWN, F. C., ZAWAD, J. and HARRALSON, J. D. (1978) Interactions of pyrazole and ethanol on norepinephrine metabolism in rat brain. *J. Pharmacol. Exp. Ther.* **206**: 75–80.

BURNS, M. and MOSKOWITZ, H. (1978) Gender related differences in impairment of performance by alcohol. In: *Currents in Alcoholism*, Vol. 3, *Biological Biochemical and Clinical Studies,* pp. 479–492, SEIXAS, F. (eds) Grune and Stratton, New York.

BURCH, G. E., HARB, J. M., COLCOLOUGH, H. H. and TSUI, C. Y. (1971) The effect of prolonged consumption of beer, wine and ethanol on the myocardium of the mouse. *Johns Hopkins Med. J.* **129**: 130–148.

BUSTOS, G. and ROTH, R. H. (1976) Effect of acute ethanol treatment on transmitter synthesis and metabolism in central dopaminergic neurons. *J. Pharmacol. Exp. Ther.* **28**: 580–582.

BUSTOS, G., ROTH, R. H. and MORGENROTH, V. H. III (1976) Activation of tyrosine hydroxylase in rat striatal slices by K^+-depolarization-effect of ethanol. *Biochem. Pharmacol.* **25**: 2493–2497.

CAMERON, D., SPENCE, M. T. and DREWERY, J. (1978) Rate of onset of drunkenness. *J. Stud. Alc.* **39**: 517–524.

CAPPELL, H. and HERMAN, C. P. (1972) Alcohol and tension reduction. A review. *Q. J. Stud. Alc.* **53**: 33–64.

CARLSSON, A. and LINDQVIST, M. (1973) Effect of ethanol on the hydroxylation of tyrosine and tryptophan in rat brain in vivo. *J. Pharm. Pharmacol.* **25**: 437–440.

CARLSSON, C. and FASTH, B.-G. (1976) A comparison of the effects of propranolol and diazepam in alcoholics. *Br. J. Addic.* **71**: 321–326.

CARLSSON, A., MAGNUSSON, T., SVENSSON, T. H. and WALDECK, B. (1973) Effect of ethanol on the metabolism of brain catecholamines. *Psychopharmacology* **30**: 30–36.

CARMICHAEL, F. J. and ISRAEL, Y. (1975) Effects of ethanol on neurotransmitter release by rat brain slices. *J. Pharmacol. Exp. Ther.* **193**: 824–834.

CARPENTER, J. A. (1963) Effects of alcohol on some psychological processes. *Q. J. Stud. Alc.* **23**: 274–314.

CARPENTER, T. M. (1929) Ethyl alcohol in fowls after exposure to alcohol vapor. *J. Pharmacol. Exp. Ther.* **37**: 217–219.

CARTER, E. A., WANDS, J. R. and ISSELBACHER, K. J. (1977) Effect of acute murine hepatitis (MHV-A-59) on ethanol oxidation *in vivo*. In: *Alcohol and Aldehyde Metabolizing Systems*, Vol. III, *Intermediary Metabolism and Neurochemistry*, pp. 251–259, Academic Press, New York.

CARTER, W. P. JR. (1976) Drug induced hypoglycemia and hypothermia. *J. Maine Med. Ass.* **67**: 272–279.

CEDERBAUM, A. I. (1983) Regulation of pathways of alcohol metabolism by the liver. *Mt. Sinai J. Med.* **47**: 317–328.

CENTER OF ALCOHOL STUDIES. Alco-calculator. *Alco-Research Documentation, Inc.* Center of Alcohol Studies, Rutgers University, New Brunswick, New Jersey.

CERDA, M. and ISRAEL, Y. (1969) Effect of ethanol on synthesis and active accumulation of γ-aminobutyric acid in rat brain slices. *Arch. Biol. Med. Exp.* **6**: 62–64.

CHAKRABORTY, J. (1980) Metabolic basis of ethanol-drug interactions. In: *Psychopharmacology of Alcohol*, pp. 191–198, SANDLER, M. (ed). Raven Press, New York.

CHAN, A. W. K. (1976) Gamma-aminobutyric acid in different strains of mice. Effect of ethanol. *Life Sci.* **19**: 597–604.

CHAN, C. H. (1983) The aging liver. In: *The Aging Gut*, pp. 21–26, TEXTER, E. C. (ed.) Masson, New York.

CHAN, T. C. K. and SUTTER, M. C. (1982) The effects of chronic ethanol consumption on cardiac function in rats. *Can. J. Physiol. Pharmacol.* **30**: 777–782.

CHAN, T. C. K. and SUTTER, M. C. (1983) Ethanol consumption and blood pressure. *Life Sci.* **33**: 1965–1973.

CHARNOCK, J. S. and BASHFORD, C. L. (1975) A fluorescent probe study on the lipid mobility of membranes containing sodium- and potassium-dependent adenosine triphosphatase. *Molec. Pharmacol.* **11**: 766–774.

CHENG, S. S. and TSENG, L.-F. (1982) Chronic administration of ethanol on pituitary and hypothalamic B-endorphin in rats and golden hamsters. *Pharmacol. Res. Commun.* **14**: 1001–1008.

CHILD, J. S., KOVICK, R. B., LEVISMAN, J. A. and PEARCE, M. L. (1979) Cardiac effects of acute ethanol ingestion unmasked by autonomic blockade. *Circulation* **59**: 120–125.

CHIN, J. M. and GOLDSTEIN, D. B. (1977a) Effects of low concentrations of ethanol on the fluidity of spin-labeled erythrocyte and brain membranes. *Molec. Pharmacol.* **13**: 435–441.

CHIN, J. M. and GOLDSTEIN, D. B. (1977b) Drug tolerance in membranes: A spin label study of the effects of ethanol. *Science* **196**: 684–685.

CHIN, J. M., PARSONS, L. M. and GOLDSTEIN, D. B. (1978) Increased cholesterol content of erythrocyte and brain membranes in ethanol-tolerant mice. *Biochem. Biophys. Acta* **513**: 358–363.

CHOPDE, C. T., BRAHMANKAR, D. M. and SHRIPAD, V. N. (1977) Neurochemical aspects of ethanol dependence and withdrawal reactions in mice. *J. Pharmacol. Exp. Ther.* **200**: 314–319.

CICERO, T. J. (1980a) Alcohol self-administration, tolerance and withdrawal in humans and animals: theoretical and methodological issues. In: *Alcohol Tolerance and Dependence*, pp. 1–51, RIGTER H. and CRABBE, J. C. (eds) Elsevier/North-Holland Biomedical Press, Amsterdam.

CICERO, T. J. (1980b) Sex differences in the effects of alcohol and other psychoactive drugs on endocrine function, clinical and experimental evidence: In: *Alcohol and Drug Problems in Women. Research Advances in Alcohol and Drug Problems*, Vol. 5, pp. 545–593, KALANT, H. (ed.) Plenum, New York.

CICERO, T. J. (1981) Neuroendocrinological effects of alcohol. *Ann. Rev. Med.* **32**: 123–142.

CICERO, T. J., SNIDER, S. R., PEREZ, V. J. and SWANSON, L. W. (1971) Physical dependence on and tolerance to alcohol in the rat. *Physiol. Behav.* **6**: 191–198.

CICERO, T. J., BERNARD, J. D. and NEWMAN, K. (1980) Effects of castration and chronic morphine administration on liver alcohol dehydrogenase and metabolism of ethanol in the male Sprague-Dawley rat. *J. Pharmacol. Exp. Ther.* **215**: 317–324.

CLARK, J. W., KALANT, H. and CARMICHAEL, F. J. (1977) Effect of ethanol tolerance on release of acetylcholine and norepinephrine by rat cerebral cortex slices. *Can. J. Physiol. Pharmacol.* **55**: 758–768.

COBB, C. F. and VAN THIEL, D. H. (1982) Mechanisms of ethanol induced adrenal stimulation. *Alcoholism Clin. Exp. Res.* **6**: 202–206.

COBB, C. F., VAN THIEL, D. H., ENNIS, M. F., GAVALER, J. S. and LESTER R. (1978) Acetaldehyde and ethanol are testicular toxins. *Gastroenterology* **75**: 958.

COCCO, K., ADLER, J., WESTRICK, E., NATHAN, P. and BRICK, J. (1986) Computerized program for the calculation of target blood alcohol levels in humans. *Proceedings and Abstracts of the Annual Meeting of the Eastern Psychological Association*, Vol. 57, p. 29.

COHEN, L., SELLERS, E. and FLATTERY, K. (1980) Ethanol and sympathetic denervation effects on rat adrenal catecholamine turnover. *J. Pharmacol. Exp. Ther.* **212**: 425–429.

COLLIER, H. O. J. (1965) A general theory of the genesis of drug dependence by induction of receptors. *Nature* **205**: 181–182.

COLLIER, H. O. J., HAMMOND, M. D. and SCHNEIDER, C. (1976) Effects of drugs affecting endogenous amines or cyclic nucleotides. *Br. J. Pharmacol.* **58**: 9–16.

COLLINS, A. C., YEAGER, T. N., LEBSACK, M. E. and PANTER, S. S. (1975) Variations in alcohol metabolism: Influence of sex and age. *Pharmacol. Biochem. Behav.* **3**: 973–978.

COLLINS, A. C., SMOLEN, A., WAYMAN, A. L. and MARKS, M. J. (1984) Ethanol and temperature effects on five membrane bound enzymes. *Alcohol* **1**: 237–246.

CONNERS, G. J. and MAISTO, S. A. (1979) Effects of alcohol, instructions and consumption rate on affect and physiological sensations. *Psychopharmacol.* **62**: 261–266.

CONNERS, G. J. and MAISTO, S. A. (1983) Methological issues in alcohol and stress research with human participants. In: *Stress and Alcohol Use*, pp. 105–120, POHORECKY, L. A. and BRICK, J. (eds.) Elsevier Science, New York.

CONWAY, N. (1968) Haemodynamic effects of ethanol alcohol in patients with coronary heart disease. *Br. Heart J.* **30**: 638–643.

COOPER, B. R., VIIK, K., FERRIS, R. M. and WHITE, H. L. (1979) Antagonism of the enhanced susceptibility to audiogenic-seizures during alcohol withdrawal in the rat by Gamma-aminobutyric acid (GABA) and GABA mimetic agents. *J. Pharmacol. Exp. Ther.* **209**: 396–403.

CORRODI, H., FUXE, K. and HOKFELT, T. (1966) The effect of ethanol on the activity of central catecholamine neurons in rat brain. *J. Pharm. Pharmacol.* **18**: 821–822.

COTT, J., CARLSSON, A., ENGEL, J. and LINDQUIST, M. (1976) Suppression of ethanol-induced locomotor stimulation by GABA-like drugs. *N.-S's Arch. Pharmacol.* **295**: 203–209.

COWAN, C. M., CARDEAL, J. O. and CAVALHEIRO, E. A. (1980) Membrane Na^+-K^+ ATPase activity: Changes using an experimental model of alcohol dependence and withdrawal. *Pharmacol. Biochem. Behav.* **12**: 333–335.

CRABBE, J. C., GRAY, D. K., YOUNG, E. R., JANOWSKY, J. S. and RIGTER, H. (1981) Initial sensitivity and tolerance to ethanol in mice: Correlations among open field activity, hypothermia, and loss of righting reflex. *Behav. Neural Biol.* **33**: 188–203.

CRABBE, J. C. and KOSOBUD, A. (1986) Sensitivity and tolerance to ethanol in mice bred to be genetically prone or resistant to ethanol withdrawal seizures. *J. Pharmacol. Exp. Ther.* **239**: 327–333.

CRABBE, J. C. and RIGTER, H. (1980) Hormones, peptides and ethanol responses. In: *Alcohol Tolerance and Dependence*, pp. 293–316, RIGTER, H. and CRABBE, J. (eds) Elsevier/North-Holland Biomedical Press, New York.

CRABBÉ, J. C., RIGTER, H., UIJLEN, J. and STRIJBOS, C. (1979) Rapid development of tolerance to the hypothermic effect of ethanol in mice. *J. Pharmacol. Exp. Ther.* **208**: 128–133.

CRABBE, J. C., JANOWSKY, J. S., YOUNG, E. R., KOSOBUD, A., STACK, J. and RIGTER, H. (1982) Tolerance to ethanol hypothermia in inbred mice: Genotypic correlations with behavioral responses. *Alcoholism: Clin. Exp. Res.* **6**: 446–458.

CRABBE, J. C., KOSOBUD, A. and YOUNG, E. R. (1983) Peak ethanol withdrawal convulsions in genetically selected mice. *Proc. West. Pharmacol. Soc.* **26**: 201–204.

CROWELL, C. R., HINSON, R. E. and SIEGEL, S. (1981) The role of conditional drug responses in tolerance to the hypothermic effects of ethanol. *Psychopharmacology* **73**: 51–54.

D'ALONZO, C. A. and PELL, S. (1968) Cardiovascular disease among problem drinkers. *J. Occup. Med.* **10**: 344–350.

DANCY, M. and MAXWELL, J. D. (1986) Alcohol and dilated cardiomyopathy. *Alc. Alcoholism* **21**: 185-198.

DAFTERS, R. and ANDERSON, G. (1982) Conditioned tolerance to the tachycardia effect of ethanol in humans. *Psychopharmacology* **78**: 365–367.

DAR, M. S. and WOOLES, W. R. (1985) GABA mediation of the central effects of acute and chronic ethanol in mice. *Pharmacol. Biochem. Behav.* **22**: 77–84.

DARDEN, J. H. and HUNT, W. A. (1977) Reduction of striatal dopamine release during an ethanol withdrawal syndrome. *J. Neurochem.* **29**: 1143–1145.

DAVE, J. R., KARANIAN, J. W. and ESKAY, R. L. (1986) Chronic ethanol treatment decreases specific nonopiate B-endorphin binding to hepatic and kidney membranes and lowers plasma B-endorphin in the rat. *Alcoholism: Clin. Exp. Res.* **10**: 161–165.

DAVIS, W. C. and TICKU, M. K. (1981) Ethanol enhances [^{3}H]-diazepam binding at the benzodiazepine-γ-aminobutyric acid receptor-ionophore complex. *Molec. Pharmacol.* **20**: 287–294.

DAVIS, V. E., BROWN, H., HUFF, J. A. and CASHAW, J. L. (1967) Ethanol-induced alterations of norepinephrine in man. *J. Lab. Clin. Med.* **69**: 787–799.

DEGANI, N. D., SELLERS, E. M. and KADZIELAWA, K. (1979) Ethanol induced spontaneous norepinephrine release from rat vas deferens. *J. Pharmacol. Exp. Ther.* **210**: 22–26.

DEMBIEC, D., MACNAMEE, D. and COHEN, G. (1976) The effect of pargyline and other monoamine oxidase inhibitors on blood acetaldehyde levels in ethanol intoxicated mice. *J. Pharmacol. Exp. Ther.* **197**: 332–339.

DESAIAH, D. and HO, I. K. (1976) Effect of biogenic amines and GABA on ATPase activities in mouse tissue. *Eur. J. Pharmacol.* **40**: 255–261.

DESAIAH, D. and HO, I. K. (1977) Kinetics of catecholamine sensitive Na^+-K^+ ATPase activity in mouse brain synaptosomes. *Biochem. Pharmacol.* **26**: 2029–2035.

DETURCK, K. H. and VOGEL, W. H. (1982) Effects of ethanol on plasma and brain catecholamine levels in stressed and unstressd rats: Evidence for an ethanol-stress interaction. *J. Pharmacol. Exp. Ther.* **223**: 348–354.

DETURCK, K. H. and POHORECKY, L. A. (1986) Development of tolerance to the inhibitory effects of ethanol in the isolated rat vas deferens. Effect of chronic ethanol administration. *Br. J. Pharmacol.* **88**: 397–403.

DETURCK, K. H. and POHORECKY, L. A. (1987a) Tolerance to ethanol in the rat vas deferens. Effect of a calcium channel antagonist. *Alcohol* **4**: 355–365.

DeTurck, K. H. and Pohorecky, L. A. (1987b) Development of tolerance to the inhibitory effects of ethanol in the isolated rat vas deferens. *Pharmacology* **34**: 337–347.

Deutsch, J. A. and Koopmans, H. S. (1973) Preference enhancement for alcohol by passive exposure. *Science* **179**: 1242–1243.

DeWied, D. (1980) Pituitary neuropeptides and behavior. In: *Central Regulation of the Endocrine System*, pp. 297–314, Fuxe, K., Hokfelt, T. and Luft, R. (eds) Plenum, New York.

Diemling, M. J. and Schnell, R. C. (1980) Circadian rhythms in the biological response and disposition of ethanol in the mouse. *J. Pharmacol. Exp. Ther.* **213**: 1–8.

Dinh, T. K. H. and Gailis, L. (1979) Effect of body temperature on acute ethanol toxicity. *Life Sci.* **25**: 547–552.

Dixon, W. E. (1907) The action of alcohol on the circulation. *J. Physiol.* **35**: 347.

Downey, J. A. and Frewin, D. B. (1970) The effect of ethyl alcohol and chlorpromazine on the response of the hand blood vessels to cold. *Br. J. Pharmacol.* **40**: 396–405.

Dubowski, K. M. (1963a) Alcohol determination: Some physiological and metabolic considerations. In: *Alcohol and Traffic Safety*, pp. 91–115, Fox, B. M. and Fox, J. H. (eds) U.S. Public Health Service Publication No. 1043, U.S. Public Health Service, National Institutes of Health, Bethesda, Maryland.

Dubowski, K. M. (1976) Human pharmacokinetics of ethanol. I. Peak blood alcohol concentrations and elimination in male and female subject. *Alc. Tech. Rep.* **5**: 55–63.

Dubowski, K. M. (1977) Human pharmacokinetics of ethanol, I. Peak blood concentrations and elimination in male and female subject. *Alc. Tech. Rep.* **5**: 27–39.

Dubowski, K. M. (1985) Absorption, distribution and elimination of alcohol: Highway safety aspects. *J. Stud. Alc. Suppl.* **10**: 98–108.

Durkin, T. P., Hashem-Zadeh, H., Mandel, P. and Ebel, A. (1982) A comparative study of the acute effects of ethanol on the cholinergic system in hippocampus and striatum of inbred mouse strains. *J. Pharmacol. Exp. Ther.* **220**: 203–208.

Dussualt, P. and Chappel, C. I. (1975) Difference in blood alcohol levels following consumption of whisky and beer in man. In: *Alcohol, Drugs and Traffic Safety*, pp. 365–370, Israel, Y., Stam, S. and Lambert, S. (eds) Addiction Research Foundation, Toronto.

Ebel, A., Vigran, R., Mack G., Durkin, T. and Mandel, P. (1979) Cholinergic involvement in ethanol intoxication and withdrawal-induced seizure susceptibility. *Psychopharmacology (Berlin)* **61**: 251–254.

Eccleston, D., Reading, W. H. and Ritchie, I. M. (1969) 5-Hydroxytryptamine metabolism in brain and liver slices and the effects of ethanol. *J. Neurochem.* **16**: 274–276.

Edelstein, C. K., Roy-Byrne, P., Fawzy, F. I. *et al.* (1983) Effects of weight loss on the dexamethasone suppression test. *Am. J. Psychiat.* **140**: 338–341.

Edes, I., Ando, A., Csanady, M., Mazarean, H. and Guba, F. (1983) Enzyme activity changes in rat heart after chronic alcohol ingestion. *Cardiovascular Res.* **17**: 691–695.

Edgarian, H. and Altura, B. M. (1976) Differential effects of ethanol on prostaglandin responses of arterial and venous smooth muscle. *Experientia* **32**: 618–619.

Edins, N. and Murray, M. M. (1924) Influence of CO_2 on the absorption of alcohol by the gastric mucosa. *J. Physiol.* (*London*) **59**: 271–275.

Edmonds, H. L. Jr., Sylvester, D. M. and Bellin, S. I. (1983) Dietary manipulation of alcohol withdrawal in the rat. *Res. Commun. Subst. Abuse* **4**: 89–92.

Edwards, G., Gross, M. M., Keller, M., Moser, J. and Room, R. (1977) Alcohol related disabilities. *WHO Offset Publication* No. 32. WHO Geneva.

Eisenhoffer, G. and Johnson, R. H. (1982) Effect of ethanol ingestion on plasma vasopressin and water balance in humans. *Am. J. Physiol.* **242**: R522–R527.

Eisenhoffer, G., Lambie, D. G., Whiteside, E. A. and Johnson, R. H. (1985) Vasopressin concentrations during alcohol withdrawal. *Br. J. Addict* **80**: 195–199.

Ellingboe, J. and Varanelli, C. C. (1979) Ethanol inhibits testosterone biosynthesis by direct action on leydig cells. *Res. Commun. Pathol. Pharmacol.* **24**: 87–102.

Ellis, F. (1966) Effect of ethanol on plasma corticosterone levels. *J. Pharmacol. Exp. Ther.* **153**: 121–127.

Engel, J. and Liljequist, S. (1976) The effect of long-term ethanol treatment on the sensitivity of the dopamine receptors in the nucleus accumbens. *Psychopharmacol.* **49**: 253–257.

Engel, J. A. and Rudberg, U. (1985) Age-dependent effects of ethanol on central monoamine synthesis in the male rate. *Acta Pharmacol. Toxicol.* **57**: 336–339.

Erickson, C. K. and Granam, D. T. (1973) Alteration of cortical and reticular acetylcholine release by ethanol in vivo. *J. Pharmacol. Exp. Ther.* **185**: 583–593.

Erickson, C. K. and Matchett, J. A. (1975) Correlation of brain amine changes with ethanol-induced sleeptime in mice. In: *Alcohol Intoxication and Withdrawal* pp. 419–430, Gross, M. M. (ed.) Plenum Press, New York.

Erickson, C. K., Koch, I. I., Mehta, C. S. and McGinity, J. W. (1978) Chronic dependence with a sustained ethanol release implant in mice. *Life Sci.* **22**: 1745–1754.

Eriksson, K. and Malmstrom, K. K. (1967) Sex differences in consumption and elimination of alcohol in albino rats. *Annu. Med. Exp. Fenn.* **45**: 389–392.

Eriksson, K., Pekkanen, L., Forsander, O. and Ahtee, L. (1975) The effect of dietary factors on voluntary ethanol intake in the albino rat. In: *The Effects of Centrally Active Drugs on Voluntary Alcohol Consumption*, Vo. 24, pp. 15–26, The Finnish Foundation for Alcohol Studies.

Erwin, V. G., Kim, J. and Anderson, A. D. (1975) Effects of aldehydes on sodium plus potassium ion-stimulated adenosine triphosphatase of mouse brain. *Biochem. Pharmacol.* **24**: 2089–2095.

Eskay, R. L., Ryback, R. S., Goldman, M. and Majchrowicz, E. (1981) Effect of chronic ethanol administration on plasma levels of LH and the estrous cycle in the female rat. *Alcoholism: Clin. Exp. Res.* **5**: 204–206.

Ettinger, P. O., Lyons, M., Oldewurtel, H. A. and Regen, T. J. (1976) Cardiac conduction abnormalities produced by chronic alcoholism. *Am. Heart J.* **91**: 66–78.

ETTINGER, P. O., WU, C. F., DE LA CRUZ, C. JR, WEISSE, A. B., AHMED, S. S. and REGAN, T. J. (1978) Arrhythmias and the "Holiday Heart": Alcohol-associated cardiac rhythm disorders. *Am. Heart J.* **95**: 555–562.

EVANS, W. (1966) Alcohol and the heart. *Practitioner* **196**: 238–246.

FADDA, F., ARGIOLAS, A., MELIS, M. R., SERRA, G. and GESSA, G. L. (1980) Differential effect of acute and chronic ethanol on dopamine metabolism in frontal cortex, caudate nucleus and substantia nigra. *Life Sci.* **27**: 979–986.

FAHN, S., KOVAL, G. J. and ALBERS, R. W. (1966) Sodium–potassium-activated adenosine triphosphatase of electrophorus electric organ. *J. Biol. Chem.* **241**: 1882–1889.

FALK, J. L., SAMSON, H. H. and WINGER, G. (1972) Behavioral maintenance of high blood ethanol and physical dependence in the rat. *Science* **177**: 811–813.

FELDSTEIN, A. (1973) Ethanol-induced sleep in relation to serotonin turnover and conversion to 5-hydroxyindoleacetaldehyde, 5-hydroxytryptophol, and 5-hydroxyindoleacetic acid. *N.Y. Acad. Sci.* **215**: 71–76.

FERKO, A. P. and BOBYOCK, E. (1977) Induction of physical dependence in rats by ethanol inhalation without the use of pyrazole. *Toxic. Appl. Pharmacol.* **40**: 269–276.

FERKO, A. P. and BOBYOCK, E. (1978) Physical dependence on ethanol: Rate of ethanol clearance from the blood and effect of ethanol on body temperature in rats. *Toxic. Appl. Pharmacol.* **46**: 235–248.

FERKO, A. P. and BOBYOCK, E. (1979) Rates of ethanol disappearance from blood and hypothermia following acute and prolonged ethanol inhalation. *Toxic. Appl. Pharmacol.* **50**: 417–427.

FERNANDEZ, J. P., O'ROURKE, R. A. and EWY, G. A. (1970) Rapid active external rewarming in accidental hypothermia. *J. Am. Med. Ass.* **212**: 153–156.

FERREIRA, A. L., SANTOS, J. C. M. and ROSSI, M. A. (1975) Effect of alcohol ingestion on the adrenergic nerve endings of rat atrioventricular valves. *Experientia* **31**: 82–83.

FEWINGS, J. D., HANNA, M. J. D., WALSH, J. A. and WHELAN, R. F. (1966) The effects of ethyl alcohol on the blood vessels of the hand and forearm in man. *Br. J. Pharmacol.* **27**: 93–106.

FISHER, F. J. and KAVALER, F. (1973) The action of ethanol upon the action potential and contraction of ventricular muscle. In: *Basic Functions of Cations and Myocardial Activity, Recent Advances in Studies on Cardiac Structure and Metabolism*, Vol. 5, FLECKENSTEIN, A. and DHALLA, A. S. (eds), University Park Press, New York.

FORBES, J. C. and DUNCAN, G. M. (1951) The effect of acute alcohol intoxication on the adrenal glands of rats and guinea pigs. *Q. J. Stud. Alc.* **12**: 355–359.

FORBES, J. C. and DUNCAN, G. M. (1961) Effect of tryptophan-niacin deficient diet in the adrenal response of rats exposed to cold and alcohol intoxication. *Q. J. Stud. Alc.* **22**: 254–260.

FORSYTH, G. A. (1979) Ethanol metabolism and indirect cardiotoxicity. *Workshop on Cardiomyopathy*, NIH Publication No. 79-1608. U.S. Dept. of Health, Education and Welfare, Public Health Service, National Institutes of Health, Washington, D.C.

FOWLER, C. J., WIBERG, A., ORELAND, L., DANIELSSON, A., PALM, U. and WINBLAD, B. (1981) Monoamine oxidase activity and kinetic properties in platelet-rich plasma from controls, chronic alcoholics, and patients with non-alcoholic liver disease. *Biochem. Med.* **25**: 356–365.

FOX, G. R., HAYWARD, J. S. and HOBSON, G. N. (1979) Effect of alcohol on thermal balance of man in cold water. *Can. J. Physiol. Pharmacol.* **57**: 860–865.

FRANKEL, D., KHANNA, J. M., KALANT, H. and LEBLANC, A. E. (1974) Effect of acute and chronic ethanol administration on serotonin turnover in rat brain. *Psychopharmacologia (Berlin)* **37**: 91–100.

FRANKEL, D., KHANNA, J. M., LEBLANC, A. E. and KALANT, H. (1975) Effect of *p*-chlorophenylalanine on the acquisition of tolerance to ethanol and pentobarbitol. *Psychopharmacologia* **44**: 247–252.

FRANKEL, D., KHANNA, J. M., BALANAT, H. and LEBLANC, A. E. (1978a) Effect of *p*-chlorophenylalanine on the loss and maintenance of tolerance in ethanol. *Psychopharmacology* **56**: 139–143.

FRANKEL, D., KHANNA, J. M., KALANT, H. and LEBLANC, A. E. (1978b) Effect of *p*-chlorophenylalanine on the acquisition of tolerance to the hypothermic effects of ethanol. *Psychopharmacology* **57**: 239–242.

FRENCH, S. W., REID, P. E., PALMER, D. S., NAROD, M. E. and RAMEY, C.W. (1974) Adrenergic subsensitivity of the rat brain during chronic ethanol ingestion. *Res. Commun. Chem. Pathol. Pharmacol.* **9**: 575–578.

FRENCH, S. W., PALMER, D. S. and NAROD, M. E. (1975) Effect of withdrawal from chronic ethanol ingestion on the cAMP response of cerebral cortical slices using the agonists histamine, serotonin, and other neurotransmitters. *Can. J. Physiol. Pharmacol.* **53**: 248–255.

FRENCH, S. W., PALMER, D. S., NAROD, M. E., REID, P. E. and RAMEY, C. W. (1975) Noradrenergic sensitivity of the cerebral cortex after chronic ethanol ingestion and withdrawal. *J. Pharmacol. Exp. Ther.* **194**: 319–326.

FRENCH, S. W., PALMER, D. S. and NAROD, M. E. (1976) Noradrenergic subsensitivity of rat liver homogenates during chronic ethanol ingestion. *Res. Commun. Chem. Path. Pharmacol.* **13**: 283–295.

FRENCH, T. A., MASSERANO, J. M. and WEINER, N. (1985) Ethanol-induced changes in tyrosine hydroxylase activity in adrenal glands in mice selectively bred for differences in sensitivity to ethanol. *J. Pharmacol. Exp. Ther.* **232**: 315–321.

FREUND, G. (1969) Alcohol withdrawal syndrome in mice. *Arch. Neurol. Chicago* **21**: 315–320.

FREUND, G. (1970) Alcohol consumption and its circadian distribution in mice. *J. Nutr.* **100**: 30–36.

FREUND, G. (1973) Hypothermia after acute ethanol and benzyl alcohol administration. *Life Sci.* **13**: 345–349.

FREUND, G. (1980a) Benzodiazepine receptor loss in brains of mice after chronic alcohol consumption. *Life Sci.* **27**: 987–992.

FREUND, G. (1980b) Physical dependence on ethanol: methodological considerations. In: *Biological Effects of Alcohol Adv. Exp. Biol. Med.*, Vol. 126, pp. 211–223, BEGLEITER, H. (ed.) Plenum Press, New York.

FREUND, G. and WALKER, D. W. (1971) Sound-induced seizures during ethanol withdrawal in mice. *Psychopharmacologia* **22**: 45–48.

FRIEDHOFF, A. J. and MILLER, J. (1973) Effect of ethanol on biosynthesis of dopamine. *Ann. N.Y. Acad. Sci.* **215**: 183–186.

FRIEDMAN, M. J., JAFFEE, J. H. and SHARPLESS, S. K. (1969) Central nervous system supersensitivity to pilocarpine after withdrawal of chronically administered scopolamine. *J. Pharmacol. Exp. Ther.* **167**: 45-55.

FRIEDMAN, H. S., MATSUZAKI, S., CHOE, S.-S., FERNANDO, H. A., CELIS, A., ZAMAN, Q. and LIEBER, C. S. (1979) Demonstration of dissimilar acute haemodynamic effects of ethanol and acetaldehyde. *Cardiovasc. Res.* **13**: 477-487.

FRIEDMAN, H. S., LOWERY, R., ARCHER, M., SHAUGHNESSY, E. and SCORZA, J. (1984) The effects of ethanol on brain blood flow in awake dogs. *J. Cardiovasc. Pharmacol.* **6**: 344-348.

FRYE, G. D. and BREESE, G. R. (1982) GABAergic modulation of ethanol-induced motor impairment. *J. Pharmacol. Exp. Ther.* **223**: 750-756.

FRYE, G. D. and ELLIS, F. W. (1977) Effects of 6-hydroxydopamine and 5,7-dihydroxytryptamine on the development of physical dependence on ethanol. *Drug Alc. Depend.* **2**: 349-359.

FRYE, G. D., ELLIS, F. W. and BREESE, G. R. (1977) Involvement of NE, DA, or 5-HT in the development of physical dependence on ethanol. *Milton M. Gross Memorial Symposium on Alcoholism, April 1-2.* Chicago, Illinois.

FRYE, G. D., VOGEL, R. A., MAILMAN, R. B., ONDRUSEK, M. G., WILSON, J. H., MUELLER, P. A. and BREESE, G. R. (1980) A comparison of behavioral and neurochemical effects of ethanol and chlordiazepoxide. In: *Alcohol and Aldehyde Metabolizing Systems*, Vol. 4, pp. 729-737, THURMAN, R. G. (ed.) Plenum Press, New York.

FRYE, G. D., MCCOWN, T. J. and BREESE, G. R. (1983a) Characterization of susceptibility to audiogenic seizures in ethanol-dependent rats after microinjection of gamma-aminobutyric acid (GABA) agonists into the inferior colliculus, substantia nigra or medial septum. *J. Pharmacol. Exp. Ther.* **227**: 663-670.

FRYE, G. D., MCCOWN, T. J. and BREESE, G. R. (1983b) Differential sensitivity of ethanol withdrawal signs in the rat to γ-aminobutyric acid (GABA)mimetics: Blockade of audiogenic seizures but not forelimb tremors. *J. Pharmacol. Exp. Ther.* **226**: 720-725.

FUHRMANN, G., BESNARD, F., KEMPF, J., KEMPF, E. and EBEL, A. (1986) Influence of mouse genotype on responses of central cholinergic neurotransmission to long term alcohol intoxication. *Alcohol* **3**: 291-298.

FUKUMORI, R., MINEGISHI, A., SATOH, T., KITAGAWA, H. and YANAURA, S. (1980) Changes in the serotonin and 5-hydroxyindoleacetic acid contents in rat brain after ethanol and disulfiram treatments. *Eur. J. Pharmacol.* **61**: 199-202.

GARLAND, T., GOLDBERG, L., GRAF, K., PERMAN, E. S., STRANDEL, T. and STROM, G. (1960) Effect of ethanol on circulatory, metabolic, and neurohormonal function during muscular work in man. *Acta Pharmacol. Toxicol.* **17**: 106-114.

GAVALER, J. S. (1983) Sex-related differences in ethanol-induced hypogonadism and sex steroid-responsive tissue atrophy: Analysis of the weanling ethanol-fed model using epidemiologic methods. In: *Ethanol Tolerance and Dependence: Endocrinological Aspects*, NIAAA Research Monograph No. 13, DHHS Publication No. (ADM) 83-1258, pp. 78-88, CICERO, T. J. (ed.) U.S. Government Printing Office, Washington, D.C.

GAVALER, J. S. (1986) Effects of alcohol on endocrine function in postmenopausal women: A review. *J. Stud. Alc.* **46**: 495-516.

GAVALER, J. S., ROSENBLUM, E. R., IMHOFF, A. F., POHL, C. R., ROSEMBLUM, E. R. and VAN THIEL, D. H. (1986) Alcoholic beverages: A source of estrogenic substances? Alcoholism: Clin. Exp. Res. **10**: 111.

GELLER, I. and HARTMANN, R. J. (1981) Blockade of 5-HTP reduction of ethanol drinking with the decarboxylase inhibitor, Ro 4-4602. *Pharmacol. Biochem. Behav.* **15**: 871-874.

GENAZZANI, A. R., NAPPI, G., FACCHINETTI, F., MAZZELLA, G. L., PARRINI, D., SINFORIANI, E., PETRAGLIA, F. and SAVOLDI, F. (1982) Central deficiency of B-endorphin in alcohol addicts. *J. Clin. Endocrinol. Metab.* **55**: 583-586.

GEORGE, F. R., JACKSON, S. J. and COLLINS, A. C. (1981) Prostaglandin synthetase inhibitors antagonize hypothermia induced by sedative hypnotics. *Psychopharmacology* **74**: 241-244.

GIANOULAKIS, C. (1983) Long term ethanol alters the binding of ^{3}H-opiates to brain membranes. *Life Sci.* **33**: 725-733.

GIANOULAKIS, C., DROUIN, S. N., SEIDAH, N. G., KALANT, H. and CHRETIEN, M. (1981) Effect of chronic morphine treatment on B-endorphin biosynthesis by the rat neurointermediate lobe. *Eur. J. Pharmacol.* **72**: 313-318.

GIANOULAKIS, C., CHAN, J. S., KALANT, H. and CHRETIEN, M. (1983) Chronic ethanol treatment alters the biosynthesis of B-endorphin by the rat neurointermediate lobe. *Can. J. Physiol. Pharmacol.* **61**: 967-976.

GILBERT, R. M. (1974) Effects of food deprivation and fluid sweetening on alcohol consumption by rats. *Q. J. Stud. Alc.* **35**: 42-47.

GILLESPIE, J. A. (1967) Vasodilator properties of alcohol. *Br. Med. J.* **ii**: 274-277.

GIMENO, A. L., GIMENO, M. F. and WEBB, J. L. (1962) Effects of ethanol on cellular membrane potentials and contractility of isolated rat atrium. *Am. J. Physiol.* **203**: 194-196.

GLIKAHRI, R. M., HOTTUNEN, M. O., HARKONER, M., LEINO, T., HELENIVS, T., LIEWENDAHL, K. and KAROWEN, S. L. (1978) Acute effects of alcohol on anterior pituitary secretion of the trophic hormones. *J. Clin. Endocrinol.* **46**: 714-720.

GODDARD, P. J. (1958) Effects on alcohol on excretion of catecholamines in conditions giving rise to anxiety. *J. Appl. Physiol.* **13**: 118-120.

GODFREY, L., KISSEN, M. D. and DOWNS, T. M. (1958) Treatment of the acute alcohol-withdrawal syndrome. *Q. J. Stud. Alc.* **19**: 118-124.

GOIST, K. and SUTKER, P. (1985) Acute alcohol intoxication and body composition in women and men. *Pharmacol. Biochem. Behav.* **22**: 811-814.

GOLDBERG, L. (1963) Quantitative studies on alcohol tolerance in man. *Acta Physiol. Scand. Suppl* **5**: 1-126 1943.

GOLDBERG, L. and RYDBERG, U. (1969) Inhibition of ethanol metabolism in vivo by administration of pyrazole. *Biochem. Pharmacol.* **18**: 1749-1754.

GOLDMAN, R. F., NEWMAN, R. N. and WILSON, O. (1973) Effects of alcohol, hot drinks, or smoking on hand and foot heat loss. *Acta Physiol. Scand.* **87**: 498-506.

GOLDMAN, H., SAPIRSTEIN, L. A., MURPHY, S. and MOORE, J. (1973) Alcohol and regional blood flow in brains of rats. *Proc. Soc. Exp. Biol. Med.* **144**: 983–988.

GOLDMAN, G. D., VOLICER, L., GOLD, B. I. and ROTH, R. H. (1981) Cerebrospinal fluid GABA and cyclic nucleotides in alcoholics with and without seizures. *Alcoholism: Clin. Exp. Res.* **5**: 431–434.

GOLDSTEIN, D. B. (1972) Relationship of alcohol dose to intensity of withdrawal signs in mice. *J. Pharmacol. Exp. Ther.* **180**: 203–215.

GOLDSTEIN, D. B. (1973) Alcohol withdrawal reactions in mice: effect of drugs that modify neurotransmission. *J. Pharmacol. Exp. Ther.* **186**: 1–9.

GOLDSTEIN, D. B. (1974) Rates of onset and decay of alcohol physical dependence in mice. *J. Pharmacol. Exp. Ther.* **190**: 377–383.

GOLDSTEIN, D. B. (1978) *Animal Studies of Alcohol Withdrawal Reactions*, pp. 77–110, ISRAEL, Y., GLASER, F. B., KALANT, H., POPHAM, R. E., SCHMIDT, W. and SMART, R. G. (eds) Plenum Press, New York.

GOLDSTEIN, D. B. (1979) Sodium bromide and sodium valproate: Effective suppressants of ethanol withdrawal reactions in mice. *J. Pharmacol. Exp. Ther.* **208**: 233–277.

GOLDSTEIN, D. B. and ARNOLD, V. W. (1976) Drinking patterns as predictors of alcohol withdrawal reactions in DBA/2J mice. *J. Pharmacol. Exp. Ther.* **199**: 408–414.

GOLDSTEIN, D. B. and GOLDSTEIN, A. (1961) Possible role of enzyme inhibition and repression in drug tolerance and addiction. *Biochem. Pharmacol.* **8**: 48–49.

GOLDSTEIN, D. B. and ISRAEL, Y. (1972) Effects of ethanol on mouse brain $(Na+K)^+$-activated adenosine triphosphatase. *Life Sci.* **11**: 957–963.

GOLDSTEIN, D. B. and PAL, N. (1971) Alcohol dependence produced in mice by inhalation of ethanol: grading the withdrawal reaction. *Science* **172**: 288–290.

GOLDSTEIN, D. B. and ZAECHELEIN, R. (1983) Time course of functional tolerance produced in mice by inhalation of ethanol. *J. Pharmacol. Exp. Ther.* **227**: 150–153.

GOMBERG, E. S. L. (1982) Alcohol use and alcohol problems among the elderly. In: *National Institute on Alcohol Abuse and Alcoholism*, pp. 263–290, Special Population Issues. Alcohol and Health Monograph No. 4, DHHS Publication No. (ADM) 82-1193, U.S. Government Printing Office, Washington, D.C.

GONZALEZ-CALVIN, J. L. SAUNDERS, J. B. and WILLIAMS, R. (1983) Effects of ethanol and acetaldehyde on hepatic plasma membrane ATPases. *Biochem. Pharmacol.* **32**: 1723–1728.

GOODKIND, M. J., GERBER, N. H., MELLEN, J. R. and KOSTIS, J. B. (1975) Altered intracardiac conduction after acute administration of ethanol in the dog. *J. Pharmacol. Exp. Ther.* **194**: 633–638.

GOODMAN, D. S. and DEYKIN, D. (1963) Fatty acid ethyl ester formation during ethanol metabolism *in vivo. Proc. Soc. Exp. Biol.* **113**: 65–67.

GOODWIN, D. W. (1980) The genetics of alcoholism. *Substance and Alcohol Actions: Misuse* **1**: 101–117.

GOODWIN, D. W. (1983) The genetics of alcoholism. *Hospital and Community Psychiatry* **34**: 1031–1034.

GORDON, E. R. (1967) The effect of ethanol on the concentration of γ-aminobutyric acid in the rat brain. *Can. J. Physiol. Pharmacol.* **45**: 915–918.

GORDON, T. and KANNEL, W.B. (1983) Drinking and its relation to smoking, BP, blood lipids, and uric acid: The Framingham study. *Arch. Intern. Med.* **143**: 1366–1374.

GORDON, G. G., SOUTHREN, A. L., VITTEK, J. and LIEBER, C. S. (1979) The effect of alcohol ingestion on hepatic aromatase activity and plasma steroid hormone in the rat. *Metabolism* **28**: 20–24.

GOTHERT, M. and THIELECKE, G. (1976) Inhibition by ethanol of noradrenaline output from peripheral sympathetic nerves: possible interaction of ethanol with neuronal receptors. *Eur. J. Pharmacol.* **37**: 321–328.

GOTHERT, M., KENNERKNECHT, E. and THIELECKE, G. (1976) Inhibition of receptor-mediated noradrenaline release from the sympathetic nerves of the isolated rabbit heart by anaesthetics and alcohols in proportion to their hydrophobic property. *N.-S. Arch. Pharmacol.* **292**: 145–152.

GOTHONI, P. and AHTEE, L. (1980) Chronic ethanol administration decreases 5-HT and increases 5-HIAA concentrations in rat brain. *Acta Pharmacol. Toxicol.* **46**: 113–120.

GOTTFRIES, C. G., ORELAND, L., WIBERG, A. and WINBLAD, B. (1975) Lowered monoamine oxidase activity in brains from alcoholic suicides. *J. Neurochem.* **25**: 667–673.

GOULD, L., COLLICA, C., ZAHIR, M. and GOMPRECHT, R. F. (1972) Ethyl alcohol: Effects on coronary blood flow in man. *Br. Heart J.* **34**: 815–820.

GOULD, L., REDDY, C. V. R., BECKER, W., OH, K. C. and KIM, S. G. (1978) Electrophysiological properties of alcohol in man. *J. Electrocardiol.* **11**: 219–226.

GOULD, L., ZAHIR, M., DEMARTINO, A. and GOMPRECHT, R. F. (1971) Cardiac effects of a cocktail. *J. Am. Med. Assoc.* **218**: 1799–1802.

GRAHAM, T. (1981) Thermal and glycemic responses during mild exercise in +5° and −15°C environments following alcohol ingestion. *Aviat. Space Environ. Med.* **52**: 517–522.

GRAHAM, T. (1983) Alcohol ingestion and sex differences on the thermal responses to mild exercise in a cold environment. *Human Biol.* **55**: 463–476.

GRAHAM, T. and BAULK, K. (1980) Effect of alcohol ingestion on man's thermoregulatory responses during cold water immersion. *Aviat. Space Environ. Med.* **51**: 155–159.

GRAHAM, T. and DALTON, J. (1980) Effect of alcohol on man's response to mild physical activity in a cold environment. *Aviat. Space Environ. Med.* **51**: 793–796.

GREENBERG, L. A. (1968) Pharmacology of alcohol and its relationship to drinking and driving. *Q. J. Stud. Alc.*, Suppl No. **4**: 252–266.

GREENBERG, D. A., COOPER, E. C., GORDON, A. and DIAMOND, I. (1984) Ethanol and the γ-aminobutyric acid-benzodiazepine receptor complex. *J. Neurochem.* **42**: 1062–1068.

GREENBLATT, D. J., SELLERS, E. M. and SHADER, R. I. (1982) Drug therapy: Drug disposition in old age. *New Engl. J. Med.* **306**: 1081–1088.

GREHANT, N. and QUINQUAUD, E. (1983) Sur l'absorption des vapeurs d'alcool absolu par les poumons. *Compt. Rend. Soc. Biol.* **35**: 426–431.

GRIEVE, S. J. and LITTLETON, J. M. (1979a) Age and strain differences in the rate of development of functional tolerance to ethanol by mice. *J. Pharm. Pharmacol.* **31**: 696–700.

GRIEVE, S. J. and LITTLETON, J. M. (1979b) Ambient temperature and the development of functional tolerance to ethanol by mice. *J. Pharm. Pharmacol.* **31**: 707–708.

GRIEVE, S. J., GRIFFITHS, P. and LITTLETON, J. (1979a) Genetic influences on the rate of development of ethanol tolerance and the ethanol physical withdrawal syndrome in mice. *Drug Alc. Depend.* **4**: 77–86.

GRIEVE, S. J., LITTLETON, J. M., JONES, P. and JOHN, G. R. (1979b) Functional tolerance to ethanol in mice: Relationship to lipid metabolism. *J. Pharm. Pharmacol.* **31**: 737–742.

GRIFFITHS, P. J., LITTLETON, J. M. and ORTIZ, A. (1974) Effect of *p*-chlorophenylalanine of brain monoamines and behavior during ethanol withdrawal in mice. *Br. J. Pharmacol.* **51**: 307–309.

GROSS, M. M., LEWIS, E. and HASTEY, J. (1974) Acute alcohol withdrawal syndrome. In: *The Biology of Alcoholism*, Vol. 3, *Clinical Pathology*, pp. 191–263, KISSIN, B. and BEGLEITER, H. (eds) Plenum Press, New York.

GROSS, M. M., LEWIS, E., BEST, S., YOUNG, N. and FEUER, L. (1975) Quantitative changes of signs and symptoms associated with acute alcohol withdrawal: Incidence, severity, and circadian effects, in experimental studies of alcoholics. *Adv. Exp. Med. Biol.* **59**: 615–631.

GUAZA, C. and BORRELL, S. (1983) Adrenomedullary response to acute and chronic ethanol administration to rats. *Biochem. Pharmacol.* **32**: 3091–3095.

GUAZA, C. and BORRELL, S. (1985) Brain catecholamines during ethanol administration, effect of naloxone on brain dopamine and norepinephrine responses to withdrawal from ethanol. *Pharmacol. Res. Commun.* **17**: 1159–1167.

GUERRI, C. and GRISOLIA, S. (1983) Chronic ethanol treatment affects synaptosomal membrane-bound enzymes. *Pharmacol. Biochem. Behav.* **11** (Suppl. 1): 45–50.

GUERRI, C., WALLACE, R. and GRISOLIA, S. (1978) The influence of prolonged ethanol intake on the levels and turnover of alcohol and aldehyde dehydrogenases and of brain (Na+K)-ATPase of rats. *Eur. J. Biochem.* **86**: 581–587.

GUERRI, C., RIBELLES, M. and GRISOLIA, S. (1981) Effects of lithium and alcohol administration on (Na^+-K^+)-ATPase. *Biochem. Pharmacol.* **30**: 25–30.

GUPTA, K. K. (1960) Effect of alcohol in cold climate. *J. Indian Med.* **35**: 211–212.

GYNTELBERG, F. and MEYERS, J. (1974) Relationship between blood pressure and physical fitness, smoking and alcohol consumption in Copenhagen males aged 40–59. *Acta Med. Scand.* **195**: 375–380.

HAGEN, D. Q. (1967) GABA levels in rat brain after prolonged ethanol intake. *Q. J. Stud. Alc.* **28**: 613–618.

HAGGARD, H. W., GREENBERG, L. A. and COHEN, L. H. (1938) Quantitative differences in the effects of alcoholic beverages. *N. Engl. J. Med.* **219**: 446–470.

HAGGARD, H. W., GREENBERG, L. A., COHEN, L. H. and TAKIETEN, N. (1941a) Studies on the absorption, distribution and elimination of alcohol. *J. Pharmacol. Exp. Ther.* **71**: 358–361.

HAGGARD, H. W., GREENBERG, L. A. and LOLLI, G. (1941b) The absorption of alcohol with specific reference to its influence on the concentration of alcohol appearing in the blood. *Q. J. Stud. Alc.* **1**: 684–726.

HAGGENDAL, J. and LINDQVIST, M. (1961) Ineffectiveness of ethanol on noradrenaline, dopamine or 5-hydroxytryptamine levels in brain. *Acta Pharmacol. Toxicol.* **18**: 278–280.

HAIGHT, J. S. J. and KEATINGE, W. R. (1973) Failure of thermoregulation in the cold during hypoglycaemia induced by exercise and ethanol. *J. Physiol.* **229**: 87–97.

HAKKINEN, H.-M. and KULONEN, E. (1961) The effect of ethanol on the amino acids of the rat brain with a reference to the administration of glutamine. *Biochem. J.* **78**: 588–593.

HAKKINEN, H.-M. and KULONEN, E. (1976) Ethanol intoxication and γ-aminobutyric acid. *J. Neurochem.* **27**: 631–633.

HAMMOND, M. D. and SCHNEIDER, C. (1973) Behavioral changes induced in mice following termination of ethanol administration. *Br. J. Pharmacol.* **47**: 667–675.

HARBURG, E., OZGOREN, F., HAWTHORNE, V. M. and SCHORK, A. (1980) Community norms of alcohol usage and blood pressure: Tecumseh, Michigan. *Am. J. Public Health* **70**: 813–820.

HARGER, R. N. and JULPIEU, H. R. (1956) The pharmacology of alcohol. In: *Alcoholism*, G. N. THOMPSON (ed.), pp. 103–232, Thomas, Springfield, IL.

HARGER, R. N. and FORNEY, R. B. (1963) Aliphatic alcohols. In: *Progress in Chemical Toxicology*, Vol. 1, p. 79, STOLMAN, A. (ed.) Academic Press, New York.

HARRIS, R. A. (1979) Alteration of alcohol effects by calcium and other inorganic cations. *Pharmacol. Biochem. Behav.* **10**: 527–534.

HARRIS, R. A. and HITZEMANN, R. J. (1981) Membrane fluidity and alcohol actions. In: *Currents in Alcoholism*, Vol. 8, pp. 379–397, GALANTER, M. (ed.) Grune and Stratton, New York.

HARRIS, R. A., BAXTER, D. M., MITCHEL, M. A. and HITZEMAN, R. J. (1984) Physical properties of brain membranes from ethanol-tolerant-dependent mice. *Molec. Pharmacol.* **25**: 401–409.

HASTILLO, A. H., POLAND, J. and HESS, M. L. (1980) Mechanical and subcellular function of rat myocardium during chronic ethanol consumption. *Proc. Soc. Exp. Biol. Med.* **164**: 415–420.

HAWKINS, R. D., KALANT, H. and KHANNA, J. M. (1966) Effects of chronic intake of ethanol on rate of ethanol metabolism. *Can. J. Physiol. Pharmacol.* **44**: 241–257.

HAWLEY, R. J., MAJOR, L. F., SCHULMAN, E., TROCHA, P. J., TAKENAGA, J. K. and CATRAVAS, G. N. (1981) Cerebrospinal fluid cyclic nucleotides and GABA do not change in alcohol withdrawal. *Life Sci.* **28**: 295–299.

HAY, W. M., NATHAN, P. E., HEERMANS, H. W. and FRANKENSTEIN, W. (1984). Menstrual cycle tolerance and blood alcohol level discrimination ability. *Addictive Behaviors* **9**: 67–77.

HAYASHI, T., NANIKAWA, R. and AMENO, K. (1978) Effect of alcohol administration levels of plasma catecholamines in injured state. *Jpn. J. Stud. Alc.* **13**: 272–280.

HEINTZELMAN, M. E., BEST, J. and SENTER, R. J. (1976) Polydipsia-induced alcohol dependency in rats: A reexamination. *Science* **191**: 482–483.

HELDERMAN, J. H., VESTAL, R. E. and ROWE, J. W. (1978) The response of arginine vasopressin to intravenous ethanol and hypertonic saline in man: The impact of aging. *J. Gerontol.* **33**: 39–47.

HIGGINS, E. S. (1962) The effect of ethanol on GABA content of rat brain. *Biochem. Pharmacol.* **11**: 394–395.

HILL, M. W. and BANGHAM, A. D. (1975) General depressant drug dependency: A biophysical hypothesis. *Adv. Exp. Med. Biol.* **59**: 1–9.

HILLBOM, M. E. (1975) The prevention of ethanol withdrawal seizures in rats by dipropylacetate. *Neuropharmacol.* **14**: 755–761.

HILLER, J., ANGEL, L. M. and SIMON, E. J. (1981) Multiple opiate receptors: Alcohol selectivity inhibits binding to delta receptors. *Science* **214**: 468–469.

HILLER, J., ANGEL, L. M. and SIMON, E. J. (1984) Characterization of the selective inhibition of the delta subclass of opioid binding sites by alcohols. *Molec. Pharmacol.* **25**: 249–255.

HINSON, R. E. and SIEGEL, S. (1980). The contribution of Pavlovian conditioning to ethanol tolerance and dependence. In: *Alcohol Tolerance, Dependence and Addiction: A Research Handbook*, pp. 181–199, RIGTER, H. and CRABBE, J. C. (eds) Elsevier/North-Holland Biomedical Press, Amsterdam.

HIROTA, Y., BING, O. H. L. and ABELMAN, W. H. (1976) Effect of ethanol on contraction and relaxation of isolated rat ventricular muscle. *J. Molec. Cell Cardiol.* **8**: 727–731.

HIRSCH, J. D. (1981) Selective inhibition of [^{3}H]lysergic acid diethylamide binding to mouse brain membranes by ethanol. *J. Pharm. Pharmacol.* **33**: 475–477.

HIRVONEN, J. (1976) Necropsy findings in fatal hypothermia cases. *Forensic Sci.* **8**: 155–164.

HIRVONEN, J. and HUTTUNEN, P. (1977) The effect of ethanol on the ability of guinea pigs to withstand severe cold exposure. In: *Drugs, Biogenic Amines and Body Temperature*, Third Symposium on the Pharmacology of Thermoregulation, Banff, Alberta, pp. 230–232, COOPER, K. E., LOMAX, P. and SCHONBAUM, E. (eds) Karger, Basel.

HOBSON, G. N. and OLLIS, M. L. (1977) The effects of alcohol upon cooling rates of humans immersed in 7-5°C water. *Can. J. Physiol. Pharmacol.* **55**: 744–746.

HOFFMAN, P. L. and TABAKOFF, B. (1977) Alterations in dopamine receptor sensitivity by chronic ethanol treatment. *Nature* (*London*) **268**: 551–553.

HOFFMAN, P. L. and TABAKOFF, B. (1979) Peptide-neurotransmitter interactions influencing ethanol tolerance. *Drug. Alc. Depend.* **4**: 249–253.

HOFFMAN, P. L. and TABAKOFF, B. (1981) Centrally acting peptides and tolerance to ethanol. In: *Currents in Alcoholism*, Vol. 8, pp. 359–378, GALANTER, M. (ed.) Grune and Stratton, New York.

HOFFMAN, P. L. and TABAKOFF, B. (1982) Effects of ethanol on Arrhenius parameters and activity of mouse striatal adenylate cyclase. *Biochem. Pharmacol.* **31**: 3101–3106.

HOFFMAN, P. L. and TABAKOFF, B. (1986) Ethanol does not modify opiate-mediated inhibition of striatal adenylate cyclase. *J. Neurochem.* **46**: 812–816.

HOFFMAN, P. L., LEVENTAL, M., FIELDS, J. Z. and TABAKOFF, B. (1980) Receptor and membrane function in the alcohol tolerant/dependent animal. In: *Alcohol and Aldehyde Metabolizing Systems—IV*, Advances in Experimental Medicine and Biology, Vol. 132, pp. 761–770, THURMAN, R. G. (ed.) Plenum Press, New York.

HOFFMAN, P. L., MELCHIOR, C. L., RITZMANN, R. F. and TABAKOFF, B. (1981) Structural requirements for neurohypophyseal peptide effects of ethanol tolerance. *Alcoholism: Clin. Exp. Res.* **5**: 154 (Abstract).

HOFFMAN, P. L., MELCHIOR, C. L. and TABAKOFF, B. (1983) Vasopressin maintenance of ethanol tolerance requires intact brain noradrenergic system. *Life Sci.* **32**: 1065–1071.

HOFFMAN, P. L., VALVERIUS, P., KWAST, M. and TABAKOFF, B. (1987) Comparison of the effects of ethanol on beta-adrenergic receptors in heart and brain. *Alcohol Suppl.* **1**: 749–754.

HOLMAN, R. B., ELLIOTT, G. R., KRAMER, A. M., SEAGRAVES, E. and BARCHAS, J. D. (1977) Stereotype and hyperactivity in rats receiving ethanol and a monoamine oxidase inhibitor. *Psychopharmacology* **54**: 237–239.

HOLMAN, R. B. and SNAPE, B. M. (1985) Effects of ethanol in vitro and in vivo on the release of endogenous catecholamines from specific regions of rat brain. *J. Neurochem.* **44**: 357–363.

HOPKINS, A. (1966) The pattern of gastric emptying: A new view of old results. *J. Physiol.* **182**: 144–149.

HORWITZ, L. D. and ATKINS, J. M. (1974) Acute effects of ethanol on left ventricular performance. *Circulation* **49**: 124–128.

HORWITZ, L. D. and MYERS, J. H. (1980) Ischemia of the pancreas due to ethanol in conscious dogs. *Circulation* **62** (Suppl. 3): 22.

HOWERTON, T. C. and COLLINS, A. C. (1984) Ethanol-induced inhibition of norepinephrine release from brain slices obtained from LS and SS mice. *Alcohol* **1**: 47–53.

HOWERTON, T. C., MARKS, M. J. and COLLINS, A. C. (1982) Norepinephrine, gamma-aminobutyric acid and choline reuptake kinetics and the effects of ethanol in long-sleep and short-sleep mice. *Subst. Alc. Actions Misuse* **3**: 89–99.

HRUSKA, R. E. and SILBERGELD, E. K. (1980) Inhibition of [^{3}H]spiroperidol binding by in vitro addition of ethanol. *J. Neurochem.* **35**: 750–752.

HUNG, C. R., TABAKOFF, B., MELCHIOR, C. L. and HOFFMAN, P. L. (1984) Intraventricular arginine vasopressin maintains ethanol tolerance. *Eur. J. Pharmacol.* **106**: 645–648.

HUNT, W. A. (1985) *Alcohol and Biological Membranes. The Guildford Press*, New York.

HUNT, W. A. and DALTON, T. K. (1976) Regional brain acetylcholine levels in rats acutely treated with ethanol or rendered ethanol-dependent. *Brain Res.* **109**: 628–631.

HUNT, W. A. and DALTON, T. K. (1981) Neurotransmitter–receptor binding in various brain regions in ethanol-dependent rats. *Pharmacol. Biochem. Behav.* **14**: 733–739.

HUNT, W. A. and MAJCHROWICZ, E. (1978) Alterations in neurotransmitter function after acute and chronic treatment with ethanol. In: *Biochemistry and Pharmacology of Ethanol*, Vol. 2, pp. 167–185, MAJCHROWICZ, E. and NOBLE, E. P. (eds) Plenum Press, New York.

HUNT, W. A. and MAJCHROWICZ, E. (1983) Studies of neurotransmitter interactions after acute and chronic ethanol administration. *Pharmacol. Biochem. Behav.* **18**: Suppl. 1, 371–374.

Hunt, G. P. and Overstreet, D. H. (1977) Evidence for a parallel development of tolerance to the hyperactivating and discoordinating effects of ethanol. *Psychopharmacology (Berlin)* **55**: 75–81.

Hunt, W. A., Majchrowicz, E. and Dalton, T. K. (1979) Alterations in high affinity choline uptake in brain after acute and chronic ethanol treatment. *J. Pharmacol. Exp. Ther.* **210**: 259–263.

Hunt, W. A., Majchrowicz, E., Dalton, T. K., Swartzwelder, H. S. and Wixon, H. (1979) Alterations in neurotransmitter activity after acute and chronic ethanol treatment: Studies of transmitters interactions. *Alcoholism Clin. Exp. Res.* **3**: 359–363.

Hunt, W. A., Redos, J. D., Dalton, T. K. and Catravas, G. N. (1977) Alterations in brain cyclic guanosine 4′,5′-monophosphate levels after acute and chronic treatment with ethanol. *J. Pharmacol. Exp. Ther.* **200**: 103–109.

Hunter, B. E., Boast, C. A., Walker, D. W. and Zornetzer, S. F. (1973) Alcohol withdrawal syndrome in rats: Neural and behavioral correlates. *Pharmacol. Biochem. Behav.* **1**: 719–725.

Hunter, B. E., Riley, J. N., Walker, D. W. and Freund, G. (1975) Ethanol dependence in the rat: A parameteric analysis. *Pharmacol. Biochem. Behav.* **3**: 619–629.

Huttunen, P. (1982) Hypothalamic catecholamines and tolerance for severe cold in ethanol-treated guinea-pigs. *Br. J. Pharmacol.* **75**: 613–616.

Huttunen, P., Penttinen, J. and Hirvonen, J. (1980) The effect of ethanol and cold-adaptation on the survival of guinea pigs in severe cold. *Z. Rechtsmed.* **85**: 289–294.

Hyatt, M. C. and Tyce, G. M. (1985) The effects of ethanol on the efflux and release of norepinephrine and 5-hydroxytryptamine from slices of rat hypothalamus. *Brain Res.* **337**: 255–262.

Ihrig, T. J., Pettit, N. B. and French, S. W. (1978) Reduced adrenergic sensitivity *in vivo* in acute ethanol-fed rats. *Res. Commun. Chem. Pathol. Pharmacol.* **21**: 149–152.

Imperato, A. and DiChiara, G. (1986) Preferential stimulation of dopamine release in the nucleus accumbens of freely moving rats by ethanol. *J. Pharmacol. Exp. Ther.* **239**: 219–228.

Ireland, M. A., Vandongen, R., Davidson, L., Beilin, L. J. and Rouse, I. L. (1984) Acute effects of moderate alcohol consumption on blood pressure and plasma catecholamines. *Clin. Sci.* **66**: 643–648.

Isbell, H., Fraser, H. F., Wikler, A., Belleville, R. E. and Eisenman, A. J. (1955) An experimental study of the etiology of “rum fits” and delerium tremens. *Q. J. Stud. Alc.* **16**: 1–33.

Israel, M. A. and Kuriyama, K. (1971) Effect of *in vivo* ethanol administration on adenosinetriphosphatase activity of subcellular fractions of mouse brain and liver. *Life Sci.* **10**: 591–599.

Israel, Y. and Salazar, I. (1967) Inhibition of brain microsomal adenosine triphosphatases by general depressants. *Arch. Biochem. Biophys.* **122**: 310–317.

Israel, M. A., Kimura, H. and Kuriyama, K. (1972) Changes in activity and hormonal sensitivity of brain adenyl cyclase following chronic ethanol administration. *Experientia* **28**: 1322–1323.

Israel, Y., Carmichael, F. J. and Macdonald, J. A. (1973) Effects of ethanol on norepinephrine uptake and electrically stimulated release in brain tissue. *Ann. N.Y. Acad. Sci.* **215**: 38–48.

Israel, Y., Carmichael, F. J. and Macdonald, J. A. (1975) Effects of ethanol on electrolyte metabolism and neurotransmitter release in the CNS. In: *Alcohol Intoxication and Withdrawal: Experimental Studies II*, pp. 55–64, Gross, M. M. (ed.) Plenum Press, New York.

Israel, Y., Kalant, H. and Laufer, I. (1965) Effects of ethanol on Na, K, Mg-stimulated microsomal ATPase activity. *Biochem. Pharmacol.* **14**: 1803–1814.

Israel, Y., Kalant, H. and LeBlanc, A. E. (1966) Effects of lower alcohols on potassium transport and microsomal adenosine-triphosphatase activity of rat cerebral cortex. *Biochem. J.* **100**: 27–32.

Israel, Y., Kalant, H., LeBlanc, A. E., Bernstein, J. C. and Salazar, I. (1970) Changes in cation transport and (Na+K)-activated adenosine triphosphatase produced by chronic administration of ethanol. *J. Pharmacol. Exp. Ther.* **174**: 330–336.

Isselbacher, K. J. and Carter, E. A. (1976) Effect of propranolol on ethanol metabolism—Evidence for the role of mitochondrial NADH oxidation. *Biochem. Pharmacol.* **25**: 169–174.

Iturriaga, H., Kelly, M., Bunout, D., Pino, M. E., Pereda, T., Berrera, R., Petermann, M. and Ugarte, G. (1986) Glucose tolerance and the insulin response in recently drinking alcoholic patients: Possible effects of withdrawal. *Metabolism* **35**: 238–243.

Jarnefet, J. (1961) Inhibition of the brain microsomal adenosinetriphosphatase by depolarizing agents. *Biochim. Biophys. Acta* **48**: 111–116.

Jeffcoate, W. J., Platts, M., Ridout, A. D., Hastings, I., Macdonald, I. and Selby, C. (1980) Effect of ethanol infusion on plasma cortisol, corticotrophin, β-lipotrophin, growth hormone and prolactin, and its modification by naloxone. *Drug. Alc. Depend.* **6**: 47.

Jellinek, E. M. (1960) *The Disease Concept of Alcoholism.* Hillhouse Press, Highland Park, New Jersey.

Jetter, W. W. (1938) Studies in Alcohol, I. The diagnosis of acute alcoholic intoxication by a correlation of clinical and chemical findings. *Am. J. Med. Sci.* **196**: 475–487.

Johnson, W. D. (1975) Impaired defense mechanisms associated with acute alcoholism. In: *Medical Consequences of Alcoholism. Annals of the New York Academy of Sciences*, Seixas, F. A., Williams, K. and Eggleston, S. (eds) New York Academy of Sciences, New York.

Jones, B. M. (1974) Circadian variation in the effects of alcohol on cognitive performance. *Q. J. Stud. Alc.* **35**: 3–10.

Jones, B. M. and Jones, M. K. (1976a) Alcohol effects in women during the menstrual cycle. *Ann. N.Y. Acad. Sci.* **273**: 567–587.

Jones, B. M. and Jones, M. K. (1976b) Women and alcohol: Intoxication, metabolism and menstrual cycle. In: *Alcoholism Problems in Women and Children*, Greenblatt, M. and Schuckit, M. A. (eds) Grune and Stratton, New York.

Jones, B. M. and Jones, M. K. (1981) Ethanol absorption, elimination and peak blood alcohol levels in male and female social drinkers as a function of age. (Abstract) *Alcoholism: Clin. Exp. Res.* **5**: 156.

Jones, M. K. and Jones, B. M. (1984) Ethanol metabolism in women taking oral contraceptives. *Alcoholism: Clin. Exp. Res.* **8**: 24–28.

Jones, B. M. and Vega, A. (1972) Cognitive performance measured on the ascending and descending limb of the blood alcohol curve. *Psychopharmacologia (Berlin)* **23**: 99–114.
Jones-Saumity, D. J., Fabian, M. S. and Parsons, O. A. (1981) Medical status and cognitive functioning in alcoholic women. *Alcoholism: Clin. Exp. Res.* **5**: 372–377.
Jorgensen, H. A. and Hole, J. (1986) Evidence from behavioral and in vitro receptor binding studies that the enkephalinergic system does not mediate acute ethanol effects. *Eur. J. Pharmacol.* **125**: 249–256.
Juchems, R. and Klobe, R. (1969) Hemodynamic effects of ethyl alcohol in man. *Am. Heart J.* **78**: 133–141.
Julkunen, R. J. K., Di Padova, C. and Lieber, C. S. (1985) First pass metabolism of ethanol—A gastrointestinal barrier against systemic toxicity of ethanol. *Life Sci.* **37**: 567–573.
Julkunen, R. J. K., Tannenbaum, L., Barona, E. and Lieber, C. S. (1985) First pass metabolism of ethanol: An important determinant of blood levels after alcohol consumption. *Alcohol* **2**: 437–441.
Jung, Y. and Russfield, A. B. (1972) Prolactin cells in the hypophysis of cirrhotic patients. *Arch. Path.* **94**: 265–269.
Kakihana, R. (1976) Adrenocortical function in mice selectively bred for different sensitivity to ethanol. *Life Sci.* **18**: 1131–1135.
Kakihana, R. and Butte, J. (1979) Ethanol and endocrine function. In: *Biochemistry and Pharmacology of Ethanol*, Vol. 2, Machrowicz, E. and Noble, E. (eds) Plenum, New York.
Kakihana, R. and Moore, J. A. (1977) Effect of alcohol on biological rhythms: body temperature and adrenocortical rhythmicities in mice. In: *Currents in Alcoholism*, Vol. 3, pp. 85–95. Seixas, F. (ed.) Grune and Stratton, New York.
Kako, K. J., Lui, M. S. and Thornton, M. J. (1973) Changes in fatty acid composition of myocardial triglyceride following a single administration of ethanol to rabbits. *J. Molec. Cell. Cardiol.* **5**: 473–489.
Kalant, H. (1971a) Alcoholism. In: *Biology of Alcoholism*, Vol. 1, *Biochemistry*, pp. 1–62, Kissin, B. and Begleiter, H. (eds) Plenum Press, New York.
Kalant, H. (1971b) Absorption, diffusion, distribution and elimination of ethanol: Effects on biological membranes. In: *The Biology of Alcoholism*, Vol. 1, *Biochemistry*, pp. 1–46, Kissin, B. and Begleiter, H. (eds) Plenum Press, New York.
Kalant, H. and Grose, W. (1967) Effects of ethanol and pentobarbital on release of acetylcholine from cerebral cortex slices. *J. Pharmacol. Exp. Ther.* **158**: 386–393.
Kalant, H. and Khanna, J. M. (1980) Environmental-neurochemical interactions in ethanol tolerance. In: *Psychopharmacology of Alcohol*, pp. 107–120, Sandler, M. (ed.) Raven Press, New York.
Kalant, H. and Le, A. D. (1984) Effects of ethanol on thermoregulation. *Pharmacol. Ther.* **23**: 313–364.
Kalant, H. and Rangaraj, N. (1981) Interaction of catecholamines and ethanol on the kinetics of rat brain (Na^++K^+)-ATPase. *Eur. J. Pharmacol.* **70**: 157–166.
Kalant, H., Woo, N. and Endrenyi, L. (1978) Effect of ethanol on the kinetics of rat brain (Na^++K^+)-ATPase and K^+-dependent phosphatase with different alkali ions. *Biochem. Pharmacol.* **27**: 1353–1358.
Kalant, H., Hawkins, R. D. and Czaja, C. (1963) Effect of acute alcohol intoxication on steroid output of rat adrenals in vitro. *Am. J. Physiol.* **204**: 849–855.
Kalant, H., Israel, Y. and Mahon, M. A. (1967) The effect of ethanol on acetylcholine synthesis, release, and degradation in brain. *Can. J. Physiol. Pharmacol.* **45**: 172–176.
Kannel, W. B. and Sorlie, P. (1974) In: *Hypertension in Framingham, Epidemiology and Control at Hypertension*, p. 553, Paul, O. (ed.) Stratton International Medical Book Corporation, New York.
Karanian, J. W., D'Souza, N. B. and Salem, N. Jr (1986) The effect of chronic alcohol inhalation on blood pressure and the pressor response to noradrenaline and the thromboxane-mimic. U46619. *Life Sci.* **39**: 1245–1255.
Karel, L. and Fleisher, J. H. (1948) Gastric absorption of ethyl alcohol in the rat. *Am. J. Physiol.* **153**: 268–276.
Karobath, M., Rogers, J., van den Berg, C. J., van der Helm, H. J. and Veldstra, H. (1965) Benzodiazepine receptors remain unchanged after chronic ethanol administration. *Neuropharmacology* **19**: 125–128.
Karoum, F., Wyatt, R. J. and Majchrowicz, E. (1976) Brain concentrations of biogenic amine metabolites in acutely treated and ethanol-dependent rats. *Br. J. Pharmacol.* **56**: 403–411.
Keatinge, W. R. and Evans, M. (1960) Effect of food, alcohol, and hyoscine on body-temperature and reflex responses of men immersed in cold water. *Lancet* **ii**: 176–178.
Keith, L. D., Crabbe, J. C., Robertson, L. M. and Young, E. R. (1983) Ethanol dependence and the pituitary adrenal axis in mice. II. Temporal analysis of dependence and withdrawal. *Life Sci.* **33**: 1889–1897.
Khanna, J. M., LeBlanc, A. E. and Le, A. D. (1979) Role of serotonin in tolerance to ethanol and barbiturates: Evidence for a specific versus nonspecific concept of tolerance. *Drug Alc. Depend.* **4**: 207–219.
Khanna, J. M., Kalant, H., Le, A. D. and LeBlanc, A. E. (1979) Effect of modification of brain serotonin (5HT) on ethanol tolerance. *Alcoholism: Clin. Exp. Res.* **3**: 353–358.
Khanna, J. M., Kalant, H., Le, A. D. and LeBlanc, A. E. (1980) Reversal of tolerance to ethanol—A possible consequence of ethanol brain damage. *Acta Physiol. Scand.* **62**: (Suppl. 286), 129–134.
Khetarpal, V. K. and Volicer, L. (1979) Effects of ethanol on blood pressure of normal and hypertensive rats. *J. Stud. Alc.* **40**: 732–736.
Kieffer, J. D. and Ketchel, M. M. (1970) Blockade of ovulation in the rat by ethanol. *Acta Endoc. Copenhagen* **65**: 117–124.
Kiianmaa, K. and Tabakoff, B. (1983) Neurochemical correlates of tolerance and strain differences in the neurochemical effects of ethanol. *Pharmacol. Biochem. Behav.* **18**: Suppl. 1, 383–388.
Kiianmaa, K., Hoffman, P. L. and Tabakoff, B. (1983) Antagonism of the behavioral effects of ethanol by naltrexone in BALB/C, C57BL/6, and DBA/2 mice. *Psychopharmacology* **79**: 291–294.
Kijima, T. (1979) Alcohol sensitivity and urinary catecholamines. *Jpn. J. Stud. Alc.* **14**: 101–117.
Kikichi, T. and Kako, K. (1970) Metabolic effects of ethanol on the rabbit heart. *Circulation Res.* **26**: 625–634.
Kimelberg, H. K. and Papahadjopoulos, D. (1974) Effects of phospholipid acyl chain fluidity, phase transitions, and cholesterol on (Na^++K^+)-stimulated adenosine triphosphatase. *J. Biol. Chem.* **249**: 1071–1080.

KIVILUOMA, K. and HASSINEN, L. (1983) Role of acetaldehyde and acetate in the development of ethanol-induced cardiac lipidosis, studied in isolated perfused rat hearts. *Alcoholism: Clin. Exp. Res.* **7**: 169–174.

KLATSKY, A. L., FRIEDMAN, G. D., SEIGELAUB, A. B. and GERARD, M. J. (1977) Alcohol consumption and blood pressure. *New Engl. J. Med.* **296**: 1194–1200.

KNOX, W. H., PERRIN, R. G. and SEN, A. K. (1972) Effect of chronic administration of ethanol on (Na^+,K^+)-activated ATPase activity in six areas of the cat brain. *J. Neurochem.* **19**: 2881–2884.

KOBAYASHI, M., FURUKAWA, Y. and CHIBA, S. (1979) Effect of ethanol on frequency-force relationship in isolated right atrial muscle of the dog. *J. Stud. Alc.* **40**: 892–895.

KONDO, K. and EBIHARA, A. (1984) Alcohol consumption and blood pressure in a rural community of Japan. *Nutritional Prevention of Cardiovascular Disease*, pp. 217–224. Academic Press, New York.

KOPUN, M. and PROPPING, P. (1977) The kinetics of ethanol absorption and elimination in twins and supplementary repetitive experiments in singleton subjects. *Eur. J. Clin. Pharmacol.* **44**: 337–344.

KOSOBUD, A. and CRABBE, J. C. (1986) Ethanol withdrawal in mice bred to be genetically prone or resistant to ethanol withdrawal seizures. *J. Pharmacol. Exp. Ther.* **238**: 170–177.

KRAMP, P., HEMMINGSEN, R. and RAFAELSEN, O. J. (1979) Delirium tremens. Some clinical features. *Acta Psychiat. Scand.* **60**: 405–422.

KURIYAMA, K. (1977) Ethanol-induced changes in activities of adenylate cyclase, guanylate cyclase and cyclic adenosine 3′,5′-monophosphate dependent protein kinase in the brain and liver. *Drug Alc. Depend.* **2**: 335–348.

KURIYAMA, K., RAUSCHER, G. E. and SZE, P. Y. (1971) Effect of acute and chronic administration of ethanol on the 5-hydroxytryptamine turnover and tryptophan hydroxylase activity in the mouse brain. *Brain Res.* **26**: 450–454.

KURIYAMA, K., MURAMATSU, M., AISO, M. and UENO, E. (1981) Alteration in β-adrenergic receptor binding in brain, lung and heart during morphine and alcohol dependence and withdrawal. *Neuropharmacology.* **20**: 659–666.

KURIYAMA, K., KANMORI, K. and YONEDA, Y. (1984) Preventive effect of alcohol against stress-induced alteration in content of monoamines in brain and adrenal gland. *Neuropharmacol.* **23**: 649–654.

KWAST, M., TABAKOFF, B. and HOFFMAN, P. (1987) Effect of ethanol on cardiac B-adrenoceptors. *Eur. J. Pharmacol.* **142**: 441–445.

LABELLA, F. S., PINSKY, C., HAVLICEK, V. and QUEEN, G. (1979) Effects of anesthetics *in vitro* on brain receptors for opiates, spiroperidol, and ouabain. In: *Endogenous and Exogenous Opiate Agonists and Antagonists*, WAY, E. L. (ed.) Pergamon Press, New York.

LAI, H., MAKOUS, W. L., HORITA, A. and LEUNG, H. (1979) Effects of ethanol on turnover and function of striatal dopamine. *Psychopharmacology* **61**: 1–9.

LAI, H., CARINO, M. A. and HORITA, A. (1980) Effects of ethanol on central dopamine functions. *Life Sci.* **27**: 299–304.

LAKE, D. A., CHILIAN, W. M. and ROBERTS, L. A. (1978) Ethanol increases rate of isolated atria. *Alcoholism: Clin. Exp. Res.* **2**: 271–275.

LANGE, L. G. (1983) Nonoxidative ethanol metabolism: Formation of fatty acid ethyl esters by cholesterol esterase. *Proc. Natl. Acad. Sci. U.S.A.* **79**: 3954–3957.

LANGE, L. G. and SOBEL, B. E. (1983) Myocardial metabolites of ethanol. *Circ. Res.* **52**: 479–482.

LANGE, L. G., BERGMANN, S. R. and SOBEL, B. E. (1981) Identification of fatty acid ethyl esters as products of rabbit myocardial ethanol metabolism. *J. Biol. Chem.* **256**: 12968–12973.

LAPORTE, R. E., CRESANTA, J. L. and KULLER, L. H. (1980) The relationship of alcohol consumption to atherosclerotic heart disease. *Prevent. Med.* **9**: 22–40.

LASKER, N., SHERROD, T. R. and KILLAM, K.F. (1955) Alcohol on coronary circulation of dog. *J. Pharmacol. Exp. Therap.* **113**: 414–420.

LE, A. D., POULOS, C. X. and CAPPELL, H. (1979) Conditioned tolerance to the hypothermic effect of ethyl alcohol. *Science* **206**: 1109–1110.

LE, A. D., KHANNA, J. M., KALANT, H. and LEBLANC, A. E. (1980) Effect of L-tryptophan on the acquisition of tolerance to ethanol-induced motor impairment and hypothermia. *Psychopharmalogy* **61**: 125–129.

LE, A. D., KHANNA, J. M., KALANT, H. and LEBLANC, A. E. (1981) Effect of modification of brain serotonin (5-HT), norepinephrine (NE), and dopamine (DA) on ethanol tolerance. *Psychopharmacology* **75**: 231–235.

LEBACH, W. K. (1975) Cirrhosis in the alcoholic and its relation to volume of alcohol abuse. In: *Medical Consequences of Alcoholism. Annals of the New York Academy of Sciences*, pp. 85–104, SEIXAS, F. A., WILLIAMS, K. and EGGLESTON, W. (eds) New York Academy of Sciences, New York.

LEBLANC, A. E., KALANT, H., GIBBINS, R. J. and BERMAN, N. D. (1969) Acquisition and loss of tolerance to ethanol by the rat. *J. Pharmacol. Exp. Ther.* **168**: 244–250.

LEBLANC, A. E., KALANT, H. and GIBBINS, R. J. (1975) Acute tolerance to ethanol in the rat. *Psychopharmacologia (Berlin)* **41**: 43–46.

LEBLANC, A. E., KALANT, H. and GIBBINS, R. J. (1976) Acquisition and loss of behaviorally augmented tolerance to ethanol in the rat. *Psychopharmacology* **48**: 153–158.

LE BOURHIS, B. and AUFRERE, G. (1983) Pattern of alcohol administration and physical dependence. *Alcoholism: Clin. Exp. Res.* **7**: 378–381.

LEDIG, M. M., M'PARIA, J.-R and MANDEL, P. (1981) Superoxide dismutase activity in the rat brain during acute and chronic alcohol intoxication. *Neurochem. Res.* **6**: 385–390.

LEE, S. L. and PHILLIS, J. W. (1977) Stimulation of cerebral cortical synaptosomal Na–K ATPase by biogenic amines. *Can. J. Physiol. Pharmacol.* **55**: 961–966.

LEPPALUOTO, J., RAPELI, M., VARIS, R. and RANTA, T. (1975) Secretion of anterior pituitary hormones in man. Effects of ethyl alcohol. *Acta Physiol. Scand.* **95**: 400–406.

LESTER, D. and FREED, E. X. (1973) Criteria for an animal model of alcoholism. *Pharmacol. Biochem. Behav.* **1**: 103–107.

LESTER, D., GREENBERG, L. A., SMITH, R. F. and CARROLL, R. P. (1951) The inhalation of ethyl alcohol by man. I. Industrial hygiene and medicolegal aspects. *Q. J. Stud. Alc.* **12**: 167–178.

LESTER, D., KEOKOSKY, W. Z. and FELZENBERG, F. (1968) Effects of pyrazoles and other compounds on alcohol metabolism. *Q. J. Stud. Alc.* **29**: 449–455.
LEVENTAL, M. and RAKIC, L. (1980) Na-K, adenosine triphosphatase activity in myelin, axoplasmic and syn aptic plasma membranes isolated from rat brain: Effect of ethanol. *Subst. Alcohol Actions Misuse* **1**: 493–506.
LEVENTAL, M. and TABAKOFF, B. (1980) Sodium-potassium-activated adenosine triphosphatase activity as a measure of neuronal membrane characteristics in ethanol tolerant mice. *J. Pharmacol. Exp. Ther.* **212**: 315–319.
LEVINE, A. S., HESS, S. and MORLEY, J. E. (1983) Alcohol and the opiate receptor. *Alcoholism: Clin. Exp. Res.* **7**: 83–84.
LEVY, R., ELO, T. and HANENSON, I. B. (1977) Intravenous fructose treatment of acute alcohol intoxication: Effects on alcohol metabolism. *Arch. Int. Med.* **137**: 1175–1177.
LI, T. K. (1977) Enzymology of human alcohol metabolism. *Adv. Enzymol. Molec. Biol.* **45**: 427–438. M. ALTON (ed.) Kneger Inc.
LI, T. K., LUMENG, L., MCBRIDE, W. J. and WALLER, M. B. (1979) Progress toward a voluntary oral consumption model of alcoholism. *Drug. Alc. Depend.* **4**: 45–60.
LIEBER, C. (1975) Liver disease and alcohol: Fatty liver, alcoholic hepatitis, cirrhosis and their interrelationships. In: *Medical Consequences of Alcoholism, Annals of the New York Academy of Sciences*, pp. 63–84, SEIXAS, F. A., WILLIAMS, K. and EGGLESTON, S. A. (eds) New York Academy of Sciences, New York.
LIEBER, C. S. (1983) Pathogenesis of alcoholic liver disease. In: *Recent Advances in the Biology of Alcoholism*, pp. 67–85, LIEBER, C. S. and STIMMEL, B. (eds) Haworth Press, New York.
LIEBER, C. S. and DECARLI, L. M. (1968) Ethanol oxidation by hepatic microsomes. Adaptive increase after ethanol feeding. *Science* **162**: 917–918.
LIEBER, C. S. and DECARLI, L. M. (1969) Hepatic microsomal ethanol-oxidizing system. *J. Biol. Chem.* **245**: 2505–2512.
LIEBER, C. S. and DECARLI, L. M. (1972) The role of the hepatic microsomal ethanol oxidizing system (MEOS) for ethanol metabolism in vivo. *J. Pharmacol. Exp. Ther.* **81**: 279–287.
LIEBER, C. S. and DECARLI, L. M. (1973) Ethanol dependence and tolerance: A nutritionally controlled experimental model in the rat. *Res. Commun. Chem. Pathol. Pharmacol.* **6**: 938–991.
LIEBER, C. S. and DECARLI, L. M. (1986) The feeding of ethanol in liquid diets. *Alcoholism: Clin. Exp. Res.* **10**: 550–553.
LIEBER, C. S. and PIROLA, R. C. (1982) Clinical relèvance of alcohol-drug interactions. In: *Recent Advances in the Biology of Alcoholism*, LIEBER, C. S. and STIMMEL, B. (eds) Haworth Press, New York.
LILJEQUIST, S. (1978) Changes in the sensitivity of dopamine receptors in the nucleus accumbens and in the striatum induced by chronic ethanol administration. *Acta Pharmacol. Toxicol.* **43**: 19–28.
LILJEQUIST, S. and ENGEL, J. (1979) The effect of chronic ethanol administration on central neurotransmitter mechanisms. *Med. Biol.* **57**: 199–210.
LILEQUIST, S. and ENGEL, J. (1980) Effect of ethanol on central GABAergic mechanisms. In: *Animal Models in Alcohol Research*, ERICKSSON, K., SINCLAIR, J. D. and KIIANMAA, K. (eds) pp. 309–315. Academic Press, New York.
LILJEQUIST, S. and ENGEL, J. (1982) Effects of GABAergic agonists and antagonists on various ethanol-induced behavioral changes. *Psychopharmacology* **78**: 71–75.
LILJEQUIST, S., AHLENIUS, S. and ENGEL, J. (1977) The effect of chronic ethanol treatment on behaviour and central monoamines in the rat. *N.-S Arch. Pharmacol.* **300**: 205–216.
LILJEQUIST, S., ANDEN, N. E., ENGEL, J. and HENNING, M. (1978) Noradrenaline receptor sensitivity after chronic ethanol administration. *J. Neural Trans.* **43**: 11–17.
LILJEQUIST, S., CULP, S. and TABAKOFF, B. (1986) Effect of ethanol on the binding of ^{35}S-T-butylbicyclophosphorothionate to mouse brain membranes. *Life Sci.* **38**: 1931–1939.
LIN, D. C. (1980) Involvements of the lipid and protein components of ($Na^{+}+K^{+}$)-adenosine triphosphatase in the inhibitory action of alcohol. *Biochem. Pharmacol.* **29**: 771–775.
LINDHOLM, J., FABRICIUS-BJEERE, N., BAHNSEN, P. and BOLESEN, L. (1978) Sex steroids and sex hormone binding globulin in males with chronic alcoholism. *Eur. J. Clin. Invest.* **8**: 273–276.
LINDROS, K. O., VAANANEN, H., SARVIHARJU, M. and HAATAJA, H. (1984) A simple procedure using 4-methylpyrazole for developing tolerance and other chronic alcohol effects. *Alcohol* **1**: 145–150.
LINDSAY, R. (1974) The effect of prolonged ethanol treatment on the sodium-plus-potassium-ion-stimulated adenosine triphosphatase content of cultured human and mouse cells. *Clin. Sci. Molec. Med.* **47**: 639–642.
LINKOLA, J., GLIKAHRI, R., FYHRQUIST, F. and WALLENIVS, M. (1978) Plasma vasopressin ethanol intoxication. *Acta Physiol. Scand.* **104**: 180–187.
LINNOILA, M., STOWELL, L., MARANGOS, P. J. and THURMAN, R. G. (1981) Effect of ethanol and ethanol withdrawal on (^{3}H)-muscimol binding and behavior in the rat: a pilot study. *Acta Pharmacol. Toxicol.* **49**: 407–411.
LIPSCOMB, T. and NATHAN, P. E. (1980) Blood alcohol discrimination: The effects of family history of alcoholism, drinking pattern and tolerance. *Arch. Gen. Psych.* **37**: 577–582.
LISTER, R.G. (1987) Interactions of Ro 15-4513 with diazepam, sodium pentobarbital and ethanol in a holeboard test. *Pharmacol. Biochem. Behav.* **28**: 75–79.
LISTER, R. G. and KARANIAN, J. W. (1987) RO 15-4513 induces seizures in DBA/2 mice undergoing alcohol withdrawal. *Alcohol* **4**: 409–411.
LITTLE, R. E. and STREISSGUTH, A. P. (1978) Drinking during pregnancy in alcoholic women. *Alcoholism: Clin. Exp. Res.* **2**: 179–183.
LITTLE, R. E., SCHULTZ, F. A. and MANDELL, W. (1976) Drinking during pregnancy. (1976) *J. Stud. Alc.* **37**: 375–379.
LITTLETON, J. M. (1980a) The assessment of rapid tolerance to ethanol. In: *Alcohol Tolerance and Dependence*, pp. 53–79, RIGTER, H. and CRABBE, J. C. (eds) Elsevier, Amsterdam.

LITTLETON, J. M. (1980b) Development of membrane tolerance to ethanol may limit intoxication and influence dependence liability. In: *Psychopharmacology of Alcohol*, pp. 121–127, SANDLER, M. (ed.) Raven Press, New York.

LITTLETON, J. M., GRIFFITHS, P. and ORTIZ, A. (1974) The induction of ethanol dependence and the ethanol withdrawal syndrome: The effects of pyrazole. *J. Pharm. Pharmacol.* **25**: 81–91.

LOCHNER, A., COWLEY, R. and BRISK, A.J. (1969) Effect of ethanol on metabolism and function of perfused rat Heart. *Am. Heart J.* **78**: 770–780.

LOEB, O. (1905) Die wirkung des alkohols auf das warmbluterherz. *Arch. Exp. Pathol. Pharmakol.* **52**: 459–480.

LOOMIS, T. A. (1952) The effect of alcohol on myocardial and respiratory function. The influence of modified respiratory function on the cardiac toxicity of alcohol. *Q. J. Stud. Alc.* **13**: 561–570.

LOOSEN, P. T. and PRANGE, A. J. (1977) Alcohol and anterior pituitary secretion. *Lancet* **2**: 985.

LOWENSTEIN, L. M., SIMONE, R., BOYLTER, P. and NATHAN, P. E. (1970) Effect of fructose on alcohol concentrations in the blood of man. *J. Am. Med. Assoc.* **213**: 1899–1901.

LUCCHI, L., LUPINI, M., GOVONI, S., COVELLI, V., SPANO, P. F. and TRABUCCHI, M. (1983) Ethanol and dopaminergic systems. *Pharmacol. Biochem. Behav.* **18**: Suppl. 1: 379–382.

LUMENG, L., HAWKINS, T. D. and LI, T.-K. (1977) New strains of rats with alcohol preference and non-preference. In: *Alcohol and Aldehyde Metabolizing Systems*, Vol. 3, pp. 537–544, THURMAN, R. G., WILLIAMSON, J. R., DROTT, H. and CHANCE, B. (eds) Academic Press, New York.

LUNDBERG, D. B. A., BREESE, G. R., MAILMAN, R. B., FRYE, G. D. and MUELLER, R. A. (1979) Depression of some drug induced *in vivo* changes of cerebellar guanosine 3′,5′-monophosphate by control of motor and respiratory responses. *Molec. Pharmacol.* **15**: 246–256.

LUNDQUIST, F. and WOLTHERS, H. (1958) The kinetics of alcohol elimination in man. *Acta Pharmacol. Toxicol.* **14**: 265–289.

LUNDY, J., RAAF, J. H., DEAKINS, S., WANEBO, H. J., JACOBS, D. A., LEE, T. JACOBOWITZ, E., SPEAR, C. and OETTGEN, H. F. (1975) The acute and chronic effects of alcohol on the human immune system. *Surg. Gyn. Obs.* **141**: 212–218.

LUTHIN, G. R. and TABAKOFF, B. (1984) Activation of adenylate cyclase by alcohols requires the nucleotide-binding protein. *J. Pharmacol. Exp. Ther.* **228**: 579–587.

LUTTINGER, D., NEMEROFF, C. B., GAU, B. and PRANGE, A. J. JR (1981) Investigation of the interactions of ethanol with neuropeptides. *Alcoholism: Clin. Exp. Res.* **5**: 348 (Abstract).

MAGOUR, S., KRISTOF, V., BAUMANN, M. and ASSMANN, G. (1981) Effect of acute treatment with cadmium on ethanol anesthesia, body temperature, and synaptosomal Na^+-K^+-ATPase of rat brain. *Environ. Res.* **26**: 381–391.

MAIER, D. M. and POHORECKY, L. A. (1986) The effect of stress on tolerance to ethanol in rats. *Alc. Drug Res.* **6**: 387–401.

MAIER, D. M. and POHORECKY, L. A. (1987) The effect of repeated withdrawal episodes on acquisition and loss of tolerance to ethanol in ethanol-treated rats. *Physiol. Behav.* **40**: 411–424.

MAILMAN, R. B., MUELLER, R. A. and BREESE, G. R. (1979a) The effect of drugs which alter GABA-ergic function on cerebellar guanosine-3′-5′-monophosphate content. *Life Sci.* **23**: 623–628.

MAILMAN, R. B., FRYE, G. E., MUELLER, R. A. and BREESE, G. R. (1978b) Thyrotropin-releasing hormone reversal of ethanol-induced decreases in cerebellar cGMP. *Nature* **272**: 832–833.

MAINES, J. E. and ALDINGER, E. E. (1967) Myocardial depression accompanying chronic consumption of alcohol. *Am. Heart J.* **73**: 55–63.

MAJCHROWICZ, E. (1973) Induction of physical dependence on alcohol and the associated metabolic and behavioral changes in rats. *Pharmacologist* **15**: 159.

MAJCHROWICZ, E. (1975) Induction of physical dependence upon ethanol and the associated behavioral changes in rats. *Psychopharmacologia* **43**: 245–254.

MAJCHROWICZ, E. (1977) Comparison of ethanol withdrawal syndrome in humans and rats. In: *Alcohol Intoxication and Withdrawal—IIb: Studies in Alcohol Dependence, Advances in Experimental Medicine and Biology Series*, Vol. 85B, pp. 15–23, GROSS, M. M. (ed.) Plenum Press, New York.

MAJCHROWICZ, E. and HUNT, W. A. (1976) Temporal relationship of the induction of tolerance and physical dependence after continuous intoxication with maximum tolerable doses of ethanol in rats. *Psychopharmacology* **50**: 107–112.

MAJOR, L. F. and MURPHY, D. L. (1978) Platelet and plasma amine oxidase activity in alcoholic individuals. *Br. J. Psychiat.* **132**: 548–554.

MAJOR, L. F., BALLENGER, J. D., GOODWIN, F. K. and BROWN, G. L. (1977) Cerebrospinal fluid homovanillic acid in male alcoholics: Effects of disulfiram. *Biol. Psychiat.* **12**: 635–642.

MAJUMDAR, S. K. (1982) Serum prolactin concentrations during the hangover phase of ethanol withdrawal syndrome. *Neuroendocrinol. Lett.* **4**: 253–259.

MALCOLM, R. D. and ALKANA, R. L. (1981) Temperature dependence of ethanol depression in mice. *J. Pharmacol. Exp. Ther.* **217**: 770–775.

MANSFIELD, J. G. and CUNNINGHAM, C. L. (1980) Conditioning the extinction of tolerance to the hypothermic effect of ethanol in rats. *J. Comp. Physiol. Psychol.* **94**: 962–969.

MANTELLI, L., CORTI, V. and LEDDA, F. (1985) Cardiodepressant effects of ethanol on guinea pig atria: Presynaptic and postsynaptic components. *J. Pharm. Pharmacol.* **37**: 651–653.

MARBACH, G. and SCHWERTZ, M.-T. (1964) Effets physiologiques de l'alcool et de la caféine au cours du sommeil chez l'homme. *Arch. Sci. Physiol.* **18**: 163–210.

MARKS, M. J., SMOLEN, A. and COLLINS, A. C. (1984) Brain Na^+K^+-ATPase in mice differentially sensitive to alcohols. *Alcoholism: Clin. Exp. Res.* **8**: 390–396.

MARSHALL, A. W., KINGSTONE, D., BOSS, M. and MORGAN, M. Y. (1983) Ethanol elimination in males and females: Relationship to menstrual cycle and body composition. *Hepatology* **3**: 701–706.

MARTIN, S. and COOPER, K. E. (1978) Alcohol and respiratory and body temperature changes during tepid water immersion. *J. Appl. Physiol.* **44**: 683–689.

MARTIN, S., DIEWOLD, R. J. and COOPER, K. E. (1977) Alcohol, respiration, skin and body temperature during cold water immersion. *J. Appl. Physiol.* **43**: 211–215.

MARTZ, A., DEITRICH, R. A. and HARRIS, R. A. (1983) Behavioral evidence for the involvement of gamma-aminobutyric acid in the actions of ethanol. *Eur. J. Pharmacol.* **89**: 53–62.

MASON, D. T., SPANN, J. F. JR, MILLER, R. R., LEE, G., ARBOGAST, R. and SEGEL, L.D. (1978) Effects of acute ethanol on the contractile state of normal and failing cat papillary muscles. *Eur. J. Cardiol.* **7**: 311–316.

MASSARELLI, R., SYAPIN, P. J. and NOBLE, E. P. (1966) Increased uptake of choline by neural cell cultures chronically exposed to ethanol. *Life Sci.* **18**: 397–404.

MASSERANO, J. M., TAKIMOTO, G. S. and WEINER, N. (1983) Tyrosine hydroxylase activity in the brain and adrenal gland of rats following chronic administration of ethanol. *Alcoholism: Clin. Exp. Res.* **7**: 294–298.

MASUR, J. and BOERNGEN, R. (1980) The excitatory component of ethanol in mice: A chronic study. *Pharmacol. Biochem. Behav.* **13**: 777–780.

MASUR, J., TUFIK, S., RIBEIRO, A. B., SARAGOCA, M. A. S. and LARANJEIRA, R. R. (1979) Alcohol consumption by patients of general hospitals: A neglected problem? *Rev. Ass. Med. Brasil* **25**: 302–306.

MATHEWS, J. D. (1976) Alcohol use, hypertension and coronary heart disease. *Clin. Sci. Molec. Med.* **51** (Suppl. 3): 661s–663s.

MATHEWS, J. D. (1979) Alcohol and hypertension. *Aust. N. Z. J. Med.* **9**: 124–128.

MATSUDA, T., IWATA, H. and COOPER, J. R. (1984) Specific inactivation of (+) molecular form of ($Na^{+}+K^{+}$)-ATPase by pyrithiamin. *J. Biol. Chem.* **259**: 3858–3863.

MCCABE, E. R., LAYNE, E. C., SAYLER, D. F., SLUSHER, N. and BESSMAN, S. P. (1971) Synergy of ethanol and a natural soporific—Gamma hydroxybutyrate. *Science* **171**: 404–406.

MCCLEARN, G. E. and KAKIHANA, R. (1981) Selective breeding for ethanol sensitivity: Short-sleep and long-sleep mice. In: G. E. MCCLEARN, R. A. DEITRICH, V. G. ERWIN (eds.) *Development of Animal Models as Pharmacogenetic Tools*, pp. 147–159, U.S. Government Printing Office, Washington, D.C.

MCGAUGH, J. L., GOLD, P. E., VAN BUSKIRK, R. and HAYCOCK, J. (1975) Modulating influences of hormones and catecholamines on memory storage processes. In: *Hormones, Homeostasis and the Brain*, pp. 151–162. GISPEN, W. H., TJ, B., VAN WIMERSMA, G., BOHUS, B. and DEWIED, D. (eds) Elsevier/North Holland, Amsterdam.

MCGAUGH, J. L., MARTINEZ, J. L. JR, JENSEN, R. A., MESSING, R. B. and VASQUEZ, B. J. (1980) Central and peripheral catecholamine function in learning and memory processes. In: *Neural Mechanisms of Goal-Directed Behavior and Learning*, pp. 75–91, THOMPSON, R. F., HICKS, L. H. and SHVYRKOV, V. B. (eds) Academic Press, New York.

MCMILLAN, D. E., LEANDER, J. D., ELLIS, F. W., LUCOT, J. B. and FRYE, G. D. (1976) Characteristics of ethanol drinking patterns under schedule-induced polydipsia. *Psychopharmacology* **49**: 49–55.

MCQUEEN, J. D., SKLAR, F. K. and POSEY, J. B. (1978) Autoregulation of cerebral blood flow during alcohol infusion. *J. Stud. Alcohol* **39**: 1477–1487.

MCSWIGAN, J. D., CRABBE, J. C. and YOUNG, E. R. (1984) Specific ethanol withdrawal seizures in genetically selected mice. *Life Sci.* **35**: 2119–2126.

MEISCH, R. A. and THOMPSON, T. (1974) Rapid establishment of ethanol as a reinforcer for rats. *Psychopharmacologia* **37**: 311–321.

MELCHIOR, C. L. and MYERS, R. D. (1976) Genetic differences in ethanol drinking of the rat following injection of 6-OHDA, 5,6-DHT or 5,7-DHT into the cerebral ventricles. *Pharmacol. Biochem. Behav.* **5**: 63–72.

MELCHIOR, C. L. and TABAKOFF, B. (1981) Modification of environmentally cued tolerance to ethanol in mice. *J. Pharmacol. Exp. Ther.* **219**: 175–180.

MELCHIOR, C. L. and TABAKOFF, B. (1985) Features of environmentally-dependent tolerance to ethanol. *Psychopharmacology* **87**: 94–100.

MELLANBY, E. (1919) Alcohol: Its absorption into and disappearance from the blood under different conditions. *Medical Research Committee Special Report Series*, No. 31, HMSO, London.

MELLO, N. K. and MENDELSON, J. H. (1978) Alcohol and human behavior. *Handbook of Psychopharmacology* **12**: 235–317.

MELLO, N. K., BREE, M. P., MENDELSON, J. H. and ELLINGBOE, J. (1983) Alcohol self administration disrupts reproduction function in female macaque monkeys. *Science* **211**: 677–679.

MELLO, N. K., BREE, M. P., SKUPNY, A. A. and MENDELSON, J. H. (1984) Blood alcohol levels as a function of menstrual cycle phase in female macaque monkeys. *Alcohol* **1**: 27–31.

MENA, M. A. and HERRERA, E. (1980) Monoamine metabolism in rat brain regions following long term alcohol treatment. *J. Neural Trans.* **47**: 227–236.

MENDELSON, J. H. (1964) Experimentally induced chronic intoxication and withdrawal in alcoholics. *Q. J. Stud. Alc.* **2**: 1–129.

MENDELSON, J. H. and MELLO, N. K. (1985) Diagnostic criteria for alcoholism and alcohol abuse. In: *The Diagnosis and Treatment of Alcoholism*, pp. 1–20, MENDELSON, J. H. and MELLO, N. K. (eds) McGraw–Hill, New York.

MENDELSON, J. H., MELLO, N. K., BAVLI, S., ELLINGBOE, J., BREE, M. P., HARVEY, K. L. KING, N. W. and SEGHAL, P. K. (1983) Alcohol efforts on female reproductive hormones. In: *Ethanol Tolerance and Dependence: Endocrinological Aspects*, NIAAA Research Monograph No. 13, DHHS Publication No (ADM) 83–1258, pp. 146–161, CICERO, T. J. (ed.) US Government Printing Office, Washington, D.C.

MENDELSON, J. H., OGATA, M. and MELLO, N. K. (1971) Adrenal function and alcoholism. I. Serum cortisol. *Psychosom. Med.* **33**: 145–157.

MENDELSON, J. H., MELLO, N. K. and ELLINGBOE, J. (1977) Effects of acute alcohol intake on pituitary-gonadal hormones in normal human males. *J. Pharmacol. Exp. Ther.* **202**: 676–682.

MENDELSON, J. H., MELLO, N. K. and ELLINGBOE, J. (1978) Effect of alcohol on pituitary-gonadal hormones, sexual function and aggression in human males. In: *Psychopharmacology: A Generation of Progress.* LIPTON, M. A., DIMASCIO, A. and KILLAM, K. F. (eds) Raven Press, New York.

MENDELSON, J. H., ROSSI, M., BERNSTEIN, J. G. and BUEHNLE, J. (1974) Propranolol and behavior of alcohol addicts after acute alcohol ingestion. *Clin. Pharmacol. Ther.* **15**: 571–578.

MENDELSON, W. B., MARTIN, J. V., WAGNER, R., ROSEBERRY, C., SKOLNICK, P., WEISSMAN, B. A. and SQUIRES, R. (1985) Are the toxicites of pentobarbital and ethanol mediated by the GABA-benzodiazepine receptor-chloride ionophore complex? *Eur. J. Pharmacol.* **108**: 63–70.

MENDOZA, L. C., HELLBERG, K., RICHARD, A. (1971) The effect of intravenous ethyl alcohol on the coronary circulation and myocardial contractility of the human and canine heart. *J. Clin. Pharmacol.* **11**: 165–176.

MERRY, J. and MARKS, V. (1972) The effect of alcohol barbituate and diazepam on hypothalamic/pituitary adrenal function in chronic alcoholics. *Lancet* **2**: 990–991.

MEYER, H. (1901) Zur theorie der alkolnarkose: Der einfuss wechseldner temperatur auf wirkung starke und theilungscoefficient der narcotica. *N. S.'s Archiv. fur Experimentelle Pathologie und Pharmakologie* **46**: 338–346.

MEZEY, E. and POTTER, J. J. (1979) Rat liver alcohol dehydrogenase activity: Effects of growth hormone and hypophysectomy. *Endocrinology* **104**: 1667–1673.

MEZEY, E. and POTTER, J. J. (1981) Effect of thyroidectomy and triiodothyronine administration on rat liver on alcohol dehydrogenase. *Gastroenterology* **80**: 566–574.

MEZEY, E., POTTER, J. J. and KVETNANSKY, R. (1979) Effect of stress by repeated immobilization on hepatic alcohol dehydrogenase activity and ethanol metabolism. *Biochem. Pharmacol.* **28**: 657–663.

MEZEY, E., POTTER, J. J., HARMON, S. M. and TSITOURAS, P. D. (1980) Effects of castration and testosterone administration on rat liver alcohol dehydrogenase activity. *Biochem. Pharmacol.* **28**: 657–663.

MIERZWIAK, D. S., WILDENTHAL, K. and MITCHELL, J. H. (1972) Acute effects of ethanol on the left ventricle in dogs. *Arch. Int. Pharmacodyn. Ther.* **199**: 43–52.

MILLER, S. L. (1961) A theory of gaseous anesthetics. *Proc. Natl. Acad. Sci.* **47**: 1515–1524.

MILLER, S. L., GOLDMAN, E., ERICKSON, C. K. and SHOREY, R. L. (1980) Induction of physical dependence on and tolerance to ethanol in rats fed a new nutritionally complete and balanced liquid diet. *Psychopharmacology* **68**: 55–59.

MILLS, K. C. and BISGROVE, E. Z. (1983) Body sway and divided attention performance under the influence of alcohol: Dose-response differences between males and females. *Alcoholism: Clin. Exp. Res.* **7**: 393–397.

MORGAN, E. P. and PHILLIS, J. W. (1975) The effects of ethanol on acetylcholine release from the brain of anesthetized cats. *Gen. Pharmacol.* **6**: 281–284.

MOSCATELLI, E. A., FUJIMOTO, K. and GILFOIL, T. C. (1975) Effects of chronic consumption of ethanol and sucrose on rat whole brain 5-hydroxytryptamine. *J. Neurochem.* **25**: 273–276.

MUCHA, R. F., PINEL, J. P. J. and VAN OOT, P. H. (1975) Simple method for producing an alcohol withdrawal syndrome in rats. *Pharmacol. Biochem. Behav.* **3**: 765–769.

MULLER, P., BRITTON, R. S. and SEEMAN, P. (1980) The effects of long-term ethanol on brain receptors for dopamine, acetylcholine, serotonin and noradrenaline. *Eur. J. Pharmacol.* **65**: 31–37.

MULLIN, M. J. and FERKO, A. P. (1981) Ethanol and functional tolerance interactions with pimozide and clonidine. *J. Pharmacol. Exp. Ther.* **216**: 459–464.

MULLIN, M. J. and FERKO, A. P. (1983) Alterations in dopaminergic function after subacute ethanol administration. *J. Pharmacol. Exp. Ther.* **225**: 694–698.

MULLINS, L. J. (1954) Some physical mechanisms of narcosis. *Chem. Rev.* **54**: 289–323.

MUNOZ, C. and GUIVERNAU, M. (1980) Antagonistic effects of propranolol upon ethanol-induced narcosis on mice. *Res. Commun. Chem. Pathol. Pharmacol.* **29**: 57–65.

MURDOCK, B. B. (1976) Item and order information in short term serial memory. *J. Exp. Psychol.* **105**: 191–206.

MURRAY, M. M. (1932) The diuretic action of alcohol and its relation to pituitrin. *J. Physiol.* **76**: 379–386.

MYERS, R. D. (1981) Alcohol's effect on body temperature hypothermia, hyperthermia or poikilothermia? *Brain Res. Bull.* **7**: 209–220.

MYERS, R. D. and CICERO, T. J. (1969) Effects of serotonin depletion on the volitional alcohol intake of rats during a condition of psychological stress. *Psychopharmacologia (Berlin)* **15**: 373–381.

MYERS, R. D. and MELCHOIR, C. L. (1975) Alcohol drinking in the rat after destruction of serotonergic and catecholaminergic neurons in the brain. *Res. Comm. Chem. Pharmacol. Pathol.* **10**: 363–378.

MYERS, R. D. and VEALE, W. L. (1968) Alcohol preference in the rat: Reduction following depletion of brain serotonin. *Science* **160**: 1469–1471.

MYRSTEN, A.-L., POST, B. and FRANKENHAEUSER, M. (1971) Catecholamine output during and after acute alocholic intoxication. *Percept. Motor Skills* **33**: 652–654.

NACHMAN, M., LESTER, D. and LEMAGNEN, J. (1970) Alcohol aversion in the rat: Behavioral assessment of noxious drug effects. *Science* **168**: 1244–1246.

NAKANO, J. and KESSINGER, J. M. (1972) Cardiovascular effects of ethanol, its congeners and synthetic bourbon in dogs. *Eur. J. Pharmacol.* **17**: 195–201.

NARANJO, C. A. and SELLERS, E. M. Clinical assessment and pharmacotherapy of the alcohol withdrawal syndrome. In: *Recent Developments in Alcoholism*, pp. 265–280, GALANTER, M. (ed.) Plenum Press, New York.

NATIONAL INSTITUTE ON ALCOHOL ABUSE AND ALCOHOLISM (NIAAA) (1978) Special population groups. In: *Alcohol and Health*, DHEW Publication No. (ADM) 78-569, pp. 17–24, Third Special Report to the Congress. U.S. Government Printing Office, Washington, D.C.

NEWLIN, D. B. (1985a) Human conditioned compensatory response to alcohol cues: Initial evidence. *Alcohol* **2**: 507–509.

NEWLIN, D. B. (1986b) The antagonistic placebo response to alcohol cues. *Alcoholism: Clin. Exp. Res.* **9**: 411–416.

NEWMAN, H. and ABRAMSON, M. (1942) Some factors influencing the intoxicating effects of alcoholic beverages. *Q. J. Stud. Alc.* **3**: 351–370.

NHAMBURO, P. T., SALATSKY, B. P., HOFFMAN, P. L. and TABAKOFF, B. (1986) Effects of short-chain alcohols and norepinephrine on brain (Na^+,K^+)ATPase activity. *Biochem. Pharmacol.* **35**: 1987–1992.

NIAURA, R., SHAPIRO, A., NATHAN, P. E. and BRICK, J. (1986) The role of conditioning and expectancy in acute tolerance to alcohol. Unpublished manuscript, Rutgers University.

NIAURA, R., NATHAN, P. E., FRANKENSTEIN, W., SHAPIRO, A. and BRICK, J. (1987) Gender differences in acute psychomotor, cognitive pharmacokinetic response to alcohol. *Addict. Behav.* (in press).

NICHOLSON, G. and PATON, A. (1983) Glucose tolerance and b-cell function in chronic alcoholism: Its relation to hepatic histology and exocrine pancreatic function. *Metabolism* **32**: 1029–1032.

NICHOLSON, W. M. and TAYLOR, H. M. (1983) The effect of alcohol on the water and electrolyte balance in man. *J. Clin. Invest.* **17**: 279–285.

NIKANDER, P. and PEKKANEN, L. (1977) An inborn alcohol tolerance in alcohol-preferring rats: The lack of relationship between tolerance to ethanol and the brain microsomal (Na^+K^+)ATPase activity. *Psychopharmacologia (Berlin)* **51**: 219–223.

NOBLE, E. P. (1971) Ethanol and adrenocortical stimulation in inbred mouse strains. In: *Recent Advances in Studies of Alcoholism*, pp. 72–106. MELLO, N. and MENDELSON, J. (eds) U.S. Government Printing Office, Washington, D.C.

NOBLE, E. P. (1973) Alcohol and adrenocortical function of animals and man. In: *Alcoholism, Progress in Research and Treatment*, pp. 1005–1035, BOURNE, P. G. and FOX, R. (eds) Academic Press, New York.

NOBLE, E. P., KAKIHANA, R. and BUTTE, J. (1971) Corticosterone metabolism in alcohol-adapted mice. In: *Biological Aspects of Alcohol*, pp. 389–412, ROACH, M. K., MCISSAC, W. N. and CREAVEN, P. J. (eds) Lea and Febiger, New York.

NOBLE, E. P., GILLIES, R., VIGRAN, R. and MANDEL, P. (1976) The modification of the ethanol withdrawal syndrome in rats by di-*n*-propylacetate. *Psychopharmacologia (Berlin)* **46**: 127–131.

NORDBERG, A. and WAHLSTROM, G. (1983) Tolerance, physical dependence and changes in muscarinic receptor binding sites after chronic ethanol treatment in the rat. *Life Sci.* **31**: 277–287.

NORDBERG, A., LARSSON, C., PERDAHL, E. and WINBLAD, B. (1983) Changes in cholinergic activity in human hippocampus following chronic alcohol abuse. *Pharmacol. Biochem. Behav.* **18**: Suppl 1: 397–400.

NOREN, G. R., STALEY, N. A., EINZING, S., MIKELL, F. L. and ASINGER, R. W. (1983) Alcohol-induced congestive cardiomyopathy: An animal model. *Cardiovasc. Res.* **17**: 81–87.

NUMAN, R. and GILROY, A. M. (1978) Induction of physical dependence upon ethanol in rats using intravenous infusion. *Pharmacol. Biochem. Behav.* **9**: 279–282.

NUMAN, R. and NAPARZEWSKA, A. M. (1984) Comparison of two intravenous infusion schedules for inducing physical dependence upon ethanol in rats. *Alcohol* **1**: 9–17.

OGATA, M., MENDELSON, J. H., MELLO, N. K. and MAJCHROWICZ, E. (1971) Adrenal function and alcoholism. II. Catecholamines. *Psychosom. Med.* **33**: 159–180.

OLIVERIA SOUZA, M. L. and MASUR, J. (1982) Does hypothermia play a relevant role in the glycemic alterations induced by ethanol? *Pharmacol. Biochem. Behav.* **16**: 903–908.

ORELAND, L., WILBERG, A., WINBLAD, B., FOWLER, C. J., GOTTFRIES, C.-G. and KIIANMAA, K. (1983) The activity of monoamine oxidase-A and -B in brains from chronic alcoholics. *J. Neural. Trans.* **56**: 73–83.

ORENBERG, E. K., RENSON, J. and BARCHAS, J. D. (1976) The effects of alcohol on cyclic AMP in mouse brain. *Neurochem. Res.* **1**: 659–667.

ORENBERG, E. K., ZARCONE, V. P., RENSON, J. F. and BARCHAS, J. D. (1976) The effects of ethanol ingestion on cyclic AMP, homovanillic acid and 5-hydroxyindoleacetic acid in human cerebrospinal fluid. *Life Sci.* **19**: 1669–1672.

ORLANDO, J., ARONOW, W. C., CASSIDY, J. and PRAKASH, R. (1976) Effect of ethanol on angina pectoris. *Ann. Intern. Med.* **84**: 652–655.

ORTIZ, A., GRIFFITHS, R. J. and LITTLETON, J. M. (1974) A comparison of the effects of chronic administration of ethanol and acetaldehyde in mice: Evidence for a role of acetaldehyde in ethanol dependence. *J. Pharm. Pharmacol.* **26**: 249–260.

OTT, J., HUNTER, B. and WALKER, D. (1985) The effect of age on ethanol metabolism and on the hypothermic and hypnotic responses to ethanol in the Fischer 344 rat. *Alcoholism: Clin. Exp. Res.* **9**: 59–65.

OVERTON, D. A. (1966) State dependency learning produced by depressant and atropine like drugs. *Psychopharmacologia (Berlin)* **10**: 6–31.

OVERTON, D. A. (1972) State dependent learning produced by alcohol and its relevance to alcoholism. In: *The Biology of Alcoholism*, Vol. 2. Physiology and Behavior, KISSIN, B. and BEGLEITER, H. (eds) Plenum Press, New York.

PACHINGER, O. M., TILLMANNS, H., MAO, J. C., FAUVEL, J. M. and BING, R. J. (1973) The effect of prolonged administration of ethanol on cardiac metabolism and performance in the dog. *J. Clin. Invest.* **52**: 2690–2696.

PADFIELD, P. L. and MORTON, J. T. (1974) Application of a sensitive radioimmunoassay for plasma arginine vasopressin to pathological conditions in man. *Clin. Sci.* **47**: 16p–17p.

PALAIC, D. J., DESATY, J., ALBERT, J. M. and PANISSET, J. C. (1971) Effect of ethanol on metabolism and subcellular distribution of serotonin in rat brain. *Brain Res.* **25**: 381–386.

PARKER, L. F. and RADOW, B. L. (1976) Effects of parachlorophenylalanine on ethanol self-selection in the rat. *Pharmacol. Biochem. Behav.* **4**: 535–540.

PATEL, G. J. and LAL, H. (1973) Reduction in brain gamma-aminobutyric acid and in barbital narcosis during ethanol withdrawal. *J. Pharmacol. Exp. Ther.* **186**: 625–629.

PATON, B. C. (1983) Accidental hypothermia. *Pharmacol. Ther.* **22**: 331–377.

PELHAM, T. W., MARQUIS, J. K., KUGELMANN, K. and MUNSAT, T. L. (1980) Prolonged ethanol consumption produces persistent alterations of cholinergic function in rat brain. *Alcoholism: Clin. Exp. Res.* **4**: 282–287.

PENNER, D. W. and COLDWELL, B. B. (1958) Car driving and alcohol consumption: Medical observations on an experiment. *Canad. Med. Assoc.* **79**: 793–800.

PENTTILA, A., TENHU, M. and KATAJA, M. (1971) Clinical examination for intoxication in cases of suspected drunken driving. *Reports from Talja* **11**: 43, Helsinki, Finland.

PERIS, J. and CUNNINGHAM, C. L. (1985) Dissociation of tolerance to the hypothermic and tachycardiac effects of ethanol. *Pharmacol. Biochem. Behav.* **22**: 973–978.

PERMAN, E. S. (1961) Observations on the effect of ethanol on the urinary excretion of histamine, 5-hydroxyindole acetic acid, catecholamines and 17-hydroxycorticosteroids in man. *Acta Physiol. Scand.* **51**: 62–67.

PETERMAN, M., BRAVO, M., VIDELA, L. and UGARTE, G. (1979) Effect of epinephrine and alprenolol on ethanol metabolism, liver cell respiration and mitochondrial function. *Pharmacology* **18**: 42–47.

PETIT, N. B., IHRIG, T. J. and FRENCH, S. W. (1980) An intragastric pairfeeding model for ethanol administration. *Fed. Proc.* **39**: 541 (Abstract).

PEUHKURINEN, K. J., KIVILUOMA, K. T., HILTUNEN, J. K., TAKALA, T. E. S. and HASSINEN, I. E. (1983) Effects of ethanol metabolites on intermediary metabolism in heart muscle. *Pharmacol. Biochem. Behav.* **18**: 279–283.

PFEIFFER, A., SEIZINGER, B. R. and HERZ, A. (1981) Chronic ethanol inhibition with delta-, but not with mu-opiate receptors. *Neuropharmacol.* **20**: 1229–1232.

PHILLIS, J. W., JIANG, Z. G. and CHELACK, B. J. (1980) Effects of ethanol on acetylcholine and adenosine efflux from the in vivo rat cerebral cotex. *J. Pharm. Pharmacol.* **32**: 871–872.

PIEPER, W. A. and SKEEN, M. J. (1972) Induction of physical dependence on ethanol in rhesus monkeys using an oral acceptance technique. *Life Sci.* **11**: (Part I): 989–997.

PITT, B., SUGISHITA, Y., GREEN, H. L. and FRIESINGER, G. C. (1970) Coronary hemodynamic effect of ethyl alcohol in the conscious dog. *Am. J. Physiol.* **219**: 175–177.

PLATONOW, N. and COLDWELL, B. B. (1966) Metaoblism of alcohol in partially hepatectomized rats exposed to cold. *Experimentia* **23**: 213–214.

PODOLSKY, E. (1963) The woman alcoholic and premenstrual tension. *J. Am. Med. Women. Assoc.* **18**: 816–818.

POHORECKY, L. A. (1974) Effects of ethanol on central and peripheral noradrenergic neurons. *J. Pharmacol. Exp. Ther.* **189**: 380–391.

POHORECKY, L. A. (1976) Withdrawal from ethanol: Simple quantitative behavioral tests for its evaluation. *Psychopharmacology* **50**: 125–129.

POHORECKY, L. A. (1978) Biphasic action of ethanol: A review. *Biol. Behav. Res.* **1**: 231–240.

POHORECKY, L. A. (1981a) Animal analog of alcohol dependence. *Fed. Proc.* **40**: 2056–2064.

POHORECKY, L. A. (1981b) Interaction of ethanol and stress. A review. *Neurosci. Biobehav. Res.* **5**: 209–229.

POHORECKY, L. A. (1985) Effect of ethanol on urine ouptut in rats. *Alcohol* **2**: 659–666.

POHORECKY, L. A. (1986) The effects of peripherally administered monoaminergic drugs on ethanol diuresis in rats. *J. Pharm. Pharmacol.* **38**: 283–287.

POHORECKY, L. A. and BRICK, J. (eds) (1983) *Stress and Alcohol Use.* Elsevier Biomedical, New York.

POHORECKY, L. A. and JAFFE, L. S. (1975) Noradrenergic involvement in the acute effects of ethanol. *Res. Commun. Chem. Pathol. Pharmacol.* **12**: 433–447.

POHORECKY, L. A. and NEWMAN, B. (1977) Effect of ethanol on dopamine synthesis in rat striatal synaptosomes. *Drug Alc. Depend.* **2**: 329–334.

POHORECKY, L. A. and PACKARD, K. (1986) Noradrenergic mechanisms in ethanol diuresis. *Alcoholism: Clin. Exp. Res.* **10**: 177–183.

POHORECKY, L. A. and RIZEK, A. E. (1981) Biochemical and behavioral effects of acute ethanol in rats at different environmental temperatures. *Psychopharmacology* **72**: 205–209.

POHORECKY, L. A. and JAFFE, L. S. and BERKLEY, H. A. (1974) Effect of ethanol on serotonergic neurons in the rat brain. *Res. Commun. Chem. Pathol. Pharmacol.* **8**: 1–11.

POHORECKY, L. A., BRICK, J. and SUN, J. Y. (1976a) Serotonergic involvement in the effect of ethanol on body temperature in rats. *J. Pharm. Pharmacol.* **28**: 157–159.

POHORECKY, L. A., CAGAN, M., BRICK, J. and JAFFE, L. S. (1976b) The startle response in rats: Effect of ethanol. *Pharmacol. Biochem. Behav.* **4**: 311–316.

POHORECKY, L. A. NEWMAN, B., SUN, J. and BAILEY. W. (1978) Acute and chronic ethanol ingestion and serotonin metabolism in rat brain. *J. Pharmacol. Exp. Ther.* **204**: 424–432.

POHORECKY, L. A., MARKOWSKI, E., NEWMAN, B. and RASSI, E. (1979) Cholinergic mediation of motor effects of ethanol in rats. *Eur. J. Pharmacol.* **55**: 67–72.

POHORECKY, L. A., BRICK, J. and CARPENTER, J. A. (1986) Assessment of the development of tolerance to ethanol using multiple measures. *Alcoholism: Clin. Exp. Res.* **10**: 616–622.

POHORECKY, L. A., BRICK, J. and CARPENTER, J. A. (1986) Assessment of the development of tolerance to ethanol using the tail-flick response. *Proceedings of the IV World Congress of Biological Psychiatry, Philadelphia, PA. September 8-13, 1985.*

POHORECKY, L. A., PETERSON, T. J. and CARPENTER, J. A. (1986) Development of tolerance to ethanol in heart rate of rats. *Alcohol Drug Res.* **6**: 431–439.

POKRAS, R. and TABAKOFF, B. (1982) On the mechanism by which dopamine inhibits prolactin release in the anterior pituitary. *Life Sci.* **31**: 2587–2593.

POLIMENI, P. I., OTTEN, M. O. and HOESCHEN, L. E. (1983) In vivo effects of ethanol on the rat myocardium: Evidence for a reversible, non-specific increase of sarcolemmal permeability. *J. Molec. Cell. Cardiol.* **15**: 113–122.

POSNER, P., BAKER, S. P., CARPENTIER, R. G. and WALKER, D. W. (1985) Negative chronotropic effect of chronic ethanol ingestion in the rat. *Alcohol* **2**: 309–311.

POST, R. M. and BALLENGER, J. C. (1981) Kindling models for the progressive development of psychopathology: Sensitization to electrical, pharmacological, and psychological stimuli. In: *Handbook of Biological Psychiatry, Part IV.* pp. 609–651, VAN PRAAG, H. M., LADER, M. H. and RAFAELSEN, O. J. (eds) Marcel Dekker, New York.

POST, M. E. and SUN, A. Y. (1973) The effect of chronic ethanol administration on the levels of catecholamines in different regions of the rat brain. *Res. Commun. Chem. Pathol. Pharmacol.* **6**: 887–894.

POTTER, D. E. and MORRIS, J. W. (1980) Ethanol-induced changes in plasma glucose, insulin and glucagon in fed and fasted rats. *Experientia* **36**: 1003–1004.

POULOS, C., WOLFF, L., ZILM, D., CAPLAN, H. and CAPPELL, H. (1981) Acquisition of tolerance to alcohol-induced memory deficits in humans. *Psychopharmacology* **73**: 176–179.

PRINZ, P. N., ROEHRS, T. A., VITALIANO, P. P. *et al.* (1980) Effect of alcohol on sleep and nighttime plasma growth hormone and cortisol concentrations. *J. Clin. Endocrinol. Metab.* **51**: 759–764.

RABIN, R. A. and MOLINOFF, P. B. (1981) Activation of adenylate cyclase by ethanol on mouse striatal tissue. *J. Pharmacol. Exp. Ther.* **216**: 129–134.

RABIN, R. A. and MOLINOFF, P. B. (1983) Multiple sites of action of ethanol on adenylate cyclase. *J. Pharmacol. Exp. Ther.* **227**: 551–556.

RABIN, R. A., WOLFE, B. B., DIBNER, M. K., ZAHNISER, N. R., MELCHOIR, C. and MOLINOFF, P. B. (1980) Effects of ethanol administration and withdrawal on neurotransmitter receptor systems in C57 mice. *J. Pharmacol. Exp. Ther.* **213**: 491–496.

RACHAMIN, G., MACDONALD, J. A., WAHID, S., CLAPP, J. J., KHANNA, J. M. and ISRAEL, Y. (1980) Modulation of alcohol dehydrogenase and ethanol metabolism by sex hormones in the spontaneously hypertensive rat. *Biochem. J.* **103**: 623–626.

RANGARAJ, N. and KALANT, H. (1978) Effects of ethanol withdrawal, stress and amphetamine on rat brain $(Na^{+}+K^{+})$-ATPase. *Biochem. Pharmacol.* **27**: 1139–1144.

RANGARAJ, N. and KALANT, H. (1979) Interaction of ethanol and catecholamines on rat brain $(Na^{+}+K^{+})$-ATPase. *Can. J. Physiol. Pharmacol.* **57**: 1098–1106.

RANGARAJ, N. and KALANT, H. (1980) α-Adrenoreceptor mediated alteration of ethanol effects on $(Na^{+}+K^{+})$-ATPase of rat neuronal membranes. *Can. J. Physiol. Pharmacol.* **58**: 1342–1346.

RANGARAJ, N. and KALANT, H. (1980) Acute and chronic catecholamine-ethanol interactions on rat brain $(Na^{+}+K^{+})$-ATPase. *Pharmacol. Biochem. Behav.* **13**: Suppl. 1, 183–189.

RANGARAJ, N. and KALANT, H. (1982) Effect of chronic ethanol treatment on temperature dependence and on norepinephrine sensitization of rat brain $(Na^{+}+K^{+})$-adenosine triphosphatase. *J. Pharmacol. Exp. Ther.* **223**: 536–539.

RANGARAJ, N. and KALANT, H. (1984) Effect of ethanol tolerance on norepinephrine-ethanol inhibition of $(Na^{+}+K^{+})$-ATPase in various regions of rat brain. *J. Pharmacol. Exp. Ther.* **231**: 416–421.

RANGARAJ, N., BEAUGE, F. and KALANT, H. (1984) Temporal correlation of changes in rat brain sialic acid and in inhibition of $Na^{+}+K^{+}$-ATPase with ethanol tolerance. *Can. J. Physiol. Pharmacol.* **62**: 899–904.

RANGARAJ, N., KALANT, H. and BEAUGE, F. (1985) α_1-Adrenergic receptor involvement in norepinephrine-ethanol inhibition of rat brain $Na^{+}-K^{+}$-ATPase and in ethanol tolerance. *Can. J. Physiol. Pharmacol.* **63**: 1075–1079.

RAPTIS, S., VON BERGER, L., DOLLINGER, H. C., GOSTOMZYK, J. G. and PFEIFFER, E. F. (1974) Influence of ethanol, caffeine, and intragastric cooling on gastrin and insulin secretion in man. *Nutr. Metab.* **17**: 352–359.

RASTOGI, S. K., THYAGARAJAN, R., CLOTHIER, J. and TICKU, M. K. (1986) Effect of chronic treatment of ethanol benzodiazepine and picrotoxin sites on the GABA receptor complex in regions of the brain of the rat. *Neuropharmacology* **25**: 1179–1184.

RATHER, L. J. (1974) Hepatic cirrhosis and testicular atrophy. *Arch. Int. Med.* **80**: 397–405.

RAWAT, A. K. (1974) Brain levels and turnover rates of presumptive neurotransmitters influenced by administration and withdrawal of ethanol in mice. *J. Neurochem.* **22**: 915–922.

RAWAT, A. K. (1979) Inhibition of cardiac protein synthesis by prolonged ethanol administration. *Res. Comm. Chem. Path. Pharmacol.* **25**: 89–102.

REDEI, E., BRANCH, B. J. and NEWMAN TAYLOR, A. (1986) Direct effect of ethanol on adrenocorticotropin (ACTH) release in vitro. *J. Pharmacol. Exp. Ther.* **237**: 59–63.

REDOS, J. D., CATRAVAS, G. N. and HUNT, W. A. (1976) Ethanol-induced depletion of cerebellar guanosine 3′,5′-cyclic monophosphate. *Science* **193**: 58–59.

REDOS, J. D., HUNT, W. A. and CATRAVAS, G. N. (1976) Lack of alteration in regional brain adenosine-3′-5′-cyclic monophosphate levels after acute and chronic treatment with ethanol. *Life Sci.* **18**: 989–992.

REGAN, T. J. (1971) Ethyl alcohol and the heart. *Circulation* **44**: 957–963.

REGAN, T. J. (1984) Alcoholic cardiomyopathy. *Prog. Cardiovasc. Dis.* **XXVII**: 141–152.

REGAN, T. J. and ETTINGER, P. O. (1979) Varied cardiac abnormalities in alcoholics. *Alcoholism: Clin. Exp. Res.* **3**: 40–45.

REGAN, T. J., KAROXENIDIS, G. and MOSCHOS, C. B. (1966) The acute metabolic hemodynamic responses of the left ventricle to ethanol. *J. Clin. Invest.* **45**: 270–280.

REGAN, T. J., LEVINSON, G. E.and OLDEWURTEL, H. A. (1969) Ventricular function in noncardiacs with alcoholic fatty liver. Role of ethanol in the production of cardiomyopathy. *J. Clin. Invest.* **48**: 397–407.

REGAN, T. J., ETTINGER, P. O. and OLDEWURTEL, H. A. (1974) Heart cell responses to ethanol. *Ann. N.Y. Acad. Sci.* **242**: 250–263.

REGAN, T. J., ETTINGER, P. O., HAIDER, B., AHMED, S. S., OLDEWURTEL, H. A. and LYONS, M. M. (1977) The role of ethanol in cardiac disease. *Annu. Rev. Med.* **28**: 393–409.

REGGIANI, A., BARBACCIA, M. L., SPANO, P. F. and TRABUCCHI, M. (1980a) Acute and chronic ethanol administration on specific ^{3}H-GABA binding in different rat brain areas. *Psychopharmacology* **67**: 261–264.

REGGIANI, A., BARBACCIA, M. L., SPANO, P. F. and TRABUCCHI, M. (1980b) Dopamine metabolism and receptor function after acute and chronic ethanol. *J. Neurochem.* **35**: 34–37.

REGGIANI, A., BARRACCIA, M. L., SPANO, P. F. and TRABUCCHI, M. (1980c) Role of dopaminergic-enkephalinergic interactions in the neurochemical effects of ethanol. *Subst. Alc. Actions Misuse* **1**: 151–158.

RICHTER, C. P. (1926) A study of the effect of moderate doses of alcohol on the growth and behavior of the rat. *J. Exp. Zool.* **44**: 397–418.

RICHTER, J. A. and WERLING, L. L. (1979) K-stimulated acetylcholine release: Inhibition by several barbiturates and chloral hydrate but not by ethanol, chlordiazepoxide or 11-OH-Δ^{9}-tetrahydrocannabinol. *J. Neurochem.* **32**: 935–941.

RIFF, D. P., JAIN, A. C. and DOYLE, J. T. (1969) Acute hemodynamic effects of ethanol on normal human volunteers. *Am. Heart J.* **78**: 592–597.

RIGTER, H., CRABBE, J. C. and SCHONBAUM, E. (1980a) Hypothermia in mice as an index of the rapid development of tolerance to ethanol. In: *Thermoregulatory mechanisms and Their Therapeutic Implications*, pp. 216–219, COX, B., LOMAX, P., MILTON, A. S. and SCHONBAUM, E. (eds) Karger, Basel.

RIGTER, H., DORTMANS, C. and CRABBE, J. C. JR (1980b) Effects of peptides related to neurohypophyseal hormones on ethanol tolerance. *Pharmacol. Biochem. Behav.* **13** (Suppl. 1): 285–290.

RIHMER, Z. and ARATO, M. (1982) Depression and diabetes mellitus. *Neuropsychobiol.* **8**: 315–318.

RIJK, H., CRABBE, J. C. and RIGTER, H. (1982) A mouse model of alcoholism. *Physiol. Behav.* **29**: 833–839.

RISBO, A., HAGELSTEN, J. O. and JESSEN, K. (1981) Human body temperature and controlled cold exposure during moderate and severe experimental alcohol-intoxication. *Acta Anaesthesiol. Scand.* **25**: 215–218.

RITZMANN, R. F. and TABAKOFF, B. (1976a) Body temperature in mice: A quantitative measure of alcohol tolerance and physical dependence. *J. Pharmacol. Exp. Ther.* **199**: 158–170.

RITZMANN, R. F. and TABAKOFF, B. (1970b) Ethanol, serotonin metabolism, and body temperature. *Ann. N.Y. Acad. Sci.* **273**: 247–255.

RIVIER, C., BRUHN, T. and VALE, W. (1984) Effect of ethanol on the hypothalamic-pituitary-adrenal axis in the rat: Role of corticotropin-releasing factor (CRF). *J. Pharmacol. Exp. Ther.* **229**: 127–131.

RIVIER, C. and VALE, W. (1987) Diminished responsiveness of the hypothalamic-pituitary-adrenal axis of the rat during exposure to prolonged stress: A pituitary-mediated mechanism. *Endocrinology* **121**: 1320–1328.

RIVIER, C. and VALE, W. (1988) Interaction between ethanol and stress on ACTH and B-endorphin secretion. *Alcohol. Clin. Exp. Res.* **12**: 206–210.

ROACH, M. K., DAVIS, D. L., PENNINGTON, W. and NORDYKE, E. (1973) Effect of ethanol on the uptake by rat brain synaptosomes of (^{3}H)DL-norepinephrine, (^{3}H)5-hydroxytryptamine, (^{3}H)GABA and (^{3}H)glutamate. *Life Sci.* **12**: 433–441.

ROACH, M. K., KHAN, M. M., COFFMAN, R., PENNINGTON, W. and DAVIS, D. L. (1973) Brain (Na^+,K^+)-activated adenosine triphosphatase activity and neurotransmitter uptake in alcohol-dependent rats. *Brain Res.* **63**: 323–329.

ROGAWSKI, M. A., KNAPP, S. and MANDELL, A. J. (1974) Effects of ethanol on tryptophan hydroxylase activity from striate synaptosomes. *Biochem. Pharmacol.* **23**: 1955–1962.

ROGERS, J., WIENER, S. G. and BLOOM, F. E. (1979) Long-term ethanol administration methods for rats: advantages of inhalation over intubation or liquid diets. *Behav. Neural Biol.* **27**: 466–486.

ROSSI, M. A. (1980) Alcohol and malnutrition in the pathogenesis of experimental alcoholic cardiomyopathy. *Pathology* **130**: 105–116.

ROSSI, M. A. and OLIVERIA, J. S. M. (1976) Effect of prolonged ethanol administration on the noradrenaline levels of rat heart. *Eur. J. Pharmacol.* **40**: 187–190.

ROSSI, M. A., OLIVERIA, J. S. M., ZUCOLOTO, S. and BECKER, P. F. L. (1976) Norepinephrine levels and morphologic alterations of myocardium in chronic alcoholic rats. *Beitr. Pathol.* **159**: 51–60.

RUBIO, M. C., PEREC, C. J., MEDINA, J. H. and TISCOMIA, O. M. (1984) Effects of chronic ethanol feeding on sympathetic innervated organs: Temporal sequence of biochemical, functional, and trophic changes. *Alcoholism: Clin. Exp. Res.* **8**: 37–41.

RUNNAR, R. M., DEMAKIS, J., RAHIMTOOLA, S. H., SINNO, M. Z. and TOBIN, J. R. (1975) Clinical signs and natural history of alcoholic heart disease. In: *Medical Consequences of Alcoholism. Ann. N.Y. Acad. Sci.* pp. 264–272, SEIXAS, F. A., WILLIAMS, K. and EGGLESTON, S. (eds) New York Academy of Sciences, New York.

RYBACK, R. S. (1977) Chronic alcohol consumption and menstruation. *J. Am. Med. Assoc.* **283**: 2143.

RYDER, S., STRAUS, E., LIEBER, C. S. and YALOW, R. S. (1981) Cholecystokinin and enkephalin levels following ethanol administration in rats. *Peptides* **2**: 223–226.

SABOUROULT, D., BAUCHES, F., GIUDICELLI, Y., NORDMANN, J. and NORDMANN, R. (1981) Alpha- and beta-adrenergic receptors in rat myocardium membranes and prolonged ethanol inhalation. *Experientia* **37**: 2–4.

SAMSON, H. H. and FALK, J. L. (1975) Pattern of daily blood ethanol elevation and the development of physical dependence. *Pharmacol. Biochem. Behav.* **3**: 1119–1123.

SANDERS, B., COLLINS, A. C. and WESLEY, V. H. (1976) Reduction of alcohol selection by pargyline in mice. *Psychopharmacologia* (*Berlin*) **46**: 159–162.

SANTAMARIA, J. N. (1975) In: *Alcohol, Drugs and Traffic Safety*, pp. 381–388, ISRAEL, I., STAM, S. and LAMBERT, S. (eds) Addiction Research Foundation, Toronto.

SARDESAI, V. M. and PROVIDO, H. S. (1978) The effect of chronic ethanol ingestion on myocardial glucose and energy metabolism. *J. Nutrition* **108**: 1907–1912.

SARGENT, W. Q., SIMPSON, J. R. and BEARD, J. D. (1975) Renal hemodynamics and electrolyte excretions after reserpine and ethanol. *J. Pharmacol. Exp. Ther.* **193**: 356–362.

SARMA, J. S. M., IKEDA, S., FISCHER, R., MARUYAMA, T., WEISHAAR, R. and BING, R. J. (1976) Biochemical and contractile properties of heart muscle after prolonged alcohol administration. *J. Molec. Cell. Cardiol.* **8**: 951–972.

SAUNDERS, J. B., BEEVERS, D. B. and PATON, A. (1979) Factors influencing blood pressure in chronic alcoholics. *Clin. Sci.* **57**: 295s–298s.

SAWYER, D. C., LUMB, W. V. and STONE, H. L. (1971) Cardiovascular effects of halothane, methoxyflurane, pentobarbitol, and thiamylal. *J. Appl. Physiol.* **30**: 36–43.

SCHMIDT, M. J., SCHMIDT, D. E. and ROBISON, G. A. (1971) Cyclic adenosine monophosphate in brain areas: microwave irradiation as a means of tissue fixation. *Science* **173**: 1142–1143.

SCHREIBER, S. S., BRIDEN, K., ORATZ, M. and ROTHSCHILD, M. A. (1972) Ethanol, acetaldehyde, and myocardial protein synthesis. *J. Clin. Invest.* **51**: 2820–2826.

SCHREIBER, S. S., ORATZ, M., ROTHSCHILD, M. A., REFF, F. and EVANS, C. (1974) Alcoholic cardiomyopathy. III. The inhibition of cardiac microsomal protein synthesis by acetaldehyde. *J. Molec. Cell. Cardiol.* **6**: 207–213.

SCHREIBER, S. S., EVANS, C. D., REFF, F., ROTHSCHILD, M. A. and ORATZ, M. (1982) Prolonged feeding of ethanol to the young growing guinea pig. I. The effect of protein synthesis in the afterloaded right ventricle measured in vitro. *Alcoholism: Clin. Exp. Res.* **10**: 531–534.

SCHREIBER, S. S., EVANS, C. D., REIFF, F., ORATZ, M. and ROTHSCHILD, M. A. (1984) Prolonged feeding of ethanol to the young growing guinea pig. II. A model to study the effects of severe ischemia on cardiac protein synthesis. *Alcoholism: Clin. Exp. Res.* **8**: 54–60.

SCHREIBER, S. S., REFF, F., EVANS, C. D., ROTHSCHILD, M. A. and ORATZ, M. (1986) Prolonged feeding of ethanol to the young growing guinea pig. II. Effect on the synthesis of the myocardial contractile proteins. *Alcoholism: Clin. Exp. Res.* **10**: 531–534.
SCHULTHEIB, H.-P., SPIEGEL, M. and BOLTE, H. D. (1985) The effects of chronic ethanol treatment on oligomycin sensitive ATPase activity in the guinea pig heart. *Basic Res. Cardiol.* **80**: 548–555.
SCHULZ, R., WUSTER, M., DUKA, T. and HERZ, A. (1980) Acute and chronic ethanol treatment changes endorphin levels in brain and pituitary. *Psychopharmacology* **68**: 221–227.
SCHWARZ, M., APPEL, K. E., SCHRENK, D. and KUNZ, W. (1980) Effect of ethanol on microsomal metabolism of dimethylnitrosamine. *J. Can. Res. Clin. Oncol.* **97**: 233–240.
SEEBER, U. and KUSCHINSKY, K. (1976) Dopamine-sensitive adenylate cyclase in homogenates of rat striata during ethanol and barbiturate withdrawal. *Arch. Toxicol.* **35**: 247–253.
SEEMAN, P. (1974) The membrane expansion theory of anesthesia: Direct evidence using ethanol and a high precision density meter. *Experientia* **30**: 759–760.
SEEMAN, P. and ROTH, S. (1972) General anesthetics expand cell membranes at surgical concentrations. *Biochim. Biophys. Acta* **225**: 171–177.
SEGEL, L., RENDIG, S., SHOQUET, Y., CHACKO, K., AMSTERDAM, E. A. and MASON, D. T. (1975) Effects of chronic graded ethanol consumption on the metabolism, ultrastructure, and mechanical function of the rat heart. *Cardiovasc. Res.* **9**: 649–663.
SEGEL, L. D., RENDIG, S. V. and MASON, D. T. (1979) Left ventricular dysfunction of isolated working rat hearts after chronic alcohol consumption. *Cardiovasc. Res.* **13**: 136–146.
SEILICOVICH, A., DUVILANSKI, B., GONZALEZ, N. N., RETTORI, V., MITRIDATE DE NOVARA, A., MAINES, V. M. and FISZER DE PLAZAS, S. (1985) The effect of acute ethanol administration on GABA receptor binding in cerebellum and hypothalamus. *Eur. J. Pharmacol.* 111: 365–369.
SEIZINGER, B. R., BOVERMANN, K., HOLLT, V. and HERZ, A. (1984) Enhanced activity of the β-endorphinergic system in the anterior and neurointermediate lobe of the rat pituitary after chronic treatment with ethanol liquid diet. *J. Pharmacol. Exp. Ther.* **230**: 455–461.
SEIZINGER, B. R., BOVERMANN, K., MAYSINGA, D., HOHT, V. and HERZ, A. (1983) Differential effects of acute and chronic ethanol treatment on particular opioid peptide systems in discrete regions of rat brain and pituitary. *Pharmacol. Biochem. Behav.* **18**: (Suppl. 1), 361–369.
SELLERS, E. M., COOPER, S. D., ZILM, D. H. and SHANKS, C. (1976) Lithium treatment during alcohol withdrawal. *Clin. Pharmacol. Ther.* **20**: 199–212.
SELLERS, E. M., COOPER, S. D. and ROY, M. L. (1978) Variations in serum dopamine β-hydroxylase in normal subjects and chronic alcoholics. *Can. J. Physiol. Pharmacol.* **56**: 806–811.
SERENY, G. and ENDRENYI, L. (1978) Mechanism and significance of carbohydrate intolerance in chronic alcoholism. *Metabolism* **27**: 1041–1046.
SEWARD, J. (1970) Conditioning theory. In: *Learning Theories*, MARX, M. (ed.) Macmillan, New York.
SHAPIRO, A. and NATHAN, P. E. (1986) Human tolerance to alcohol: The role of Pavlovian conditioning processes. *Psychopharmacology* **88**: 90–95.
SHARMA, V. K. and BANERJEE, S. P. (1979) Effect of chronic ethanol treatment on specific [^{3}H]ouabain binding to (Na^++K^+)-ATPase in different areas of cat brain. *Eur. J. Pharmacol.* **56**: 297–304.
SHARMA, V. K., KLEE, W. A. and NIRENBERG, M. (1975) Dual regulation of adenylate cyclase accounts for narcotic dependence and tolerance. *Proc. Natl. Acad. Sci.* **72**: 3092–3096.
SHARMA, V. K., NAGARAJ, M. G. and BANERJEE, S. P. (1977) Effect of ethanol on [^{3}H]ouabain binding to different regions of the cat brain. *Brain Res.* **129**: 183–186.
SHAW, S., HELLER, E. A., FRIEDMAN, H. S., BARAONA, E. and LIEBER, C. S. (1977) Increased hepatic oxygenation following ethanol administration in the baboon. *Proc. Soc. Exp. Biol. Med.* **156**: 509–513.
SHEN, A., JACOBYANSKY, A., SMITH, T., PATHMAN, D. and THURMAN, R. G. (1977) Cyclic adenosine 3′,5′-monophosphate, adenylate cyclase and physical dependence on ethanol: studies with tranylcypromine. *Drug. Alc. Depend.* **2**: 431–440.
SHEN, A., JACOBYANSKY, A., PATHMAN, D. and THURMAN, R. G. (1983) Changes in brain cyclic AMP levels during chronic ethanol treatment and withdrawal in the rat. *Eur. J. Pharmacol.* **89**: 103–110.
SHIOHARA, E., TSUKADA, M., CHIBA, S., YAMAZAKI, H., NISCHIGUCHI, K., MIYAMOTO, R. and NAKANISHI, S. (1984) Effect of prolonged ethanol consumption of (Na^++K^+)-ATPase activity of rat brain membranes. *Jpn. J. Alcohol Drug Depend.* **19**: 302–308.
SIEGEL, S. (1978) A Pavlovian conditioning analysis of morphine. In: *Behavioral Tolerance; Research and Treatment Implications*, NIDA Research Monograph 18; pp. 27–53, KRASNEGOR, N. A. (ed.) U.S. Government Printing Office, Washington, D.C.
SIMLER, S., CLEMENT, J., CIESIELSKI, L. and MANDEL, P. (1986) Brain γ-aminobutyric acid turnover rates after spontaneous chronic ethanol intake and withdrawal in discrete brain areas of C57 mice. *J. Neurochem.* **47**: 1942–1947.
SIMPER, P., SAVARD, G., BAUCE, L. and COOPER, K. E. (1983) The effect of alcohol ingestion on body temperature following cross-country skiing. *Can. J. Physiol. Pharmacol.* **61**: A29–A30.
SIMPSON, L. (1980) Evidence that there are subcellular pools of norepinephrine and that there is flux of norepinephrine between these pools. *J. Pharmacol. Exp. Ther.* **214**: 410–416.
SMITH, A. A., GITLOW, S. B., GALL, E., WORTIS, S. B. and MENDLOWITZ, M. (1960) Effect of disulfiram and ethanol on the metabolism of dl-B-H^3-norepinephrine. *Clin. Res.* **8**: 367–376.
SMITH, B. R., ARAGON, C. M. G. and AMIT, Z. (1985) A time-dependent biphasic effect of an acute ethanol injection on 3-methoxy 4-hydroxyphenylethylene glycol sulfate in rat brain. *Biochem. Pharmacol.* **34**: 1311–1314.
SMITH, J. (1951) The effect of alcohol on the adrenal ascorbic acid and cholesterol of the rat. *J. Clin. Endocrinol.* **11**: 792.
SMITH, T. L. (1983) Influence of chronic ethanol consumption on muscarinic cholinergic receptors and their linkage to phospholipid metabolism in mouse synaptosomes. *Neuropharmacology* **22**: 661–663.
SMITH, T. L., JACOBYANSKY, A., SHEN, A., PATHMAN, D. and THURMAN, R. G. (1981) Adaptation of cyclic AMP

generating system in rat cerebral cortical slices during chronic ethanol treatment and withdrawal. *Neuropharmacology* **20**: 67–72.

Snoy, F. J., Harker, R. J., Thies, W. and Greenspan, K. (1980) Ethanol-induced electrophysiological alterations in canine cardiac purkinje fibers. *J. Stud. Alc.* **41**: 1023–1029.

Sokol, R. J., Miller, S. I., Debanne, S., Golden, N., Collins, G., Kaplan, J. and Martier, S. (1981) The Cleveland NIAAA prospective alcohol-in-pregnancy study. The first year. *Neurobehav. Tox. Terat.* **3**: 203–209.

Solarz, A. (1974) Medical conclusions from the clinical tests of drunken drivers with high blood alcohols. In: *Alcohol, Drugs and Traffic Safety*, pp. 391–393, Israelstam, S. and Lambert, S. (eds). Proceedings of the Sixth International Conference on Alcohol, Drugs and Traffic Safety, Toronto, September 8–13, 1974. Toronto, Addiction Research Foundation on Ontario.

Soliman, K. F. A. and Walker, C. A. (1979) Diurnal rhythm of ethanol metabolism in the rat. *Experientia.* **35**: 808–809.

Somer, J. B., Colley, P. W., Pirola, R. C. and Wilson, J. S. (1981) Ethanol-induced changes in cardiac lipid metabolism. *Alcoholism: Clin. Exp. Res.* **5**: 536–539.

Specht, S. C. (1984) Development and regional distribution of two molecular forms of the catalytic subunit of the Na,K-ATPase in rat brain. *Biochem. Biophys. Res. Commun.* **212**: 208–212.

Speisky, M. B. and Kalant, H. (1985) Site of interaction of serotonin and desglycinamide-arginine-vasopressin in maintenance of ethanol tolerance. *Brain Res.* **326**: 281–290.

Stein, J. W., Wayner, M. J. and Tilson, H. A. (1977) The effect of parachlorophenylalanine on the intake of ethanol and saccharin solutions. *Pharmacol. Biochem. Behav.* **6**: 117–122.

Stenstrom, S. and Richelson, E. (1982) Acute effect of ethanol on prostaglandin E_1-mediated cyclic. AMP formation by a murine neuroblastoma clone. *J. Pharmacol. Exp. Ther.* **221**: 334–341.

Stratton, R., Dormer, K. J. and Zeiner, A. R. (1981) The cardiovascular effects of ethanol and acetaldehyde in exercising dogs. *Alcoholism: Clin. Exp. Res.* **5**: 56–63.

Straus, B. and Berenyi, M. R. (1973) Infection and immunity in alcoholic cirrhosis. *Mt. Sinai J. Med.* **40**: 631–640.

Strong, R. and Wood, W. G. (1984) Membrane properties and aging: In vivo and in vitro effects of ethanol on synaptosomal γ-aminobutyric acid (GABA) release. *J. Pharmacol. Exp. Ther.* **229**: 726–730.

Sturtevant, R. P. and Garber, S. L. (1980) Light-dark and feeding regimens affect circadian phasing of blood-ethanol decay rates. *Pharmacol. Biochem. Behav.* **13**: 637–642.

Sullivan, J. L., Stanfield, C. N., Maltbie, A. A., Hammett, E. and Cavenar, J. (1978a) Stability of low blood platelet monoamine oxidase activity in human alcoholics. *Biol. Psychiat.* **13**: 391–397.

Sullivan, J. L., Stanfield, C. N., Schanberg, S. and Cavenar, J. (1978b) Platelet monoamine oxidase and serum dopamine-B-hydroxylase activity in chronic alcoholics. *Arch. Gen. Psychiat.* **35**: 1209–1212.

Sun, A. Y. (1974) Effect of phospholipases in the active uptake of norepinephrine by synaptosomes isolated from the cerebral cortex of guinea pig. *J. Neurochem.* **22**: 551–556.

Sun, A. Y. (1983) The kindling effect of ethanol on neuronal membranes. In: *Neural Membranes*, pp. 317–340, Sun, G. Y., Bazan, N., Wu, J.-Y., Porcellati, G. and Sun, A. Y. (eds) The Humana Press, Clifton, N.J.

Sun, A. Y. and Samorajski, T. (1970) Effects of ethanol on the activity of adenosine triphosphatase and acetylcholinesterase in synaptosomes isolated from guinea-pig brain. *J. Neurochem.* **17**: 1365–1372.

Sun, A. Y. and Samorajski, T. (1975) The effects of age and alcohol on (Na^++K^+)-ATPase activity of whole homogenate and synaptosomes prepared from mouse and human brain. *J. Neurochem.* **24**: 161–164.

Sun, A. Y. and Seaman, P. (1980) Physicochemical approaches to the alcohol-membrane interaction in brain. *Neurochem. Res.* **5**: 537–545.

Sunahara, G. I. and Kalant, H. (1980) Effect of ethanol on potassium-stimulated and electrically stimulated acetylcholine release in vitro from rat cortical slices. *Can. J. Physiol. Pharmacol.* **58**: 706–711.

Supavilai, P. and Karobath, M. (1980) Ethanol and other CNS depressants decrease GABA synthesis in mouse cerebral cortex and cerebellum *in vivo. Life Sci.* **27**: 1035–1040.

Sutker, P. B., Allain, A. N., Brantley, P. S. and Randall, C. L. (1982) Acute alcohol intoxication, negative affect, and autonomic arousal in women and men. *Addict. Behav.* **7**: 17–25.

Sutker, P. B., Goist, K. C. and King, A. (1987) Acute alcohol intoxication in women: Relationship to dose and menstrual cycle phase. *Alcoholism: Clin. Exp. Res.* **11**: 74–79.

Sutker, P. B., Goist, K. D., Allain, A. N. and Bugg, F. (1987) Acute alcohol intoxication: Sex comparisons on pharmacokinetic and mood measures. *Alcohol, Clin. Exp. Res.* **11**: 507–512.

Sutton, I. and Simmonds, M. A. (1973) Effects of acute and chronic ethanol on the γ-aminobutyric acid system in rat brain. *Biochem. Pharmacol.* **22**: 1685–1692.

Suzdak, P. D., Schwartz, R. D., Skolnick, P. and Paul, S. M. (1986) Ethanol stimulates γ-aminobutyric acid receptor-mediated chloride transport in rat brain synaptoneurosomes. *Proc. Natl. Acad. Sci. U.S.A.* **83**: 4071–4075.

Svensson, T. H. and Waldeck, B. (1973) Significance of acetaldehyde ethanol-induced effects on catecholamine metabolism and motor activity in the mouse. *Psychopharmacologia* **31**: 229–238.

Svenssen, T. H., Hartling, D. and Trap-Jensen, J. (1978) Effect of adrenergic beta receptor blockade on ethanol elimination and on ethanol-induced changes in carbohydrate and lipid metabolism in man. *Eur. J. Clin. Pharmacol.* **13**: 91–95.

Swann, A. C. (1983) Brain (Na^+,K^+)-ATPase. Opposite effects of ethanol and dimethyl sulfoxide on temperature dependence of enzyme conformation and univalent cation binding. *J. Biol. Chem.* **258**: 11780–11786.

Swann, A. C. (1984) Free fatty acids and (Na^+,K^+)-ATPase: Effects on cation binding, enzyme conformation, and interactions with ethanol. *Arch. Biochem. Biophys.* **233**: 354–361.

Swann, A. C. (1985) Chronic ethanol and (Na^+,K^+)-adenosine triphosphate: Apparent adaptation in cation binding and enzyme conformation. *J. Pharmacol. Exp. Ther.* **232**: 475–479.

Swann, A. C. (1986) Brain Na^+,K^+-ATPase: Alteration of ligand affinities and conformation by chronic ethanol and noradrenergic stimulation in vito. *J. Neurochem.* **47**: 707–714.

SWANN, A. C. and ALBERS, R. W. (1981) Temperature effects on cation affinities of the (Na^+,K^+)-ATPase of the mammalian brain. *Biochim. Biophys. Acta* **644**: 36–40.

SWARTZ, C. M. and DUNNER, F. J. (1982) Dexamethasone suppression testing of alcoholics. *Arch. Gen. Psychiat.* **39**: 1309–1312.

SWARTZ, M. H., REPKE, D. I., KATZ, A. M. and RUBIN, E. (1974) Effects of ethanol on calcium binding and calcium uptake by cardiac microsomes. *Biochem. Pharmacol.* **23**: 2369–2376.

SWEANDER, K. J. (1979) Two molecular forms of (Na^++K^+)-stimulated ATPase in brain. *J. Biol. Chem.* **254**: 6060–6067.

SYAPIN, P. J., STEFANOVIC, V., MANDEL, P. and NOBLE, E. P. (1976) The chronic and acute affects of ethanol on adenosine triphosphatase activity in cultured astroblast and neuroblastoma cells. *J. Neurosci. Res.* **2**: 147–155.

SYTINSKY, I. A., GUZIKOV, B. M., GOMANKO, M. V., EREMIN, V. P. and KONOVALOVA, N. N. (1975) The gamma-aminobutyric acid (GABA) system in brain during acute and chronic ethanol intoxication. *J. Neurochem.* **25**: 43–48.

SZE, P. Y. (1975) The permissive effect of glucocorticoids in the liver alcohol dehydrogenase by ethanol. *Biochem. Med.* **14**: 156–161.

SZE, P. Y. and NECKERS, L. (1974) Requirement for adrenal glucocorticoid in the ethanol-induced increase of tryptophan hydroxylase activity in mouse brain. *Brain Res.* **72**: 375–378.

TABAKOFF, B. (1974) Inhibition of sodium, potassium, and magnesium activated ATPases by acetaldehyde and "biogenic" aldehydes. *Res. Comm. Chem. Pathol. Pharmacol.* **7**: 621–624.

TABAKOFF, B. (1977) Neurochemical aspects of ethanol dependence. In: *Alcohol and Opiates: Neurochemical and Behavioral Mechanisms*, pp. 21–37, BLUM, K. (ed.) Academic Press, New York.

TABAKOFF, B. and BOGGAN, W. O. (1974) Effects of ethanol on serotonin metabolism in brain. *J. Neurochem.* **22**: 759–764.

TABAKOFF, B. and HOFFMAN, P. L. (1978) Alterations in receptors controlling dopamine synthesis after chronic ethanol ingestion. *J. Neurochem.* **31**: 1223–1229.

TABAKOFF, B. and HOFFMAN, P. L. (1979) Development of functional dependence on ethanol in dopaminergic systems. *J. Pharmacol. Exp. Ther.* **208**: 216–222.

TABAKOFF, B. and HOFFMAN, P. L. (1983a) Alcohol interactions with brain opiate receptors. *Life Sci.* **32**: 197–204.

TABAKOFF, B. and HOFFMAN, P. L. (1983b) Neurochemical aspects of tolerance to and physical dependence on alcohol. In: *The Biology of Alcoholism*, Vol. 7, p. 199–252, KISSIN, B. and BEGLEITER, H. (eds) Plenum Press, New York.

TABAKOFF, B. and KIIANMAA, K. (1982) Does tolerance develop to the activating, as well as to depressant effects of ethanol? *Pharmacol. Biochem. Behav.* **17**: 1073–1076.

TABAKOFF, B. and RITZMANN, R. F. (1977) The effects of 6-hydroxydopamine on tolerance to and dependence on ethanol. *J. Pharmacol. Exp. Ther.* **203**: 319–321.

TABAKOFF, B. and RITZMANN, R.F. (1979) Acute tolerance to inbred and selected lines of mice. *Drug Alc. Depend.* **4**: 87–90.

TABAKOFF, B., HOFFMAN, P. L. and MOSES, F. (1977) Neurochemical correlates of ethanol withdrawal: Alterations in serotoninergic function. *J. Pharm. Pharmacol.* **29**: 471–476.

TABAKOFF, B., JAFFE, R. C. and RITZMAN, R. F. (1978) Corticosterone concentrations in mice during ethanol drinking and withdrawal. *J. Pharm. Pharmacol.* **30**: 371–374.

TABAKOFF, B., MUNOZ-MARCUS, M. and FIELDS, J. Z. (1979) Chronic ethanol feeding produces an increase in muscarinic cholinergic receptors in mouse brain. *Life Sci.* **25**: 2173–2180.

TABAKOFF, B., RITZMAN, R. F. and BOGGAN, W. O. (1975) Inhibition of the transport of 5-hydroxyindoleacetic acid from brain by ethanol. *J. Neurochem.* **24**: 1043–1051.

TABAKOFF, B., RITZMANN, R. F., RAJU, T. S. and DEITRICH, R. A. (1980) Characterization of acute and chronic tolerance to mice selected for inherent differences in sensitivity to ethanol. *Alcoholism: Clin. Exp. Res.* **4**: 70–73.

TABAKOFF, B., URWYLER, S. and HOFFMAN, P. L. (1981) Ethanol alters kinetic characteristics and function of striatal morphine receptors. *J. Neurochem.* **37**: 518–521.

TAKAHASHI, S., TANI, N. and YAMANE, H. (1976) Monoamine oxidase activity in blood platelets in alcoholism. *Folia Psychiatrica et Neurologica Japonica* **30**: 455–462.

TEPLIN, L. A. and LUTZ, G. Q. (1985) Measuring alcohol intoxication: The development, reliability and validity of an observational instrument. *Q. J. Stud. Alc.* **46**: 459–466.

TERAVAINEN, H. and LARSEN, A. (1976) Effect of propranolol on acute withdrawal tremor in alcoholic patients. *J. Neurol. Neurosur. Psych.* **39**: 607–612.

THADANI, P., KULIG, B. M., BROWN, F. C. and BEARD, J. D. (1976) Acute and chronic ethanol-induced alterations in brain norepinephrine metabolites in the rat. *Biochem. Pharmacol.* **25**: 93–94.

THADANI, P. and TRUITT, E. B., JR. (1977) Effect of acute ethanol or acetaldehyde administration on the uptake, release, metabolism and turnover of norepinephrine in rat brain. *Biochem. Pharmacol.* **26**: 1147–1150.

THIEDEN, H. I. D. and LUNDQUIST, F. (1967) The influence of fructose and its metabolites on ethanol metabolism in vitro. *Biochem. J.* **102**: 177–180.

THOMAS, G., HAIDER, H., OLDEWURTEL, H. A., LYONE, M. M., YEH, C. K. and REGAN, T. J. (1980) Progression of myocardial abnormalities in experimental alcoholism. *Am. J. Cardiol.* **46**: 233–240.

THOMAS, H. M. and TREMOLIERES, J. (1968) Dose lethale 50 de l'ethanol; influence de la temperature, de la voie d'introduction et des regimes. *Rev. Alcoholisme.* **14**: 215–228.

THOMPSON, W. L., JOHNSON, A. D. and MADDREY, W. L. (1975) Diazepam and paraldehyde for treatment of severe delirium tremens: A controlled trial. *Ann. Intern. Med.* **82**: 175–180.

THURMAN, R. G., OSHINO, N. and CHANCE, B. (1977) The role of hydrogen peroxide production and catalase in hepatic ethanol metabolism. In: *Alcohol Intoxication and Withdrawal, Experimental Studies II*, pp. 163–183, GROSS, M. M. (ed.) Plenum Press, New York.

TICKU, M. K. (1980) The effects of acute and chronic ethanol administration and its withdrawal on γ-aminobutyric acid receptor binding in rat brain. *Br. J. Pharmacol.* **70**: 403–410.
TICKU, M. K. and BURCH, T. (1980) Alterations in γ-aminobutyric acid receptor sensitivity following acute and chronic ethanol treatments. *J. Neurochem.* **34**: 417–423.
TICKU, M. J. and DAVIS, W. C. (1981) Evidence that ethanol and pentobarbital enhance [^{3}H]-diazepam binding at the BDZ-GABA receptor-ionophore complex indirectly. *Eur. J. Pharmacol.* **71**: 521–522.
TICKU, M. K., LOWRIMORE, P. and LEHOULLIER, P. (1986) Ethanol enhances GABA-induced ^{36}Cl-influx in primary spinal cord cultured neurons. *Brain Res. Bull.* **17**: 123–126.
TIFFANY, S. T. and BAKER, T. B. (1986) Tolerance to alcohol: Psychological models and their application to alcoholism. *Ann. Behav. Med.* **8**: 7–12.
TOBON, F. and MEZEY, E. (1971) Effect of ethanol administration on hepatic ethanol and drug-metabolizing enzymes and on rates of ethanol degradation. *J. Lab. Clin. Med.* **77**: 110–121.
TRAN, V. T., SNYDER, S. H., MAJOR, L. F. and HAWLEY, R. J. (1981) GABA receptors are increased in brains of alcoholics. *Ann. Neurol.* **9**: 289–292.
TRELL, E., KRISTENSON, H. and PETERSON, B. (1981) Two hour glucose and insulin responses after a standardized oral glucose load in relation to serum gamma-glutamyl transferase and alcohol consumption. *Acta Diabetol. Lat.* **18**: 311–317.
TSUJI, M., IWASE, N., TAKAHASHI, S., FUJITA, T., SHIMOMURA, H. and WAKE, R. (1982) Measurement of platelet monoamine oxidase activity using three different substrates in chronic alcoholics. *Jpn. J. Alcohol Drug. Depend.* **17**: 87–100.
TSUKAMOTO, H., FRENCH, S., REIDELBERGER, R. and LARGMAN, C. (1985) Cyclical pattern of blood alcohol levels during continuous intragastric ethanol infusion in rats. *Alcoholism: Clin. Exp. Res.* **9**: 31–37.
TYCE, G. M., FLOCK, E. V. and OWEN, C. A. JR. (1968) 5-Hydroxytryptamine metabolism in brains of ethanol-intoxicated rats. *Mayo Clin. Proc.* **43**: 668–673.
TYCE, G. M., FLOCK, E. V., TAYLOR, W. F. and OWEN, C. A. JR (1970) Effect of ethanol on 5-hydroxytryptamine turnover in rat brain. *Proc. Soc. Exp. Biol. Med.* **134**: 40–44.
UMEZU, K., BUSTOS, G. and ROTH, R. H. (1980) Regional inhibitory effect of ethanol on monoamine synthesis regulation within the brain. *Biochem. Pharmacol.* **29**: 2477–2483.
UNWIN, J. W. and TABERNER, P. V. (1980) Sex and strain differences in GABA receptor binding after chronic ethanol drinking in mice. *Neuropharmacology* **19**: 1257–1259.
VALIMAKI, M., HARKONEN, M. and YLIKAHRI, R. (1983) Acute effects of alcohol on female sex hormones. *Alcoholism: Clin. Exp. Res.* **7**: 289–293.
VALIMAKI, M., PELKONEN, R., HARKONEN, M., *et al.* (1984) Hormonal changes in noncirrhotic male alcoholics during ethanol withdrawal. *Alc. Alcoholism* **19**: 235–242.
VAN THIEL, D. H. (1980) Alcohol and its effect on endocrine functioning. *Alcoholism: Clin. Exp. Res.* **4**: 44–49.
VAN THIEL, D. H. (1983) Adrenal response to stress: A stress response? In: *Stress and Alcohol Use*, pp. 23–28, POHORECKY, L. A. and BRICK, J. (eds) Elsevier Science, New York.
VAN THIEL, D. H. and LESTER, R. (1976) Alcoholism: Its effect on hypothalamic-pituitary-gonadal function. *Gastroenterology* **71**: 318–327.
VAN THIEL, D. H., GAVALER, J. S. and LESTER, R. (1977) Ethanol: A gonadal toxin in the female. *Drug Alc. Depend.* **2**: 373–380.
VAN THIEL, D. H., GAVALER, J. S., LESTER, R. and SHERINS, R. J. (1978) Alcohol induced ovarian failure in the rat. *J. Clin. Invest.* **61**: 624–632.
VAN THIEL, D. H., GAVALER, J. S., WIGHT, C., SMITH, W. I. and ABUID, J. (1978) Thyrotropin-releasing hormone (TRH)-induced growth hormone (hGH) responses in cirrhotic men. *Gastroenterology* **75**: 66–70.
VAN THIEL, D. H., GAVALER, J. S., COBB, C. F., SHERINS, R. J. and LESTER, R. (1979) Alcohol induced testicular atrophy in the adult male rat. *Endocrinology* **105**: 888–895.
VEALE, W. L. and MYERS, R. D. (1970) Decrease in ethanol intake in rats following administration of p-chlorophenylalanine. *Neuropharmacology* **9**: 317–326.
VICTOR, M. (1966) Treatment of alcoholic intoxication and the withdrawal syndrome; a critical analysis of the use of drugs and other forms of therapy. *Psychosom. Med.* **25**: 636–650.
VICTOR, M. and ADAMS, R. D. (1953) The effect of alcohol on the nervous system. *Research Publications—Association for Research in Nervous and Mental Disease* **32**: 526–573.
VIDELA, L., FLATTERY, K. V., SELLERS, E. A. and ISRAEL, Y. (1975) Ethanol metabolism and liver oxidative capacity in cold acclimation. *J. Pharmacol. Exp. Ther.* **192**: 575–582.
VOGEL-SPROTT, M. (1979) Acute recovery and tolerance to low doses of alcohol: Differences in cognitive and motor skill performance. *Psychopharmacology* **61**: 287–291.
VOGEL-SPROTT, M. and BARRETT, P. (1984) Age, drinking habits and the effects of alcohol. *J. Stud. Alc.* **45**: 517–521.
VOGEL-SPROTT, M., ROWANA, E. and WEBSTER, R. (1984) Mental rehearsal of a task under ethanol facilitates tolerance. *Pharmacol. Biochem. Behav.* **21**: 329–331.
VOLICER, L. (1980) GABA levels and receptor binding after acute and chronic ethanol administration. *Br. Res. Bull.* **5 (Suppl. 2)**: 809–813.
VOLICER, L. and BIAGIONI, T. M. (1982a) Effect of ethanol administration and withdrawal on benzodiazepine receptor binding in the rat brain. *Neuropharmacology* **21**: 283–286.
VOLICER, L. and BIAGIONI, T. M. (1982b) Presence of two benzodiazepine binding sites in the rat hippocampus. *J. Neurochem.* **38**: 591–593.
VOLICER, L. and GOLD, B. I. (1973) Effects of ethanol on cyclic AMP levels in the rat brain. *Life Sci.* **13**: 269–280.
VOLICER, L. and HURTER, B. P. (1977) Effects of acute and chronic ethanol administration and withdrawal on adenosine 3′,5′-monophosphate and guanosine 3′-5′-monophosphate levels in the rat brain. *J. Pharmacol. Exp. Ther.* **200**: 298–305.
VOLICER, L., HURTER, B. P., WILLIAMS, R. and PURI, S. K. (1976) Effects of acute and chronic ethanol admin-

istration and ethanol withdrawal on guanosine 3′,5′-monophosphate and gamma-aminobutyric acid levels in rat brain. *Fed. Proc.* **35**: 467.

VOLICER, L., MIRIN, R. and GOLD, B. I. (1977a) Effect of ethanol on the cyclic AMP system in rat brain. *J. Stud. Alc.* **38**: 11–24.

VOLICER, L., PURI, S. K. and HURTER, B. P. (1977b) Role of cyclic nucleotides in drug addiction and withdrawal. In: *Clinical Aspects of Cyclic Nucleotides*, pp. 361–371, VOLICER, L. (ed.) Spectrum Publications, Inc.

VON WARTHBURG, J. P. (1982) Polymorphism of human alcohol and aldehyde dehydrogenase. In: *Recent Advances in the Biology of Alcoholism*, LIEBER, C. S. and STIMMEL, B. (eds) Haworth Press, New York.

VUORIEN, I., HEINONEN, J. and ROSENBERG, P. (1976) The effect of ethanol on the duration of toxic action of lidocaine: An experimental study on rats and mice. *Acta Pharmacol. Toxicol.* **38**: 31–37.

WAGNER, J. G., WILKINSON, P. K., SEDMAN, A. J., KAY, D. R. and WEIDLER, D. J. (1976) Elimination of alcohol from human blood. *J. Pharmac. Sci.* **65**: 152–154.

WAJDA, I. J., MANIGUALT, I. and HUDICK, J. P. (1977) Dopamine levels in the striatum and the effect of alcohol and reserpine. *Biochem. Pharmacol.* **26**: 653–655.

WALLACE, R. B., LYNCH, C. F., POMREHN, P. R., CRIQUI, M. H. and HEISS, G. (1981) Alcohol and hypertension: Epidemiologic and experimental considerations. The lipid research clinics program. *Circulation* **64 (Suppl. III)**: 31–41.

WALLER, M. B., MCBRIDE, W. J., LUMENG, L. and LI, T.-K. (1982a) Induction of dependence on ethanol by free-choice drinking in alcohol-preferring rats. *Pharmacol. Biochem. Behav.* **16**: 501–507.

WALLER, M. B., MCBRIDE, W. J., LUMENG, L. and LI, T.-K. (1982b) Effects of intravenous ethanol and of 4-methylpyrazole on alcohol drinking in alcohol-preferring rats. *Pharmacol. Biochem. Behav.* **17**: 763–768.

WALLER, M. B., MCBRIDE, W. J., GATTO, G. J., LUMENG, L. and LI, T.-K. (1984) Intragastric self-infusion of ethanol by ethanol-preferring and -nonpreferring lines of rats. *Science* **225**: 78–80.

WALLGREN, H. and LINDBOHM, R. (1961) Adaptation to ethanol in rats with special reference to brain tissue respiration. *Biochem. Pharmacol.* **8**: 423–424.

WALLGREN, H., KOSUNEN, A.-L. and AHTEE, L. (1973) Technique for producing an alcohol withdrawal syndrome in rats. *Israel J. Med. Sci.* **9**: 63–71.

WALLGREN, H., NIKANDER, P. and VIRTANEN, P. (1975) Ethanol-induced changes in cation-stimulated adenosine triphosphatase activity and lipid-proteolipid labeling of brain microsomes. In: *Alcohol Intoxication and Withdrawal Adv. Exp. Med. Biol.* **59**: 23–36; GROSS, M. M. (ed.) Plenum Press, New York.

WALSHE, W. H. (1873) *Diseases of the Heart and Great Vessels*, Smith Elder, London.

WALTERS, J. K. (1977) Effects of PCPA on the consumption of alcohol, water and other solutions. *Pharmacol. Biochem. Behav.* **6**: 377–383.

WATSON, P. E., WATSON, I. D. and BUTT, R. D. (1981) Prediction of blood alcohol concentrations in human subjects: Updating the Widmark equation. *J. Stud. Alc.* **42**: 547–556.

WEBB, W. R., GUPTA, D N., COOK, W. A., SUGG, W. L., BASHOUR, F. A. and UNAL, M. O. (1967) Effects of alcohol on myocardial contractility. *Dis. Chest* **52**: 602.

WEINER, H., MYERS, R. D., SIMPSON, C. W. and THURMAN, J. A. (1980) The effect of alcohol on dopamine metabolism in the caudate nucleus of an unanesthetized monkey. *Alcoholism: Clin. Exp. Res.* **4**: 427–429.

WEISHAAR, R., BERTUGGLIA, S., ASHIKAWA, K., SARMA, J. S. M. and BING, R. J. (1978) Comparative effects of chronic ethanol and acetaldehyde exposure on myocardial function in rats. *J. Clin. Pharm.* **18**: 377–387.

WEITBRECHT, W.-U. and CRAMER, H. (1980) Depression of cyclic AMP and cyclic GMP in the cerebrospinal fluid of rats after acute administration of ethanol. *Brain Res.* **200**: 478–480.

WELTE, J. W. and GREIZERSTEIN, H. B. (1984) Alcohol consumption and systolic blood pressure in the general population. *Subst. Alc. Actions/Misuse* **5**: 299–306.

WENGER, J. R., TIFFANY, S. T., BOMADIER, C., NICHOLLS, K. and WOODS, S. C. (1981) Ethanol tolerance in the rat is learned. *Science* **213**: 575–577.

WHITMAN, V., SCHULER, H. G. and MUSSELMAN, J. (1980) Effects of chronic ethanol consumption on the myocardial hypertrophic response to a pressure overload in the rat. *J. Molec. Cell. Cardiol.* **12**: 519–525.

WIBERG, A., WAHLSTROM, G. and ORELAND, L. (1977) Brain monoamine oxidase activity after chronic ethanol treatment of rats. *Psychopharmacology* **52**: 111–113.

WIDMARK, E. (1932) *Die theoretischen Grundlagen und die praktische Verwendbarkeit der gerichtlich—medizinischen Alkoholbestimmung*. Urban and Schwarzenberg, Berlin.

WILKINS, J. N., CARLSON, H. E., VAN VUNAKIS, H. *et al.* (1982) Nicotine from cigarette smoking increases circulating levels of cortisol, growth hormone and prolactin in male chronic smokers. *Psychopharmacology* **78**: 305–308.

WILKINSON, C. W., CRABBE, J. C., KEITH, L. D., KENDALL, J. W. and DORSA, D. M. (1986) Influence of ethanol dependence on regional brain content of B-endorphin in the mouse. *Brain Res.* **378**: 107–114.

WILLENBRING, M. L., MORLEY, J. E., NIEWOEHNER, C. B. *et al.* (1984) Adrenocortical hyperactivity in newly admitted alcoholics: Prevalence, course and associated variables. *Psychoneuroendocrinology* **9**: 415–422.

WILLIAMS, E. S. and LI, T. K. (1977) The effect of chronic alcohol administration on fatty acid metabolism and pyruvate oxidation of heart mitochondria. *J. Molec. Cell Cardiol.* **12**: 1003–1011.

WILSON, G. T. (1987) Alcohol use and abuse: A social learning analysis. In: *Theories of Alcoholism*, CHAUDRON, C. D. and WILKINSON, D. A. (eds) Toronto Addiction Research Foundation (in press).

WILSON, R. H. L., NEWMAN, E. J. and NEWMAN, H. S. (1956) Diurnal variation in rate of alcohol metabolism. *J. App. Physiol.* **8**: 556–558.

WIMBISH, G. H., MARTZ, R. and FORNEY, R. B. (1977) Combined effects of ethanol and propranolol on sleep time in the mouse. *Life Sci.* **20**: 65–72.

WIXON, H. N. and HUNT, W. A. (1980) Effect of acute and chronic ethanol treatment on gamma-aminobutyric acid levels and on aminooxyacetic acid-induced GABA accumulation. *Subst. Alc. Actions/Misuse* **1**: 481–491.

WONG, M. (1973) Depression of cardiac performance by ethanol unmasked during autonomic blockade. *Am. Heart J.* **86**: 508–515.

WOOD, J. M. and LAVERTY, R. (1977) Effect of brain catecholamine depletion on the development of ethanol tolerance and dependence in the rat. *Proc. Univ. Otago Med. Sch.* **55**: 57–59.

WOOD, W., ARMBRECHT, H. and WISE, R. (1982) Ethanol intoxication and withdrawal among three age groups of C57Bl/6NNIA mice. *Pharmacol. Biochem. Behav.* **17**: 1037–1041.

YAMAMOTO, H. and HARRIS, R. A. (1983) Effects of ethanol and barbiturates on Ca^{2+}-ATPase activity of erythrocyte and brain membranes. *Biochem. Pharmacol.* **32**: 2787–2791.

YAMAMOTO, H., SUTOO, D. and MISAWA, S. (1981) Effect of cadmium on ethanol induced sleeping time in mice. *Life Sci.* **28**: 2917–2923.

YAMANAKA, Y. and KONO, S. (1974) Brain serotonin turnover in alcoholic mice. *Jpn. J. Pharmacol.* **24**: 247–252.

YAMAWAKI, S., LAI, H. and HORITA, A. (1984) Effects of dopaminergic and serotonergic drugs on ethanol-induced hypothermia. *Life Sci.* **34**: 467–474.

YESAVAGE, J. A. and LEIRER, V. O. (1986) Hangover effects on aircraft pilots 14 hours after alcohol ingestion: A preliminary report. *Am. J. Psychiat.* **143**: 1546–1550.

YLIKAHRI, R. H., HUTTUNEN, M. O. and HARKONEN, M. (1976) Effect of alcohol on anterior-pituitary secretion of trophic hormones. *Lancet* **1**: 1353.

YLIKAHRI, R. H., HUTTUNEN, M. O. and HARKONEN, M. (1980) Hormonal changes during alcohol intoxication and withdrawal. *Pharmacol. Biochem. Behav.* **13**: 131–137.

YORK, J. L. (1982) The influence of age upon the physiological response to ethanol. In: *Alcoholism and Aging: Advances in Research*, pp. 99–113, WOOD, W. G. and ELIAS, M. F. (eds) CRC Press, Boca Raton, Florida.

YORK, J. L. (1983) Increased responsiveness to ethanol with advancing age in rats. *Pharmacol. Biochem. Behav.* **19**: 687–691.

YOSHIDA, K., ENGEL, J. and LILJEQUIST, S. (1982) The effect of chronic ethanol administration on high affinity ^{3}H-nicotinic binding in rat brain. *N.-S. Arch. Pharmacol.* **321**: 74–76.

YOSHIMURA, K. (1973) Activation of Na-K activated ATPase in rat brain by catecholamine. *J. Biochem.* **74**: 389–391.

ZABIK, J. E., LIAO, S.-S., JEFFREYS, M. and MAICKEL, R. P. (1978) The effects of DL-5-hydroxytryptophan on ethanol consumption by rats. *Res. Commun. Chem. Pathol.* **20**: 69–78.

ZACCHIA, C., PIHL, R. O., YOUNG, S. and ERVIN, F. (1986) Sugar reduces impairment without altering blood alcohol levels in males. Paper presented at 94th Annual Convention of American Psychological Association, Washington, D.C.

ZARCONE, V., BARCHAS, J., HODDES, E., MONTPLAISIR, J., SACK, R. and WILSON, R. (1975) Experimental ethanol ingestion: Sleep variables and metabolites of dopamine and serotonin in the cerebrospinal fluid. In: *Alcohol Intoxication and Withdrawal. Experimental Studies II*, pp. 431–452, GROSS, M. M. (ed.) Plenum Press, New York.

ZEINER, A. R. and FERRIS, J. J. (1978) Male-female and birth control pill effects on ethanol pharmacokinetics in American Indians. *Alcoholism: Clin. Exp. Res.* **2**: 179–183.

ZEINER, A. R. and KEGG, P. S. (1980) Menstrual cycle and oral contraceptive effects on alcohol pharmacokinetics in caucasian females. *Alcoholism: Clin. Exp. Res.* **4**: 233–237.

ZILM, D. H. (1981) Ethanol-induced spontaneous and evoked EEG, heart rate and respiration rate changes in man. *Clin. Toxicol., N.Y.* **18**: 549–563.

ZILM, D. H., KAPLAN, H. L. and CAPPELL, H. (1981) Electroencephalographic tolerance and abstinence phenomena during repeated alcohol ingestion by non-alcoholics. *Science* **212**: 1175–1177.

ZUSMAN, M. E. and HUBER, J. D. (1979) Multiple measures and the validity of response in research on drinking drivers. *J. Saf. Res.* **11**: 132–137.

ZYSSET, T., SUTHERLAND, E. and SIMON, F. R. (1983) Studies on the differences in Na-K ATPase and lipid properties of liver plasma membranes in long sleep and short sleep mice. *Alcoholism: Clin. Exp. Res.* **7**: 85–92.

CHAPTER 9

TREATMENT OF ALCOHOL PROBLEMS: WITH SPECIAL REFERENCE TO THE BEHAVIORAL APPROACH

NICK HEATHER
National Drug and Alcohol Research Centre, University of New South Wales, Australia

1. INTRODUCTION

This is not intended as an exhaustive review of the results of treatment for alcohol problems. The astronomical number of outcome studies of treatment now available in the literature makes this an almost impossible task and, in any event, it is far from clear what value there is in such an exercise. Nor is the aim to list all the various methods which are commonly used in treatment in order to make a detailed estimate of the effectiveness of each, since this information is already available (Miller and Hester, 1980, 1986a). Only a brief summary of major treatment categories will be provided, before devoting more attention to the development and application of behavioral treatment methods. It is also intended to describe the general developments in treatment philosophies and methods over the last twenty years or so, to isolate the more important areas of disagreement between alcohol treatment specialists, and to attempt very speculatively a projection of a few current themes into the future.

1.1. CHANGES IN THE SCIENTIFIC BASIS OF TREATMENT

The last 20 years have seen fundamental and dramatic changes in the scientific basis for the treatment of alcohol problems. This has partly been caused by the more systematic use of the scientific method to examine previously unchallenged assumptions about what was effective. As a consequence, several comfortable dogmas have been shattered. Another factor has been the growing influence of professions other than medicine: psychologists have developed theories and methods which are often directly at odds with the thinking behind conventional, medically-based treatments and sociologists have widened the discussion of the overall response to alcohol problems away from a narrow concentration on the clinic. Some of the controversies in the alcohol field, particularly that involving the possibility of controlled drinking by persons previously dependent on alcohol, have been accompanied by considerable acrimony. Moreover, progress in the scientific understanding of alcohol problems and their treatment has not been accompanied by a concomitant improvement in treatment practice, as we shall discover.

Underlying these changes there has been a radical transformation in the theoretical understanding of alcohol dependence and its associated problems. Having been launched in the 1930s in the United States and promoted chiefly by the Fellowship of Alcoholics Anonymous and its sympathizers, the 'disease concept' of alcoholism appears to have acquired a growing acceptance among the general public ever since. Paradoxically, however, it has at the same time become increasingly unpopular with researchers, academics and many treatment specialists alike owing to a growing body of evidence which is simply incompatible with its major tenets (see, e.g. Heather and Robertson, 1986). These inadequacies of the disease theory have been enthusiastically greeted by psychologists and sociologists, but many psychiatrists would also now accept that to regard alcohol problems as diseases is unhelpful.

1.2. Definitions of Alcohol Problems

It is against this background that a discussion of the treatment of alcohol problems must proceed. Indeed, the very term 'alcohol problems' has some theoretical significance, since it implies an abandonment of the older term 'alcoholism'. The evidence suggests that there is no convenient cut-off point, either in terms of severity of problems caused by alcohol or degree of alcohol dependence, which justifies the postulation of a discrete and qualitatively distinct group of drinkers who may be termed 'alcoholics'. Other more neutral and more encompassing terms, such as 'problem drinking' and 'problem drinkers' are now often preferred (Heather and Robertson, 1986).

In this article, the term 'alcohol problems' will be used to describe any disabilities—physical, psychological or social—which are related to the consumption of ethyl alcohol, including the particular disability of dependence on the drug. Anyone suffering from such problems will be referred to generically as a 'problem drinker'. Where necessary, distinctions will be made with respect to levels of severity of problems or dependence and to specific types of problem. The older terms, 'alcoholism' and 'alcoholics', will be retained for convenience where they were used in the original publications referred to or where they are demanded by the particular context of the discussion.

1.3. Definitions of Treatment

In the light of the demise of the disease view of alcohol problems, it is ironical that the term 'treatment' continues to be used in discussions of attempts to ameliorate such problems. Thorley (1983) has argued that, as it is usually understood, treatment implies an activity characterized by an individual focus and by the use of specific modalities of intervention aimed at identified symptoms or problems; it is perceived as being directed towards largely passive recipients and is normally short-term in nature. For the alcohol problems field, Thorley prefers to think in terms of 'rehabilitation', since it contains the implication of "a much more active and extended process, with the patient or client being encouraged to shed the passivity of the sick role and to take responsibility himself for his improved functioning" (p. 86). This is a well-made point and a useful distinction. Nevertheless, in this article, for the sake of convenience, treatment will be taken to mean any direct attempt to improve the quality of the lives of problem drinkers by any group of helping agents, using any kind of approach. Thus 'counselling', which normally refers to the helping responses of paraprofessional workers using less intrusive methods of intervention, is included in the remit of this article.

The only related activity which is specifically excluded is 'detoxification'—the removal of the short-term, toxic effects of alcohol consumption—which will not be covered in any detail here. All that will be said on this subject is that detoxification is now a relatively straightforward procedure, that for the majority of those dependent on alcohol, inpatient detoxification is unnecessary (Rada and Kellner, 1979) and that detoxification, in hospital or elsewhere, without continuing attempts at rehabilitation is virtually useless (Thorley, 1980).

1.4. Types of Alcohol Problem

Another disadvantage of the term 'treatment' is that it is often taken to mean the treatment of specifically alcohol dependence. Thorley (1980) has suggested that there are basically three types of problem caused by alcohol which deserve the attention of helping agents. These are problems caused (i) by regular excessive consumption, (ii) by intoxication and (iii) by alcohol dependence. The first involves mainly health and financial problems, although legal and employment difficulties may also emerge; the second results in problems for public order, such as accidents and personal violence, although there are health, social, legal and employment implications too; the third type, problems of dependence as such, will normally involve the medical complications of withdrawal, with associated psychological problems and subjective distress, but problems in the social and other spheres need not necessarily be present. Each type of problem is logically and empirically independent of the others, although in many cases more than one type may be present, and in the stereotypical 'alcoholic' all three may simultaneously occur. This is illustrated in Fig. 1. The thinking underlying Thorley's 'three balls' model of alcohol problems, which reflects a desire to move away from a narrow and exclusive preoccupation with alcohol dependence in treatment and a shift to a more 'problem-oriented' approach, has gained wide acceptance among workers in the field.

2. THE DEVELOPMENT OF TREATMENT SERVICES IN BRITAIN

In a general sense, the activities of the many mutual-aid societies for habitual drunkards which existed in Victorian Britain and were part of the Temperance Movement can be seen as the first attempts to treat problem drinkers in this country. Towards the end of the 19th Century, too, there emerged a network of 'inebriate asylums' in which the treatment effort became more formalized. However, owing to a change in temperance concerns away from individual drunkards and also to the considerable reduction in alcohol consumption in Britain following World War I, interest in the treatment of problem drinkers was virtually extinguished during the earlier part of the 20th Century. Indeed, when in 1951 a consultant psychiatrist applied for funds to attend a WHO conference on alcoholism, this was rejected on the ground that "there was no alcoholism in England or Wales" (Orford and Edwards, 1977, p. 6)! Medical and scholarly involvement in the treatment of alcoholism was almost entirely due to energetic stimulation from Alcoholics Anonymous (AA) which reached the U.K. in 1948.

2.1. Modern Developments

The modern evolution of services in Britain began with the establishment of a specialized, self-contained, inpatient unit at Warlingham Park Hospital near London by Dr. Max Glatt in the early 1950s. This has subsequently served as the model for many Alcoholism Treatment Units (ATUs) under the control of psychiatrists throughout the country. A memorandum issued by the Ministry of Health in 1962 recommended the setting-up of at least one ATU in every region of Britain and there are now over 30 such units in existence.

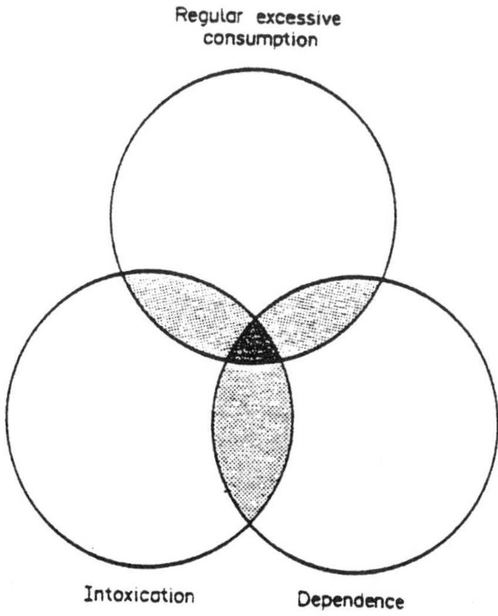

Fig. 1. Three aspects of alcohol consumption which can cause problems. (Adapted from Thorley, 1980, p. 1817.)

Although the character of ATUs varies to some extent, they are mainly associated with a strong emphasis on group therapy, close links with AA and a commitment to total abstinence as the goal of treatment for all alcoholics.

Orford and Edwards (1977) have commented that this formula for the treatment of alcoholics was applied before any good evidence was available for its effectiveness. Moreover, it ran counter to the shift towards out-patient and community involvement which occurred in the mainstream of psychiatric treatment. In 1973, however, the Department of Health and Social Security (DHSS) produced a circular entitled *Community Services for Alcoholics* and this was followed by an expansion in the number of community-based hostels, intended primarily for homeless alcoholics. More recently, some hostels have catered to a wider client group and included individuals who are not necessarily 'down-and-out' but who may need special accommodation for rehabilitation to take place. At the same time, there has been an increasing tendency for ATUs to offer outpatient and day clinic facilities as well as inpatient treatment.

Another important development during the 1970s was the steady expansion of local Councils on Alcoholism around the country. These are nonstatutory, voluntary organizations funded mainly from local sources. Initially, they were usually staffed by 'recovering alcoholics' and counselling was carried out by volunteers along AA lines. Over the last 10 years, however, local councils have changed considerably in staffing and outlook; the director is now usually someone with a professional background who has never had a personal drinking problem; the types of counselling methods used are much more flexible and may include behavioral methods (see below) and a controlled drinking goal; and more attention is paid to preventative and educational work. Significantly, many have changed their names from Councils on Alcoholism to Councils on Alcohol. They are to be found in nearly all areas of Britain and represent an important arm of the nation's overall treatment response.

2.2. Community Alcohol Teams

The latest major development was stimulated by a report of the DHSS Advisory Committee on Alcoholism in 1978, entitled *The Pattern and Range of Services for Problem Drinkers* (Department of Health and Social Security, 1978). The report recommended a downgrading of specialist treatment in ATUs and a greater emphasis on services provided by 'front-line' professionals, like general practitioners, social workers and community nurses. In the same year, an influential book entitled *Responding to Drinking Problems* (Shaw, *et al.*, 1978) described the development and evaluation of a Community Alcohol Team (CAT) in the London borough of Camberwell and this has been followed by the setting-up of a number of CATs in other parts of the country. Although concepts of what is meant by a CAT have varied (see Stockwell and Clement, 1987), they are characterized principally by three elements: (1) the integration of previously disparate services, such as psychiatric treatment, local voluntary councils, and hostel accommodation; (2) a multidisciplinary approach which includes psychiatrists, nurses, clinical psychologists and social workers; and (3) the provision of training and support for professional groups in direct contact with problem drinkers. As well as treatment for severe problems, there is an emphasis on early intervention and secondary prevention using some of the methods which will be described later (see pp. 305–307).

2.3. Summary

Summing up the changes which have occurred in treatment services since the 1950s, we may say that there has been a process of 'demedicalization'. In accordance with the view that problem drinking cannot profitably be described as a disease, its treatment is no longer seen as lying exclusively within the special expertise of psychiatrists, although psychiatrists continue, of course, to have a most important role. Today, much of the treatment, counselling, rehabilitation, or whatever term is preferred, of problem drinkers is carried out by people with no medical training, using methods derived from other sources than medical science. Paradoxically, there has recently been a greater willingness to become involved with the response to problem drinking on the part of branches of medicine besides psychiatry, as witnessed by the publication of two reports by the Royal College of General Practitioners (1986) and the Royal College of Physicians (1987).

3. DOES TREATMENT FOR ALCOHOL PROBLEMS WORK?

The very fact that this question has been seriously addressed over the last 10 to 15 years gives some indication of the state of uncertainty existing in the field of alcohol treatment. Although there is a great deal of evidence which is relevant to this issue, two studies published during the 1970s were mainly responsible for undermining the assumption, rarely questioned till then, that offering treatment to those suffering from alcohol problems was to improve their chances of recovery.

The first study was that of Emrick (1975) who reviewed a total of 384 reports of outcome of psychologically oriented treatment for alcohol problems published between 1952 and 1973. Emrick's first conclusion from this herculean effort reinforced a rough and ready estimate of treatment effectiveness widely held by workers in the field and known as 'the rule of the thirds'; about one third of treated clients were abstinent at follow-up, another third were still drinking but had improved in varying degrees, while the remaining third were unimproved or worse than before treatment. It should be noted, however, that these estimates were derived mainly from studies using only relatively short-term follow-up (3 or 6 months); when follow-up is extended for longer periods, the proportion of successful outcomes drops considerably. For example, in a very large study of outcome from many different centers, Polich *et al.* (1980) found that only 7% of clients had been consistently abstinent during a 4-year period following treatment. Apart from this difficulty, it might also be claimed that the very attempt to arrive at an average success rate for alcohol treatment is misguided, since client populations and the type and quality of treatment offered vary widely.

Emrick also attempted to answer the question, whether any particular form of treatment was superior to others, by confining attention to 72 studies with randomly assigned or adequately matched treatment groups and follow-up extended to 6 months or longer. The conclusion was that differences in treatment methods did not significantly affect long-term outcome, and this too became part of recent folklore of alcohol treatment: irrespective of the type of treatment method used, results are about the same. Finally, Emrick looked at studies comparing treatment with no treatment or, at least, only minimal treatment contact. He found no evidence that treatment improved abstinence rates and it was this conclusion that contributed strongly to skepticism over the real effectiveness of treatment. However, Emrick also noted that more treated than untreated clients showed some improvement in their drinking problems, suggesting that formal treatment does at least increase the probability of some amelioration in the adverse consequences of drinking. Unfortunately, even this conclusion is made suspect by the possible existence of selective client characteristics which may have biassed the comparison between formally and minimally treated groups.

The second influential study was Orford and Edwards' (1977) controlled comparison of treatment and advice among 100 married, male alcoholics seen at the Maudsley Hospital, London. Following a comprehensive 3 hr assessment, clients were randomly assigned either to a group which received a single counselling session together with their wives and were then told, in constructive and sympathetic terms, that the responsibility for solving their problem lay in their own hands or to a group which received a mixture of outpatient and inpatient, psychiatric and social work care representing the standard package of help available at any well-supported treatment center. At follow-up 12 months after initial assessment, there was no evidence of any significant differences between these groups in drinking behavior, alcohol-related problems, social adjustment or any other outcome measure. Once more, these results induced a widespread feeling of pessimism about alcoholism treatment, despite the author's own warnings against a nihilistic interpretation of their results. However, as in the case of Emrick's review, a closer inspection of the data revealed grounds for more confidence in the effects of conventional treatment. Thus, a 2-year follow-up of the same cohort suggested that those with more severe levels of alcohol dependence were more likely to attain the stated goal of abstinence if they had received treatment than if they had received advice (Orford *et al.*, 1976). Moreover, it is often pointed out that the married and socially stable alcoholics without psychiatric disturbance studied by Orford and Edwards had a generally good prognosis and may therefore have been more likely to benefit from the brief intervention than unmarried or less socially stable individuals frequently seen in treatment (Kissin, 1977).

It will be convenient to mention here a recently completed study by Chick *et al.* (1988) based on Orford and Edwards' design but with a few important modifications. One hundred and fifty-two attenders at an alcohol problems clinic in Edinburgh were randomly assigned to receive extended inpatient or outpatient treatment typical of that offered in British treatment centers or alternatively one session of advice. The advice group was itself randomly divided into subgroups receiving very brief advice or a more comprehensive advice session lasting an hour. Unlike Orford and Edwards' sample, this included women and unmarried patients. The results showed that, at 2-year follow-up, there was no difference between extended treatment and advice groups in abstinence rates or in terms of employment or intact marriages. However, the extended group showed evidence of less alcohol-related damage since intake. There was no difference in outcome between the very brief and the comprehensive advice groups. This study thus supported Emrick's (1975) suggestion that, compared with brief intervention, extended treatment does not affect the likelihood of successful abstinence but may reduce the amount of harm caused by drinking.

3.1. Spontaneous Remission

As might be expected, the effectiveness of treatment for alcohol problems has been judged in relation to evidence on 'spontaneous remission' among untreated samples of problem drinkers. This is a difficult area of research, partly because of uncertainties in defining what is to count as remission and partly because there are obvious grounds for believing that problem drinkers who do not seek treatment, or who drop out right at the beginning, differ in important ways from those who complete treatment. As with a standard figure for average outcome rates, a standard rate of spontaneous remission is elusive and may even be a meaningless statistic. Nevertheless, Roizen *et al.* (1978) have shown that, depending on the criterion used, remission rates could be made to vary between 11% and 71%. Another difficulty is differences between studies in the time period during which evidence of naturally-occurring recovery is looked for. In two long-term follow-ups of 15 years each, Ojesjo (1981) in Sweden found a spontaneous abstinence rate of 30% and Vaillant (1983) in the USA found a rate of 35%, rates which are clearly similar to the averaged abstinence rates derived from Emrick's review of treatment (see above). Indeed, in Vaillant's study, which allowed a direct comparison with the effects of treatment, the author concluded that they were no better than the natural history of the disease. Another estimate from a review of the literature (Roizen *et al.*, 1978) suggests an abstinence rate of 15%, with a much higher rate of general improvement of about 40%.

What is clear from longitudinal household surveys (Clark and Cahalan, 1975) is that 'alcoholism' is not the progressive and fairly inexorable condition it was thought of as being in the disease perspective and that changes in remission category, both into and out of problem status, commonly occur in the natural environment. It is also clear that, in evaluating the impact of treatment, this must be judged against a rate of natural recovery which is variably estimated but relatively high.

3.2. Client Characteristics

Other, more indirect lines of evidence have also cast doubt on the importance of treatment in the recovery process. First, there is the possibility that the main determinants of outcome following treatment are not characteristics of the treatment regime itself but, rather, characteristics of the clients entering treatment. Thus, in a 'meta-analysis' of 58 studies of treatment outcome, Costello (1975a,b) found that the main predictor of how effective a particular program was likely to be was its selection policy; programs which selected out unpromising candidates, such as vagrants, transients or those with serious mental or physical illness, produced the best results, whereas programs which admitted 'all-comers' gave the poorest. In a subsequent analysis, Costello (1980) showed that the major determinant of outcome variance was client social stability, defined in this case as simply whether or not the client was married and/or in employment.

In his review of treatment methods for chronic alcoholism, Baekeland (1977) was also impressed by the dominant role played by client rather than treatment factors, both in persistence in treatment and eventual outcome. Higher socio-economic status and higher social stability were the main variables associated with good prognosis. No differences were found in the effectiveness of different treatment regimes.

3.3. Post-Treatment Factors

Secondly, Moos and his colleagues from Stanford University have conducted an extensive research program in which the contributions to recovery of treatment factors and external, psychosocial factors have been compared (Cronkite and Moos, 1978, 1980). For example, Billings and Moos (1983) found that, compared with clients who had relapsed after treatment, those with successful outcome showed significantly higher levels of family cohesiveness, more effective coping skills for dealing with personal problems and had experienced fewer stressful life events in the period following treatment. The general tendency of these findings is to place more emphasis on the importance of post-treatment factors in the recovery process and less on treatment or pre-treatment characteristics.

The same kind of picture emerges when clients are actually asked what they regard as the most telling contributions to their recovery. For example, Orford and Edwards (1977), in the Maudsley study described above, found that the four items rated highest by their clients at follow-up did not include inpatient or outpatient care, AA or any other helping agency. Rather, it was changes in external reality (e.g., work or housing), intrapsychic changes (e.g., mood or self-appraisal) and improvements in the marital relationship which were rated most highly. The only aspect of treatment or advice to receive a high rating was the intake interview. Interestingly, this evidence fits well with data collected from those who have achieved spontaneous recovery (Saunders and Kershaw, 1979; Tuchfeld, 1976); events like changing jobs, getting married or forming new relationships, changing house to a different environment and other broad changes in life circumstances are repeatedly mentioned as the main reasons for recovery. Taken together, all this evidence suggests that, compared with the normal vicissitudes of human life, treatment as such has little impact on the fate of problem drinkers. Nevertheless, it is possible to envisage a form of 'treatment' which attempts to modify these crucial environmental influences (see pp. 295–297 below).

3.4. Rejoinders from Treatment Providers

As might be expected, this onslaught of evidence against the effectiveness of treatment has not gone without rejoinders by those involved in providing treatment. One sort of response has been to argue that the evidence is mainly based on an inappropriate model of treatment evaluation drawn from clinical medicine. The standard methodology of the controlled trial, it is claimed, obscures relevant therapeutic processes and effects, such as the quality of the therapeutic relationship, and also confounds subtle but important client–treatment interactions. Cartwright (1985), for example, has adduced evidence to show that, when the therapeutic relationship is of high quality and when treatment is geared to the needs and expectations of the client, recovery is the rule rather than the exception. Another kind of response is to assert that clients enter treatment with widely differing needs and that, when a broader conception of treatment aims is adopted, including perhaps the acknowledgement that many people enter treatment simply for shelter or for a respite from the ravages of heavy drinking, treatment can be said to work (Yates, 1985). Furthermore, Gawlinski and Otto (1985) have suggested that when treatment does not work, it is usually because the vehicle delivering it is beset by low morale, ill-defined goals, poor working relationships or other aspects of 'organizational melancholia'.

Probably the strongest rejoinder to a blanket rejection of treatment effectiveness has become known as 'the matching hypothesis' (Glaser, 1980). This begins with the assumption that different clients respond differentially to different kinds of treatment method and, indeed, to different treatment goals, such as total abstinence or controlled drinking (see p. 303 below). The hypothesis is that clients who are appropriately matched in treatment will show superior outcome to those who are unmatched or mismatched. In this way, the failure to demonstrate clear evidence of the superiority of treatment results over rates of spontaneous remission is explained by failure to match in the past, as is the uniformity of results across different methods. Miller and Hester (1986b) review evidence which they interpret as showing that clients fare better when the treatment allocated takes account of particular kinds of alcohol problem, varying levels of alcohol dependence, and different cognitive styles. There is also evidence that, when clients are allowed to participate in the choice of treatment approach and goals, greater acceptance of, compliance with and improvement following treatment can be demonstrated (see Miller and Hester, 1986b, p. 193).

It is likely that the controversy over whether treatment for alcohol problems works has been based on several misunderstandings. All writers who have been critical of treatment effectiveness have denied the charge of 'therapeutic nihilism'; their stated aim is invariably to stimulate a re-appraisal of treatment objectives and methods in order to render it more effective or, at least, more cost-effective. Although there has been a great deal of research in this area, it is still possible that some specific treatment methods or, more relevantly, certain broad approaches to treatment, such as the range of methods deriving from the cognitive-behavioral perspective to be described in a later section, have not yet been fully evaluated and may well result eventually in a significant improvement to success rates. Certainly, it cannot be denied that, whether or not we regard treatment as statistically effective from the point of view of national alcohol policy, many sufferers from alcohol problems and their families demand expert help and it is simply inconceivable that their requests should be ignored.

3.5. Effects of the Treatment Debate

This much having been conceded, it is nevertheless true that the treatment effectiveness debate has had the useful function of tempering uncritical enthusiasm for conventional treatment methods and of channelling the attention of scholars, researchers and policy makers into the area of primary prevention. It is salutary now to recall that when President Nixon established the National Institute on Alcohol Abuse and Alcoholism in 1970, and thus provided for a massive injection of money into treatment centers in the United States, it was confidently expected that more and supposedly better treatment would actually solve the nation's alcohol problem. Similar illustrations of faith in the power of treatment may be traced in Britain and in the pronouncements of various WHO Committees dating back to 1951 (World Health Organization, 1951). With the benefit of hindsight, this unthinking commitment to treatment as the main weapon against the spread of alcohol problems now seems extraordinarily naive; the increase in treatment resources has signally failed to contain the rise in alcohol-related problems, let alone reduce them. More recently, skepticism over the true effectiveness of treatment was one of the crucial factors in the emergence of much-needed lobbies and pressure groups, such as Action on Alcohol Abuse in the U.K., urging governments to check the rise in per capita alcohol consumption by fiscal controls, as the only possible way of making any significant impact on the prevalence of alcohol problems in our society (Kendell, 1979; Saunders, 1985).

At the same time, while it has been recognized that treatment must continue to be offered to those who request it, there has been a definite move away from prolonged and expensive inpatient regimes, since the evidence clearly shows that, at the very least, they are no more effective than cheaper outpatient programs (Edwards and Guthrie, 1967). More generally, there is now a great deal of interest in the potential of brief and inexpensive 'minimal interventions' for alcohol problems.

The debate has also led to an enrichment of criteria of improvement, to a consequent rethinking of treatment aims and the sorts of problem to which it should be directed, to a move away from a narrow hospital-based conception of treatment and to a serious consideration of what problem drinkers and their families themselves expect and desire of treatment. Rather than marking a nihilistic attitude to helping problem drinkers or a withdrawal of humanitarian concern, the critical re-evaluation of treatment witnessed over the last decade has been essential if genuine progress is ever to be made.

4. TREATMENT APPROACHES AND METHODS

In the light of the confused state of treatment for alcohol problems, it is likely that the most promising treatments will be those founded on some attempt at a theoretical understanding of the nature of alcohol problems and their development. Unfortunately, a sound and empirically-grounded theoretical underpinning is the exception rather than the rule.

4.1. Drug Treatments

Medically-based treatments have included a range of drug therapies for alcoholism. Among those which have been tried are minor tranquilizers, antidepressants, tranquilizer/antidepressant combinations, antipsychotics, and lithium. None of these medications has been shown to be an effective treatment for alcohol problems in randomized, controlled trials with adequate follow-up, although they may have some success in alleviating associated psychological disorders, such as anxiety and depression, in some appropriate cases (Baekeland and Lundwall, 1975; Rada and Kellner, 1979).

The 1960s and early 1970s witnessed a period of enthusiasm for the use of hallucinogens, especially LSD, but, again, controlled trials have not supported the effectiveness of this method (see Miller and Hester, 1986a, p. 130). Here, as least, practice appears to have been influenced by research findings and the use of LSD has now been virtually discontinued. Apart from general justifications derived from their use in other branches of psychiatry, there is no specific rationale for these drug treatments for alcohol problems.

The same cannot be said of a special class of drug treatments—the 'deterrent' drugs, disulfiram (Antabuse) and cyanamide (Abstem). These have the simple justification that they deter the problem drinker from drinking by producing a violently unpleasant reaction, caused by a massive arousal of the autonomic nervous system, when mixed with beverage alcohol. They are thought to work by blocking the action of the enzyme, aldehyde dehydrogenase, leading to a build up of acetaldehyde in the bloodstream. Cyanamide is apparently associated with less toxic side-effects than disulfiram and may also place less stress on the cardiovascular system if alcohol is consumed. However, disulfiram, in particular, enjoyed a wave of popularity during the 1950s and 1960s. After a period of relative neglect, disulfiram shows signs of renewed popularity and the rationale for this will be described below (p. 297).

4.2. Psychotherapy

Another general approach to treatment comes under the heading of psychotherapy. As noted above, group psychotherapy represents the dominant mode of treatment response in British ATUs but types of psychotherapeutic method used in the treatment of problem drinking range all the way from full-blown psychoanalysis to transactional analysis, client-centered counselling and encounter groups. Although the theoretical justifications for offering psychotherapy to problem drinkers are many and varied, a prominent tradition is associated with a psychodynamic formulation that sees the problem drinker as having an 'oral personality', characterized by a lack of self-control, passive dependence on others, self-destructive impulses and a tendency to use the mouth as a primary means of gratification (Blum, 1966). However, the concept of the oral personality is used to explain many other kinds of disorder commonly encountered by psychotherapists and it is not clear in what way it is thought to be specific to problem drinking. Moreover, research has failed to demonstrate the existence of premorbid personality differences marking out alcoholics as a group (Barry, 1974).

Research on the effectiveness of psychotherapy has not produced encouraging results. For example, in a well-known study, Levinson and Sereny (1969) found that clients who had received insight psychotherapy showed a significantly lower rate of improvement at follow-up than those who had received only occupational and recreational therapy. Other studies have not arrived at quite such negative conclusions, but none has found good evidence for the effectiveness of psychotherapy compared with less intensive interventions (see Miller and Hester, 1986a, pp. 131–3). In view of the lack of evidence to substantiate its use, it is curious, but perfectly typical of the alcohol problems field, that psychotherapy in various guises should have been such a popular approach to treatment for so long.

4.3. Other Treatments

A few other types of treatment have been used and should briefly be mentioned. Hypnosis has been tried on occasion but, again, there is no good research evidence for its effectiveness (Edwards, 1966). The same applies to videotape self-confrontation, in which clients are shown videotapes of themselves recorded when they were in a drunken state. Although this procedure appears to have some impact on drinking behavior, it is also thought to lead to lowered self-esteem and depression and should therefore be used with caution (Schaefer *et al.*, 1971). Finally, marital and family therapy have been shown in a few studies to result in improvements at follow-up compared with controls, but this appears to evaporate over more extended time-periods (McCrady *et al.*, 1982; O'Farrell *et al.*, 1985). Nevertheless, the involvement of spouse and family in treatment should certainly be encouraged in principle and this forms part of the behavioral approach to be described below.

4.4. Alcoholics Anonymous

No outline of treatment in the area could be complete without mentioning Alcoholics Anonymous, although it would be more accurate to describe what AA offers as a new way of life, rather than another type of treatment. It is possible to discover in AA writings a kind of implicit theory of alcoholism, centered around the notion of an incurable 'allergy' to alcohol which means that the individual can never drink safely and that total and life-long abstinence is the only solution. It is probably fair to say, however, that this 'theory' was employed only to buttress a particular kind of pragmatic approach to alcoholism, perhaps best described as 'quasi-religious'. It is on this pragmatic level that AA must be evaluated.

Unfortunately, it has proved extremely difficult to conduct research on the effectiveness of AA. This is because of the anonymity which prevents the keeping of records and the fact that the Fellowship itself has been reluctant to cooperate in research. This has not prevented AA from making startling claims as to its own effectiveness, with success rates of over 75% being put forward (Alcoholics Anonymous, 1955). Some professionals and academics in the field have accepted such claims and there are many psychiatrists and general practitioners who regard the Fellowship as the best hope of success for their patients (Moore and Buchanan, 1966; Jones and Heldrich, 1972). Moreover, the penetration of AA affiliates themselves in the treatment of alcohol problems is extensive although, as noted above, this has become less pronounced recently, at least in the U.K.

One recent study did succeed in randomly assigning problem drinkers to either AA, individual psychotherapy from a professional, two types of behavior therapy also carried out by professionals and a no-treatment control group (Brandsma *et al.*, 1981). At one year follow-up, it was found that, although all treatments given were better than no treatment, AA produced success rates inferior to the other treatment regimes. The main reservation in interpreting this finding is that the clients involved were court-referred and there are grounds for supposing that such clients are less than ideally suited to the kind of approach AA has to offer.

This suggests that successful AA affiliates differ systematically from other problem drinkers and, indeed, there is good evidence that AA is suited to individuals of a more authoritarian type of personality (Ogborne and Glaser, 1981). Other evidence suggests that they tend to have a stronger need for affiliation than most people and are overtly religious in orientation. Although AA groups differ across different cultures, there is also evidence that it appeals more to white, socially stable, middle- to upper-class problem drinkers than to lower-class individuals or those from other ethnic backgrounds. Thus it is likely that some problem drinkers are put off by their first experience of AA and this tends to be confirmed by findings that only about 20% of those who are referred ever attend meetings regularly, the rest either attending on an irregular basis or dropping out completely (Robinson, 1979).

Although it is thus possible to be skeptical of AA claims of success and although there is good evidence for the operation of selective factors, research may eventually confirm that AA is a successful resource for those problem drinkers who are suited to it. Its advantage over formal treatment is that it provides a source of help which is continuous over time and far more readily accessible. There is no doubt, also, that a great many 'recovering alcoholics' owe their lives to AA. On the other hand, as we shall see below, the image of alcoholism which has been successfully promoted by AA can be seen as a barrier to progress in the fields of early intervention and secondary prevention.

5. THE BEHAVIORAL APPROACH TO TREATMENT

In a recent review of research on the effectiveness of alcohol problems treatment, Miller and Hester (1986a) concluded with two lists of treatment methods: (i) those whose effectiveness was supported by empirical research, and (ii) those most commonly in use in the U.S.A. (see Table 1). What is striking about these lists is that there is no overlap between them; none of the treatments for which research support is available is commonly in use and none of those most commonly in use is supported by empirical data. This is a neat summary of the gap between research evidence and treatment practice in the field. The situation is somewhat less irrational in Britain, where there has been a greater willingness to respond to new developments in treatment and where the dominance of traditional views is less pronounced than in America. Nevertheless, the same general conclusion applies: the evidence strongly suggests that behavioral treatment methods offer the best prospects for successful outcome but treatment providers appear strangely reluctant to make full use of them.

TABLE 1. *A Comparison of Treatment Methods Commonly Used in the U.S.A. and Those for which Research Support Exists*

Methods supported by research	Methods commonly in use
Aversion therapy	Alcoholics Anonymous
Behavioral self-control training	Alcoholism education
Community reinforcement approach	Confrontation
Marital and family therapy	Disulfiram
Social skills training	Group therapy
Stress management	Individual counselling

(Adapted from Miller and Hester, 1986a, p. 162.)

5.1. Advantages of the Behavioral Approach

The main advantage of the behavioral approach to treatment is that it is firmly grounded in a theoretical account of the problem in question. The behavioral formulation of the development and maintenance of alcohol problems is supported by laboratory research, involving the use of both human and infrahuman subjects (Nathan and Briddell, 1977; Marlatt and Nathan, 1978). Moreover, because they are related to a wider body of theory and empirical findings, behavioral treatment methods which have proved efficacious with one type of disorder may be modified for use with another. To be sure, the particular theoretical principles on which a treatment method is based may eventually be found to be faulty or the treatment method itself may be discovered not to work as it should on theoretical grounds. However, when this does occur, research links between theory and practice allow both to be revised in the light of experience. This potential for the integration of theory, research and practice is unique among approaches to alcohol problems treatment.

A common criticism of earlier, stimulus-response behavioral theories was that they were too 'mechanistic' and were based almost entirely on experiments with lower organisms, ignoring the qualitatively distinct aspects of human behavior. Whatever force this criticism may have had 30 or 40 years ago, it is inappropriate now. The modern behavioral perspective is best described by the umbrella term, social learning theory (Bandura, 1977). It is characterized, first, by the recognition that many important aspects of human learning take place by imitating the behavior of others (i.e. by 'modelling') and, secondly, by a much greater attention to cognitive processes in specifically human learning. This does not mean that earlier learning paradigms, namely classical (Pavlovian) or operant (Skinnerian) conditioning, are no longer applicable to, for example, alcohol consumption. As this section will show, they are. Rather, these more primitive forms of learning have been placed in a more complex and adequate theory embracing social and cognitive learning processes, including thoughts, expectations, attitudes and self-images. Also fully incorporated in the theory is the human capacity for self-regulation, as opposed to the idea of passive control by the environment.

5.2. Aversion Therapy

The first behavioral method to be applied to alcohol problems was aversion therapy, or 'aversive counterconditioning', which was used as early as the 1920s in Russia following the work of Pavlov on the conditioned reflex (Kantorovich, 1930). The principle of aversion therapy is simply the attempt to create an aversive conditioned response to alcohol by pairing stimuli associated with drinking (sight, smell and taste of alcohol) with powerfully unpleasant unconditioned stimuli, such as nausea or electric shock. An extensive program of research on aversion therapy was carried out in Seattle in the 1940s using nausea induced by emetine as the conditioned response (Voegtlin *et al.*, 1941). Reported success rates at one year follow-up were high, being mostly between 60% and 70% (Voegtlin *et al.*, 1942). However, the authors stressed the importance of selecting clients with good prognosis in terms of intact marriages, high occupational status and high motivation as shown by willingness to pay fees (Voegtlin and Broz, 1949). As suggested earlier, it is probable that these characteristics make problem drinkers good bets for almost any form of treatment.

Since these pioneering studies, further research on aversion therapy has produced mixed results and firm conclusions are difficult (see Miller and Hester, 1980, pp. 31–40). For reasons which are not fully understood, it appears that this form of treatment results unintentionally in more moderate drinking outcomes than other methods. There has also been some debate about which technique for inducing the aversive reaction is preferable, chemically-produced nausea or punishment by electric shock (Rachman, 1965). The latter is much more controllable in terms of onset and intensity, but the former is more likely to produce an aversion to the taste of alcohol which appears to be the crucial change in successful cases (Revusky *et al.*, 1979). One alternative to these procedures is the use of an injection of succinylcholine resulting in the terrifying experience of total paralysis and apnea for about 60 sec (Sanderson *et al.*, 1963), although this method is no longer in use. Another issue is why precisely aversion therapy works when it does. There is some evidence to suggest that classical conditioning as such may not be the crucial element and that cognitive factors, such as a cognitive restructuring of the desire for alcohol, are at least partly responsible (Lovibond and Caddy, 1970). Aversion therapy can be criticized because of the difficulty in generalizing changes made in the clinic to the home environment and also because it merely weakens the drinking response without offering any alternative behavior to replace it.

5.3. Covert Sensitization

Despite the early promise of aversion therapy, it is now no longer in widespread use in Britain. This is chiefly because there are less painful, dangerous and unpleasant methods of achieving the same results. One such method is similarly based on the Pavlovian, classical conditioning paradigm—the procedure known as covert sensitization, in which the pairing of aversive scenes with drinking is conducted, under guidance, entirely in imagination (Cautela, 1970). This has the clear advantage of avoiding the undesirable aspects of aversion therapy while allowing some generalization to the home environment, since the client can simply carry the method with him. Some controlled studies have produced promising results (Ashem and Donner, 1968; Hedberg and Campbell, 1974), although, again, covert sensitization appears to produce more moderation outcomes than expected, rather than total abstinence. One refinement of the approach has been to bolster the aversive imagery by the foul-smelling liquid, valeric acid (Maletzky, 1974). Careful work by Elkins (1980) has shown that outcome may be predicted by degree of conditioning measured immediately after treatment, thus suggesting that conditioning factors are responsible for success in this procedure.

5.4. Operant Conditioning

In addition to methods deriving from the classical conditioning paradigm, behavioral treatments have also been based on the principles of instrumental learning (or operant conditioning), as described originally by Skinner (1938). These principles describe the way in which behavior is shaped and maintained by its environmental consequences and they can be used to modify problem behavior by altering the reinforcement contingencies applying to it. A great number of laboratory studies have demonstrated that the drinking behavior of problem drinkers, even those labelled as 'chronic alcoholics' showing high levels of alcohol dependence, can be modified by altering the environmental consequences of drinking (Heather and Robertson, 1983). In contrast to the disease view of alcoholism, which sees alcoholic drinking as a largely uncontrollable activity subject to abnormal, internal urges, this learning perspective regards problem drinking as goal-directed activity, similar in kind and modifiable according to the same laws as normal drinking.

In spite of this extensive backing from the laboratory, there have been few direct applications of instrumental learning to treatment for alcohol problems. One notable exception, however, began with research published by Hunt and Azrin (1973) from Illinois, using what they termed the Community Reinforcement Approach (CRA). The basic idea of this approach was to arrange environmental contingencies so that vocational, familial, social and recreational reinforcements would predictably and consistently occur only when the client was abstinent and not if he were drinking. This involved a massive effort in enlisting the cooperation of employers, wives and friends of the client, as well as other community agencies. For those without families, a 'foster family' was arranged and, to encourage an active social life without alcohol, a special 'dry club' was set up where clients could meet friends and engage in a large number of recreational activities. Clients were also provided, where appropriate, with training in job-seeking, marital and family counselling and even financial assistance to buy cars, telephones, newspaper subscriptions, etc. They were visited twice a week by a counsellor during the first month after discharge and on an average of twice per month thereafter.

CRA was added to a full inpatient treatment program and eight diagnosed chronic alcoholics with multiple problems were compared with a group of carefully matched controls. At 6-month follow-up, the experimental group showed a large superiority to controls on numerous measures. They had drunk on 14% of days compared with 79% in the controls; the control group had a 12 times higher rate of unemployed days and had spent 15 times more days in institutions; and all the marriages in the experimental group were still intact whereas 25% had ended in divorce or separation in the control group. These are some of the most impressive results ever reported for alcohol problems treatment.

Azrin (1976) reported the results of an improved CRA. The improvements consisted in the use of disulfiram to inhibit impulsive drinking, together with special motivational procedures for its continued use, an early warning system to alert the counsellor that problems were developing, the use of a neighborhood friend/advisor (the 'buddy' system) to provide support after counselling had ended, and group counselling procedures to reduce total counselling time. A group of 20 alcoholics receiving CRA was compared with 20 matched controls. At 6-month follow-up, the experimental group had drunk on only 2% of days compared with 56% in the controls, had spent 7% of days away from home (cf. 67%), had 20% of days unemployed (cf. 56%), and had no days institutionalized (cf. 45%). These are even more impressive results and, on this occasion, were found to persist to 2-years follow-up, with over 90% days abstinent in the experimental group, all of whom were located. Further, Azrin reports that the improved CRA was less time-consuming to run than the previous version.

Lastly, Azrin *et al.* (1982) reported a study examining the specific contribution made to their successful results by disulfiram. Forty-three outpatient alcoholics were randomly assigned to (1) a traditional disulfiram treatment program; (2) a group in which disulfiram was taken under supervision by relatives, plus special training for clients in solving problems associated with its regular use; and (3) a group given supervised disulfiram as above combined with CRA. Overall, the results showed that group 3 was superior to group 2 which was superior to group 1. However, there was an important interaction between drinking outcome and marital status which is shown in Table 2. This suggests that for single clients, supervised disulfiram alone was ineffective, but that behavior therapy, in the form of CRA, led to a significant improvement, whereas for married clients there was no additional benefit from CRA since abstinent days had already reached a ceiling. This makes sense if one assumes that the social support of a partner is necessary for successful disulfiram treatment and that married clients already had access to many of the reinforcements provided by CRA.

The outcome results in this series of studies are the best ever reported in adequately controlled research in this area. It might be wondered, then, why treatment providers all over the world have not switched to offering the Community Reinforcement Approach and its associated methods. One reason is clearly that the full CRA is extremely expensive and labor-intensive, both in terms of counsellors' time and the commitment of community agencies and individuals. However, there appears no good reason why elements of the approach should not be more widely applied. Depending on an analysis of the drinking be-

TABLE 2. *Mean Number of Days of Abstinence during the 30 Days before Interview for Single and Married Clients*

	Single	Married
Traditional disulfiram	6.8	17.4
Supervised disulfiram	8.0	30.0
Supervised disulfiram + CRA	28.3	30.0

(Adapted from Azrin *et al.*, 1982, p. 110.)

havior and particular problems of an individual client, an attempt could be made to arrange environmental contingencies so that excessive drinking is not reinforced and abstinence, or moderate drinking, is systematically rewarded. For example, the approach known as 'marital contracting' (Stuart, 1969) entails the drawing up of a contract between problem drinker and spouse specifying the agreed consequences of drinking and abstaining. The same principles can be applied, on a somewhat larger scale, to family situations or to groups of friends, employing organizations, etc. Probably more important is a secure grasp of the principles of instrumental learning by therapists and counsellors and their consistent application in treatment. This applies as much to the organizational behavior of treatment agencies, which often reward undesirable drinking behavior by paying attention to a client only when he is in trouble and ignoring him otherwise, as it does to individual therapists.

5.5. Disulfiram as a Behavioral Treatment

Azrin's work described above has been one of the principal influences leading to a resurgence of interest in disulfiram, championed in the U.K. mainly by Colin Brewer (Brewer and Smith, 1983; Brewer, 1986). Earlier research on disulfiram had not produced especially promising results (Lundwall and Baekeland, 1971), largely owing to problems of compliance with taking the drug at home and a consequently high rate of drop-out from treatment. Those problem drinkers who were compliant were probably those with a good prognosis for any form of treatment. It was for this reason that surgical implants of disulfiram in the lower abdomen were tried, but experience showed that blood levels were unreliable (see Miller and Hester, 1980, p. 20). Brewer argues that this situation has been changed by the recent emphasis on supervised disulfiram, in which a relative supervises and records the client's daily ingestion of disulfiram, usually accompanied by a contract drawn up by client, relative and counsellor. There is evidence that this procedure increases compliance and lowers drop-out (Keane *et al.*, 1984). Brewer (1984) also argues that, in the past, doses given have often been too low to prevent many clients from drinking and that the adverse side-effects and dangers of disulfiram have been greatly exaggerated.

There are at least three ways of seeing disulfiram as a behavioral technique. First, when a challenge dose is administered to demonstrate to the client the disulfiram–ethanol reaction, this may be regarded as a classical conditioning trial leading to a learned aversive response to drinking. One trial learning may sometimes occur if the unconditioned stimulus is sufficiently powerful. More importantly, the use of the drug is clearly in line with the range of devices used to alter the contingencies of drinking under an operant conditioning paradigm, leading in this case to immediate and powerful punishment if drinking is attempted. Finally, it has recently been suggested (Brewer, C. personal communication, published with permission) that disulfiram can be viewed as a 'response prevention' technique, like those commonly used in the treatment of obsessive/compulsive and phobic disorders. During the period in which disulfiram prevents the consumption of alcohol, there may occur extinction of conditioned craving responses to cues previously associated with drinking (see p. 301 below). At the same time, this may also lead to increased 'self-efficacy' or, in other words, the client's increased confidence in his ability to cope with high-risk situations, such as social pressure to drink, without relapse. These interesting suggestions deserve further exploration.

5.6 Broad Spectrum Treatment

One of the basic tenets of the behavioral approach is that each client's particular alcohol problem must be subjected to a 'functional analysis' to discover the specific antecedents and consequences of drinking in the individual case. This follows from the view that alcohol problems are functionally related to a variety of other problems in living and that an effective treatment program must offer a 'cafeteria' range of methods to enable the client to cope with his problems without drinking. It is assumed that such programs will be more effective than those which concentrate on drinking behavior alone. This summarizes the 'broad spectrum' approach to treatment which first became popular in the early 1970s (Hamburg, 1975).

While the broad spectrum approach in its entirety does not appear to have been evaluated, some of the typical ingredients of these 'multimodal' programs have been researched. For example, anxiety and stress have often been proposed as antecedents of excessive drinking and the value of relaxation training as an adjunct to conventional treatment was explored by Freedberg and Johnston (1978). At 1 year follow-up, there were no differences on drinking measures between a group given relaxation training in addition to conventional inpatient treatment and another given inpatient treatment alone, but the relaxation group was superior in terms of employment status and a measure of depression. However, Rosenberg (1979) showed that, if clients high on anxiety were distinguished from those low on this variable, significant improvements in drinking behavior among the high group could be obtained. The effectiveness of systematic desensitization, a procedure used to treat phobic reactions, has also been examined. Hedberg and Campbell (1974) evaluated this procedure in a method in which phobic situations included interpersonal anxieties, authority and family problems, and anxieties related to the absence of alcohol. They found systematic desensitization to be equivalent in effectiveness to family therapy but superior to covert desensitization and electrical aversion therapy.

Another type of broad spectrum ingredient may be included under the category of 'skills training', where clients are trained in behavioral skills to cope with specific situations which in the past have led to excessive drinking. For example, Jackson and Oei (1978) from New Zealand investigated social skills training, in which clients are taught to be more assertive in interpersonal contacts, and cognitive restructuring, a procedure derived from the treatment of depression in which distorted and irrational beliefs are examined and clients taught to modify their beliefs in appropriate ways. The authors found that, among problem drinkers low on assertiveness skills, both these procedures were superior in effectiveness to a traditional supportive therapy. In a later study, Oei and Jackson (1980) showed that a combined social skills/cognitive restructuring method was superior to either alone, although all behavioral treatments were better than supportive therapy.

Skills training of a somewhat different kind was investigated by Chaney *et al.* (1978). These authors used a method known as 'problem-solving skills training' (D'Zurilla and Goldfried, 1971) to teach problem drinkers to cope with situations identified as those likely to lead to relapse, such as social pressure to drink or negative mood states. In a group setting, the therapist first modelled a response to the high-risk situation that did not involve drinking, and the client then decided on his own coping response, rehearsed it in front of the group and received feedback about its appropriateness. The rules for generating and evaluating coping strategies were summarized by a member of the group at the end of each session. Two control groups were used: one encouraged to discuss personal feelings about the same situations as used in the experimental group but without practising new skills, and another given conventional hospital treatment only. At 1-year follow-up, the skills training group showed a significantly greater improvement on various measures of drinking behavior than both control groups. The results of this well-designed study can be interpreted as confirmation of a basic assumption of social learning theory—that 'performance-based' methods, involving the practice and rehearsal of new skills, will be superior to 'verbally-based' treatments relying merely on discussion and verbal persuasion, such as those employed in traditional psychotherapeutic and counselling approaches (Bandura, 1977).

There thus appears to be good evidence that behavioral methods aimed at teaching problem drinkers specific coping skills can be effective adjuncts to treatment. However, the value of these methods in practice will depend on accurate assessment designed to reveal the particular deficits of each client, so that treatment may be appropriately matched to individual needs (see p. 290 above).

5.7. Stages of Change

A major recent development in thinking about alcohol problems has been an integration of theory and practice with other 'addictive behaviors', such as drug dependence, cigarette smoking, forms of eating disorder, compulsive gambling, forms of sexual disorder and a wide range of appetitive behaviors which appear to have a compulsive element. It is assumed that the learning processes underlying all the diverse behaviors are similar in kind and that, therefore, similar methods may be used to modify them. Moreover, it is also assumed that the change processes occurring during treatment are the same as those which are responsible for 'spontaneous' change in the natural environment and that by studying naturally-occurring change processes, we may learn something about what is necessary for treatment to be successful.

These assumptions form the basis for a model of change in the addictive behaviors, developed by Prochaska and DiClemente (1986), which has become rapidly influential in the last few years (see Fig. 2). This simple model proposes that change in the addictive behaviors—say, reducing alcohol consumption to safer levels—may be seen as involving four stages: a Precontemplation stage, in which the individual is not aware of any problems connected with the addictive behavior and has no desire to change; a Contemplation stage, in which there is some awareness of problems and the individual may be seen as weighing up the respective advantages and disadvantages of changing the addictive behavior as against continuing with it; an Action stage in which practical efforts are made to change the behavior in question; and a Maintenance stage, in which the individual is engaged in an attempt to retain the changes that have been made. In the event that maintenance is unsuccessful, relapse occurs and the individual returns to the Precontemplation and Contemplation stages. There is some empirical evidence from the cigarette smoking area to support the existence of these separate stages (Prochaska *et al.*, 1985), but it is as a simple heuristic device to assist thinking about the modification of addictive behaviors that the model has become popular. The complete model is more complex than this short description and also involves associated levels and processes of change (see Prochaska and DiClemente, 1986) but it is the idea of stages of change which has proved most influential.

5.8. Motivational Interviewing

Clearly, most of this chapter has been concerned with the Action stage and has discussed the relative merits of various methods which have been used to facilitate action. The Maintenance stage has been relatively neglected in thinking about alcohol problems, but this will

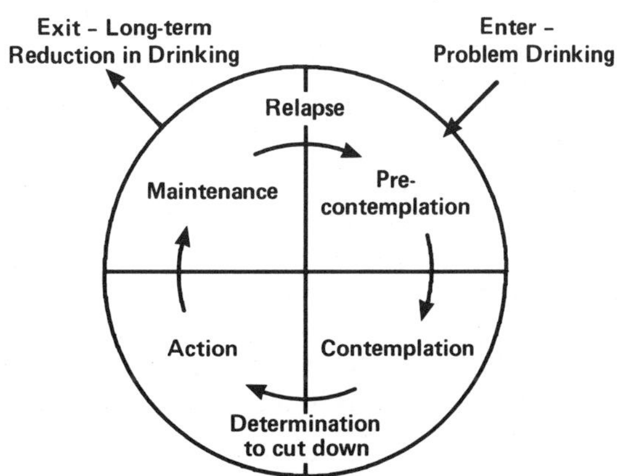

Fig. 2. Stages of change in problem drinking. (Adapted from Prochaka and DiClemente, 1986, p. 6.)

form the subject matter of the next section on 'relapse prevention'. Even more neglected, however, has been the transition onwards from the Precontemplation and Contemplation stages. One of the most widely acknowledged facts about the treatment of alcohol problems is that it is difficult because the client is often 'unmotivated' to change. However, the implications of this basic observation have rarely been pursed to their logical conclusions.

Miller (1983a) has argued that the mistake in the past has been to explain poor motivation and lack of compliance in treatment by personality traits and other inadequacies of the client himself. By contrast, when treatment succeeds, it is usually seen as being due to the quality of the treatment program or the skill of the therapist. Rather, says Miller, motivational problems must be seen in the context of an interpersonal process between client and therapist. Miller uses well-established principles from social psychology to show how the traditional confrontational approach to problem drinkers is likely to lead to 'denial', 'resistance' and low client self-esteem. As an alternative, Miller describes his own approach as 'motivational interviewing'. This de-emphasizes the labelling of drinking problems and instead places heavy emphasis on individual responsibility and internal, rather than external, attribution of change. A deliberate attempt is made to create 'cognitive dissonance' in the client by subtly contrasting the current problem behavior with an awareness of its negative consequences. The therapeutic principle of 'empathic listening', derived from client-centered counselling, combined with social psychological principles of attitudinal change and the feedback of the results of objective assessments, are used to channel dissonance towards the desired behavior change.

Based as it is in a body of sound psychological findings and a great deal of practical experience and common-sense, motivational interviewing is proving highly attractive to many workers in the alcohol problems field. As yet, however, there is no good evidence for its superior effectiveness compared with the traditional approach, although it uses specifiable and testable processes and is eminently suited to research evaluation. It may transpire that motivational interviewing works best with certain types of problem drinker, particularly those with relatively less serious problems, but that the confrontational approach is still best for severely deteriorated individuals.

5.9. Relapse Prevention

Another commonly acknowledged fact about the treatment of alcohol problems and other addictive behaviors is that the initiation of change is a relatively simple and straightforward matter; it is the maintenance of these initial changes over time—in other words, the prevention of relapse—which presents the major difficulties. Although the inpatient problem drinker may be confident of having overcome his problem when in hospital and may experience little or no craving for alcohol, it is when he returns to the home environment and, for example, encounters situations and moods associated with excessive drinking in the past that a return to problem drinking will often occur. Even for outpatients treated in the community, relapse sooner or later is the rule rather than the exception. From a learning theory standpoint, this is perfectly understandable. Deeply-ingrained habits which have taken years to build up cannot be extinguished or significantly modified in the short period usually devoted to treatment as such; rather, the necessary 'relearning' process may take many months, or even years, before it becomes firmly established in the behavioral repertoire. It is for this reason that much attention is now being paid to issues stemming from Prochaska and DiClemente's Maintenance stage in the change process (see Fig. 2 above) and that a model of relapse prevention developed by Marlatt and his colleagues in Seattle (Marlatt and George, 1984; Marlatt and Gordon, 1985) has become extremely popular. Indeed, of all the recent developments in the alcohol treatment field, this has been the most influential.

The Marlatt model of relapse is based on research showing that, in retrospective accounts by problem drinkers, the most frequently cited relapse precipitants may be grouped as follows: (1) negative emotional states (frustration, anger, anxiety, depression, boredom etc.); (2) interpersonal conflict (e.g. in marital, family, friendship, employer-employee relationships); and (3) social pressure (either with or without direct persuasion). Thus, the major relapse precipitants are all described by social or psychological variables. The first task in a relapse prevention program is to train the client to identify such precipitants as 'high risk situations', stressing those types of situation which are assessed as being especially relevant to the individual client. Further, the problem drinker is assumed to be deficient in skills which could be used to cope with high-risk situations without relapse and past failures to cope are assumed to have led to decreased 'self-efficacy' (Bandura and Adams, 1977) or loss of confidence in the ability to cope. This, combined with positive learned expectations regarding the psychotropic effects of alcohol, will lead to initial use. The program therefore devotes much attention to training skills such as relaxation, assertiveness, problem solving etc., to changing positive expectations about alcohol and to developing alternative ways of responding to high-risk situations. Finally, if alcohol is taken there occurs a process dubbed by Marlatt the 'abstinence violation effect', in which, because of beliefs derived from the disease theory of alcoholism, the individual feels powerless to control further consumption. The program therefore attempts a cognitive restructuring of such beliefs and encourages the client to view the initial 'slip' as a learning experience which could be used to guard against future relapse. The basic relapse prevention model is shown schematically in Fig. 3.

In fact, the model is more complex than it is possible to convey in this short summary and the interested reader is referred to the original publications (Cummings *et al.*, 1980; Marlatt and George, 1984). In more recent work, Marlatt and Gordon (1985) have added to the model by emphasizing the importance of broad life-style changes, as well as the training in specific coping skills. The use of relapse prevention programs in the alcohol problems field has received some empirical support from the study by Chaney *et al.* (1978) described above (p. 298). However, its current popularity owes less to this empirical backing than to the fact that it fits so well with the experience of many workers in the field and has provided a sophisticated and well-grounded solution to an obvious inadequacy of the conventional treatment approach. Some important criticisms of the model have already been developed (see Saunders and Allsop, 1987) but there is no doubt that Marlatt's work represents an important turning point in our understanding of how to modify problem drinking.

5.10. Cue Exposure

The very latest treatment method to be developed along behavioral principles is known as cue exposure. This method is itself based on recent advances in our understanding of the nature of tolerance and withdrawal from addictive drugs—in particular the idea that both tolerance and withdrawal are partly conditioned processes (MacCrae *et al.*, 1987). It

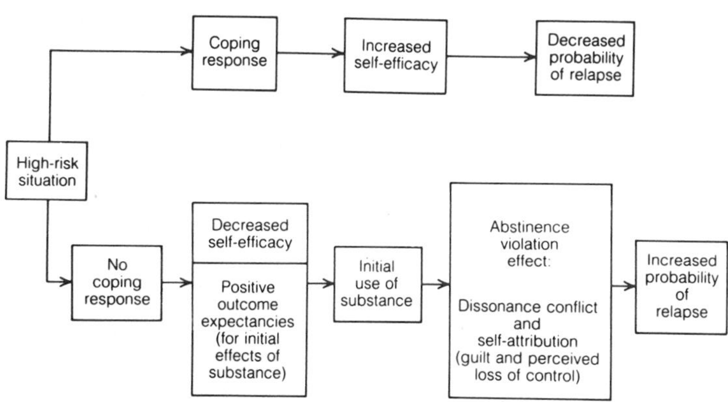

Fig. 3. A model of relapse and relapse prevention. (From Marlatt and Gordon, 1985, p. 38, with permission.)

has been demonstrated that stimuli associated with administration of a drug can come to elicit conditioned responses opposite in the direction of physiological effect to that of the drug and these conditioned responses have been called drug compensatory CRs. They act to preserve homeostatis when a drug is taken and, as such, play an important role in tolerance. It has been shown in many experiments that animals made tolerant to a drug in a specific environmental setting retain that tolerance if later tested in the same setting but lose it if tested in a different environment (Siegel, 1983).

Drug withdrawal is explained in the same way by the fact that drug compensatory CRs are anticipatory in nature, i.e., they occur before the expected onset of a drug as part of the attempted regulation of drug effects. Thus, anticipatory drug compensatory CRs are experienced as withdrawal symptoms if they have been elicited by drug-related stimuli but no drug administration occurs. As in the case of tolerance, there have been many experimental demonstrations of the environmental specificity of conditioned withdrawal in animals. In the case of alcohol, since this drug is a CNS depressant, anticipatory CRs take the form of CNS excitation, thus accounting for the major aspects of alcohol withdrawal. In this formulation, the presence of subclinical conditioned withdrawal leads to the experience of craving.

The implications for treatment of this model of conditioned tolerance and withdrawal are obvious. If tolerance, withdrawal and craving are conditioned phenomena, it follows that they can, in principle, be extinguished. In other words, if problem drinkers are exposed to cues for drinking but discouraged or prevented from drinking, the cues in question should lose their power to evoke a desire to consume alcohol and should also lead to lowered tolerance in response to those cues. This hypothesis was tested by Blakey and Baker (1980) in Aberdeen. They interviewed problem drinkers to assess which situations would lead to a desire to drink and then asked them to rank these situations in order of how 'tempting' they would find them. Starting with the least difficult item, say, walking past a favorite pub, clients were given practice, at first supervised but later on their own, at facing up to the tempting situations while resisting the urge to drink. Eventually, clients were encouraged to go into pubs where alcohol was placed in front of them. Most reported that many of the situations that had previously made them want to drink had largely lost that power. The results of the study were therefore very promising, although this was not a controlled clinical trial. As well as extinguishing classically conditioned withdrawal symptoms, this type of exposure procedure probably weakens the instrumental response of drinking to escape or avoid withdrawal discomfort.

A powerful class of drinking cues is the interoceptive stimuli associated with a rising blood alcohol level. If such stimuli become cues for further drinking, this may explain the process of 'loss of control' over drinking which is traditionally linked with chronic alcoholism. Thus, a most important type of cue exposure procedure is to give dependent problem drinkers a strong priming dose of alcohol and then prevent further drinking in the presence of alcohol-related cues. After case-reports (Hodgson and Rankin, 1976, 1982), this method was put to test in a controlled trial by Rankin *et al.* (1983). These authors randomly divided ten severely dependent problem drinkers into two groups, one of which received only six sessions of *in vivo* cue exposure and response prevention, while the other received six sessions of a control procedure in which cue exposure was conducted in imagination followed by a further six sessions of *in vivo* cue exposure and response prevention. In each experimental session, subjects were given a priming dose which produced blood alcohol levels of between 65 and 100 mg% and then resisted a further drink for 45 min. Temptation was maximized by asking subjects to hold the glass of alcohol in their hands, put it to their lips and smell the alcohol. The results showed that the *in vivo* cue exposure method produced significant decrements on behavioral and subjective variables measuring 'desire to drink' and 'difficulty to resist alcohol', whereas the imaginal cue exposure produced trivial changes on these measures. In discussing how these changes took place, the authors point out that, as well as extinction of classically conditioned and instrumental responses, it is possible that cognitive changes in subjects' confidence in coping with feelings of craving without relapse were partly responsible. They also point out that the cue exposure method could be aimed equally well at total abstinence or at a goal of controlled drinking (see next section). No follow-up data have been reported for the subjects of this study and there has as yet been no controlled comparison with a more conventional form of treatment in a clinical trial.

Nevertheless, although in early days of development, the cue exposure method is of the greatest importance for the future of behavioral treatments in this area. It is little exaggeration to claim that it is potentially capable of 'unlocking' alcohol dependence. Attention is now being paid to the refinement and testing of the cue exposure method in several research centers throughout the world.

6. ABSTINENCE VERSUS CONTROLLED DRINKING TREATMENT GOALS

Of all the controversies in the alcohol field, none has been so bitter and so protracted as that concerning the possibility that individuals dependent on alcohol can sometimes return to a controlled, harmfree pattern of drinking. As will be readily appreciated, this suggestion runs directly counter to the central postulate of the disease theory of alcoholism, that total and lifelong abstinence is essential for recovery. There is no intention here to review the complete history and many facets of this dispute, since this has been covered several times already (Heather and Robertson, 1983; Miller, 1983b; Marlatt, 1983). All that will be attempted is a brief outline of the development of the controversy and some indication of current thinking about it.

Although the issue of abstinence versus moderation was argued for a time among the ranks of Temperance supporters during the last Century, in modern times the debate began with the publication by Davies (1962) of observations that seven male patients formerly treated for 'alcohol addiction' at the Maudsley Hospital, London, had resumed harmfree drinking after periods ranging from 7 to 11 years. This article provoked a storm of protest from subscribers to the *Quarterly Journal of Studies on Alcohol*. Nevertheless, during the remainder of the decade, several studies appeared which essentially confirmed Davies' findings and it also became clear that such observations had not infrequently been made before Davies wrote (see Heather and Robertson, 1983, pp. 21–77). Indeed, with the benefit of hindsight, we may say that the existence of 'resumed normal drinkers' began to be observed as soon as even moderately well-designed follow-up studies of alcoholism treatment were conducted.

The next major development was the appearance in 1976 of the so-called Rand Report, a follow-up study of the results of treatment from 44 Alcohol Treatment Centers throughout the United States (see Armor *et al.*, 1978). This study, which represents the largest follow-up ever conducted in the field, was commissioned by the U.S. Government. In their summary, the authors stated that their findings suggested "the possibility that for some alcoholics moderate drinking is not necessarily a prelude to a full relapse and that some alcoholics can return to moderate drinking with no greater chance of relapse than if they abstained" (p. 294). As we have seen, this finding was by no means novel, but the difference this time was that it became widely reported in the national press. This had the effect of bringing the conflict between the two opposing camps of alcohol treatment specialists out into the open, with much hostility and irrationality on view. Four years later, the authors of the Rand Report produced the results of an extended follow-up of some of the same cohort with more rigorous definitions of what was to count as 'nonproblem drinking' (Polich *et al.*, 1980). Despite considerable misrepresentation, this later report confirmed the findings of its predecessor with respect to nonproblem drinking.

It is important to note that all the studies referred to above were concerned with outcome after treatment directed at total abstinence. Thus, if problem drinkers returned to harmfree drinking they were acting in defiance of the advice they had probably received. However, in the early 1970s and after an increase in the number of clinical psychologists interested in alcohol treatment, research began to be directed at evaluating treatment methods aimed at a controlled drinking goal, since there is nothing in a learning theory conception of problem drinking to suggest that the condition is permanently irreversible. The most famous, or in some circles infamous, of these studies was carried out by Sobell and Sobell (1973, 1976) in California. These researchers showed that a group of randomly-assigned 'gamma' alcoholics (i.e., those showing evidence of physical dependence on alcohol), given what they termed 'individualized behavior therapy' aimed at controlled drinking, had a superior outcome at follow-up to a group given conventional, hospital-based treatment aimed at abstinence. Roughly 10 years later, there appeared an article in *Science* which claimed, in effect, that the Sobells' reported findings were fraudulent (Pendery *et al.*, 1982), thus engendering the most acrimonious episode in the long history of this dispute.

It will not be possible here to enter into the details of what has become known as 'the Sobell affair' (but see Heather and Robertson, 1983, pp. 259–281). What can be said is that the Sobells have been cleared of fraud by at least three committees set up to investigate the charges against them and that, at the time of writing, no convincing evidence of scientific malpractice has ever been produced. Despite this exoneration, however, the effect of the Sobell affair has been to virtually halt all further research and practical applications of controlled drinking methods in the United States, where it seems obvious that the dispute has very little to do with scientific evidence and everything to do with ideological commitment. Fortunately, the situation is better in the United Kingdom and, despite some continued opposition, there is a much greater acceptance of the use of the controlled drinking goal for certain types of problem drinker.

6.1. Criteria for Goal Allocation

There is an emerging consensus in Britain that, although some problem drinkers with high levels of dependence can sometimes return to harmfree drinking, it is usually extremely difficult for them to do so and that the best advice is to direct such problem drinkers towards abstinence. This is not because high-dependence problem drinkers have an 'allergy' to alcohol which prevents them from drinking moderately in principle, as AA would suggest, but merely that the complete change in lifestyle and attitudes towards alcohol which is necessary to break free of a strongly ingrained, habitual pattern of excessive drinking is more easily achieved by complete avoidance of the drug. Nor does it mean that level of alcohol dependence is the only variable which should be taken into account in the decision about treatment goals. There are some circumstances in which controlled drinking might be the better option for a highly dependent individual, especially where the client himself refuses to consider abstinence and would previously have been turned away as 'unmotivated'. Conversely, there are circumstances where the abstinence option may be more suited to a low-dependence problem drinker, owing perhaps to particular family or occupational circumstances or to medical complications.

Nevertheless, it is low-dependence problem drinkers that the controlled drinking goal has become mainly associated. Miller and Baca (1983), reviewing the accumulated results from a controlled drinking treatment method which they term Behavioral Self-control Training, found an improvement rate of over 70% among low-dependence problem drinkers followed up 2 years after treatment. This shows that a controlled drinking goal is eminently suitable for such a population. Moreover, there is evidence that directing such problem drinkers towards total abstinence is actually counter-productive (Sanchez-Craig and Lei, 1986). Using behavioral methods adjusted to the needs of each client, Robertson *et al.* (1986) showed that controlled drinking treatment produced superior results compared with minimal assessment and advice. Unfortunately, however, there was a very slow rate of referral to this project, presumably because individuals with relatively less serious problems were reluctant to attend a hospital-based clinic.

6.2. Minimal Interventions

It is in the response to alcohol problems conducted outside the clinical setting that the controlled drinking goal has found its niche. More specifically, the emergence of controlled drinking treatment has coincided with an upsurge of interest in early intervention and secondary prevention of alcohol problems. In the last few years much research attention has been paid to developing and evaluating community-based 'minimal interventions' for problem drinkers using a variety of occupational groups to deliver them. Clearly, the empirical justification for minimal interventions relies to a great extent on the evidence covered earlier of the relative ineffectiveness of traditional, intensive treatments (pp. 287–291) and to the demonstrably higher cost-effectiveness of brief, inexpensive ways of communicating help and advice.

The controlled drinking goal has come into its own in the area of minimal interventions because of the obvious fact that low-dependence problem drinkers will be deterred from attempting to change their drinking behavior and, indeed, from even admitting that problems exist, if they believe that total and lifelong abstinence is the only solution to a drinking problem. Until quite recently, however, there have been no formal services available aimed at assisting problem drinkers to reduce consumption to safer levels before their problems get worse. It is in this respect that the image of alcoholism portrayed by AA, directly through their own promotional activities and through numerous fictional portrayals of alcohol problems, has been a considerable hindrance to progress. The AA concept of 'rock bottom' suggests that the problem drinker has to reach a very low ebb indeed, with complete disintegration of health, job and family life, before he will recognize his disease and seek a cure. Given the belief that abstinence is the only alternative, this view is probably correct and this leads to the situation where problem drinkers will say to themselves, "I'm not as bad as that, I can't be an alcoholic and I don't need help." It is not surprising that the evidence shows that AA has not succeeded in its aim of attracting younger problem drinkers or those earlier in the course of their problem (Robinson, 1979). The typical AA affiliate is still someone of middle age with a very high level of alcohol dependence and severe alcohol-related problems. However, once the principle of the controlled drinking goal is accepted and once the definition of an alcohol problem is expanded to include less severe forms of damage and lower degrees of dependence, the possibility arises of making a real impact on the prevalence of alcohol problems in the community.

The most direct method of delivering minimal interventions is simply through self-help manuals, either commercially on sale, sent through the post to those who request them or available in GPs' waiting rooms, public libraries etc. A series of studies by Miller and his colleagues in Albuquerque, New Mexico (Miller, 1978; Miller and Taylor, 1980; Miller *et al.*, 1980, 1981) showed that self-help manuals were no less effective in helping low-dependence problem drinkers to reduce drinking than individual or group behavior therapy. However, some degree of therapist contact was always present in these studies and it remained to be demonstrated that self-help manuals would work in conditions more closely similar to their intended widespread use, i.e. without any therapist contact. This was the issue examined by Heather *et al.* (1986, 1987a) in a study of problem drinkers recruited via the Scottish national press. Seven hundred eighty-five individuals who responded to newspaper advertisements were sent either a behaviorally-based self-help manual (Robertson and Heather, 1985) or a general advice and information booklet. Results for 6-month and 1-year follow-up are shown in Fig. 4. The greater mean reduction in consumption among the manual group was statistically significant at the 6-month follow-up and, if respondents who had received other forms of help were excluded, at the 1-year follow-up. However, the high rate of sample attrition in this study introduces some problems of interpretation and this line of research is continuing. Also, it is intended to explore an interesting hypothesis which emerged from the results of the above study—that some degree of supplementary telephone contact may improve the effectiveness of self-help procedures.

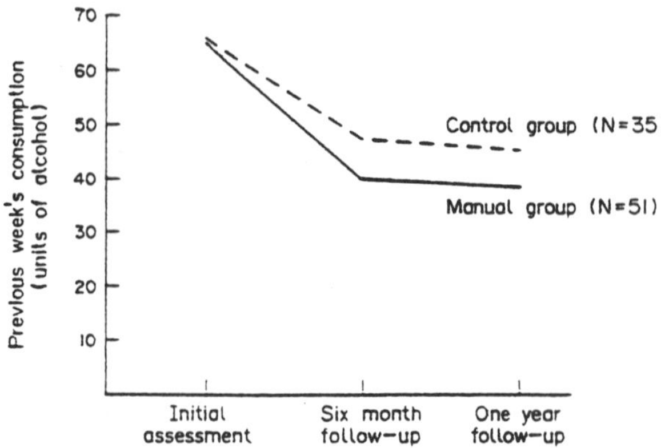

FIG. 4. Changes in mean alcohol consumption for subjects sent a behaviourally-based self-help manual (Manual Group) or an advice and information booklet (Control Group).

Apart from self-help manuals, the most intensively researched area of minimal intervention is the effectiveness of brief interventions by general practitioners. There are currently four major projects underway in the U.K. investigating somewhat different means of delivering brief advice to problem drinkers from a general practice setting. One project (Heather *et al.*, 1987b) has evaluated the effectiveness of a package developed by the Scottish Health Education Group called DRAMS (Drinking Reasonably and Moderately with Self-control). Patients identified as excessive and/or problem drinkers by a waiting-room screening procedure were randomly assigned to groups given DRAMS, simple advice to cut down by the GP or a nonintervention control. At 6-month follow-up there were no significant differences between groups in drinking behavior but the DRAMS group showed a significantly greater reduction in gamma-glutamyltransferase (GGT), a liver enzyme known to reflect recent alcohol consumption. The disappointingly low rate of referral to this project may have been responsible for the failure to observe more positive effects of DRAMS. Moreover, the sample overall showed significant improvements in drinking, GGT and physical health and it may be that all three groups benefitted to some extent from a form of minimal intervention, including the group who merely had their attention directed to their drinking by the fairly lengthy assessment procedure. Without a nonassessment control group, of course, this must remain speculation. Nevertheless, brief intervention among early and low-dependence problem drinkers in general practice remains a potentially very valuable means of effecting change, provided GPs themselves can be persuaded to overcome the reluctance to become involved with this work which previous research has demonstrated (Clement, 1986; Thom and Tellez, 1986).

Another potentially valuable mode of intervention could occur on general hospital wards. The proportion of male inpatients found to have illnesses related, either directly or indirectly, to excessive alcohol consumption has been variably estimated at between 10% and 30% and much attention has been paid to improving the recognition of such cases by hospital doctors. Chick *et al.* (1985) in Edinburgh randomly assigned 156 problem drinkers from various types of ward to a group given a single session of counselling about their drinking from a nurse or one given only routine medical care. At 1-year follow-up, both groups reported a reduction in drinking but the counselling group had a superior outcome in terms of drinking measures, alcohol-related problems and GGT. The implications of this finding are being pursued in Dundee in two studies, one directed at reduced drinking and the other at abstinence, where this is indicated on grounds of physical health rather than a high level of alcohol dependence. The object of the research is to discover the most cost-effective level of intervention, with input ranging all the way from a group given pre-discharge counselling only to one given counselling, a self-help manual to take home, periodic home visits from a nurse and feedback of GGT results. It is hoped that the results will have implications for the work of doctors, ward nurses, community nurses, and health visitors.

GGT feedback formed a crucial element in perhaps the most impressive piece of research in this area. As part of a population health screening exercise, Kristenson *et al.* (1982, 1983) in Malmö, Sweden randomly allocated middle-aged, male heavy drinkers to either a group given counselling and GGT feedback or a nonintervention control. At successive contacts up to 6 years later, significantly greater improvements in the experimental group were found for GGT levels, sickness absenteeism from work, hospitalizations, and mortality. In France, early detection and secondary prevention of alcohol problems are carried out by the Centres Alimentaires d'Hygiene, with encouraging results (Babor *et al.*, 1983; Chick, 1984).

Minimal interventions need not be confined to medical settings. For example, Robertson and Heather (1982) described the model for an 'alcohol education course' for young offenders with alcohol problems referred from the courts. Of course, in this context, alcohol education refers to much more than information-giving and includes a range of behavioral self-management procedures. This type of course has become very popular and is currently being offered in over 20 centers in Britain by social workers and probation officers (Baldwin and Heather, 1987). However, it has never been properly evaluated in controlled research and this is now proceeding in Dundee.

There is no space here to describe all the many possibilities that arise from the concept of minimal intervention. Suffice it to say that self-help procedures need not be confined to the written word but could be delivered by audiotapes, videotapes and even home computer programs. A wide variety of types of supplementary contact could be used to bolster the effectiveness of brief interventions and a range of professional and paraprofessional groups could be involved. Specific types of problem drinkers, such as drunk-drivers or problem drinkers identified in the workplace, could form the targets of intervention and methods could be adjusted to match the particular situation in which they are used. Indeed, this area is currently one which allows great ingenuity in the design, application and evaluation of minimal interventions.

7. FUTURE PROSPECTS

When making prognostications about the future, it is often difficult to separate out realistic assessments of what is likely to happen from pious hopes as to what ought to occur. This is especially true of the alcohol treatment field, where so much will depend on the extent to which future developments proceed on rational lines, involving a close correspondence between theory, research and practical application, or are mainly determined by sociopolitical changes, the interests of occupational groupings and other less predictable sorts of influence. As a result, the following paragraphs will no doubt contain a mixture of accurate prediction and wishful thinking.

One thing which seems fairly clear is that the days when it was believed that treatment is capable of providing a solution to the national alcohol problem, in the same manner in which a new treatment can provide a cure for a specific disease in the realm of organic medicine, are over. Owing to the great complexity and diversity of alcohol problems and to the general difficulties inherent in changing human behavior inextricably linked to lifestyles and personal philosophies, much less is to be expected from treatment in the future. If one is serious about the ideal of a wholescale reduction in the number of alcohol problems in our society, it must be recognized that the only way this can be achieved is by primary prevention at source. And although education has a vital role to play in this, the only way in which preventive measures can be truly effective is if supported by fiscal policies designed to increase or, at least, stabilize the real price of alcohol. However unpopular with the general public and however electorally risky, these palpable facts must eventually be recognized by government.

While it will thus be necessary to continue to downgrade the relative importance of treatment in national alcohol policy, this does not mean, of course, that efforts to improve the effectiveness of treatment, in the wider sense it has been defined in this article, should be abandoned. On the contrary, several recent broad developments in thinking about treatment promise much for the future once they are fully implemented. Chief among these is the recent emphasis on secondary prevention and early intervention. In moving such attempts at intervention away from the hospital setting and out into the community, and by aiming them at a goal of drinking reduced to safer levels of consumption, this tendency may be fully integrated with new public health initiatives and mass media campaigns on the medical and social dangers of heavy drinking. By such means it may be possible to promote the same kind of change in the public consciousness of excessive alcohol consumption as has happened with cigarette smoking. The message is slightly more complex and difficult to get over, since complete abandonment of the drug is not being urged and the types of damage incurred are considerably more diverse, but these are surely not insuperable problems.

As with nicotine dependence, however, there will remain many individuals who will need specialized help to overcome their dependence on alcohol; there will still be a need to improve intensive treatment for alcohol problems and to find ways of appropriately matching individuals to optimal methods and treatment goals. In this article, there has been no attempt to disguise the view that behavioral treatment methods offer the best prospects in this regard. Besides the methods which have already been shown to be effective, such as the Community Reinforcement Approach (see p. 295) and skills training (see p. 298), and the flexibility of the broad spectrum approach to treatment (p. 298), it is possible that future evaluations of methods based on the principles of relapse prevention (p. 300) and on motivational interviewing (p. 299) will demonstrate a marked improvement in treatment effectiveness. So too, the cue-exposure method (p. 301), when it is fully developed and tested in controlled trials, offers the promise of a highly rational and empirically supported approach to the extinction of alcohol dependence.

These recent reformulations of the change process mark a liberation from the lingering constraints of the disease view of alcohol problems and, in particular, the implicit equation of treatment in the area with a kind of specific, medical procedure. At the same time, they mark the first fully logical explorations of the view that alcohol problems are essentially learned behaviors which can only be permanently modified by a long-term program of cognitive and behavioral relearning. Much remains to be discovered about the determinants of change in such an obstinate and complex behavior as problem drinking but the social learning paradigm represents the most fruitful setting in which such discoveries may be made.

REFERENCES

ALCOHOLICS ANONYMOUS (1955) *The Story of How Thousands of Men and Women Have Recovered from Alcoholism*, AA World Services, New York.

ARMOR, D. J., POLICH, J. M. and STAMBUL, H. B. (1978) *Alcoholism and Treatment*, Wiley, New York.

ASHEM, B. and DONNER, L. (1968) Covert sensitization with alcoholics: a controlled replication. *Behav. Res. Ther.* **6**: 7–12.

AZRIN, N. H. (1976) Improvements in the community reinforcement approach to alcoholism. *Behav. Res. Ther.* **14**: 339–348.

AZRIN, N. H., SISSON, R. W., MEYERS, R. and GODLEY, M. (1982) Alcoholism treatment by disulfiram and community reinforcement therapy. *J. Behav. Ther. Exp. Psychiat.* **13**: 105–112.

BABOR, T. F., TREFFARDIER, M., WEILL, J., FEGEUR, L. and FERRANT, J. P. (1983) The early detection and secondary prevention of alcoholism in France. *J. Stud. Alcohol* **44**: 600–616.

BAEKELAND, F. (1977) Evaluation of treatment methods in chronic alcoholism. In: *The Biology of Alcoholism, (Vol. 5), Treatment and Rehabilitation of the Chronic Alcoholic*, pp. 385–440, KISSIN B. and BEGLEITER, H. (Eds). Plenum Press, New York.

BAEKELAND, F. and LUNDWALL, L. K. (1975) Effects of discontinuity of medication on the results of a double-blind drug study in outpatient alcoholics. *J. Stud. Alcohol* **36**: 1268–1272.

BALDWIN, S. and HEATHER, N. (1987) Alcohol education courses for offenders: a survey of British agencies. *Alcohol Alcohol.* **22**: 79–82.

BANDURA, A. (1977) *Social Learning Theory*, Prentice Hall, Englewood Cliffs, NJ.

BANDURA, A. and ADAMS, N. E. (1977) Analysis of self-efficacy theory of behavioral change. *Cog. Ther. Res.* **1**: 287–310.

BARRY, H. III. (1974) Psychological factors in alcoholism. In: *The Biology of Alcoholism*, Vol. **3**, *Clinical Pathology*, pp. 53–108, KISSIN, B. and BEGLEITER, H. (Eds). Plenum Press, New York.

BILLINGS, A. G. and MOOS, R. H. (1983) Psychosocial processes of recovery among alcoholics and their families: implications for clinicians and program evaluators. *Addict. Behav.* **8**: 205–218.

BLAKEY, R. and BAKER, R. (1980) An exposure approach to alcohol abuse. *Behav. Res. Ther.* **18**: 319–326.

BLUM, E. M. (1966) Psychoanalytic views of alcoholism: a review. *Q. J. Stud. Alcohol* **27**: 259–299.

BRANDSMA, J. M., MAULTSBY, M. C. and WELSH, R. J. (1981) *The Outpatient Treatment of Alcoholism: A Review and Comparative Study*. University Park Press, Baltimore.

BREWER, C. (1984) How effective is the standard dose of disulfiram? A review of the alcohol-disulfiram reaction in practice. *Br. J. Psychiat.* **144**: 200–202.

BREWER, C. (1986) Supervised disulfiram in alcoholism. *Br. J. Hosp. Med.* **35**: 116–119.

BREWER, C. and SMITH, J. (1983) Probation linked supervised disulfiram in the treatment of habitual drunken offenders: results of a pilot study. *Br. Med. J.* **287**: 1282–1283.

CARTWRIGHT, A. (1985) Is treatment an effective way of helping clients resolve difficulties associated with alcohol? In: *The Misuse of Alcohol: Crucial Issues in Dependence, Treatment and Prevention*, pp. 117–134, HEATHER, N., ROBERTSON, I. and DAVIES, P. (Eds). Croom Helm, London.

CAUTELA, J. R. (1970) The treatment of alcoholism by covert sensitization. *Psychotherapy: Theory Res. Pract.* **7**: 86–90.

CHANEY, E. F., O'LEARY, M. R. and MARLATT, G. A. (1978) Skill training with alcoholics. *J. Consult. Clin. Psychol.* **46**: 1092–1104.

CHICK, J. (1984) Secondary prevention of alcoholism and the Centres D'Hygiene Alimentaire. *Br. J. Addict.* **79**: 221–225.

CHICK, J., LLOYD, G. and CROMBIE, E. (1985) Counselling problem drinkers in medical wards: a controlled study. *Br. Med. J.* **290**: 965–967.

CHICK, J., RITSON, B., CONNAUGHTON, J., STEWART, A. and CHICK, J. (1988) Advice versus extended treatment for alcoholism: a controlled study. *Br. J. Addict.* **83**: 159–170.

CLARK, W. B. and CAHALAN, D. (1976) Changes in problem drinking over a four year span. *Addict. Behav.* **1**: 251–260.

CLEMENT, S. (1986) The identification of alcohol-related problems by general practitioners. *Br. J. Addict.* **81**: 257–264.

COSTELLO, R. M. (1975a) Alcoholism treatment and evaluation: in search of methods. *Int. J. Addict.* **10**: 251–275.

COSTELLO, R. M. (1975b) Alcoholism treatment and evaluation: in search of methods. II. Collation of two year follow-up studies. *Int. J. Addict.* **10**: 857–867.

COSTELLO, R. M. (1980) Alcoholism treatment effectiveness: slicing the outcome variance pie. In: *Alcoholism Treatment in Transition*, pp. 113–127, EDWARDS, G. and GRANT, M. (Eds). Croom Helm, London.

CRONKITE, R. C. and MOOS, R. H. (1978) Evaluating alcoholism treatment programs: an integrated approach. *J. Consult. Clin. Psychol.* **46**: 1105–1119.

CRONKITE, R. C. and MOOS, R. H. (1980) Determinants of the posttreatment functioning of alcoholic patients: a conceptual framework. *J. Consult. Clin. Psychol.* **48**: 305–316.

CUMMINGS, C., GORDON, J. R. and MARLATT, G. A. (1980) Relapse: strategies of prevention and prediction. In: *The Addictive Behaviors: Treatment of Alcoholism, Drug Abuse, Smoking and Obesity*, pp. 291–321, MILLER, W. R. (Ed.). Pergamon, Oxford.

DAVIES, D. L. (1962) Normal drinking in recovered alcohol addicts. *Q. J. Stud. Alcohol.* **23**: 93–104.

DEPARTMENT OF HEALTH AND SOCIAL SECURITY (1973) *Community Services for Alcoholics* (Circular 21/73) HMSO, London.

DEPARTMENT OF HEALTH AND SOCIAL SECURITY (1978) *The Pattern and Range of Services for Problem Drinkers*. (Report of Advisory Committee on Alcoholism) HMSO, London.

D'ZURILLA, J. and GOLDFRIED, M. (1971) Problem solving and behavior modification. *J. Abnorm. Psychol.* **78**: 107–126.

EDWARDS, G. (1966) Hypnosis in the treatment of alcohol addiction. *Q. J. Stud. Alcohol.* **27**: 221–241.

EDWARDS, G. and GUTHRIE, S. (1967) A controlled trial of inpatient and outpatient treatment of alcohol dependence. *Lancet* **i**: 555–559.

ELKINS, R. L. (1980) Covert sensitization treatment of alcoholism: contributions of successful conditioning to subsequent abstinence maintenance. *Addict. Behav.* **5**: 67–89.

EMRICK, C. (1975) A review of psychologically oriented treatment of alcoholism. II. The relative effectiveness of different treatment approaches and the effectiveness of treatment versus no treatment. *J. Stud. Alcohol.* **36**: 88–108.

FREEDBERG, E. J. and JOHNSTON, W. E. (1978) The effects of relaxation training within the context of a multimodal alcoholism treatment program for employed alcoholics (Substudy no. 988) Alcoholism and Drug Addiction Research Foundation, Toronto, Ontario.

GAWLINSKI, G. and OTTO, S. (1985) The anatomy of organizational melancholia, or why treatment works on some occasions and not on the others. In: *The Misuse of Alcohol: Crucial Issues in Dependence, Treatment and Prevention*, pp. 178–187, HEATHER, N., ROBERTSON, I. and DAVIES, P. (Eds). Croom Helm, London.

GLASER, S. B. (1980) Anybody got a match? Treatment research and the matching hypothesis. In: *Alcoholism Treatment in Transition*, pp. 178–196, EDWARDS, G. and GRANT, M. (Eds). Croom Helm, London.

HAMBURG, S. (1975) Behavior therapy in alcoholism: a critical review of broad spectrum approaches. *J. Stud. Alcohol.* **36**: 69–87.

HEATHER, N. and ROBERTSON, I. (1983) *Controlled Drinking* (Revised edition) Methuen, London.

HEATHER, N. and ROBERTSON, I. (1986) *Problem Drinking*, Penguin Books, Harmondsworth.

HEATHER, N., WHITTON, B. and ROBERTSON, I. (1986) Evaluation of a self-help manual for media-recruited problem drinkers: six month follow-up results. *Br. J. Clin. Psychol.* **25**: 19–34.

HEATHER, N., ROBERTSON, I., MACPHERSON, B., ALLSOP, S. and FULTON, A. (1987a) Effectiveness of a controlled drinking self-help manual: one year follow-up results. *Br. J. Clin. Psycohl.* **26**: 279–287.

HEATHER, N., CAMPION, P. D., NEVILLE, R. G. and MACCABE, D. (1987b) Evaluation of a controlled drinking minimal intervention for problem drinkers in general practice (the DRAMS Scheme). *J. R. Coll. Gen. Pract.* **37**: 358-363.

HEDBERG, A. G. and CAMPBELL, L. M. (1974) A comparison of four behavioral treatment approaches to alcoholism. *J. Behav. Ther. Exp. Psychiat.* **5**: 251-256.

HODGSON, R. J. and RANKIN, H. J. (1976) Modification of excessive drinking by cue exposure. *Behav. Res. Ther.* **14**: 305-307.

HODGSON, R. J. and RANKIN, H. J. (1982) Cue exposure and relapse prevention. In: *Clinical Case Studies in the Behavioral Treatment of Alcoholism*, pp. 207-226, NATHAN, P. and HAY, W. (Eds). Plenum Press, New York.

HUNT, G. M. and AZRIN, N. H. (1973) A community reinforcement approach to alcoholism. *Behav. Res. Ther.* **11**: 91-104.

JACKSON, T. R. and OEI, T. P. S. (1978) Social skills training and cognitive restructuring with alcoholics. *Drug Alcohol. Depend.* **3**: 369-374.

JONES, R. W. and HELDRICH, A. R. (1972) Treatment of alcoholism by physicians in private practice: a national survey, *Q. J. Stud. Alcohol.* **33**: 117-131.

KANTOROVICH, N. (1930) An attempt at associative-reflex therapy in alcoholism. *Psych. Abs.* **4**: 493.

KEANE, T. M., FOY, D. W., NUNN, B. and RYCHTARIK, R. G. (1984) Spouse contracting to increase antabuse compliance in alcoholic veterans. *J. Clin. Psychol.* **40**: 340-344.

KENDELL, R. E. (1979) Alcoholism: a medical or political problem? *Br. Med. J.* **283**: 367-371.

KISSIN, B. (1977) Comments on "Alcoholism: a controlled trial of 'treatment' and 'advice'". *J. Stud. Alcohol.* **38**: 1804-1808.

KRISTENSON, H., OHLIN, H., HULTEN-NOSSLIN, M., TRELL, E. and HOOD, B. (1983) Identification and intervention of heavy drinking in middle-aged men: results and follow-up of 24:60 months of long-term study with randomized controls. *J. Alcohol. Clin. Exp. Res.* **20**: 203-209.

KRISTENSON, H., TRELL, E. and HOOD, B. (1982) Serum of glutamyl-transferase in screening and continuous control of heavy drinking in middle-aged men. *Am. J. Epidemiol.* **114**: 862-872.

LEVINSON, T. and SERENY, G. (1969) An experimental evaluation of "insight therapy" for the chronic alcoholic. *Can. Psychiat. Ass. J.* **14**: 143-145.

LOVIBOND, S. H. and CADDY, G. (1970) Discriminated aversive control in the moderation of alcoholics' drinking behaviour. *Behav. Ther.* **1**: 437-444.

LUNDWALL, L. and BAEKELAND, F. (1971) Disulfiram treatment of alcoholism. *J. Nerv. Ment. Dis.* **153**: 381-394.

MACCRAE, J. R., SCOLES, M. T. and SIEGEL, S. (1987) The contribution of Pavlovian conditioning to drug tolerance and dependence. *Br. J. Addict.* **82**: 371-380.

MALETZSKY, B. M. (1974) Assisted covert sensitization for drug abuse. *Int. J. Addict.* **9**: 411-429.

MARLATT, G. A. (1983) The controlled drinking controversy: a commentary. *Am. Psychol.* **38**: 1097-1110.

MARLATT, G. A. and GEORGE, W. H. (1984) Relapse prevention: introduction and overview of the model. *Br. J. Addict.* **79**: 261-274.

MARLATT, G. A. and GORDON, J. R. (Eds) (1985) *Relapse Prevention: Maintenance Strategies in the Treatment of Addictive Behaviors*, Guilford, New York.

MARLATT, G. A. and NATHAN, P. E. (Eds) (1978) *Behavioral Approaches to Alcoholism*, Rutgers Center of Alcohol Studies, New Brunswick NJ.

MCCRADY, B. S., MOREAU, J., PAOLINO, T. J., JR. and LONGABOUGH, R. (1982) Joint hospitalization and couples therapy for alcoholism: a four-year follow-up study. *J. Stud. Alcohol.* **43**: 1244-1250.

MILLER, W. R. (1978) Behavioral treatment of problem drinkers: a comparative outcome study of three controlled drinking therapies. *J. Consult. Clin. Psychol.* **46**: 74-86.

MILLER, W. R. (1983a) Motivational interviewing with problem drinkers. *Behav. Psychotherapy* **11**: 147-172.

MILLER, W. R. (1983b) Controlled drinking: a history and critical review. *J. Stud. Alcohol.* **44**: 68-82.

MILLER, W. R. and BACA, L. M. (1983) Two-year follow-up of bibliotherapy and therapist-directed controlled drinking training for problem drinkers. *Behav. Ther.* **14**: 441-448.

MILLER, W. R. and HESTER, R. K. (1980) Treating the problem drinker: modern approaches. In: *The Addictive Behaviors: Treatment of Alcoholism, Drug Abuse, Smoking and Obesity*, pp. 11-141. MILLER, W. R. (Ed.). Pergamon Press, New York.

MILLER, W. R. and HESTER, R. K. (1986a) The effectiveness of alcoholism treatment: what research reveals. In: *Treating Addictive Behaviors: Process of Change*, pp. 121-174, MILLER, W. R. and HEATHER, N. (Eds). Plenum Press, New York.

MILLER, W. R. and HESTER, R. K. (1986b) Matching problem drinkers with optimal treatments. In: *Treating Addictive Behaviors: Processes of Change*, pp. 175-203, MILLER, W. R. and HEATHER, N. (Eds). Plenum Press, New York.

MILLER, W. R. and TAYLOR, C. A. (1980) Relative effectiveness of bibliotherapy, individual and group self-control training in the treatment of problem drinkers. *Addict. Behav.* **5**: 13-24.

MILLER, W. R., TAYLOR, C. S. and WEST, J. C. (1980) Focused versus broad spectrum behavior therapy for problem drinkers. *J. Consult. Clin. Psychol.* **48**: 590-601.

MILLER, W. R., GRIBSKOV, C. and MORTELL, R. (1981) The effectiveness of a self-control manual for problem drinkers with and without therapist contact. *Int. J. Addict.* **16**: 829-839.

MOORE, R. A. and BUCHANAN, T. K. (1966) State hospitals and alcoholism: a nationwide survey of treatment techniques and results. *Q. J. Stud. Alcohol.* **27**: 459-468.

NATHAN, P. E. and BRIDDELL, D. W. (1977) Behavioral assessment and treatment of alcoholism. In: *The Biology of Alcoholism*, Vol. 5, *Treatment and Rehabilitation of the Chronic Alcoholic*, pp. 301-349, KISSIN, B. and BEGLEITER, H. (Eds). Plenum Press, New York.

OEI, T. P. S. and JACKSON, P. (1980) Long-term effects of group and individual social skills training with alcoholics. *Addict. Behav.* **5**: 129-136.

OGBORNE, A. C. and GLASER, F. B. (1981) Characteristics of affiliates of Alcoholics Anonymous: a review of the literature. *J. Stud. Alcohol.* **42**: 661-675.

O'Farrell, T. J., Cutter, H. S. G. and Floyd, F. J. (1985) Evaluating marital therapy for male alcoholics: effects on marital adjustment and communication before to after treatment. *Behav. Ther.* **16**: 147–167.
Ojesjo, L. (1981) Long-term outcome in alcohol abuse and alcoholism among males in the Lundby general population, Sweden. *Br. J. Addict.* **76**: 391–400.
Orford, J. and Edwards, G. (1977) *Alcoholism* (Maudsley Monographs no. 26). Oxford University Press, Oxford.
Orford, J., Oppenheimer, E. and Edwards, E. (1976) Abstinence or control: the outcome for excessive drinkers two years after consultation. *Behav. Res. Ther.* **14**: 409–418.
Pendery, M. L, Maltzman, I. M. and West, L. J. (1982) Controlled drinking by alcoholics? New findings and a reevaluation of a major affirmative study. *Science* **217**: 169–175.
Polich, J. M., Armor, D. J. and Braiker, H. B. (1980) *The Course of Alcoholism: Four Years After Treatment.* The Rand Corporation, Santa Monica CA.
Prochaska, J. O. and DiClemente, C. C. (1986) Toward a comprehensive model of change. In: *Treating Addictive Behaviors: Processes of Change*, pp. 3–27, Miller W. R. and Heather, N. (Eds). Plenum Press, New York.
Prochaska, J. O., DiClemente, C., Velicer, W. F., Ginpil, S. and Norcross, J. (1985) Predicting change in smoking status for self-changers. *Addict. Behav.* **10**: 395–406.
Rachman, S. (1965) Aversion therapy: chemical or electrical. *Behav. Res. Ther.* **2**: 289–299.
Rada, R. T. and Kellner, R. (1979) Drug treatment in alcoholism. In: *Recent Developments in Psychopharmacology*, pp. 105–144, Davis, J. and Greenblatt, D. J. (Eds). Grune and Stratton, New York.
Rankin, H., Hodgson, R. and Stockwell, T. (1983) Cue exposure and response prevention with alcoholics: a controlled trial. *Behav. Res. Ther.* **21**: 435–446.
Revusky, S., Taukulis, H. K., Parker, L. A. and Coombes, S. (1979) Chemical aversion therapy: rat data suggest it may be countertherapeutic to pair an addictive drug state with sickness. *Behav. Res. Ther.* **17**: 177–188.
Robertson, I. and Heather, N. (1982) An alcohol education course for young offenders: preliminary report. *Br. J. Alcohol Alcohol.* **17**: 32–38.
Robertson, I. and Heather, N. (1985) *So You Want to Cut Down Your Drinking? A Self-help Guide to Sensible Drinking.* Scottish Health Education Group, Edinburgh.
Robertson, I., Heather, N., Dzialdowski, A., Crawford, J. and Winton, M. (1986) A comparison of minimal versus intensive controlled drinking treatment interventions for problem drinkers. *Br. J. Clin. Psychol.* **22**: 185–194.
Robinson, D. (1979) *Talking Out of Alcoholism: The Self-Help Process of Alcoholics Anonymous*, Croom Helm, London.
Roizen, R. Cahalan, D. and Shanks, P. (1978) "Spontaneous remission" among untreated problem drinkers. In: *Longitudinal Research on Drug Use*, pp. 197–221, Kandel, D. (Ed.). Wiley, New York.
Rosenberg, S. D. (1979) Relaxation Training and Differential Assessment of Alcoholism (Unpublished doctoral dissertation) Cited in Miller, W. R. and Hester, R. K. (1986a, op. cit., p. 151).
Royal College of General Practitioners (1986) *Alcohol: A Balanced View*, RCGP, London.
Royal College of Physicians (1987) *A Great and Growing Evil*, Tavistock, London.
Sanchez-Craig, M. and Lei, H. (1986) Disadvantages of imposing the goal of abstinence on problem drinkers: an empirical study. *Br. J. Addict.* **81**: 505–512.
Sanderson, R. E., Campbell, D. and Laverty, S. G. (1963) An investigation of a new aversive conditioning treatment for alcoholism. *Q. J. Stud. Alcohol* **24**: 261–275.
Saunders,W. (1985) The case for controlling alcohol comsumption. In: *The Misuse of Alcohol: Crucial Issues in Dependence, Treatment and Prevention*, pp. 214–231, Heather, N., Robertson, I. and Davies, P. (Eds). Croom Helm, London.
Saunders, W. and Allsop, S. (1987) Relapse: a psychological perspective. *Br. J. Addict.* **82**: 417–429.
Saunders, W. and Kershaw, P. (1979) Spontaneous remission from alcoholism: results from a community survey. *Br. J. Addict.* **74**: 251–265.
Schaefer, H. H., Sobell, M. B. and Miller, K. C. (1971) Some sobering data on the use of self-confrontation with alcoholics. *Behav. Ther.* **2**: 28–39.
Shaw, S., Cartwright, A., Spratley, T. and Harwin, J. (1978) *Resonding to Drinking Problems*, Croom Helm, London.
Siegel, S. (1983) Classical conditioning, drug tolerance and drug dependence. In: *Recent Advances in Alcohol and Drug Problems* (Vol. 7), pp. 207–246, Israel, Y., Glaser, H., Kalant, H., Popham, R. E., Schmidt, W. and Smart, R. G. (Eds). Plenum Press, New York.
Skinner, B. F. (1938) *The Behavior of Organisms*, Appleton-Century, New York
Sobell, M. B. and Sobell, L. C. (1973) Individualized behavior therapy for alcoholics. *Behav. Ther.* **4**: 49–72.
Sobell, M. B. and Sobell, L. C. (1976) Second-year treatment outcome of alcoholics treated by individualized behavior therapy: results. *Behav. Res. Ther.* **14**: 195–215.
Stockwell, T. and Clement, S. (1987) *Helping the Problem Drinker: New Initiatives in Community Care.* Croom Helm, London.
Stuart, R. B. (1969) Operant-interpersonal treatment for the marital discord. *J. Consult. Clin. Psychol.* **33**: 675–682.
Thom, B. and Tellez, C. (1986) A difficult business: detecting and managing alcohol problems in general practice. *Br. J. Addict.* **81**: 405–418.
Thorley, A. (1980) Medical responses to problem drinking. *Medicine (3rd Ser.)* **35**: 1816–1822.
Thorley, A. (1983) Rehabilitation of problem drinkers and drug takers. In: *Theory and Practice of Psychiatric Rehabilitation*, pp. 83–114, Watts, F. N. and Bennett, D. H. (Eds). Wiley, London.
Tuchfeld, B. (1976) *Changes in Patterns of Alcohol Use Without the Aid of Formal Treatment.* Center for Health Studies, Research Triangle Institute, North Carolina.
Vaillant, G. E. (1983) *The Natural History of Alcoholism*, Harvard University Press, Cambridge.

VOEGTLIN, W. L. and BROZ, W. R. (1949) The conditioned reflex treatment of chronic alcoholism. X. An analysis of 3125 admissions over a period of ten and a half years. *Ann. Intern. Med.* **30**: 580–597.

VOEGTLIN, W. L., LEMERE, F., BROZ, W. R. and O'HOLLARAN, P. (1941) Conditioned reflex therapy of chronic alcoholism. IV. A preliminary report on the value of reinforcement. *Q. J. Stud. Alcohol.* **2**: 505–511.

VOEGTLIN, W. L., LEMERE, F., BROZ, W. R. and O'HOLLARAN, P. (1942) Conditioned reflex therapy of chronic alcoholism. V. Follow-up report of 1042 cases. *Am. J. Med. Sci.* **203**: 525–528.

WORLD HEALTH ORGANIZATION (1951) Report of the First Session of the Alcoholism Subcommittee (Public Health Paper no. 3) WHO, Geneva.

YATES, F. (1985) Does treatment work? Yes, but not always in the way we plan it. In: *The Misuse of Alcohol: Crucial Issues in Dependence, Treatment and Prevention*, pp. 148–157, HEATHER, N., ROBERTSON, I. and DAVIES, P. (Eds). Croom Helm, London.

CHAPTER 10

ELECTROPHYSIOLOGY OF PSYCHOTOMIMETIC DRUGS

KURT RASMUSSEN AND GEORGE K. AGHAJANIAN

Department of Psychiatry and Pharmacology, Yale University School of Medicine, Connecticut Mental Health Center and the Abraham Ribicoff Research Facilities, 34 Park Street, New Haven, CT 06508, U.S.A.

1. PSYCHEDELICS

There are two major classes of psychedelic hallucinogenic drugs, the indoleamines and the phenethylamines. Despite differences in chemical structures between the two groups a common site of action has been proposed. This hypothesis is supported by behavioral studies showing that (1) cross-tolerance develops between the two groups of hallucinogens (Appel and Freedman, 1968); (2) phenethylamines and indoleamines generalize to each other in drug-discrimination tests (Glennon *et al.*, 1979, 1983b); (3) the two groups have similar effects on autonomic function and behavior in man (Hollister, 1978; Wolbach *et al.*, 1962); and (4) both have affinity for the 5-HT_2 receptor which correlates with their psychotomimetic potency (see below). However, until recently, a common site of action for the two groups has been difficult to demonstrate using electrophysiological techniques. This section will describe electrophysiological evidence for the major hypotheses of the mechanism of action of psychedelic hallucinogens, including a discussion of some common sites of action.

1.1. SEROTONIN DISINHIBITORY HYPOTHESIS

1.1.1. *LSD and Other Indoleamines*

Partly because of its structural similarity to the endogenous indoleamine serotonin (5-hydroxytryptamine; 5-HT), it was thought that LSD might act upon 5-HT receptors in the CNS (Gaddum, 1953; Woolley and Shaw, 1954; Freedman, 1961). The first direct evidence for an effect of LSD on the 5-HT neuronal system came with the demonstration that small intravenous doses of LSD inhibit the firing of 5-HT neurons in the raphe nuclei of rats (Aghajanian *et al.*, 1968, 1970). Initially, it was suggested that LSD might inhibit 5-HT neurons through a negative feedback circuit by acting as an agonist on postsynaptic neurons (Aghajanian *et al.*, 1968; Anden *et al.*, 1968). However, subsequent studies have shown that LSD has a powerful direct inhibitory action upon 5-HT neurons in the raphe when applied by microiontophoresis (Aghajanian *et al.*, 1972; Bramwell and Gonye, 1976). Moreover, the inhibition of 5-HT neurons by LSD is more pronounced than its inhibitory effect upon neurons receiving an identified serotonergic input in several visual and limbic areas (Haigler and Aghajanian, 1974b; deMontigny and Aghajanian, 1977). In contrast, 5-HT itself shows no such preferential activity. The 2-bromo derivative of LSD, which has minimal hallucinogenic effects, also fails to show such preferential action (Aghajanian, 1976). From these results it was hypothesized that, by inhibiting 5-HT neurons directly, LSD could release postsynaptic neurons from a tonic inhibitory 5-HT influence; such a release or disinhibition might account for the sensory, cognitive, and other disturbances caused by LSD. The finding of increased activity of some neurons in the lateral geniculate nucleus, amygdala, and other areas after low doses of LSD was consistent with this idea (Mouriz-Garcia *et al.*, 1969; Guilbaud *et al.*, 1973; Horn and McKay, 1973; Haigler and Aghajanian, 1974b).

Studies using three other indoleamine hallucinogenic drugs, psilocin (4-hydroxy-*N,N*-dimethyltryptamine), DMT (*N,N*-dimethyltryptamine), and 5-methoxy-*N,N*-dimethyltryptamine supported this disinhibitory hypothesis; these three hallucinogens also had a preferential inhibitory action upon 5-HT neurons as compared to postsynaptic neurons in the lateral geniculate (ventral nucleus) and amygdala (Aghajanian and Haigler, 1975; deMontigny and Aghajanian, 1977). On the other hand, there was only a slight difference between the pre- and postsynaptic actions of bufotenine (5-hydroxy-*N,N*-dimethyltryptamine). In general, these results paralleled the known hallucinogenic (or psychotogenic) actions of these compounds. Except for LSD and some of its congeners, psilocin is the most potent of the indoleamine hallucinogens that have been tested in human subjects (Wolbach *et al.*, 1962). The effects of another powerful indoleamine hallucinogen, psilocybin (4-phosphoryl-*N,N*-dimethyltryptamine) are most probably mediated through its rapid metabolic conversion to psilocin (Horita, 1963). The physiologic effects of DMT are similar to those of LSD and psilocin except for its lesser potency (Szara, 1956; Rosenberg *et al.*, 1964). On the other hand, even high doses of bufotenine have little hallucinogenic action (Fabing and Hawkins, 1956; Turner and Merlis, 1959).

The actions of one indoleamine, the ergoline lisuride, did not fit with this disinhibitory hypothesis. Lisuride is an ergoline derivative which is structurally similar to LSD. However, unlike LSD, lisuride does not produce hallucinations in man and, in fact, has been evaluated for use in the prophylaxis of migraine headache (Herrman *et al.*, 1977) and in the treatment of hyperprolactinemic states (Liuzzi *et al.*, 1978); Horowski *et al.*, 1978). In common with some but not all chemically related ergot alkaloids (Burki *et al.*, 1978; Fuxe *et al.*, 1978), lisuride reduces 5-HT and dopamine (DA) turnover and, at higher doses, increases NE turnover (Kehr, 1977; Pieri *et al.*, 1978). However, as previously demonstrated for LSD, extremely small doses of lisuride have been found to produce a rapid, dose-dependent suppression of 5-HT neuronal activity (Rogawski and Aghajanian, 1979). In microiontophoretic experiments, both lisuride and LSD produce a complete suppression of most raphe units studied, but, for equivalent iontophoretic currents the recovery with lisuride is more prolonged. These results suggest that lisuride, like LSD, has a direct agonist action at 5-HT autoreceptors.

Electrophysiological and behavioral studies of LSD in unanesthetized cats have also failed to support the disinhibitory hypothesis (Trulson and Jacobs, 1978; Trulson *et al.*, 1981). The behavioral effects of hallucinogenic drugs in awake, freely moving cats were examined while simultaneously recording the activity of 5-HT neurons. Both LSD and 5-methoxy-*N,N*-dimethyltryptamine decreased the activity of 5-HT neurons in a dose-dependent manner in association with increases in behaviors that are characteristically produced by hallucinogenic drugs in cats (e.g. the limb flick response). In the case of 5-methoxy-*N,N*-dimethyltryptamine, the onset, offset, and peak of the behavioral effects were temporally correlated with changes in neuronal activity. The results of LSD were in general similar to those seen with 5-methoxy-*N,N*-dimethyltryptamine. However, in the case of LSD the behavioral effects outlasted the depression of 5-HT neuronal activity. Furthermore, when LSD was readministered the next day, it produced little or no behavioral effect, but the depression in 5-HT cell activity was as large as that on the first day. In addition, pretreatment of animals with the serotonin antagonist mianserin was able to completely block the behavioral effects of LSD, but failed to alter the LSD-induced depression of 5-HT neuronal activity (Heym *et al.*, 1984).

1.1.2. *Mescaline and Other Phenethylamines*

Systemic administration of mescaline (2-4 mg/kg, i.v.) has been found to inhibit a subpopulation of 5-HT neurons located within the ventral portion of the dorsal raphe nucleus and adjacent areas of the median raphe nucleus (Aghajanian *et al.*, 1970). A similar subpopulation of raphe neurons are inhibited by 2,5-dimethoxy-4-methylamphetamine (DOM), a potent phenethylamine hallucinogen. When LSD is administered systemically in doses comparable to those that produce behavioral effects, the firing of serotonergic neurons in the raphe nuclei of the brainstem is reversibly inhibited (see above). When LSD is administered microiontophoretically a similar inhibition is obtained (Aghajanian *et al.*, 1972). These data, coupled with the fact that after the systemic administration of mescaline a subpopulation of raphe neurons is inhibited (Aghajanian *et al.*, 1970), indicate that there may exist a subpopulation of raphe neurons that would be inhibited by the microiontophoretic application of mescaline. However, this expectation was not borne out by studies in which the effects of microiontophoretically and systemically applied mescaline are compared (Haigler and Aghajanian, 1973). Although some raphe neurons are partially depressed by the microiontophoretic application of mescaline, this effect may represent a local anesthetic action and is not correlated with the inhibition produced by mescaline given intravenously. On the other hand, some raphe cells are unaffected by the microiontophoretic application of mescaline, but are completely inhibited by the systemic administration of mescaline. The failure to obtain a response to mescaline, even under extreme conditions, from cells that are very sensitive to systemic mescaline does not support the view that the action of systemic mescaline on these raphe neurons is a direct one. In contrast, certain cortical neurons are highly responsive to the direct application of mescaline with no reported local anesthetic effect (Bradshaw *et al.*, 1971). In the raphe there is no correlation between the response to mescaline and NE administered microiontophoretically (Haigler and Aghajanian, 1973) as has been reported for cortical cells (Bradshaw *et al.*, 1971). Moreover, in the raphe there is no relationship between responses to i.v. mescaline and responses to NE given iontophoretically. In addition, the administration of DOM or mescaline does not produce consistent effects on raphe unit activity in unanesthetized cats (Trulson *et al.*, 1981). Thus, the actions of phenethylamine hallucinogens in the raphe do not support the serotonin disinhibitory hypothesis.

1.2. Psychedelics as 5-HT$_2$ Agonists

1.2.1. *Background*

The possibility that multiple 5-HT receptors exist in the CNS was first suggested by microiontophoretic studies in the cerebral cortex (Roberts and Straughan, 1967) and subcortical regions (Haigler and Aghajanian, 1974a). In these early experiments, putative 5-HT antagonists such as methysergide and cinanserin blocked excitatory but not inhibitory effects of 5-HT, indicating that at least two types of 5-HT receptors may be present in the brain, one for excitation and one for inhibition. Subsequently, radioligand binding techniques disclosed the presence of multiple 5-HT binding sites in the brain, termed 5-HT$_1$ and 5-HT$_2$ (Peroutka and Snyder, 1979).

Recently, a group of studies has shown that indoleamine and phenethylamine hallucinogens share the common property of interacting with 5-HT$_2$ receptors. (Indoleamines also act as 5-HT$_1$ agonists—which accounts for their inhibition of raphe cell firing—see below.) Receptor binding studies have shown that there is a strong correlation between the 5-HT$_2$ binding affinities of indoleamine and phenethylamine hallucinogens and hallucinogenic potency in humans (Glennon *et al.*, 1984) and behavioral studies have shown that selective 5-HT$_2$ antagonists block the effects of either indoleamine or phenethylamine hallucinogens (Colpaert *et al.*, 1985; Mokler *et al.*, 1985; Glennon *et al.*, 1983a; Heym *et al.*, 1984). The role of hallucinogens as 5-HT$_2$ agonists has also been supported by electrophysiological studies.

1.2.2. *Actions of Psychedelic Hallucinogens in the Locus Coeruleus*

The locus coeruleus (LC) is one of the few places in the rat brain where indoleamine and phenethylamine hallucinogens have been demonstrated to have a common electrophysiological action. In anesthetized rats, systemically administered mescaline or LSD induces a decrease in the spontaneous activity of noradrenergic cells in the LC but, paradoxically, facilitates the activation of these cells by tactile stimuli (Aghajanian, 1980). That the effects of LSD and mescaline on LC neurons are mediated by 5-HT$_2$ receptors is suggested by the fact that they can be reversed not only by the classical 5-HT antagonists such as cinanserin (Aghajanian *et al.*, 1987) but also by the newer, more selective 5-HT$_2$ antagonists such as ritanserin and LY-53857 (Rasmussen and Aghajanian, 1986; Figs. 1, 2).

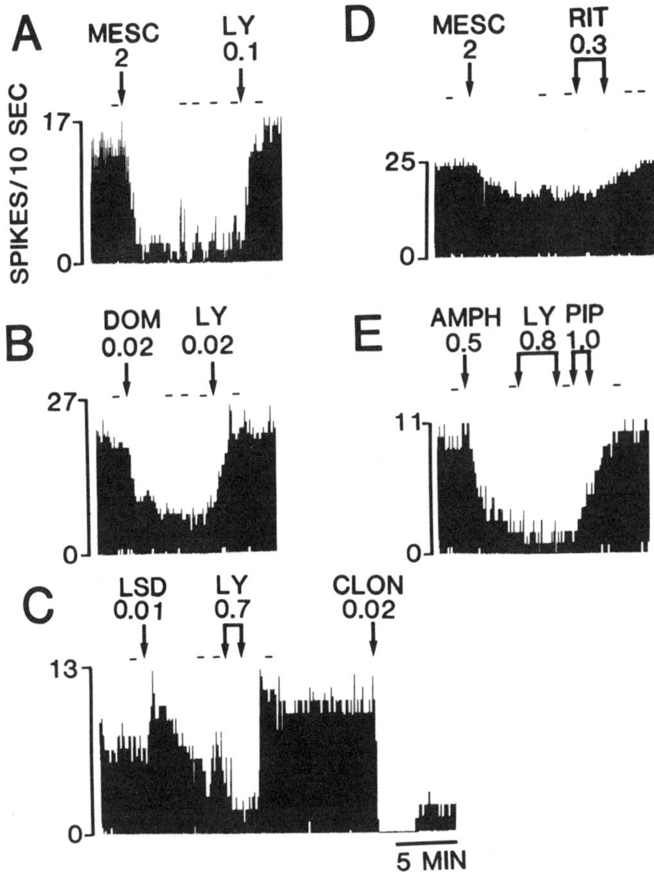

FIG. 1. Effects of mescaline (MESC; A), DOM (B), and LSD (C) followed by LY 53857 (LY); mescaline followed by ritanserin (RIT; D); and (+)-amphetamine (AMPH; E) followed by LY 53857 and piperoxane (PIP) on LC unit activity. In C clonidine was administered after the test drugs as an additional confirmation of the noradrenergic identity of the cell and to demonstrate that the drugs previously administered did not affect the α_2 receptors on the LC neurons. Drugs were given by slow i.v. infusion (arrows: numbers refer to dose in mg/kg). Bars represent periods of sciatic nerve stimulation. Reprinted by permission of publisher from Rasmussen and Aghajanian (1986). Copyright 1986 by Elsevier Science Publishing Co., Inc.

In addition, 1-(2,5-dimethoxy-4-methylphenyl)-2-aminopropane (DOM) and two hallucinogenic structural analogs of DOM [(+) and (−)DOB] have extremely potent mescaline-like action on LC neurons, while a nonhallucinogenic structural analog of DOM (SL-7161) has no effect on LC neurons (Rasmussen *et al.*, 1986; Fig. 3). Thus, the relative potencies of hallucinogens in their action on LC neurons correlates with their affinity for 5-HT_2 receptors (Glennon *et al.*, 1984). However, this action of hallucinogens is not a direct one as the effects of these drugs given systemically are not mimicked by their iontophoretic application onto LC cell bodies (Aghajanian, unpublished observations). Moreover, the systemic administration of mescaline or LSD does not enhance the excitation of LC neurons evoked by microiontophoretically applied acetylcholine, glutamate or substance P (Aghajanian, 1980). These results imply that the hallucinogens are acting on afferents to the LC, afferents that are affected directly, or indirectly, by 5-HT_2 receptors. When these 5-HT_2 receptors are activated they facilitate the response of the LC to peripheral stimuli. Presumably, the relevant afferents to the LC arise from various sensory relay nuclei in the spinal cord and lower brainstem. However, since 5-HT_2 receptors are not located in high densities in these nuclei (Pazos *et al.*, 1985), it is possible that other areas of the brain which are rich in 5-HT_2 receptors send efferents to these sensory relay nuclei and/or directly to the LC.

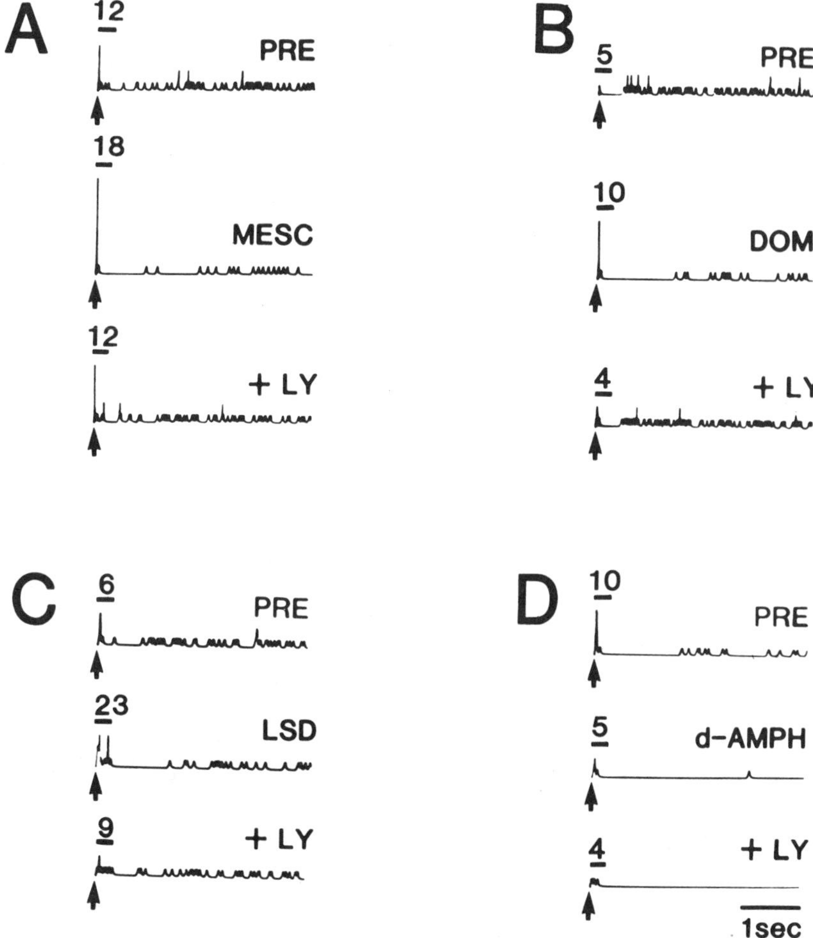

FIG. 2. Post-stimulus time histograms during locus coeruleus cell recordings before and after the administration of mescaline (MESC; A). DOM (B), LSD (C), or (+)-amphetamine (d-AMPH; D) and again after the administration of LY 53857 (LY). Each histogram was generated from 10 sweeps initiated by sciatic nerve stimulation (arrows). Evoked spikes occurred during the first 250 msec of each histogram (bars); the total number of evoked spikes occurring during this period is given above the bars. Note both the increased number of spikes evoked by sciatic nerve stimulation (initial 250 msec of histogram) and the decrease in spontaneous activity (remainder of histogram) after LSD, DOM, or mescaline administration. In addition, following hallucinogen administration, the increased number of spikes evoked by sciatic nerve stimulation, combined with the decrease in spontaneous activity, leads to a prolonged period of post-activation inhibition. Also note the reversal of these effects after LY 53587 administration. After (+)-amphetamine administration both the spontaneous activity and the number of evoked spikes are decreased; the subsequent administration of LY 53857 does not reverse either of these effects. Reprinted by permission of publisher from Rasmussen and Aghajanian (1986). Copyright 1986 by Elsevier Science Publishing Co., Inc.

1.2.3. *Antipsychotic Drugs: A 5-HT$_2$ Component of Their Actions*

Recent studies have shown that the 5-HT$_2$ receptor may play a role in antipsychotic drug action. Binding studies have shown that most antipsychotics have affinity for 5-HT$_2$ receptors in addition to dopamine receptors (Peroutka and Snyder, 1980). In fact, a few antipsychotics (e.g. clozapine) have a much higher affinity for 5-HT$_2$ receptors than dopamine receptors. This potency at 5-HT$_2$ receptors may be important for the lack of extrapyramidal side effects seen with some antipsychotics (Altar *et al.*, 1986). Using electrophysiological techniques we have been able to demonstrate functional activity of some antipsychotics at 5-HT$_2$ receptors. In the locus coeruleus (see above) selective 5-HT$_2$ antagonists reverse the actions of 5-HT$_2$ agonists (i.e. hallucinogens; Fig. 4). Antipsy-

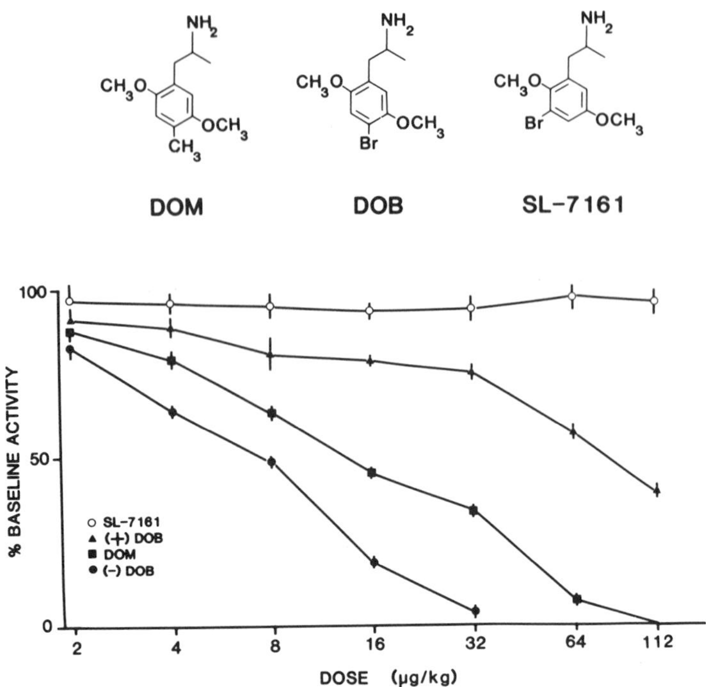

FIG. 3. Structure DOM, DOB and SL-7161 and the effects of systemic administration of these compounds on LC unit activity in anesthetized rats. Each point represents the geometric mean of 3-11 cells, and vertical bars are S.D. of the geometric mean. Reprinted by permission of the publisher from Rasmussen *et al.* (1986). Copyright 1986 by Elsevier Science Publishing Co., Inc.

chotics with 5-HT_2 binding affinity (including spiperone—a compound that has relatively low affinity for the 5-HT_{ic} receptor) are also able to reverse the actions of hallucinogens in the locus coerulus independent of their actions at dopamine and adrenoceptors (Rasmussen and Aghajanian, 1988). In addition, 5-HT_2 antagonists have been shown to reverse the depression of A9 to A10 dopamine neurons caused by *d*-amphetamine administration, an effect that is characteristic of antipsychotic drugs, raising the possibility that 5-HT_2 antagonists may display a form of antipsychotic action in man (Goldstein *et al.*, 1986).

1.2.4. *Actions of Psychedelic Hallucinogens in the Facial Motor Nucleus*

While there generally are very few 5-HT_2 binding sites in the brainstem, one exception is the facial motor nucleus (Pazos *et al.*, 1985). In this nucleus the microiontophoretic application of 5-HT or norepinephrine does not by itself induce firing in quiescent facial motoneurons but does facilitate the subthreshold and threshold excitatory effects of iontophoretically applied glutamate (McCall and Aghajanian, 1979a). A similar effect of 5-HT and norepinephrine on glutamate excitation of spinal motoneurons has also been documented (White and Neuman, 1980). Activation of 5-HT receptors on facial motoneurons has since been shown to cause a slow depolarization, increased input resistance and increased excitability, probably through a decrease in resting membrane conductance to potassium (VanderMaelen and Aghajanian, 1982a,b).

The facilitation of glutamate excitation by the activation of 5-HT receptors on facial motoneurons appears to be physiologically relevant since: (1) the facial nucleus receives a dense and uniform 5-HT input (Fuxe, 1965; Palkovits *et al.*, 1974); (2) the release of endogenous 5-HT following iontophoresis of the 5-HT releasing agent *p*-chloroamphetamine mimics the effects of iontophoretic 5-HT (McCall and Aghajanian, 1979a); (3) the destruction of the 5-HT terminals with 5,7-dihydroxytryptamine significantly decreases the ejecting current of 5-HT required to excite facial motoneurons (McCall and Aghajanian, 1979b); (4) the activation of facial motoneurons produced by electrical stimulation of the motor

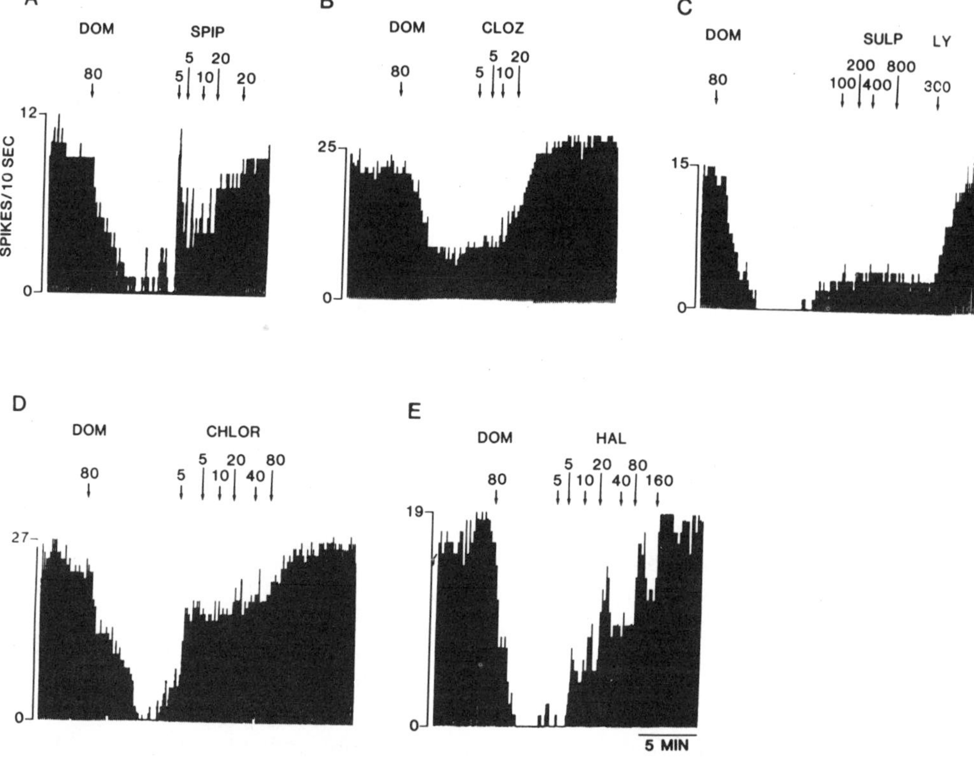

FIG. 4. Effects of DOM followed by spiperone (SPIP; A), clozapine (CLOZ; B), sulpiride (SULP; C), haloperidol (HAL; D), and chlorpromazine (CHLOR; E) on LC unit activity. Note that in some cases administration of the antipsychotic drug produced a transient increase in activity of the LC cell. Such transient increases may be related to the local irritant effects of the injection. In C a selective 5-HT_2 antagonist that is known to reverse the effects of DOM (Rasmussen and Aghajanian, 1986) (LY 53857) was administered after sulpiride. Drugs were given by slow i.v. infusion (arrows; numbers refer to doses in μg/kg). Reprinted by permission of the publisher from Rasmussen and Aghajanian (1987). Copyright 1987 by Elsevier Science Publishing Co., Inc.

cortex or red nucleus is potentiated by the microiontophoretic application of 5-HT (McCall and Aghajanian, 1979a).

An action of 5-HT on 5-HT_2 receptors would appear to be mainly responsible for producing 5-HT-mediated headshakes since these behavioral effects can be blocked by the selective 5-HT_2 antagonists ketanserin and pipamperone (Lucki *et al.*, 1984). The action of iontophoretically applied 5-HT in the facial nucleus can be blocked by the classical 5-HT antagonists metergoline, methysergide, cyproheptadine and cinanserin (McCall and Aghajanian, 1980a). However, as all of these antagonists have been shown to interact with both the 5-HT_1 and 5-HT_2 receptors, with greater affinity for 5-HT_2 receptors (Leysen *et al.*, 1981), it is conceivable that the action of 5-HT in the facial motor nucleus involves 5-HT_2 receptors. As mentioned above, a large number of studies, using behavioral as well as binding techniques, have shown that indoleamine and phenethylamine hallucinogens share the property of interacting with 5-HT_2 receptors (Buckholtz *et al.*, 1985; Colpaert *et al.*, 1985; Glennon *et al.*, 1983a, 1984; Heym *et al.*, 1984; Mokler *et al.*, 1985). Therefore, one would expect members of both classes of hallucinogens to have direct effects in the facial motor nucleus. Thus, it is of interest that the iontophoretic administration of LSD, mescaline or psilocin, although having relatively little effect by itself at low doses, markedly enhances the facilitation of facial motoneuron excitation produced by iontophoretically applied 5-HT and norepinephrine (McCall and Aghajanian, 1980b); curiously, the enhancement can persist for several hours after only a single application of a hallucinogen. In essence, the hallucinogens facilitate the facilitation produced by 5-HT and norepinephrine. Two nonhallucinogenic ergot derivatives, lisuride and methysergide, do not enhance the facilitatory effects of 5-HT and norepinephrine, suggesting that the phenomenon is specific to hallucinogens.

1.2.5. *Indoleamine Hallucinogens as 5-HT$_{1A}$ Agonists*

Binding studies have shown that the 5-HT$_1$ receptor can be subdivided into 5-HT$_{1A}$, 5-HT$_{1B}$. 5-HT$_{1C}$ and 5-HT$_{1D}$ subtypes. A 5-HT agonist 8-hydroxy-2-(di-*n*-propylamino) tetralin (8-OH-DPAT; Arvidsson *et al.*, 1981) possesses an almost 1000-fold selectivity for the 5-HT$_{1A}$ binding site (Middlemiss and Fozard, 1983) and both small intravenous doses and iontophoretic application of this compound were found to inhibit the firing rate of 5-HT neurons in the dorsal raphe of the chloral hydrate anesthetized rat (Fallon *et al.*, 1983; deMontigny *et al.*, 1984). In addition, buspirone, a purported non-benzodiazepine anxiolytic which displays 5-HT$_{1A}$ binding properties (Peroutka, 1985), also has been shown in extracellular recordings to potently inhibit the firing of 5-HT dorsal raphe neurons when administered systemically, microiontophoretically, or added to media bathing brain slices (VanderMaelen *et al.*, 1986). Buspirone has also been shown to slow dorsal raphe cell firing when it is administered to awake, freely moving cats (Trulson and Trulson, 1986; Wilkinson *et al.*, 1987). Selective 5-HT$_{1B}$ compounds, when applied by microiontophoresis, are only weak autoreceptor agonists, and do not strongly affect the firing rate of dorsal raphe neurons (Sprouse and Aghajanian, 1987).

Binding studies have indicated that indoleamine, but not phenethylamine, hallucinogens have affinity for 5-HT$_1$ sites (Glennon *et al.*, 1984) and that indoleamines are selective for the 5-HT$_{1A}$ site (Peroutka, 1986). Given the actions of 5-HT$_{1A}$ selective compounds on dorsal raphe firing, this difference could explain why indoleamine hallucinogens but not phenethylamine hallucinogens, are able to inhibit the firing of dorsal raphe neurons (where a high density of 5-HT$_{1A}$ receptors are located—Pazos and Palacios, 1985).

PHENCYCLIDINE

2.1. ACTIONS ON MONOAMINE-CONTAINING NEURONS

Phencyclidine (PCP) is a dissociative anesthetic that is a widely abused street drug ('angel dust'). In man, PCP is capable of producing psychotic symptoms which resemble some features of schizophrenia (Snyder, 1980; Pradhan, 1984). Partly due to this ability to mimic some aspects of psychosis, a great deal of attention has been focused on PCP's interactions with dopamine-containing neurons.

On dopamine-containing cell bodies, PCP has been found to have a variety of actions. For substantia nigra dopamine neurons (A9) one study reports an increase in firing rate of a subpopulation of cells (Raja and Guyenet, 1980), while another reports biphasic responses (increases followed by decreases with increasing dose) (Freeman and Bunney, 1984) following intravenous administration of PCP. Iontophoretic application of PCP onto substantia nigra cells has only weak inhibitory actions (Freeman and Bunney, 1984). For ventral tegmental area dopamine neurons (A10) one study reports either increases or decreases in firing rate (French, 1986), while another study reports biphasic responses (increases followed by decreases with increasing dose—as seen for A9 cells) (Freeman and Bunney, 1984) following intravenous administration of PCP. Iontophoretic application of PCP has been reported to inhibit a subset (Freeman and Bunney, 1984) or the vast majority (French, 1986) of A10 cells. Some of these results may be explained by an indirect action of PCP on the dopamine system. This hypothesis states that PCP increases the postsynaptic effects of dopamine either by augmenting the release of dopamine or by blocking its reuptake. This indirect dopamine agonist property of PCP may be more apparent at dopamine nerve terminals and has been demonstrated by electrophysiological studies in the rat caudate nucleus (Johnson *et al.*, 1984) and prefrontal cortex (Gratton *et al.*, 1987).

PCP's effects on serotonin and norepinephrine neurons have also been examined. Intravenous administration of PCP was found to have little effect on the activity of serotonergic neurons of the dorsal raphe (Raja and Guyenet, 1980), indicating that PCP may not interact with autoreceptors on serotonin cell bodies (i.e. the 5-HT_1 receptor). However, several recent behavioral studies have suggested that PCP produces its behavioral effects via an agonistic interaction with the 5-HT_2 receptor (Nabeshima *et al.*, 1986; 1987a,b). An interaction with 5-HT_2 receptors could be one possible mechanism for PCP evoked hallucinations. PCP administered either intravenously (Raja and Guyenet, 1980) or iontophoretically (Marwaha, 1982) to anesthetized rats decreases the firing rate of norepinephrine-containing locus coeruleus neurons. However, intracellular recordings of locus coeruleus neurons in the brain slice preparation showed that PCP had no effect on membrane potential, input resistance or spontaneous activity, but did decrease the response of locus coeruleus neurons to *N*-methyl-D-aspartic acid (NMDA), norepinephrine and enkephalin (Lacey and Henderson, 1986).

2.2. Interaction with the NMDA-Linked Ion Channel

PCP's blockade of NMDA-induced excitation seen in locus coeruleus neurons has been seen in other types of cells and may be important for the actions of PCP and other dissociative anesthetics (e.g. ketamine). Extracellular *in vivo* recordings have shown that PCP (and ketamine) selectively block the excitation of rat and cat spinal neurons produced by the iontophoretic application of NMDA (Anis *et al.*, 1983). Biochemical studies support this hypothesis and have shown that PCP selectively inhibits NMDA-induced release of norepinephrine in the hippocampus (Jones *et al.*, 1987b) and NMDA-induced release of acetylcholine and dopamine in the nucleus accumbens (Jones *et al.*, 1987a) and the striatum (Snell and Johnson, 1986).

While PCP may block the excitation produced by NMDA, it probably does not directly bind to the NMDA receptor. Instead, it has been hypothesized that the PCP binding site may be part of a macromolecular complex that includes the NMDA receptor and that PCP interacts with the voltage-sensitive cation channel of the receptor complex (Honey *et al.*, 1985; Foster and Wong, 1987; Snell and Johnson, 1986). Originally this PCP binding site was hypothesized to be the same as the sigma opiod binding site; however, recent studies have shown that the PCP and sigma opiate receptors have different ligand selectivity profiles and different anatomical distributions (Adams *et al.*, 1987; Largent *et al.*, 1986).

An interaction with the NMDA macromolecular complex in parts of the brain where PCP binding sites are densest could explain some of the behavioral actions of the drug. For example, the highest concentrations of PCP binding sites are found in the hippocampus and the cerebral cortex (Contreras *et al.*, 1986). As NMDA receptors in the hippocampus have been shown to play an important role in long-term potentiation (Harris *et al.*, 1984), blockade of NMDA-linked ion channels by PCP may account for the drug's effects on memory. Further, blockade of NMDA-linked ion channels in the cerebral cortex may play a role in the cognitive and sensory disturbances seen during PCP intoxication.

3. CONCLUSIONS

The original serotonin disinhibitory hypothesis proposed for psychedelic hallucinogenic drug action was based largely on the actions of indoleamine hallucinogens in anesthetized rats. These studies showed that indoleamine hallucinogens were more potent at inhibiting the activity of serotonin-containing cells in the dorsal raphe than at mimicking the serotonin-induced depression of post-synaptic cells in areas that received serotonergic projections. Thus, it was hypothesized that psychedelic hallucinogens exerted their actions by inhibiting the serotonergic system, which in turn released postsynaptic cells from a tonic inhibition produced by serotonin. However, subsequent studies revealed that phenethylamine hallucinogens do not share this depressant action on serotonin cells with the indoleamines. Also, studies done in unanesthetized animals showed that there are important dissociations between the behavioral effects of indoleamine hallucinogens and their actions on serotonin cell bodies. (The action of indoleamines on serotonergic cell bodies has since been shown to be due to an agonist action at 5-HT_{1A} receptors.) The advent of selective 5-HT_2 antagonists has led to a great number of experiments, using a variety of techniques, supporting the hypothesis that psychedelic hallucinogens exert their actions through an agonist interaction at 5-HT_2 receptors. In addition, there is recent biochemical (Sanders-Bush et al., 1988) and electrophysiological (Rasmussen and Aghajanian, in preparation) evidence that the psychedelic hallucinogens act as partial agonists at the 5-HT_2 receptor. Similarly, the actions of PCP have been linked to activity at one specific receptor in the ion channel of the NMDA macromolecular complex. Whether activity at this receptor will be able to explain all the actions of PCP awaits further experimentation.

Acknowledgments—Supported in part by PHS Grant MH-17871 and the State of Connecticut. The authors wish to thank Nancy Margiotta and Leslie Fields for their excellent technical assistance.

REFERENCES

ADAMS, J. T., TEAL, P. M., SONDERS, M. S., TESTER, B., ESHERICK, J. S., SCHEREZ, M. W., KEANA, J. F. W. and WEBER, E. (1987) Synthesis and characterization of an affinity label for brain receptors to psychotomimetic benzomorphans; differentiation of *o*-type and phencyclidine receptors. *Eur. J. Pharmac.* **142**: 61–71.

AGHAJANIAN, G. K. (1976) LSD and 2-Bromo-LSD: Comparison of effects of serotonergic neurones and neurones in two serotonergic projection areas, the ventral lateral geniculate and amygdala. *Neuropharmacology* **15**: 521–528.

AGHAJANIAN, G. K. (1980) Mescaline and LSD facilitate the activation of locus coeruleus neurons by peripheral stimuli. *Brain Res.* **186**: 492–498.

AGHAJANIAN, G. K. (1981) Neurophysiologic Properties of Psychotomimetics. In: *Handbook of Experimental Pharmacology*, pp. 89–109, HOFFMEISTER, F. and STILLE, G. (eds) Springer–Verlag, New York.

AGHAJANIAN, G. K. and HAIGLER, H. J. (1975) Hallucinogenic indoleamines: preferential action upon presynaptic serotonin receptors. *Psychopharmac. Commun.* **1**: 619–629.

AGHAJANIAN, G. K., FOOTE, W. E. and SHEARD, M. H. (1968) Lysergic acid diethylamide sensitive neuronal units in the midbrain raphe. *Science* **161**: 706–708.

AGHAJANIAN, G. K., FOOTE, W. E. and SHEARD, M. H. (1970) Action of psychotogenic drugs on single midbrain raphe neurons. *J. Pharmac. Exp. Ther.* **171**: 178–187.

AGHAJANIAN, G. K., HAIGLER, H. J. and BLOOM, F. E. (1972) Lysergic acid diethylamide and serotonin: direct actions on serotonin-containing neurons. *Life Sci.* **11**: 615–622.

AGHAJANIAN, G. K., SPROUSE, J. S. and RASMUSSEN, K. (1987) Physiology of the midbrain serotonin system. In: *Psychopharmacology: The Third Generation of Progress*, pp. 141–149, MELTZER, H. Y. (ed.) Raven Press, New York.

ALTAR, C. A., WASLEY, A. M., NEALE, R. F. and STONE, G. A. (1986) Typical and atypical antipsychotic occupancy of D_2 and S_2 receptors: an autoradiographic analysis in rat brain. *Brain Res. Bull.* **16**: 517–525.

ANDEN, N. E., CORRODI, H., FUXE, K. and HOKFELT, T. (1968) Evidence for a central 5-hydroxytryptamine receptor stimulation by lysergic acid diethylamide. *Br. J. Pharmac.* **34**: 1–7.

ANIS, N. A., BERRY, S. C., BURTON, N. R. and LODGE, D. (1983) The dissociative anaesthetics, ketamine and phencyclidine, selectively reduce excitation of central mammalian neurones by *N*-methyl-aspartate. *Br. J. Pharmac.* **79**: 565–575.

APPELL, J. B. and FREEDMAN, D. X. (1968) Tolerance and cross-tolerance among psychotomimetic drugs. *Psychopharmacology* **13**: 267–274.

ARVIDSSON, L., HACKSELL, U., NILSSON, J. L. G., HJORTH, S., CARLSSON, A., LINDBERG, P., SANCHEZ, D. and WIKSTROM, H. (1981) 8-Hydroxy-2-(di-*n*-propylamino)tetralin, a new centrally acting 5-hydroxtryptamine receptor agonist. *J. Med. Chem.* **24**: 921–923.

BRADSHAW, C. M., ROBERTS, M. H. T. and SZABDI, E. (1971) Effect of mescaline on single cortical neurones. *Br. J. Pharmac.* **43**: 871–873.

BRAMWELL, G. J. and GONYE, T. (1976) Response of midbrain neurones to microiontophoretically applied 5-hydroxytryptamine: comparison with the response to intraventrously administered lysergic acid diethylamide. *Neuropharmacology* **15**: 457–461.

BUCKHOLTZ, N. S., FREEDMAN, D. X. and MIDDAUGH, L. D. (1985) Daily LSD administration selectively decreases $serotonin_2$ receptor binding in rat brain. *Eur. J. Pharmac.* **109**: 421–425.

BURKI, H. R., ASPER, H., RUCH, W. and ZUGER, P. B. (1978) Bromocriptine, dihydroergotoxine, methysergide, d-LSD, CF 25-397, and 29-712; effects on the metabolism of the biogenic amines in the brain of the rat. *Psychopharmacology* **57**: 227–337.

COLPAERT, F. C., MEERT, T. F., NIEMEGEERS, C. J. E. and JANSSEN, P. A. J. (1985) Behavioral and 5-HT antagonist effect of ritanserin: a pure and selective antagonist of LSD discrimination in rat. *Psychopharmacology* **86**: 45–54.

CONTRERAS, P. C., QUIRION, R. and O'DONOHUE, T. L. (1986) Autoradiographic distribution of phencyclidine receptors in the rat brain using $[^3H]$1-((1-(2-Thienlyl)cyclohexyl)piperidine ($[^3H]$TCP). *Neurosci. Lett.* **67**: 101–106.

DEMONTIGNY, C. and AGHAJANIAN, G. K. (1977) Preferential action of 5-methoxytryptamine and 5-methoxydimethyltryptamine on presynaptic serotonin receptors: a comparative iontophoretic study with LSD and serotonin. *Neuropharmacology* **16**: 811–818.

deMontigny, C., Blier, P. and Chaput, Y. (1984) Electrophysiologically-identified serotonin receptors in the rat CNS. *Neuropharmacology* **23**: 1511–1520.

Fabing, H. D. and Hawkins, R. J. (1956) Intravenous bufotenine injection in human being. *Science* **123**: 886–887.

Fallon, S. L., Kim, H. S. and Welch, J. J. (1983) Electrophysiological evidence for modulation of dopamine neurons by 8-hydroxy-2(di-*n*-propylamino)tetralin. *Soc. Neurosci. Abstr.* **9**: 716.

Foster, A. C. and Wong, E. H. F. (1987) The novel anticonvulsant MK-801 binds to the activated state of the N-methyl-D-aspartate receptor in rat brain. *Br. J. Pharmac.* **91**: 403–409.

Freedman, D. X. (1961) Effects of LSD-25 on brain serotonin. *J. Pharmac. Exp. Ther.* **134**: 160–166.

Freeman, A. S. and Bunney, B. S. (1984) The effects of phencyclidine and *N*-allylnormtazocine on midbrain dopamine neuronal activity. *Eur. J. Pharmac.* **104**: 287–293.

French, E. D. (1986) Effects of phencyclidine on ventral tegmental A_{10} dopamine neurons in the rat. *Neuropharmacology* **25**: 241–248.

Fuxe, K. (1965) Evidence for the existence of monoamine neurons in the central nervous system. II. Distribution of monoamine nerve terminals in the central nervous system. *Acta Physiol. Scand.* **64** (Suppl. 247): 41–85.

Fuxe, K., Fredholm, B. B., Ogren, S. O., Agnati, L. F., Hokfelt, T. and Gustafsson, J. A. (1978) Ergot drugs and central monoaminergic mechanisms: a histochemical, biochemical, and behavioral analysis. *Fed. Proc.* **37**: 2181–2191.

Gaddum, J. H. (1953) Antagonism between lysergic acid diethylamide and 5-hydroxy-tryptamine. *J. Physiol., Lond.* **121**: 15.

Glennon, R. A., Rosecrans, J. A., Young, R. and Gaines, J. (1979) Hallucinogens as a discriminative stimuli: generalization of DOM to a 5-methoxy-*N-N*-dimethyltryptamine stimulus. *Life Sci.* **24**: 993–998.

Glennon, R. A., Young, R. and Rosecrans, J. A. (1983a) Antagonism of the effects of the hallucinogen DOM and the purported 5-HT agonist quipazine by 5-HT_2 antagonists. *Eur. J. Pharmac.* **91**: 189–196.

Glennon, R. A., Young, R., Jacyno, J. M., Slusher, M. and Rosecrans, J. A. (1983b) DOM-stimulus generalization to LSD and other hallucinogenic indolealkylamines. *Eur. J. Pharmac.* **86**: 453–459.

Glennon, R. A., Titeler, M. and McKenney, J. D. (1984) Evidence for 5-HT_2 involvement in the mechanism of action of hallucinogenic agents. *Life Sci.* **35**: 2505–2511.

Goldstein, J. M., Litwin, L. C., Sutton, E. B. and Malick, J. B. (1986) The role of 5-HT_2 receptor blockade on amphetamine (AMP) inhibition of dopamine (DA) cell firing. *Fed. Proc.* **45**: 436.

Gratton, A., Hoffer, B. J. and Freedman, R. (1987) Electrophysiological effects of phenycyclidine in the medial prefrontal cortex of the rat. *Neuropharmacology* **26**: 1275–1283.

Guilbaud, G., Besson, J. M., Oliveras, J. L. and Liebeskind, J. C. (1973) Suppression by LSD of the inhibitory effect exerted by dorsal raphe stimulation on certain spinal cord interneurons in the cat. *Brain Res.* **61**: 417–422.

Haigler, H. J. and Aghajanian, G. K. (1973) Mescaline and LSD: direct and indirect effects on serotonin-containing neurons in brain. *Eur. J. Pharmac.* **21**: 53–60.

Haigler, H. J. and Aghajanian, G. K. (1974a) Peripheral serotonin antagonists: failure to antagonize serotonin in brain areas receiving a prominent serotonergic input. *J. Neural Trans.* **35**: 257–273.

Haigler, H. J. and Aghajanian, G. K. (1974b) Lysergic acid diethylamide and serotonin: a comparison of effects of serotonergic neurons and neurons receiving a serotonergic input. *J. Pharmac. Exp. Ther.* **188**: 688–699.

Harris, E. W., Ganong, A. H. and Cotman, C. W. (1984) Long-term potentiation in the hippocampus involves activation of *N*-methyl-D-aspartate receptors. *Brain Res.* **323**: 132–137.

Herrmann, W. M., Horowski, R., Dannehl, U., Kramer, U. and Lurati, K. (1977) Clinical effectiveness of lisuride hydrogen maleate: a double-blind trial versus methysergide. *Headache* **17**: 54–60.

Heym, J., Rasmussen, K. and Jacobs, B. L. (1984) Some behavioral effects of hallucinogens are mediated by a postsynaptic serotonergic action: evidence from single unit studies in free moving cats. *Eur. J. Pharmac.* **101**: 57–68.

Hollister, S. D. (1978) Psychotomimetic drugs in man. In: *Handbook of Psychopharmacology*, pp. 389–424, L. L. Iversen, S. D. Iversen and S. H. Snyder (eds) Plenum Press, New York.

Honey, C. R., Miljkovic, Z. and MacDonald, J. F. (1985) Ketamine and phencyclidine cause a voltage-dependent block of responses to L-aspartic acid. *Neurosci. Lett.* **61**: 135–139.

Horita, A. (1963) Some biochemical studies on psilocybin and psilocin. *J. Neuropsychiat.* **4**: 270–273.

Horn, G. and McKay, J. M. (1973) Effect of lysergic acid diethylamide on the spontaneous activity and visual receptive fields of cells in the lateral geniculate nucleus of the cat. *Exp. Brain Res.* **17**: 271–284.

Horowski, R., Wendt, H. and Graf, K. J. (1978) Prolactin-lowering effect of low doses of lisuride in man. *Acta Endocrinol. (Kbh.)*. **87**: 234–240.

Johnson, S. W., Haroldsen, P. E., Hoffer, B. J. and Freedman, R. (1984) Presynaptic dopaminergic activity of phencyclidine in rat caudate. *J. Pharmac. Exp. Ther.* **229**: 322–332.

Jones, S. M., Snell, L. D. and Johnson, K. M. (1987a) Inhibition by phencyclidine of excitatory amino acid-stimulated release of neurotransmitter in the nucleus accumbens. *Neuropharmacology* **26**: 173–179.

Jones, S. M., Snell, L. D. and Johnson, K. M. (1987b) Phencyclidine selectively inhibits *N*-methyl-D-aspartate-induced hippocampal (^{3}H) norepinephrine release. *J. Pharmac. Exp. Ther.* **240**: 492–497.

Kehr, W. (1977) Effect of lisuride and other ergot derivatives on monoaminergic mechanisms in rat brain. *Eur. J. Pharmac.* **41**: 261–273.

Lacey, M. G. and Henderson, G. (1986) Actions of phencyclidine on rats locus coeruleus neurons *in vitro*. *Neuroscience* **17**: 485–494.

Largent, B. L., Gundlach, A. L. and Snyder, S. H. (1986) Pharmacological and autoradiographic discrimination of sigma and phencyclidine receptor binding sites in brain with (+)-(3H) SKF 10.047, (+)-(3H)-3-(3-hydroxyphenyl)-*N*-(1-propyl)piperidine and (3H)-1-(1-(2-thienyl)cyclohexyl)piperdine. *J. Pharmac. Exp. Ther.* **238**: 739–748.

Leysen, J. E., Awouters, F., Kennis, L., Laduron, P. M., Vandenberk, J. and Janssen, P. A. J. (1981) Receptor binding profile of R 41 468, a novel antagonist at 5-HT_2 receptors. *Life Sci.* **28**: 1015–1022.

Lizzui, A., Chiodini, P. G., Oppizzi, G., Botalla, L., Verde, G., Destefano, L., Colussi, G., Graff, K. J. and Horowski, R. (1978) Lisuride hydrogen maleate: evidence for a long lasting dopaminergic activity in humans. *J. Clin. Endocr. Metab.* **46**: 196–202.

Lucki, I., Nobler, M. S. and Frazer, A. (1984) Differential actions of serotonin antagonists on two behavioral models of serotonin receptor activation in the rat. *J. Pharmac. Exp. Ther.* **228**: 133–139.

Marwaha, J. (1982) Candidate mechanisms underlying phencyclidine-induced psychosis: an electrophysiological, behavioural and biochemical study. *Biol. Psychiat.* **17**: 155–198.

McCall, R. B. and Aghajanian, G. K. (1979a) Serotonergic facilitation of facial motoneuron excitation. *Brain Res.* **169**: 11–27.

McCall, R. B. and Aghajanian, G. K. (1979b) Denervation supersensitivity to serotonin in the facial nucleus. *Neuroscience* **4**: 1501–1510.

McCall, R. B. and Aghajanian, G. K. (1980a) Pharmacological characterization of serotonin receptors in the facial motor nucleus: a microiontophoretic study. *Eur. J. Pharmac.* **65**: 175–183.

McCall, R. B. and Aghajanian, G. K. (1980b) Hallucinogens potentiate responses to serotonin and norepinephrine in the facial motor nucleus. *Life Sci.* **26**: 1149–1156.

Middlemiss, D. N. and Fozard, J. R. (1983) 8-Hydroxy-2-(di-n-propylamino) tetralin discriminates between subtypes of the 5-HT_1 recognition site. *Eur. J. Pharmac.* **90**: 151–153.

Mokler, D. J., Stoudt, K. W. and Rech, R. H. (1985) The 5-HT_2 antagonist pirenperone reverses disruption of FR-40 by hallucinogenic drugs. *Pharmacol. Biochem. Behav.* **22**: 677–682.

Mouriz-Garcia, A., Schmidt, R. and Arlazoroff, A. (1969) Effects of LSD on the spontaneous and evoked activity of retinal and geniculate ganglion cells. *Psychopharmacology* **15**: 382–391.

Nabeshima, T., Ishikawa, K., Yamaguchi, K., Furukawa, H. and Kameyama, T. (1986) Methysergide-induced precipitated withdrawal syndrome in phencyclidine-dependent rats. *Neurosci. Lett.* **69**: 275–278.

Nabeshima, T., Ishikawa, K., Yamaguchi, K., Furukawa, H. and Kameyama, T. (1978a) Phencyclidine-induced head-twitch responses as 5-HT_2 receptor-mediated behavior in rats. *Neurosci. Lett.* **76**: 335–338.

Nabeshima, T., Ishikawa, K., Yamaguchi, K., Furukawa, H. and Kameyama, T. (1987b) Phencyclidine-induced head-weaving observed in mice after ritanserin treatment. *Eur. J. Pharmac.* **139**: 171–178.

Palkovits, M., Brownstein, M. and Saavedra, J. M. (1974) Serotonin content of the brain stem nuclei in the rat. *Brain Res.* **80**: 237–249.

Pazos, A. and Palacios, J. M. (1985) Quantitative autoradiographic mapping of serotonin receptors in the rat brain. I. Serotonin-I-receptors. *Brain Res.* **346**: 205–230.

Pazos, A., Cortes, R. and Palacios, J. M. (1985) Quantitative autoradiographic mapping of serotonin receptors in the rat brain. II. Serotonin-2 receptors. *Brain Res.* **346**: 231–249.

Peroutka, S. J. (1985) Selective interaction of novel anxiolytics with 5-$hydroxytryptamine_{1A}$ receptors. *Biol. Psychiat.* **20**: 971–979.

Peroutka, S. J. (1986) Pharmacological differentiation and characterization of 5-HT_{1A}, 5-HT_{1B}, and 5-HT_{1C} binding sites in rat frontal cortex. *J. Neurochem.* **47**: 529–540.

Peroutka, S. J. and Snyder, S. H. (1979) Multiple serotonin receptors: differential binding of ^{3}H-serotonin. ^{3}H-lysergic acid diethylamide and ^{3}H-spiroperidol. *Molec. Pharmac.* **16**: 687–699.

Peroutka, S. J. and Snyder, S. H. (1980) Relationship of neuroleptic drug effects at brain dopamine, serotonin, α-adrenergic, and histamine receptors to clinical potency. *Am. J. Psychiat.* **137**: 1518–1522.

Pieri, L., Keller, H. H., Burkhard, W. and Daprada, M. (1978) Effects of lisuride and LSD on cerebral monoamine systems and hallucinosis. *Nature* 272: 278–280.

Pradham, S. N. (1984) Phencyclidine (PCP): some human studies. *Neurosci. Biobehav. Revs.* **8**: 493–501.

Raja, S. N. and Guyenet, P. G. (1980) Effects of phencyclidine on the spontaneous activity of monoaminergic neurons. *Eur. J. Pharmac.* **63**: 229–233.

Rasmussen, K. and Aghajanian, G. K. (1986) Effect of hallucinogens on spontaneous and sensory-evoked locus coeruleus unit activity in the rat: reversal by selective 5-HT_2 antagonists. *Brain Res.* **385**: 395–400.

Rasmussen, K. and Aghajanian, G. K. (1988) Potency of antipsychotics in reversing the effects of a hallucinogenic drug on locus coeruleus neurons correlates with 5-HT_2 binding affinity. *Neuropsychopharmacology* **1**: 101–107.

Rasmussen, K., Glennon, R. A. and Aghajanian, G. K. (1986) Phenethylamine hallucinogens in the locus coeruleus: potency of action correlates with rank order of 5-HT_2 binding affinity. *Eur. J. Pharmac.* **132**: 79–82.

Roberts, M. H. T. and Straughan, D. W. (1967) Excitation and depression of cortical neurones by 5-hydroxytryptamine. *J. Physiol.* **193**: 269–294.

Rogawski, M. A. and Aghajanian, G. K. (1979) Response of central monoaminergic neurons to lisuride: comparison with LSD. *Life Sci.* **24**: 1289–1298.

Rosenberg, D. E., Isbell, H., Miner, E. J. and Logan, C. R. (1964) The effect of *N,N*-dimethyltryptamine in human subjects tolerant to lysergic acid diethylamide. *Psychopharmacology* **5**: 217–227.

Sanders-Bush, E., Burns, K. D. and Knoth, K. (1988) Lysergic acid diethylamide and 2,5-dimethoxy-4-methylamphetamine are partial agonists at serotonin receptors linked to phosphoinositide hydrolysis. *J. Pharmac. Exp. Ther.* **246**: 924–928.

Snell, L. D. and Johnson, K. M. (1986) Characterization of the inhibition of excitatory amino acid-induced neurotransmitter release in the rat striatum by phencyclidine-like drugs. *J. Pharmac. Exp. Ther.* **238**: 938–946.

Snyder, S. H. (1980) Phencyclidine. *Nature* **285**: 355–356.

Sprouse, J. S. and Aghajanian, G. K. (1987) Electrophysiological responses of serotonergic dorsal raphe neurons to 5-HT_{1a} and 5-HT_{1b} agonists. *Synapse* **1**: 3–9.

Szara, S. (1956) Dimethyltryptamine: its metabolism in man; the relation of its psychotic effect to the serotonin metabolism. *Experientia* **12**: 441–442.

Trulson, M. E. and Jacobs, B. L. (1978) Effects of LSD on behavior and raphe unit activity in freely moving cats. *Fed. Proc.* **37**: 346.

TRULSON, M. E. and TRULSON, T. J. (1986) Buspirone decreases the activity of serotonin-containing neurons in the dorsal raphe in freely-moving cats. *Neuropharmacology* **25**: 1263–1266.

TRULSON, M. E., HEYM, J. and JACOBS, B. L. (1981) Dissociations between the effects of hallucinogenic drugs on behavior and raphe unit activity in freely moving cats. *Brain Res.* **215**: 275–293.

TURNER, W. J. and MERLIS, S. (1959) Effect of some indolealkylamines on man. *Arch. Neurol. Psychiat.* **81**: 121–129.

VANDERMAELEN, C. P. and AGHAJANIAN, G. K. (1982a) Intracellular studies on the effects of systemic administration of serotonin agonists on rat facial motoneurons. *Eur. J. Pharmac.* **78**: 233–236.

VANDERMAELEN, C. P. and AGHAJANIAN, G. K. (1982b) Serotonin-induced depolarization of rat facial motoneurons *in vivo*: comparison with amino acid transmitters. *Brain Res.* **239**: 139–152.

VANDERMAELEN, C. P., MATHESON, G. K., WILDERMAN, R. C. and PATTERSON, L. A. (1986) Inhibition of serotonergic dorsal raphe neurons by systemic and iontophoretic administration of buspirone, a non-benzodiazepine anxiolytic drug. *Eur. J. Pharmac.* **129**: 123–130.

WHITE, S. R. and NEUMAN, R. S. (1980) Facilitation of spinal motoneurone excitability by 5-hydroxytryptamine and nonadrenaline. *Brain Res.* **188**: 119–127.

WILKINS, L. O., ABERCROMBIE, E. D., RASMUSSEN, K. and JACOBS, B. L. (1987) Effect of buspirone on single unit activity in locus coeruleus and dorsal raphe nucleus in behaving cats. *Eur. J. Pharmac.* **136**: 123–127.

WOLBACH, A. B., JR., MINER, E. J. and ISBELL, H. (1962) Comparison of psilocin with psilocybin, mescaline and LSD-25. *Psychopharmacologia. Berl.* **3**: 219–223.

WOOLLEY, D. W. and SHAW, E. (1954) A biochemical and pharmacological suggestion about certain mental disorders. *Proc. Natl. Acad. Sci. U.S.A.* **40**: 228–231.

CHAPTER 11

THE BEHAVIORAL PHARMACOLOGY OF STIMULANTS AND HALLUCINOGENS: DRUG DISCRIMINATION AND SELF-ADMINISTRATION PROCEDURES

J. Broadbent and J. B. Appel

Behavioral Pharmacology Laboratory, Department of Psychology, University of South Carolina, Columbia, S.C., U.S.A.

1. INTRODUCTION

Since the beginnings of recorded history, stimulants and hallucinogens have been among the most widely used and abused of all psychoactive substances (Caldwell, 1978). Indeed, despite repeated warnings as to their toxic and possibly fatal effects, a dramatic increase in the abuse of cocaine (a potent psychomotor stimulant and, when administered chronically, psychotomimetic) has recently been observed (Kozel and Adams, 1985). Such facts point to an important problem: many drugs have powerful reinforcing properties that cannot be altered readily (either by social sanctions or 'therapeutic' interventions). It is equally unfortunate that the (neuronal) mechanisms which may be responsible for the altered subjective states that presumably mediate these properties, continue to elude precise delineation.

Assessment of the subjective effects of drugs and the etiology of drug-seeking behavior in humans has been valuable in analyzing some of the factors involved in drug abuse (Henningfield *et al.*, 1986). However, many of the experimental manipulations that may be required to disentangle the relative importance of biological, pharmacological, physiological, and socioeconomic variables on such complex behavior cannot be undertaken readily in this species. Fortunately, the subjective properties of drugs can and have been analyzed in animals using methods such as drug discrimination and self administration; the results of such studies are the subject of the present review. In the interest of space, only *prototypic* psychomotor stimulants (amphetamine and cocaine), hallucinogens (LSD, lysergic acid-diethylamide and mescaline), and substituted phenylisopropylamines (MDA, 3,4-methylenedioxyamphetamine and MDMA, *N*-methyl-1-(3,4-methylenedioxyamphetamine)) which, purportedly have both stimulant *and* hallucinogenic properties (Glennon and Young, 1984a,c), will be discussed; research that promises to shed some light on neuronal mechanisms through which these substances might act *in vivo* will receive particular attention.

2. PSYCHOMOTOR STIMULANTS

2.1. Discriminative Stimulus Properties of Psychomotor Stimulants

In humans, *d*-amphetamine and cocaine appear to cause similar alternations in affect or mood. Thus, subjects sometimes confuse *d*-amphetamine with cocaine and cocaine with *d*-amphetamine (Fischman and Schuster, 1982). The results of drug discrimination experiments indicate that a similar lack of discriminability between these substances occurs in other animals.

All drug discrimination procedures analyze the effects of drugs directly by training subjects to make an appropriate response (e.g. press the left of two levers) contingent on the administration of a particular drug and to make a different response following either vehicle or some other, active compound in order to obtain food or water or, less frequently, avoid aversive stimuli such as electric shock (Fig. 1). Thus, the drug functions as a discriminative stimulus or 'cue' which signals the availability of reinforcement contingent on the occurrence of an appropriate choice response. The method has become quite popular

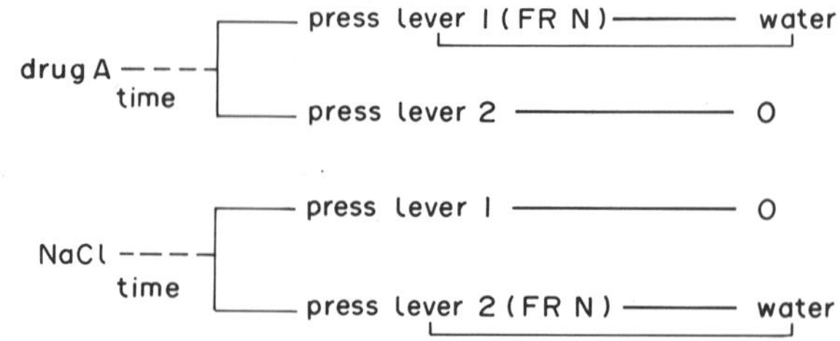

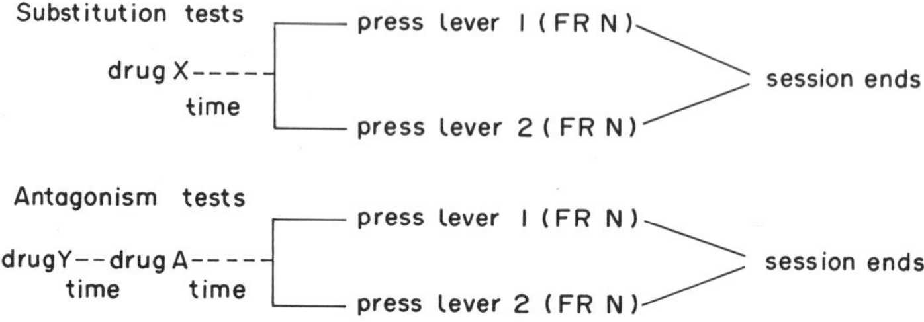

FIG. 1. Drug discrimination training and testing procedures. Animals are trained to complete a fixed ratio (FR N) or lever 1 after drug A administration or lever 2 following vehicle injection to obtain water; inappropriate responding is not reinforced. Animals demonstrating acccurate discrimination (e.g. exceeding 80% appropriate responses during the first FR over several sessions) receive substitution (generalization) or antagonism (combination) tests. Drug X (a 'novel' compound) is injected in place of drug A during substitution tests; putative antagonists (drug Y) are injected in combination with drug A in combination tests. During both types of tests, completion of the FR on either lever terminates the session without reinforcement. Reprinted with permission of Pergamon Press Ltd.

in behavioral pharmacology during recent years (Colpaert and Slangen, 1982) because it is: (1) *sensitive* (animals are able to discriminate very small doses of most psychoactive drugs); (2) pharmacologically *specific* (only the effects of the drug with which the animal has been trained or those of closely related compounds are identified as drug-like); and (3) *reliable*, in that it is relatively unaffected by the effects of drugs on motor behavior (since it is primarily concerned with response choice rather than response rate) (Appel *et al.*, 1982; Glennon and Rosecrans, 1981; Young and Glennon, 1986).

Cross-generalization or substitution between cocaine and *d*-amphetamine has been a consistent finding in drug discrimination studies; this occurs across different species, training doses, types of reinforcers, and schedules of reinforcement [Table 1(a)]. In addition to their similar stimulus properties, *d*-amphetamine (or methamphetamine) and cocaine show cross-tolerance (Wood and Emmett-Oglesby, 1986; Wood *et al.*, 1984), suggesting that these substances act through common mechanisms. Because of their cross-generalization and reports that many, if not most, of the neurochemical and neurophysiological effects of *d*-amphetamine are the result of preferential actions on dopamine (DA) neurotransmitter systems (Iversen and Iversen, 1981), it has been suggested that DA systems are involved in both the *d*-amphetamine and cocaine cues (Colpaert *et al.*, 1979a). Because the peripherally active amphetamine derivative parahydroxyamphetamine has no stimulant-like, discriminable properties (Colpaert *et al.*, 1979a), these DA systems are probably central. However, the local anesthetic properties of cocaine may also contribute to its discriminability (Huang and Wilson, 1982). Indeed, the subjective effects of cocaine have been described as similar to those of other local anesthetics (Van Dyke *et al.*, 1979) and, in some drug discrimination experiments, procaine substitutes, at least partially, for cocaine (De la Garza and Johanson, 1983; Jarbe, 1984); however, this result is not obtained consistently (Colpaert *et al.*, 1979a; De la Garza and Johanson, 1985; Huang and Wilson, 1982; Jarbe, 1981; McKenna and Ho, 1980).

Even if, as is the case with other psychoactive substances, the stimulus properties of psychomotor stimulants are mediated centrally, a variety of neuronal mechanisms may be involved in their subjective effects. For example, both amphetamine and cocaine cause nonselective increases in concentrations of noradrenaline (NE) and serotonin (5-HT) as well as DA (Kuczenski, 1983; Moore, 1978; Ross and Renyi, 1967a,b). However, monoamine oxidase inhibitors (MAOIs) of the A configuration (which preferentially block the catabolism of 5-HT, NE and, to some extent, DA) do not mimic either *d*-amphetamine or cocaine in drug discrimination experiments (Colpaert *et al.*, 1980; Porsolt *et al.*, 1982). Mixed Type A and B MAOIs (which, in addition to their effects on NE, DA, and 5-HT concentrations reduce the degradation of phenylethylamine and benzylamine) have stimulus properties that can best be described as puzzling: although tranylcypromine, pargyline and pheniprazine appear to substitute for psychomotor stimulants and have similar interoceptive effects, other, functionally related compounds such as iproniazid and nialamide, act quite differently (Huang and Ho, 1974a; Colpaert *et al.*, 1980). The amphetamine-like actions of tranylcypromine (Youdim and Finberg, 1983) may explain the fact that this substance mimics stimulants; similarly, generalization of stimulant cues to deprenyl (Colpaert *et al.*, 1980; Porsolt *et al.*, 1984), a specific MAOB inhibitor (Knoll *et al.*, 1965), may be the result of the metabolic conversion of deprenyl to amphetamine (Reynolds *et al.*, 1978). Thus, studies with MAOIs have provided no clear evidence as to the nature of the neural substrates of the subjective effects of either *d*-amphetamine or cocaine.

Cathinone, a stimulant which increases synaptic concentrations of DA, NE, and 5-HT by blocking their re-uptake, has been reported to mimic both *d*-amphetamine and cocaine (De la Garza and Johanson, 1983, 1985; Huang and Wilson, 1986). Similarly, methylphenidate, which inhibits DA re-uptake (Braestrup, 1977), engenders *d*-amphetamine appropriate responding at doses of 2.5 mg/kg (Huang and Ho, 1974b); lower doses of this stimulant substitute only partially for *d*-amphetamine (Porsolt *et al.*, 1982). Selective elevation of DA concentration also appears to be the common factor in the substitutions of the antidepressants amineptine, bupropion, nomifensine and amantidine for *d*-amphetamine (Porsolt *et al.*, 1982; Schechter, 1977). Since amantidine and nomifensine induce partial and complete generalization respectively in animals trained to discriminate cocaine from saline (Colpaert *et al.*, 1979a) while methylphenidate substitutes at least partially for this substance (Colpaert *et al.*, 1979a; Emmett-Oglesby *et al.*, 1983; McKenna and Ho, 1980), synaptic concentrations of DA may be of importance in the subjective effects of cocaine as well as *d*-amphetamine.

Unfortunately, other efforts to use substitution paradigms to delineate the neuronal substrates of the stimulus properties of psychomotor stimulants have not been particularly successful. Findings that DA receptor agonists such as piribedil and *n*-propylnoraporphine substitute as much as 80% for *d*-amphetamine (Schechter, 1977) while piribedil induces only 57% drug appropriate responding in cocaine-trained animals (Colpaert *et al.*, 1979a), imply that *d*-amphetamine has more DA-like activity than cocaine. However, results with apomorphine are confusing [Table 1(b)]; in some studies, this DA (D-2) agonist has been reported to elicit 80% drug-appropriate responding in *d*-amphetamine-trained animals (Schechter and Cook, 1975; Schechter, 1977) but this substitution has not been replicated in other laboratories (Bueno *et al.*, 1976; Hernandez *et al.*, 1978; Ho and Huang, 1975; Jarbe and Kroon, 1980; Nielsen and Jepsen, 1985). While inconsistent results with apomorphine can sometimes be explained by the use of different test doses and routes of administration, the lack of substitution of 2 mg/kg of this compound for *d*-amphetamine (Ho and Huang, 1975) is difficult to reconcile with data from Schechter's laboratory. However, amount of cross-generalization may also depend on *training* dose; for example, complete substitution of apomorphine for *d*-amphetamine only occurs at doses of at least 1.6 mg/kg of the training drug (Stolerman and D'Mello, 1981).

Similarities between the stimulus properties of cocaine and apomorphine (1 mg/kg) have been reported (McKenna and Ho, 1980; Stolerman and D'Mello, 1981). In addition, apomorphine has been found to potentiate the discriminable effect of a low dose of cocaine (Cunningham and Appel, 1982). Unfortunately, another D-2 agonist, bromocriptine does not seem to mimic cocaine and has not yet been tested in *d*-amphetamine-trained animals

Table 1 *Results of Substitution (Generalization) Tests in Animals Trained to Discriminate* d-*Amphetamine (A) or Cocaine (C) from Saline*

(a) *Complete Substitution* (≥80%)		
(A)	Amantidine	Schechter (1977)
(A)	Amineptine	Porsolt *et al.* (1982)
(C)	*d*-Amphetamine	Colpaert *et al.* (1979a), De La Garza and Johanson (1983, 1985), Emmett-Oglesby *et al.* (1983), Huang and Wilson (1986), McKenna and Ho (1980), Stolerman and D'Mello (1981), Wood and Emmett-Oglesby (1986)
(C) (A)	*l*-Amphetamine	Colpaert *et al.* (1979a), Huang and Ho (1974b), Schechter and Rosecrans (1973)
(C) (A)	Apomorphine	McKenna and Ho (1980), Schechter (1977), Schechter and Cook (1975), Stolerman and D'Mello (1981)
(C) (A)	Cathinone	Colpaert *et al.* (1978), De La Garza and Johanson (1983, 1985), Huang and Wilson (1986)
(A)	Cocaine	Ho *et al.* (1976), Kilbey and Ellinwood (1979), Porsolt *et al.* (1982), Stolerman and D'Mello (1981)
(C) (A)	Deprenyl	Colpaert *et al.* (1980), Porsolt *et al.* (1982, 1984)
(A)	*l*-Dopa	Ho and Huang (1975)
(A)	Ephedrine	Huang and Ho (1974b)
(A)	Ly-171555	Nielsen and Scheel-Kruger (1988)
(C) (A)	Methamphetamine	Colpaert *et al.* (1979a), Huang and Ho (1974b), Kuhn *et al.* (1974)
(C) (A)	Methylphenidate	Colpaert *et al.* (1979a) Emmett-Oglesby *et al.* (1983), Ho *et al.* (1976), Huang and Ho (1974b)
(A)	Nisoxetine	Snoddy and Tessel (1983)
(C) (A)	Nomifensine	Colpaert *et al.* (1979a), Porsolt *et al.* (1982)
(C)	Pargyline	Colpaert *et al.* (1980)
(A)	Pergolide	Nielsen and Scheel-Kruger (1988)
(C)	Phencyclidine	Colpaert *et al.* (1979a)
(C)	Pheniprazine	Colpaert *et al.* (1980)
(A)	Phenylethylamine	Huang and Ho (1974a)
(A)	Piribedil	Schechter (1977)
(C)	Procaine	De La Garza and Johanson (1983), Jarbe (1984)
(A)	Propylnoraporphine	Schechter (1977)
(A)	Tetrahydrocannibol	Bueno *et al.* (1976)
(C)	Tranylcypromine	Colpaert *et al.* (1980)
(b) *Partial Substitution* (60–79%)		
(C)	Amantidine	Colpaert *et al.* (1979a)
(C) (A)	Apomorphine	Bueno *et al.* (1976), De La Garza and Johanson (1985), Nielsen and Jepsen (1985)
(C)	Benztropine	Colpaert *et al.* (1979a)
(A)	Bupropion	Porsolt *et al.* (1982)
(C)	Clonidine	Wood *et al.* (1985)
(C)	Fentanyl	Colpaert *et al.* (1979a)
(C)	Lidocaine	Woolverton and Balster (1982)
(C)	Methamphetamine	Wood *et al.* (1984)
(C)	Methylphenidate	Hernandez *et al.* (1978), Porsolt *et al.* (1982)
(A)	Methoxyamphetamine	Huang and Ho (1974b)
(C)	Phenylethylamine	Wood *et al.* (1984)
(A)	Tranylcypromine	Porsolt *et al.* (1982)

continued

TABLE 1 *continued.*

(c) *No Substitution* (≤59%)		
(A)	Apomorphine	Hernandez *et al.* (1978), Jarbe and Kroon (1980)
(C)	Bromocriptine	Colpaert *et al.* (1979a)
(C)	Chlordiazepoxide	Colpaert *et al.* (1979a)
(C)	Clorgyline	Colpart *et al.* (1980)
(A)	Caffeine	Kuhn *et al.* (1974)
(A)	Cimoxatone	Porsolt *et al.* (1982)
(C) (A)	Desipramine	Colpaert *et al.* (1979a), Porsolt *et al.* (1982), Schechter (1980)
(A)	Doet	Huang and Ho (1974b)
(A)	DPI	Nielsen and Jepsen (1985)
(A)	Ethanol	Bueno *et al.* (1976)
(C) (A)	Fenfluramine	McKenna and Ho (1980), Schechter and Rosecrans (1973)
(C) (A)	Imipramine	Colpaert *et al.* (1979a), McKenna and Ho (1980), Schechter (1980)
(A)	Iproniazid	Huang and Ho (1974a)
(C)	Isoproterenol	Colpaert *et al.* (1979a)
(C)	Lidocaine	Colpaert *et al.* (1979a), De La Garza and Johanson (1985)
(A)	Lisuride	Nielsen and Jepsen (1985)
(C) (A)	LSD	Colpaert *et al.* (1979a), Kuhn *et al.* (1974), Schechter and Rosecrans (1973)
(C) (A)	Mescaline	Colpaert *et al.* (1979a), Kuhn *et al.* (1974), McKenna and Ho (1980)
(C) (A)	Morphine	Colpaert *et al.* (1979a), Hernandez *et al.* (1978), Kilbey and Ellinwood (1979)
(C)	Nialamide	Colpaert *et al.* (1980)
(C) (A)	Nicotine	De La Garza and Johanson (1983), Ho and Huang (1975), Schechter and Rosecrans (1973)
(A)	Nortryptiline	Schechter (1980)
(C)	Oxazepam	De La Garza and Johanson (1985)
(C)	Oxotremorine	Colpaert *et al.* (1979a)
(C) (A)	*p*-OH-Amphetamine	Colpaert *et al.* (1979a), Jarbe and Kroon (1980), Stolerman and D'-Mello (1981)
(C)	Pentobarbital	De La Garza and Johanson (1983, 1985)
(A)	Pentazocine	Hernandez *et al.* (1978)
(C)	Pentylenetetrazol	Emmett-Oglesby *et al.* (1983)
(C)	Phencyclidine	Cunningham and Appel (1982)
(C)	Piribedil	Colpaert *et al.* (1979a)
(C)	Procaine	Colpaert *et al.* (1979a), De La Garza and Johanson (1985), Huang and Wilson (1982), Jarbe (1981)
(C)	Propranolol	Colpaert *et al.* (1979a)
(C)	Pseudococaine	McKenna and Ho (1980)
(A)	Psilocybin	Kuhn *et al.* (1974)
(C)	Salbutamol	Colpaert *et al.* (1979a)
(C)	Strychnine	McKenna and Ho (1980)
(A)	SKF-38393	Nielsen and Scheel-Kruger (1988)
(A)	SKF-75670	Nielsen and Scheel-Kruger (1988)
(A)	STP (4-Methyl-2,5-Dimethoxyamphetamine)	Huang and Ho (1974a)
(A)	Tetrahydrocannibol	Jarbe and Kroon (1980), Kuhn *et al.* (1974)

[Table 1(c)]. Subjects trained on either the selective D-1 agonist SKF 38393 or the D-2 agonist LY-171555 do not respond significantly on the drug lever after challenge injections of either cocaine or *d*-amphetamine (Appel *et al.*, 1988), although LY-171555 does generalize in *d*-amphetamine trained animals (Nielsen and Scheel-Kruger, 1988).

More convincing evidence that central DA systems are critically involved in the behavioral effects of *d*-amphetamine and, less certainly, cocaine, comes from combination testing (Fig. 1) with neuroleptics (which act primarily as DA receptor antagonists). For example when given in combination with the training drug, fluphenazine and trifluoperazine block the *d*-amphetamine cue [Table 2(a)] while thioridazine attenuates this cue partially [Table 2(b)]. Similar antagonism may occur with clozapine (Kilbey and Ellinwood, 1979; Nielsen and Jepsen, 1985), although this result is not always reported (Schechter, 1980). Low doses of haloperidol (0.08–0.5 mg/kg), which purportedly block D-2 receptors selectively, are also effective antagonists of both *d*-amphetamine and cocaine (Colpaert *et al.*, 1978; Jarbe and Kroon, 1980; McKenna and Ho, 1980; Nielsen and Jepsen, 1985; Schechter and Cook, 1975), although haloperidol-induced blockade of the cocaine cue is not complete except, perhaps, at relatively high (and, consequently, less selective) doses (Jarbe, 1978, 1984). Pimozide, another neuroleptic that blocks D-2 receptors, also antagonizes the stimulus properties of *d*-amphetamine and cocaine (Ho and Huang, 1975; Jarbe, 1978; Nielsen and Jepsen, 1985), as does chlorpromazine, a less selective D-2 antagonist (Jarbe, 1978).

Further evidence implicating central DA systems in the subjective effects of *d*-amphetamine involves pretreatment with alpha-methyl-*para*-tyrosine (AMPT; Schechter and Cook, 1975); this agent, which depletes catecholamine concentrations by at least 80% by blocking their synthesis, reduces the ability to discriminate a 0.5 mg/kg dose of *d*-amphetamine from 76% to 40% (Kuhn *et al.*, 1974).

Generalization testing with compounds that act on nondopaminergic neuronal systems indicate that such systems are not critical to the mediation of the stimulus properties of psychomotor stimulants, although they may play some, as yet undefined, role in these effects. For example, the NE agonists salbutamol and isoproterenol fail to elicit significant cocaine responding over a wide range of doses (Colpaert *et al.*, 1979a) and, although the alpha-adrenoceptor agonist clonidine appears to mimic cocaine partially, when subjects are tested with cocaine after training with clonidine they do not respond on the drug-appropriate lever (Wood *et al.*, 1985). Surprisingly, the effects of NE agonists have not yet been tested extensively in subjects trained to discriminate *d*-amphetamine from saline. Nevertheless, the role of NE in the stimulus properties of both stimulants warrants further study since some generalization of *d*-amphetamine for the specific NE uptake inhibitors desipramine and nisoxetine has been reported (Shearman *et al.*, 1978; Snoddy and Tessel, 1983).

Antagonists of nondopaminergic neurotransmitters are not as effective as neuroleptics in blocking the stimulus effects of psychomotor stimulants [Table 2(c)], with the possible exception of the beta-adrenergic antagonist propranolol, which reduces *d*-amphetamine responding to 33% (Jarbe and Kroon, 1980). The lack of effect of disulfiram, which inhibits dopamine-beta-hydroxylase (the enzyme which converts DA to NE) and therefore depletes NE levels more selectively than AMPT, also suggests that NE systems do not play an important role in the *d*-amphetamine cue (Schechter and Cook, 1975). Interestingly, humans report an inhibition of the euphoric effects of *d*-amphetamine following treatment with AMPT, chlorpromazine (when given chronically), and pimozide (Gunne *et al.*, 1972); in the same clinical study, the alpha-adrenoceptor antagonist phenoxybenzamine increased the effects of *d*-amphetamine slightly; propranolol had no effect.

Although the role of 5-HT in the cocaine cue has not yet been explored systematically enough to reach any definite conclusions, this neurotransmitter does not appear to be significant in the effects of *d*-amphetamine (Jarbe and Kroon, 1980; Schechter and Rosecrans, 1973).

In a recent study, an attempt was made to more precisely define sites within the CNS which may be involved in the stimulus properties of *d*-amphetamine (Nielsen and Scheel-Kruger, 1986). Animals trained to discriminate peripheral injections of this compound from saline were tested for generalization following intracerebral microinjections of *d*-amphetamine into the nucleus accumbens and anterior ventrolateral striatum. While nucleus accumbens microinjections elicited drug appropriate responding, striatal injections did not. Further, blockade of D-2 receptors in the nucleus accumbens with sulpiride, reversed the

TABLE 2. *Results of Combination (Antagonism) Tests in Animals Trained to Discriminate d-Amphetamine (A) or Cocaine (C) from Saline*

(a) *Complete Antagonism* (≤40%)		
(A)	AMPT	Kuhn *et al.* (1974), Schechter and Cook (1975)
(C) (A)	Chlorpromazine	Jarbe (1978), Nielsen and Jepsen (1985)
(A)	Clozapine	Kilbey and Ellinwood (1979), Nielsen and Jepsen (1985)
(A)	Fluphenthixol	Nielsen and Jepsen (1985)
(A)	Fluphenazine	Schechter (1980)
(C) (A)	Haloperidol	Colpaert *et al.* (1978), Jarbe (1978), Nielsen and Jepsen (1985), Schechter and Cook (1975)
(A)	Metoclopromide	Nielsen and Jepsen (1985)
(A)	Molindone	Nielsen and Jepsen (1985)
(A)	Perphenazine	Nielsen and Jepsen (1985)
(A)	Pimozide	Ho and Huang (1975), Nielsen and Jepsen (1985)
(A)	Propranolol	Jarbe and Kroon (1980)
(A)	SCH-23390	Nielsen and Jepsen (1985)
(A)	Spiroperidol	Nielsen and Jepsen (1985)
(A)	Sulpiride	Nielsen and Jepsen (1985)
(A)	Trifluoperazine	Nielsen and Jepsen (1985), Schechter (1980)
(b) *Partial Antagonism* (41–79%)		
(A)	Chloropromazine	Schechter (1980)
(C)	Clozapine	Kilbey and Ellinwood (1979)
(C)	Haloperidol	Colpaert *et al.* (1978), Cunningham and Appel (1982), Huang and Wilson (1986), McKenna and Ho (1980), Schechter (1980)
(C)	Pimozide	Jarbe (1978)
(C)	Reserpine	McKenna and Ho (1980)
(A)	Thioridazine	Neilsen and Jepsen (1985), Schechter (1980)
(c) *No Antagonism* (≥80%)		
(C)	AMPT	Jarbe (1978)
(C)(A)	Atropine	Ho and Huang (1975), McKenna and Ho (1980)
(C)(A)	Cinanserin	Ho and Huang (1975), McKenna and Ho (1980)
(A)	PCPA	Schechter and Cook (1975)
(A)	Clozapine	Schechter (1980)
(C)	Diazepam	Emmett-Oglesby *et al.* (1983)
(A)	Disulfiram	Schechter and Cook (1975)
(C)	Haloperidol	Huang and Wilson (1986)
(A)	Methysergide	Ho and Huang (1975)
(C)	Naloxone	Cunningham and Appel (1982)
(A)	Naltrexone	Hernandez *et al.* (1978)
(C)(A)	Phenoxybenzamine	Jarbe (1978), Kilbey and Ellinwood (1979), McKenna and Ho (1980)
(A)	Phentolamine	Ho and Huang (1975)
(C)	Physostigmine	Jarbe (1978)
(A)	Promethazine	Nielsen and Jepsen (1985)
(C)(A)	Propranolol	Ho and Huang (1975), Jarbe (1978), Schechter and Cook (1975)
(C)	Sotalol	McKenna and Ho (1980)

substitution of the microinjections for systemic *d*-amphetamine, suggesting that D-2 receptors in the nucleus accumbens play a critical role in the *d*-amphetamine cue.

In summary, the most striking finding of the drug discrimination literature concerns the similarity between the discriminable effects of cocaine and *d*-amphetamine. The relatively consistent antagonism of the cues by DA receptor antagonists, especially those that act primarily at D-2 binding sites, indicates an involvement of DA in the subjective effects of both psychomotor stimulants; however, the results of generalization tests require clarification, perhaps by testing selective D-1 and D-2 agonists more extensively (Appel *et al.*, 1988). The identification of specific CNS sites through which these compounds exert their complex actions must be pursued vigorously; Nielsen and Scheel-Kruger (1986) have provided the first intriguing results in the identification of such sites.

2.2. Self-Administration of Psychomotor Stimulants

Although studies utilizing drug discrimination procedures have provided valuable information about *d*-amphetamine and cocaine, other procedures must be employed to identify those aspects of the states induced by stimulants (and other compounds) that are reinforcing and may therefore explain their liability for abuse. While it is true that the reinforcing effects (of drugs or any other stimuli) are usually discriminable, the discriminable properties are not necessarily reinforcing. Fortunately, the reinforcing effects of many substances can and have been assessed directly in experiments involving self-administration: in this procedure animals are, most often, trained to press a lever in order to obtain an infusion of a substance through a catheter which has been implanted surgically into a jugular vein.

Psychomotor stimulants maintain self-administration behavior in a variety of different species including rhesus monkeys (Balster and Schuster, 1973; Deneau *et al.*, 1969; Goldberg *et al.*, 1971; Hoffmeister and Schlichting, 1972; Wilson and Schuster, 1972, 1973a,b; Wilson *et al.*, 1971; Woods and Schuster, 1968), squirrel monkeys (Goldberg, 1973), dogs (Risner, 1975; Risner and Jones, 1975) and rats (Davis and Smith, 1975; Davis *et al.*, 1975; Ettenberg *et al.*, 1982; Pickens 1968; Roberts and Vickers, 1984; Yokel and Pickens, 1973). In many of these experiments, reliance has been placed on rate of lever pressing to indicate the reinforcing efficacy of the infusion; questions concerning the effects of the drug on motor activity and, hence, ability or disposition to respond therefore have been raised (Davis *et al.*, 1975). The use of chambers containing an 'active' lever, depression of which results in the delivery of a reinforcing substance such as *d*-amphetamine or cocaine, and an 'inactive' lever, depression of which has no scheduled consequences, has answered some of these concerns; thus, when two levers are provided; both accurate discrimination and a preference for the 'active' lever, which is not disrupted by reversing the position of the 'active' lever, occurs (Pickens and Harris, 1968; Pickens and Thompson, 1968). Additional evidence that it is the reinforcing, rather than some other property of the drug that maintains self-administration stems from observations that the *contingency* between the response and the infusion of the drug is critically important in maintaining lever pressing behavior; thus, infusing substances automatically (at rates comparable to those determined previously by the subjects' response rate) normally results in the complete cessation of lever-pressing (Pickens and Thompson, 1968). Most importantly, a correlation exists between those drugs that are abused (voluntarily) by humans and those that are self-administered by other animals (Schuster, 1975).

As mentioned previously, some psychomotor stimulants (most notably, cocaine) have local anesthetic effects that could contribute to their reinforcing (as well as discriminative) properties. This possibility was assessed in several studies of cocaine derivative such as procaine, norcocaine and chloroprocaine (Ford and Balster, 1977; Hammerbeck and Mitchell, 1978; Johanson, 1980; Risner and Jones, 1980; Woolverton and Balster, 1982). It has been suggested that the processes underlying the reinforcing properties of cocaine and procaine differ, since pretreatment with DA receptor antagonists *increase* responding for cocaine but *decrease* responding for procaine (De la Garza and Johanson, 1982); unfortunately, the different response rates maintained by infusions of the different substances may have affected the results of this study. Since procaine is known to inhibit MAO (Macfarlane, 1973), which is partially responsible for the metabolism of DA, NE and 5-HT (Iversen and Iversen, 1981), elevations in the concentrations of these neurotransmitters may be sufficient to maintain self-administration. Moreover, self-administration is not maintained by local anesthetics such as proparacaine (Johanson, 1980), tetracaine, lidocaine and procainamide (Woolverton and Balster, 1979), suggesting that the reinforcing effects of procaine, norcocaine and chloroprocaine are not due to the local anesthetic actions of these compounds. Furthermore humans do not appear to abuse either procaine or local anesthetics other than cocaine (Hammerbeck and Mitchell, 1978; Woolverton and Balster, 1982).

Since both cocaine and *d*-amphetamine are thought to act mainly by increasing the synaptic availability of catecholamines (above), the involvement of both DA and NE in the reinforcing efficacy of these compounds has been examined in some detail. Studies with DA antagonists suggest that DA neuronal systems play a significant role in the self-administration of *d*-amphetamine. For example, pimozide, a selective D-2 antagonist, has been found to increase responding on a lever associated with infusions of this drug in a manner resembling reward reduction while having no effect on the rate of pressing an inactive lever; a second DA antagonist (+) butaclamol has similar effects (Yokel and Wise, 1975, 1976). Following the highest doses of pimozide, a response pattern characteristic of extinction was seen, suggesting that DA antagonists block the reinforcing properties of *d*-amphetamine completely. The possibility that these results are due to direct effects of the DA antagonists on the ability to perform the operant response seems unlikely since another D-2 antagonist, haloperidol, was found to block both the reacquisition of *d*-amphetamine self-administration following an extinction session and the establishment of a conditioned response based on the reinforcing effects of *d*-amphetamine (Davis and Smith, 1975).

The effects of pimozide on the self-administration of *d*-amphetamine have also been examined in dogs (Risner and Jones, 1976). Again, this compound was found to increase the number of infusions except, at high doses, when rate of self-administration decreased. Further, relatively low doses of the less selective DA antagonist, chlorpromazine, also increased response rates in this species (Risner and Jones, 1976; Wilson and Schuster, 1972).

The effects of NE antagonists on *d*-amphetamine self-administration appear to be less consistent than those of DA antagonists. Phentolamine and propranolol have been found to decrease drug-maintained response rates, an effect that could be due to a variety of nonspecific actions of the antagonists (Yokel and Wise, 1975, 1976); another NE antagonist, phenoxybenzamine did not alter *d*-amphetamine self-administration except, perhaps, at high doses (Risner and Jones, 1976; Yokel and Wise, 1976). In a conditioned reinforcement paradigm, dopamine-beta-hydroxylase inhibitors such as U-14,624 and diethyldithiocarbamate, were found to block both the reinforcing properties of *d*-amphetamine and the reacquisition of *d*-amphetamine-maintained behavior following an interposed session of extinction (Davis *et al.*, 1975); however, the possibility that the enzyme inhibitors may have induced a conditioned aversion through actions of their own must be considered. Davis and Smith (1975) also provided evidence to suggest that central cholinergic systems may be involved in the reinforcing properties of *d*-amphetamine since atropine, but not methylatropine (which is only peripherally active), increased reacquisition rates (Davis and Smith, 1975); visual observation of these animals ruled out any effects of atropine on motor activity in animals working for *d*-amphetamine infusions.

If DA and, possibly, NE systems are involved in the reinforcing effects of *d*-amphetamine, DA and NE agonists should maintain behavior required for their administration; such results have been reported with apomorphine, piribedil and clonidine (Davis and Smith, 1977). More importantly, haloperidol blocks apomorphine and piribedil self-administration while phenoxybenzamine inhibits responding maintained by clonidine (Davis and Smith, 1977). Thus, activation of both DA and NE receptors appears to be reinforcing, although further assessment of this possibility is necessary because contradictory results have been obtained. For example, the direct alpha-adrenergic agonist, methoxamine does not maintain *d*-amphetamine self-administration (Risner and Jones, 1976).

The effects of many DA receptor antagonists also have been analyzed in animals trained to self-administer cocaine; thus, in studies that parallel those already considered, chlorpromazine (Roberts and Vickers, 1984; Wilson and Schuster, 1972), trifluoperazine (Wilson and Schuster, 1973a), haloperidol, fluphenthixol, thioridazine, sulpiride, metaclopramide, and pimozide (Roberts and Vickers, 1984; Woolverton, 1986) have been found to increase rates of responding maintained by i.v. cocaine administration. However, no evidence eliminating the possibility of drug-induced increases in motor activity or changes in cocaine metabolism is presented in any of this research. One study does indicate some specificity in the effects of perphenazine, since this compound increased rates of cocaine but not pentobarbital infusions (Johanson *et al.*, 1976). Similarly, the DA antagonist alpha-fluphenthixol increased responding for cocaine but not heroin (Ettenberg *et al.*, 1982); the opiate antagonist naltrexone increased heroin but not cocaine intake (Ettenberg *et al.*, 1982). Since the purportedly selective D-1 antagonist SCH 23390 (Iorio *et al.*, 1983) does not seem to alter cocaine self-administration (Woolverton, 1986), all of these results can be interpreted to indicate that DA (specifically, the D-2 receptors), is involved in the reinforcing (as well as the discriminative) properties of cocaine.

The effects of compounds that act primarily through NE mechanisms on behavior maintained by cocaine closely parallel their effects on *d*-amphetamine self-administration. Thus, NE antagonists such as phenoxybenzamine and phentolamine (De Witt and Wise, 1977; Wilson and Schuster, 1974), have no effects on responding for cocaine. Furthermore, the alpha-adrenergic antagonist prazosin does not alter responding for cocaine while the NE uptake inhibitor nisoxetine fails to maintain self-administration (Woolverton, 1987). In contrast, propranolol decreases responding for cocaine but not for food reinforcement (Goldberg and Gonzales, 1976); however, the specificity of this effect is uncertain because this drug is known to alter the pharmacodynamics of several other compounds (Goldberg and Gonzales, 1976).

The effects of cholinergic compounds on the behavior of rhesus monkeys trained under a continuous reinforcement schedule of cocaine self-administration have also been evaluated; 0.25 mg/kg of atropine significantly increased response rates while methylatropine did not (Wilson and Schuster, 1973b). Physostigmine, an anticholinesterase, decreased response rates, an effect that is associated with toxic reactions and is therefore likely to be nonspecific (Wilson and Schuster, 1973b). Obviously, more data must be gathered before any definitive conclusions regarding the role of noncatecholaminergic systems in the reinforcing effects of either amphetamine or cocaine can be drawn.

In summary, the studies reviewed thus far highlight striking similarities in the effects of neurotransmitter antagonists on the self-administration of psychomotor stimulants. Among other things, this suggests that the reinforcing action of cocaine may not be due to its local anesthetic effects. Dopamine antagonists consistently increase responding for both cocaine and *d*-amphetamine; this characteristic appears to be common to different D-2, but not D-1 antagonists. However, the possibility that D-1 receptor activation may modulate D-2 mediated effects (Waddington *et al.*, 1986) needs further investigation. In any event, the results that have been replicated consistently do not appear to result from nonspecific effects of test compounds on performance. While, the reported effects of NE antagonists on both amphetamine and cocaine reinforcement need clarification, the fact that DA and NE agonists are self-administered suggests that catecholaminergic receptor stimulation may be reinforcing. Indeed, Dackis and Gold (1985) have hypothesized that the post-synaptic actions of the DA released by cocaine may induce cocaine 'euphoria' while chronic cocaine abuse leads to DA depletion which results in 'dysphoria' and cocaine 'craving'.

Although central nervous system manipulations might not be comparable to systemic pharmacological interventions (above), various sorts of direct manipulations of central neurotransmitter systems have provided valuable information about the neuronal substrates of the reinforcing effects of *d*-amphetamine and cocaine. For example, the influence of catecholamine depletion on self-administration behavior has been examined in the conditioned reinforcement paradigm (Davis and Smith, 1973); treatment with AMPT abolished the reacquisition of *d*-amphetamine self-administration following an extinction session and prevented the establishment of a conditioned response based on the reinforcing properties of *d*-amphetamine and, thus, could not have been the result of drug-induced, motor incapacitation (Davis and Smith, 1973). These findings support the hypothesis that catecholamines play a role in the reinforcing properties of *d*-amphetamine.

DA neuronal systems have been more specifically implicated in the effects of *d*-amphetamine by research in which the functional activity of discrete brain areas has been altered. In one such study, electrolytic lesions of the ventral tegmentum which selectively destroy meso-cortico-limbic DA pathways, did not alter saline self-administration (in rats, tested 1 month later) but caused a response maintained by *d*-amphetamine infusions to be acquired more rapidly and induced faster than normal response rates (Le Moal *et al.*, 1979). Lesions of the same area with the catecholaminergic neurotoxin 6-hydroxydopamine (6-OHDA) also enhanced the rate of acquisition and response rate; importantly, this effect occurred in animals tested 1 month after treatment, when DA concentrations in the nucleus accumbens and frontal cortex (both of which are terminal areas of fibers originating in the ventral tegmentum) are considerably reduced (Deminiere *et al.*, 1984). However, specific lesions of the nucleus accumbens with microinjections of 6-OHDA have also been reported to abolish lever pressing in animals previously trained to self-administer *d*-amphetamine but not food (Lyness *et al.*, 1979). During the period when responding had ceased, nucleus accumbens DA concentrations were reduced to 5% of control values. Furthermore, drug naive animals given 6-OHDA lesions did not acquire a response reinforced with i.v. infusions of 0.125 mg/kg *d*-amphetamine in 19 days (control animals responded within 7-10 days). While the apparently contradictory results of Deminiere *et al.* (1984) and Lyness *et al.* (1979) may be attributed to the actions of ventral tegmental lesions on many terminal areas, further study is required to clarify the role of the nucleus accumbens in the reinforcing effects of psychotomotor stimulants.

A true test of the reinforcing efficacy of a drug at a particular site lies in the ability of the drug to maintain behavior when it is injected directly into that site. Responding for direct injection of *d*-amphetamine into the nucleus accumbens has been reported (Hoebel *et al.*, 1983; Monaco *et al.*, 1980) and animals were found to regulate the quantity of drug self-administered (Hoebel *et al.*, 1983). Since infusing the drug into the lateral ventricle or into the caudate nucleus did not similarly maintain responding (Hoebel *et al.*, 1983), amphetamine-induced activation of areas surrounding the ventricular system could not have been responsible for its reinforcing effect. Thus, the meso-cortico-limbic DA system, and more specifically, the nucleus accumbens, may be involved in the reinforcing properties of *d*-amphetamine, an inference also made on the basis of the results of drug discrimination experiments (above).

The effects of lesions of the 5-HT system have also been examined on *d*-amphetamine self-administration. In one experiment, intraventricular injections of the neurotoxin 5,7-dihydroxytryptamine (5,7-DHT) into drug naive animals did not alter the rate of acquisition of self-administration behavior but did induce consistently higher response rates than appropriate controls (Lyness *et al.*, 1980). Similarly, chemical lesions of the medial forebrain bundle also elevated response rates for *d*-amphetamine while having no effect on acquisition rates (Leccese and Lyness, 1984). These results may indicate a role of 5-HT in the aversive properties of *d*-amphetamine, although further analysis of this effect is required (Lyness *et al.*, 1980). Surprisingly, similar lesions of the nucleus accumbens did not alter either the acquisition or rate of self-administration in drug naive animals (Lyness *et al.*, 1980).

The meso-cortico-limbic DA system may be involved in the reinforcing effects of psychomotor stimulants other than *d*-amphetamine. For example, cocaine self-administration was reduced over a significant period of time by 6-OHDA lesions of the ventral tegmentum in a study in which extensive intersubject variation also occurred. However, the correlation between DA levels in the nucleus accumbens and rate of self-administration was not significant (Roberts and Koob, 1982). These results may be attributed to the effects of ventral tegmental area lesions on other terminal regions; specific lesions of the nucleus accumbens reduced cocaine intake to 30% of controls, an effect that persisted for more than 14 days and did not occur when self-administration behavior was reinforced with food (Roberts *et al.*, 1977). Moreover, a good correlation between DA levels in the nucleus accumbens and rate of self-administration was observed in another experiment, despite the spread of the lesions to the septal, cortical and olfactory areas (Roberts *et al.*, 1980). The possibility that this correlation may be due to a motor deficit induced by DA depletion in the accumbens appears unlikely since the 6-OHDA-induced lesions blocked self-administration of cocaine but not heroin (Pettit *et al.*, 1984).

The destruction of both nerve terminals and fibers of passage by 6-OHDA raises questions concerning the role of neurons passing through the nucleus accumbens in the effects of the lesions. Kainic acid, a compound which leaves fibers of passage intact while selectively destroying nerve terminals also decreases the rate of responding for cocaine with the extent of damage correlating well with rate of responding (Zito *et al.*, 1985). However, infusions of apomorphine do not reinstate responding following kainic acid lesions and animals trained to self-administer heroin are also disrupted. Thus, the possibility that the lesions alter self-administration behavior because of their many nonspecific effects cannot be ruled out entirely. Interestingly, reducing catecholamine levels less selectively by pretreating with either AMPT or reserpine appears to *increase* the amount of cocaine self-administered (Wilson and Schuster, 1974), an effect that may reflect a partial decrease in the reinforcing properties of cocaine. NE does not, however, appear to play a major role in the maintenance of self-administration behavior since protection of NE neurons from the toxic effects of 6-OHDA does not prevent the disruption of responding (Roberts *et al.*, 1980). Furthermore, 6-OHDA lesions of the dorsal or ventral nonadrenergic bundles (which decrease NE concentrations in hippocampus, cortex and hypothalamus) do not alter responding maintained by cocaine infusions (Roberts *et al.*, 1977).

While the studies mentioned thus far imply that the meso-cortico-limbic DA system is involved in the reinforcing effects of cocaine (although possible nonspecific deficits in performance cannot be ignored), neither the nucleus accumbens nor the ventral tegmental area were implicated in this phenomenon by research in which cocaine was infused directly into different brain areas (Goeder and Smith, 1983). Rather, responding for injections of cocaine into the medial prefrontal cortex was observed, even when drug-reinforced lever-pressing was maintained under an FR schedule and when the positions of 'active' and 'inactive' levers were reversed in two lever operant chambers (Goeders and Smith, 1983). In these studies, spread of the infused cocaine appeared to be restricted to the medial prefrontal cortex, although the low recovery rates of the labelled infusion suggest that cocaine was removed rapidly from the injection site (Goeders and Smith, 1984, 1986). Concomitant infusions of sulpiride and cocaine reduced the rate of cocaine-maintained responding (Goeders and Smith, 1983, 1984); other receptor antagonists (e.g. atropine, propranolol, SCH 23390) had no effect on the day of the infusion (Goeders and Smith, 1984; Goeders *et al.*, 1986). However, SCH 23390 and atropine and delayed depressant effects indicating indirect actions. Self-administration of cocaine into the medial prefrontal cortex was abolished by lesions of this area with 6-OHDA and was restored by DA, but not 5-HT, infusions; addition of sulpiride to the DA solution once again reduced responding (Goeders and Smith, 1986). While these data suggest that cocaine may exert its reinforcing effects by increasing cortical DA concentrations at this site which, in turn acts on post synaptic D-2 receptors, these results require clarification since 6-OHDA lesions of the medial prefrontal cortex had no effect on intravenous cocaine self-administration despite the fact that the lesions significantly reduced DA concentrations in this area (Martin-Iverson *et al.*, 1986).

Thus, direct manipulations of CNS neurotransmitter systems have revealed both similarities and differences in the mechanisms subserving *d*-amphetamine and cocaine reinforcement. Specific lesions of the nucleus accumbens abolished *d*-amphetamine self-administration while infusions of *d*-amphetamine directly into this nucleus maintained responding, suggesting an important role of the nucleus accumbens in *d*-amphetamine reinforcement. The role of the nucleus accumbens in cocaine self-administration is less clear. Although lesions of this nucleus appear to abolish cocaine-maintained behavior, injections of cocaine directly into this site are not reinforcing. It is possible that the effects of the lesions may involve more rostral brain regions such as the prefrontal cortex. In all of this research, however, there is a need to eliminate nonspecific motor deficits that may be caused by lesions and other direct interventions.

In conclusion, the results of drug discrimination and self-administration studies are generally parallel: DA antagonists block psychomotor stimulant cues and increase response rates for intravenous drug infusions, an effect which is probably due to the decreased reinforcing value of the drug states. Although the drug discrimination data are not always clear, DA agonists generally appear to mimic *d*-amphetamine and, less certainly, cocaine. Such receptor agonists are also reinforcing in that they maintain self-administration behavior. NE systems appear to be less important than DA systems in the discrimination or self-administration of psychomotor stimulants. The self-administration of *d*-amphetamine into the nucleus accumbens directly parallels the discriminative cue induced by this drug in the same area. Unfortunately, the central cocaine cue has not yet been examined directly in drug discrimination procedures; such studies are presently in progress in the Behavioral Pharmacology Laboratory (BPL) (Department of Psychology, University of South Carolina).

3. HALLUCINOGENS: THE DISCRIMINATIVE STIMULUS PROPERTIES OF LSD AND MESCALINE

In spite of many differences in their chemical structures, compounds classified as 'hallucinogens' have subjective effects that are both (qualitatively) different from those of other drugs and similar to each other (Jacobs, 1987). For example, humans report similar feelings of happiness, loss of control, detachment, anxiety, and euphoria following ingestion of the phenylalkylamine mescaline or the ergot derivative LSD (Katz and Waskow, 1968; Rosenberg *et al.*, 1963; Wolbach *et al.*, 1962); moreover, cross-tolerance to many of these effects is reported consistently (Wolbach *et al.*, 1962). Drug discrimination experiments have shown that similar relationships occur in other animals [Table 3(a)]; that is, the effects of mescaline and LSD cross-generalize (Colpaert *et al.*, 1979b, 1982; Hirschhorn and Winter, 1971; Schechter and Rosecrans, 1972; Winter, 1978) and are blocked by the same (serotonergic) agents [Table 4(a)]. As with humans, many of the effects of these substances show cross-tolerance (Appel and Freedman, 1968) that is not related to drug-induced increases in metabolism (Winter, 1971). While these observations probably mean that structurally different hallucinogens act through similar mechanisms, it is unlikely that these mechanisms are restricted to the hallucinogenic properties of these substances, since agents that are not known to be hallucinogenic (e.g. TMPEA, DOET, lisuride, BL-3912 and quipazine) mimic substances such as LSD (Winter, 1973, 1975a, 1980).

While the neuronal mechanisms responsible for the subjective effects of hallucinogens will probably never be fully known, it is likely that they involve 5-HT neuronal systems and, more specifically, 5-HT-2 receptors (Appel *et al.*, 1982; Hamon, 1984). The evidence in support of this hypothesis has been the focus of considerable recent attention (Appel and Cunningham, 1986; Jacobs, 1987) and will be summarized here. Relatively nonselective central 5-HT antagonists such as cinanserin, methysergide, BC 105 and cyproheptadine have been known for some time to block the discriminable properties of both LSD and mescaline (Browne and Ho, 1975; Cunningham and Appel, 1987; Kuhn *et al.*, 1978; White and Appel, 1982b; Winter, 1975b, 1978). In addition, BC-105 antagonizes the substitution of LSD for mescaline, but does not affect the discriminability of non-hallucinogenic compounds such as *d*-amphetamine (Winter, 1978). Xylamidine, a 5-HT antagonist that acts peripherally, does not generally block the mescaline or LSD cues [Table 4(c)]. However, discrepancies in the effects of some of these antagonists have been reported; in one study, neither cyproheptadine (3 mg/kg) nor methysergide (10 mg/kg) blocked the LSD cue completely (Hirschhorn and Rosecrans, 1974) and, in another, only partial antagonism of LSD was induced by metergoline, bromo-LSD, cinanserin, metitepine, methysergide, cyproheptadine and mianserin (Colpaert *et al.*, 1982). Interestingly, such

TABLE 3. *Results of Substitution (Generalization) Tests in Animals Trained to Discriminate LSD (L) or Mescaline (M) from Saline*

(a) *Complete Antagonism* (≥80%)		
(L)	BL-3912	Winter (1980)
(L)	Clonidine	Colpaert (1984)
(M)	Doet	Winter (1975a)
(M)	Dom	Winter (1975a)
(L)	Fenfluramine	Winter (1980)
(L)	Lisuride	Holohean *et al.* (1982), White and Appel (1982a)
(M)	LSD	Hirschhorn and Winter (1971), Winter (1978)
(L)	5-MEODMT	White and Appel (1982b)
(L)	Mescaline	Colpaert *et al.* (1979b), Colpaert *et al.* (1982), Schechter and Rosecrans (1972)
(L)	Methysergide	Colpaert *et al.* (1982)
(L)	Mianserin	Colpaert *et al.* (1979b, 1982)
(L)	MK-212	White and Appel (1982b)
(L)	Psilocybin	Schechter and Rosecrans (1972)
(L)	Quipazine	Colpaert *et al.* (1979b, 1982), Cunningham and Appel (1987), White and Appel (1982a,b)
(M)	TMPEA	Winter (1973)
(L)	Yohimbine	Colpaert (1984)
(b) *Partial Substitution* (60–79%)		
(L)	Cyproheptadine	Colpaert *et al.* (1979b, 1982)
(L)	Ergonovine	Holohean *et al.* (1982)
(L)	5-MOEDMT	Rosecrans and Glennon (1979)
(L)	Methysergide	Colpaert *et al.* (1979b)
(L)	Quipazine	Kuhn *et al.* (1978)
(L)	SCH-12679	Winter (1980)
(L)	Xylazine	Colpaert (1984)
(c) *No Substitution* (≤59%)		
(M) (L)	Amphetamine	Schechter and Rosecrans (1972), White and Appel (1982b), Winter (1975a)
(L)	Apomorphine	Holohean *et al.* (1982), Kuhn *et al.* (1978), White and Appel (1982b)
(L)	BC-105	Colpaert *et al.* (1982), Cunningham and Appel (1987)
(L)	Bromocriptine	Holohean *et al.* (1982)
(L)	Bromo-LSD	Colpaert *et al.* (1982), Cunningham and Appel (1987)
(L)	Chlorimipramine	Kuhn *et al.* (1978)
(L)	Cinanserin	Colpaert *et al.* (1982)
(M)	Cocaine	Winter (1975a)
(L)	Fluoxetine	Kuhn *et al.* (1978)
(L)	8 OHDPAT	Cunningham and Appel (1987)
(L)	L-5-HTP	Cunningham *et al.* (1985)
(L)	Ketanserin	Cunningham and Appel (1987)
(L)	Lergotrile	Holohean *et al.* (1982)
(L)	LY-53857	Cunningham and Appel (1987)
(L)	MCPP	Cunningham and Appel (1987)
(L)	Metergoline	Colpaert *et al.* (1982, Cunningham and Appel (1987)
(L)	Morphine	Hirschhorn and Rosecrans (1974)
(L)	Metitepine	Colpaert *et al.* (1982)
(L)	Pirenperone	Colpaert *et al.* (1982), Cunningham and Appel (1987)
(L)	R-56413	Colpaert *et al.* (1985)
(L)	Ritanserin	Colpaert *et al.* (1985)
(L)	RU-24969	Cunningham and Appel (1987)
(L)	Spiperone	Cunningham and Appel (1987)
(L)	TFMPP	Cunningham and Appel (1987)
(L)	Trazodone	Cunningham and Appel (1987)
(L)	L-Tryptophan	Kuhn *et al.* (1978)

TABLE 4. *Results of Combination (Antagonism) Tests in Animals Trained to Discriminate LSD (L) or Mescaline (M) from Saline*

(a) *Complete Antagonism* (≤40%)		
(M) (L)	BC-105	Colpaert *et al.* (1982), Cunningham and Appel (1987), Holohean *et al.* (1982), Nielsen *et al.* (1985), Winter (1978)
(L)	Bromo-LSD	Cunningham and Appel (1987)
(M)	Cinanserin	Browne (1978), Browne and Ho (1975), Winter (1975b, 1978)
(M) (L)	Cyproheptadine	Browne (1978), Browne and Ho (1975), Kuhn *et al.* (1978) White and Appel (1982b)
(L)	Ketanserin	Cunningham and Appel (1987), Nielsen *et al.* (1985)
(L)	LY-53857	Cunningham and Appel (1987)
(L)	Metergoline	Cunningham and Appel (1987)
(L)	Methiothepin	Kuhn *et al.* (1978)
(L)	Methysergide	Kuhn *et al.* (1978)
(L)	Pirenperone	Colpaert *et al.* (1982), Cunningham and Appel (1987), Nielsen *et al.* (1985)
(L)	Ritanserin	Colpaert *et al.* (1985)
(L)	Trazodone	Cunningham and Appel (1987)
(b) *Partial Antagonism* (41–79%)		
(L)	Bromo-LSD	Colpaert *et al.* (1982), Kuhn *et al.* (1978)
(L)	Cinanserin	Colpaert *et al.* (1982), Kuhn *et al.* (1978)
(L)	Cyproheptadine	Colpaert *et al.* (1982), Kuhn *et al.* (1978)
(M) (L)	Metergoline	Browne (1978), Colpaert *et al.* (1982)
(M) (L)	Methysergide	Browne and Ho (1975), Colpaert *et al.* (1982), Hirschhorn and Rosecrans (1974)
(L)	Metitepine	Colpaert *et al.* (1982)
(L)	Mianserin	Colpaert *et al.* (1982)
(L)	Naloxone	Hirschhorn and Rosecrans (1974)
(L)	Methiothepin	White and Appel (1982b)
(c) *No Antagonism* (≥80%)		
(M) (L)	Atropine	Browne and Ho (1975), Hirschhorn and Rosecrans (1974), Kuhn *et al.* (1978)
(L)	(+)Butaclamol	Kuhn *et al.* (1978)
(L)	Chlorimipramine	Kuhn *et al.* (1978)
(L)	Cyproheptadine	Hirschhorn and Rosecrans (1974)
(L)	Fluoxetine	Kuhn *et al.* (1978)
(L)	Fluphenazine	Kuhn *et al.* (1978)
(L)	(Alpha)-Fluphenthixol	Kuhn *et al.* (1978)
(L)	Haloperidol	Colpaert *et al.* (1982), Holohean *et al.* (1982), Kuhn *et al.* (1978), Nielsen *et al.* (1985), White and Appel (1982b)
(L)	8-OHDPAT	Cunningham and Appel (1987)
(L)	Naloxone	Colpaert *et al.* (1982)
(L)	Phenoxybenzamine	Colpaert *et al.* (1982)
(M) (L)	Phentolamine	Browne and Ho (1975), Kuhn *et al.* (1978)
(M)	Pimozide	Browne and Ho (1975)
(L)	Promethazine	Kuhn *et al.* (1978)
(M) (L)	Propranolol	Browne and Ho (1975), Colpaert *et al.* (1982), Kuhn *et al.* (1978)

continued

TABLE 4 *continued.*

(c) *No Antagonism (≥80%) continued*		
(L)	Pyrilamine	Colpaert *et al.* (1982)
(L)	R-56413	Colpaert *et al.* (1985)
(L)	Spiperone	Colpaert *et al.* (1982), Cunningham and Appel (1987)
(L)	Trifluoperazine	Kuhn *et al.* (1978)
(L)	L-Tryptophan	Kuhn *et al.* (1978)
(M) (L)	Xylamidine	Browne (1978), Browne and Ho (1975), White and Appel (1982b)

'antagonists' as methysergide, cyproheptadine and mianserin have been reported to *substitute* for the LSD cue when administered alone. [Tables 3(a) and 3(b)]. However, the doses required for this effect exceed those used for antagonism; thus, an assessment of the changing effects of these antagonists over a range of doses may provide information concerning the mechanisms subserving hallucinogenic drugs.

More recent findings suggest that antagonists which act selectively at the 5-HT-2 receptor subtype are particularly and consistently effective in antagonizing LSD. For example, ritanserin, and pirenperone [which do not have any agonist properties; Table 3(c)], ketanserin, and LY 53857, block the discriminable effects of this substance (Colpaert *et al.*, 1982, 1985; Cunningham and Appel, 1987; Nielsen *et al.*, 1985); in addition, pretreatment with pirenperone shifts the LSD dose response curve to the right (Colpaert and Janssen, 1983) and ketanserin blocks the substitution of LSD for L-5-HTP (Cunningham *et al.*, 1985). Recent experiments have examined the effects of these 5-HT-2 antagonists on the mescaline cue (Appel and Callahan, 1987). Relatively low doses of ketanserin, LY 53857, and pirenperone completely block both the discrimination of 10 mg/kg of this compound from saline and the drug-induced suppression of responding; Xylamidine does not antagonize the mescaline cue. Thus, the effects of 5-HT-2 antagonists on LSD and mescaline are remarkably similar; if anything, mescaline is a more 'pure' 5-HT-2 agonist than LSD.

Depletion of central 5-HT concentrations by pretreatment with the tryptophan hydroxylase inhibitor *para*-chlorophenylalanine (PCPA) enhances the discriminability of both mescaline and LSD (Browne, 1978; Browne and Ho, 1975; Cameron and Appel, 1973; White *et al.*, 1980). This may be caused either by PCPA-induced receptor supersensitivity or decreased competition of hallucinogens with endogenous substances (e.g. 5-HT) for serotonergic receptor sites. The effects of PCPA on the mescaline cue seem to be specific, since this treatment does not alter either CNS concentrations of mescaline or the ability of rats to discriminate other active compounds (e.g. pentobarbital) from saline (Browne, 1978); unfortunately, other investigators have not always obtained similar results (Winter, 1980).

While 5,7-DHT, like PCPA, has been found to enhance the LSD cue (White *et al.*, 1980), another serotonergic neurotoxin, *para*-chloroamphetamine (PCA) does not have comparable effects on sensitivity to LSD (White *et al.*, 1980), despite the fact that it causes similar depletions in 5-HT concentrations. It has been suggested that differences in the patterns of neurochemical lesions may account for this inconsistency; that is, PCA, in contrast to other neurotoxins, has relatively selective actions on B9 cells (bilateral pontine raphe nuclei) and does not decrease 5-HT throughout the neuron as do PCPA and 5,7-DHT (White *et al.*, 1980). Similarly, although 5,7-DHT lesions do not appear to have any effect on the discriminability of LSD in neonatal rats (Minnema and Rosecrans, 1984), the depletion of 5-HT was not complete in this study, thus compensatory activity in the remaining intact 5-HT neurons could have occurred.

Since 5-HT antagonists (particularly those that act selectively at 5-HT-2 subtypes) block, and 5-HT depletion enhances, the discriminability of both LSD and mescaline, it is likely that these compounds act, at least in part, by directly stimulating post-synaptic 5-HT-2 receptors (Jacobs, 1987). Therefore, directly acting 5-HT agonists should substitute for hallucinogenic drug cues; indeed, compounds that purportedly act at 5-HT-2 receptors, quipazine DOI and DOM, engender LSD- and mescaline-like responding (Colpaert *et al.*, 1979b, 1982; Cunningham and Appel, 1987; Friedman *et al.*, 1984; Kuhn *et al.*, 1978; White and Appel, 1982a, 1982b). Another putative 5-HT agonist, MK 212 also mimics the LSD cue (White and Appel, 1982b) but the receptor subtype at which this substance acts is not clear (Cunningham *et al.*, 1986). Interestingly, 5-HT agonists that act at other serotonergic receptor subtypes (e.g. 8-OHDPAT, RU24969 and TFMPP) elicit a maximum of only 50% LSD- or mescaline-like responding in virtually identical experimental situations (Cunningham and Appel, 1987; unpublished data) and disrupt response rates at higher doses. Moreover, complete generalization to LSD does not occur in animals trained to discriminate either 8-OHDPAT (Cunningham *et al.*, 1987) or TFMPP (Cunningham and Appel, 1986) from saline.

The specificity of the mechanisms underlying the discriminable effects of hallucinogens is demonstrated further by the fact that drugs such as 5-HTP, chlorimipramine and fluoxetine, which have indirect (presynaptic) actions at 5-HT receptors do not mimic LSD (Cunningham *et al.*, 1985; Kuhn *et al.*, 1978); unfortunately, in some cases, only a few doses of these substances have been tested. However, fenfluramine, a compound which releases 5-HT, does induce as much as 80% drug-like responding, but only at very disruptive doses (Winter, 1980). All of these compounds increase synaptic 5-HT concentrations at a variety of receptors (5-HT-1, 5-HT-2, etc.) which may mask their actions at 5-HT-2 receptor subtypes. In addition, 5-HTP is known to displace catecholamines (Fuxe *et al.*, 1971).

Although postsynaptic 5-HT receptors have been implicated many times in hallucinogenic drug effects (Appel *et al.*, 1982; Jacobs, 1987), experiments designed to identify the particular brain regions that are directly involved in the actions of these substances have not yet been undertaken with sufficient frequency to yield definitive conclusions. Both systemic and microiontopheretic applications of LSD are known to inhibit the activity of neurons in the site from which many 5-HT neurons arise, the dorsal raphe nucleus (Haigler and Aghajanian, 1974). Systemic injections of mescaline also suppress the firing rate of some of these neurons but microiontophoresis of this compound does not have comparable effects to those of LSD (Haigler and Aghajanian, 1973). Thus, ability to inhibit raphe firing rate probably does not account for the similar effects of these compounds and, indeed, may not be involved in the *in vivo* effects of LSD (Kuhn *et al.*, 1978; White and Appel, 1982a). In another interesting experiment involving the electrical activity of 5-HT cell bodies animals were trained to emit a response based on the presence or absence of dorsal raphe stimulation (Hirschhorn *et al.*, 1975). Systemic injections of 0.05 mg/kg of LSD induced 65% stimulation–appropriate responding; however, no such generalization occurred when LSD was injected directly into the dorsal raphe nucleus (Rosecrans and Glennon, 1979) suggesting the involvement of 5-HT in rostral brain regions in the stimulus properties of dorsal raphe stimulation.

The nucleus accumbens is another region that may be involved in the LSD cue. Nielsen and Scheel-Kruger (1986) demonstrated that microinjections of LSD (1 μg) directly into this area produced drug-appropriate responding in animals trained to discriminate peripheral injections of LSD (0.16 mg/kg) from saline; moreover, this generalization was found to be specific since injection of LSD into the caudate nucleus did not mimic the training drug.

Another approach to the problem of which brain sites might be involved in the subjective effects of hallucinogens explored by Nielsen *et al.*, (1985) involved combining drug discrimination and receptor binding procedures. By comparing the potencies of antagonists in blocking the LSD cue to their abilities to displace [^{3}H]spiroperidol from 5-HT receptors in the frontal cortex, striatum, and cerebellum, these investigators demonstrated that pirenperone, ketanserin, and BC-105 inhibited spiroperidol binding in the frontal cortex at doses which blocked the LSD cue; haloperidol was ineffective against both spiroperidol binding and the drug cue. Unfortunately, LSD itself did not inhibit spiroperidol binding at doses that had discriminable effects, perhaps because this compound has multiple actions at other receptor sites; alternatively, LSD may occupy only a small number of 5-HT receptors due to its high efficacy, thereby displacing little spiroperidol.

Thus, although a large body of evidence implicates 5-HT, particularly 5-HT-2 receptors in hallucinogenic drug cues, possible interactions with other neurotransmitter systems must also be considered. Some studies have, for example, suggested that LSD has weak dopaminergic properties. DA agonists such as lisuride (Holohean *et al.*, 1982; White and Appel, 1982a) and apomorphine (White and Appel, 1982a) substitute for the training drug, at least partially, in animals trained to discriminate LSD (0.08 mg/kg) from saline and, in animals trained to discriminate apomorphine from saline, 70% generalization occurs to LSD (Holohean *et al.*, 1982). Moreover, depletion of catecholamines with 6-OHDA enhances the discriminability of low doses of LSD (but not *d*-amphetamine), at least in neonatal rats (Minnema and Rosecrans, 1984). On the other hand, the LSD and mescaline cues are not blocked to any extent by DA antagonists [Table 4(c)]; thus, if they are in any way involved in the actions of hallucinogens, DA neurons may play a secondary or indirect role to 5-HT. Antagonists of acetylcholine, NE, histamine and opiate receptors also appear to be ineffective in altering the subjective effects of both LSD and mescaline [Table 4(c)], although more research needs to be conducted with mescaline as well as other phenylalkylamines. Indeed, it is interesting the alpha-2-adrenoceptor antagonist, yohimbine, which has anxiogenic properties (in humans), has been reported to substitute for LSD (Colpaert, 1984), suggesting that the subjective effects of hallucinogens may include anxiety.

4. THE BEHAVIORAL PHARMACOLOGY OF 3,4-METHYLENEDIOXYAMPHETAMINE (MDA) AND 3,4-METHYLENEDIOXYMETHAMPHETAMINE (MDMA)

Neither the pharmacological actions nor the behavioral effects of MDA (the so-called 'love' drug) or MDMA ('ecstasy') have been studied extensively. Nevertheless, the abuse of these substances, which was first reported in the early 1970s (Jackson and Reed, 1970; Richards, 1972), led to their being placed under Schedule 1 restrictions by the Drug Enforcement Agency (DEA), United States Department of Justice; several fatalities have also been attributed to MDA (Thiessen and Cook, 1973).

In humans, the effects of oral ingestion of 500 mg of MDA include muscular spasms and clonic convulsions, increased heart rate, temperature, and blood pressure (Richards and Borgstedt, 1971). However, the severity of these and other symptoms varies dramatically among individuals, even following identical doses (Richards and Borgstedt, 1971). On a more quantitative level, the effects of MDA (40–150 mg, p.o.) begin 30 to 60 min after administration, peak within the first 2 hr, and continue for as long as 12 hr (Naranjo *et al.*, 1967; Turek *et al.*, 1974).

The subjective effects of MDA are difficult to characterize precisely. In one study, 80 mg (p.o.) of this compound was reported to *enhance* sensory perception, particularly of auditory stimuli (Alles, 1959); however, MDA (75 mg, p.o.) has also been found to *decrease* ability to perform a visual motor task, and to increase the amount of perceived effort required to concentrate (Turek *et al.*, 1974). Subjects given his 'hallucinogen' report drug-induced feelings of peace, joy, gentleness, and closeness to others, in addition to an *enhanced* sense of taste and *reduced* sense of time, but not of control, over their perceived environment (Jackson and Reed, 1970; Turek *et al.*, 1974). A drug-induced need to be close to and talk with others (Jackson and Reed, 1970) has prompted some authors to argue that MDA may be a useful adjunct to psychotherapy (Yensen *et al.*, 1976). Although MDA is often regarded as an hallucinogen (Richards, 1972), studies conducted thus far do not support such a classification (Alles, 1959; Turek *et al.*, 1974); however, it is likely that much higher doses of this drug are used outside the laboratory and that substances obtained 'on the street' are likely to contain many impurities, some of which may be hallucinogenic. The subjective effects of MDMA have not been extensively studied; however, Shulgin and Nichols (1978) have described the effects of MDMA as comparable to those of PCP, low doses of MDA, and marijuana.

The appearance of MDA and MDMA on the 'underground' drug market and reports of their apparently toxic side effects prompted a comparative assessment of these compounds in animals. In spinally transected dogs, the effects of intravenous injections of MDA (2.0 mg/kg) on flexor reflexes, respiration rate, body temperature, and eye tracking were found to be similar to those of LSD (10 μg/kg); effects on stereotypy, the nictitating membrane response, and pupillary dilatation resembled those of 3.2 mg/kg of *d*-amphetamine (Nozaki *et al.*, 1977). Further, animals tolerant to LSD showed a partial cross-tolerance to MDA. Thus, MDA appears to resemble both LSD and *d*-amphetamine. However, the mechanisms mediating the effects of phenylisopropylamines appear to be closer to those of *d*-amphetamine than to those of LSD; for example, several of the effects of MDA, like *d*-amphetamine, are blocked by the alpha-adrenergic antagonist phenoxybenzamine but are unaffected by the 5-HT antagonist cyproheptadine, while those of LSD are diminished by cyproheptadine and unaffected by phenoxybenzamine (Nozaki *et al.*, 1977).

All of the studies discussed thus far involve racemic (+/−) MDA; Marquardt *et al.* (1978) described the differential effects of the (+) and (−) isomers of MDA in mice. In this experiment, the (+) isomer appeared to be more potent in eliciting convulsions autonomic activities such as salivation and increased respiration, and such motor activities as hyperreactivity and stereotypy; all of these effects resemble those of *d*-amphetamine. However, apparent hallucinations were said to be present following either (+/−) or (−)MDA, since animals appeared to hide from, fight, or stare at 'objects' that were not present. Thus, the stimulant properties of this drug appear to be elicited by the (+) isomer while hallucinogenic-like activity is induced by the (−) isomer.

Since replacement of cocaine solutions with MDA engenders similar rates of lever-pressing in self-administration sessions, MDA has been said to be reinforcing, at least in baboons (Griffiths *et al.*, 1976). However, the doses necessary to maintain this behavior (1, 2 or 5 mg/kg per infusion) indicate that MDA is 20 times less potent in this regard than *d*-amphetamine. Access to infusions of MDMA also maintains self-administration behavior in baboons previously trained to self-administer cocaine (Beardsley *et al.*, 1986; Lamb and Griffiths, 1987). Response rates for MDMA were found to be both lower (Lamb and Griffiths, 1987) and higher than those induced by cocaine (Beardsley *et al.*, 1986); thus, there is a need to examine these effects further.

While its putatively reinforcing properties may account for its 'street' abuse, Richards (1972) has suggested that drug users in Toronto cannot distinguish between the effects of MDA and those of other 'psychedelics'. The stimulus properties of MDA and MDMA have been assessed further (in animals) with drug discrimination procedures [Tables 5(a), (b), and (c)]. Using a foot-shock avoidance task, Shannon (1980) examined the MDA cue in rats trained to discriminate 1 mg/kg *d*-amphetamine from saline; despite the testing of an extensive range of doses, (+/−)MDA did not induce responding on the training drug lever. However, in a more standard situation involving food reinforcement, generalization of (+/−)amphetamine has been reported to occur to (+/−)MDA and generalization of (+/−)MDA occurs to *d*-amphetamine (Glennon and Young, 1984a); substitution of (+/−)MDA for *d*-amphetamine has also been demonstrated in pigeons (Evans and Johanson, 1986) and monkeys (Kamien *et al.*, 1986). Surprisingly, cross-generalization also occurs between the hallucinogen (+/−)DOM and (+/−)MDA (Glennon *et al.*, 1982); (+/−)DOM does not engender *d*-amphetamine responding (Glennon and Young, 1984a). In another study, animals trained to discriminate 1.5 mg/kg (+/−)MDA from saline responded on the drug lever when given either LSD (0.075 mg/kg) or cocaine (9.15 mg/kg) (Glennon and Young, 1984b). Thus, despite differences in the stimulant (i.e. *d*-amphetamine or cocaine) and hallucinogen (i.e. DOM or LSD) cues, (+/−)MDA appears to have stimulus properties that are similar to both groups of compounds. However, the small number of subjects used in these studies must be considered before such conclusions can be supported.

Glennon and Young have extended their examination of the subjective effects of MDA to those of the separate isomers. Initially, generalization of the (−), but not the (+) iso-

TABLE 5. *Results of Substitution (Generalization) Tests*

(a) *In Animals Trained to Discriminate* d-*Amphetamine from Saline*		
(±)2,3-MDA	X	Glennon *et al.* (1984)
(±)3,4-MDA	X	Glennon and Young (1984b)
	C	Evans and Johanson (1986), Glennon and Young (1984a), Kamien *et al.* (1986)
(+)3,4-MDA	C	Glennon and Young (1984c)
(−)3,4-MDA	X	Glennon and Young (1984c)
(±)3,4-MDMA	C	Glennon and Young (1984c), Kamien *et al.* (1986)
(b) *In Animals Trained to Discriminate (±)3,4-MDA from Saline*		
(±) Amphetamine	C	Glennon and Young (1984a)
Cocaine	C	Glennon and Young (1984b)
LSD	C	Glennon and Young (1948b)
(±)2,3-MDA	C	Glennon *et al.* (1984)
(+)3,4-MDA	C	Glennon and Young (1984c)
(−)3,4-MDA	C	Glennon and Young (1984c)
(±)3,4-MDMA	C	Glennon and Young (1984c)
(c) *In Animals Trained to Discriminate (±) DOM from Saline*		
(±)2,3-MDA	X	Glennon *et al.* (1984)
(±)3,4-MDA	C	Glennon *et al.* (1982)
(+)3,4-MDA	X	Glennon *et al.* (1982)
(−)3,4-MDA	C	Glennon *et al.* (1982)
(±)3,4-MDMA	X	Glennon *et al.* (1982)
(+)3,4-MDMA	X	Glennon *et al.* (1982)
(−)3,4-MDMA	X	Glennon *et al.* (1982)

Symbols: X = no substitution (≤59%), P = partial substitution (60–79%), C = complete substitution (≥80%)

mer of MDA, was observed to occur to (+/−)DOM (Glennon *et al.*, 1982). In addition, the (+) isomer of MDA was reported to substitute for the training drug in animals exposed to a *d*-amphetamine–saline discrimination; (−)MDA did not have comparable effects (Glennon and Young, 1984c). The effects of (+/−)MDA appear to more closely resemble those of (+)MDA than (−)MDA, since higher doses were required of the (−) than the (+) isomer to substitute for the (+/−)MDA cue (Glennon and Young, 1984c). Thus, these studies indicate that the stimulant-like properties of (+/−)MDA result from the actions of the (+) isomer while the hallucinogenic properties result from the (−) isomer, a hypothesis that agrees with the results of Marquardt *et al.* (1978).

Recent data from the BPL have indicated that (−)MDA also substitutes for another hallucinogenic compound, mescaline (Callahan and Appel, 1987). However, in the BPL study, animals trained to discriminate 10 mg/kg of mescaline from saline also responded on the drug-appropriate lever when given (+)MDA. These results suggest that the disassociation of the stimulant and hallucinogenic properties of the (+) and (−) isomers of MDA may not extend to all hallucinogens.

Unfortunately, the different isomers of MDMA have not been tested to the same extent as those of MDA. Glennon *et al.*, (1982) did not find generalization between (+/−)DOM and (+/−)MDMA or its separate isomers, suggesting that, unlike MDA, MDMA has no hallucinogenic properties. However, recent data from the BPL indicate that both (+) and (−)MDMA substitute for mescaline; surprisingly, the (+) isomer substitutes at a lower dose than the (−) isomer. Racemic MDMA is also known to generalize to both fenfluramine and tetra-hydrobetacarboline (Schechter, 1986), compounds that interact with the 5-HT neurotransmitter system (which is, as mentioned previously, thought to be involved in the hallucinogenic cues). Interactions between MDMA and DA receptors have also been reported; for example, racemic MDMA substitutes for *d*-amphetamine in both rats (Glennon and Young, 1984c) and monkeys (Kamien *et al.*, 1986). In addition, (+/−)MDMA substitutes partially for the DA agonists apomorphine and *l*-cathinone (Schechter, 1986).

Neurochemical studies, like those involving drug discrimination, have generally supported the view that MDA and MDMA interact with both 5-HT and catecholaminergic neuronal systems. Indeed, MDA and MDMA potently release 5-HT from rat whole brain synaptosomes (Johnson *et al.*, 1986; Nichols *et al.*, 1982; Schmidt, 1987); an action which may explain the substitution of MDMA for fenfluramine and tetra-hydrobetacarboline (Schechter, 1986). In addition, chronic treatment with (+/−)MDA reduces the number of 5-HT uptake sites in hippocampal synaptosomes (Ricaurte *et al.*, 1985). Furthermore, both MDA nd MDMA decrease 5-HT levels in many brain regions after chronic administration (Ricaurte *et al.*, 1985; Stone *et al.*, 1986). A recent observation that the isomers of MDMA have neurotoxic effects on 5-HT neurons after acute administration raises concern over the abuse of this compound (Schmidt, 1987). The neurotoxic actions of these substances appear to be selective for 5-HT neurons. While relatively few effects on catecholamines have been reported, the competitive inhibition of NE uptake into hypothalamic synaptosomes by MDA (Marquardt *et al.*, 1978) and the release of DA from rat brain slices by (+)MDA, and less potently, (+)MDMA (Johnson *et al.*, 1986) suggest that some actions of MDA and MDMA may involve nonserotonergic systems.

With regard to the hypothesis concerning the stimulant and hallucinogenic properties of (+) and (−)MDA respectively, Lyon *et al.* (1986) have now demonstrated a greater affinity of (−)MDA for 5-HT-1 and 5-HT-2 receptors than that of either (+/−) or (+)MDA. Similarly, (−)MDMA also has greater affinity for 5-HT receptors than the (+) isomer; this affinity for 5-HT receptors has previously been associated with the hallucinogenic properties of drugs in humans (Glennon and Rosecrans, 1981). However, the potency of (+)MDMA exceeds that of the (−) isomer in eliciting subjective effects (Anderson *et al.*, 1978), a steroselective property that resembles the effects of amphetamine rather than those of hallucinogenic substances. Further studies may therefore be expected to reveal more amphetamine-like actions of MDMA. Indeed, (+/−)MDMA has a greater affinity for DA receptor sites than MDA although the affinity of (+/−)MDMA for these sites is still poor (Lyon *et al.*, 1986).

Acknowledgments—Preparation of this chapter was supported by USPHS Research Grant R01 DA02543, from the National Institute on Drug Abuse. The authors would like to thank E. Michael, D. Escue, P. Bowden, and C. Scott for their assistance in preparing this manuscript.

REFERENCES

ALLES, G. A. (1959) Some relations between chemical structive and physiological action of mescaline and related compounds. In: *Neuropharmacology*, pp. 181–268, ABRAMSON, H. A. (ed.) Josiah Macey Jr. Foundation, New York.

ANDERSON, G. M., BRAUN, G., BRAUN, U. and NICHOLS, D. (1978) Absolute configuration and psychotomimetic activity. *NIDA Res. Monogr. Ser.* **22**: 8–15.

APPEL, J. B. and CALLAHAN, P. M. (1987) Involvement of 5-HT receptor subtypes in the discriminative stimulus properties of mescaline. Paper presented at meeting of the Society for Neuroscience (Satellite session of the Society for the Stimulus Properties of Drugs), New Orleans.

APPEL, J. B. and CUNNINGHAM, K. A. (1986) The use of drug discrimination procedures to characterize hallucinogenic drug actions. *Psychopharmac. Bull.* **22**: 959–967.

APPEL, J. B. and FREEDMAN, D. X. (1968) Tolerance and cross-tolerance among psychotomimetic drugs. *Psychopharmacology* **13**: 267–274.

APPEL, J. B., WHITE, F. J. and HOLOHEAN, A. M. (1982) Analyzing mechanism(s) of hallocinogenic drug action with drug discrimination procedures. *Neurosci. Biobehav. Rev.* **6**: 529–536.

APPEL, J. B., WEATHERSBY, R. T., CUNNINGHAM, K. A., CALLAHAN, P. M. and BARRETT, R. L. (1988) Stimulus properties of dopaminergic drugs: effects of putatively selective agonists and antagonists. In: *Transduction Mechanisms of Drug Stimuli*, pp.44–56. COLPAERT, F. C. and BALSTER, R. L. (eds) Springer-Verlag, Berlin.

BALSTER, R. L. and SCHUSTER, C. R. (1973) A comparison of *d*-amphetamine, *l*-amphetamine, and methamphetamine self-administration in rhesus monkeys. *Pharmac. Biochem. Behav.* **1**: 67–71.

BEARDSLEY, P. M., BALSTER, R. L. and HARRIS, L. S. (1986) Self-administration of methylenedioxymethamphetamine (MDMA) by rhesus monkeys. *Drug Alcohol Depend.* **18**: 149–157.

BRAESTRUP, C. (1977) Biochemical differentiation of amphetamine vs methylphenidate and nomifensine in rats. *J. Pharm. Pharmac.* **29**: 463–470.

BROWNE, R. G. (1978) The role of serotonin in the discriminative stimulus properties of mescaline. In: *Drug Discrimination and State Dependent Learning*, pp. 79–101, HO, B. T., RICHARDS, D. W. and CHUTE, D. L. (eds) Academic Press, New York.

BROWNE, R. G. and HO, B. T. (1975) Role of serotonin in the discriminative stimulus properties of mescaline. *Pharmac. Biochem. Behav.* **3**: 429–435.

BUENO, O. F. A., CARLINI, E. A., FINKELFARB, E. and SUZUKI, J. (1976) Δ^9-tetrahydrocannabinol, ethanol, and amphetamine as discriminative stimuli-generalization tests with other drugs. *Psychopharmacology* **46**: 235–243.

CALDWELL, A. E. (1978) History of psycopharmacology. In: *Principles of Psychopharmacology*, pp. 9–40, CLARK, W. G. and DEL GIUDICE, J. (eds) Academic Press, New York.

CALLAHAN, P. M. and APPEL, J. B. (1987) Differences in the stimulus properties of 3,4-methylenedioxyamphetamine (MDA) and 3,4-methylenedioxymethamphetamine (MDMA) in animals trained to discriminate hallucinogens from saline. *Neurosci. Abstr.* **13**: 1720.

CAMERON, O. G. and APPEL, J. B. (1973) A behavioral and pharmacological analysis of some discriminable properties of d-LSD in rats. *Psychopharmacology* **3**: 117–134.

COLPAERT, F. C. (1984) Cross generalization with LSD and yohimbine in the rat. *Eur. J. Pharmac.* **102**: 541–544.

COLPAERT, F. C. and JANSSEN, P. A. J. (1983) A characterization of LSD-antagonist effects of pirenperone in the rat. *Neuropharmacology* **22**: 1001–1005.

COLPAERT, F. C. and SLANGEN, J. L. (1982) *Drug Discrimination: Applications in CNS Pharamacology.* Elsevier Biomedical.

COLPAERT, F. C., NIEMEGEERS, C. J. E. and JANSSEN, P. A. J. (1978) Discriminative stimulus properties of cocaine and *d*-amphetamine, and antagonism by haloperidol: A comparative study. *Neuropharmacology* **17**: 937–942.

COLPAERT, F. C., NIEMEGEERS, C. J. E. and JANSSEN, P. A. J. (1979a) Discriminative stimulus properties of cocaine: Neuropharmacological characteristics as derived from stimulus generalization experiments. *Pharmac. Biochem. Behav.* **10**: 535–546.

COLPAERT, F. C., NIEMEGEERS, C. J. E. and JANSSEN, P. A. J. (1979b) *In vivo* evidence of partial agonist activity exerted by purported 5-hydroxytryptamine antogonists. *Eur. J. Pharmac.* **58**: 505–509.

COLPAERT, F. C., NIEMEGEERS, C. J. E. and JANSSEN, P. A. J. (1980) Evidence that a preferred substrate for type B monoamine oxidase mediates stimulus properties of MAO inhibitors: A possible role for β-phenylethylamine in the cocaine cue. *Pharmac. Biochem. Behav.* **13**: 513–517.

COLPAERT, F. C., NIEMEGEERS, C. J. E. and JANSSEN, P. A. J. (1982) A drug discrimination analysis of lysergic acid diethylamide (LSD): *In vivo* agonist and antagonist effects of purported 5-hydroxytryptamine antagonists and of pirenperone, a LSD-antagonist. *J. Pharmac. Exp. Ther.* **221**: 206–214.

COLPAERT, F. C., MEERT, T. F., NIEMEGEERS, C. J. E. and JANSSEN, P. A. J. (1985) Behavioral and 5-HT antagonist effects of ritanserin: A pure and selective antagonist of LSD discrimination in rat. *Psychopharmacology* **86**: 45–54.

CUNNINGHAM, K. A. and APPEL, J. B. (1982) Discriminative stimulus properties of cocaine and phencyclidine: Similarities in the mechanism of action. In: *Drug Discrimination: Applications in CNS Pharamacology*, pp. 181–192, COLPAERT, F. C. and SLANGEN, J. L. (eds.) Elsevier Biomedical.

CUNNINGHAM, K. A. and APPEL, J. B. (1986) Possible 5-hydroxytryptamine-1 (5HT1) receptor involvement in the stimulus properties of 1-(*m*-trifluoromethylphenyl)piperazine (TFMPP). *J. Pharmac. Exp. Ther.* **237**: 369–377.

CUNNINGHAM, K. A. and APPEL, J. B. (1987) Neuropharmacological reassessment of the discriminative stimulus properties of *d*-lysergic acid diethylamide (LSD). *Psychopharmacology* **91**: 67–73.

CUNNINGHAM, K. A., CALLAHAN, P. M. and APPEL, J. B. (1985) Differentiation between the stimulus effects of L-5-hydroxytryprophan and LSD. *Eur. J. Pharmac.* **108**: 179–186.

CUNNINGHAM, K. A., CALLAHAN, P. M. and APPEL, J. B. (1986) Discriminative stimulus properties of the serotonin agonist MK 212. *Psychopharmacology* **90**: 193–197.

CUNNINGHAM, K. A., CALLAHAN, P. M. and APPEL, J. B. (1987) Discriminative stimulus properties of 8-hydroxy-2-(di-*n*-propylamino)tetralin (8-OHDPAT): Implications for understanding the actions of novel anxiolytics. *Eur. J. Pharmac.* **138**: 29–36.

DACKIS, C. A. and GOLD, M. S. (1985) New concepts in cocaine addiction: The dopamine depletion hypothesis. *Neurosci. Biobehav. Rev.* **9**: 469–477.

DAVIS, W. M. and SMITH, S. G. (1973) Blocking effect of α-methyltyrosine on amphetamine based reinforcement. *J. Pharm. Pharmac.* **25**: 174–177.

DAVIS, W. M. and SMITH, S. G. (1975) Central cholinergic influence on self-administration of morphine and amphetamine. *Life Sci.* **16**: 237–246.

DAVIS, W. M. and SMITH, S. G. (1977) Catecholaminergic mechanisms of reinforcement: Direct assessment by drug self-administration. *Life Sci.* **20**: 483–492.

DAVIS, W. M., SMITH, S. G. and KHALSA, J. H. (1975) Noradrenergic role in the self-administration of morphine or amphetamine. *Pharmac. Biochem. Behav.* **3**: 477–484.

DE LA GARZA, R. and JOHANSON, C. E. (1982) Effects of haloperidol and physostigmine on self-administration of local anaesthetics. *Pharmac. Biochem. Behav.* **17**: 1295–1299.

DE LA GARZA, R. and JOHANSON, C. E. (1983) The discriminative stimulus properties of cocaine in the rhesus monkey. *Pharmac. Biochem. Behav.* **19**: 145–148.

DE LA GARZA, R. and JOHANSON, C. E. (1985) Discriminative stimulus properties of cocaine in pigeons. *Psychopharmacology* **85**: 22–30.

DEMINIERE, J. M., SIMON, H., HERMAN, J. P. and LE MOAL, M. (1984) 6-Hydroxydopamine lesions of the dopamine mesocorticolimbic cell bodies increases (+)-amphetamine self-administration. *Psychopharmacology* **83**: 281–284.

DENEAU, G., YANAGITA, T. and SEEVERS, M. H. (1969) Self-administration of psychoactive substances by the monkey. *Psychopharmacology* **16**: 30–48.

DE WITT, H. and WISE, R. A. (1977) Blockade of cocaine reinforcement in rats with the dopamine receptor blocker pimozide, but not with the noradrenergic blockers phentolamine or phenoxybenzamine. *Can. J. Psychol.* **31**: 195–203.

EMMETT-OGLESBY, M. W., WURST, M. and LAL, H. (1983) Discriminative stimulus properties of a small dose of cocaine. *Neuropharmacology* **22**: 97–101.

ETTENBERG, A., PETTIT, H. O., BLOOM, F. E. and KOOB, G. F. (1982) Heroin and cocaine intravenous self-administration in rats: Mediation by separate neural systems. *Psychopharmacology* **78**: 204–209.

EVANS, S. M. and JOHANSON, C. E. (1986) Discriminative stimulus properties of (+/−)-3,4-methylenedioxymethamphetamine and (+/−)-3,4-methylenedioxyamphetamine in pigeons. *Drug Alcohol Depend.* **18**: 159–164.

FISCHMAN, M. W. and SCHUSTER, C. R. (1982) Cocaine self-administration in humans. *Fed. Proc.* **41**: 241-246.

FORD, R. D. and BALSTER, R. L. (1977) Reinforcing properties of intravenous procaine in rhesus monkeys. *Pharmac. Biochem. Behav.* **6**: 289–296.

FRIEDMAN, R. L. , BARRETT, R. J. and SANDERS-BUSH, E. (1984) Discriminative stimulus properties of quipazine: Mediation by serotonin-2 binding sites. *J. Pharmac. Exp. Ther.* **228**: 628–635.

FUXE, K., BUTCHER, L. L. and ENGEL, J. (1971) DL-5-Hydroxytryptophan induced changes in the central monoamine neurons after peripheral decarboxylase inhibition. *J. Pharm. Pharmac.* **23**: 420–424.

GLENNON, R. A. and ROSECRANS, J. A. (1981) Speculations on the mechanism of action of hallucinogenic indolealkylamines. *Neurosci. Biobehav. Rev.* **5**: 197–207.

GLENNON, R. A. and YOUNG, R. (1984a) MDA: A psychoactive agent with dual stimulus effects *Life Sci.* **34**: 379–383.

GLENNON, R. A. and YOUNG, R. (1984b) MDA: An agent that produces stimulus effects similar to those of 3,4 DMA, LSD and Cocaine. *Eur. J. Pharmac.* **99**: 249–250.

GLENNON, R. A. and YOUNG, R. (1984c) Further investigation of the discriminative stimulus properties of MDA. *Pharmac. Biochem. Behav.* **20**: 501–505.

GLENNON, R. A., YOUNG, R., ROSECRANS, J. A. and ANDERSON, G. M. (1982) Discriminative stimulus properties of MDA analogs. *Biol. Psychiat.* **17**: 807–814.

GLENNON, R. A., YOUNG, R. and STONE, W. (1984) 1-(2,3-Methylenedioxyphenyl)-2-aminopropane (2,3-MDA): A preliminary investigation. *Gen. Pharmac.* **15**: 361–362.

GOEDERS, N. E. and SMITH, J. E. (1983) Cortical dopaminergic involvement in cocaine reinforcement. *Science* **221**: 773–775.

GOEDERS, N. E. and SMITH, J. E. (1984) Parameters of intracranial self-administration of cocaine into the medial prefrontal cortex. *NIDA Res. Monogr. Ser.* **55**: 132–137.

GOEDERS, N. E. and SMITH, J. E. (1986) Reinforcing properties of cocaine in the medial prefrontal cortex: Primary action on presynaptic dopaminergic terminals. *Pharmac. Biochem. Behav.* **25**: 191–199.

GOEDERS, N. E., DWORKIN, S. I. and SMITH, J. E. (1986) Neuropharmacological assessment of cocaine self-administration into the medial prefrontal cortex. *Pharmac. Biochem. Behav.* **24**: 1429–1440.

GOLDBERG, S. R. (1973) Comparable behavior maintained under fixed-ratio and second-order schedules of food presentation, cocaine injection or *d*-amphetamine injection in the squirrel monkey. *J. Pharmac. Exp. Ther.* **186**: 18–30.

GOLDBERG, S. R. and GONZALES, F. A. (1976) The effects of propranolol on behavior maintained under fixed-ratio schedules of cocaine injection or food presentation in squirrel monkeys. *J. Pharmac. Exp. Ther.* **198**: 626–634.

GOLDBERG, S. R., HOFFMEISTER, F., SCHLICHTING, V. V. and WUTIKE, W. (1971) A comparison of pentobarbital and cocaine self-administration in rhesus monkeys: Effects of dose and fixed-ratio parameter. *J. Pharmac. Exp. Ther.* **179**: 277–283.

GRIFFITHS, R. R., WINGER, G., BRADY, J. V. and SNELL, J. D. (1976) Comparison of behavior maintained by infusions of eight phenylethylamines in baboons. *Psychopharamacology* **50**: 251–258.

GUNNE, L. M., ANGGARD, E. and JONSSON, L. E. (1972) Clinical trials with amphetamine-blocking drugs. *Psychiat. Neurol. Neurochir.* **75**: 225–226.

HAIGLER, H. J. and AGHAJANIAN, G. K. (1973) Mescaline and LSD: Direct and indirect effects on serotonin-containing neurons in brain. *Eur. J. Pharmac.* **21**: 53–60.

HAIGLER, H. J. and AGHAJANIAN, G. K. (1974) Lysergic acid diethylamide and serotonin: A comparison of effects on serotonergic neurons and neurons receiving a serotonergic input. *J. Pharmac. Exp. Ther.* **188**: 688–699.

HAMMERBECK, D. M. and MITCHELL, C. L. (1978) The reinforcing properties of procaine and *d*-amphetamine compared in rhesus monkeys. *J. Pharmac. Exp. Ther.* **204**: 558–569.

HAMON, M. (1984) Common neurochemical correlates to the action of hallucinogens. In: *Hallucinogens: Neurochemical, Behavioral and Clinical Perspectives*, JACOBS, B. L. (eds) Raven Press, New York.

HENNINGFIELD, J. A., LUKAS, S. E. and BIGELOW, G. E. (1986) Human studies of drugs as reinforcers. In: *Behavioral Analysis of Drug Dependence*, pp. 69–122, GOLDBERG, S. R. and STOLERMAN, I. P. (eds) Academic Press, New York.

HERNANDEZ, L. L., HOLOHEAN, A. M. and APPEL, J. B. (1978) Effects of opiates on the discriminative stimulus properties of dopamine agonists. *Pharmac. Biochem. Behav.* **9**: 459–463.

HIRSCHHORN, I. D. and ROSECRANS, J. A. (1974) A comparison of the stimulus effects of morphine and lysergic acid diethylamide (LSD). *Pharmac. Biochem. Behav.* **2**: 361–366.

HIRSCHHORN, I. D. and WINTER, J. C. (1971) Mescaline and lysergic acid diethylamide (LSD) as discriminative stimuli. *Psychopharmacology* **22**: 64–71.

HIRSCHHORN, I. D., HAYES, R. L. and ROSECRANS, J. A. (1975) Discriminative control of behavior by electrical stimulation of the dorsal raphe nucleus: Generalization to lysergic acid diethylamide (LSD). *Brain Res.* **86**: 134–138.

Ho, B. T. and Huang, J. (1975) Role of dopamine in *d*-amphetamine-induced discriminative responding. *Pharmac. Biochem. Behav.* **3**: 1085–1092.

Ho, B. T., McKenna, M. and Huang, J. (1976) Common discrimination stimulus properties for psychomotor stimulants. *Res. Commun. Psychol. Psychiat. Behav.* **1**: 249–255.

Hoebel, B. G., Monaco, A. P., Hernandez, L., Aulisi, E. F., Stanley, B. G. and Lenard, L. (1983) Self-injection of amphetamine directly into the brain. *Psychopharmacology* **81**: 158–163.

Hoffmeister, F. and Schlichting, V. V. (1972) Reinforcing properties of some opiates and opioids in rhesus monkeys with histories of cocaine and codeine self-administration. *Psychopharmacology* **23**: 55–74.

Holohean, A. M., White, F. J. and Appel, J. B. (1982) Dopaminergic and serotonergic mediation of the discriminable effects of ergot alkaloids. *Eur. J. Pharmac.* **81**: 595–602.

Huang, D. snd Wilson, M. C. (1982) Comparative stimulus properties of cocaine and other local anesthetics in rats. *Res. Commun. Substances Abuse* **3**: 129–140.

Huang, D. and Wilson, M. C. (1986) Comparative discriminative stimulus properties of dl-cathinone, d-amphetamine and cocaine in rats. *Pharmac. Biochem. Behav.* **24**: 205–210.

Huang, J. and Ho, B. T. (1974a) The effect of pretreatment with iproniazid on the behavioral activities of *β-phenylethylamine in rats. Psychopharmacology* **35**: 77–81.

Huang, J. and Ho, B. T. (1974b) Discriminative stimulus properties of *d*-amphetamine and related compounds in rats. *Pharmac. Biochem. Behav.* **2**: 669–673.

Iorio, L. C., Barnett, A., Leitz, F. H., Houser, V. P. and Korduba, C. A. (1983) SCH 23390, a potential benzazepine antipsychotic with unique interactions on dopaminergic systems. *J. Pharmac. Exp. Ther.* **226**: 462–468.

Iversen, S. D. and Iversen, L. L. (1981) *Behavioral Pharmacology*. Oxford University Press.

Jackson, B. and Reed, A. (1970) Another abusable amphetamine. *J. Am. Med. Ass.* **221**: 830.

Jacobs, B. L. (1987) How hallucinogenic drugs work. *Am. Sci.* **75**: 386–392.

Jarbe, T. U. C. (1978) Cocaine as a discriminative cue in rats: Interactions with neuroleptics and other drugs. *Psychopharmacology* **59**: 183–187.

Jarbe, T. U. C. (1981) Cocaine cue in pigeons: Time course studies and generalization to structurally related compounds (norcocaine, win 35, 428 and 35,065-2) and (+)-amphetamine. *Br. J. Pharmac.* **73**: 843–852.

Jarbe, T. U. C. (1984) Discriminative stimulus properties of cocaine. Effects of apomorphine, haloperidol, procaine and other drugs. *Neuropharmacology* **23**: 899–907.

Jarbe, T. U. C. and Kroon, E. R. (1980) Discriminative properties of *d*-amphetamine in gerbils: Tests for drug generalization and antagonism. *Gen. Pharmac.* **11**: 153–156.

Johanson, C. E. (1980) The reinforcing properties of procaine, chloroprocaine and proparacaine in rhesus monkeys. *Psychopharmacology* **67**: 189–194.

Johanson, C. E., Kandel, D. A. and Bonese, K. (1976) The effects of perphenazine on self-administration behavior. *Pharmac. Biochem. Behav.* **4**: 427–433.

Johnson, M. P., Hoffman, A. J. and Nichols, D. E. (1986) Effects of the enantiomers of MDA, MDMA and related analogues on [3H]serotonin and [3H]dopamine release from superfused rat brain slices. *Eur. J. Pharmac.* **132**: 269–276.

Kamien, J. B., Johanson, C. E. and Schuster, C. R. (1986) The effects of (+/−)methylenedioxymethamphetamine and (+/−)methylenedioxyamphetamine in monkeys trained to discriminate (+)amphetamine from saline. *Drug Alcohol Depend.* **18**: 139–147.

Katz, M. M. and Waskow, I. E. (1968) Characterizing the psychological state produced by LSD. *J. Abnorm. Psychol.* **73**: 1–14.

Kilbey, M. M. and Ellinwood, E. H. (1979) Discriminative stimulus properties of psychomotor stimulants in the cat. *Psychopharmacology* **63**: 151–153.

Kozel, N. J. and Adams, E. H. (1985) Cocaine use in America: Epidemiologic and clinical perspectives. In: *NIDA Res. Monogr. Ser.* **61**.

Knoll, J., Ecseri, Z., Kelemen, K., Nievel, J. and Knoll, B. (1965) Phenylisopropylmethylpropinylamine (E-250), a new spectrum psychic energizer. *Arch. Int. Pharmacodyn. Ther.* **155**: 154–164.

Kuczenski, R. (1983) Biochemical actions of amphetamine and other stimulants. In: *Stimulants: Neurochemical, Behavioral, and Clinical Perspectives*, pp. 31–61, Creese, I. (ed.) Raven Press, New York.

Kuhn, D. M., Appel, J. B. and Greenburg, I. (1974) An analysis of some discriminative properties of *d*-amphetamine. Psychopharmacology **39**: 57–66.

Kuhn, D. M., White, F. J. and Appel, J. B. (1978) The discriminative stimulus properties of LSD: Mechanisms of action. *Neuropharmacology* **17**: 257–263.

Lamb, R. J. and Griffiths, R. R. (1987) Self-injection of *d, l*-3,4-methylenedioxymethamphetamine (MDMA) in the baboon. *Psychopharmacology* **91**: 268–272.

Leccese, A. P. and Lyness, W. H. (1984) The effects of putative 5-hydroxytryptamine receptor active agents on *d*-amphetamine self-administration in controls and rats with 5,7-dihydroxytryptamine median forebrain bundle lesions. *Brain Res.* **303**: 153–162.

Le Moal, M., Stinus, L. and Simon, H. (1979) Increased sensitivity to (+)amphetamine self-administered by rats following mesocortico-limbic dopamine neurone destruction. *Nature* **280**: 156–158.

Lyness, W. H., Friedle, N. M. and Moore, K. E. (1979) Destruction of dopaminergic nerve terminals in nucleus accumbens: Effect on *d*-amphetamine self-administration. *Pharmac. Biochem. Behav.* **11**: 553–556.

Lyness, W. H., Friedle, N. M. and Moore, K. E. (1980) Increased self-administration of *d*-amphetamine after destruction of 5-hydroxytryptaminergic neurons. *Pharmac. Biochem. Behav.* **12**: 937–941.

Lyon, R. A., Glennon, R. A. and Titeler, M. (1986) 3,4-Methylenedioxymethamphetamine (MDMA): Stereoselective interactions at brain 5-HT1 and 5-HT2 receptors. *Psychopharmacology* **88**: 525–526.

MacFarlane, M. D. (1973) Possible rationale for procaine (Gerovital H3) therapy in geriatrics: Inhibitor of monoamine oxidase. *J. Am. Geriatr. Soc.* **216**: 414–418.

Marquardt, G. M., Distefano, V. and Ling, L. (1978) Pharmacological effects of (+/−), (*S*) and (*R*) MDA.

In: *Psychopharmacology of Hallucinogens*, pp. 84–104, Stillman, R. C. and Willette, R. E. (eds) Pergamon Press, Oxford.

Martin-Iverson, M. T., Szostak, C. and Fibiger, H. C. (1986) 6-Hydroxydopamine lesions of the medial prefrontal cortex fail to influence intravenous self-administration of cocaine. *Psychopharmacology* **88**: 310–314.

McKenna, M. L. and Ho, B. T. (1980) The role of dopamine in the discriminative stimulus properties of cocaine. *Neuropharmacology* **19**: 297–303.

Minnema, D. J. and Rosecrans, J. A. (1984) Amphetamine and LSD as discriminative stimuli: Alterations following neonatal monoamine reductions. *Pharmac. Biochem. Behav.* **20**: 95–101.

Monaco, A. P., Hernandez, L. and Hoebel, B. G. (1980) Nucleus accumbens site of amphetamine self-injection: Comparison with lateral ventricle. In: *The Neurobiology of the Nucleus Accumbens*, pp. 338–343. Chronister, R. B. and DeFrance, J. F. (eds) Haer Institute, Brunswick, ME.

Moore, K. (1978) Biochemical and behavioral actions in animals. In: *Handbook of Psychopharmacology*, Vol. 11, pp. 41–98, Iversen, L. L., Iversen, S. D. and Snyder, S. H. (eds) Plenum Press, New York.

Naranjo, C., Shulgin, A. T. and Sargent, T. (1967) Evaluation of 3,4-methylenedioxyamphetamine (MDA) as an adjunct to psychotherapy. *Med. Pharmac. Exp.* **17**: 359.

Nichols, D. E., Hoyd, D. H., Hoffman, A. J., Nichols, M. B. and Yim, G. K. W. (1982) Effects of certain hallucinogenic amphetamine analogues on the release of 3-H serotonin from rat brain synaptosomes. *J. Med. Chem.* **25**: 530–353.

Nielsen, E. B. and Jepsen, S. A. (1985) Antagonism of the amphetamine cue by both classical and atypical antipsychotic drugs. *Eur. J. Pharmac.* **11**: 167–176.

Nielsen, E. B. and Scheel-Kruger, J. (1986) Cueing effects of amphetamine and LSD: Elicitation by direct microinjection of the drugs into the nucleus accumbens. *Eur. J. Pharmac.* **125**: 85–92.

Nielsen, E. B. and Scheel-Kruger, J. (1988) CNS stimulants: Neuropharmacological mechanisms. In: *Transduction Mechanisms of Drug Stimuli*, pp. 57–72. Balster, R. L. and Colpaert, F. C. (eds.) Springer-Verlag, Berlin.

Nielsen, E. B., Ginn, S. R., Cunningham, K. A. and Appel, J. B. (1985) Antagonism of the LSD cue by putative serotonin antagonists: Relationship to inhibition of *in vivo* [3-H]spiroperidol binding. *Behav. Brain Res.* **16**: 171–176.

Nozaki, M., Vaupel, D. B. and Martin, W. R. (1977) Pharmacological comparison of 3,4-methylenedioxyamphetamine and LSD in the chronic spinal dog. *Eur. J. Pharmac.* **46**: 339–349.

Pettit, H. O., Ettenberg, A., Bloom, F. E. and Koob, G. F. (1984) Destruction of dopamine in the nucleus accumbens selectively attenuates cocaine but not heroin self-administration in rats. *Psychopharamacology* **84**: 167–173.

Pickens, R. (1968) Self-administration of stimulants by rats. *Int. J. Addict.* **3**: 215–221.

Pickens, R. and Harris, W. C. (1968) Self-administration of *d*-amphetamine by rats. *Psychopharmacology* **12**: 158–163.

Pickens, R. and Thompson, T. (1968) Cocaine-reinforced behavior in rats: Effects of reinforcement magnitude and fixed ratio size. *J. Pharmac. Exp. Ther.* **161**: 122–129.

Porsolt, R. D., Pawelec, C. and Jalfre, M. (1982) Use of a drug discrimination procedure to detect amphetamine-like effects of antidepressants. In: *Drug Discrimination: Applications in CNS Pharmacology*. pp. 193–202, Colpaert, F. C. and Slangen, J. L. (eds) Elsevier Biomedical, Amsterdam.

Porsolt, R. D., Pawelec, C., Roux, S. and Jalfre, M. (1984) Discrimination of the amphetamine cue. Effects of A, B and mixed inhibitors of monoamine oxidase. *Neuropharmacology* **23**, 569–573.

Ratcliffe, B. E. (1974) MDA. *Clin. Tox.* **7**: 409–411.

Reynolds, G. P., Elsworth, J. D., Blau, K., Snadler, M., Lees, A. J. and Stern, G. M. (1978) Deprenyl is metabolized to methamphetamine and amphetamine in man. *Br. J. Clin. Pharmac.* **6**: 542–544.

Ricaurte, G., Bryan, G., Strauss, L., Seiden, L. and Schuster, C. (1985) Hallucinogenic amphetamine selectively destroys brain serotonin nerve terminals. *Science* **229**: 986–988.

Richards, K. C. and Borgstedt, H. H. (1971) Near fatal reaction to ingestion of the hallucinogenic drug MDA. *J. Am. Med. Ass.* **218**: 1826–1827.

Richards, R. N. (1972) Experience with MDA. *Can. Med. Ass. J.* **106**: 256–259.

Risner, M. E. (1975) Intravenous self-administration of *d*- and *l*-amphetamine by dog. *Eur. J. Pharmac.* **32**: 344–348.

Risner, M. E. and Jones, B. E. (1975) Self-administration of CNS stimulants by dog. *Psychopharmacology* **43**: 207–213.

Risner, M. E. and Jones, R. E. (1976) Role of noradrenergic and dopaminergic processes in amphetamine self-administration. *Pharmac. Biochem. Behav.* **5**: 477–482.

Risner, M. E. and Jones, R. E. (1980) Intravenous self-administration of cocaine and norcocaine by dogs. *Psychopharmacology* **71**: 83–89.

Roberts, D. C. S. and Koob, G. F. (1982) Disruption of cocaine self-administration following 6-hydroxydopamine lesions of the ventral tegmental area in rats. *Pharmac. Biochem. Behav.* **17**: 901–904.

Roberts, D. C. S. and Vickers, G. (1984) Atypical neuroleptics increase self-administration of cocaine: An evaluation of a behavioral screen for antipsychotic activity. *Psychopharmacology* **82**: 135–139.

Roberts, D. C. S., Corcoran, M. E. and Fibiger, H. C. (1977) On the role of ascending catecholaminergic systems in intravenous self-administration of cocaine. *Pharmac. Biochem. Behav.* **6**: 615–620.

Roberts, D. C. S., Koob, G. F., Klonoff, P. and Fibiger, H. C. (1980) Extinction and recovery of cocaine self-administration following 6-hydroxydopamine lesions of the nucleus accumbens. *Pharmac. Biochem. Behav.* **12**: 781–787.

Rosecrans, J. A. and Glennon, R. A. (1979) Drug-induced cues in studying mechanisms of drug actions. *Neuropharmacology* **18**: 981–989.

Rosenberg, D. E., Wolbach, A. B., Miner, E. J. and Harris, I. (1963) Observation on direct and cross tolerance with LSD and *d*-amphetamine in man. *Psychopharmacology* **5**: 1–5.

Ross, S. B. and Renyi, A. L. (1967a) Accumulation of tritiated 5-hydroxytryptamine in brain slices. *Life Sci.* **6**: 1407–1415.

Ross, S. F. and Renyi, A. L. (1967b) Inhibition of the uptake of tritiated catecholamines by antidepressant and related agents. *Eur. J. Pharmac.* **2**: 181–186.

Schechter, M. D. (1977) Amphetamine discrimination as a test for antiparkinsonism drugs. *Eur. J. Pharmac.* **44**: 51–56.

Schechter, M. D. (1980) Effect of neuroleptics and tricyclic antidepressants upon *d*-amphetamine discrimination. *Pharmac. Biochem. Behav.* **12**: 1–5.

Schechter, M. D. (1986) Discriminative profile of MDMA. *Pharmac. Biochem. Behav.* **24**: 1533–1537.

Schechter, M. D. and Cook, P. G. (1975) Dopaminergic mediation of the interoceptive cue produced by *d*-amphetamine in rats. *Psychopharmacology* **42**: 185–193.

Schechter, M. D. and Rosecrans, J. A. (1972) Lysergic acid diethylamide (LSD) as a discriminative cue: Drugs with similar stimulus properties. *Psychopharmacology* **26**: 313–316.

Schechter, M. D. and Rosecrans, J. A. (1973) *d*-Amphetamine as a discriminative cue: Drugs with similar discriminative properties. *Eur. J. Pharmac.* **21**: 212–216.

Schmidt, C. J. (1987) Neurotoxicity of the psychedelic amphetamine methylenedioxymethamphetamine. *J. Pharmac. Exp. Ther.* **240**: 1–7.

Schuster, C. R. (1975) Drugs as reinforcers in monkeys and man. *Pharmac. Rev.* **27**: 511–521.

Shannon, H. E. (1980) MDA and DOM: Substituted amphetamines that do not produce amphetamine-like discriminative stimuli in the rat. *Psychopharmacology* **67**: 311–312.

Shearman, G., Miksic, S. and Lal, H. (1978) Discriminative stimulus properties of desipramine. *Neuropharmacology* **17**: 1045–1048.

Shulgin, A. T. and Nichols, D. E. (1978) Characterization of three new psychotomimetics. In: *Psychopharmacology of Hallucinogens*, pp. 74–83, Stillman, R. C. and Willette, R. E. (eds) Pergamon Press, Oxford.

Snoddy, A. M. and Tessel, R. E. (1983) Nisoxetine and amphetamine share discriminative stimulus properties in mice. *Pharmac. Biochem. Behav.* **19**: 205–210.

Stolerman, I. P. and D'Mello, G. D. (1981) Role of training conditions in discrimination of central nervous system stimulants by rats. *Pyschopharmacology* **73**: 295–303.

Stone, D. M., Stahl, D. C., Hanson, G. R. and Gibb, J. W. (1986) The effects of 3,4-methylenedioxymethamphetamine (MDMA) and 3,4-methylenedioxyamphetamine (MDA) on monoaminergic systems in the rat brain. *Eur. J. Pharmac.* **128**: 41–48.

Thiessen, P. N. and Cook, D. A. (1973) The properties of 3,4-methylenedioxyamphetamine (MDA) 1. A view of the literature. *Clin. Tox.* **6**: 45–52.

Turek, I. S., Soskin, R. A. and Kurkland, A. A. (1974) Methylenedioxyamphetamine (MDA) subjective effects. *J. Psyched. Drugs* **6**: 7–14.

Van Dyke, C., Jatlow, P., Ungerer, J., Barash, P. and Byck, R. (1979) Cocaine and lidocaine have similar psychological effects after intranasal application. *Life Sci.* **24**: 271–274.

Waddington, J. L., Molloy, A. G., O'Boyle, K. M. and Mashurano, M. (1986) Enantiomeric analogues of SCH 23390 as new probes for behavior interactions between D1 and D2 dopaminergic function. In: *Neurobiology of Central D1-Dopamine Receptors*, pp. 125–136, Breese, G. R. and Creese, I. (eds) Plenum Publishing.

White, F. J. and Appel, J. B. (1982a) Lysergic acid diethylamide (LSD) and lisuride: Differentiation of their neuropharmacological actions. *Science* **216**: 535–537.

White, F. J. and Appel, J. B. (1982b) Training dose as a factor in LSD-saline discrimination. *Psychopharmacology* **76**: 20–25.

White, F. J., Simmons, M. A., West, K. B., Holohean, A. M. and Appel, J. B. (1980) The effect of serotonin depletion on the discrimination of LSD. *Pharmac. Biochem. Behav.* **13**: 569–574.

Wilson, M. C. and Schuster, C. R. (1972) The effects of chlorpromazine on psychomotor stimulant self-administration in the rhesus monkey. *Psychopharmacology* **26**: 115–126.

Wilson, M. C. and Schuster, C. R. (1973a) The effects of stimulants and depressanats on cocaine self-administration behavior in the rhesus monkey. *Psychopharmacology* **31**: 291–304.

Wilson, M. C. and Schuster, C. R. (1973b) Cholinergic influence on intravenous cocaine self-administration by rhesus monkeys. *Pharmac. Biochem. Behav.* **1**: 643–649.

Wilson, M. C. and Schuster, C. R. (1974) Aminergic influences on intravenous cocaine self-administration by rhesus monkeys. *Pharmac. Biochem. Behav.* **2**: 563–571.

Wilson, M. C., Hitomi, M. and Schuster, C. R. (1971) Psychomotor stimulant self-administration as a function of dosage per injection in the rhesus monkey. *Psychopharmacology* **22**: 271–281.

Winter, J. C. (1971) Tolerance to a behavorial effect of lysergic acid diethylamide and cross-tolerance to mescaline in the rat: Absence of a metabolic component. *J. Pharmac. Exp. Ther.* **178**: 625–630.

Winter, J. C. (1973) A comparison of the stimulus properties of mescaline and 2,3-trimethoxyphenylethylamine. *J. Pharmac. Exp. Ther.* **185**: 101–107.

Winter, J. C. (1975a) The effects of 2,5-dimethoxy-4-methylamphetamine (DOM), 2,5-dimethoxy-4-ethylamphetamine (DOET), *d*-amphetamine, and cocaine in rats trained with mescaline as a discriminative stimulus. *Psychopharmacology* **44**: 29–32.

Winter, J. C. (1975b) Blockade of the stimulus properties of mescaline by a serotonin antagonist. *Arch. Int. Pharmacodyn.* **214**: 250–253.

Winter, J. C. (1978) Stimulus properties of phenylethylamine hallucinogens and lysergic acid diethylamide: The role of 5-hydroxytryptamine. *J. Pharmac. Exp. Ther.* **204**: 416–423.

Winter, J. C. (1980) Effects of the phenethylamine derivatives, BL-3912, fenfluramine, and SCH-12679 in rats trained with LSD as a discriminative stimulus. *Psychopharmacology* **68**: 159–162.

Wolbach, A. B., Isabell, H. and Miner, E. J. (1962) Cross tolerance between mescaline and LSD 25 with a comparison of the mescaline and LSD reactions. *Psychopharmacology* **3**: 1–14.

WOOD, D. M. and EMMETT-OGLESBY, M. W. (1986) Characteristics of tolerance, recovery from tolerance and cross-tolerance for cocaine used as a discriminative stimulus. *J. Pharmac. Exp. Ther.* **237**: 120–125.

WOOD, D. M., LAL, H. adn EMMETT-OGLESBY, M. (1984) Acquisition and recovery of tolerance to the discriminative stimulus properties of cocaine. *Neuropharmacology* **23**: 1419–1423.

WOOD, D. M., LAL, H., YADEN, S. and EMMETT-OGLESBY, M. W. (1985) One way generalization of clonidine to the discriminative stimulus produced by cocaine. *Pharmac. Biochem. Behav.* **23**: 529–533.

WOODS, J. H. and SCHUSTER, C. R. (1968) Reinforcement properties of morphine, cocaine and SPA as a function of unit dose. *Int. J. Addict.* **3**: 231–237.

WOOLVERTON, W. L. (1986) Effects of a D1 and a D2 dopamine antagonist on the self-administration of cocaine and piribedil by rhesus monkeys. *Pharmac. Biochem. Behav.* **24**: 531–535.

WOOLVERTON, W. L. (1987) Evaluation of the role of norepinephrine in the reinforcing effects of psychomotor stimulants in rhesus monkeys. *Pharmac. Biochem. Behav.* **26**: 835–839.

WOOLVERTON, W. L. and BALSTER, R. L. (1979) Reinforcing properties of some local anesthetics in rhesus monkeys. *Pharmac. Biochem. Behav.* **11**: 669–672.

WOOLVERTON, W. L. and BALSTER, R. L. (1982) Behavioral pharmacology of local anesthetics: Reinforcing and discriminative stimulus effects. *Pharmac. Biochem. Behav.* **16**: 491–500.

YENSEN, R., DILEO, F. B., RHEAD, J. C., RICHARDS, W. A., SOSKIN, R. A., TUREK, B. and KURLAND, A. A. (1976) MDA-assisted psychotherapy with neurotic outpatients: A pilot study. *J. Nerv. Ment. Dis.* **163**: 233-245.

YOKEL, R. A. and PICKENS, R. (1973) Self-administration of optical isomers of amphetamine and methylamphetamine by rats. *J. Pharmac. Exp. Ther.* **187**: 27–33.

YOKEL, R. A. and WISE, R. A. (1975) Increased lever pressing for amphetamine after pimozide in rats: Implications for a dopamine theory of reward. *Science* **187**: 547–549.

YOKEL, R. A. and WISE, R. A. (1976) Attenuation of intravenous amphetamine reinforcement by central dopamine blockade in rats. *Psychopharmacology* **48**: 311–318.

YOUDIM, M. B. H. and FINBERG, J. P. M. (1983) Implication of MAO-A and MAO-B inhibition for antidepressant therapy. In: *Modern Problems in Pharmacopsychiatry*, pp. 63–74, BECKMANN, H. and RIEDERER, P. (eds) Karger Press, Basel.

YOUNG, R. and GLENNON, R. A. (1986) Discriminative stimulus properties of amphetamine and structurally related phenalkylamines. *Med. Res. Rev.* **6**: 99–130.

ZITO, K. A., VICKERS, G. and ROBERTS, D. C. S. (1985) Distruption of cocaine and heroin self-administration following kainic acid lesions of the nucleus accumbens. *Pharmac. Biochem. Behav.* **23**: 1029–1036.

CHAPTER 12

THE CENTRAL NEUROPHARMACOLOGY OF PSYCHOTROPIC CANNABINOIDS

R. G. PERTWEE
Department of Pharmacology, Marischal College, University of Aberdeen, Aberdeen, AB9 1AS Scotland

1. INTRODUCTION

Since the identification in 1964 of delta-9-tetrahydrocannabinol (delta-9-THC) as the main psychically active constituent of cannabis (see Mechoulam 1973, for a review), most studies directed at establishing the mechanisms responsible for the psychotropic effect of cannabis have been carried out with delta-9-THC or other constituents of cannabis, rather than with the crude plant material itself. It is with these studies that this review is primarily concerned. Several important areas of research can be identified. One is the study of cannabinoids at the electrophysiological level, and another the study of the part played by putative central neurotransmitters in the psychopharmacology of cannabis. Other areas of importance are the study of interactions between constituents of cannabis and membranes and the study of effects of cannabis constituents on the activity of centrally located membrane-bound enzymes. All these areas are reviewed in this chapter. The chapter also contains a section which considers current thoughts about the molecular basis for the psychotropic activity of cannabis. Two sections in this chapter deal primarily with the human pharmacology of cannabis. One briefly outlines the therapeutic potential of cannabis constituents and related compounds and the other contains a short account of the central effects of cannabis in man and a more detailed discussion about the psychotropic activity of those constituents of cannabis whose neuropharmacology is discussed elsewhere in the chapter. Where possible, review articles have been cited in both these sections. There is also a section concerned with the solubility of delta-9-THC and related compounds. This is an important subject; the high lipid solubility and low water solubility of these substances markedly influencing their pharmacology and also giving rise to formidable practical and interpretational difficulties in the laboratory. The chapter ends with a general discussion and summary. It is important to note that apart from brief references to the existence of cannabis tolerance and dependence, discussions in this review have been limited to effects of single drug administration.

2. THE PSYCHOPHARMACOLOGICAL EFFECTS OF CANNABIS IN MAN

The effects of cannabis which make up a 'high' consist essentially of changes in perception, mood, emotion and cognition (Paton and Pertwee, 1973b; Hollister, 1986). Thus, after cannabis has been taken, there are reports that colors seem brighter and music more pleasant and that 'felt time' passes more slowly than 'clock time.' Effects on mood and emotion vary. Usually there is some euphoria. Sometimes, however, particularly in the inexperienced, mood may be unaffected or there may be dysphoria or anxiety. More serious adverse psychopharmacological responses can also occur, in particular, panic reactions and psychoses (Paton *et al.*, 1973; Hollister, 1986). Signs of changed cognitive function include difficulty in concentrating and thinking and impairment of memory (Miller, 1984). The 'high' is usually followed by a period of drowsiness. Associated with the 'high' are reductions in psychomotor coordination and performance and changes in autonomic processes. The most prominent autonomic changes are cardiovascular, in particular, tachycardia, postural hypotension and supine hypertension (Jones, 1985; Hollister, 1986). There is also evidence, largely but not exclusively from animal studies, that cannabis can induce changes in thermoregulation (Pertwee, 1985a; Dewey, 1986) and in endocrine and reproductive function (Pertwee, 1985b; Rosenkrantz, 1985; Dewey, 1986; Hollister, 1986). On repeated administration, to animals or man, cannabis can give rise to tolerance and dependence (Pertwee, 1983; Agurell *et al.*, 1986; Beardsley *et al.*, 1986; Dewey, 1986; Hollister, 1986). The tolerance seems to be mainly pharmacodynamic in nature, resulting far more from adaptive changes within the brain than from changes in disposition or metabolism.

Like other natural cannabinoids, the main psychically active constituent of cannabis, (−) delta-9-6a,10a-*trans*-tetrahydrocannabinol (delta-9-THC), is a C_{21} compound, contains only carbon, hydrogen and oxygen and occurs naturally, exclusively in the plant *Cannabis sativa*. The term 'cannabinoid' is also used to describe the transformation products and synthetic analogs of natural cannabinoids. The structure of delta-9-THC is shown in Fig. 1. Also shown in this figure are two numbering systems for tetrahydrocannabinol, both of which are still used. The dibenzopyran numbering system is the one that now appears most often in neuropharmacological papers and it is this system which has been adopted in this review. The structures of many of the other cannabinoids discussed in this article are shown in Figs. 2 to 4.

Present knowledge about the psychoactive potencies in man of cannabinoids mentioned later in this review is summarized in Table 1. More complete accounts of structure-activity relationships of cannabinoids are to be found in recent reviews by Razdan (1986) and by

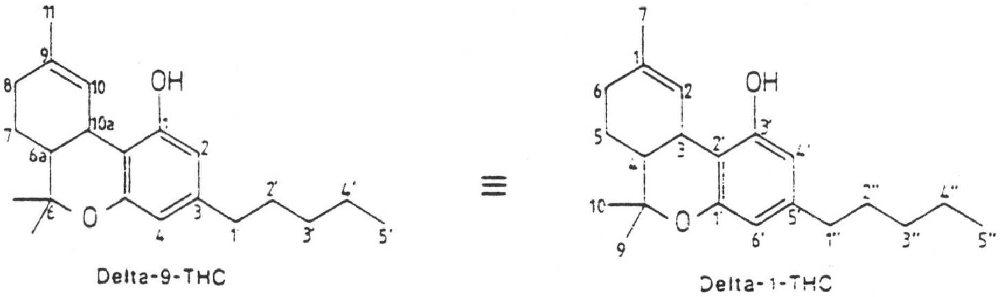

Delta-9-THC ≡ Delta-1-THC

FIG. 1. The structure of the main psychically active constituent of cannabis showing the dibenzopyran numbering system on the left and the monoterpenoid system on the right.

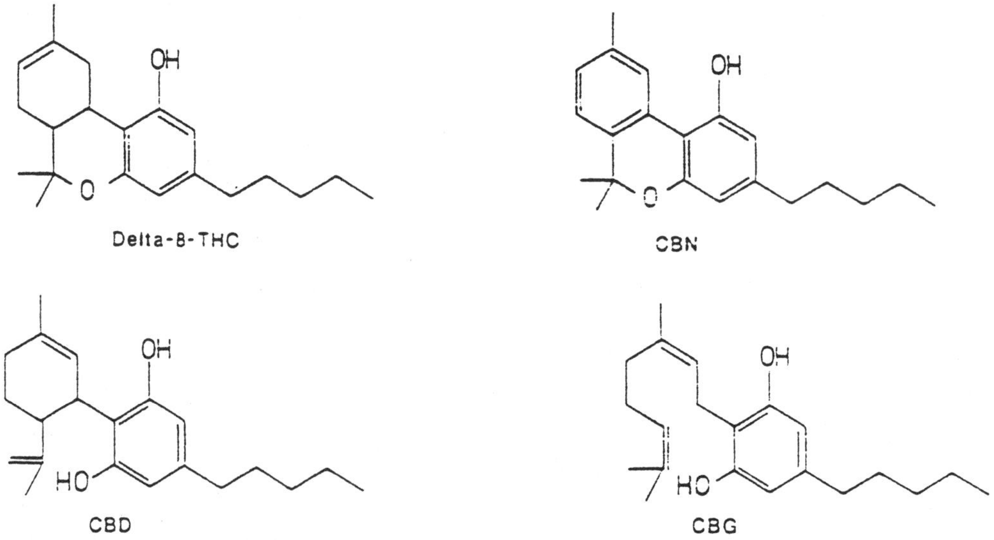

Delta-8-THC CBN CBD CBG

FIG. 2. The structure of four constituents of cannabis, delta-8-tetrahydrocannabinol (delta-8-THC), cannabinol (CBN), cannabidiol (CBD) and cannabigerol (CBG).

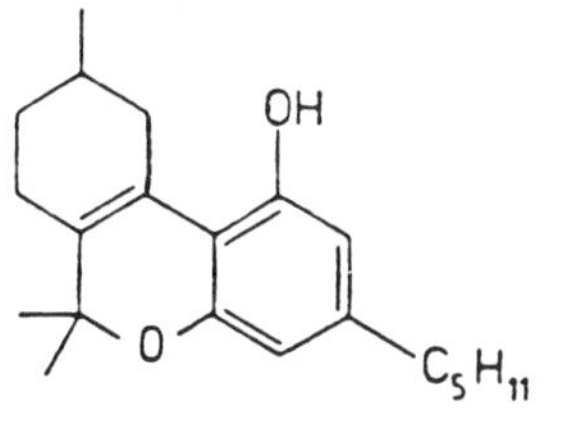

OH C_5H_{11} O

Delta-6a,10a-THC

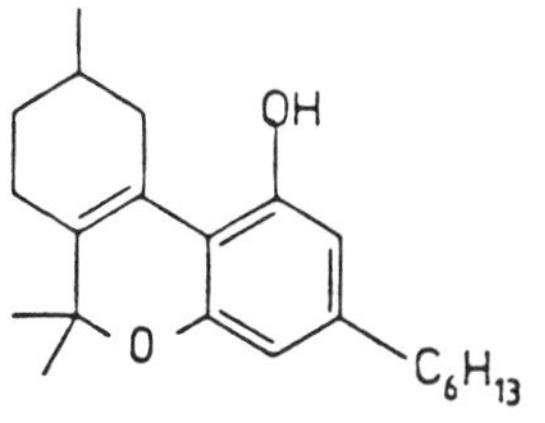

OH C_6H_{13} O

Delta-6a,10a-hexyl-THC
= synhexyl = pyrahexyl

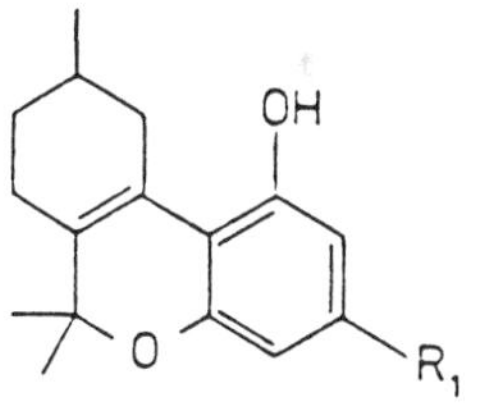

OH R_1 O

Delta-6a,10a-dimethylheptyl-THC

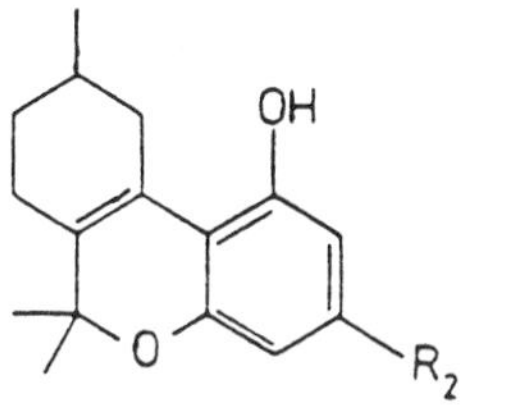

OH R_2 O

Delta-6a,10a-methyloctyl-THC

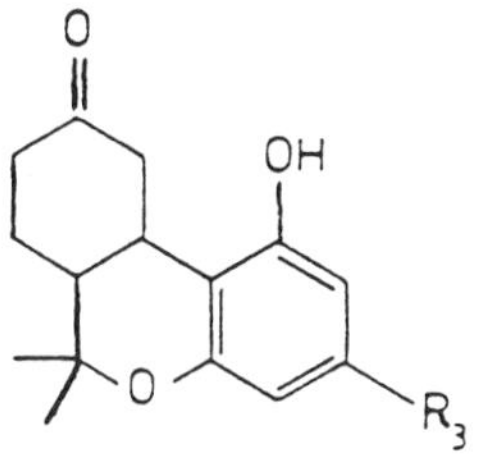

O OH R_3 O

Nabilone

OH O C CH_3 N OR_4

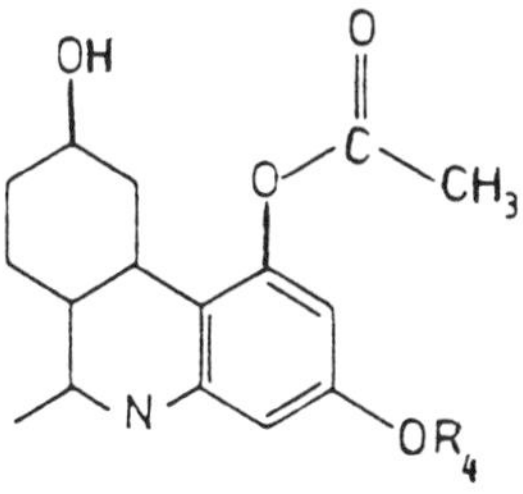

Levonantradol

FIG. 3. The structure of several synthetic analogs of delta-9-tetrahydrocannabinol. $R_1 = CH(CH_3)CH(CH_3)C_5H_{11}$; $R_2 = CH(CH_3)C_7H_{15}$; $R_3 = C(CH_3)_2C_6H_{13}$; $R_4 = CH(CH_3)CH_2CH_2CH_2(C_6H_5)$.

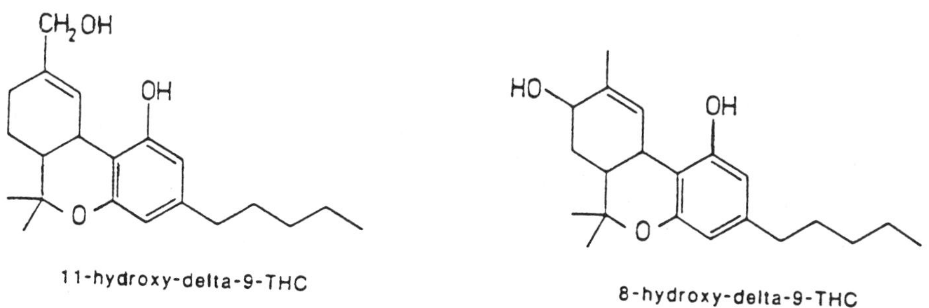

FIG. 4. The structure of two hydroxylated metabolites of delta-9-tetrahydrocannabinol.

Martin (1986). As shown in Table 1, there is evidence that psychological changes in human subjects similar to those experienced recreationally with cannabis can be produced by delta-9-THC at doses of about 30 to 50 μg/kg given intravenously, at a dose of about 50 μg/kg inhaled in smoke and at a dose of about 120 μg/kg taken orally. The naturally occurring (−) delta-8-tetrahydrocannabinol (delta-8-THC) has been shown to be only slightly less potent (Hollister and Gillespie, 1973). However, it probably contributes little to cannabis-induced 'highs' since it is only present in the plant in relatively small amounts. Cannabidiol (CBD) has been found to be psychically inactive when administered orally or

TABLE 1. *The Psychoactivity of Cannabinoids in Human Subjects*

Cannabinoid	Dose (μg/kg)	n	Route	Presence of "high"	Potency ratio	Reference
Δ^9-THC	50	10 to 40	i.h.	+*	1	1
	171†	6	i.h.	+	1	2
	120	10 to 40	p.o.	+*	1	1
	341 to 946	16	p.o.	+	1	3
	286†	6	p.o.	+	1	4
	29†	4	i.v.	+*	1	4
	14 to 16	3	i.v.	+	1	5
	13 to 14	6	i.v.	+	1	5
	50	15	i.v.	+	1	6
	41	6	i.v.	+*	1	7
	53	21	i.v.	+*	1	8,9
	14 to 43†	4	i.v.	+*	1	10
Δ^8-THC	286†	6	p.o.	+	0.7	4
	571†	6	p.o.	+	0.7	4
	29†	3	i.v.	+	0.7	4
	43†	3	i.v.	+	0.7	4
$\Delta^{6a,10a}$-THC	214†	6	i.h.	+	0.2 to 0.3	2
	400	10 to 40	i.h.	0	<0.25	1
9S-$\Delta^{6a,10a}$-THC	57 to 229†	6	i.v.	+*	0.2 to 0.3	10
9R-$\Delta^{6a,10a}$-THC	114 to 457†	6	i.v.	0	10	10
Synhexyl	214†	6	i.h.	+	0.2 to 0.3	2
	633 to 2666	13	p.o.	+	0.3	3
DMH-THC (Rac)	3	3	i.v.	0/+	?	11
(Rac)	0.5 to 8.3	33	i.v.	0	?	12
(2)	0.5 to 2.8	16	i.v.	0/+	?	12
Nabilone	43 to 71†	6	p.o.	+*	2 to 3	13
11-OH-Δ^9-THC	14 to 16	3	i.v.	+	>3.5	5,14
	13 to 14	6	i.v.	+	>3.5	5
	32	6	i.v.	+*	1	7
	47	11	i.v.	+*	1	8
8α-OH-Δ^9-THC	>186	5	i.v.	0	<0.3	8
8β-OH-Δ^9-THC	183	9	i.v.	+	<0.3	8
CBN	286 to 5714†	6	p.o.	0	<0.02	15
	270	6	i.v.	+	<0.2	9
CBD	286 to 1429†	5	p.o.	0	<0.08	15
	71 to 429†	4	i.v.	0	<0.1	15
	>268	6	i.v.	0	<0.2	9

Psychoactive potency of each cannabinoid is expressed relative to that of delta-9-THC given by the same route and, where possible, in the same study. The values given in the table are the ratios of doses producing approximately the same intensity of "high" (delta-9-THC/other cannabinoid). The presence (+) or absence (0) of a "high" is also shown.

*Indicates that the "high" (nature and intensity) was judged similar to "highs" experienced previously with cannabis. (In most studies, the subjects used had had prior recreational experience of cannabis).

†Indicates that the dose shown has been calculated assuming a body weight of 70 kg.

Inhalation (i.h.) indicates that the cannabinoid was inhaled in smoke.

DMH-THC (delta-6a,10a-dimethylheptyl-THC) has 3 asymmetric carbon atoms and can exist as one or other of 8 optical isomers (numbered 1 to 8) or as a racemic mixture (Rac).

References. 1, Isbell et al., 1967; 2, Hollister, 1970; 3, Hollister et al., 1968; 4, Hollister and Gillespie, 1973; 5, Lemberger et al., 1973; 6, Hollister and Gillespie, 1975; 7, Perez Reyes et al., 1972; 8, Perez Reyes et al., 1973b; 9, Perez Reyes et al., 1973a; 10, Hollister et al., 1987; 11, Lemberger et al., 1974; 12, Sidell et al., 1973; 13, Lemberger and Rowe, 1975; 14, Lemberger et al., 1972; 15, Hollister, 1973.

intravenously at doses well above those at which delta-9-THC is known to produce its psychic effects (Hollister, 1973; Perez Reyes *et al.*, 1973a). Experiments in which high doses of cannabinol (CBN) were administered orally yielded similar results (Hollister, 1973). However, when CBN was injected intravenously, it was found to produce a cannabis-like 'high' (Perez Reyes *et al.*, 1973a). The maximum dose of CBN used, 270 μg/kg i.v., produced a 'high' less intense than that produced by delta-9-THC at a dose of 53 μg/kg i.v., suggesting that the i.v. delta-9-THC/CBN potency ratio exceeds five. 11-Hydroxy-delta-9-THC and 8-beta-hydroxy-delta-9-THC, both metabolites of delta-9-THC, have also been shown to possess cannabis-like psychoactive properties (Table 1). The 11-hydroxy-compound has been found to be particularly potent, and indeed there is evidence that it can contribute significantly to the psychopharmacological effects of delta-9-THC. The extent of this is thought to depend on the route by which delta-9-THC is administered since this can affect the ratio of 11-hydroxy-delta-9-THC to its parent compound in the blood (Agurell *et al.*, 1986). The contribution made by the 11-hydroxy metabolite is probably far greater in man when delta-9-THC has been given orally than when it has been inhaled in smoke or injected intravenously (Agurell *et al.*, 1986).

The synthetic cannabinoid, delta-6a,10a-dimethylheptyl-THC, has so far been studied in man only at rather low doses, 3 to 6 times less than those at which delta-9-THC is known to produce a 'recreational high' (Sidell *et al.*, 1973; Lemberger *et al.*, 1974). These doses have been reported to produce euphoria or a mild 'high' in some subjects and to have no psychic effects in others. Other synthetic cannabinoids shown to have psychic activity in man are synhexyl which was 3 to 6 times less potent than delta-9-THC (Hollister, 1970; Hollister *et al.*, 1968) and nabilone which was somewhat more potent than delta-9-THC (Lemberger and Rowe, 1975). Delta-6a,10a-THC was reported to be approximately equipotent with synhexyl in one study (Hollister, 1970) but to be psychically inactive in another (Isbell *et al.*, 1967). More recently, experiments with the 9R- and 9S-enantiomers of delta-6a,10a-THC showed that the psychoactivity of this cannabinoid could be attributed to its 9S configuration (Hollister *et al.*, 1987). Although animal experiments have already established that cannabinoids exhibit stereoselectivity (see below), this is the first time that the phenomenon has been demonstrated in man.

The ability of several of the cannabinoids mentioned in this review to produce behavioral changes in rhesus monkeys, squirrel monkeys or dogs is summarized in Table 2. On

TABLE 2. *Delta-9-THC/Cannabinoid Potency Ratios in Three Behavioral Tests*

Cannabinoid	Rhesus monkey test (i.v.)	Squirrel monkey test (i.p.)	Dog ataxia test (i.v.)
$(-)\Delta^9$-THC	1 (0.1 mg/kg)	1 (1.0 mg/kg)	1 (0.2 mg/kg)
11-OH-Δ^9-THC	ND	5	4
Δ^8-THC	0.1 to 0.2	ND	0.4
$\Delta^{6a,10a}$-THC	0.2	ND	ND
Δ^8-DMH-THC	2	ND	ND
8α-OH-Δ^9-THC	0.05	ND	ND
R-3′-OH-Δ^9-THC	ND	ND	<1
S-3′-OH-Δ^9-THC	ND	ND	>1
R/S-3′-OH-Δ^9-THC	ND	ND	>1
1′-OH-Δ^8-THC	<0.01	ND	ND
2′-OH-Δ^8-THC	0.05	ND	ND
3′-OH-Δ^8-THC	0.5	ND	ND
4′-OH-Δ^8-THC	0.2 to 0.4	ND	ND
5′-OH-Δ^8-THC	0.2	ND	ND
$(+)\Delta^9$-THC	<0.1*	ND	<0.1*
$(+)\Delta^8$-THC	<0.1*	ND	ca.0.1
CBN	Inactive	0.04	ca.0.2
CBD	Inactive	<0.01*	ND
CBG	<0.02*	ND	ND

In the squirrel monkey assay, cannabinoids were given to animals that had been trained to respond on a chain fixed-interval 4 min fixed-ratio 50 schedule of food presentation. The potency ratios shown have been calculated after inspection of dose-response curves (Carney *et al.*, 1979). In the other assays, the potency of 'test' cannabinoid relative to that of delta-9-THC was either the reported value (when given) or the value obtained by comparing doses required to produce a particular pattern of behavior. In the rhesus monkey assay (Grunfeld and Edery, 1969; Edery *et al.*, 1971; Mechoulam and Edery, 1973; Ohlsson *et al.*, 1979) the end point has been taken as behavior which the authors have scored ++ ('stupor, ataxia, suppression of motor activity, full ptosis, typical crouched posture kept for up to three hours and presence of reaction to external stimuli). In the dog assay (Martin *et al.*, 1981, 1984a, b) the end point has been taken as behavior which the authors have scored 3 ('tail is often tucked, some loss of tone in hind legs as evidenced by a semi-squatting position, static ataxia...seen after dog stands in one position for 1–2 min and nodding may be observed 30–60 min after injection'). CBG and DMH are abbreviations for cannabigerol and dimethylheptyl respectively.

*Indicates inactive at the doses used. ND = not determined.

the whole, the data in this Table are consistent with those obtained from human psychopharmacological studies (Table 1). Thus the animal data show that 11-hydroxy-delta-9-THC is more potent than delta-9-THC, than delta-8-THC, delta-6a,10a-THC and 8-alpha-hydroxy-delta-9-THC are all less potent than delta-9-THC and that CBD is inactive. CBN was reported to elicit no behavioral effects in rhesus monkeys (Mechoulam and Edery, 1973) but did produce delta-9-THC-like behavioral changes in squirrel monkeys and dogs (Carney *et al.*, 1979; Martin *et al.*, 1984a). As in the human studies of Perez Reyes *et al.*, 1973a) it was markedly less potent than delta-9-THC in both tests. The data in Table 2 also show that the unnatural (+) isomer of delta-9-THC was at least 10 times less potent than its naturally occurring (−) isomer in both rhesus monkey and dog tests. The stereoselectivity of delta-9-THC has been demonstrated in numerous other animal experiments, both *in vivo* and *in vitro* (Pertwee, 1983; Martin, 1986), and it is likely that (−) delta-9-THC will also be much more potent than (+) delta-9-THC in producing cannabis-like 'highs' in human subjects. This has still to be confirmed. Also still to be confirmed in man is the evidence from animal data (Table 2) that delta-8-dimethylheptyl-THC and certain side chain hydroxylated metabolites of delta-8- and delta-9-THC possess marked psychic activity and that cannabigerol is psychically inactive.

One important synthetic analog of delta-9-THC not included in Tables 1 or 2 is levonantradol. Clinical trials directed at assessing the antiemetic activity of this drug in cancer patients undergoing chemotherapy have shown that it can produce affective, emotional, perceptual and cognitive changes and that it does so at oral doses (0.5 to 2 mg every 4 hr) well below those at which delta-9-THC is known to produce its psychopharmacological effects (Diasio *et al.*, 1981; Laszlo *et al.*, 1981; see also references cited by Pertwee, 1985b). There is also evidence that levonantradol (0.03 to 0.3 mg/kg i.v.) can produce delta-9-THC-like changes in the behavior of rhesus monkeys (Young *et al.*, 1981). The behavioral changes elicited by a levonantradol dose of 0.3 mg/kg i.v. were similar to those produced by delta-9-THC at a dose of 3 mg/kg i.v. These data suggest that levonantradol is a highly potent psychoactive cannabinoid. However, confirmatory controlled experiments with healthy human subjects are still required, there being a need for qualitative as well as quantitative comparisons to be made between the psychopharmacological properties of levonantradol and those of delta-9-THC or cannabis.

The results of experiments conducted with cannabis can be particularly difficult to interpret. There are three main reasons for this. First, cannabis contains a number of compounds, both cannabinoid and non-cannabinoid, having different pharmacological properties (Pertwee, 1983; 1985b). Second, the chemical composition of cannabis is not always the same (Paton, 1975; Pertwee, 1983). It is affected by heat when smoked and by storage and also depends on the geographical origin of the plant material. Third, there is evidence that the effects of delta-9-THC can be intensified or attenuated by CBN, CBD and other constituents of cannabis (Pertwee, 1983; Dewey, 1986; Martin, 1986). For these reasons, the remainder of this review follows the practice of many recent neuropharamacological studies and deals only with effects produced by individual cannabinoids.

Before proceeding to the next section it is important to note that like cannabis, delta-9-THC and many of the other cannabinoids referred to in this review have the ability to produce quite large falls in deep-body temperature (Pertwee, 1985a). A few neuropharmacological studies with whole animals have taken this into account, using ambient temperatures sufficiently high to prevent hypothermia. However, most have been conducted at normal room temperature and therefore presumably often with hypothermic animals. This must be borne in mind when results are being interpreted since brain function is markedly affected by hypothermia.

3. THE THERAPEUTIC POTENTIAL OF CANNABINOIDS

Cannabis has a long history not only as a recreational drug but also as a therapeutic agent. Although its traditional uses have been taken over by more effective and selective agents there has recently been an upsurge of interest in the possible clinical uses of individual cannabinoids. Experiments have been directed both at examining the therapeutic potential of existing cannabinoids and at producing new analogs with improved selectivity (Lemberger, 1980, 1985; Pertwee, 1985b; Hollister *et al.*, 1986; Mechoulam 1986). The ability of delta-9-THC and two of its synthetic analogs, nabilone and levonantradol, to suppress nausea and vomiting associated with cancer chemotherapy has attracted particular interest. Indeed, nabilone (cesamet) can now be prescribed in the United Kingdom for this purpose. Also of interest is the possible use of the psychically inactive cannabinoid, CBD, in the treatment of epilepsy. Other potential therapeutic applications which show some degree of promise include the use of delta-9-THC or its synthetic analogs as analgesics, as muscle relaxants and in the treatment of glaucoma.

4. THE SOLUBILITY OF CANNABINOIDS

Cannabinoids are very lipophilic. They have extremely low water solubilities, high lipid solubilities and high membrane/water and organic solvent/water partition coefficients. The values of the organic solvent/water coefficients vary somewhat from cannabinoid to cannabinoid. However, there is no correlation between these values and psychoactive potency. The octanol/water and benzene/water partition coefficients of delta-9-THC have both been reported to be about 6000 (Gill and Jones, 1972; Ho *et al.*, 1973). For delta-8-THC, the corresponding values are only slightly less, about 5000 (Ho *et al.*, 1973; Ohlsson *et al.*, 1980). Gill *et al.*, (1973) found that the octanol/water partition coefficient of the more polar cannabinoid, 11-hydroxy-delta-9-THC, was about 3500. The 11-hydroxy metabolite of delta-8-THC was shown to have octanol/water and benzene/water partition coefficients of about 1500 and CBN had a benzene/water partition coefficient of 1175 (Ho *et al.*, 1973; Ohlsson *et al.*, 1980). The octanol/water partition coefficients of side chain hydroxylated derivatives of delta-8-THC were found to range from 1500 to 4000 (Ohlsson *et al.*, 1980).

Binder *et al.*, (1984) studied the distribution of delta-9-THC in a system consisting of egg phosphatidylcholine, glycerol trioleate and phosphate buffer. The cannabinoid distributed almost equally between the two lipids and none of it was detectable in the aqueous phase. Seeman *et al.*, (1972) measured the membrane/phosphate buffer partition coefficient of delta-9-THC using both guinea-pig brain synaptosomes and human erythrocyte ghosts. They reported that the partition coefficient varied inversely with the free concentration of delta-9-THC. It ranged from about 500 to 40 for the synaptosomal membranes and from about 800 to 35 for the erythrocyte membranes. More recently, Roth and Williams (1979) found the partition coefficient of delta-9-THC between rat brain synaptosomes and Krebs solution or phosphate buffer to be of the order of 12 000 to 14 000. They also reported that the value of the partition coefficient did not vary with the free concentration of delta-9-THC. These results are clearly quite different from those of Seeman *et al.* (1972). One possible explanation for this difference is that the latter group overestimated the concentration of delta-9-THC remaining in free solution. Whereas Roth and Williams (1979) used concentrations of delta-9-THC in the range 0.01 to 1 μM, Seeman *et al.*, (1972) reported the use of concentrations of 4 to 40 μM, a range which extends well beyond the aqueous solubility of delta-9-THC (less than 10 μM; see below).

Because of their low solubility in water, cannabinoids are usually administered dissolved or dispersed in agents such as ethanol, dimethyl sulfoxide, Tween 80, Cremophor E. L. or polyvinylpyrrolidone. Most studies making use of vehicles of this kind have not included experiments to test for an effect of the vehicle (relative to an untreated group) or for the existence of synergistic or antagonistic interactions between cannabinoid and vehicle. (For further discussion on this point, see Burstein *et al.*, 1986a and the review by Dewey, 1986).

Although the administration of cannabinoids is facilitated by dissolving them in organic solvents, there is no guarantee that such solutions will not precipitate out immediately after administration. When Banerjee *et al.* (1975b) added 0.33 μmoles of delta-9-THC dissolved in dimethyl sulfoxide to 10 mls of Krebs-Henseleit buffer (final 'nominal' concentration = 33 μM), they found that only about 2% of the cannabinoid remained in solution (actual concentration = 0.63 μM). The same result was obtained when the buffer also contained rat brain synaptosomes. When delta-8-THC or CBD was added to the buffer (final 'nominal' concentrations = respectively 37 and 28 μM), 1% of delta-8-THC and 4.4% of CBD remained in solution. Only 0.3 to 0.5% of delta-9-THC remained in solution at 'nominal' concentrations in buffer ranging from 0.1 to 1 mM. Johnson *et al.* (1976a) added delta-9-THC dissolved in polyvinylpyrrolidone to Krebs-Henseleit buffer and found that 3.9% of the drug remained in solution (final 'nominal' concentration = 0.1 mM). The results obtained by Banerjee *et al.* (1975a), by Johnson *et al.* (1976a) and by Roth and Williams (1979) suggest that aqueous solutions of delta-9-THC become saturated at concentrations of about 1 to 4 μM. Consistent with this conclusion is the observation by Bach *et al.* (1976a) that delta-9-THC and CBD precipitated out of 0.15 M aqueous NaCl and KCl solutions at a concentration of about 8 μM and the report by Garrett and Hunt (1974) that the solubilities of delta-9-THC in water and in aqueous 0.15 M NaCl solutions are respectively 9 and 2.5 μM.

Some vehicles, for example Tween 80 and Cremophor E. L., combine with cannabinoids in aqueous media to form micelles, the vehicle-cannabinoid-water mixture existing in a dispersion rather than as a true solution. It is likely that after administration to animals or to *in vitro* preparations, such micelles remain intact so that the cannabinoids stay homogeneously dispersed. There is evidence that, at least in some media, the transfer of delta-9-THC from micelles to tissue is much slower and less complete than tissue absorption of delta-9-THC from free solution. Thus Roth and Williams (1979) found that Tween 80 markedly reduced the synaptosomal membrane/buffer partition coefficient of delta-9-THC, the size of the reduction increasing with the amount of Tween 80 present. Similar results were obtained with Cremophor E. L. Interestingly, ethanol also reduced the partition coefficient of delta-9-THC. However, its effect was much smaller than that of the other vehicles.

Reports about *in vitro* experiments with cannabinoids often give a value for the concentration used that implies uniform and complete dissolution in the aqueous bathing medium. For the want of more accurate values, such 'nominal' concentrations are also given in the Tables and text of this review. It is likely, however, that when, as is frequently the case, the vehicle used is an organic solvent, the final actual free concentration of cannabinoid in the medium will only equal the 'nominal' concentration when the latter is of the order of 1 μM or less (see above), an increasing proportion of added cannabinoid coming out of solution as the 'nominal' concentration is raised above 1 μM. Even when low concentrations of cannabinoids are used, the actual free concentration in the medium will probably be less than expected. This is because delta-9-THC and presumably other cannabinoids bind avidly to the surfaces of the vessels in which they are contained (Garrett and Hunt, 1974; Kujtan *et al.*, 1983) and also because the drug will be readily taken up by the tissue present in the medium (see above). It follows that the dose of delta-9-THC that must be added to an *in vitro* preparation to produce a given effect may well increase if the amount of biological material is increased. Such a relationship has been demonstrated by Vaysse *et al.* (1987) and by Sung and Jakubovic (1987). The extent to which precipitation of cannabinoids into aqueous media affects their ability to reach and interact with a responsive tissue is not certain. Complete loss of this ability is unlikely, however, and indeed Banerjee *et al.* (1975b) found that when delta-9-THC was dissolved in dimethyl sulfoxide and then added to an aqueous suspension of synaptosomes, it produced 'concentration dependent' inhibition of neurotransmitter uptake at 'nominal' concentrations ranging from 1 to 100 μM (Section 6).

Many of the experiments described in this review have involved addition of delta-9-THC directly to preparations of brain tissue suspended in aqueous media. In order to assess the importance of delta-9-THC-induced changes detected in such experiments, it would be helpful to know how the tissue concentrations achieved in these *in vitro* experiments compare with the concentrations of delta-9-THC reached in brain tissue after the drug has been administered *in vivo* at doses known to elicit pharmacological responses. This is an extremely complex task and indeed the data at present available are insufficient to make comparisons of this kind with any degree of accuracy. Gill and Jones (1972) measured whole brain levels of ^{3}H-delta-9-THC at various times after the drug had been injected intravenously into mice. The dose used, 2 mg/kg, produced detectable behavioral changes and is also known to lower body temperature (Pertwee and Tavendale, 1977). The maximum concentration of delta-9-THC found in the brain was 1.46 μmoles/kg. Ryrfeldt *et al.* (1973) showed that mouse brain concentrations of delta-9-THC rose to about 3.2 μmoles/kg following intravenous injection of this cannabinoid at a dose of 12 mg/kg. In rats, intravenous injections of delta-9-THC at doses of 4 and 5 mg/kg were reported to produce peak brain levels of 5.1 and 11.2 μmoles/kg, respectively (Klausner and Dingell, 1971; Ho *et al.*, 1973). These brain concentrations were all determined per unit wet weight of whole brain and, given the high lipid/water partition coefficient of delta-9-THC, it is likely that the drug reached higher concentrations in the lipid phase of neuronal membranes. [Roth and Williams (1979) estimated that a dose of delta-9-THC known to elicit behavioral changes in mice would give rise to a brain membrane concentration of about 20 μmoles/kg dry membrane.] Metabolites of delta-9-THC are thought to make a significant contribution towards the responses evoked by *in vivo* administration of delta-9-THC (Section 2) and this too must be taken into account when calculating the concentration of delta-9-THC required in brain tissue to bring about pharmacological changes.

Roth and Williams (1979) obtained values for the membrane concentration of delta-9-THC in various *in vitro* systems from the equation membrane concentration = free concentration × membrane/buffer partition coefficient. The equation is of limited value in interpreting the data described in this review since the amount of delta-9-THC added to *in vitro* systems has often exceeded its aqueous solubility. Another problem can be the selection of an appropriate value for the partition coefficient because, as already discussed, the partition coefficient of delta-9-THC can vary considerably not only with the vehicle used but also with vehicle concentration. For example, if the concentration of delta-9-THC in the aqueous medium of an *in vitro* preparation were 1 μM, then depending on the vehicle used, the membrane concentration of the drug might be as low as 0.1 or 0.5 mmoles/kg dry membrane or as high as 10 or 12 mmoles/kg dry membrane (Roth and Williams, 1979). Nonetheless, these calculations do suggest that, irrespective of the vehicle used, a 'nominal' delta-9-THC concentration in the medium of less than 1 μM will be sufficient to achieve a tissue concentration (20 μmoles/kg dry membrane) which will, when present in the brain, give rise to behavioral changes (see above). This conclusion is supported by evidence firstly that delta-9-THC can elicit responses in several *in vitro* preparations when present in the medium at 'nominal' concentrations ranging from 10 pM to 300 nM and secondly that the ability of cannabinoids to produce changes at such concentrations does, in several preparations, correlate with psychoactive potency (see, for example, Sections 10.1.1. and 10.2.

5. ELECTROPHYSIOLOGICAL STUDIES

Delta-9-THC, 50 to 500 μM, has been shown to decrease the amplitude of the action potential in the desheathed cervical vagus nerve of the rabbit (Byck and Ritchie, 1973). In addition, at concentrations of 0.1 to 1.0 mM it has been found to reduce voltage-dependent sodium conductance in single myelinated fibers of frog sciatic nerve (Strichartz *et al.*, 1978). In the same preparation, the drug also reduced potassium conductance, albeit to a smaller extent. One preparation in which delta-9-THC has been reported to have no effect on impulse conduction is the giant squid axon (Brady and Carbone, 1973). Interestingly, its primary metabolite, 11-hydroxy-delta-9-THC, was found to be highly active in this preparation, concentrations as low as 5 nM reducing both the amplitude of the action potential and conduction velocity (Brady and Carbone, 1973).

There is evidence that as well as reducing the excitability of some isolated nerve preparations, delta-9-THC can depress the excitability of nerve cells in isolated buccal and parieto-visceral ganglia of *Aplysia californica* (Acosta-Urquidi and Chase, 1975) and decrease the activity of prejunctional neurons in isolated preparations of rat phrenic nerve-diaphragm (Kayaalp *et al.*, 1974; Hoekman *et al.*, 1976), frog sciatic nerve-sartorius muscle

(Kumbaraci and Nastuk, 1980), crayfish neuromuscular junction (Aldridge and Pomeranz, 1977) and guinea-pig ileum (Table 3). Thus, for example, experiments with the rat phrenic nerve-diaphragm preparation showed that when just a portion of the phrenic nerve was exposed to delta-9-THC (95 μM), there was a marked reduction in the size of the twitch evoked by electrical stimulation of the nerve (Kayaalp *et al.*, 1974). In experiments with isolated preparations of the guinea-pig ileum, delta-9-THC was shown to decrease the size of the twitches induced by repetitive electrical stimulation (Table 3). The twitches observed in these experiments were produced by electrically stimulated prejunctional release of acetylcholine rather than by direct stimulation of ileal smooth muscle and it was found that delta-9-THC could reduce the size of these twitches at concentrations at which it had no effect on contractions induced by the addition of acetylcholine (Gill *et al.*, 1970; Layman and Milton, 1971; Roth, 1978). It was also found that concentrations of delta-9-THC known to reduce the twitch response, decreased the output of acetylcholine from resting strips of whole ileum (Layman and Milton, 1971) or of ileal longitudinal muscle (Paton *et al.*, 1972). Interestingly, the effect of delta-9-THC was greatest when the initial spontaneous release of acetylcholine had been high, suggesting that the drug acted to reduce acetylcholine output to a basal level (Paton *et al.*, 1972). It is noteworthy that CBD, which had no detectable effect on the twitch response, was reported by Layman and Milton

Table 3. *Effects of Cannabinoids on the Twitch Response Evoked in Isolated Preparations of the Guinea-pig Ileum by Repetitive Electrical Stimulation*

Procedure	Cannabinoid	Concentration	Twitch amplitude	Reference
Transmural stimulation of whole ileum	Δ^9-THC	3.18 μM upwards	–	1
	Δ^9-THC	0.16 μM (=ED_{50})	–	2
	CBD	3.18 μM	0	2
Supramaximal stimulation of whole ileum at 0.1 Hz (cannabinoid vehicle when named was ethanol)	(−)Δ^9-THC	c.a. 79.5 nM	–	3
	(−)Δ^8-THC	79.5 nM	–	3,4
	(+)Δ^8-THC	318 nM	0	3
	(−)11-OH-Δ^9-THC	c.a. 3 nM upwards	–	3
	(+)11-OH-Δ^9-THC	76 nM	0	3
	(−)11-OH-Δ^8-THC	3 nM upwards	–	3,4
	(−)1′-OH-Δ^8-THC	75.6 nM	–/0	5
	(−)2′-OH-Δ^8-THC	75.6 nM	–/0	5
	(−)3′-OH-Δ^8-THC	75.6 nM	–	5
	(−)4′-OH-Δ^8-THC	75.6 nM	–/0	5
	(−)5′-OH-Δ^8-THC	75.6 nM	–	5
	CBD	318 nM	0	3,4
	CBN	322 nM	0	3,4
Stimulation of whole ileum at 0.1 Hz (cannabinoid vehicle was ethanol)	(−)Δ^9-THC	100 nM (=ED_{50})	–	6
	(+)Δ^9-THC	2 μM	0	6
	(−)Δ^8-THC	100 nM (=ED_{50})	–	6
	11-OH-Δ^9-THC	15 nM (=ED_{50})	–	6
	1′-OH-Δ^9-THC (A)	1.1 μm (=ED_{50})	–	6
	1′-OH-Δ^9-THC (B)	2.3 μm	0	6
	2′-OH-Δ^9-THC	500 μM (=ED_{50})	–	6
	3′-OH-Δ^9-THC	20 nM (=ED_{50})	–	6
	4′-OH-Δ^9-THC	80 nM (=ED_{50})	–	6
	5′-OH-Δ^9-THC	110 nM (=ED_{50})	–	6
	Nabilone	100 nM (=ED_{50})	–	6
	Levonantradol	10 nM (=ED_{50})	–	6
	CBN	2 μM	0	6
	CBD	2 μM	0	6
	CBG	2 μM	0	6
Supramaximal field stimulation of longitudinal muscle strip at 0.2 Hz (cannabinoid vehicle was Cremophor E. L.)	(−)Δ^9-THC	6.4 nM to 0.64 μM*	–	7
	(+)Δ^9-THC	64 nM to 6.4 μM**	–	7

*Indicates ED_{50} = 0.125 μM and ** indicates ED_{50} = 3.1 μM. CBG is an abbreviation for cannabigerol.
References: 1, Gill *et al.*, 1970; 2, Layman and Milton, 1971; 3, Rosell *et al.*, 1976; 4, Rosell and Agurell, 1975; 5, Rosell *et al.*, 1979; 6, Nye *et al.*, 1985; 7, Roth, 1978.

(1971) to be more effective than delta-9-THC in reducing spontaneous acetylcholine output from lengths of whole ileum.

The ability of cannabinoids to decrease the size of electrically evoked twitches in the isolated guinea-pig ileum correlates well with psychoactive potency (see Table 3 for references). For example, (−) delta-8-THC and (−) delta-9-THC have been found to be approximately equipotent as inhibitors of the twitch response (Rosell *et al.*, 1976; Nye *et al.*, 1985). Both were less potent than their 11-hydroxy metabolites but markedly more potent than their (+) isomers (Rosell and Agurell, 1975; Rosell *et al.*, 1976; Roth, 1978; Nye *et al.*, 1985). CBN and CBD were reported not to attenuate the twitch response even at relatively high concentrations (Layman and Milton, 1971; Rosell and Agurell, 1975; Rosell *et al.*, 1976; Nye *et al.*, 1985).

Rosell and Agurell (1975) found that like delta-9-THC (see above), concentrations of delta-8-THC or 11-hydroxy-delta-8-THC known to decrease the size of the twitch response in the isolated guinea-pig ileum, did not reduce contractions elicited by the addition of acetylcholine. They also found that the 11-hydroxy compound did not attenuate the response of guinea-pig ileum to histamine which acts directly on the smooth muscle but did reduce the response to 5-hydroxytryptamine which acts prejunctionally to increase acetylcholine release.

During their experiments with the isolated sciatic nerve-sartorius muscle preparation of the frog, Kumbaraci and Nastuk (1980) obtained evidence that delta-9-THC (30 μM) markedly decreased prejunctional release of acetylcholine per nerve impulse and suggested that the drug might have acted not only by diminishing prejunctional action potentials but also by reducing prejunctional Ca^{2+} influx. It is noteworthy, therefore, that Harris and Stokes (1982) have shown that *in vitro* addition of delta-9-THC can inhibit depolarization-dependent Ca^{2+} uptake into synaptosomes prepared from mouse whole brain or from rat cerebral cortex, striatum, cerebellum or brain stem. Effective concentrations ranged upwards from 10 nM and varied depending on the brain area from which the synaptosomes had been prepared. Delta-9-THC inhibited Ca^{2+} uptake at concentrations at which it had no apparent effect on Ca^{2+} efflux or on synaptosomal membrane potentials and it was concluded that it had altered Ca^{2+} uptake by interacting with voltage-dependent Ca^{2+} channels. The psychically inactive cannabinoid, CBD, was as potent as delta-9-THC as an inhibitor of Ca^{2+} uptake, albeit only in the experiments with mouse brain synaptosomes. 11-hydroxy-delta-9-THC was less potent than delta-9-THC, and CBN was inactive. Like delta-9-THC, CBD also inhibited Ca^{2+} uptake into rat brain stem synaptosomes. However, in contrast to delta-9-THC, it had no detectable effect on Ca^{2+} uptake into synaptosomes prepared from rat cerebral cortex or cerebellum. In more recent studies, Turkanis and Karler (1986a) found that psychically active cannabinoids can exert both depressant and excitant effects on transmission across the neuromuscular junction of the frog sartorius muscle. Using extracellular recording techniques, they obtained evidence that, at concentrations of 0.1 to 1.0 μM, delta-9-THC and its 11-hydroxy metabolite could act prejunctionally, initially to enhance transmitter release (an increase in the mean quantum content of the end plate potential) and subsequently to depress release. CBD, on the other hand, had only a depressant effect on release. All three cannabinoids also depressed the amplitude of miniature end-plate potentials, presumably a postjunctional effect. In addition, it was found that the frequency of the miniature end plate potentials was increased by delta-9-THC, unaffected by 11-hydroxy-delta-9-THC and decreased by CBD.

Niemi (1979) studied the effect of delta-9-THC on the electrical excitability of innervated electric eel electroplaques. At a concentration of 50 μM, the drug reduced the action potential elicited by direct stimulation of the electroplaque. Delta-9-THC also suppressed transmission across the nerve-electroplaque junction without altering the ability of carbamylcholine to depolarize the postjunctional membrane. It was concluded that, in this preparation, the drug can reduce the electrical excitability of the postjunctional membrane and that it can also act prejunctionally to reduce the size of the action potential or to impair excitation–secretion coupling.

Cannabinoids have been shown to alter transmission along central synaptic pathways in a variety of mammalian preparations (Tables 4 to 8). Their effects on spinal reflexes may well involve sites of action in the brain. Thus Dagirmanjian and Boyd (1962) found that although delta-6a, 10a-dimethylheptyl-THC could suppress the polysynaptic flexion and linguomandibular reflexes in unanesthetized cats sectioned at the level of the midbrain, it had no effect on the flexion reflex in animals with low spinal sections. Low spinal sections did not, however, abolish the effect of delta-6a, 10a-dimethylheptyl-THC on the linguomandibular reflex. In further experiments (Boyd and Meritt, 1965), delta-6a, 10a-dimethylheptyl-THC was shown in 6/10 cats to depress facilitation of the flexion reflex induced by electrical stimulation of the brain stem reticular formation. Similarly, facilitation of the knee jerk produced by brain stem stimulation was attenuated or abolished by the cannabinoid in 9/20 cats. In contrast to the earlier experiments, it was found that delta-6a, 10a-dimethylheptyl-THC was able to suppress the flexion reflex (5/8 cats) as well as the linguomandibular reflex in cats with low spinal sections. It would seem, therefore, that the drug can suppress spinal reflexes both by acting at the level of the brain stem to reduce motor facilitation and by interacting directly with the reflex system itself.

Campbell *et al.* (1986a; 1986b) have investigated effects of delta-9-THC on potentials evoked in the hippocampal dentate gyrus of unanesthetized rats by sound stimuli during an auditory two-tone discrimination task. Doses impairing performance in the behavioral test (1 and 2 mg/kg i.p.), were found to decrease the firing rate of granule cells, both spontaneous and sound-evoked activity being affected. Changes in the amplitude of sound-evoked potentials were also detected (Table 6). Unlike the other electrophysiological changes induced by THC, suppression of the sound-evoked activity of granule cells outlasted the behavioral response. In several experiments, the psychically active cannabinoids delta-9-THC, delta-8-THC and delta-6a,10a-dimethylheptyl-THC have been found to have an excitatory effect on neuronal transmission at low doses and an inhibitory effect at higher doses. This is so for one or other of these drugs in experiments concerned with effects on spinal reflexes (Table 4), on the amplitude of potentials evoked in various parts of the brain (Tables 5 and 6) and on post-tetanic potentiation in cat spinal cord and rat hippocampus (Table 7). Delta-9-THC has also been shown to elicit both excitatory and inhibitory changes in behavioral and electrophysiological models of epilepsy, the drug possessing a mixture of convulsant and anticonvulsant properties (Feeney, 1979; Karler and Turkanis, 1979; Turkanis and Karler, 1981a; Pertwee, 1985b).

The effect of delta-9-THC on evoked activity in the brain varies not only with dose but also with the recording site and with the type of stimulus used to evoke a response (Table 5). Results from experiments with anesthetized cats suggest that thalamocortical sensory pathways are particularly sensitive to the drug's actions, raising the possibility that

TABLE 4. *Effects of Cannabinoids on Monosynaptic (Mono) and Polysynaptic (Poly) Spinal Reflexes*

Cannabinoid	Dose (mg/kg i.v.)	Preparation	Type of reflex	Effect	Reference
$\Delta^{6a,10a}$-DMH-THC	0.05	Anesthetized cat	Poly (Flexion)	0	1
	0.10	Anesthetized cat	Poly (Flexion)	−	1,2
	0.05 and 0.10	Anesthetized cat	Poly (Linguomandibular)	−	1,2
	0.20	Anesthetized cat	Mono (Patellar)	0	1
$\Delta^{6a,10a}$-MO-THC	0.20 to 0.40	Anesthetized cat	Poly (Flexion)	−	1
	0.20 to 0.40	Anesthetized cat	Poly (Linguomandibular)	−	1
Δ^9-THC	0.01 to 0.10	Anesthetized spinal cat	Mono	+	3
Δ^9-THC	0.05 to 0.15	Unanesthetized spinal cat	Mono	+	4
	0.20 to 0.75		Mono	−	4
CBD	0.05 to 14.0	Unanesthetized spinal cat	Mono	−	4

DMH and MO are abbreviations for dimethylheptyl and methyloctyl, respectively.

References: 1, Dagirmanjian and Boyd, 1962; 2, Boyd and Meritt, 1965; 3, Turkanis and Karler, 1983; 4, Tramposch *et al.*, 1981.

TABLE 5. *Effects of Cannabinoids on the Amplitude of Potentials Evoked at Sites in the Sensory Cortex, Thalamus, Midbrain and Hindbrain*

Cannabinoid	Dose (mg/kg)	Route	Preparation	Stimulation site	Recording site	Effect	Reference
Δ^8- & Δ^9-THC	0.25 to 1.5	i.v.	Unanesthetized squirrel monkey (cerveau isolé)	Somatosensory cortex	Postarcuate polysensory cortex	+	1
	0.50 to 1.5	i.v.				−	1
Δ^9-THC	0.065 to 2.5	i.v.	Unanesthetized squirrel monkey (spinal or pontine)	Somatosensory cortex	Postarcuate polysensory cortex	+	2,3
Δ^9-THC	0.032 to 1.0	i.v.	Unanesthetized squirrel monkey	Ear (stimulus = tone cue)	Postarcuate polysensory cortex	−	4
Δ^9-THC	0.1 to 1.0	i.p.	Unanesthetized rat	Parietal cortex	Parietal cortex (contralateral to stimulation site)	+	5
	1.2 to 6.0	i.p.				−	
CBD	0.1 to 40.0	i.p.	Unanesthetized rat	Parietal cortex		−	5
Δ^9-THC	0.1 to 0.3*	*	Anesthetized rat	Eye (stimulus = light)	Lateral geniculate nucleus	−	6
Δ^9-THC	0.1 to 0.3*	*	Anesthetized rat	Optic nerve	Lateral geniculate nucleus	− (5/8 rats)	6
THC	0.80 to 1.0†	i.v.	Anesthetized cat	Trigeminal afferent nerve	Superior sensory nucleus of trigeminal nerve	−	7
THC	0.80 to 1.0†	i.v.	Anesthetized cat	Trigeminal afferent nerve	Trigeminal afferent nerve	−	7
Δ^9-THC	4.0	i.v.	Anesthetized cat	Radial nerve or ventral posterolateral nucleus	Somatosensory cortex	−	8
Δ^9-THC	2.0 to 4.0	i.v.	Anesthetized cat	Radial nerve, ear (stimulus = sound) or eye (stimulus = light)	Polysensory cortex	−	9,10
CBD	2.0 to 8.0	i.v.	Anesthetized cat		Polysensory cortex	+	9
Δ^9-THC	2.0 to 4.0	i.v.	Anesthetized cat	Radial nerve or eye (stimulus = light)	Mesencephalic reticular formation or n. centralis lateralis	0	10
Δ^9-THC	2.0 4.0	i.v.	Anesthetized cat	Ear (stimulus = sound)	Mesencephalic reticular formation	+ 0	10
Δ^9-THC	2.0 4.0	i.v.	Anesthetized cat	Ear (stimulus = sound)	N. centralis lateralis	0 +	10
Δ^9-THC	2.0	i.v.	Anesthetized cat	Mesencephalic reticular formation	Polysensory cortex and n. centralis lateralis	−	10
Δ^9-THC	2.0 to 4.0	i.v.	Anesthetized cat	Mesencephalic reticular formation	Caudate nucleus	0	10
Δ^9-THC	2.0 to 4.0	i.v.	Anesthetized cat	N. centralis lateralis	Polysensory cortex	−	10
Δ^9-THC	2.0 to 4.0	i.v.	Anesthetized cat	N. centralis lateralis	Caudate nucleus	0	10
Δ^9-THC	0.5 to 2.0	i.p.	Unanesthetized cat	Ear (stimulus = sound)	Auditory cortex	+	11
$\Delta^{6a,10a}$-DMH-THC	0.2	i.v.	Unanesthetized cat	Radial nerve	Mesencephalic medial lemniscus	0	12
$\Delta^{6a,10a}$-DMH-THC	0.2	i.v.	Unanesthetized cat	Radial nerve	Ventrobasal complex of thalamus	+ (2/7 cats) − (1/7 cats)	12
$\Delta^{6a,10a}$-DMH-THC	0.2	i.v.	Unanesthetized cat	Radial nerve	Mesencephalic reticular formation	− (6/14 cats)	12

DMH is an abbreviation for dimethylheptyl.

*Indicates administration by close arterial injection (catheter in internal carotid artery; dose in mg).

†Indicates that these doses had no effect on tibialis nerve action potentials.

References. 1, Boyd et al., 1971; 2, Boyd et al., 1974; 3, Boyd et al., 1975; 4, Boyd et al., 1976; 5, Turkanis and Karler, 1981b; 6, Bieger and Hockman, 1973; 7. Lapa et al., 1968; 8, Wilkison et al., 1982; 9, Pontzer et al., 1986; 10, Pontzer and Wilkison, 1987; 11, Guha and Pradhan, 1974; 12, Boyd and Meritt, 1966.

TABLE 6. *Effects of Cannabinoids on the Amplitude of Potentials Evoked at Sites in the Hippocampus*

Cannabinoid	Dose*	Preparation	Stimulation site	Recording site	Effect	Reference
In vivo experiments						
Δ^9-THC	2.5 to 10	Anesthetized rat	Fornix	Hippocampal surface	0	1
Δ^8-THC	2.5 to 10				0	
CBD	1.25 to 5	Anesthetized rat	Fornix	Hippocampal surface	0	1
CBN	2.5 to 10				0	
SP-111	10	Unanesthetized rat	Hippocampus	Hippocampus (contralateral to stimulation site)	–	2
Δ^9-THC	2 to 8	Unanesthetized rat	Afferents to CA1 pyramidal cells	CA1 pyramidal cell body layer	+	3,4
	16				–	4
Δ^9-THC	0.5 and 1.0	Unanesthetized rat	Ear (stimulus = sound)	Dentate gyrus	0	5
	2.0				–/+	
In vitro experiments						
Δ^9-THC†	0.001 nM	Rat hippocampal slices	Afferents to CA1 pyramidal cells	CA1 pyramidal cell body layer		6
	0.01 nM				0	
	0.1 to 10 nM				+	
					–	
Δ^9-THC†	0.01 nM	Rat hippocampal slices	Afferents to CA1 pyramidal cells	CA1 pyramidal cell body layer	+	7
	0.1 & 1.0 nM				–	
Δ^9-THC‡	0.01 μM	Guinea-pig hippocampal slices	Afferents to CA1 pyramidal cells	CA1 pyramidal cell body layer	0	8
	0.1 μM				+	
	1.0 μM				–	
Δ^9-THC‡	0.1 μM	Guinea-pig hippocampal slices	Afferents to dentate granule cells	Dentate granule cells	+	8
	1.0 μM				–	

*Dose expressed as mg/kg i.p. (in vivo) or in molar terms (in vitro).
†Indicates that the vehicle used was polyvinylpyrrolidone.
‡Indicates that no "solubilizer" was used.
SP-111 is a water soluble derivative of delta-9-THC.
References. 1, Izquierdo et al., 1973; 2, Segal, 1978; 3, Vardaris et al., 1977; 4, Weisz et al., 1982; 5, Campbell et al., 1986a; 6, Foy et al., 1982; 7, Nowicky et al., 1987; 8, Kujtan et al., 1983.

this brain region mediates the perceptual changes produced by delta-9-THC (Pontzer *et al.*, 1986; Pontzer and Wilkison, 1987). It has also been found that delta-9-THC can decrease both spontaneous and sound-evoked neuronal activity in the hippocampus of the unanesthetized rat at doses having no detectable effect on such activity in the inferior colliculus, pointing to a selective action on the hippocampus (Campbell *et al.*, 1986b).

The effect of delta-9-THC on paired pulse inhibition in rat hippocampal CA1 pyramidal cells (Table 8) was found by Weisz *et al.* (1982) to depend on the interval between the initial 'conditioning' pulse and the subsequent 'test' pulse. When this interval lay in the range 60 or 80 to 500 ms, delta-9-THC (2 to 16 mg/kg i.p.) produced dose-dependent increases in paired pulse inhibition. However, when the interval was above or below this range (20 to 60 or 750 to 2000 ms), the drug had no effect. These results are different from those of an earlier study in which delta-9-THC (2 mg/kg i.p.) was found to reduce paired pulse inhibition when the pulse interval was 40 ms (Vardaris *et al.*, 1977).

A number of mechanisms have been put forward to explain the effects of delta-9-THC on paired pulse inhibition in hippocampal CA1 pyramidal cells (Weisz *et al.*, 1982; Kujtan *et al.*, 1983). Among these is the hypothesis that delta-9-THC acts by altering feedback inhibition of these cells. When CA1 cells are stimulated, recurrent axon collaterals from CA1 cells are thought to activate gamma-aminobutyric acid-releasing interneurons. These in turn exert a feedback inhibition on the CA1 neurons. Paired pulse inhibition of CA1 cells probably arises because the first pulse triggers feedback inhibition so that the response to the second pulse is reduced. It is possible, therefore, that delta-9-THC alters paired pulse

TABLE 7. *Effects of Cannabinoids on Post-tetanic Potentiation (PTP)*

Cannabinoid	Dose*	Preparation	Stimulation site	Recording site	Effect on PTP	Reference
In vivo experiments						
Δ^9-THC	0.05 to 0.15 i.v. 0.20 to 0.75 i.v.	Unanesthetized spinal cat	Dorsal root	Ventral root	+ –	1
CBD	0.05 to 14 i.v.	Unanesthetized spinal cat	Dorsal root	Ventral root	–	1
Δ^9-THC	2 and 4 i.p. 8 i.p. 16 i.p.	Unanesthetized rat	Afferents to hippocampal CA1 pyramidal cells	CA1 pyramidal cell body layer	+ 0 –	2
In vitro experiments						
Δ^9-THC†	1 to 25 μM	Isolated paravertebral ganglia X of bull frog	Preganglionic neurons	Ganglia	0	3‡
11-OH-Δ^9-THC	0.1 to 0.33 μM				–	
8α,11-diOH-Δ^9-THC	0.1 to 0.25 μM				–	
CBD	60 to 100 μM				–	
Δ^9-THC**	10 pM	Rat hippocampal slices	Afferents to CA1 pyramidal cells	CA1 pyramidal cell body layer	0 (PTP) + (LTP)	4
	100 and 1000 pM				0 (PTP) – (LTP)	

*Dose expressed as mg/kg (in vivo) or in molar terms (in vitro).
†Indicates that cannabinoids were dispersed in Pluronic F68.
**Indicates that the vehicle used was polyvinylpyrrolidone.
‡All the cannabinoids in this study reduced the amplitude of pretetanic potentials (delta-9-THC at 25 to 100 μM).
LTP = long-term potentiation, a component of the potentiation induced by tetanic stimulation that decays more slowly than PTP.
References. 1, Tramposch et al., 1981; 2, Weisz et al., 1982; 3, Turkanis and Karler, 1975; 4, Nowicky et al., 1987.

inhibition of these cells by interfering with feedback inhibition, perhaps by altering the release or fate of gamma-aminobutyric acid or perhaps by altering the sensitivity of CA1 neurons to this amino acid (Weisz *et al.*, 1982; Kujtan *et al.*, 1983; see also Section 6.6.1). Consistent with the latter possibility is an observation by Segal (1978) that reductions in the spontaneous activity of rat cerebellar cells induced by iontophoretic administration of gamma-aminobutyric acid could be enhanced by simultaneous iontophoretic administration of SP-111, a water soluble derivative of delta-9-THC.

There are two early reports that neither delta-9-THC nor delta-6a, 10a-dimethylheptyl-THC suppress transmission in the cat superior cervical ganglion (Dagirmanjian and Boyd, 1962; Dewey *et al.*, 1970). However, there is also some albeit rather weak, less direct evidence from other early electrophysiological experiments to suggest not only that cannabinoids may alter transmission across some synapses but also that these synapses are more susceptible than axons to the effects of cannabinoids. Thus (i) Dagirmanjian and Boyd (1962) found that polysynaptic reflexes of the cat were more sensitive than the monosynaptic patellar reflex to the depressant effect of delta-6a, 10a-dimethylheptyl-THC and (ii) Boyd and Meritt (1966) found that delta-6a, 10a-dimethylheptyl-THC was particularly effective in reducing the amplitude of responses evoked by radial nerve stimulation in the mesencephalic reticular formation, a brain area rich in synapses. Consistent with these observations is the evidence that delta-9-THC can augment or suppress transmission along synaptic pathways in the hippocampus at concentrations far lower than those at which it has been shown to block axonal conduction along peripheral nerves (Byck and Ritchie, 1973; Tables 6 and 8).

Further evidence that cannabinoids can alter synaptic transmission comes from the more recent experiments of Turkanis and Karler (1983) in which it was found that delta-9-THC could increase the amplitude of excitatory postsynaptic potentials in cat spinal cord without

TABLE 8. *Effects of Cannabinoids on Paired Pulse Facilitation (f) and Inhibition (i)*

Cannabinoid	Dose*	Preparation	Stimulation site	Recording site	Effect	Reference
In vivo experiments						
Δ^8 and Δ^9-THC	0.5 to 1.5 i.v.	Unanesthetized squirrel monkey (cerveau isolé)	Somatosensory cortex	Postarcuate polysensory cortex	0/−(f)	1
CBD	3.5 i.p.	Anesthetized rat	Fornix or alveus of hippocampus	Alveus (contralateral to stimulated alveus)	− (f)	2
SP-111	10 i.p.	Unanesthetized rat	Hippocampus	Hippocampus (contralateral to stimulation site)	− (f) − (i)	3
Δ^9-THC	2 i.p.	Unanesthetized rat	Afferents to hippocampal CAl pyramidal cells	CAl pyramidal cell body layer	− (i)	4
Δ^9-THC	2 to 16 i.p.	Unanesthetized rat	Afferents to hippocampal CAl pyramidal cells	CAl pyramidal cell body layer	+ (i)	5
In vitro experiments						
Δ^9-THC†	0.1 and 1.0 μM	Guinea-pig hippocampal slices	Afferents to hippocampal CAl pyramidal cells	CAl pyramidal cell body layer	0 (f)	6
Δ^9-THC†	0.1 and 1.0 μM	Guinea-pig hippocampal slices	Afferents to hippocampal dentate granule cells	Dentate granule cells	0 (f)	6
Δ^9-THC†	0.1 μM 1.0 μM	Guinea-pig hippocampal slices	Alveus (conditioning pulse) and stratum radiatum (test pulse)	CAl pyramidal cell body layer	− (i) 0 (i)	6

*Dose expressed as mg/kg (*in vivo*) or in molar terms (*in vitro*).
†Indicates that no 'solubilizer' was used.
SP-111 is a water soluble derivative of delta-9-THC.
Stimuli were applied in pairs, the size of the response to the second stimulus (test pulse) being either greater (facilitation, f) or less (inhibition, i) than the response to the first stimulus (conditioning pulse).
References: 1, Boyd *et al.*, 1971; 2, Izquierdo and Nasello, 1973; 3, Segal, 1978; 4, Vardaris *et al.*, 1977; 5, Weisz *et al.*, 1982; 6, Kujtan *et al.*, 1983.

producing detectable changes in afferent input to the cord. This evidence is not conclusive, however, since it was also found that the drug raised the membrane resistance of the postsynaptic spinal motoneurons, an effect which could have accounted for the enhancement of excitatory postsynaptic potentials. Interestingly, at the same dose levels, (0.01 to 0.1 mg/kg i.v.), delta-9-THC also had a depressant effect, raising the firing threshold for the motoneuron action potential. It also decreased the amplitude of inhibitory postsynaptic potentials demonstrating that its stimulatory properties may stem in part from an ability to reduce inhibition. In the same experimental model, CBD was found to have only a depressant effect (Turkanis and Karler, 1986b).

6. STUDIES CONCERNED WITH PUTATIVE CENTRAL NEUROTRANSMITTERS

This section contains a detailed account of the effects of cannabinoids on the concentration and turnover of putative transmitters in the central nervous system. Evidence that cannabinoids can alter the neuronal uptake and storage of certain transmitters is also presented. The section concludes with an account of the ability of cannabinoids to change the specific binding to brain tissue of various ligands, including benzodiazepines. The latter were included in this section because of the intimate functional relationship that is thought to exist between benzodiazepine receptors and receptors for the putative transmitter, gamma-aminobutyric acid. Effects of cannabinoids on monoamine oxidase activity and on prostaglandin production are discussed in Section 7.

6.1. Norepinephrine

6.1.1. *Brain Levels of Norepinephrine*

Delta-9-THC has been shown to alter brain levels of norepinephrine (NE) in rats, mice and squirrel monkeys. There is evidence that the direction as well as the degree of change in NE concentrations produced by delta-9-THC in rat or mouse brain may be dose dependent. Consider, for example, the effect of intraperitoneal administration of delta-9-THC on NE levels in rat whole brain (Table 9). The lowest dose studied, 10 mg/kg, depressed NE concentrations whereas the highest dose used, 100 mg/kg, had the opposite effect. Intermediate doses either lowered NE levels or had no effect. A similar biphasic effect of intraperitoneally administered delta-9-THC has been observed in experiments with mice (Holtzman *et al.*, 1969). Dose-dependent biphasic effects on NE levels in rat brain (Table 10) or mouse brain (Ho *et al.*, 1972) have also been detected when the drug was given intravenously. In these experiments, however, NE levels were elevated by low doses and depressed or unaffected by higher doses. In squirrel monkeys only decreases in NE concentrations have been observed after intravenous administration of delta-9-THC (Ho *et al.*, 1972). These decreases occurred in the hypothalamus with doses of 0.5, 2 and 10 mg/kg and in the cerebral cortex, midbrain and pons/medulla with a dose of 10 mg/kg. None of the doses used produced statistically significant changes in NE concentrations in squirrel monkey whole brain or cerebellum. In mice, an intraperitoneal dose of delta-9-THC, 10 mg/kg, reported to depress NE concentrations in whole brain (Holtzman *et al.*, 1969) had no detectable effect on NE levels in the telencephalon or brain stem (Welch *et al.*, 1971). Effects of intraperitoneal injection of delta-9-THC on NE levels in discrete areas of rat brain are summarized in Table 9.

Although delta-9-THC has been shown to alter brain levels of NE after intraperitoneal or intravenous administration, experiments in which the drug was given orally or sub-

Table 9. *The Effect of Intraperitoneal Administration of Delta-9-THC on Rat Brain Levels of Norepinephrine*

Dose (mg/kg)	Time after injection (hr)	Brain area	Effect	Reference
20	1 to 1.5	Olfactory bulb	+	1
20	1 to 1.5	Diencephalon	+	1
100	0.75	Whole brain	+	2
5 and 50	0.5, 1 and 2	Hypothalamus	0	3
5	0.5, 1 and 2	Pons/medulla	0	3
10	2, 4 and 6	Brain stem	0	4
10	2, 4 and 6	Hypothalamus	0	4
10	1 to 2.5	Midbrain/diencephalon	0	5
20	0.5 to 1.5	Whole brain	0	6
25 and 30	2	Whole brain	0	7,8
30	1 to 4	Whole brain	0	9
80	0.75	Whole brain	0	10
10	1	Pons/medulla	−	5
10	0.75 to 6	Whole brain	−	2
10	2	Hypothalamus	−	11
40	0.75	Whole brain	−	6
50	0.5	Pons/medulla	−	3

References: 1, Shiomi *et al.*, 1979; 2, Poddar and Ghosh, 1976a; 3, Yagiela *et al.*, 1974; 4, Hattendorf *et al.*, 1977; 5, Bhattacharyya *et al.*, 1980; 6, Bensemana and Gascon, 1974; 7, Maître *et al.*, 1970; 8, Maître *et al.*, 1972; 9, Filipovic and Trkovnik, 1980; 10, Schildkraut and Efron, 1971; 11, Steger *et al.*, 1983.

cutaneously have so far yielded only negative results. Maître *et al.*, (1970) failed to detect an effect on rat whole brain levels of NE after an oral dose of 75 mg/kg or after subcutaneous doses of 25 or 100 mg/kg. However, they also reported the absence of an effect when the drug was given intraperitoneally (Table 9). Bracs *et al.* (1975) reported that oral administration of 20 mg/kg of delta-9-THC to rats kept at 31°C to prevent hypothermia had no effect on NE levels measured 1 hr later in whole brain, striatum, cerebellum, pons/medulla or hypothalamus/midbrain/thalamus. NE levels in rat striatum have also been reported to be unaltered by an oral dose of 10 mg/kg (Moss *et al.*, 1984). It is noteworthy that Fennessy and Taylor (1977) found that when delta-9-THC was given intravenously to rats kept at 31°C, a dose of 2 mg/kg produced a small but significant fall in whole brain NE levels (Table 10).

Experiments with delta-8-THC have shown that it too can alter brain levels of NE at least in squirrel monkeys and mice. In squirrel monkeys, intravenous administration of the drug was found to lower NE levels in several brain areas although it did not have a significant effect on whole brain NE (Ho *et al.*, 1972). Intravenous injection of delta-8-THC was, however, found to alter NE levels in mouse whole brain (Ho *et al.*, 1972). In contrast to delta-9-THC (see above) it was found to decrease mouse brain NE levels at low doses and to increase them at a higher dose. Rat experiments with delta-8-THC have produced only negative results, intraperitoneal doses of 10, 30 or 100 mg/kg having been reported to have no effect on NE levels in whole brain, striatum, or hypothalamus (Leonard, 1971; Maître *et al.*, 1972; Maclean and Littleton, 1977).

6.1.2. *Norepinephrine Turnover*

Delta-9-THC has been shown to increase the accumulation of ^{3}H-NE in the whole brains of rats (Maître *et al.*, 1970, 1972) and mice (Bloom *et al.*, 1978b; Bloom and Kiernan, 1980) injected intraveneously with ^{3}H-tyrosine (after delta-9-THC). In rats, similar increases in ^{3}H-NE specific activity have been detected following pretreatment with delta-8-THC, 10 or 30 mg/kg i.p., both in whole brain and in hypothalamus, striatum and pons/medulla (Maître *et al.*, 1972; Maclean and Littleton, 1977). Increases in whole brain levels of ^{3}H-NE were also observed in rats injected with delta-6a, 10a-dimethylheptyl THC (Maître *et al.*, 1972). Interestingly, the effect of delta-8-THC on the conversion of tyrosine to NE in striatum and hypothalamus was no longer observed when the drug was administered to rats which had been stressed by isolation and food deprivation (Maclean and Littleton, 1977). In mice, increases in the accumulation of ^{3}H-NE have been observed after administration of delta-9-THC, 9-nor-9-beta-hydroxy-hexahydrocannabinol (beta-HHC) and 11-hydroxy-delta-9-THC (Bloom *et al.*, 1978b). CBN and CBD did not alter ^{3}H-NE levels and none of the cannabinoids studied affected brain levels of ^{3}H-tyrosine (Bloom *et al.*, 1978b). The doses of delta-9-THC, beta-HHC and 11-hydroxy-delta-9-THC used in the mouse studies were hypothermic. It is unlikely, however, that their effect on

TABLE 10. *Rat Brain Levels of Norepinephrine One Hour After Intravenous Injection of Delta-9-THC*

Dose (mg/kg)	Ambient temperature (°C)	Brain area	Effect	Reference
0.05 to 0.5	21	Whole brain	0	1
1	21	Whole brain	+	1
2 and 5	21	Whole brain	0	1,2
2	21	Whole brain	−	3
2	31	Whole brain	−	2
2	4	Whole brain	0	2
2	37	Whole brain	0	2
2	21	Hypothalamus	0	3
2	21	Medulla	0	3

References: 1, Taylor and Fennessy, 1977; 2, Fennessy and Taylor, 1977; 3. Taylor and Fennessy. 1979b.

the accumulation of ^{3}H-NE in mouse brain was caused by a fall in body temperature since the ability of delta-9-THC to elevate brain ^{3}H-NE levels was not impaired when the drug was given to mice kept at an ambient temperature (31°C) sufficiently high to prevent hypothermia (Bloom and Kiernan, 1980). Moreover, Bloom (1982) found that delta-9-THC could increase the conversion of ^{3}H-tyrosine to ^{3}H-NE when it was added to a crude synaptosomal preparation obtained from mouse whole brain or brain stem.

The *in vitro* experiments of Bloom (1982) support the hypothesis that delta-9-THC can increase brain levels of ^{3}H-NE in ^{3}H-tyrosine-treated animals by interacting directly with NE-releasing neurons to stimulate NE synthesis. This it might do by reducing feedback inhibition of tyrosine hydroxylase (Bloom, 1982). There is little evidence in favor of alternative mechanisms such as inhibition of ^{3}H-NE metabolism (Bloom, 1982), suppression of the neuronal release of newly synthesized NE or facilitation of the neuronal uptake of released NE. Thus, concentrations of delta-9-THC effective in augmenting the conversion of ^{3}H-tyrosine to ^{3}H-NE in mouse synaptosomes (3 to 30 μM; Bloom, 1982) were found to fall within the delta-9-THC concentration range known to have an inhibitory effect on the synaptosomal uptake of both NE (Table 11) and tyrosine (Bloom, 1982). Consider also the effect of delta-9-THC on the ability of the tyrosine hydroxylase inhibitor, alpha-methyl-*para*-tyrosine, to lower rat brain levels of NE. Although delta-9-THC has been shown to reduce this effect of alpha-methyl-*para*-tyrosine in some experiments, a sign that the cannabinoid may indeed reduce NE release, in other experiments it has been shown to augment the effect of alpha-methyl-*para*-tyrosine on NE levels or to have no effect (Table 12). The absence of an effect on alpha-methyl-*para*-tyrosine-induced falls in rat brain levels of NE has also been noted in experiments with delta-8-THC (Leonard, 1971; Maclean and Littleton, 1977). Other evidence against the proposal that delta-9-THC can increase the rate at which ^{3}H-NE accumulates after ^{3}H-tyrosine injection by suppressing NE release comes from the experiments of Maître *et al.* (1972) in which it was found that delta-9-THC enhanced the disappearance rate of ^{3}H-NE from the brains of rats that had been preloaded with ^{3}H-tyrosine (before delta-9-THC administration).

6.1.3. *Synaptosomal Uptake and Storage of Norepinephrine*

In vitro administration of delta-9-THC has been found to alter the uptake of ^{3}H-NE into synaptosomal preparations obtained from rat forebrain, striatum or hypothalamus or from mouse whole brain (Table 11). The effect on uptake was biphasic, increases in up-

TABLE 11. *Effects of Delta-9-THC on the Uptake of Norepinephrine into Mouse and Rat Brain Synaptosomes*

Species	Vehicle	Concentration of Δ^9-THC	Brain area	Effect	Reference
Mouse	Ethanol	1 and 5 μM	Whole brain	0	1
		10 μM		0/–	
		50 μM		–*	
Rat	PVP/saline	30 μM	Forebrain	–	2
Rat	PVP/saline	10 and 50 nM	Striatum	0	3
		0.1 μM		+	
		0.2 and 1 μM		0	
		10 and 100 μM		–	
Rat	PVP/saline	10 and 50 nM	Hypothalamus	0	3
		0.1 and 0.2 μM		+	
		1 μM		0	
		10 and 100 μM		–	
Rat	DMSO	1 μM	Hypothalamus	c.a.0	4
		50 and 100 μM		–**	

DMSO and PVP are abbreviations for dimethyl sulfoxide and polyvinylpyrrolidone respectively.
*Indicates that synaptosomes were severely damaged by 50 μM delta-9-THC.
**Indicates $K_i = 20$ μM.
References: 1, Hershkowitz *et al.*, 1977; 2, Johnson *et al.*, 1976b; 3, Poddar and Dewey, 1980; 4, Banerjee *et al.*, 1975b.

Table 12. *Effects of Delta-9-THC on Norepinephrine Turnover in Mouse and Rat Brain*

Species	Dose and Route (mg/kg)	Brain area	Method of measuring NE turnover	Effect	Reference
Mouse	10 to 100 s.c.	Whole brain	Rise in ^{3}H-NE after ^{3}H-tyrosine (i.v.)	+	1
Mouse	2 to 16 i.v.	Whole brain*	Rise in ^{3}H-NE after ^{3}H-tyrosine (i.v.)	+	2
Rat	10 and 30 i.p.	Whole brain	Rise in ^{3}H-NE after ^{3}H-tyrosine (i.v.)	+	3
Rat	25 i.p.	Whole brain	Rise in ^{3}H-catecholamines after ^{3}H-tyrosine (i.v.)	+	4
	25 s.c.	Whole brain		+	
	75 p.o.	Whole brain		+	
Rat	c.a. 80 i.p.	Whole brain	Fall in ^{3}H-NE after intracisternal ^{3}H-NE	+	5
	c.a. 80 i.p.	Whole brain	Rise in ^{3}H-NM after intracisternal ^{3}H-NE	+	
Rat	10 i.p.	Whole brain	Fall in NE after α-methyl-*para*-tyrosine (i.v.)	+	6
	100 i.p.	Whole brain		–	
Rat†	20 and 60 p.o.	Whole brain	Fall in NE after α-methyl-*para*-tyrosine (i.p.)	0	7
Rat	10 i.p.	Hypothalamus	Fall in NE after α-methyl-*para*-tyrosine (i.p.)	–	8
Rat	5 and 50 i.p.	Hypothalamus	Fall in NE after α-methyl-*para*-tyrosine (i.v.)	0	9
Rat†	20 and 60 p.o.	Hypothalamus/ midbrain/ thalamus	Fall in NE after α-methyl-*para*-tyrosine (i.p.)	0	7
Rat	5 and 50 i.p.	Pons/medulla	Fall in NE after α-methyl-*para*-tyrosine (i.v.)	0	9
Rat†	20 and 60 p.o.	Pons/medulla	Fall in NE after α-methyl-*para*-tyrosine (i.p.)	0	7
Rat†	20 and 60 p.o.	Striatum	Fall in NE after α-methyl-*para*-tyrosine (i.p.)	0	7

*Indicates whole brain minus cerebellum.
†Indicates experiments conducted at an ambient temperature of 31°C.
NM is an abbreviation for normetanephrine.
References: 1, Bloom *et al.*, 1978b; 2, Bloom and Kiernan, 1980; 3, Maître *et al.*, 1972; 4, Maître *et al.*, 1970; 5, Schildkraut and Efron, 1971; 6, Poddar and Ghosh, 1976a; 7, Bracs *et al.*, 1975; 8. Steger *et al.*, 1983; 9, Yagiela *et al.*, 1974.

take being induced by delta-9-THC concentrations of 0.1 or 0.2 μM and decreases by concentrations of 10 μM or more. The cannabinoid exhibited a similar concentration-dependent biphasic effect on ^{3}H-NE release from preloaded rat brain synaptosomes. Release of ^{3}H-NE was decreased by a delta-9-THC concentration of 0.1 μM, was unaffected by a concentration of 10 μm and increased by concentrations of 75 and 100 μm (Poddar and Dewey, 1980; Johnson *et al.*, 1976b). The changes in uptake and release produced by delta-9-THC at the higher concentrations used (50 μM or more) may well have been a reflection of its ability to damage synaptosomes (Hershkowitz *et al.*, 1977). Some of these *in vitro* findings are consistent with an earlier report that *in vivo* pretreatment with delta-9-THC, 10 mg/kg i.v., can increase NE uptake into mouse brain synaptosomes (Hershkowitz and Szechtman, 1979). The *in vitro* data are also consistent with the observation by Schildkraut and Efron (1971) that *in vivo* administration of delta-9-THC (ca. 80 mg/kg i.p.) increased the rate of disappearance of ^{3}H-NE from rat brains which had been preloaded with the tritiated catecholamine. It is noteworthy that at the same dose, delta-9-THC was reported to have no effect on uptake into rat brain of intracisternally administered ^{3}H-NE (Schildkraut and Efron, 1971).

The synaptosomal uptake of ^{3}H-NE has been reported to be inhibited by the *in vitro* administration not only of delta-9-THC but also of delta-8-THC and of the 11-hydroxy metabolites of delta-8- and delta-9-THC, all psychically active compounds (Banerjee *et al.*, 1975b; Poddar and Dewey, 1980). However, experiments with CBD (Banerjee *et al.*, 1975b; Hershkowitz *et al.*, 1977; Poddar and Dewey, 1980) and also some (Poddar and Dewey, 1980) but not all experiments (Banerjee *et al.*, 1975b) with CBN indicated that these cannabinoids can also decrease ^{3}H-NE uptake into rat or mouse brain synaptosomes. CBD has no psychic activity and CBN has been reported to be significantly less potent than delta-9-THC as a psychotropic agent or, like CBD, to be inactive (Section 2). Hence there is little support for a link between psychic activity and the ability to inhibit the neuronal uptake of NE. Similarly, there seems to be little correlation between psychic activity and the ability to enhance the release of ^{3}H-NE from preloaded synaptosomes (Poddar and

Dewey, 1980). In contrast, the ability of delta-9-THC to increase synaptosomal ^{3}H-NE uptake and to decrease synaptosomal ^{3}H-NE release has been shown to be shared by delta-8-THC but not by CBN or CBD (Hershkowitz and Szechtman, 1979; Poddar and Dewey, 1980) supporting a link between these actions and the psychotropic properties of delta-8- and delta-9-THC.

6.2. Dopamine

6.2.1. *Brain Levels of Dopamine*

There are only a few reports that delta-9-THC can alter brain concentrations of dopamine (DA). Graham *et al.*, (1974) found that oral administration of delta-9-THC (10 mg/kg) decreased DA concentrations both in rat whole brain and rat heart. Bhattacharyya *et al.* (1980) found that delta-9-THC, 10 mg/kg i.p., had a time-dependent biphasic effect on DA concentrations in rat caudate nucleus and diencephalon/midbrain (Table 13). In both brain areas, there was an initial fall in DA concentrations followed by a marked increase.

Poddar and Ghosh (1976a) found that DA concentrations in rat whole brain were increased by delta-9-THC at doses of both 10 and 100 mg/kg i.p., the effect being greater at the lower dose. A slight increase in DA concentration was also reported to occur in rat brain stem following delta-9-THC administration at a dose of 10 mg/kg i.p. (Hattendorf *et al.*, 1977). On the other hand, Maître *et al.* (1970, 1972) reported that at doses of 25 or 30 mg/kg i.p., delta-9-THC had no effect on DA concentration in rat whole brain. Similarly, intraperitoneal administration of delta-8-THC was reported to have no effect on rat striatal or hypothalamic DA concentrations at a dose of 10 mg/kg (Maclean and Littleton, 1977) and to have no effect on rat whole brain DA concentrations at doses of 30 or 100 mg/kg (Leonard, 1971; Maître *et al.*, 1972). The absence of an effect on DA concentrations was also noted (i) in rat whole brain after administration of delta-9-THC at doses of 0.5 to 5 mg/kg i.v. (Fennessy and Taylor, 1977; Taylor and Fennessy, 1977, 1979b), 25 mg/kg s.c. (Maître *et al.*, 1970) or 75 mg/kg p.o. (Maître *et al.*, 1970), (ii) in rat hypothalamus after administration of delta-9-THC at doses of 2 mg/kg i.v. (Taylor and Fennessy, 1979b) or 10 mg/kg i.p. (Steger *et al.*, 1983) (iii) in rat striatum after administration of delta-9-THC at doses of 10 or 100 mg/kg p.o. (Lew and Richardson, 1981; Moss *et al.*, 1984) and (iv) in rat medulla oblongata after administration of delta-9-THC at a dose of 2 mg/kg i.v. (Taylor and Fennessy, 1979b). These experiments were all carried out at 'normal' room temperature. However, there are also reports that delta-9-THC had no effect on brain levels of DA when given orally or intravenously to rats kept at high or low ambient temperatures (Bracs *et al.*, 1975; Fennessy and Taylor, 1977).

Table 13. *The Effect of Intraperitoneal Administration of Delta-9-THC on Rat Brain Levels of Dopamine*

Dose (mg/kg)	Time after injection (hr)	Brain area	Effect	Reference
10	0.5 to 6	Whole brain	+	1
10	1.5 and 2	Caudate nucleus	+	2
10	1.5 and 2	Midbrain/diencephalon	+	2
100	0.5 to 6	Whole brain	+	1
10	2	Brain stem	+/0	3
10	2, 4 and 7	Hypothalamus	0	4
25	2	Whole brain	0	5
30	2	Whole brain	0	6
30	1 to 4	Whole brain	0	7
10	1	Caudate nucleus	−	2
10	1	Midbrain/diencephalon	−	2

References: 1, Poddar and Ghosh, 1976a; 2, Bhattacharyya *et al.*, 1980; 3, Hattendorf *et al.*, 1977; 4, Steger *et al.*, 1983; 5, Maître *et al.*, 1970; 6, Maître *et al.*, 1972; 7, Filipovic and Trkovnik, 1980.

In experiments with mice, delta-9-THC was found to have no effect on whole brain levels of DA when injected subcutaneously at doses of 1 to 100 mg/kg (Bloom *et al.*, 1978b). The drug was also found to have no effect on DA concentration in mouse telencephalon when injected intraperitoneally at a dose of 10 mg/kg (Welch *et al.*, 1971).

6.2.2. *Dopamine Turnover*

There are several reports that delta-9-THC can increase the accumulation of ^{3}H-DA in the brains of rats or mice injected intravenously with ^{3}H-tyrosine (Table 14). It is unlikely that this increase was caused by delta-9-THC-induced falls in body temperature, since it could be demonstrated in experiments with mice kept at an ambient temperature (31°C) sufficiently high to prevent hypothermia (Bloom and Kiernan, 1980). Increases in ^{3}H-DA levels in animals pretreated with ^{3}H-tyrosine have also been observed in response to other psychically active cannabinoids. In rats, for example, delta-6a, 10a-dimethylheptyl-THC (30 mg/kg i.p.) increased ^{3}H-DA levels in whole brain, hypothalamus and striatum although not in pons/medulla (Maître *et al.*, 1972). Rat whole brain, striatal and hypothalamic levels of ^{3}H-DA were also increased by delta-8-THC, again at a dose of 30 mg/kg i.p. (Maître *et al.*, 1972). A lower dose of delta-8-THC, 10 mg/kg i.p., was found to have no effect on striatal or hypothalamic ^{3}H-DA levels (Maclean and Littleton, 1977). In mice, whole brain levels of ^{3}H-DA were increased by 11-hydroxy-delta-9-THC and by 9-

Table 14. *Effects of Delta-9-THC on Dopamine Turnover in Mouse and Rat Brain*

Species	Dose and route (mg/kg)	Brain area	Method of measuring DA turnover	Effect	Reference
Mouse	10 to 100 s.c.	Whole brain	Rise in ^{3}H-DA after ^{3}H-tyrosine (i.v.)	+	1
Mouse	2 to 16 i.v.	Whole brain*	Rise in ^{3}H-DA after ^{3}H-tyrosine (i.v.)	+	2
Rat	10 and 30 i.p.	Whole brain	Rise in ^{3}H-DA after ^{3}H-tyrosine (i.v.)	+	3
Rat	25 i.p.	Whole brain	Rise in ^{3}H-catecholamines after ^{3}H-tyrosine (i.v.)	+	4
	25 s.c.			+	
	75 p.o.			+	
Rat	10 and 30 i.p.	Whole brain	Rise in ^{3}H-DOPAC after ^{3}H-tyrosine (i.v.)	+	3
Rat	10 and 100 i.p.	Whole brain	Fall in DA after α-methyl-*para*-tyrosine (i.v.)	−	5
Rat†	20 and 60 p.o.	Whole brain	Fall in DA after α-methyl-*para*-tyrosine (i.p.)	0	6
Rat	10 i.p.	Anterior hypothalamus	Fall in DA after α-methyl-*para*-tyrosine (i.p.)	0	7
Rat	10 i.p.	Medial basal hypothalamus	Fall in DA after α-methyl-*para*-tyrosine (i.p.)	−	7
Rat†	20 and 60 p.o.	Striatum	Fall in DA after α-methyl-*para*-tyrosine (i.p.)	0	6
Rat	10 i.v.	Striatum	Rise in DOPA after haloperidol plus NSD-1024 or NSD-1015	−	8
Mouse	40 i.p.	Striatum	Concentrations of DOPAC and HVA	0	9
Rat	5 and 10 i.p.	Caudate nucleus	Concentration of HVA	0	10
	20 and 40 i.p.			+	
Rat	5 i.p.	Olfactory tubercle	Concentration of HVA	0	10
	10 to 40 i.p.			+	
Rat	5 i.p.	Prefrontal cortex	Concentration of HVA	0	10
	10 to 40 i.p.			+	

*Indicates whole brain minus cerebellum.
†Indicates experiment conducted at an ambient temperature of 31°C
DOPA, DOPAC and HVA are abbreviations for dihydroxyphenylalanine, dihydroxyphenylacetic acid and homovanillic acid, respectively. NSD-1024 and NSD-1015 are aromatic amino acid decarboxylase inhibitors.
References: 1, Bloom *et al.*, 1978b; 2, Bloom and Kiernan, 1980; 3, Maître *et al.*, 1972; 4, Maître *et al.*, 1970; 5, Poddar and Ghosh, 1976a; 6, Bracs *et al.*, 1975; 7, Steger *et al.*, 1983; 8, Koe, 1981; 9, Osgood and Howes, 1974; 10, Bowers and Hoffman, 1986.

nor-9-beta-hydroxyhexahydrocannabinol but not by CBN or CBD, even at a dose of 200 mg/kg s.c. (Bloom *et al.*, 1978b).

Maître *et al.*, (1970) found that a dose of delta-9-THC increasing ^{3}H-catecholamine levels in the brains of rats injected intravenously with ^{3}H-tyrosine also decreased plasma concentrations of endogenous tyrosine. This raises the possibility that the cannabinoid increased ^{3}H-catecholamine levels in the brain by reducing 'background' levels of unlabeled tyrosine so as to increase the specific activity of the intravenously injected ^{3}H-tyrosine. It is noteworthy, however, that delta-9-THC has been found not to affect brain concentrations of endogenous tyrosine in either rats (Maître *et al.*, 1970) or mice (Bloom *et al.*, 1978b). Furthermore, Bloom (1982) found that delta-9-THC could increase ^{3}H-DA accumulation in crude synaptosomal preparations obtained from mouse whole brain or striatum to which ^{3}H-tyrosine had been added. The cannabinoid was effective at concentrations known also to impair the ability of synaptosomes to retain DA (Section 6.2.3) and to inhibit the synaptosomal uptake of both DA (Table 15) and tyrosine (Bloom, 1982). It is unlikely, therefore, that delta-9-THC increased ^{3}H-DA accumulation in synaptosomes by attenuating DA efflux or facilitating reuptake. It is also unlikely that the drug acted by inhibiting DA metabolism (Bloom, 1982). Hence, there is good evidence that delta-9-THC can act directly to stimulate the synthesis of both DA and NE (Section 6.1.2). Possible mechanisms are discussed in the paper by Bloom (1982) and also, briefly, in Section 6.1.2.

Results from *in vivo* experiments suggest that in addition to stimulating DA synthesis, delta-9-THC may also increase DA release. Maître *et al.* (1972) showed that delta-9-THC enhanced the disappearance rate of ^{3}H-DA from the brains of rats pretreated 2 hr earlier with intravenous injections of ^{3}H-tyrosine. They obtained similar results in experiments with delta-8-THC and delta-6a, 10a-dimethylheptyl-THC. Osgood and Howes (1974) reported that delta-9-THC (10 to 40 mg/kg i.p.) enhanced the ability of L-DOPA to increase mouse striatal concentrations of 3,4-dihydroxyphenylacetic acid (DOPAC) and homovanillic acid (HVA). However, the cannabinoid had no effect on DOPAC or HVA levels in the absence of L-DOPA. On the other hand, in a more recent study with rats, Bowers and Hoffman (1986) found that delta-9-THC could increase HVA levels in several brain areas including the corpus striatum (Table 14). Interestingly, the drug was more potent in its effects on HVA levels in the prefrontal cortex and olfactory tubercle than in its effect on striatal HVA. More direct evidence for a stimulatory effect of delta-9-THC on striatal DA release has recently been obtained in experiments with anesthetized rats, using microdialysis (Taylor *et al.*, 1988). A dose of 2 mg/kg, given intravenously, was reported to produce a 7 to 8 fold increase in the amount of DA collected from the microdialysis probe. No changes were detected in the levels of DA metabolites (DOPAC and HVA) and it was therefore concluded that the cannabinoid had not acted by inhibiting tissue uptake of DA. Against the hypothesis that delta-9-THC increases DA release are reports that falls in brain levels of DA induced by the tyrosine hydroxylase inhibitor, alpha-methyl-*para*-tyrosine, are either unaffected or else reduced by delta-9-THC (Table 14) and delta-8-THC (Maclean and Littleton, 1977).

6.2.3. *Synaptosomal Uptake and Storage of Dopamine*

The uptake of ^{14}C-DA or ^{3}H-DA into synaptosomal preparations obtained from rat hypothalamus, rat or mouse striatum or mouse whole brain has been shown in several studies to be markedly affected by delta-9-THC (Table 15). Drug concentrations of 5 μM or more have been found to inhibit uptake. In one study (Howes and Osgood, 1974), a slight inhibitory effect was also noted at concentrations of 0.1 and 1 μM. In another study, however, concentrations ranging from 0.05 to 0.2 μM were found to stimulate ^{3}H-DA uptake (Poddar and Dewey, 1980).

Cannabinoids other than delta-9-THC that have been reported to inhibit ^{3}H-DA uptake into rat or mouse brain synaptosomal preparations are delta-8-THC, CBN and CBD (Hershkowitz *et al.*, 1977; Poddar and Dewey, 1980). Like delta-9-THC, delta-8-THC was

TABLE 15. *Effects of Delta-9-THC on the Uptake of Dopamine into Mouse and Rat Brain Synaptosomes*

Species	Vehicle	Concentration of Δ^9-THC	Brain area	Effect	Reference
Mouse	Ethanol	5 to 100 μM	Whole brain	–*	1
Mouse	Ethanol	0.1 to 100 μM	Striatum	–**	2
Rat	DMSO	100 μM	Striatum	–	3
Rat	PVP/saline	10 nM	Striatum	0	4
		0.05 to 0.2 μM		+	
		1 μM		0	
		10 and 100 μM		–	
Rat	PVP/saline	10 nM	Hypothalamus	0	4
		0.05 and 0.1 μM		+	
		0.2 and 1 μM		0	
		10 and 100 μM		–	

DMSO and PVP are abbreviations for dimethyl sulfoxide and polyvinylpyrrolidone respectively.
*Indicates that synaptosomes were severely damaged by 50 μM delta-9-THC.
**Indicates $IC_{50} = 5.4$ μM.
References: 1, Hershkowitz *et al.*, 1977; 2, Howes and Osgood, 1974; 3, Banerjee *et al.*, 1975b; 4, Poddar and Dewey, 1980.

found to exert a concentration-dependent biphasic effect on ^{3}H-DA uptake (Poddar and Dewey, 1980). It was stimulatory at a concentration of 10 nM and inhibitory at concentrations of 1 and 10 μM. CBN and CBD were at least as potent as delta-8- or delta-9-THC as inhibitors of ^{3}H-DA uptake (Hershkowitz *et al.*, 1977; Poddar and Dewey, 1980). However, there was no sign of a stimulatory effect when sub-inhibitory concentrations were used (Poddar and Dewey, 1980).

Effects of cannabinoids on ^{3}H-DA uptake have also been observed in experiments in which drug administration was made *in vivo*. Maclean and Littleton (1977) reported that there was a marked increase in ^{3}H-DA uptake into striatal homogenates prepared from isolated, food-deprived rats that had been injected with delta-8-THC (10 mg/kg i.p.). On the other hand, the drug had no effect on ^{3}H-DA uptake when given to animals kept under normal environmental conditions. Hershkowitz and Szechtman (1979) detected an enhancement of ^{3}H-DA uptake into synaptosomes prepared from the cerebral cortices or striata of mice which had been injected with delta-9-THC at doses of 5 or 10 mg/kg i.v. The effect of delta-9-THC on cortical uptake of ^{3}H-DA was greater than its effect on striatal uptake. At the same doses, CBD had a smaller but nonetheless significant stimulatory effect on ^{3}H-DA uptake. Intravenous injection of the psychically inactive isomer, (+) delta-8-THC, had no effect on ^{3}H-DA uptake.

There is evidence that as well as affecting the synaptosomal uptake of DA, delta-9-THC can alter tyrosine uptake. Delta-9-THC concentrations ranging from 3 to 100 μM were found to inhibit uptake of ^{3}H-tyrosine into crude synaptosomal preparations obtained from mouse whole brain, striatum and brain stem (Bloom, 1982). Several cannabinoids have also been shown to alter the release of radioactively labeled DA from preloaded synaptosomes. Howes and Osgood (1974) reported a significant increase in ^{14}C-DA release from mouse striatal synaptosomes in the presence of delta-9-THC (1 μM). Poddar and Dewey (1980) detected decreased ^{3}H-DA release from a rat striatal synaptosomal preparation at a delta-9-THC concentration of 0.1 μM and increased release at 10 and 100 μM. At a concentration of 100 μM, delta-9-THC also increased ^{3}H-DA release from a hypothalamic preparation. However, it had no effect on DA release from this preparation at lower concentrations. In the same study, delta-8-THC increased ^{3}H-DA release from hypothalamic and striatal synaptosomal preparations at concentrations of 10 and 100 μM and decreased ^{3}H-DA release from the striatal preparation at lower concentrations (0.01 and 0.1 μM). It did not inhibit ^{3}H-DA release from the hypothalamic preparation at any of the concentrations used. CBN and CBD had a stimulatory effect on ^{3}H-DA release at concentrations of 10 and 100 μM but did not inhibit release at lower concentrations.

6.3. 5-Hydroxytryptamine

6.3.1. *Brain Levels of 5-Hydroxytryptamine*

Delta-9-THC has been reported to increase, to decrease or to have no effect on the concentration of 5-hydroxytryptamine (5-HT) in the brain. These differences can to a large extent be attributed to the use of different routes of administration and species and to the study of different brain areas.

In rats, intracerebroventricular injection of delta-9-THC (50 μg) increased concentrations of 5-HT and 5-hydroxyindoleacetic acid (5-HIAA) in the forebrain (Gallagher *et al.*, 1972). When given to rats by the intraperitoneal route, delta-9-THC at doses of 6 mg/kg or more increased the concentration of 5-HT and sometimes also of 5-HIAA in whole brain and cerebellum (Table 16). The drug either did not affect or else decreased concentrations of 5-HT or 5-HIAA in the rat forebrain, hypothalamus and brain stem (Table 16). In some areas, for example the diencephalon and midbrain, there were signs of an initial delta-9-THC-induced increase in 5-HT levels followed by a later depression. Intraperitoneal injection of delta-8-THC at a dose of 100 mg/kg had no effect on rat brain 5-HT or 5-HIAA (Leonard, 1971). Delta-9-THC given orally at a dose of 20 mg/kg to rats kept at an ambient temperature of 31°C to avoid hypothermia, was without effect on 5-HT levels in whole brain, striatum, hypothalamus/midbrain/thalamus or pons/medulla (Bracs *et al.*, 1975). 5-HT levels in rat striatum have also been found to be unaltered by an oral dose of 10 mg/kg (Moss *et al.*, 1984).

In mice, intraperitoneal or subcutaneous administration of delta-9-THC at doses ranging upwards from 10 mg/kg increased 5-HT concentrations in whole brain (Holtzman *et al.*, 1969), in whole brain minus the olfactory bulbs and cerebellum (Johnson and Dewey, 1978a) and in the telencephalon and brain stem (Welch *et al.*, 1971). CBN given intraperitoneally at a dose of 10 mg/kg also elevated 5-HT concentrations in mouse telencephalon although it had no effect on brain stem 5-HT levels (Welch *et al.*, 1971).

The effects of intravenous administration of delta-9-THC on rat brain levels of 5-HT and 5-HIAA are summarized in Table 17. It is noteworthy that the drug had a dose-related

Table 16. *The Effect of Intraperitoneal Administration of Delta-9-THC on Rat Brain Levels of 5-Hydroxytryptamine (5-HT) and 5-Hydroxyindoleacetic Acid (5-HIAA)*

Dose (mg/kg)	Time after injection (hr)	Brain area	Effect: 5-HT	Effect: 5-HIAA	Reference
6 to 80	0.5 to 4	Whole brain	+	ND	1, 2, 3
10	1	Whole brain*	+	+	4
20	0.5	Cerebellum	+	ND	1
20	0.5	Hypothalamus/midbrain	+	ND	1
20	1 to 1.5	Diencephalon	+	+	5
5 to 50	0.5 to 4	Hypothalamus	0	ND	6
5 to 50	0.5 to 4	Pons/medulla	0	ND	1,6
5 to 5.5	0.5 to 4	Forebrain	0	0	7,8
5.5	0.5 to 4	Brain stem	0	0	8
10	2 to 7	Hypothalamus	0	–	9
20	0.5	Cerebral cortex	0	ND	1
5 to 50	3 and 24	Brain stem	–	ND	10
10	1.5 and 2	Pons/medulla	–	ND	11
10	1.5 and 2	Midbrain/diencephalon	–	ND	11
20	1 to 1.5	Olfactory bulb	–	–	5
50	3	Cerebral cortex	–	ND	10

*Indicates whole brain minus cerebellum.
ND = not determined.
References: 1, Sofia *et al.*, 1971a; 2, Schildkraut and Efron, 1971; 3, Filipovic and Trkovnik, 1980; 4, Segawa *et al.*, 1976; 5, Shiomi *et al.*, 1979; 6, Yagiela *et al.*, 1974; 7, Gallager *et al.*, 1971; 8, Gallager *et al.*, 1972; 9, Steger *et al.*, 1983; 10, Ouellet *et al.*, 1973; 11, Bhattacharyya *et al.*, 1980.

TABLE 17. *Rat Brain Levels of 5-Hydroxytryptamine (5-HT) and 5-Hydroxyindoleacetic Acid (5-HIAA) after Intravenous Injection of Delta-9-THC*

Dose of Δ^9-THC (mg/kg)	Ambient temperature (°C)	Time after injection (hr)	Brain area	Effect		Reference
				5-HT	5-HIAA	
2	4	1	Whole brain	+	0	1
2	37	1	Whole brain	+	+	1
2	21	1	Medulla	+	0	2
0.05	21	1	Whole brain	0	−	3
0.1 to 0.5	21	1	Whole brain	0	0	3
1	?	4, 7 and 19	Whole brain	0	ND	4
1	?	0.1 to 4	Brain stem	0	0	5
1	?	0.1 to 4	Forebrain	0	0	5,6
2	21	1	Whole brain	0	0	2
2	21	1	Hypothalamus	0	+	2
2	31	1	Whole brain	0	+	1
1 to 5	21	1	Whole brain	0	+	1,3
0.1 to 10	?	0.75, 3 and 24	Brain stem	0	0	7
0.1 to 1	?	0.75	Cerebral cortex	−	ND	7

ND = not determined.
References: 1, Fennessy and Taylor, 1977; 2, Taylor and Fennessy, 1979b; 3, Taylor and Fennessy, 1977; 4, Englert *et al.*, 1973; 5, Gallager *et al.*, 1972; 6, Gallager *et al.*, 1971; 7, Ouellet *et al.*, 1973.

biphasic effect on 5-HIAA levels which were depressed by low doses and elevated by higher doses (Taylor and Fennessy, 1977). A similar biphasic effect was observed in experiments with mice injected intravenously with either delta-8- or delta-9-THC (Ho *et al.*, 1972). In contrast, intravenous administration of delta-8- or delta-9-THC to squirrel monkeys at doses of 0.5, 2 or 10 mg/kg produced only falls in brain 5-HT levels (Ho *et al.*, 1972).

There is evidence that the ability of delta-9-THC to alter rat brain levels of 5-HT and 5-HIAA depends on ambient temperature (Table 17). Fennessy and Taylor (1977) reported that at a dose of 2 mg/kg i.v., the cannabinoid had no effect on rat whole brain 5-HT levels in experiments carried out at 21° or 31°C but increased 5-HT levels at high or low ambient temperatures (37° and 4°C). They also detected delta-9-THC-induced increases in rat brain 5-HIAA levels at 21°, 31° and 37°C but not at 4°C.

6.3.2. *5-Hydroxytryptamine Turnover (Table 18)*

In experiments in which mice were injected intravenously with ^{3}H-tryptophan, Johnson and Dewey (1978a) found that pretreatment with delta-9-THC at doses known to augment endogenous brain levels of 5-HT increased the specific activity of ^{3}H-5-HT in the brain and concluded that the cannabinoid had increased the rate of 5-HT synthesis. In the same experiments, delta-9-THC also increased (i) the specific activity of ^{3}H-tryptophan in the brain, (ii) the brain to plasma ratio of ^{3}H-tryptophan and (iii) endogenous brain levels of tryptophan. It was therefore proposed that delta-9-THC can accelerate 5-HT synthesis by augmenting tryptophan uptake from blood to brain thereby increasing the quantity of brain tryptophan available for metabolism to 5-HT. Johnson and Dewey (1978a) found that delta-9-THC reduced total levels of endogenous plasma tryptophan without affecting free plasma levels of this amino acid. In experiments with rats, however, a dose of delta-9-THC elevating brain levels of 5-HT was shown to increase tryptophan concentrations in both brain and blood (Filipovic and Trkovnik, 1980). On the other hand, in another rat study, delta-8-THC was found to lower blood levels of tryptophan (Leonard, 1971). Effects of delta-8-THC on brain levels of tryptophan or 5-HT were not detected.

Although it would seem that delta-9-THC can increase the synthesis of 5-HT by increasing the brain concentration of its amino acid precursor, there is no evidence that the drug can also increase the proportion of brain tryptophan converted to 5-HT. Thus, delta-9-THC did not affect the ratio of ^{3}H-5-HT to ^{3}H-tryptophan in the brains of mice injected

TABLE 18. *Effects of Delta-9-THC on 5-Hydroxytryptamine Turnover in Mouse and Rat Brain*

Species	Dose and route (mg/kg)	Brain area	Method of measuring 5-HT turnover	Effect	Reference
Mouse	10 to 100 s.c.	Whole brain*	Rise in ^{3}H-5-HT after ^{3}H-tryptophan (i.v.)	+	1
Mouse	3 to 100 s.c.	Whole brain	^{3}H-5-HT/^{3}H-tryptophan after ^{3}H-tryptophan (i.v.)	0	1
Mouse	10 s.c.	Whole brain	^{3}H-5-HIAA/^{3}H-tryptophan after ^{3}H-tryptophan (i.v.)	–	1
Rat	2 i.v.	Whole brain	Rise in ^{3}H-5-HT after ^{3}H-tryptophan (i.c.v.)	0	2
Rat	2 i.v.	Whole brain	Rise in ^{3}H-5-HIAA after ^{3}H-tryptophan (i.c.v.)	0	2
Rat	2 i.v.	Whole brain	Fall in 5-HIAA after pargyline	+	2
Rat	2 i.v.	Whole brain	Rise in 5-HT after pargyline	0	2
Rat	5 to 10 i.p.	Whole brain**	Rise in 5-HT after pheniprazine	–	3
Rat	20 i.p.	Whole brain	Rise in 5-HT after pargyline	–	4
Rat	5.5 i.p.	Forebrain	Rise in 5-HT after pargyline	0	5
Rat	5 and 50 i.p.	Pons/medulla	Rise in 5-HT after pargyline	0	6
Rat	5 and 50 i.p.	Hypothalamus	Rise in 5-HT after pargyline	0	6
Rat	2 i.v.	Whole brain	Rise in 5-HIAA after probenecid	0	2
Rat	20 i.p.	Whole brain**	Rise in 5-HIAA after probenecid	0	7
Rat	1 i.v.	Forebrain	Rise in 5-HIAA after probenecid	0	5
Rat	1 i.v.	Brain stem	Rise in 5-HIAA after probenecid	0	5
Rat	5.5 i.p.	Forebrain	Rise in 5-HIAA after probenecid	0	5
Rat	5.5 i.p.	Brain stem	Rise in 5-HIAA after probenecid	0	5

*Indicates whole brain minus cerebellum and olfactory bulbs.
**Indicates whole brain minus cerebellum.
5-HIAA is an abbreviation for 5-hydroxyindoleacetic acid and i.c.v. indicates intracerebroventricular administration.
References: 1, Johnson and Dewey, 1978a; 2, Taylor and Fennessy, 1979a; 3, Segawa *et al.*, 1977; 4, Sofia *et al.*, 1971a; 5, Gallager *et al.*, 1972; 6, Yagiela *et al.*, 1974; 7, Segawa *et al.*, 1976.

intravenously with ^{3}H-tryptophan (Johnson and Dewey, 1978a). Nor did it affect the rates of fall in the specific activities of ^{3}H-tryptophan and ^{3}H-5-HT in the brains of rats which had been injected intracerebroventricularly with ^{3}H-tryptophan (Taylor and Fennessy, 1979a). Moreover, *in vivo* administration of delta-9-THC has been reported to inhibit rat brain tryptophan hydroxylase, albeit only in the brain stem (Ouellet *et al.*, 1973). The activity of this enzyme in the cerebral cortex was not affected.

The mechanism by which delta-9-THC enhances the uptake of ^{3}H-tryptophan from blood to brain in mice remains to be elucidated since delta-9-THC has been found to inhibit rather than to facilitate uptake of ^{3}H-tryptophan into mouse brain synaptosomes (Johnson and Dewey, 1978b) and since *in vivo* pretreatment of mice with the cannabinoid has been found to have no effect on subsequent synaptosomal uptake of ^{3}H-tryptophan (Johnson and Dewey, 1978a,b). Interestingly, the effect of delta-9-THC on the uptake of ^{3}H-tryptophan from blood to brain has been shown to be abolished in mice by adrenalectomy (Johnson *et al.*, 1981). Now, delta-9-THC can elevate plasma corticosterone levels in rats and mice (Johnson *et al.*, 1981; Pertwee, 1985b) and since there is evidence that corticosteroids can facilitate the synaptosomal uptake of tryptophan, it is possible that delta-9-THC may enhance tryptophan uptake into the brain indirectly through its effect on corticosterone release (Johnson *et al.*, 1981).

At a dose (10 mg.kg s.c.) known to enhance the uptake of ^{3}H-tryptophan from blood to brain (see above), delta-9-THC has been shown to decrease the ratio in the brain of ^{3}H-5-HIAA to ^{3}H-tryptophan suggesting that it can either reduce the neuronal release of 5-HT or increase the transport of 5-HIAA from brain to blood (Johnson and Dewey, 1978a). Segawa *et al.* (1977) studied the effect of delta-9-THC on the accumulation of 5-HT in rat brain (whole brain minus cerebellum) induced by *in vivo* administration of the monoamine oxidase inhibitor, pheniprazine. The cannabinoid was found to reduce the ability of pheniprazine to elevate 5-HT levels in 'muricide positive' rats, an observation also consistent with the proposal that delta-9-THC can reduce the neuronal release of 5-HT.

Similarly, delta-9-THC was found to reduce the rise in rat whole brain 5-HT concentrations produced by the monoamine oxidase inhibitor, pargyline (Sofia *et al.*, 1971a). In this case, however, the dose of delta-9-THC used, 20 mg/kg i.p., was reported to increase brain 5-HT levels when given by itself, making its effect on 5-HT levels in the presence of pargyline difficult to interpret.

Not all studies with rats have yielded results supporting an effect of delta-9-THC on the neuronal release of 5-HT. In experiments in which delta-9-THC was injected intravenously or in which 5-HT concentrations were measured in discrete brain areas (forebrain, hypothalamus and brain stem), the cannabinoid was found not to alter monoamine oxidase inhibitor-induced increases in central 5-HT levels (Gallager *et al.*, 1971, 1972; Yagiela *et al.*, 1974; Taylor and Fennessy, 1979a). In addition, the cannabinoid was reported not to enhance increases in brain 5-HIAA induced by probenecid, a drug known to inhibit the efflux of 5-HIAA from brain to blood (Gallager *et al.*, 1971, 1972; Segawa *et al.*, 1976; Taylor and Fennessy, 1979a). Taylor and Fennessy (1979a) found that delta-9-THC, 2 mg/kg i.v., enhanced pargyline-induced depletion of rat brain 5-HIAA without affecting pargyline-induced elevation of brain 5-HT, providing support for the hypothesis (see above) that delta-9-THC can accelerate the transport of 5-HIAA from brain to blood. It is also noteworthy that delta-8-THC, 100 mg/kg i.p., had no effect on the degree of rat brain 5-HT depletion induced by *para*-chlorophenylalanine, an inhibitor of 5-HT synthesis (Leonard, 1971).

6.3.3. *Synaptosomal Uptake and Storage of 5-Hydroxytryptamine*

There is good evidence from experiments with synaptosomal preparations obtained from rat or mouse brain that delta-9-THC can alter the neuronal uptake of 5-HT (Table 19). The drug has been found to inhibit ^{14}C-5-HT or ^{3}H-5-HT uptake into crude synaptosomal preparations derived from rat whole brain (Sofia *et al.*, 1971b), forebrain (Johnson *et al.*, 1976a, b) or hypothalamus (Banerjee *et al.*, 1975b). Kinetic analysis of data derived from experiments with the hypothalamic tissue revealed that the inhibition was non-competitive (Banerjee *et al.*, 1975b).

Cannabinoids other than delta-9-THC have also been found to inhibit the synaptosomal uptake of 5-HT. The results of experiments with synaptosomal preparations derived from rat hypothalamus (Banerjee *et al.*, 1975b) or forebrain (Johnson *et al.*, 1976a) suggest that there is not a good correlation between psychic activity *in vivo* and the ability to inhibit 5-HT uptake *in vitro*. For example, even when solubility differences were taken into account, the psychically inactive CBD seemed to be no less potent than delta-9-THC as an inhibitor of 5-HT uptake (Banerjee *et al.*, 1975b; Johnson *et al.* (1976a).

Using a relatively pure synaptosomal preparation derived from mouse brain, Hershkowitz *et al.* (1977) detected a concentration related biphasic effect of delta-9-THC on 5-

TABLE 19. *Effects of Delta-9-THC on the Uptake of 5-Hydroxytryptamine into Mouse and Rat Brain Synaptosomes*

Species	Vehicle	Concentration of Δ^9-THC	Brain area	Effect	Notes	Reference
Mouse	Ethanol	1 μM	Whole brain	+	Synaptosomes	1
		10 and 50 μM		0	damaged by	
		100 μM		–	Δ^9-THC (50 μM)	
Rat	PG	1 and 10 nM	Whole brain	0		2
		0.1 and 1 μM		–		
Rat	PVP/saline	10 μM	Forebrain	0		3
		30 and 100 μM		–	$IC_{50} = 39\ \mu$M	
Rat	PVP/saline		Forebrain	–	$IC_{50} = 29.3\ \mu$M	4
Rat	DMSO	1 μM	Hypothalamus	0/–		5
		50 and 100 μM		–	$K_i = 25\ \mu$M	

PG, PVP and DMSO are abbreviations for propylene glycol, polyvinylpyrrolidone and dimethyl sulfoxide, respectively.

References: 1, Hershkowitz *et al.*, 1977; 2, Sofia *et al.* 1971b; 3, Johnson *et al.*, 1976b; 4, Johnson *et al.*, 1976a; 5, Banerjee *et al.*, 1975b.

HT uptake. At a concentration of 1 μM, the drug increased 5-HT uptake. There was no effect at 10 or 50 μM and inhibition of uptake at 100 μM. The uptake of 5-HT was also inhibited but not enhanced by CBD. The synaptosomes showed signs of severe morphological damage in the presence of 50 μM delta-9-THC or CBD but no detectable damage when exposed to either cannabinoid at a concentration of 10 μM. Interestingly, the uptake of 5-HT into a crude synaptosomal preparation obtained from the cerebral cortices of mice was enhanced when the animals had been pretreated *in vivo* with delta-9-THC albeit with the rather high intravenous dose of 10 mg/kg (Hershkowitz and Szechtman, 1979). In contrast, *in vivo* pretreatment with CBD (10 mg/kg i.v.) did not affect synaptosomal uptake of 5-HT.

Johnson *et al.* (1976b) investigated the effect of delta-9-THC on synaptosomal retention of 5-HT. It was found that at concentrations greater than those required to inhibit 5-HT uptake, delta-9-THC reduced the ability of a rat forebrain crude synaptosomal preparation to retain preloaded ^{3}H-5-HT. Although the amount of ^{3}H-5-HT in the synaptosomes was reduced by delta-9-THC, there was no corresponding increase in the medium. An increase in ^{3}H-5-HIAA was detected in the medium, however, implying that the cannabinoid had increased the loss of ^{3}H-5-HT from synaptosomal storage vesicles to the surrounding cytosol, thereby (i) increasing the amount of free ^{3}H-5-HT available for metabolism to ^{3}H-5-HIAA within the cytosol and hence (ii) increasing the synaptosomal concentration of ^{3}H-5-HIAA and therefore its transfer to the medium by passive diffusion. Consistent with the hypothesis that delta-9-THC impairs vesicular storage of 5-HT is a report that 4 to 7 hr after intravenous administration of this cannabinoid the subcellular distribution of 5-HT is altered, there being a shift of 5-HT from the particulate or 'bound' fraction to the supernatant or 'free' fraction (Englert *et al.*, 1973). No such a change in the subcellular distribution of 5-HT was detected in rat brain 10 or 60 min after intravenous injection of delta-9-THC (Taylor and Fennessy, 1979b). However, at 10 min (but not at 60 min) after its intravenous administration, the drug was found to shift 5-HIAA from the 'free' to the 'bound' fraction.

6.4. Histamine and Spermidine

6.4.1. *Histamine*

In experiments with rats, Fennessy *et al.* (1983) detected marked reductions in histamine (HA) concentrations in the cerebral cortex, hypothalamus and midbrain 30 min after intravenous injection of delta-9-THC (2 mg/kg) and in the pons/medulla 120 min after delta-9-THC. The drug had no effect on HA concentrations in the cerebellum. Further experiments are needed to determine whether the drug acted to reduce concentrations of HA in neurons and also to determine whether the drug acted to alter HA synthesis, release or metabolism. In more recent experiments, Oishi *et al.* (1985) found that intravenous administration of delta-9-THC at doses of 2 or 5 mg/kg had no detectable effect on HA concentrations in rat whole brain. The absence of an effect on whole brain concentrations of HA has also been noted in mice receiving delta-9-THC at doses of 1 to 50 mg/kg i.v. (Oishi *et al.*, 1985) or 20 mg/kg i.p. (Taylor and Snyder, 1972). At a dose of 5 mg/kg i.v., however, delta-9-THC has been found to reduce rat brain concentrations of the HA metabolite, tele-methylhistamine (Oishi *et al.*, 1985). Consistent with this observation, Oishi *et al.* (1985) also found that delta-9-THC, given intravenously at doses of 2, 5 or 10 mg/kg, could attenuate pargyline-induced increases in rat brain concentrations of tele-methylhistamine. Other signs of a delta-9-THC-induced decrease in the turnover of brain HA were observed in mice, albeit only at a very high intravenous dose (50 mg/kg) and in experiments with guinea-pig hypothalamic slices in which the drug (30 and 100 μM) was found to produce a small but significant inhibition of K^+-induced HA release.

6.4.2. *Spermidine*

Lewis *et al.* (1986) have recently reported that 30 min after intravenous injection of delta-9-THC (2 mg/kg) concentrations of the aliphatic polyamine, spermidine, were reduced in rat cerebral cortex and midbrain although not in hypothalamus, cerebellum or pons/medulla. They proposed that some effects of delta-9-THC including its hypothermic effect may result at least in part from delta-9-THC-induced spermidine release within the brain.

6.5. ACETYLCHOLINE

6.5.1. *Brain Levels of Acetylcholine*

Tripathi *et al.* (1987) reported that intraperitoneal injection of delta-9-THC at a dose of 30 mg/kg increased concentrations of acetylcholine (ACh) in mouse hippocampus, striatum, midbrain and pons/medulla. The same treatment did not increase cerebral cortical levels of ACh above control levels although it did raise ACh levels in the cerebral cortex to values significantly above those observed in mice treated with 1 or 10 mg/kg doses of the drug. When lower doses of delta-9-THC were used (1 or 10 mg/kg i.p.) no significant change in the concentration of ACh was detected. Levels of ACh were increased in hippocampus, striatum and midbrain by 11-hydroxy-delta-9-THC (10 or 30 mg/kg i.p.) and in cerebral cortex and hippocampus by delta-8-THC (10 or 30 mg/kg i.p.). However, other cannabinoids given intraperitoneally at doses of up to 30 mg/kg [9-nor-9-beta-hydroxy-hexahydrocannabinol (beta-HHC), CBD and CBN] or 100 mg/kg [9-nor-9-alpha-hydroxy-hexahydrocannabinol (alpha-HHC) and delta-8-THC methyl ether], had no detectable effect on ACh levels in any of the brain areas investigated. Choline levels were increased in cerebral cortex by delta-9-THC, 11-hydroxy-delta-9-THC and beta-HHC (30 mg/kg i.p.), in striatum by beta-HHC (30 mg/kg i.p.), in midbrain by delta-9-THC (30 mg/kg i.p.) and by 11-hydroxy-delta-9-THC and beta-HHC (10 and 30 mg/kg i.p.) and in pons/medulla by beta-HHC (30 mg/kg i.p.). None of the cannabinoids used in this study altered choline levels in the hippocampus. Domino (1981) found that delta-9-THC increased concentrations of ACh in rat whole brain when injected intraperitoneally at a dose of 32 mg/kg. Intraperitoneal administration of delta-9-THC at lower dose levels has also been reported to elevate ACh levels in rat amygdala and striatum, although not in other brain areas (Table 20). Friedman *et al.* (1976) found that neither delta-9-THC nor delta-8-THC altered ACh or choline concentrations in the striata of rats (10 mg/kg; route not given).

Askew *et al.* (1974) reported that after intravenous administration of delta-9-THC at a dose of 5 mg/kg, there was a decrease in ACh concentration in rat whole brain. A similar result was obtained in experiments with delta-8-THC but not with 11-hydroxy-delta-8-THC. Askew *et al.* (1974) also found that synaptosomes prepared from the brains of rats which had been pretreated with delta-8-THC (5 mg.kg i.v.) contained reduced amounts of ACh. In other studies, intravenous injection of delta-9-THC was found to have no effect

TABLE 20. *The Effect of Intraperitoneal Administration of Delta-9-THC on Rat Brain Levels of Acetylcholine*

Dose (mg/kg)	Time after injection (hr)	Brain area	Effect	Reference
6	1	Amygdala	+	1
6	1	Striatum	+	1
32	0.5	Whole brain	+	2
3.2 and 10	0.5 and 1	Whole brain	0	2
6	1	Cerebral cortex	0	1
6	1	Diencephalon	0	1
6	1	Brain stem	0	1
10	1	Thalamus	0	2
10	1	Hippocampus	0	2
10	1	Hypothalamus	0	2
10	1	Caudate nucleus	0	2
10	1 to 2.5	Caudate nucleus	0	3

References: 1, Yoshimura *et al.*, 1974; 2, Domino, 1981; 3, Bhattacharyya *et al.*, 1980.

on ACh concentrations either in rat whole brain (5 mg/kg; Domino, 1981) or in rat parietal cortex, hippocampus or striatum (0.2 to 10 mg/kg; Revuelta *et al.*, 1978, 1979, 1980). Similarly, delta-8-dimethylheptyl-THC had no effect on ACh or choline concentrations in rat parietal cortex or striatum when injected intravenously at doses of 0.12 to 1 mg.kg (Revuelta *et al.*, 1980). It did, however, elevate rat hippocampal concentrations of ACh at a dose of 1 mg/kg, although not at lower doses. In the same study, (+) and (−) delta-8-THC (1 to 20 mg/kg i.v.) had no effect on cortical, striatal or hippocampal levels of ACh. Nabilone too (0.1 to 1.0 mg/kg i.v.) was found to have no effect on ACh or choline concentrations in rat parietal cortex, striatum or hippocampus (Revuelta and Cheney, 1981). Similar experiments with levonantradol (0.3 and 3 mg/kg s.c.) also yielded negative results (Costa *et al.*, 1981).

6.5.2. *Acetylcholine Turnover*

Effects of delta-9-THC on ACh turnover in cat, rat and mouse brain are summarized in Table 21. In experiments with rats, the drug was found to produce signs of reduced ACh turnover in hippocampus and striatum. The cannabinoid was markedly more potent in reducing ACh turnover in hippocampus than striatum and had no detectable effect on ACh turnover in any other area of rat brain studied. Essentially similar results were obtained in experiments with delta-8-dimethylheptyl-THC and levonantradol (Table 22). The (−) isomer of delta-8-THC also reduced ACh turnover in rat hippocampus although not in the cerebral cortex or striatum whereas nabilone affected ACh turnover in rat hippocampus, striatum and cerebral cortex (Table 22). In contrast, the psychically inactive cannabinoids,

TABLE 21. *Effects of Delta-9-THC on Acetylcholine Turnover or Release in Mouse, Rat and Cat Brain*

Species	Dose & route (mg/kg)	Brain area	Method of measuring ACh turnover	Effect	Reference
Mouse	1.0 i.p.	Cerebral cortex	Rise in ^{3}H-ACh relative to ^{3}H-choline and endogenous choline after ^{3}H-choline (i.v.)	+	1
		Hippocampus		0	
		Striatum		0	
		Midbrain		+	
		Pons/medulla		0	
	10 i.p.	Cerebral cortex		0	
		Hippocampus		0	
		Striatum		0	
		Midbrain		0	
		Pons/medulla		+	
	30 i.p.	Cerebral cortex		0	
		Hippocampus		−	
		Striatum		0	
		Midbrain		0	
		Pons/medulla		0	
Rat	0.2 to 10 i.v.	Parietal cortex	Rise in ^{3}H-ACh relative to ^{3}H-choline and endogenous choline after ^{3}H-choline (i.v.)	0	2
	0.2 to 10 i.v.	Hippocampus		−	2,3,4
	0.2 & 0.5 i.v.	Striatum		0	2
	5 & 10 i.v.	Striatum		−	
Mouse	10 s.c.	Whole brain	Fall in ACh after ASHC-3 (i.c.v.)	0	5
	32 & 56 s.c.	Whole brain		−	
Rat	10 & 30 i.p.	Whole brain	Fall in ACh after ASHC-3 (i.c.v.)	−	5
	1 i.p.	Hippocampus		0	
	3.2 to 32 i.p.	Hippocampus		−	
	1 to 32 i.p.	Thalamus		0	
		Caudate nucleus		0	
		Hypothalamus		0	
Cat*	1 to 11 i.v.	Somatosensory cortex	ACh release (collecting cups)	−	6

*Brain stem transected animals.

ASHC-3 is an abbreviation for acetylsecohemicholinium-3 and i.c.v. for intracerebroventricular administration.

References. 1, Tripathi et al., 1987; 2, Revuelta et al., 1978; 3, Revuelta et al., 1979; 4, Revuelta et al., 1980; 5, Domino, 1981; 6, Domino and Bartolini, 1972.

TABLE 22. *Effects of Various Cannabinoids on Acetylcholine Turnover in Three Areas of Rat Brain*

Cannabinoid	Dose and route (mg/kg)	Effect on ACh turnover*			Reference
		Parietal cortex	Striatum	Hippocampus	
(−)Δ⁹-THC	0.2 i.v.	ND	0	−	1
	0.5 i.v.	0	0	−	
	5 and 10 i.v.	0	−	−	
(−)Δ⁸-THC	1.0 i.v.	0	0	0	2
	5 to 20 i.v.	0	0	−	
(−)Δ⁸-DMH-THC	0.025 i.v.	ND	ND	0	2
	0.05 i.v.	ND	ND	−	
	0.12 to 0.5 i.v.	0	0	−	
	1.0 i.v.	0	−	−	
Nabilone	0.1 i.v.	−	0	−	3
	1.0 i.v.	−	−	−	
Levonantradol	0.3 to 3.0 s.c.	0	−	−	4
(+)Δ⁸-THC	1.0 to 20 i.v.	0	0	0	2
CBD	10 i.v.	0	0	0	1
	20 i.v.	0	−	0	

*ACh turnover measured using the method described by Revuelta *et al.*, 1979.
ND = not determined.
References: 1, Revuelta *et al.*, 1978; 2, Revuelta *et al.*, 1980; 3, Revuelta and Cheney, 1981; 4, Costa *et al.*, 1981.

CBD and (+) delta-8-THC, did not alter ACh turnover in rat hippocampus or cerebral cortex. CBD did alter ACh turnover in the striatum, however, albeit only at a rather high dose, whereas the (+) isomer of delta-8-THC had no effect on ACh turnover in this area (Table 22). In brain stem transected cats, delta-9-THC administered intravenously at doses of 1 to 11 mg/kg produced dose-related falls in ACh release from the sensorimotor cortex (Domino and Bartolini, 1972). In the same study, a dose of 0.5 mg/kg i.v. of delta-9-THC either had no effect on ACh release or caused a slight increase. In mice, delta-9-THC was found by Tripathi *et al.* (1987) to decrease ACh turnover in the hippocampus (as with rats) and whole brain. However, unlike the changes reported to occur in rat brain, increases as well as decreases in ACh turnover were detected in mouse brain and there was no change in ACh turnover in the striatum (Table 21). Several other cannabinoids have also been shown to alter ACh turnover in mouse brain, usually in the same direction as delta-9-THC (Tripathi *et al.*, 1987). In pons/medulla, ACh turnover was increased by 11-hydroxy-delta-9-THC (10 mg/kg i.p.). Decreases in ACh turnover were detected in cerebral cortex (delta-8-THC, 30 mg/kg i.p.), in hippocampus (11-hydroxy-delta-9-THC, delta-8-THC, CBN and beta-HHC, 30 mg/kg i.p.; alpha-HHC and delta-8-THC methyl ether, 100 mg.kg i.p.), in striatum (alpha-HHC, 100 mg/kg i.p.) and in midbrain (delta-8-THC methyl ether, 100 mg/kg i.p.). Alpha-HHC and delta-8-THC methyl ether are thought to possess little or no psychoactivity (Tripathi *et al.*, 1987). However, rather large doses of these two agents were needed to alter ACh turnover in mouse brain; the experimental data, in both rat and mouse, therefore indicating that it is psychically active cannabinoids which are most effective in altering ACh turnover in the brain.

Signs of cannabinoid-induced alterations in the functioning of central ACh-releasing neurons have been observed not only with *in vivo* techniques but also in studies using brain slices or synaptosomes. Thus non-competitive inhibition of choline uptake has been reported to occur after *in vitro* addition of delta-9-THC in experiments with crude synaptosomal preparations obtained from rat hippocampus ($IC_{50} = 4.6\ \mu M$; Lindamood and Colasanti, 1980) or mouse forebrain ($IC_{50} = 16\ \mu M$; Johnson and Dewey, 1978b). *In vivo* pretreatment with delta-9-THC has also been found to reduce choline uptake into certain synaptosomal preparations. Inhibition was observed in rat hippocampal and hypothalamic preparations (Lindamood and Colasanti, 1980) but not in preparations obtained from rat cerebral cortex, striatum, midbrain or pons/medulla (Friedman *et al.*, 1976; Lindamood and Colasanti, 1980) or from mouse forebrain (Johnson and Dewey, 1978b).

Like delta-9-THC, CBD has been found to inhibit choline uptake when added directly to a rat hippocampal synaptosomal preparation (IC_{50} = 16 μM; Lindamood and Colasanti, 1980). However, *in vivo* pretreatment with CBD had no effect on choline uptake into synaptosomal preparations obtained from rat cerebral cortex, striatum, hippocampus, hypothalamus, midbrain or pons/medulla (Lindamood and Colasanti, 1980).

Friedman *et al.* (1976) studied the effect of *in vivo* pretreatment with delta-8-THC, delta-9-THC (5 to 40 mg/kg) and CBD (20 and 40 mg/kg) on ^{3}H-ACh formation from ^{3}H-choline in slices of rat hypothalamus and striatum. Delta-8- and delta-9-THC were both inhibitory, the former cannabinoid producing the greater inhibition, whereas CBD had no detectable effect. *In vivo* pretreatment with delta-8- and delta-9-THC also reduced ^{3}H-ACh accumulation in rat cortical slices.

Observations that *in vivo* administration of delta-9-THC can produce decreases in central ACh turnover, in choline uptake into synaptosomes and in the synthesis of ACh in brain slices have been taken to indicate that the drug can reduce the firing rate of central ACh-releasing neurons (Friedman *et al.*, 1976; Revuelta *et al.*, 1978; Lindamood and Colasanti, 1980). The evidence for this hypothesis can be summarized as follows.

(i) Reductions in choline uptake, in ACh synthesis and in ACh turnover are all expected consequences of a reduction in impulse flow along cholinergic pathways.

(ii) Alternative hypotheses that delta-9-THC acts by inhibiting choline acetyltransferase or by increasing the activity of acetylcholinesterase are unlikely to be true since no such changes in enzyme activity have been detected in rat brain after *in vivo* administration of delta-8 or delta-9-THC (Askew *et al.*, 1974; Yoshimura *et al.*, 1974; Friedman *et al.*, 1976; Moss *et al.*, 1978). Moreover, reductions in ACh synthesis provoked in rat brain slices by *in vivo* pretreatment with delta-8- or delta-9-THC occurred in the presence of physostigmine (Friedman *et al.*, 1976).

(iii) The effect of *in vivo* injection of delta-8-THC on ACh synthesis in rat brain slices could be prevented by using a K^+-rich incubation medium (Friedman *et al.*, 1976).

(iv) The effects of *in vivo* injection of delta-9-THC on hippocampal turnover of ACh and on ^{3}H-choline uptake by hippocampal synaptosomes could be mimicked by surgical or electrolytic procedures expected to reduce the neuronal activity of a septal-hippocampal cholinergic pathway (Revuelta *et al.*, 1979; Lindamood and Colasanti, 1981a). Conversely, electrical stimulation of the same pathway has been shown to increase the hippocampal turnover of ACh (Moroni *et al.*, 1978).

(v) The ability of delta-9-THC, administered *in vivo*, to reduce ACh turnover in rat hippocampus or to reduce uptake of ^{3}H-choline into hippocampal synaptosomes was abolished by surgical or electrolytic procedures expected to reduce impulse flow in septal-hippocampal cholinergic neurons (Revuelta *et al.*, 1979; Lindamood and Colasanti, 1981a).

Two hypotheses have been put forward to explain how delta-9-THC might act to reduce the firing rate of central ACh-releasing neurons. In one, it is proposed that delta-9-THC acts directly on cholinergic neurons to interfere with the propagation of action potentials or with the depolarization process (Friedman *et al.*, 1976). This hypothesis leaves unanswered the question of why delta-9-THC seems to alter ACh turnover in only a few brain areas. In the other hypothesis, put forward to account for the effect of delta-9-THC on ACh turnover in the hippocampus, it is proposed that delta-9-THC interacts with pathways that serve to regulate the activity of septal-hippocampal cholinergic neurons (Revuelta *et al.*, 1978). According to this hypothesis, possible sites of action include (i) septal GABA-releasing interneurons thought to exert an inhibitory influence on septal-hippocampal cholinergic neurons and (ii) dopamine and beta-endorphin-releasing neurons thought to decrease ACh release in the hippocampus by acting on septal GABA-ergic interneurons (Revuelta *et al.*, 1979). An involvement of GABA in the effect of delta-9-THC on hippocampal turnover of ACh is supported by the observation that this effect of delta-9-THC could be prevented by intraseptal injection of the GABA antagonist, bicuculline (Revuelta *et al.*, 1979). Also consistent with an involvement of GABA is the finding that delta-9-THC can increase GABA turnover in the septum (Revuelta *et al.*, 1979; see also Section 6.6.1). There is, however, no evidence for an involvement of DA or beta-endorphin releasing neurons in the effect of delta-9-THC on ACh turnover (Revuelta *et al.*, 1979; Lindamood and Colasanti, 1981b) or indeed for an involvement of NE or 5-HT (Lindamood and Colasanti, 1981b).

6.6. Amino Acids and Peptides

6.6.1. *Gamma-aminobutyric Acid*

Revuelta *et al.* (1979) studied the effects of delta-9-THC and CBD on central gamma-aminobutyric acid (GABA) turnover rate by simultaneous measurement of endogenous GABA and ^{13}C-GABA levels in the brains of rats which had been given an intravenous infusion of ^{13}C-glucose. At a dose of 5 mg/kg i.v., delta-9-THC was reported to double GABA turnover in the septum. At higher doses, respectively 10 and 20 mg/kg i.v., delta-9-THC and CBD increased GABA turnover in the substantia nigra. Neither drug affected the concentration of endogenous GABA. Nor did they alter GABA turnover in the caudate nucleus or nucleus accumbens.

In further studies with rats, Revuelta *et al.* (1982) found that (−) delta-8-dimethylheptyl-THC reduced GABA turnover both in the septum (1 mg/kg i.v.) and in the nucleus accumbens (0.25 and 1 mg/kg i.v.). Septal turnover of GABA was also reduced by nabilone at a dose of 1 mg/kg i.v. (Revuelta and Cheney, 1981). Neither cannabinoid altered endogenous brain concentrations of GABA. The dimethylheptyl compound had no detectable effect on GABA turnover in the caudate nucleus, globus pallidus or substantia nigra and the psychically inactive (+) isomer of delta-8-THC had no effect on GABA turnover in the septum, even at a dose of 5 mg/kg i.v. (Revuelta *et al.*, 1982). Clearly additional experiments are required to determine why delta-9-THC had the opposite effect on GABA turnover to other psychically active cannabinoids. It would, for example, be interesting to test whether these differences reflect a dose-dependent biphasic effect, GABA turnover perhaps being reduced by low doses of delta-9-THC and increased by higher doses.

Edery and Gottesfeld (1975) reported that at a dose of 20 mg/kg i.p., delta-8-THC had no effect on GABA concentrations in the rat cerebellum, striatum or cerebral cortex. Delta-8-THC was also reported to have no effect on GABA concentrations in rat whole brain (minus cerebellum) when injected at a dose of 50 mg/kg i.p. (Leonard, 1971). In the same study, a long-lasting fall in GABA concentration was detected when the dose of delta-8-THC used was increased to 100 mg/kg i.p.

In vitro administration of delta-9-THC at concentrations of 10 to 100 μM was found to inhibit the uptake of ^{3}H-GABA into synaptosomal preparations obtained from rat cerebral cortex or mouse whole brain (Banerjee *et al.*, 1975b; Hershkowitz *et al.*, 1977). Other cannabinoids found to inhibit ^{3}H-GABA uptake include delta-8-THC, the 11-hydroxy metabolites of delta-8- and delta-9-THC, CBN, CBD and cannabigerol (Banerjee *et al.*, 1975b; Hershkowitz *et al.*, 1977). The inhibition of ^{3}H-GABA uptake by delta-9-THC, delta-8-THC and CBD was reported to be non-competitive (Banerjee *et al.*, 1975b). When administered *in vivo* at a dose of 10 mg/kg i.v., delta-9-THC was found to increase the uptake of ^{3}H-GABA into a mouse brain synaptosomal preparation (Hershkowitz and Szechtman, 1979). CBD injected at the same dose level, had no effect on ^{3}H-GABA uptake.

6.6.2. *Opioid Peptides*

In experiments with rats, Weigant *et al.* (1987) have found that delta-9-THC (c.a. 12 mg/kg i.p.) can elevate the concentration of beta-endorphin-like immunoreactivity in plasma and hypothalamus. These changes were only detected in rats which had been habituated to the injection procedure. Similar changes were not detected in response to CBD (c.a. 24 mg/kg i.p.). Neither cannabinoid altered the level of beta-endorphin-like immunoreactivity in the hippocampus. However, unlike plasma and hypothalamus, the hippocampus was found to contain higher levels of immunoreactivity when obtained from "habituated" rats injected with the drug vehicle than when obtained from "non-habituated" vehicle-treated animals.

6.7. Binding Studies

6.7.1. *Neurotransmitters*

There is evidence from experiments with mouse brain preparations that when administered *in vitro*, delta-9-THC can alter binding to adrenoceptors, to dopamine receptors and to opioid receptors (Table 23).

Hillard and Bloom (1982, 1984) reported that delta-9-THC (3 and 10 μM) and its 11-hydroxy metabolite (10 μM) could facilitate specific binding of the beta-adrenoceptor antagonist, ^{3}H-dihydroalprenolol, to mouse brain tissue by increasing the affinity of the tritiated ligand for its binding sites. Both cannabinoids had a concentration-dependent biphasic effect, producing no significant changes in binding at concentrations below 3 μM or above 10 μM. Concentrations of CBD ranging from 1 to 100 μM had no effect on ^{3}H-dihydroalprenolol binding. It was also found that delta-9-THC could enhance the ability of several unlabeled beta-adrenoceptor antagonists to displace ^{3}H-dihydroalprenolol from its binding sites (Hillard and Bloom, 1984; Bloom and Hillard, 1985). In contrast, the ability of beta-adrenoceptor agonists to displace ^{3}H-dihydroalprenolol was unaffected or decreased by delta-9-THC. The experimental data suggest that delta-9-THC acted to induce a second population of binding sites with a particularly high affinity for beta-adrenoceptor antagonists (Hillard and Bloom, 1984; Bloom and Hillard, 1985). In other experiments with mouse brain tissue, Bloom and Hillard (1985) found that delta-9-THC decreased specific binding of ^{3}H-naloxone. The cannabinoid had no effect on the binding of the delta opioid ligand, ^{3}H-D-Ala-D-Leu-enkephalin, to mouse brain tissue suggesting that it has a selective effect on mu opioid binding sites. Delta-9-THC has also been reported to have no effect on the specific binding of ^{3}H-D-Ala-D-Leu-enkephalin to delta opioid sites located on neuroblastoma cell membranes (Devane *et al.*, 1986). In experiments with neuronal membranes prepared from rat whole brain, Vaysse *et al.* (1987) have confirmed that delta-9-THC can decrease specific *in vitro* binding of mu opioid ligands ($IC_{50} = 2$ to 19μM). Their results suggest that delta-9-THC decreases binding site density and has no effect on binding affinity. The results also suggest that the drug alters mu opioid binding by interacting directly with opioid binding site protein or protein/lipid rather than by perturbing the lipid bilayer of the membrane. Experiments with a range of cannabinoids showed that there was no correlation between ability to inhibit mu opioid binding and psychoactive potency. For example, CBD had the same potency as delta-9-THC whereas levonantradol and 11-hydroxy-delta-9-THC were markedly less potent. The results obtained by Vaysse *et al.* (1987) do not support the notion that delta-9-THC has a selective effect on sites which preferentially bind mu opioid ligands (see above), since the drug was found to be as effective in decreasing specific binding of the delta opioid ligand, ^{3}H-D-Pen^2,D-Pen^5-enkephalin (IC_{50} = 16 μM), as it was in decreasing mu opioid binding. Vaysse *et al.* (1987) did, however, find the drug to show some degree of selectivity; concentrations of delta-9-THC of up to 100 μM having no detectable effect on specific binding at kappa opioid sites or, indeed, at sigma/phencyclidine sites, muscarinic sites or D_2 DA sites.

The finding by Vaysse *et al.* (1987) that delta-9-THC fails to inhibit specific binding to D_2 DA sites disagrees with results of earlier experiments performed with membrane preparations obtained from mouse corpus striatum (Bloom, 1984; Bloom and Hillard, 1985). In the mouse experiments, delta-9-THC, 11-hydroxy-delta-9-THC and CBD were all reported to decrease specific binding of ^{3}H-spiperone to D_2 DA sites and of ^{3}H-ADTN (2-amino-6,7-dihydroxy-1,2,3,4-tetrahydronaphthalene) to D_3 DA sites. Interestingly, whereas the reductions in ^{3}H-spiperone binding were caused mainly by a decrease in the apparent affinity of D_2 sites for ^{3}H-spiperone, the reductions in ^{3}H-ADTN binding resulted largely from a decrease in the number of binding sites. Neither delta-9-THC nor CBD altered the ability of haloperidol or (+)butaclamol to displace ^{3}H-spiperone from its binding sites. However, delta-9-THC (unlike CBD) did enhance the ability of DA and apomorphine to displace ^{3}H-spiperone, raising the possibility that this cannabinoid can selectively increase the affinity of D_2 DA receptors for agonists. In view of these findings, it is noteworthy that Agrawal *et al.* (1985) have recently reported increased ^{3}H-spiperone binding in striatal tissue obtained from mice pretreated intraperitoneally 24 hr earlier with cannabis.

Leader *et al.* (1981) investigated the effects of *in vitro* administration of delta-9-THC and levonantradol on specific GABA binding to rat whole brain synaptic membranes. Levonantradol reduced GABA binding (IC_{50} = 4 μM) whereas delta-9-THC had no effect at concentrations of up to 400 μM.

6.7.2. *Benzodiazepine Binding Sites*

Braestrup and Squires (1978) have reported that at a concentration of 3 μM, nabilone had little or no effect on specific ^{3}H-diazepam binding to rat forebrain membranes. Using much higher drug concentrations, Koe and Weissman (1981) found that ^{3}H-diazepam binding to rat cerebral cortical membranes was enhanced by levonantradol (50 and 100 μM)

TABLE 23. *Effects of Delta-9-THC on the Binding of Various Compounds to Mouse or Rat Brain Tissue*

Concentration (μM)	Vehicle	Experiment	Effect: Binding/ Displacement	Effect: Affinity constant	Effect: Number of binding sites	Reference
1	Emulphor/ ethanol/ buffer	Specific binding of ^{3}H-dihydroalprenolol (mouse cerebral cortex)	0			1,2
3 & 10			+	+	0	
30 & 100			0			
10	Emulphor/ ethanol	Ability of (±) propranolol and other beta-adrenoceptor antagonists to displace ^{3}H-dihydroalprenolol (mouse cerebral cortex)	+			2,3
10	Emulphor/ ethanol	Ability of (−) isoprenaline and other beta adrenoceptor agonists to displace ^{3}H-dihydroalprenolol (mouse cerebral cortex)	0/−			2,3
30	Emulphor/ ethanol	Specific binding of ^{3}H-spiperone (mouse striatum)	−	−	0	2,4
30	Emulphor/ ethanol	Ability of haloperidol & (+) butaclamol to displace ^{3}H-spiperone (mouse striatum)	0			2,4
30	Emulphor/ ethanol	Ability of dopamine & apomorphine to displace ^{3}H-spiperone (mouse striatum)	+			2,4
20 & 30	PVP/ saline	Specific binding of ^{3}H-ADTN* (mouse striatum)	−	0	−	4
0.6 to 3	Emulphor/ ethanol	Specific binding of ^{3}H-naloxone (mouse brain minus cerebellum)	0			2
5 to 40			−	−	0	
0.6 to 40	Emulphor/ ethanol	Specific binding of ^{3}H-D-Ala-D-Leu enkephalin (mouse brain minus cerebellum)	0			2
1 to 50	Ethanol/ albumin/ buffer	Specific binding of ^{3}H-D-Ala^2-D-Leu^5-enkephalin (neuroblastoma cell membranes)	0			5

continued

and dextronantradol (100 μM). Both cannabinoids also enhanced ^{3}H-diazepam binding to mouse brain tissue after *in vivo* administration, levonantradol at a dose of 0.47 mg/kg s.c. and dextronantradol at a dose of 1.5 mg/kg s.c. (Koe and Weissman, 1981). When ^{3}H-flunitrazepam was injected intravenously, increased benzodiazepine binding was only detected in brain tissue obtained from mice pretreated with levonantradol (0.05 to 1.5 mg/kg s.c.), dextronantradol (1.4 to 15 mg/kg s.c.) having no effect (Koe and Weissman, 1981; Koe *et al.*, 1985). In the same series of experiments, increased '*in vivo* binding' of ^{3}H-flunitrazepam was noted in mice pretreated subcutaneously with several other cannabinoids including delta-9-THC (32 mg/kg) and nabilone (1 to 12 mg/kg). CBD reduced ^{3}H-flunitrazepam binding at a dose of 10 mg/kg but had no effect on binding at higher doses (32 and 100 mg/kg). Sung and Jakubovic (1987) have carried out experiments with SP-111A, a water soluble compound which is thought to be hydrolysed to delta-9-THC after its administration. They found that the drug produced concentration-related decreases in the specific binding of ^{3}H-diazepam and ^{3}H-flunitrazepam to rat brain membranes and that it did so by decreasing the affinity of these benzodiazepines for their binding sites. There was no detectable change in binding site density. SP-111A was more potent as an inhibitor of ^{3}H-diazepam binding (IC_{50} = 7.5 μM) than as an inhibitor of the binding of ^{3}H-flunitrazepam (IC_{50} = 15 μM).

TABLE 23. *continued.*

Concentration (μM)	Vehicle	Experiment	Effect: Binding/ Displacement	Effect: Affinity constant	Effect: Number of binding sites	Reference
2 to 10 (IC_{50})†	Ethanol	Specific binding of ^{3}H-dihydromorphine (rat brain)	–	0	–	6
10 (IC_{50})	Ethanol	Specific binding of ^{3}H-naloxone (rat brain)	–			6
16 (IC_{50})	Ethanol	Specific binding of ^{3}H-D-Pen^2,D-Pen^5-enkephalin (rat brain)	–			6
10 (IC_{50})	Ethanol	Specific binding of ^{3}H-etorphine (rat brain)	–			6
100	Ethanol	Specific binding of ^{3}H-ethylketocyclazocine (μ and δ blockers present) (rat brain)	0			6
100	Ethanol	Specific binding of ^{3}H-N-(1-[2-thienyl]cyclohexyl) piperidine (rat brain)	0			6
100	Ethanol	Specific binding of ^{3}H-quinuclidinyl benzilate (rat brain)	0			6
100	Ethanol	Specific binding of ^{3}H-spiperone (rat brain)	0			6
400	Emulphor/ ethanol/ saline	Specific binding of ^{3}H-GABA (rat brain)	0			7

†IC_{50} value affected by protein concentration in medium.
*2-amino-6,7-dihydroxy-1,2,3,4-tetrahydronaphthalene, a D_3 dopamine ligand.
Dihydromorphine, D-Pen^2, D-Pen^5-enkephalin, N-(1-[2-thienyl]cyclohexyl)piperidine, quinuclidinyl benzilate and spiperone are ligands for μ opioid, δ opioid, σ/phencyclidine, muscarinic and D_2 dopamine binding sites respectively. Etorphine is a non-selective opioid ligand and ethylketocyclazocine serves as a ligand in κ opioid binding site experiments provided μ and δ sites are occupied by other ligands. PVP is an abbreviation for polyvinylpyrrolidone.
References. 1, Hillard and Bloom, 1982; 2, Bloom and Hillard, 1985; 3, Hillard and Bloom, 1984; 4, Bloom, 1984; 5, Devane et al., 1986; 6, Vaysse et al., 1987; 7, Leader et al., 1981.

7. STUDIES WITH MEMBRANE-BOUND ENZYMES

7.1. Monoamine Oxidase

Both increases and decreases in monoamine oxidase activity have been detected following administration of delta-9-THC. The increases in activity have been observed after *in vivo* administration of the drug to rats and also in two *in vitro* studies, one with eye tissue in which very low (picomolar) concentrations of delta-9-THC were used and the other with hypothalamic tissue. Decreases in monoamine oxidase activity have been observed only after *in vitro* administration of delta-9-THC, the inhibitory concentrations of the drug lying in the micromolar range. The effect of delta-9-THC on monoamine oxidase activity has been shown to vary not only with dose but also with species and with the tissue and substrate used to measure the activity of the enzyme.

In rats, increases in the activity of whole brain monoamine oxidase activity have been detected 6 hr after intraperitoneal administration of delta-9-THC although not at other times after injection (Table 24). Increases in monoamine oxidase activity have also been detected after intraperitoneal injection of delta-9-THC (10 and 50 mg/kg) in rat blood platelets and in mitochondrial preparations of rat hypothalamus and heart (Banerjee *et al.*, 1975a, 1977) and, 45 min after intravenous administration of the cannabinoid (10 mg/kg), in rat cerebral cortex although not in rat brain stem (Ouellet *et al.*, 1973). Banerjee *et al.* (1977) found that direct addition of delta-9-THC to their hypothalamic preparation also increased monoamine oxidase activity (Table 25). However, *in vitro* administration of delta-9-THC decreased monoamine oxidase activity in the rat heart preparation and had no effect on the activity of this enzyme in the rat platelet preparation (Banerjee *et al.*, 1977). Intraperitoneal administration of delta-9-THC at doses in the range 1 to 50 mg/kg had no detectable effect on monoamine oxidase activity in preparations obtained from rat liver (Sofia *et al.*, 1971a; Banerjee *et al.*, 1975a), rat kidney (Banerjee *et al.*, 1975a) or rat lung (Clarke and Jandhyala, 1977). In experiments with human blood platelets, delta-9-THC (3 to 30 μM) was reported to inhibit monoamine oxidase (Mazor *et al.*, 1982). The inhibition was non-competitive. In the same study, (−) delta-8-THC was shown to be a less potent inhibitor of monoamine oxidase than delta-9-THC. The psychically active (−) delta-8-dimethylheptyl-THC and the psychically inactive CBD and (+) delta-8-THC had no inhibitory effect.

In bovine eye preparations, delta-9-THC was reported to stimulate monoamine oxidase activity at concentrations ranging from 0.01 pM to 10 nM and to produce a slight inhibition at a concentration of 1 μM (Gawienowski *et al.*, 1982). On the other hand, in human brain and liver mitochondria, delta-9-THC (2.5 μM to 0.4 mM) was found to have no effect on monoamine oxidase activity (Schurr and Rigor, 1984, and Table 25). Similarly, the drug (0.1 mM) had no effect on the activity of the enzyme in porcine liver mitochondria (Schurr and Livne, 1976).

In porcine brain mitochondria, *in vitro* administration of delta-9-THC was found to inhibit monoamine oxidase (Table 25). The inhibition was non-competitive (Schurr *et al.*,

Table 24. *The Effect of Intraperitoneal Administration of Delta-9-THC on Rat Brain Monoamine Oxidase Activity*

Dose (mg/kg)	Time after injection (hr)	Brain area	Substrate	Effect	Reference
10 and 50	6	Whole brain	Tyramine	+	1
10 and 50	6	Hypothalamus	Tyramine	+	1,2
20	0.5	Whole brain	Tryptamine	0	3
1 and 14	18 to 22	Whole brain	Tryptamine	0	4

References: 1, Banerjee *et al.*, 1975a; 2, Banerjee *et al.*, 1977; 3, Sofia *et al.*, 1971a; 4, Clarke and Jandhyala, 1977.

TABLE 25. *Effects of* In Vitro *Administration of Delta-9-THC on Brain Monoamine Oxidase Activity*

Species	Vehicle	Concentration of Δ^9-THC*	Brain area	Substrate	Effect	Reference
Man	Ethanol	1 to 100 μg/mg (2.5 to 398 μM)	Whole brain	2-phenyl-ethylamine	0	1
			Whole brain	5-hydroxy-tryptamine	0	1
Pig	Ethanol	3 μg/mg (3.2 μM)	Whole brain	Benzylamine	0/−	2
		10 to 300 μg/mg (10.6 to 318 μM)	Whole brain	Benzylamine	−	2
		3 and 10 μg/mg (3.2 and 10.6 μM)	Whole brain	Tyramine	0	2
		30 to 300 μg/mg (32 to 318 μM)	Whole brain	Tyramine	−	2
		158 μg/mg (84 to 168 μM)	Whole brain	Dopamine	−[1]	3
			Whole brain	Benzylamine	−[1]	3
			Whole brain	5-hydroxy-tryptamine	−[2]	3
			Whole brain	Tyramine	−[2]	3
			Whole brain	Dimethylamino-benzylamine	−[2]	3
			Whole brain	Tryptamine	−[3]	3
Rat	Propylene glycol	10 to 40 μg/ml (32 to 127 μM)	Whole brain	Tryptamine	0	4
	Tween/saline	2 to 8 μg/mg	Hypothalamus	Tyramine	+	5

*μg/mg protein or μg/ml medium. The concentrations shown in parentheses have been calculated from the published values which were given in terms of μg/mg or μg/ml. The numbers in square brackets show how the degree of delta-9-THC-induced enzyme inhibition varied with substrate, [1] indicating the greatest degree of inhibition and [3] the least.

References: 1, Schurr and Rigor, 1984; 2, Schurr and Livne, 1976; 3, Schurr *et al.*, 1978; 4, Sofia *et al.*, 1971a; 5, Banerjee *et al.*, 1977.

1978). Interestingly, the degree of inhibition observed varied not only with the dose of delta-9-THC added to the incubation medium but also with the substrate used in the enzyme assay (Schurr and Livne, 1976; Schurr *et al.*, 1978). Inhibition was greatest with benzylamine or DA as substrate and least with tryptamine. Intermediate degrees of inhibition were observed when the substrate was 5-HT, tyramine or dimethylaminobenzylamine. With benzylamine as substrate, signs of monoamine oxidase inhibition were detected at delta-9-THC concentrations of about 10 μM and more (Table 25). When the substrate was tryptamine, the drug inhibited porcine brain monoamine oxidase at concentrations of 84 to 168 μM (Table 25). In contrast, delta-9-THC concentrations of 32 to 127 μM had no effect on tryptamine deamination in rat brain or liver (Sofia *et al.*, 1971a, and Table 25).

The effect of CBD on monoamine oxidase activity has also been found to vary with the substrate used. With tyramine as substrate, CBD produced a slight inhibition of the enzyme, albeit only at a rather high concentration (Schurr and Livne, 1976). However, in marked contrast to delta-9-THC, CBD had no detectable effect on monoamine oxidase activity when the substrate was benzylamine. Interestingly, although lacking an effect when given by itself, CBD completely abolished the inhibitory effect of delta-9-THC on benzylamine deamination (Schurr and Livne, 1976).

In further experiments, Schurr *et al.* (1978) found that delta-9-THC could still markedly reduce the activity of porcine brain mitochondrial monoamine oxidase after the enzyme had been solubilized by sonication to separate it from the mitochondrial membrane, suggesting that the cannabinoid must interact either with the enzyme itself or with some phospholipid component bound to it. It was also found that the ability of delta-9-THC to inhibit monoamine oxidase was reduced after chloroform (in the presence of delta-9-THC or CBD) had been used to extract lipid material from the solubilized enzyme. The effect could be largely reversed by the addition of phosphatidylcholine and was not seen when the chloroformic extraction was performed in the absence of a cannabinoïd. These findings led Schurr *et al.* (1978) to propose that delta-9-THC inhibits brain monoamine oxidase by interacting with phospholipids associated with the enzyme to induce a conformational change.

7.2. ATPases

In experiments with mice, intraperitoneal administration of delta-9-THC at a dose of 10 mg/kg has been reported to produce a 27% increase in whole brain ATPase activity (Jain *et al.*, 1974). More recently, Dalterio *et al.* (1987) investigated the effect of oral administration of delta-9-THC on Ca^{2+}-ATPase activity in tissues obtained from pubertal and adult male mice. At a dose of 50 mg/kg, the drug reduced activity of the enzyme in pubertal hypothalamic tissue and increased it in pubertal testicular tissue. The same treatment decreased Ca^{2+}-ATPase activity in adult testicular tissue and had no significant effect on enzyme activity in adult hypothalamic tissue. In pubertal and adult pituitary tissue, the activity of the enzyme was decreased by the drug (5 and 50 mg/kg). *In vivo* pretreatment with delta-9-THC (5 and 50 mg/kg) was also found to abolish inhibition of pituitary Ca^{2+}-ATPase by *in vitro* administration of luteinizing hormone releasing hormone. In contrast to its effects on Ca^{2+}-ATPase activity, delta-9-THC (50 mg/kg) had no detectable effect on hypothalamic, pituitary or testicular Mg^{2+}- or Na^{+}-K^{+}-ATPases or on cerebellar Na^{+}-K^{+}-ATPase (Dalterio *et al.*, 1987). In rats, doses of 10 and 100 mg/kg i.p. of delta-9-THC have been found to increase brain microsomal Mg^{2+}- and Na^{+}-K^{+}-ATPase activity, to decrease synaptosomal Na^{+}-K^{+}-ATPase activity and to have no effect on synaptosomal Mg^{2+}-ATPase activity (Poddar and Ghosh, 1976b). The drug has also been reported to inhibit synaptosomal Na^{+}-K^{+}-ATPase when given to rats at doses of 1 or 2 mg/kg i.p. (Lee and Olmsted, 1976).

When delta-9-THC was added directly to various preparations obtained from rat or mouse brains, concentrations in the low micromolar range were found to inhibit Na^{+}-K^{+}- and Mg^{2+}-Ca^{2+}-ATPases (Table 26). In rat brain synaptosomes and synaptic vesicles, delta-9-THC concentrations of 3 μM or more were also found to inhibit Mg^{2+}-ATPase (Table 26). However, a delta-9-THC concentration of 1 μM increased Mg^{2+}-ATPase activity in the vesicular preparation. *In vitro* administration of the drug also increased Mg^{2+}-ATPase activity in synaptosomal and mitochondrial fractions of mouse whole brain (Table 26).

In vitro administration of delta-9-THC has been shown to affect the activity of various ATPases not only in brain tissue but also in other types of preparation. Thus it has been found to increase ATPase activity in rat liver mitochondria in the presence and absence of Mg^{2+} (Chari-Bitron and Bino, 1971; Bino *et al.*, 1972) and to have an inhibitory effect on Na^{+}-K^{+}- and Mg^{2+}-ATPases in rat ileum microsomes (Laurent *et al.*, 1974, Laurent and Roy, 1975), on Ca^{2+}-ATPase activity in mouse heart microsomes (Collins and Haavik, 1979) and on Na^{+}-K^{+}-ATPase activity in an electric eel preparation and in Ehrlich ascites tumor cells (Toro-Goyco *et al.*, 1978).

There is no reason for believing that the ability of delta-9-THC to inhibit ATPases is linked with its ability to produce changes in mood and behavior. Thus CBN and CBD have been found to be as potent as delta-9-THC in inhibiting Na^{+}-K^{+}- and Mg^{2+}-ATPases in mouse or rat brain synaptosomes (Olmsted, 1976; Hershkowitz and Szechtman, 1979). Moreover, 11-hydroxy-delta-9-THC has been reported to be less effective than delta-9-THC as an inhibitor of Na^{+}-K^{+}- and Mg^{2+}-ATPases in rat brain synaptosomes (Olmsted, 1976) and CBD has been shown to be more potent than delta-9-THC as an inhibitor of Mg^{2+}-ATPase in rat brain synaptic vesicles (Gilbert *et al.*, 1977). Similarly, in experiments with mouse heart microsomes, the order of potency for inhibition of Ca^{2+}-ATPase has been found to be CBD > delta-9-THC > delta-6a,10a-dimethylheptyl-THC (Collins and Haavik, 1979).

TABLE 26. *Effects of* In Vitro *Administration of Delta-9-THC on Brain ATPase Activity*

Species	Vehicle	Concentration of Δ^9-THC (μM)	Preparation	ATPase	Effect	Reference
Rat	Ethanol	1	Synaptic vesicles from cerebral cortex	Mg^{2+}-	+	1
		3 to 1000			−	
Rat	Tween/ saline	3.2 to 12.7	Whole brain synaptosomes	Mg^{2+}-	−	2
			Whole brain microsomes		−	
Rat	Ethanol	3.2 to 95	Whole brain synaptosomes	Mg^{2+}-	−	3
		3.2 to 31.6	Cerebral cortex synaptosomes		−	
Mouse	Ethanol	5 to 50	Whole brain synaptosomes	Mg^{2+}-	−	4
Mouse	PVP	10 to 20	Whole brain synaptosomes	Mg^{2+}-	+	5
		5 to 20	Whole brain mitochondria		+	
		5 to 40	Whole brain microsomes		−(26 μM)	
		20 and 40	Whole brain myelin fraction		−46 μM)	
Rat	Tween/ saline	3.2 to 12.7	Whole brain synaptosomes	Na^+-K^+-	−	2
			Whole brain microsomes		−	
Rat	Water/ acetone	3 and 30	'Lipoprotein fraction' of whole brain minus cerebellum	Na^+-K^+-	−	6
Rat	Ethanol	1.6 to 95	Whole brain synaptosomes	Na^+-K^+-	−	3
		1.6 to 31.6	Cerebral cortex synaptosomes		−	
Mouse	Ethanol	5 to 50	Whole brain synaptosomes	Na^+-K^+-	−	4
Mouse	PVP	1 to 40	Whole brain synaptosomes	Na^+-K^+-	−(8 μM)	5
		1 to 40	Whole brain mitochondria		−(7 μM)	
		2.5 to 40	Whole brain microsomes		−(11 μM)	
		10 to 40	Whole brain myelin fraction		−(23 μM)	
Mouse	PVP	20 and 40	Whole brain synaptosomes	Mg^{2+}-Ca^{2+}-	−(25 μM)	5
		40	Whole brain mitochondria		−(15 μM)	
		5 to 40	Whole brain microsomes		−(8 μM)	
		40	Whole brain myelin fraction		−(51 μM)	

PVP is an abbreviation for polyvinylpyrrolidone.
Numbers in parentheses are IC_{50} values.
References: 1, Gilbert *et al.*, 1977; 2, Poddar and Ghosh, 1976b; 3, Olmsted, 1976; 4, Hershkowitz *et al.*, 1977; 5, Bloom *et al.*, 1978a; 6, Toro-Goyco *et al.*, 1978.

7.3. ADENYLATE CYCLASE AND GUANYLATE CYCLASE

In mice, *in vivo* administration of delta-9-THC has been shown to have a dose-dependent multi-phasic effect on brain levels of cyclic adenosine 3′,5′-monophosphate (cyclic AMP), the direction of the change produced in whole brain and in various brain areas varying with dose (Table 27). A dose-dependent effect of delta-9-THC on mouse brain adenylate cyclase activity has also been observed (Dolby and Kleinsmith, 1977). In contrast, CBN did not alter the activity of this enzyme. In rats, delta-9-THC injected intravenously at a dose of 10 mg/kg was reported to have no effect on brain concentrations of cyclic AMP (Table 27). At the same dose, delta-8-THC increased cyclic AMP levels in midbrain although not in cerebral cortex, hypothalamus, cerebellum or medulla (Askew and Ho, 1974). Delta-8-THC was also shown by Askew and Ho (1974) to decrease the activities of adenylate cyclase and cyclic nucleotide phosphodiesterase in the midbrain and to increase cyclic nucleotide phosphodiesterase activity in the cerebellum.

Leader *et al.*, (1981) reported that delta-9-THC, at doses of 32 and 100 mg/kg i.p., attenuated increases in rat cerebellar cyclic guanosine 3′,5′-monophosphate (cyclic GMP) concentrations induced by isoniazid, an inhibitor of glutamic acid decarboxylase and therefore of GABA synthesis. Levonantradol had the same effect at markedly lower doses whereas dextronantradol was inactive (Leader *et al.*, 1981; Koe *et al.*, 1985). Levonantradol was also shown to attenuate increases in cerebellar cyclic GMP levels induced by apomorphine and to depress basal cerebellar cyclic GMP levels (Leader *et al.*, 1981). The ability of delta-9-THC and levonantradol to oppose isoniazid-induced increases in cyclic GMP levels was taken as evidence in favor of the hypothesis that these cannabinoids can facilitate GABA function in the brain.

TABLE 27. *The Effect of Intraperitoneal Administration of Delta-9-THC on Rat or Mouse Brain Cyclic AMP Levels*

Species	Dose and route (mg/kg)	Time after injection (hr)	Brain area	Effect	Reference
Rat	10 i.v.	1	Cerebral cortex	0	1
			Hypothalamus	0	
			Midbrain	0	
			Cerebellum	0	
			Medulla	0	
Mouse	0.1 to 1 i.p.	0.5	Whole brain	+	2
	2 to 10 i.p.			−	
	50 i.p.			0	
Mouse	0.1 and 0.25 i.p.	0.5	Cerebral cortex	+	2
	0.5 i.p.			0	
	1 i.p.			+	
	2 to 10 i.p.			−	
	50 i.p.			0	
Mouse	0.1 and 0.25 i.p.	0.5	Hypothalamus	−	2
	0.5 and 1 i.p.			0	
	10 i.p.			+	
	2 and 50 i.p.			−	
Mouse	0.1, 0.5 and 1 i.p.	0.5	Cerebellum	+	2
	0.25 and 2 i.p.			0	
	10 and 50 i.p.			−	
Mouse	0.1 to 0.5 i.p.	0.5	Medulla	+	2
	1 and 10 i.p.			0	
	2 i.p.			−	
	50 i.p.			+	
Mouse	0.25 i.p.	0.5	Whole brain	ND*	3
	10 i.p.			ND**	

ND = not determined.
*Indicates that adenylate cyclase activity was increased or unaffected.
**Indicates that adenylate cyclase activity was decreased or unaffected.
References: 1, Askew and Ho, 1974; 2, Dolby and Kleinsmith. 1974; 3, Dolby and Kleinsmith, 1977.

Several experiments have been carried out to test whether *in vitro* administration of delta-9-THC can alter either basal adenylate cyclase activity or the ability of a range of drugs to activate this enzyme. The experiments have yielded somewhat variable results, micromolar concentrations of delta-9-THC being without effect in some preparations and having stimulant or depressant effects in others (Table 28).

In experiments with mouse brain homogenates, Dolby and Kleinsmith (1977) reported that *in vitro* administration of delta-9-THC enhanced the ability of norepinephrine to stimulate adenylate cyclase. This effect of norepinephrine was also enhanced by CBN and 11-hydroxy-delta-9-THC, both of which were more potent than delta-9-THC. None of these cannabinoids changed the basal activity of adenylate cyclase or the activity of phosphodiesterase. Hillard and Bloom (1983) found that delta-9-THC could enhance the formation of cyclic AMP initiated in homogenates of mouse cerebral cortex by the addition of ATP and GTP. The delta-9-THC concentration-response curve was bell-shaped, concentrations above as well as below the effective concentration (30 μM) having no detectable effect on cyclic AMP synthesis. Similar results were obtained with CBD and levonantradol, which were both more potent than delta-9-THC and with CBN and 11-hydroxy-delta-9-THC. Dextronantradol, the (+) isomer of levonantradol, had no detectable effect on cyclic AMP formation. In further experiments with the same preparation, Bloom and Hillard (1985) found that delta-9-THC could also enhance the formation of cyclic AMP induced by isoprenaline. Again, the delta-9-THC concentration-response curve was bell-shaped. More recently, Hillard *et al.*, (1986) showed that delta-9-THC could enhance the ability of glucagon to increase cyclic AMP concentrations in rat liver plasma membranes and in isolated rat hepatocytes. Glucagon stimulation of cyclic AMP production in liver plasma membranes was also enhanced by 11-hydroxy-delta-9-THC (30 μM) but not by CBN or

TABLE 28. *Effects of* In Vitro *Administration of Delta-9-THC on the Activities of Adenylate Cyclase and Phosphodiesterase*

Concentration of Δ^9-THC (μM)	Vehicle	Tissue	Measured effect	Change produced	Reference
0.02, 2 and 212	Ethanol	Mouse brain homogenate	Basal levels of cyclic AMP	0	1
0.02	Ethanol	Mouse brain homogenate	Norepinephrine-induced rise in cyclic AMP level	0	1
2 and 212				+	
1 to 10	Emulphor/ ethanol/ water	Mouse cerebral cortex homogenate	Basal rise in cyclic AMP level (GTP present)	0	2
30				+	
100				0	
1 and 3	Emulphor/ ethanol	Mouse cerebral cortex homogenate	Isoprenaline-induced rise in cyclic AMP level	0	3
10				+	
30 and 100				0	
1 to 50	Emulphor/ ethanol	Rat liver plasma membranes	Basal levels of cyclic AMP	0	4
1 and 3	Emulphor/ ethanol	Rat liver plasma membranes	Glucagon-induced rise in cyclic AMP level	0	4
10 and 30				+	
1 and 30	Emulphor/ ethanol	Rat liver plasma membranes	Rises in cyclic AMP levels induced by various drugs*	0	4
30	Emulphor/ ethanol	Rat isolated hepatocytes	Glucagon-induced rise in cyclic AMP level	+	4
29 and 72	PVP/ saline	Ventricular homogenate of rat heart	Basal cyclic AMP level	0	5
145 to 578				–	
1160				0	
3.2	Ethanol	Cultured human lung fibroblasts (intact)	Epinephrine-induced rise in cyclic AMP level	–	6
1.1 and 5.5	Ethanol	Cultured human lung fibroblasts (intact)	Basal cyclic AMP level	+	7
0.32 to 32	Ethanol	Cultured human lung fibroblasts (intact)	Prostaglandin E_1-induced rise in cyclic AMP level	–	6,7
1 and 30	Ethanol	Cultured mouse neuro-blastoma cells (intact)	Basal cyclic AMP level	0	8
1 and 30	Ethanol	Cultured mouse neuro-blastoma cells (intact)	Prostacyclin-induced rise in cyclic AMP level	–	8
10	Ethanol	Neuroblastoma cell membranes	Basal cyclic AMP level	–	8
0.1 to 10	Ethanol	Neuroblastoma cell membranes	Rises in cyclic AMP levels induced by various drugs†	–	8,9
1	Ethanol	S49 lymphoma cell membranes	Forskolin, isoprenaline or Mn^{2+}-induced rise in cyclic AMP level	0	10
1	Ethanol	C6 glioma cell membranes	Prostaglandin E_1-induced rise in cyclic AMP level	0	10
1	Ethanol	Soluble adenylate cyclase from rat sperm	Mn^{2+}-induced rise in cyclic AMP level	0	10
9.6	Ethanol	Synchronously dividing Tetrahymena pyriformis	Levels of cyclic AMP and cyclic GMP	–	11
0.02 and 212	Ethanol	Mouse brain homogenate	Phosphodiesterase activity	0	1
5 and 30	Ethanol	Neuroblastoma cell membranes	Phosphodiesterase activity	0	8

*Drugs: Forskolin, guanosine triphosphate (GTP), guanosine 5′-(beta, gamma-amino)-triphosphate and sodium fluoride.

†Drugs: prostacyclin, prostaglandin E_1, secretin, vasoactive intestinal peptide and forskolin.

Delta-9-THC did not inhibit activation of adenylate cyclase by guanosine 5′-(beta, gamma-imino)-triphosphate or sodium fluoride (Howlett, 1984).

PVP is an abbreviation for polyvinylpyrrolidone.

References: 1, Dolby and Kleinsmith, 1977; 2, Hillard and Bloom, 1983; 3, Bloom and Hillard, 1985; 4, Hillard *et al.*, 1986; 5, Li and Ng, 1984; 6, Kelly and Butcher, 1973; 7, Kelly and Butcher, 1979; 8, Howlett, 1984; 9, Howlett and Fleming, 1984; 10, Howlett *et al.*, 1986; 11, Zimmerman *et al.*, 1981.

CBD. Indeed, CBD attenuated the effect of glucagon. None of the cannabinoids affected the basal production of cyclic AMP. Li and Ng (1984) reported that adenylate cyclase activity in ventricular tissue of rat heart could be reduced by delta-9-THC although not by delta-8-THC. As in the experiments of Hillard and Bloom (1983), the concentration-response curve was bell-shaped, the greatest degree of inhibition being produced by a delta-9-THC concentration of 145 μM.

Kelly and Butcher (1979) showed that delta-9-THC could increase the accumulation of cyclic AMP in human cultured diploid lung fibroblasts. In the same preparation, the drug was found to attenuate the ability of epinephrine or prostaglandin E_1 to increase cyclic AMP concentrations either in the incubation medium or within the cells (Kelly and Butcher, 1973, 1979). The response to prostaglandin E_1 was also reduced by CBD and CBN.

In experiments with intact or broken mouse neuroblastoma cells, delta-9-THC was found to reduce the ability of prostaglandin E_1, prostacyclin, secretin, vasoactive intestinal protein and forskolin to stimulate adenylate cyclase (Howlett, 1984; Howlett and Fleming, 1984). The cannabinoid had no detectable effect on basal adenylate cyclase activity in intact neuroblastoma cells but reduced basal enzyme activity in a broken cell preparation (Howlett, 1984). Forskolin-induced activation of neuroblastoma cell membrane adenylate cyclase was also attenuated by levonantradol and, to a lesser extent, by delta-8-THC, CBN and CBD (Howlett and Fleming, 1984). Secretin-induced activation of the enzyme was attenuated by levonantradol, delta-8-THC and CBN but slightly enhanced by CBD (Howlett and Fleming, 1984).

Receptor-mediated activation of adenylate cyclase is thought to take place as follows (for reviews see Helmreich and Pfeuffer, 1985; Taylor and Merritt, 1986): (i) the agonist binds to its receptor, (ii) the receptor associates with a guanine nucleotide-dependent protein, G_s, (iii) GTP displaces GDP from the alpha subunit of the G_s protein, (iv) the G_s protein dissociates into its alpha and beta–gamma subunits and (v) the GTP-alpha subunit complex combines with adenylate cyclase to produce an active enzyme complex. According to the same hypothesis, GTP bound to the alpha subunit is later hydrolysed, causing deactivation of the adenylate cyclase and allowing reassociation of the alpha and beta–gamma subunits of the G_s protein. A similar GTP-dependent mechanism may be responsible for receptor-mediated inhibition of adenylate cyclase, the receptor combining with a G_i protein to trigger binding of GTP to G_i and subsequent enzyme inhibition.

Forskolin is thought to exert its stimulatory effect on adenylate cyclase by interacting directly with the enzyme rather than through G_s protein. Hence the finding that cannabinoids can inhibit forskolin-induced activation of adenylate cyclase (in the absence of stimulatory drugs acting through G_s protein) suggests that they may interact directly with the enzyme (Howlett and Fleming, 1984). It is also possible that the ability of cannabinoids to attenuate drug-induced activation of neuroblastoma cell membrane adenylate cyclase is mediated by G_i protein (Howlett, 1984, 1985; Howlett and Fleming, 1984; Howlett *et al.*, 1986). The most direct evidence for this hypothesis is that pertussis toxin, which is thought to act by blocking the action of G_i protein, abolished the inhibitory effects of delta-9-THC and desacetyllevonantradol on secretin-induced activation of adenylate cyclase in neuroblastoma cells (Howlett *et al.*, 1986). Hillard and Bloom (1983) observed that increases in cyclic AMP levels induced by delta-9-THC in mouse brain homogenate took place only in the presence of exogenously added GTP. This too points to an involvement of G protein. They also observed that the effect of delta-9-THC on cyclic AMP levels in this preparation could be prevented by the phospholipase A_2 inhibitor, quinacrine, and by the cyclo-oxygenase inhibitors, acetyl salicylic acid and indomethacin. Since there is evidence that delta-9-THC can increase prostaglandin synthesis (Section 7.4) and that prostaglandins can stimulate the production of cyclic AMP, they proposed that delta-9-THC enhanced cyclic AMP formation in mouse brain by increasing prostaglandin levels, the prostaglandins binding to receptors and thereby activating G_s protein and adenylate cyclase. A hypothesis has also been put forward to explain the ability of delta-9-THC to enhance glucagon-stimulated cyclic AMP production in rat liver plasma membranes (Hillard *et al.*, 1986). In this case, no mention is made of a possible involvement of prostaglandins. The hypothesis proposes that the cannabinoid acts by increasing the efficiency with which glucagon-occupied receptors interact with G_s protein. Support for the hypothesis comes from data that rule out likely alternative mechanisms. In essence, the data suggest that the delta-9-THC-induced increases in cyclic AMP production (i) require the presence of glucagon and (ii) occur after glucagon receptor occupation but before G_s protein activation (Hillard *et al.*, 1986).

Devane *et al.* (1986) have obtained evidence that cannabinoids do not inhibit adenylate cyclase in neuroblastoma cells by acting on opioid receptors. Concentrations of naloxone and naltrexone antagonizing the inhibitory effect of opioid agonists on adenylate cyclase activity in neuroblastoma cell membranes had no detectable effect on inhibition of the enzyme by delta-9-THC or its analog, desacetyllevonantradol. Furthermore, at a concentration known to inhibit adenylate cyclase (1 μM), neither cannabinoid altered the binding of D-Ala^2-D-Leu^5-enkephalin to neuroblastoma cell membranes. It was also demonstrated that the two cannabinoids did not alter adenylate cyclase activity in all neuronal cell lines sensitive to the inhibitory effect of opioids. Finally, there was no sign of an additive, synergistic, or antagonistic interaction between desacetyllevonantradol and etorphine when the effect on adenylate cyclase activity of a mixture of the two drugs was examined.

Howlett (1987) has shown that there is a good correlation between the psychoactive potency of cannabinoids and their ability to inhibit the activity of adenylate cyclase in neuroblastoma cells. Thus, the following orders of potency for inhibition of secretin-stimulated adenylate cyclase in neuroblastoma cell membrane preparations were established (c.f. Section 2 and Table 3): (i) delta-9-THC > delta-8-THC > CBN, (ii) 11-hydroxy-delta-9-THC > delta-9-THC, (iii) 11-hydroxy-delta-8-THC > delta-8-THC, (iv) delta-9-THC > 3′-hydroxy-delta-9-THC > 4′hydroxy-delta-9-THC = 5′-hydroxy-delta-9-THC > 2′-hydroxy-delta-9-THC. It was also found that the psychically inactive cannabinoids, 8-alpha-11-dihydroxy-delta-9-THC, CBD, CBG and cannabichromene, lacked detectable inhibitory activity when applied at concentrations at least 100-fold higher than inhibitory concentrations of delta-9-THC. The correlation was not perfect, since delta-9,11-THC, a drug which appears to be psychically inactive (Binder *et al.*, 1979; Beardsley *et al.*, 1987), was found to possess significant inhibitory activity and since high concentrations of 8-alpha- and 8-beta-delta-9-THC, both of which are psychoactive cannabinoids (albeit only at rather large doses), failed to inhibit adenylate cyclase.

7.4. Phospholipases A_2 and C, Cyclo-Oxygenase, Lipoxygenase and Thromboxane Synthetase

Results from experiments with a variety of cellular and subcellular preparations (Table 29) suggest that delta-9-THC can raise the concentration of free arachidonic acid thereby increasing the availability of this acid for conversion to a number of products including prostaglandins, prostacyclins, thromboxanes and leukotrienes. The cannabinoid is thought to act by stimulating phospholipase A_2 which catalyses the hydrolysis of acylester bonds of phospholipids in the 2-position and hence brings about the release of phospholipid-bound fatty acids including arachidonic acid (Burstein and Hunter, 1984; Martin *et al.*, 1986; Evans *et al.*, 1987a). Results from recent experiments with a crude synaptosomal preparation derived from mouse brain suggest that delta-9-THC may also stimulate phospholipase C (Hunter *et al.*, 1986). This enzyme catalyses the conversion of phosphoinositides to diacylglycerol and inositol triphosphate. Diacylglycerol is thought to be hydrolysed subsequently to its constituent fatty acids (usually stearic acid and arachidonic acid) and glycerol by the action of diacylglycerol lipase and it is noteworthy that delta-9-THC has been reported to be an inhibitor of this lipase (Hunter *et al.*, 1986). There is evidence that inositol triphosphate and diacylglycerol function as second messengers (see Abdel-Latif, 1986, for a recent review). Thus it is thought that interactions between agonists and certain types of receptor, for example the alpha$_1$-adrenoceptor, can lead to the activation of phospholipase C and hence to an increase in the production of inositol triphosphate and diacylglycerol, the former subsequently triggering intracellular Ca^{2+} mobilization and the latter activation of Ca^{2+}/phospholipid-dependent protein kinase. It is too early, however, to comment on the possible consequences of any interactions between cannabinoids and this putative second messenger system. Another way in which delta-9-THC could increase the availability of free arachidonic acid is by inhibiting lipoxygenase, an enzyme which catalyses the conversion of this fatty acid to hydroperoxyeicosatetraenoic acids, the immediate precursors of the leukotrienes. It is noteworthy, therefore, that Evans *et al.* (1987b) have shown that delta-9-THC can inhibit soybean lipoxygenase activity at concentrations in the low μM range ($IC_{50} = 3.2\ \mu$M). These results conflict with those of White and Tansik (1980) who reported human platelet arachidonate lipoxygenase activity to be unchanged by delta-9-THC, albeit in a somewhat higher concentration range (10 to 80 μM).

Although delta-9-THC has been shown to increase the synthesis of prostaglandins in some *in vitro* preparations, in others it has been reported to inhibit prostaglandin synthesis (Table 29). This inhibitory effect probably reflects an ability to inhibit cyclo-oxygenase since, in some experiments, delta-9-THC has been found to reduce prostaglandin synthesis from added free arachidonic acid. There is also evidence from experiments with lysed human platelets that delta-9-THC can inhibit thromboxane synthetase (White and Tansik, 1980). Hence delta-9-THC seems to have two opposing effects on the synthesis of prostaglandins, prostacyclins and thromboxanes. In some systems its stimulatory effect on the activity of phospholipases appears to predominate whereas in other systems, the drug may act primarily to inhibit cyclo-oxygenase and (at least in some systems) thromboxane synthetase and diacylglycerol lipase.

There is evidence that cannabinoids other than delta-9-THC, including CBN, CBD, can-

TABLE 29. *Effects of* In Vitro *Administration of Delta-9-THC on the Production of Free Arachidonic Acid and Prostaglandins in Cellular and Subcellular Preparations*

Concentration of Δ^9-THC (μM)	Vehicle	Preparation	Measured effect	Change produced	Reference
16 and 160	Ethanol	HeLa cells	Release of phospholipid-bound ^{14}C-arachidonic acid	+	1,2
3.2 to 32	Ethanol	Human lung WI-38 fibroblasts	Release of phospholipid-bound ^{14}C-arachidonic acid	+	3,4,5
8 to 32	Ethanol	Mouse peritoneal macrophages	Release of phospholipid-bound ^{14}C-arachidonic acid	+	6
80	Ethanol	Intact platelets from human blood	Release of phospholipid-bound ^{14}C-arachidonic acid	+	7
64	Ethanol	Mouse C1300 neuroblastoma cells (NBA_2)	Release of phospholipid-bound ^{14}C-arachidonic acid	+	7
3.2 to 32	Ethanol	Rat testis Leydig cells	Release of phospholipid-bound ^{14}C-arachidonic acid	+	2
32	Ethanol	Neuroblastoma cells (N2a)	Release of phospholipid-bound ^{14}C-arachidonic acid	+	8
32	Ethanol	C-6 glioma cells	Release of phospholipid-bound ^{14}C-arachidonic acid	+	8
32	Ethanol	Mouse brain synaptosomal fraction	Release of phospholipid-bound ^{14}C-arachidonic acid	+	9
1.6, 8 and 16	Ethanol	Mouse brain synaptosomal fraction	Production of ^{14}C-arachidonic acid from ^{14}C-arachidonyl-phosphatidylcholine	+	9
1.6 to 16	Ethanol	Mouse brain myelin fraction	Production of ^{14}C-arachidonic acid from ^{14}C-arachidonyl-phosphatidylcholine	+	9
1.6 to 16	Ethanol	Mouse brain mitochondrial fraction	Production of ^{14}C-arachidonic acid from ^{14}C-arachidonyl-phosphatidylcholine	+	9
8	Ethanol	Human lung WI-38 fibroblasts	Production of ^{14}C-PGE_2 from phospholipid-bound ^{14}C-arachidonic acid	+	10
0.8 to 320	Ethanol	Human lung WI-38 fibroblasts	Production of PGE or PGE_2	+	3,5,10
c.a. 0.16 to 1.6	Ethanol	Human lung WI-38 fibroblasts	Production of PGE_2	+	4

continued

nabichromene, cannabicyclol and hydroxylated metabolites of delta-9-THC, share the ability of delta-9-THC to stimulate phospholipase A_2 (Burstein and Hunter, 1978, 1981; White and Tansik, 1980; Burstein *et al.*, 1982a, 1983, 1984, 1985a,b, 1986a; Barrett *et al.*, 1985; Hunter *et al.*, 1986; Evans *et al.*, 1987a) and to inhibit cyclo-oxygenase (Burstein *et al.*, 1973; Spronck *et al.*, 1978; Dalterio *et al.*, 1978; White and Tansik, 1980; Reich *et al.*, 1982; Evans *et al.*, 1987b), lipoxygenase (Evans *et al.*, 1987b) and thromboxane synthetase (White and Tansik, 1980). The ability to interact with each of these enzymes has been shown to vary from cannabinoid to cannabinoid. Thus, for example, White and Tansik (1980) reported that CBD was almost 4 times less potent than delta-9-THC as an inhibitor of thromboxane synthetase in lysed human platelets. With regard to the other three enzymes, there is little sign of any correlation between the ability of cannabinoids to alter enzyme activity and psychoactive potency.

In a recent study with human lung fibroblasts, Burstein *et al.* (1986b) showed that the delta-9-THC metabolite, delta-9-THC-11-oic acid, could reduce the stimulant effect of delta-9-THC on prostaglandin E_2 synthesis. Results from additional experiments suggested that the two cannabinoids were interacting with different enzymes, delta-9-THC acting primarily to stimulate phospholipase A_2 and its metabolite to inhibit cyclo-oxygenase. It has also been found that repeated exposure of human lung fibroblast cultures to cannabinoids (delta-9-THC, CBD or cannabicyclol) rapidly rendered the cells tolerant to cannabinoid-induced stimulation of prostaglandin E_2 synthesis (Burstein *et al.*, 1985b). Tolerance also developed to cannabinoid-induced stimulation of release of phospholipid-

TABLE 29. *continued.*

Concentration of Δ^9-THC (μM)	Vehicle	Preparation	Measured effect	Change produced	Reference
32	Ethanol	Neuroblastoma cells (N2a)	Production of PGE	+	8
32	Ethanol	C-6 glioma cells	Production of PGE	+	8
19.1 (=EC_{50})	Ethanol	Naja naja venom	Phospholipase A_2 activity	+	11
64	Ethanol	Human cultured rheumatoid synovial cells	Production of PGE_2	+	12
64 >64	Ethanol	Human cultured rheumatoid synovial cells	TPA*-induced PGE_2 production	+ –	12
40 100 (=IC_{50})	Ethanol	Lysed platelets from human blood	Production of labeled PGE_2 and $PGF_{2\alpha}$ from ^{14}C-arachidonic acid	+ –	7
9.6	Propylene glycol/ ethanol	Ovine seminal vesicle microsomal fraction	Production of ^{14}C-PGE_2 from ^{14}C-arachidonic acid	–	13
318 (=IC_{50})	Ethanol	Bovine seminal vesicle microsomal fraction	Production of ^{14}C-PGE_1 from ^{14}C-8,11,14-eicosatrienoic acid	–	14
110 (=IC_{50})	?	Ovine seminal vesicle microsomal fraction	Rate of metabolism of 8,11,14-eicosatrienoic acid	–	15
31.8 (=IC_{50})	?	Ovine seminal vesicle microsomal fraction	Rate of metabolism of arachidonic acid	–	16
39.8	Ethanol	Decapsulated mouse testis	Production of PGE and PGF in the presence of human chorionic gonadotropin	–	17
50 to 200	Ethanol	Rat ovary cultured Graafian follicles	Production of PGE in the presence of luteinizing hormone	–	18
750 (=IC_{50})	?	Rat brain crude synaptosomal fraction	Release of $PGF_{2\alpha}$	–	19

*TPA = 12-O-tetradecanoylphorbol-13-acetate, a proinflammatory agent.

References. 1, Burstein and Hunter, 1978; 2, Burstein and Hunter, 1981; 3, Burstein et al., 1982a; 4, Burstein et al., 1985b; 5, Burstein et al., 1986b; 6, Burstein et al., 1984; 7, White and Tansik, 1980; 8, Burstein et al., 1985a; 9, Hunter et al., 1986; 10, Burstein et al., 1983; 11, Evans et al., 1987a; 12, Barrett et al., 1985; 13, Burstein and Raz, 1972; 14, Burstein et al., 1973; 15, Spronck et al., 1978; 16, Evans et al., 1987b; 17, Dalterio et al., 1978; 18, Reich et al., 1982; 19, Raffel et al., 1976.

bound arachidonic acid, suggesting that the cells had become tolerant to the stimulant effect of the cannabinoids on phospholipase activity.

Most *in vitro* experiments directed at investigating the effect of cannabinoids on prostaglandin synthesis have been performed with cellular or subcellular preparations, often obtained from non-neuronal tissues (Table 29). Recently, however, Reichman *et al.* (1987) reported changes in prostaglandin production induced by cannabinoids in guinea-pig brain slices. At a concentration of 0.8 μM, (−) delta-9-THC was found to exert an inhibitory effect on prostaglandin E and F formation in cerebral cortical slices, to stimulate production of these prostaglandins in striatal slices and to have no effect in hippocampal slices. The same treatment also decreased ACh-stimulated prostaglandin formation in cerebral cortical slices although not in slices obtained from cerebellum. The ability to inhibit prostaglandin E formation in cerebral cortical tissue was shared by delta-8-THC, which was equipotent with (−) delta-9-THC and by the psychically inactive cannabinoids, CBD and (+) delta-9-THC, both of which were markedly less potent than (−) delta-9-THC. Cerebral cortical prostaglandin F formation was inhibited by delta-8-THC [equipotent with (−) delta-9-THC] but enhanced by CBD and (+) delta-9-THC. These data suggest that there may be a link between the ability to alter prostaglandin synthesis in the brain and psychoactivity. The basis for the regional specificity of cannabinoids reported by Reichman *et al.* (1987) remains to be determined. One possibility is that the "mix" of enzymes in the brain catalysing the mobilization of arachidonic acid and its subsequent conversion to prostaglandins and other eicosanoids varies from area to area, causing the effect of cannabinoids on prostaglandin synthesis to range from stimulatory in some parts of the brain to inhibitory in others. Thus a cannabinoid might act mainly on phospholipase A_2 (stimulation) in one brain area but on cyclo-oxygenase (inhibition) in another. It is also possible that there are sub-types of prostaglandin-synthesizing enzymes in the brain which differ from one another in how they respond to cannabinoids and in how they are distributed. A third possibility is that cannabinoids can alter prostaglandin production indirectly. For example, the cannabinoids might act by altering the release, action or fate of a transmitter whose effects are mediated by prostaglandins. Consistent with such a mechanism is evidence firstly that delta-9-THC can decrease ACh-stimulated prostaglandin formation in the cerebral cortex (see above) and secondly that the ability of delta-9-THC to interact with central neurotransmitter systems is not uniform throughout the brain (Section 6).

In line with the results from *in vitro* experiments, there are a number of reports concerning changes in prostaglandin production induced by delta-9-THC *in vivo*. Thus a dose of delta-9-THC (2 mg i.p.) which prevented the proestrous rise in rat plasma levels of luteinizing hormone, follicle-stimulating hormone and prolactin and which delayed rat ovulation was found to prevent rises in rat ovarian prostaglandin E content normally occurring on the evening of proestrus (Ayalon *et al.*, 1977). In the same study, delta-9-THC was shown to have no effect on hypothalamic concentrations of prostaglandin E. However, in other rat experiments, Coupar and Taylor (1982) found that a dose of delta-9-THC producing marked hypothermia and catatonia (2 mg/kg i.v.) reduced the concentration of 'prostaglandin E_2-like material' in the hypothalamus. Concentrations in whole brain, cerebral cortex, midbrain, cerebellum and pons/medulla were not altered. More recently, Bhattacharya (1986) found that at a dose of 2 mg/kg i.p., delta-9-THC increased concentrations of prostaglandins E_2 and $F_{2\alpha}$ in rat whole brain. Prostaglandin levels (prostaglandin E_2 and I_2) have also been reported to increase in rat plasma after oral administration of delta-9-THC at doses of 50 or 100 mg/kg (Hunter *et al.*, 1988). In the same study, delta-9-THC was found to increase the conversion of arachidonic acid to prostaglandin E_2 in the brains of mice pretreated with ^{14}C-arachidonic acid (intracerebrally) and probenecid. Signs of delta-9-THC-induced increases in prostaglandin synthesis have also been detected in isolated perfused guinea-pig lung (Kaymakcalan *et al.*, 1975) and, *in vivo*, in the uteri of progesterone pretreated ovariectomized rats injected simultaneously with estradiol (Jordan and Castracane, 1976). In addition, they have been detected in mouse peritoneal macrophages taken from animals given delta-9-THC before removal of the cells (Burstein *et al.*, 1985a). It is noteworthy that in this study *in vivo* pretreatment with the psychically inactive cannabinoid CBD did not stimulate prostaglandin synthesis.

Fairbairn and Pickens (1979, 1980) proposed that the cataleptic effect of delta-9-THC in mice may depend on the presence of prostaglandin E_2. They found that delta-9-THC-induced catalepsy could be abolished by inhibitors of cyclo-oxygenase and that the effect of these inhibitors on this response to delta-9-THC could be reversed by administration of prostaglandin E_2. They also found that the cataleptic response to delta-9-THC was reduced in mice that had been maintained on a diet deficient in arachidonic acid. Arachidonic acid administration restored the response. Results from other studies have confirmed that catalepsy induced in mice by delta-9-THC (or cannabis) can be attenuated by cyclo-oxygenase inhibitors (Bhattacharya *et al.*, 1980; Burstein *et al.*, 1987, 1988). In addition, it has been found that prostaglandin E_2 and I_2 can induce catalepsy in mice (Burstein *et al.*, 1987, 1988) and that repeated pretreatment with prostaglandin E_2 can attenuate the cataleptic response of mice to delta-9-THC (Burstein *et al.*, 1988). Interestingly, the same pretreatment did not render the animals tolerant to the cataleptic effect of the prostaglandin. Further support for the hypothesis that prostaglandins have a role in delta-9-THC-induced catalepsy comes from the finding by Reichman *et al.* (1987) that this cannabinoid can increase prostaglandin formation in slices obtained from a region of the brain (the striatum) which may well be involved in the production of catalepsy by delta-9-THC (Gough and Olley, 1978). Also consistent with the hypothesis is an observation by Burstein *et al.* (1987) that the cataleptic response to delta-9-THC can be inhibited by delta-9-THC-11-oic acid, a drug which has been shown to oppose the stimulant effect of delta-9-THC on prostaglandin synthesis in fibroblasts (see above). It is not yet clear whether delta-9-THC-11-oic acid inhibits delta-9-THC-induced catalepsy by acting primarily within or outwith the central nervous system (Burstein *et al.*, 1987). In other experiments, Burstein *et al.* (1982b) found that the hypotensive effect of delta-9-THC in anesthetized dogs could be reduced by aspirin pretreatment and suggested that delta-9-THC decreases dog blood pressure by stimulating the production of a vasoactive metabolite of arachidonic acid, possibly prostacyclin.

8. MEMBRANE STUDIES

Experiments using a variety of physical methods have yielded results which suggest that delta-9-THC can produce small but significant changes in the 'fluidity' of phospholipid-containing membranes (Table 30). In some experiments (Lawrence and Gill, 1975; Bach *et al.*, 1976b; Bruggemann and Melchior, 1983), delta-9-THC was incorporated into the membranes while they were being prepared and the results obtained from these studies suggested that the drug could increase membrane fluidity. In other experiments (Tamir and Lichtenberg, 1983; Hillard *et al.*, 1985), delta-9-THC was added after the membranes had been prepared. In these studies the effect on membrane fluidity was shown to vary both with the concentration of delta-9-THC used and with membrane composition. For example, when added to rat brain synaptic plasma membranes, delta-9-THC had a concentration-dependent biphasic effect on polarization of the fluorescence emission of 1,6-diphenyl-1,3,5-hexatriene (DPH; Hillard *et al.*, 1985). At delta-9-THC concentrations of 1 to 10 μM, polarization decreased (a sign of increased fluidity) whereas at a concentration of 30 μM, polarization increased. In contrast, only decreases in fluorescence polarization of DPH were detected when delta-9-THC was added to vesicles prepared from cholesterol plus egg yolk phosphatidylcholine or dimyristoylphosphatidylcholine or from dimyristoylphosphatidylcholine alone. These decreases occurred at delta-9-THC concentrations ranging from about 1 μM to 30 μM.

In experiments with mice, Leuschner *et al.* (1984) studied the effect of *in vivo* administration of delta-9-THC on the fluidity of erythrocyte membranes. Intravenous doses of 3.2, 10 and 16 mg/kg all increased membrane fluidity as measured by electron spin resonance. When the dose used was 10 mg/kg, the plasma concentration of delta-9-THC at the

TABLE 30. *The Effect of Delta-9-THC on the 'Fluidity' of Phospholipids and Phospholipid-containing Membranes*

Phospholipid or membrane preparation	Technique	Fluidity change	Reference
Egg yolk phosphatidylcholine/cholesterol spin-labeled vesicles	Electron spin resonance	+	1
Dipalmitoylphosphatidylcholine	Differential scanning calorimetry	+	2
Dipalmitoylphosphatidylcholine bilayers	Differential scanning calorimetry	+	3
Dioleoylphosphatidylcholine bilayers	Differential scanning calorimetry	+	3
Dipalmitoylphosphatidylcholine/ distearoylphosphatidylcholine bilayers	Differential scanning calorimetry	+	3
Dioleoylphosphatidylcholine/ distearoylphosphatidylcholine bilayers	Differential scanning calorimetry	+	3
Dipalmitoylphosphatidylcholine/ cholesterol bilayers	Differential scanning calorimetry	+	3
Egg yolk phosphatidylcholine vesicles	Nuclear magnetic resonance	0	4
Egg yolk phosphatidylcholine/ cholesterol vesicles	Nuclear magnetic resonance	+	4
Egg yolk phosphatidylcholine vesicles	Fluorescence polarization	–	5
Egg yolk phosphatidylcholine/ cholesterol vesicles	Fluorescence polarization	+	5
Dimyristoylphosphatidylcholine vesicles	Fluorescence polarization	+	5
Dimyristoylphosphatidylcholine/ cholesterol vesicles	Fluorescence polarization	+	5
Synaptic plasma membranes	Fluorescence polarization	+/–*	5

*'Fluidity' was increased by delta-9-THC concentrations of 1 to 10 μM but decreased by a concentration of 30 μM. Delta-9-THC was either premixed with phospholipids (Refs. 1, 2 and 3) or added to vesicular preparations in which case the drug was dissolved in dimethyl sulfoxide (Refs. 4 and 5).

References: 1, Lawrence and Gill, 1975; 2, Bach *et al.*, 1976b; 3, Bruggemann and Melchior, 1983; 4, Tamir and Lichtenberg, 1983; 5, Hillard *et al.*, 1985.

time of blood sampling (+60 min) was about 1 μM. The membrane concentrations of delta-9-THC ranged from 1 to 10 μmoles per kg dry membrane and it was calculated that for each delta-9-THC molecule in the membrane there were about 20 000 phospholipid molecules.

In addition to delta-9-THC, several other cannabinoids have been shown to alter membrane fluidity. Bach *et al.* (1976b) showed that like delta-9-THC, CBD affected the transition of dipalmitoylphosphatidylcholine from the gel to the liquid crystalline state by decreasing both the melting temperature and the enthalpy of melting. Similarly, in fluorescence experiments with vesicles prepared from cholesterol plus egg yolk phosphatidylcholine or dimyristoylphosphatidylcholine or from dimyristoylphosphatidylcholine alone, Hillard *et al.* (1985) obtained evidence that CBD acted like delta-9-THC to increase membrane fluidity. In both of these studies, CBD was no less potent or effective than delta-9-THC as a fluidizing agent. In other experiments, however, important differences between CBD and delta-9-THC have been detected, the results obtained not only with CBD and delta-9-THC but also with other cannabinoids demonstrating a correlation between the ability to increase the fluidity of phospholipid-containing membranes and psychoactive potency. For example, using an electron spin resonance technique, Lawrence and Gill (1975) found that the ability to fluidize egg yolk phosphatidylcholine/cholesterol vesicles decreased in the order (–) delta-9-dimethylheptyl-THC, 11-hydroxy-delta-9-THC, (–) delta-9-THC and (+) delta-9-THC. CBN and CBD both reduced membrane fluidity. It was suggested by Lawrence and Gill (1975) that the stereoselectivity observed in their experiments was due to the presence of cholesterol which, being optically active, imposed asymmetry on the lipid bilayer of the vesicles. In experiments with the fluorescent probe, DPH, Hillard *et al.* (1985) showed that 11-hydroxy-delta-9-THC was more effective although not more potent than delta-9-THC in fluidizing rat brain synaptic plasma membranes, that CBN was less potent than delta-9-THC and that CBD did not increase membrane fluidity at all. Interestingly, at a concentration of 30 μM, CBD and CBN, like delta-9-THC at the same concentration (see above), decreased fluidity in this membrane preparation. Tamir and Lichtenberg (1983), using nuclear magnetic resonance spectrometry, found that (−) delta-8-dimethylheptyl-THC was slightly more effective than (−) delta-9-THC in fluidizing egg yolk phosphatidylcholine/cholesterol vesicles. (−) Delta-8-THC was less potent than (−) delta-9-THC whereas (+) delta-9-dimethylheptyl-THC and CBD reduced fluidity. The correlation between ability to increase membrane fluidity and psychoactive potency was not perfect in this study, however, since the psychically active cannabinoid, nabilone, was found to reduce membrane fluidity.

Lawrence and Gill (1975) observed that the fluidizing effect of delta-9-THC in vesicles prepared from egg yolk phosphatidylcholine and cholesterol rapidly leveled off as the drug concentration in the vesicular membrane was increased. A similar leveling off of effect was detected in the same study both with other cannabinoids and with the 'partial' anesthetics, hexadecanol and tetradecane. It was also detected in studies concerning the effects of cannabinoids on rat brain synaptic plasma membrane fluidity (Hillard *et al.*, 1985).

To investigate the role of membrane proteins in the effect of cannabinoids on the fluidity of synaptic membranes, Hillard *et al.* (1985) studied the ability of 11-hydroxy-delta-9-THC and CBD to alter fluorescence polarization of DPH in total lipid extracts of mouse brain synaptic plasma membranes. As in intact synaptic membranes, DPH polarization was increased by CBD and decreased by the 11-hydroxy compound, demonstrating that cannabinoids can produce their effects on synaptic membrane fluidity in the absence of membrane proteins.

The effect of cannabinoids on lipid membrane fluidity has been shown to be markedly influenced by cholesterol content. In experiments with vesicles containing egg yolk phosphatidylcholine, phosphatidic acid and cholesterol, Pang and Miller (1978) found that CBN decreased membrane fluidity when the cholesterol content of the vesicles was 20 mole% or less. However, when the cholesterol content was raised to 25 mole% or more, CBN had a fluidizing effect. In agreement with these findings, CBN decreased fluidity in rat liver mitochondrial membranes (cholesterol content 6 mole%) and increased fluidity in human erythrocyte ghost membranes (cholesterol content 40 mole%). In more recent studies, the addition of cholesterol to dipalmitoylphosphatidylcholine bilayers was found to enhance the ability of delta-9-THC to increase membrane fluidity (Bruggemann and Melchior, 1983; Tamir and Lichtenberg, 1983). Hillard *et al.*, (1985) found that several cannabinoids, including delta-9-THC, increased fluidity in egg yolk phosphatidylcholine vesicles containing cholesterol but decreased fluidity in vesicles consisting entirely of phosphatidylcholine. Egg yolk phosphatidylcholine forms relatively fluid bilayers that are far less rigid than those formed by phosphatidylcholine mixed with cholesterol (Pang and Miller, 1978) and indeed there is evidence to suggest that cannabinoids tend to decrease the ordering of molecules in rigid phospholipid bilayers and to increase ordering in bilayers that are more fluid (Pang and Miller, 1978; Hillard *et al.*, 1985).

Other evidence that cannabinoids can alter the physical properties of membranes derives from reports concerning the effects of cannabinoids on the stability or morphology of individual cells, subcellular organelles and model membranes. As shown in Table 31, there are signs from such experiments that delta-9-THC can stabilize membranes. Several of the studies referred to in Table 31 included experiments with CBN (Sofia *et al.*, 1974) or CBD (Raz *et al.*, 1972, 1973; Sofia *et al.*, 1974; Raz and Goldman, 1976; Hershkowitz *et al.*, 1977) and both of these were found to behave much like delta-9-THC. In some experiments, a concentration-dependent biphasic effect of cannabinoids on membrane stability has been observed. Thus, in their experiments with rat erythrocytes, Sofia *et al.* (1974) found that delta-9-THC protected against hemolysis at concentrations of 20 to 50 μM and promoted hemolysis at a concentration of 75 μM. Essentially similar results were obtained with CBN and CBD. Other erythrocyte studies with delta-9-THC or CBD (0.1 to 100 μM) revealed only an antihemolytic effect (Chari-Bitron, 1971; Ray *et al.*, 1972). It is noteworthy, however, that in one of these studies (Raz *et al.*, 1972) the antihemolytic effect of CBD diminished when the concentration was raised above 20 μM. Raz *et al.* (1973) found that delta-9-THC and CBD reduced leakage of acid phosphatase from rat liver lysosomes at a concentration of 2 μM but enhanced the leakage at concentrations of 50 and 100 μM. These results are supported by those of Britton and Mellors (1974) who also detected increases in acid phosphatase release from rat liver lysosomes in the presence of high concentrations of delta-9-THC (Table 31). Bino *et al.* (1972) showed that the degree of mitochondrial swelling induced by delta-9-THC increased with concentration in the range 17 to 56 μM but decreased in response to higher concentrations. Similarly, Alhanaty and Livne (1974) found that egg yolk phosphatidylcholine vesicles were protected against osmotic lysis by delta-9-THC concentrations of about 6 to 12 μM but were not protected by concentrations of 20, 40 or 60 μM. Hershkowitz *et al.* (1977) found that at a concentration of 50 μM both delta-9-THC and CBD severely disrupted mouse brain synaptosomes. This observation must be borne in mind when interpreting neuropharmacological data from experiments with synaptosomes.

In view of the evidence that cannabinoids can alter the physical properties of membranes it is noteworthy that there is also evidence that delta-9-THC can alter membrane composition within the brain and affect the biosynthesis of membrane lipids.

Six hours after intraperitoneal injection of delta-9-THC at a dose of 10 mg/kg, Sarkar and Ghosh (1975) detected changes per unit weight of protein in rat brain levels of total lipid, total phospholipid and total cholesterol. There were increases in the amounts of these lipid components in a microsomal fraction and decreases in mitochondrial, synaptosomal and myelin fractions of the brain. The changes in phospholipid content were attributed to

TABLE 31. *Effects of* In Vitro *Administration of Delta-9-THC on Membrane Stability and Organelle Morphology*

Concentration of Δ^9-THC (μM)	Vehicle	Preparation or organelle	Measured effect	Response	Reference
c.a. 1 to 80	Ethanol	Rat erythocytes	Hemolysis	Protection	1
c.a. 0.5 to 100	?	Human erythrocytes	Hemolysis	Protection	2
c.a. 10 to 50	Phosphate buffer	Rat erythrocytes	Hemolysis	Protection	3
c.a. 6 to 12	Ethanol	Egg yolk phosphatidylcholine vesicles	Osmotic lysis	Slight protection	4
c.a. 2 to 80	Ethanol	Erythrocyte lipid vesicles	Osmotic lysis	Protection	4
c.a. 2 to 40	Ethanol	Lamb brain lipid vesicles	Osmotic lysis	Protection	4
2 50 and 100	Methanol	Rat liver lysosomes	Release of acid phosphatase	Reduction Enhancement	5
250 to 1000	Ethanol + DMSO	Rat liver lysosomes	Release of acid phosphatase	Enhancement	6
10 to 16	Ethanol	Rat liver mitochondria	Release of malate dehydrogenase	Enhancement	7
10 to 16	Ethanol	Rat liver mitochondria	Morphology	Swelling	7
17 to 150	Ethanol	Rat liver mitochondria	Morphology	Swelling	8
200 to 300	Ethanol	Bull sperm mitochondria	Morphology	Swelling	9
100	Ethanol	Mouse peritoneal macrophage mitochondria	Morphology	Some swelling	10
100	Ethanol	Mouse peritoneal macrophages	Morphology	Extensive vacuolization	10
10	Ethanol	Mouse brain synaptosomes	Morphology	No detectable change	11
50	Ethanol	Mouse brain synaptosomes	Morphology	Disruption	11
10	Ethanol	Rat erythrocytes	Morphology	No detectable change	12
15 to 35	Ethanol	Rat erythrocytes	Morphology	Invagination of cells	12

DMSO is an abbreviation for dimethyl sulfoxide.

References: 1, Chari-Bitron, 1971; 2, Raz *et al.*, 1972; 3, Sofia *et al.*, 1974; 4, Alhanaty and Livne, 1974; Raz *et al.*, 1973; 6, Britton and Mellors, 1974; 7, Mahoney and Harris, 1972; 8, Bino *et al.*, 1972; 9, Shahar and Bino, 1974; 10, Raz and Goldman, 1976; 11 Hershkowitz *et al.*, 1977; 12, Chari-Bitron and Shahar, 1979.

changes in phosphatidylcholine, phosphatidylethanolamine and phosphatidylserine, the amount of sphingomyelin present remaining unaltered. In some fractions, changes in ganglioside and sialoglycoprotein content were also detected (Sarkar and Ghosh, 1976). None of the fractions studied showed any change in total cerebroside content.

In experiments with mice, delta-9-THC given intraperitoneally 30 min before an intravenous injection of [methyl^{14}C]-choline was found to alter the amount of radioactive label incorporated into the brain (Wing and Paton, 1979). At an ambient temperature of 22°C, the incorporation of radioactivity into a brain lipid fraction was reduced by a dose of 15 mg/kg although unaffected by a dose of 3.75 mg/kg. Incorporation of radioactivity into an aqueous fraction of the brain was not reduced by either dose. The effect of the larger dose was attenuated but not abolished when the experiment was repeated at a higher ambient temperature (33.5°C) to prevent hypothermia. Under these conditions, 3.75 mg/kg of delta-9-THC increased incorporation of label into both the brain lipid fraction and the aqueous fraction.

In experiments with mouse spleen lymphocytes, Greenberg and Mellors (1978) showed that delta-9-THC, at a concentration of 10 μM, significantly inhibited ^{14}C-acetate incorporation into the membrane lipids phosphatidylcholine, phosphatidylethanolamine, phosphatidylinositol and triglyceride. In the same preparation, delta-9-THC was shown to inhibit lysophosphatidylcholine acyltransferase, an enzyme catalysing the formation of phosphatidylcholine from lysophosphatidylcholine and coenzyme A-activated fatty acids (Greenberg *et al.*, 1977; Greenberg and Mellors, 1978; Mellors, 1979). It also inhibited lysophosphatidate acyltransferase which catalyses the conversion of lysophosphatidic acid to phosphatidic acid, a precursor of phospholipids and triglycerides (Mellors, 1979). Lysophosphatidylcholine acyltransferase was inhibited by concentrations of delta-9-THC ranging from 0.2 to 10 μM, the concentration for half maximal inhibition (K_i) being 0.35 μM. The K_i for the other enzyme was 6 μM. Inhibition of lysophosphatidylcholine acyltransferase was also detected in mouse brain synaptosomes after *in vitro* administration of delta-9-THC ($K_i = 0.3$ μM) and in mouse spleen lymphocytes and mouse brain synaptosomes 2 hr after *in vivo* administration of delta-9-THC, albeit with doses (20 to 70 mg/kg i.v.) far higher than are required to produce behavioral changes in mice (Huszar *et al.*, 1977; Greenberg *et al.*, 1978; Mellors, 1979). In addition to delta-9-THC, a number of other cannabinoids were found to inhibit lysophosphatidylcholine acyltransferase when added directly to lymphocytes or synaptosomes. The most potent inhibitors were psychically active, the ability to inhibit the enzyme decreasing in the order delta-9-THC, delta-8-THC, 11-hydroxy-delta-9-THC, synhexyl and CBN (Greenberg and Mellors, 1978; Greenberg *et al.*, 1978; Mellors, 1979). The psychically inactive cannabinoid, cannabigerol, was equipotent with synhexyl.

At concentrations ranging upwards from about 3 μM, cannabinoids have been reported to inhibit cholesterol esterase activity in preparations obtained from brain, adrenal gland, liver, pancreas, ovary and testis and in cultures of human dermal fibroblasts and of human aortic medial cells (Burstein *et al.*, 1978, 1979a,b, 1980; Shoupe *et al.*, 1980; Cornicelli *et al.*, 1981). In a microsomal preparation obtained from rat brain, the ability of cannabinoids to inhibit the enzyme decreased in the order delta-9-THC, CBN and 11-hydroxy-delta-9-THC (Burstein *et al.*, 1980). In cultured human aortic medial cells, however, CBN and CBD were reported to be more potent than delta-9-THC as inhibitors of the enzyme (Cornicelli *et al.*, 1981). From studies with a purified cholesterol esterase preparation, Shoupe *et al.* (1980) concluded that delta-9-THC is a competitive inhibitor of this enzyme and that it can compete with cholesterol esters for a position on the active site of the enzyme because its structure is somewhat similar to that of cholesterol. Cornicelli *et al.* (1981) found that in cultured human fibroblasts, although delta-9-THC, CBN and CBD reduced the incorporation of ^{14}C-oleate into cholesterol esters, they did not alter the incorporation of label into cellular phospholipid or triglyceride.

Finally, there is evidence that as well as inhibiting the production of membrane phospholipids, cannabinoids can also hasten their metabolism by stimulating phospholipases A_2 and C (Section 7.4).

9. MOLECULAR MECHANISMS

There is strong evidence that the primary sites of action of delta-9-THC reside in neuronal cellular and subcellular membranes. Thus, as discussed elsewhere in this review, the drug has been shown to alter the transport of transmitters and ions across membranes, to change the activities of important membrane-bound enzymes and to affect the physical properties of membranes.

The ability of cannabinoids to interact with neuronal membranes, like their ability to produce changes in mood and behavior is markedly influenced by their chemical shape and structure. This raises the possibility that there might be a specific cannabinoid receptor (Binder and Franke, 1982; Binder *et al.*, 1979, 1984; Harris *et al.*, 1978; Nye *et al.*, 1985) and has led to a search for binding sites in the brain. In studies with rat brain tissue, Harris *et al.* (1978) were unable to detect saturable, high affinity binding sites for ^{3}H-delta-8-THC. They did, however, detect such sites in intact hepatoma cells. These contained two populations of binding site, one of which had a very high affinity for the tritiated ligand.

The cannabinoids are particularly difficult substances with which to carry out binding studies. Their low water solubility introduces the need for a special vehicle (Section 4) and their high lipid solubility gives rise to a considerable amount of non-specific binding (Harris *et al.* 1978). In addition, delta-9-THC has been shown to bind avidly to glass, plastic, rubber, stainless steel and filter paper (Garrett and Hunt, 1974; Kujtan *et al.*, 1983). In order to circumvent some of these difficulties, Nye *et al.* (1985) carried out binding studies with ^{3}H-5′-trimethylammonium delta-8-THC (TMA), a positively charged, hydrophilic analog of delta-8-THC. Their experiments with TMA demonstrated the presence of single populations of saturable, high affinity binding sites both in various regions of rat brain (affinity constant = 0.01 liters/nmole in crude cerebral cortical membrane homogenates) and in a number of peripheral organs. They also showed that like delta-8- and delta-9-THC, TMA could reduce the size of the twitch response induced in the isolated guinea-pig ileum by electrical stimulation. Its ED_{50} was 10 times greater than that of delta-9-THC. The correlation between the ability of cannabinoids to displace TMA from its binding sites and psychoactive potency was poor, however, suggesting that TMA binding sites do not mediate effects of cannabinoids on mood or behavior. An alternative interpretation, yet to be fully explored, is that psychically inactive cannabinoids with a high affinity for TMA binding sites are delta-9-THC antagonists. It is also possible that the TMA binding sites mediate actions of the cannabinoids other than those which are responsible for psychoactivity (Nye *et al.*, 1985).

The finding that there is a correlation between psychoactive potency and the ability to produce changes in the physical properties of artificial membranes containing only cholesterol and phospholipid (Section 8) weakens the main argument for the existence of a specific cannabinoid receptor. Indeed, Lawrence and Gill (1975) have proposed that psychoactive cannabinoids do not interact with a specific receptor but rather with the lipid phase of the cell membrane and that the pharmacological activity of these substances results from a structure-dependent ability to disorder membrane lipids. According to this hypothesis, pharmacological activity depends on 'awkwardness of fit into the hydrocarbon matrix' rather than on goodness of fit between drug and site of action (Gill and Lawrence, 1976). Differences in the abilities of cannabinoids to alter membrane fluidity can be attributed to the presence of cholesterol, which being chiral, would be expected to impose asymmetry on the lipid phase of the membrane (Lawrence and Gill, 1975; Gill and Lawrence, 1976). Burstein and Hunter (1981) have pointed out that delta-9-THC is a competitive inhibitor of cholesterol esterase (Section 8) and have speculated that the cannabinoid may be able to 'mimic' membrane cholesterol. More recently, Bruggemann and Melchior (1983) proposed that delta-9-THC acts by forming a complex with some specific membrane lipid to produce changes in membrane function these changes possibly resulting from an alteration in membrane organization. In addition, they suggested that membrane cholesterol could influence the interaction of delta-9-THC with the membrane lipid, the cholesterol having either an inhibitory or a facilitatory effect depending on its concentration in the membrane. It has also been suggested that cannabinoids may induce conformational changes in membrane proteins or modify interactions between membrane proteins and lipids (Leuschner *et al.*, 1984).

Further support for the notion that the psychoactivity of delta-9-THC is mediated by mechanisms which require a particular chemical structure comes from evidence that non-specific molecular interactions of the sort that probably underlie anesthesia do not contribute significantly towards delta-9-THC's psychoactive properties. Thus, unlike general anesthetics, there is no correlation among the cannabinoids between psychoactive potency and lipid solubility (Section 4). Moreover, the cannabis 'high' is quite different from the collection of signs and symptoms experienced after the taking of alcohol or other general anesthetics at subanesthetic doses (Paton and Pertwee, 1973a, 1973b). There is also evidence from several studies (Seeman *et al.*, 1972; Roth and Williams, 1979; Leuschner *et al.*, 1984) to suggest that delta-9-THC can elicit pharmacological responses when its concentration in cell membranes is markedly less than that which is needed, according to the Meyer-Overton rule, to produce either local anesthesia (about 40 mmoles/kg dry membrane) or general anesthesia (about 3 mmoles/kg dry membrane; Seeman, 1972). For example, Roth and Williams (1979) using data produced by Gill and Lawrence (1974), calculated that behaviorally effective doses of delta-9-THC would give rise to membrane concentrations in mouse brains of about 20 μmoles/kg dry membrane. Similarly, Leuschner *et al.* (1984) calculated that the concentration of delta-9-THC in erythrocyte membranes taken from mice pretreated with behaviorally effective doses of the drug ranged from 1 to 10 μmoles/kg dry membrane. It is also noteworthy that some psychically active cannabinoids have been reported to be far more potent in inhibiting lymphocytic or synaptosomal lysophosphatidylcholine acyltransferase than was to be expected from their anesthetic activity as measured by their molar volume or their ability to protect erythrocytes against hemolysis (Greenberg and Mellors, 1978; Greenberg *et al.*, 1978). This is of interest because the ability of cannabinoids to inhibit lysophosphatidylcholine acyltransferase has been found to correlate with psychoactive potency (Section 8).

Since cannabinoids are highly lipid soluble compounds, they should, according to the Meyer-Overton rule, have anesthetic properties (Seeman, 1972). Indeed, delta-9-THC has been shown to decrease the amplitude of action potentials in isolated preparations of rabbit vagus nerve and rat phrenic nerve (Section 5). However, the action potentials were by no means abolished. Moreover, in whole animals, delta-9-THC has never been shown to produce general anesthesia. It has been proposed, therefore, that delta-9-THC is a 'partial anesthetic,' unable in spite of its high lipid solubility to reach a concentration in nerve membranes sufficiently large to produce complete anesthesia (Paton *et al.*, 1972). This may be because it has such a low solubility in water, the maximum concentration that any substance can attain in membrane lipid being a function not only of its membrane/extracellular fluid partition coefficient but also of its solubility in extracellular fluid (Seeman, 1972).

Even though delta-9-THC cannot itself produce general anesthesia, there is evidence that it can, at relatively low doses, decrease the concentrations of conventional general anesthetics or barbiturates required to produce antinociception or loss of consciousness. Vitez *et al.* (1973) showed that delta-9-THC could reduce the minimum alveolar concentration (MAC) of cyclopropane required to abolish the motor response of rats to clamping of the tail. MAC was reduced about 15% by 1 mg/kg i.p. of delta-9-THC and about 25% by 2 mg/kg i.p. of the cannabinoid. Using the rat tail flick test, Novelli *et al.* (1983) found that delta-9-THC (10 mg/kg i.p.) could potentiate the antinociceptive effect of nitrous oxide. Both drugs were active in the test when given by themselves. When given together they had a super-additive effect. In experiments with mice, Morrison and Pertwee (1985) found that delta-9-THC (20 mg/kg i.p.) brought about a reduction (about 40%) in the dose of sodium barbital needed to abolish the righting response, the dose required to abolish this response in 50% of a group of mice (ED_{50}) decreasing from approximately 230 mg/kg s.c. to 140 mg/kg s.c.* In an earlier study with mice, Pertwee (unpublished) found that doses of delta-9-THC ranging from 2 to 20 mg/kg i.v. reduced the loss of right-

*Loss of the righting response is often used as an end point for light anesthesia in mice.

ing response ED_{50} of diethyl ether (inhaled) by 10% (see also Paton, 1974). The mechanism by which delta-9-THC can augment the antinociceptive or hypnotic effects of general anesthetics and barbiturates remains to be elucidated. It is possible that these interactions reflect the ability of delta-9-THC to act as a 'partial anesthetic' and it would be of interest, therefore, to determine if other cannabinoids can also augment the effects of anesthetics and, if they do, whether this ability correlates best with chemical structure or with lipid solubility.

Reports that the ability of cannabinoids to increase the 'fluidity' of membranes correlates with psychoactive potency (Section 8) raise the possibility that such fluidity changes may underlie important cannabinoid-induced changes in membrane function. It is noteworthy, therefore, that delta-9-THC has been shown to increase membrane fluidity only at concentrations well above those at which it can produce functional changes in membranes, in particular, facilitation of the synaptosomal uptake of NE and DA (Sections 6.1.3 and 6.2.3). Either such changes in membrane function do not arise from delta-9-THC-induced increases in membrane fluidity or they are produced by fluidity changes that are too subtle to detect.

Several of the neuropharmacological changes produced by delta-9-THC, *in vivo* or *in vitro*, seem to be biphasic in nature, the direction of change depending on the dose used. Often, there is evidence that the ability of low doses of cannabinoids to produce a change in one direction correlates with psychoactive potency whereas the ability of higher doses to produce the opposite effect is independent of cannabinoid structure. Examples include effects on the amplitude of potentials evoked in the cerebral cortex (Section 5), on the synaptosomal uptake of NE and DA (Sections 6.1.3 and 6.2.3) and on the fluidity of synaptic plasma membranes (Section 8). The existence of such biphasic effects implies that, at least at some sites, cannabinoids have two types of action, one that is structure-dependent and detectable at low doses, and the other that is non-specific and detectable only at higher doses. It is noteworthy that the ability of cannabinoids to produce changes at low doses does not always parallel psychic activity. For example, both delta-9-THC and CBD have been reported to be highly potent as inhibitors of depolarization-dependent Ca^{2+} uptake into brainstem synaptosomes (Section 5). Indeed, this action has been postulated to account for the anticonvulsant properties of delta-9-THC and CBD (Harris and Stokes, 1982). It is also noteworthy that not all 'high dose' effects of cannabinoids are independent of chemical structure, an example in this case being the hypothermic effect of cannabinoids (Pertwee, 1985a).

In conclusion, in spite of its high lipid solubility, the psychic activity of delta-9-THC probably depends on an ability to undergo structure-dependent interactions with neuronal membranes rather than on non-specific membrane interactions of the sort which are thought to underlie general anesthesia. There is still no detailed information either about the molecular basis of these interactions or about the way in which they alter membrane function. Thus, it is not yet known whether delta-9-THC interacts with a specific delta-9-THC receptor or undergoes some other kind of structure-dependent interaction with membrane phospholipids or proteins. The receptor hypothesis has little experimental support at present since no one has yet developed a satisfactory selective delta-9-THC antagonist (Martin, 1986) or demonstrated the presence of specific delta-9-THC binding sites in the brain. The failure to detect such binding sites may of course simply reflect the extra practical difficulties associated with delta-9-THC binding studies rather than an absence of receptors.

10. GENERAL DISCUSSION AND SUMMARY

10.1. The Role of Transmitters in the Psychopharmacology of Cannabinoids

10.1.1. *Norepinephrine, Dopamine and 5-Hydroxytryptamine*

In vivo experiments directed at examining the ability of delta-9-THC to alter turnover of NE, DA or 5-HT by measuring its effects on changes in the brain levels of these amines induced by inhibition of their synthesis or metabolism have yielded variable results (Sections 6.1, 6.2 and 6.3). In some experiments, delta-9-THC had no apparent effect on turnover whereas in others either increases or decreases in turnover were detected. Equally variable results were obtained when effects of delta-9-THC were measured on levels of NE, DA or 5-HT in the brains of animals that had not received a second drug treatment. Brain levels rose or fell in some experiments and remained unchanged in others. This variability is no doubt due in part to the study of different brain areas and to the use of different species, different ambient temperatures and different doses of delta-9-THC.

In vivo and *in vitro* experiments designed to detect delta-9-THC-induced changes in the rates of synthesis or release of NE, DA or 5-HT in the brain have yielded more consistent data (Sections 6.1, 6.2 and 6.3). The results suggest that delta-9-THC can accelerate the rate of formation of NE and DA from tyrosine, that it can increase 5-HT synthesis by raising brain levels of the 5-HT precursor, tryptophan, and that it can stimulate DA release. There is also evidence from *in vitro* experiments with brain tissue that delta-9-THC can alter the neuronal uptake or storage of NE, DA, 5-HT and tyrosine (Sections 6.1.3, 6.2.3 and 6.3.3), inhibit monoamine oxidase (Section 7.1), increase the affinity of DA D_2 receptors for DA agonists (Section 6.7) and enhance the coupling of central beta-adrenoceptors to adenylate cyclase (Section 7.3).

Effects most likely to contribute to the psychoactivity of delta-9-THC are those which can be produced *in vitro* by concentrations of 1 μM or less (Section 4). These include (i) facilitation of synaptosomal uptake of ^{3}H-NE and ^{3}H-DA, (ii) increased retention of ^{3}H-NE and ^{3}H-DA by preloaded synaptosomes and (iii) inhibition of synaptosomal uptake of ^{3}H-5-HT (Table 32). The first of these effects is of special interest since *in vivo* administration of delta-9-THC has also been shown to facilitate *in vitro* uptake of NE and DA into brain synaptosomes (Section 6.1.3 and 6.2.3). The doses used were rather high and further *in vivo* experiments are required to test whether delta-9-THC can produce similar changes in synaptosomal uptake when given at lower doses. Also noteworthy is evidence from *in vitro* studies with synaptosomes, albeit with only a limited number of cannabinoids, that the ability to facilitate ^{3}H-NE and ^{3}H-DA uptake and to increase ^{3}H-NE and ^{3}H-DA retention correlates with psychoactive potency. Correlations with psychoactive potency have also been observed for some effects so far detected *in vitro* only at concentrations of 1μM or above (Table 32).

The extent to which interactions of delta-9-THC with central NE, DA or 5-HT releasing neurons can account for its effects in man, for example the production of mood changes or psychoses (Section 2) or the suppression of nausea and vomiting induced by anticancer drugs (Section 3), remains to be established. There is evidence, however, for an involvement of NE or DA in certain behavioral effects produced by delta-9-THC in animals. For example, results obtained by Conti and Musty (1984) from experiments with rats suggest that delta-9-THC may increase dopaminergic transmission in the nucleus accumbens, this in turn giving rise to increases in locomotor activity. In more recent studies, Sakurai *et al.* (1985) found that delta-9-THC shared the ability of methamphetamine to elicit ipsilateral circling behavior in rats with unilateral lesions in the substantia nigra. This circling behavior could be prevented by haloperidol, supporting the hypothesis that delta-9-THC had acted by increasing dopaminergic transmission in the surviving nigro-striatal pathway. Kataoka *et al.* (1987) have obtained evidence that central NE-releasing pathways may have a role in delta-9-THC-induced catalepsy. Depletion of brain NE brought about by destruction of the locus coeruleus or by intracerebroventricular pretreatment with 6-hydroxydopamine was associated with a marked reduction in the cataleptic response of rats to delta-9-THC, measured using a bar test. When desipramine was used to restrict the catecholaminergic depleting action of 6-hydroxydopamine to DA-releasing neurons, no subsequent suppression of delta-9-THC-induced catalepsy was detected.

10.1.2. *Acetylcholine*

Delta-9-THC has been shown to reduce ACh release both in cat somatosensory cortex (Section 6.5) and in peripheral nerve-containing preparations (Section 5). It has also been shown to reduce ACh turnover in rat brain. In mouse brain, however, increases as well as decreases in ACh turnover have been detected. ACh turnover has been found to be altered by delta-9-THC only in some areas of rat or mouse brain. For example, the drug has been reported to reduce ACh turnover in rat and mouse hippocampus and in rat striatum but to have no effect on turnover in mouse striatum or in rat parietal cortex. Given the findings that changes in ACh turnover can be elicited by relatively low doses of delta-9-THC and that these changes occur in general most readily in response to psychoactive cannabinoids, the possibility arises that the psychic activity of delta-9-THC depends at least in part on an ability to alter transmission along central ACh-releasing pathways. More specifically, the observation that delta-9-THC can reduce ACh turnover in the hippocampus, raises the possibility that suppression of cholinergic transmission in this part of the brain could account for the ability of delta-9-THC and cannabis to impair memory (Miller and Branconnier, 1983). Data obtained from electrophysiological experiments also point to an inhibitory effect of delta-9-THC on hippocampal function (Section 5).

10.1.3. *Gamma-aminobutyric Acid*

GABA turnover has been shown to be increased by delta-9-THC in rat septum and substantia nigra but not in rat caudate nucleus or nucleus accumbens (Section 6.6). So far only rather high doses of delta-9-THC have been used to study its effect on GABA turnover and

TABLE 32. *The Lowest Concentrations at which Delta-9-THC Has Been Shown to be Active in* In Vitro *Studies with Brain Tissue or with Peripheral Nerve Preparations*

Concentration	Preparation or tissue	Measured effect and direction of change (±)	Correlation with psychoactivity*	Section
A. *Delta-9-THC concentrations below 1 μM*				
0.01 nM	Rat hippocampal cells	Amplitude of evoked potential (+)	ND	5
0.1 nM	Rat hippocampal cells	Amplitude of evoked potential (−)	ND	5
6.4 nM	Guinea-pig ileum	Electrically evoked twitch amplitude (−)	Yes	5
10 nM	Rat brain stem synaptosomes	Depolarization-dependent Ca^{2+} uptake (−)	No	5
50 nM	Rat brain synaptosomes	^{3}H-DA uptake (+)	Yes	6.2.3
100 nM	Rat brain synaptosomes	^{3}H-DA retention (+)	Yes	6.2.3
	Rat brain synaptosomes	^{3}H-NE uptake (+)	Yes	6.1.3
	Rat brain synaptosomes	^{3}H-NE retention (+)	Yes	6.1.3
	Rat brain synaptosomes	^{3}H-5-HT uptake (−)	No	6.3.3
	Rat striatal synaptosomes	^{14}C-DA uptake (−)	ND	6.2.3
	Guinea-pig hippocampal cells	Amplitude of evoked potential (+)	ND	5
	Guinea-pig hippocampal cells	Paired pulse inhibition (−)	ND	5
200 nM	Guinea-pig cerebrocortical slices	Prostaglandin formation (−)	Yes	7.4
300 nM	Mouse brain synaptosomes	Lysophosphatidylcholine acyltransferase activity (−)	Yes	8
B. *Delta-9-THC concentrations of 1 to 10 μM*				
1 μM	Mouse brain synaptosomes	^{3}H-5-HT uptake (+)	Yes	6.3.3
	Rat brain synaptosomes	^{3}H-DA retention (−)	No	6.2.3
	Rat brain synaptic vesicles	Mg^{2+}-ATPase activity (+)	ND	7.2
	Rat/mouse brain synaptosomes	Na^+-K^+-ATPase activity (−)	No	7.2
	Guinea-pig hippocampal cells	Amplitude of evoked potential (−)	ND	5
	Rat brain synaptic plasma membranes	Membrane fluidity (+)	Yes	8
2 μM	Mouse brain homogenate	Activation of adenylate cyclase by NE (+)	No	7.3
	Mouse brain synaptosomes	Activity of phospholipases (+)	ND	7.4
3 μM	Mouse brain synaptosomes	^{3}H-Tyrosine uptake (−)	ND	6.2.2
	Mouse brain synaptosomes	Conversion of ^{3}H-tyrosine to ^{3}H-NE (+)	ND	6.1.2
	Mouse striatal synaptosomes	Conversion of ^{3}H-tyrosine to ^{3}H-DA (+)	ND	6.2.2
	Mouse cerebral cortex	^{3}H-dihydroalprenolol binding (+)	Yes	6.7.1
**	Rat brain membranes	^{3}H-dihydromorphine binding (−)	No	6.7.1
	Rat/mouse brain synaptosomes	Mg^{2+}-ATPase activity (−)	No	7.2
	Rat brain microsomes	Cholesterol esterase activity (−)	No	8

continued

there is some reason for expecting that at lower doses, the drug may reduce turnover (Section 6.6). Indeed the hypothesis that delta-9-THC has a dose-dependent biphasic effect on transmission along certain GABA-releasing pathways is supported by the evidence that at low doses, it can oppose recurrent inhibition in the hippocampus, whereas at higher doses it has the opposite effect (Section 5). Delta-9-THC is known to produce a mixture of excitant and depressant effects, both behavioral and electrophysiological, a good example being its ability to act both as a convulsant and as an anticonvulsant (Section 5). It would therefore be of interest to know whether low doses of delta-9-THC can indeed reduce GABA turnover in the brain since this might well reflect an ability to reduce GABA release, an effect which could account for at least some of the excitant properties of this cannabinoid. Similarly, the finding that delta-9-THC can increase GABA turnover could reflect an ability to enhance GABA release. Such an effect might account for the anticonvulsant action of delta-9-THC and could possibly also explain reports that the drug has anxiolytic, analgesic, cataleptic, hypnotic and muscle relaxant properties (Paton and Pertwee, 1973a; Musty, 1984; Hollister, 1986). Interestingly, CBD, which shares the ability of delta-9-THC to increase GABA turnover in the substantia nigra, has also been reported to be anxiolytic (Musty, 1984) and anticonvulsant (Section 5). Indeed, Consroe *et al.* (1982)

TABLE 32. *continued.*

Concentration	Preparation or tissue	Measured effect and direction of change (±)	Correlation with psychoactivity*	Section
B. *Delta-9-THC concentrations of 1 to 10 μM (continued)*				
5 μM	Rat/mouse brain synaptosomes	Choline uptake (−)	No	6.5.2
	Mouse brain	^{3}H-naloxone binding (−)	ND	6.7.1
10 μM	Rabbit vagus nerve	Amplitude of action potential (−)	ND	5
	Rat/mouse brain synaptosomes	^{3}H-NE uptake (−)	No	6.1.3
	Rat/mouse brain synaptosomes	^{3}H-DA uptake (−)	No	6.2.3
	Rat/mouse brain synaptosomes	^{3}H-GABA uptake (−)	No	6.6.1
	Rat striatal synaptosomes	^{3}H-DA retention (−)	No	6.2.3
	Pig brain	Monoamine oxidase activity (−)	Yes	7.1
	Mouse brain synaptosomes	Mg^{2+}-ATPase activity (+)	ND	7.2
	Mouse cerebral cortex	Activation of adenylate cyclase by isoprenaline (+)	ND	7.3
	Mouse cerebral cortex	Attenuation of ^{3}H-dihydroalprenolol binding by beta-adrenoceptor antagonists (+)	ND	6.7.1
C. *Delta-9-THC concentrations above 10 μM*				
16 μM**	Rat brain membranes	^{3}H-D-Pen^2, D-Pen^5-enkephalin binding (−)	ND	6.7.1
20 μM	Mouse brain synaptosomes	Mg^{2+}-Ca^{2+}-ATPase activity (−)	ND	7.2
30 μM	Mouse brain synaptosomes	^{3}H-ADTN (D_3) binding (−)	No	6.7.1
	Mouse brain homogenate	Basal activity of adenylate cyclase (+)	No	7.3
	Mouse striatum	^{3}H-spiperone (D_2) binding (−)	No	6.7.1
	Mouse striatum	DA-induced attenuation of ^{3}H-spiperone binding (+)	Yes	6.7.1
	Rat brain synaptic plasma membranes	Membrane fluidity (−)	No	8
50 μM	Mouse brain synaptosomes	Morphological integrity (−)	No	8
100 μM	Rat brain synaptosomes	^{3}H-NE retention (−)	No	6.1.3
	Rat brain synaptosomes	^{3}H-5-HT retention (−)	ND	6.3.3
	Mouse brain synaptosomes	^{3}H-5-HT uptake (−)	No	6.3.3
	Frog sciatic nerve	Voltage-dependent Na^+ conductance (−)	ND	5
750 μM	Mouse brain synaptosomes (crude preparation)	Release of prostaglandin $F_{2\alpha}$ (−)	ND	7.4

*The evidence is usually based on studies with very few cannabinoids and must therefore be interpreted with caution.
** IC_{50}.
ND = not determined.

have found that CBD could prevent tonic convulsions produced in mice by drugs thought to act by reducing GABAergic transmission but did not inhibit tonic convulsions induced by the glycine antagonist, strychnine. An ability to enhance GABA release could also help to explain why delta-9-THC produces a mixture of excitant and depressant responses in whole animals since increased GABA release can lead to reductions in transmission along both excitatory and inhibitory pathways.

Several mechanisms can be envisaged to account for an effect of delta-9-THC on GABAergic transmission. One possibility is that the drug interacts directly with GABA-containing neurons to alter the release, neuronal uptake and/or metabolism of GABA. Indeed there is already evidence that delta-9-THC can inhibit GABA uptake (Section 6.6.1). Another possibility is that delta-9-THC facilitates or inhibits the interaction of GABA with its receptors. However, although it is not yet known whether the cannabinoid can alter GABA efficacy, there is evidence from binding studies that it has no effect on GABA affinity (Section 6.7.1). Changes in GABAergic transmission could also be achieved indirectly, the primary site of action then being some non-GABAergic system whose effects are mediated by GABA-releasing pathways.

In view of the evidence that delta-9-THC can facilitate GABAergic transmission in the brain, it is noteworthy that the cannabinoid has also been reported to undergo synergistic interactions with benzodiazepines, drugs which are thought to produce many of their effects by enhancing the response to neuronally released GABA. Thus delta-9-THC (100 mg/kg s.c.) has been shown in experiments with mice to enhance the ability of diazepam to suppress pentylenetetrazol-induced convulsions (Koe *et al.*, 1985). In addition, at much lower doses (5 to 20 mg/kg i.p.), delta-9-THC has been found to abolish the righting response of mice pretreated with doses of flurazepam or chlordiazepoxide well below those required to abolish this response in the absence of the cannabinoid (Morrison and Pertwee, 1985; Pertwee and Greentree, 1988a). There is also evidence that delta-9-THC and benzodiazepines have a super-additive hypothermic effect in rats and mice (Pryor *et al.*, 1977; Morrison and Pertwee, 1985). It is worth noting, therefore, that delta-9-THC retained the ability to abolish the righting response in mice pretreated with subhypnotic doses of flurazepam or chlordiazepoxide when the ambient temperature was kept at 34°C to prevent hypothermia (Morrison and Pertwee, 1985; Pertwee and Greentree, 1988a). Loss of the righting response is often used as an end point for light anesthesia in mice. Nonetheless, it is likely that the loss of righting response observed in mice given a benzodiazepine followed by delta-9-THC does not indicate onset of general anesthesia but rather the occurrence of intense catalepsy. Thus, animals receiving such a drug regimen, showed a marked degree of catalepsy (immobility in a wire grip test and a "waxy flexibility" of the hind legs) but no detectable reduction in skeletal muscle tone or loss of consciousness (Greentree and Pertwee, 1987; Pertwee and Greentree, 1988a, b). It has also been found that flurazepam and chlordiazepoxide can greatly enhance the ability of delta-9-THC to produce catalepsy in a bar test (Greentree and Pertwee, 1987; Pertwee and Greentree, 1988a, b).

Although the finding that delta-9-THC can undergo synergistic interactions with benzodiazepines is consistent with the notion that certain responses to this cannabinoid are mediated by GABA-releasing pathways, other equally tenable hypotheses can be put forward to account for these interactions. It is possible, for example, that the benzodiazepine-THC interaction stems from an ability of one drug to interfere with the metabolism or disposition of the other. It is also possible that the synergism arises because delta-9-THC has an ability to promote the interaction of benzodiazepines with their receptors. In line with this possibility, is the report that a dose of delta-9-THC potentiating the anticonvulsant effect of diazepam can enhance the "*in vivo*" binding of ^{3}H-flunitrazepam to mouse brain (Section 6.7.2; Koe *et al.*, 1985). Similar results have been obtained with levonantradol. In these experiments, all the drugs were administered *in vivo* so that it is possible that delta-9-THC and levonantradol could have acted by increasing the entry of ^{3}H-flunitrazepam into the brain rather than by augmenting ^{3}H-flunitrazepam binding. Levonantradol has also been reported to enhance benzodiazepine binding in experiments in which the benzodiazepine was added directly to brain tissue (Section 6.7.2). Dextronantradol, which is pharmacologically less active than levonantradol, produced a similar enhancement. However, both cannabinoids were studied at rather high concentrations. Other delta-9-THC derivatives, applied at much lower concentrations, have been found either to have little or no effect on the *in vitro* binding of benzodiazepines (nabilone) or to reduce it (SP111A). The effect of delta-9-THC itself on benzodiazepine binding *in vitro* has yet to be studied.

In recent experiments using the bar test, Pertwee *et al.* (1988) showed that the benzodiazepine antagonist, flumazenil, could prevent the enhancement of delta-9-THC-induced catalepsy by flurazepam and it is likely, therefore, that this effect of flurazepam is benzodiazepine receptor mediated. They also found that the cataleptic response of mice to delta-9-THC could be increased not only by pretreatment with benzodiazepines but also by pretreatment with drugs expected to enhance GABAergic transmission either by acting as agonists at $GABA_A$ or $GABA_B$ receptors (muscimol and baclofen) or by acting as inhibitors of the metabolism or neuronal uptake of GABA (amino-oxyacetic acid and NO-328). In the same study, enhancement of delta-9-THC-induced catalepsy by flurazepam, muscimol, amino-oxyacetic acid and NO-328 was found to be prevented by bicuculline but not by strychnine. Bicuculline and strychnine are both convulsants but whereas bicuculline is a selective GABA antagonist, strychnine is primarily an antagonist of glycine. These results provide convincing evidence for a cause and effect relationship between ability to enhance GABAergic transmission and ability to increase delta-9-THC-induced catalepsy. Consequently they reduce the likelihood that synergism between benzodiazepines and delta-9-THC is caused by a pharmacokinetic or metabolic interaction between these two classes of drug or by some delta-9-THC-induced alteration in the benzodiazepine receptor.

Further experiments are required to establish in more detail how drugs which stimulate or facilitate GABAergic transmission (GABA-mimetic drugs) are able to increase the cataleptic response to delta-9-THC. That interactions of this kind occur because delta-9-THC can itself enhance transmission along GABA-releasing pathways to produce catalepsy still remains a possibility, there being good evidence that GABA has an important role in the production of catalepsy (Scheel-Krüger, 1986). Because extrapyramidal GABAergic pathways are arranged in series, they can mediate excitatory as well as inhibitory changes in motor function. Indeed, extrapyramidal motor function is thought to depend to some extent on an interaction between an inhibitory GABAergic pathway, the striato-pallidal pathway, and two excitatory GABAergic pathways, the striato-nigral and striato-entopeduncular pathways. It has been suggested that the first of these pathways is normally less active than the other two (Scheel-Krüger, 1986). This could well explain why an enhancement of GABAergic transmission by delta-9-THC would trigger a cataleptic response since any drug which elicits behavioral changes through such a mechanism is likely to have a greater effect on a pathway which is normally quiescent than on one which is already quite active. It is also possible to explain enhancement of delta-9-THC-induced catalepsy by GABA-mimetic drugs without invoking a stimulatory effect of delta-9-THC on GABAergic transmission. Thus Moss *et al.* (1984) have postulated that "the THC influence on extrapyramidal motor function is normally a minor subtle effect, probably on a non-dopaminergic system, that is masked by the function of the major extrapyramidal DA system. In the absence of the regulatory effect of the main DA system, however, the normal (occult) effect(s) of THC become observable." According to this hypothesis, drugs such as the benzodiazepines could enhance delta-9-THC-induced catalepsy by exerting a depressant effect on the putative dopaminergic "masking system." This might be achieved by the enhancement of transmission along some GABAergic pathway projecting to the "masking system," there being evidence that DA release from nigro-striatal neurons can be inhibited by GABA released from neurons terminating in the zona compacta of the substantia nigra (Scheel-Krüger, 1986). It should also be possible to overcome the effect of the putative "masking system" by stimulating GABA receptors at sites located "downstream" of the system. In rat or mouse brain, likely locations for such receptors include (i) certain areas receiving GABAergic inputs from the entopeduncular nucleus or from the zona reticulata of the substantia nigra (e.g. the ventro-medial nucleus of the thalamus), (ii) the globus pallidus which contains receptors for GABA released by neurons projecting from the corpus striatum and (iii) the corpus striatum which contains receptors for GABA released by interneurons innervated by DA-releasing neurons. At all these sites there are thought to be receptors ($GABA_A$ and/or $GABA_B$) at which GABA can trigger catalepsy and/or oppose the behavioral effects of striatal dopaminergic stimulation (Scheel-Krüger, 1986). One problem with this notion (that GABA-mimetics enhance the cataleptic response to delta-9-THC by increasing GABAergic transmission along pathways under dopaminergic control) is that as it stands, it leaves unanswered the question of why doses of GABA-mimetics which can enhance delta-9-THC-induced catalepsy are not also able to produce the same behavioral response in the absence of delta-9-THC. Moreover, it takes no account of the existence of sites in the brain at which GABA release brings about an increase in locomotor activity (e.g. the entopeduncular nucleus and the zona reticulata of the substantia nigra).

The hypothesis that the inhibitory effect of delta-9-THC on extrapyramidal motor function is normally opposed by a dopaminergic "masking system" is based on the finding that hypokinesia induced by reserpine in rats subjected to a bar test could be greatly enhanced by either delta-9-THC or levonantradol (Moss *et al.*, 1981, 1984; Montgomery *et al.*, 1985). The hypokinetic rats showed postural rigidity but no sign of "waxy flexibility" and were therefore not regarded as being cataleptic. CBD also enhanced the hypokinetic response to reserpine, albeit to a lesser extent than delta-9-THC, whereas cannabichromene was without effect (Moss *et al.*, 1984). Similar synergistic interactions have been observed in rats between delta-9-THC and both haloperidol and fluphenazine (Moss *et al.*, 1984; Moss *et al.*, 1988) and, in mice, the cataleptic response to delta-9-THC has been shown to be enhanced by the active isomer of flupentixol (Pertwee *et al.*, 1988). Several brain areas are implicated, levonantradol having been shown in rat experiments to interact with reserpine synergistically when injected bilaterally into the substantia nigra, corpus striatum or dorsomedial nucleus of the thalamus (Montgomery *et al.*, 1985). The hypothesis implies the existence of ongoing dopaminergic activity in the basal ganglia of delta-9-THC treated animals and there is evidence that the drug does stimulate DA release (Sections 6.2.2 and 10.1.1). There is also evidence from rat experiments with amphetamine that delta-9-THC-induced catalepsy in the bar test can be reduced by increased release of DA in the striatum (Gough and Olley, 1978). Although the hypothesis serves as a useful model, it is important to note that some drugs possessing the ability to reduce central dopaminergic transmission do not seem to undergo a synergistic interaction with delta-9-THC in the bar test. Thus no interaction has been detected in rats between delta-9-THC and chlorpromazine (Moss *et al.*, 1984). Moreover, doses of 6-hydroxydopamine and desipramine producing a selective depletion of brain DA, have been reported to have no effect on the cataleptic response of rats to delta-9-THC (Kataoka *et al.*, 1987). There is some evidence for an involvement of cholinergic (nicotinic) pathways in the interaction between delta-9-THC and dopamine antagonists/reserpine. For example, the hypokinesia produced in rats by combined administration of delta-9-THC and reserpine has been reported by Moss *et al.* (1981) to be slightly enhanced by physostigmine and to be attenuated by ethopropazine although not by scopolamine (or naloxone). In addition, experiments with rats have shown that the synergistic interaction between delta-9-THC and fluphenazine can be reduced by mecamylamine (Moss *et al.*, 1988) and that nicotine, injected either peripherally or directly into the corpus striatum, can markedly increase hypokinesia in animals which have been pretreated with reserpine or fluphenazine (Montgomery *et al.*, 1985; Moss *et al.*, 1988). An involvement of ACh is also supported by a report that the cataleptic response of rats to delta-9-THC can be potentiated by a central cholinergic stimulant (RS-86), injected either peripherally or directly into the globus pallidus or corpus striatum (Gough and Olley 1977, 1978).

Although the experiments described in this section suggest that stimulation or facilitation of GABAergic transmission can significantly modify certain responses to delta-9-THC, the question of whether or not any of the cannabinoid's effects are directly mediated by GABA-releasing pathways remains to be answered. The observation that delta-9-THC and drugs such as flurazepam or haloperidol have a synergistic inhibitory effect on extrapyramidal motor function raises the possibility that cannabinoids could come to have a role in the management of hyperkinetic motor disorders such as tardive dyskinesia and Huntington's disease. Either disorder might be successfully treated by drugs which enhance the inhibitory component of GABA's effect on motor function without simultaneously augmenting the excitatory component and this objective might well be achieved if delta-9-THC or some other cannabinoid were administered to patients together with a directly or indirectly acting GABA-mimetic. Cannabinoids might also be used to increase the effectiveness of dopamine antagonists in the management of hyperkinetic motor disorders (Moss *et al.*, 1981, 1984). Further studies are required to investigate the role of cannabinoids in the treatment of such extrapyramidal disorders. More research is also needed to determine whether interactions between cannabinoids and GABA-mimetic drugs might be exploited therapeutically in other ways, for example, in the treatment of epilepsy and anxiety.

10.2. The Synapse—A Primary Site of Action?

There are several reasons for believing that the synapse is an important site of action for delta-9-THC. These may be summarized as follows.

(i) After entry into the brain there is evidence that delta-9-THC and its metabolites accumulate in the grey matter (Kennedy and Waddell, 1972; Shannon and Fried, 1972) and may be particularly tightly bound to nerve endings (Hattori and McGeer, 1977).

(ii) There is some indirect evidence from electrophysiological experiments that delta-9-THC can alter synaptic transmission in the central nervous system and that it does so at doses lower than those required to impair impulse conduction along peripheral axons (Section 5).

(iii) Results from *in vitro* experiments suggest that delta-9-THC can produce a number of important changes at nerve terminals. Thus it has been shown to affect the synthesis, storage and/or fate of NE, DA, 5-HT and GABA in synaptosomes (Section 6), the depolarization-dependent uptake of Ca^{2+} into synaptosomes (Section 5), the activities of ATPases present in synaptosomal or synaptic vesicular membranes (Section 7.2), the activity of synaptosomal lysophosphatidylcholine acyltransferase (Section 8) and the 'fluidity' of brain synaptic plasma membranes (Section 8). Of particular interest are effects which can be produced by delta-9-THC at concentrations of 1 μM or less (Section 4), especially if in addition they can only be produced by psychically active cannabinoids. Among such effects are certain delta-9-THC-induced changes in the synaptosomal uptake and storage of NE and DA and delta-9-THC-induced inhibition of lysophosphatidylcholine acyltransferase (Table 32). Delta-9-THC has also been shown to be highly potent in its inhibitory effect on depolarization-dependent synaptosomal uptake of Ca^{2+}. Results from experiments with CBN, CBD and 11-hydroxy-delta-9-THC (Section 5) have suggested that the ability of cannabinoids to produce this effect does not correlate with psychoactive potency.

(iv) There is evidence that as well as interacting with nerve terminals, delta-9-THC may act postsynaptically, altering the ability of certain transmitters to bind to their receptors (Section 6.7) or to elicit a response after binding (Sections 7.3 and 7.4).

10.3. Final Comments

It is clear from the material presented in this review that the central effects of delta-9-THC are mediated by more than one transmitter and that it can produce neuropharmacological changes in many areas of the brain (Section 10.1). There is good evidence for an involvement of NE, DA, 5-HT, ACh and GABA. Further studies are required to investigate the roles of other substances, in particular opioid peptides, prostaglandins and HA. Experiments are also needed to test whether non-opioid peptides or amino acids other than

GABA have a part to play in the psychopharmacology of delta-9-THC. The synergism between delta-9-THC and GABA-mimetic drugs is intriguing. Not only could it throw light on the mode of action of delta-9-THC but it could also come to be exploited clinically.

The synapse seems to be a particularly important target for delta-9-THC and there are signs that it can act presynaptically to alter neurotransmitter synthesis, storage, release and fate and postsynaptically to alter neurotransmitter receptor-mediated events both at the level of the recognition site and at the level of second messenger systems (Sections 7.4 and 10.2). The extent to which each of these changes contributes towards the psychological, behavioral, physiological and neuropharmacological effects of delta-9-THC in the whole organism remains to be determined.

It is likely that the neuropharmacological basis for each of the numerous effects produced by delta-9-THC *in vivo* is not always the same and that the part played by particular transmitters and brain areas varies from effect to effect. The possible roles of hippocampal ACh-releasing neurons in the effect of delta-9-THC on memory and of DA-releasing neurons of the nucleus accumbens in the effect of the drug on locomotor activity have already been mentioned (Sections 10.1.1 and 10.1.2). There is also evidence that delta-9-THC produces its effects on heart rate, blood pressure and respiration by interacting with the brain stem (Hosko *et al.*, 1984), that its cataleptic effect involves an interaction with the striatum (Gough and Olley, 1978) and that its effects on thermoregulation involve interactions with both brain stem and hypothalamus (Pertwee, 1985a).

Little is known about the nature of the molecular events underlying the effects of delta-9-THC other than that many, including psychic activity, probably depend on the ability of the drug to undergo structure-dependent interactions with neuronal membranes rather than on its high lipid solubility (Section 9). In particular, it is not yet known whether there is a specific delta-9-THC receptor. Also unknown is the extent to which membrane fluidity changes produced by delta-9-THC account for its psychopharmacological properties. The dose-dependent biphasic nature of many of the responses to delta-9-THC points to the existence of more than one mode of action. Consistent with this conclusion is the evidence that the relationship between cannabinoid structure and pharmacological activity is not the same for all responses.

The observation that the effect of cannabinoids on membrane fluidity can be altered by changing the chemical composition of the membrane (Section 8) raises the possibility that slight differences in the composition of neuronal membranes within the brain could impose some degree of selectivity on cannabinoids by causing them to interact more readily with some neuronal pathways than with others. Since there is evidence that delta-9-THC can change the lipid composition of brain membranes (Section 8) the question also arises as to whether changes in membrane composition could lead to delta-9-THC tolerance. Indeed, it has been suggested that changes in membrane lipid composition could have accounted for the development of tolerance to the stimulatory effect of cannabinoids on arachidonic acid release and prostaglandin production in lung fibroblasts (Burstein *et al.*, 1985b and Section 7.4). A similar 'membrane lipid adaptation' mechanism has been proposed to account for ethanol tolerance (Littleton, 1978; Little and Wing, 1983).

The extent to which some of the actions of delta-9-THC, for example those which affect the rate of removal of neurotransmitter from the synapse, alter transmission along a particular pathway probably depends on the pathway's 'ongoing activity'. The observations that changes in ambient temperature can alter the effect of delta-9-THC on brain levels of 5-HT (Section 6.3.1) and that stress can influence the effect of *in vivo* administration of delta-9-THC on the conversion in the brain of tyrosine to NE (Section 6.1.2) support this view since ambient temperature and stress are both expected to influence central neuronal activity. Because ongoing neuronal activity in the brain is highly variable, dependence on it could be one reason why the effect of delta-9-THC on central transmitter turnover appears to vary from brain area to brain area. Another reason for this could be that some of the changes in transmitter turnover produced by delta-9-THC are initiated indirectly, 'upstream' of the sites at which they are detected.

In conclusion, research into the central neuropharmacology of psychically active cannabinoids has led to advances in our understanding of how cannabinoids act at the electrophysiological level and has provided knowledge about the effects of these drugs on the synthesis, storage, release, actions and fate of central neurochemicals. It has also provided convincing evidence that the cannabinoids exert their central effects through interactions with targets located in cellular and/or subcellular membranes. There is still much to be learned about the central effects of cannabinoids especially with regard to the underlying molecular mechanisms and with regard to the part played by individual neurotransmitters. Cannabinoid research would be greatly facilitated if a selective delta-9-THC antagonist were to be developed and it is therefore important to establish the basis of the stereoselectivity shown by cannabinoids and, in particular, to resolve the question of whether or not there is a specific delta-9-THC receptor. The wide-ranging neuropharmacological properties of psychically active cannabinoids form a unique pharmacological spectrum that distinguishes the cannabinoids from all other centrally active drugs and, consequently, the notion that cannabinoids could be the prototypes of important novel therapeutic agents, is well worth pursuing. Although some modest advances have already been made in the search for roles for the cannabinoids in modern medicine, further basic preclinical research with these drugs is required if their therapeutic potential is to be fully explored.

REFERENCES

Abdel-Latif, A. A. (1986) Calcium-mobilizing receptors, polyphosphoinositides, and the generation of second messengers. *Pharmac. Rev.* **38**: 227–272.

Acosta-Urquidi, J. and Chase, R. (1975) The effects of delta-9-tetrahydrocannabinol on action potentials in the mollusc Aplysia. *Can. J. Physiol. Pharmac.* **53**: 793–798.

Agrawal, A. K., Kumar, P., Singh, N., Seth, P. K. and Bhargava, K. P. (1985) Cannabis and central dopaminergic transmission: effect on receptor sensitivity and behavioral modulation. *Res. Commun. Subst. Abuse* **6**: 11–22.

Agurell, S., Halldin, M., Lindgren, J.-E., Ohlsson, A., Widman, M., Gillespie, H. and Hollister, L. (1986) Pharmacokinetics and metabolism of delta-1-tetrahydrocannabinol and other cannabinoids with emphasis on man. *Pharmac. Rev.* **38**: 21–43.

Aldridge, J. W. and Pomeranz, B. (1977) Delta-1-tetrahydrocannabinol derivative enhances excitatory synaptic potentials through a presynaptic mechanism in crayfish neuromuscular junction. *Comp. Biochem. Physiol.* **57C**: 75–77.

Alhanaty, E. and Livne, A. (1974) Osmotic fragility of liposomes as affected by anti-hemolytic compounds. *Biochim. Biophys. Acta.* **339**: 146–155.

Askew, W. E. and Ho, B. T. (1974) Effects of tetrahydrocannabinols on cyclic AMP levels in rat brain areas. *Experientia* **30**: 879–880.

Askew, W. E., Kimball, A. P. and Ho, B. T. (1974) Effect of tetrahydrocannabinols on brain acetylcholine. *Brain Res.* **69**: 375–378.

Ayalon, D., Nir, I., Cordova, T., Bauminger, S., Puder, M., Naor, Z., Kashi, R., Zor, U., Harell, A. and Lindner, H. R. (1977) Acute effect of delta-1-tetrahydrocannabinol on the hypothalamo-pituitary-ovarian axis in the rat. *Neuroendocrinology* **23**: 31–42.

Bach, D., Raz, A. and Goldman, R. (1976a) The interaction of hashish compounds with planar lipid bilayer membranes (BLM). *Biochem. Pharmac.* **25**: 1241–1244.

Bach, D., Raz, A. and Goldman, R. (1976b) The effect of hashish compounds on phospholipid phase transition. *Biochim. Biophys. Acta.* **436**: 889–894.

Banerjee, A., Poddar, M. K., Saha, S. and Ghosh, J. J. (1975a) Effect of delta-9-tetrahydrocannabinol on monoamine oxidase activity of rat tissues in vivo. *Biochem. Pharmac.* **24**: 1435–1436.

Banerjee, S. P., Snyder, S. H. and Mechoulam, R. (1975b) Cannabinoids: Influence on neurotransmitter uptake in rat brain synaptosomes. *J. Pharmac. Exp. Ther.* **194**: 74–81.

Banerjee, A., Poddar, M. K. and Ghosh, J. J. (1977) Action of delta-9-tetrahydrocannabinol on membrane-bound monoamine oxidase activity. *Toxicol. Appl. Pharmac.* **40**: 347–354.

Barrett, M. L., Gordon, D. and Evans, F. J. (1985) Isolation from Cannabis sativa L. of cannflavin—a novel inhibitor of prostaglandin production. *Biochem. Pharmac.* **34**: 2019–2024.

Beardsley, P. M., Balster, R. L. and Harris, L. S. (1986) Dependence on tetrahydrocannabinol in rhesus monkeys. *J. Pharmac. Exp. Ther.* **239**: 311–319.

Beardsley, P. M., Scimeca, J. A. and Martin, B. R. (1987) Studies on the agonistic activity of delta-9,11-tetrahydrocannabinol in mice, dogs and rhesus monkeys and its interactions with delta-9-tetrahydrocannabinol. *J. Pharmac. Exp. Ther.* **241**: 521–526.

Bensemana, D. and Gascon, A. L. (1974) Effect of delta-9-THC on the distribution uptake and release of catecholamine in rats. *Rev. Can. Biol.* **33**: 269–278.

Bhattacharya, S. K. (1986) Delta-9-tetrahydrocannabinol (THC) increases brain prostaglandins in the rat. *Psychopharmacology* **90**: 499–502.

BHATTACHARYA, S. K., GHOSH, P. and SANYAL, A. K. (1980) Effects of prostaglandins on some central pharmacological actions of cannabis. *Indian J. Med Res.* **71**: 955–960.

BHATTACHARYYA, A. K., AULAKH, C. S., PRADHAN, S., GHOSH, P. and PRADHAN, S. N. (1980) Behavioral and neurochemical effects of delta-9-tetrahydrocannabinol in rats. *Neuropharmacology* **19**: 87–96.

BIEGER, D. and HOCKMAN, C. H. (1973) Differential effects produced by delta-1-tetrahydrocannabinol on lateral geniculate neurones. *Neuropharmacology* **12**: 269–273.

BINDER, M. and FRANKE, I. (1982) Is there a THC receptor? Current perspectives and approaches to the elucidation of the molecular mechanisms of action of the psychotropic constituents of Cannabis sativa L. In: *Neuroceptors*, pp. 151–161. HUCHO, F. (ed.) Walter de Gruyter, Berlin.

BINDER, M., EDERY, H. and PORATH, G. (1979) Delta-7-tetrahydrocannabinol, a non-psychotropic cannabinoid: structure activity considerations in the cannabinoid series. In: *Marihuana: Biological Effects*, pp. 71–80, NAHAS, G. G. and PATON, W. D. M. (eds) Pergamon Press, Oxford.

BINDER, M., WITTELER, F.-J., SCHMIDT, B., FRANKE, I., BOHNENBERGER, E. and SANDERMANN, H. (1984) Triglyceride/phospholipid partitioning and pharmacokinetics of some natural and semi-synthetic cannabinoids: further evidence for the involvement of specific receptors in the mediation of the psychotropic effects of delta-1-THC and delta-6-THC. In: *The Cannabinoids: Chemical, Pharmacologic and Therapeutic Aspects*, pp. 709–727. Agurell, S., Dewey, W. L. and WILLETTE, R. E. (eds) Academic Press, New York.

BINO, T., CHARI-BITRON, A. and SHAHAR, A. (1972) Biochemical effects and morphological changes in rat liver mitochondria exposed to delta-1-tetrahydrocannabinol. *Biochim. Biophys. Acta.* **288**: 195–202.

BLOOM, A. S. (1982) Effect of delta-9-tetrahydrocannabinol on the synthesis of dopamine and norepinephrine in mouse brain synaptosomes. *J. Pharmac. Exp. Ther.* **221**: 97–103.

BLOOM, A. S. (1984) Effects of cannabinoids on neurotransmitter receptors in the brain. In: *The Cannabinoids: Chemical, Pharmacologic and Therapeutic Aspects*, pp. 575–589, AGURELL, S., DEWEY, W. L. and WILLETTE, R. E. (eds) Academic Press, New York.

BLOOM, A. S. and HILLARD, C. J. (1985) Cannabinoids, neurotransmitter receptors and brain membranes. In: *Marihuana '84*, pp. 217–231, HARVEY, D. J. (ed.) IRL Press, Oxford.

BLOOM, A. S. and KIERNAN, C. J. (1980) Interaction of ambient temperature with the effects of delta-9-tetrahydrocannabinol on brain catecholamine synthesis and plasma corticosterone levels. *Psychopharmacology* **67**: 215–219.

BLOOM, A. S., HAAVIK, C. O. and STREHLOW, D. (1978a) Effects of delta-9-tetrahydrocannabinol on ATPases in mouse brain subcellular fractions. *Life Sci.* **23**: 1399–1404.

BLOOM, A. S., JOHNSON, K. M. and DEWEY, W. L. (1978b) The effects of cannabinoids on body temperature and brain catecholamine synthesis. *Res. Commun. Chem. Path. Pharmac.* **20**: 51–57.

BOWERS, M. B. and HOFFMAN, F. J. (1986) Regional brain homovanillic acid following delta-9-tetrahydrocannabinol and cocaine. *Brain Res.* **366**: 405–407.

BOYD, E. S. and MERITT, D. A. (1965) Effects of a tetrahydrocannabinol derivative on some motor systems in the cat. *Arch. Int. Pharmacodyn. Ther.* **153**: 1–12.

BOYD, E. S. and MERITT, D. A. (1966) Effects of barbiturates and a tetrahydrocannabinol derivative on recovery cycles of medial lemniscus, thalamus and reticular formation in the cat. *J. Pharmac. Exp. Ther.* **151**: 376–384.

BOYD, E. S., BOYD, E. H., MUCHMORE, J. S. and BROWN, L. E. (1971) Effects of two tetrahydrocannabinols and of pentobarbital on cortico-cortical evoked responses in the squirrel monkey. *J. Pharmac. Exp. Ther.* **176**: 480–488.

BOYD, E. S., BOYD, E. H. and BROWN, L. E. (1974) The effects of some drugs on an evoked response sensitive to tetrahydrocannabinols. *J. Pharmac. Exp. Ther.* **189**: 748–758.

BOYD, E. H., BOYD, E. S. and BROWN, L. E. (1975) Differential effects of a tetrahydrocannabinol and pentobarbital on cerebral cortical neurones. *Neuropharmacology* **14**: 533–536.

BOYD, E. S., BOYD, E. H. and BROWN, L. E. (1976) Effects of delta-9-tetrahydrocannabinol and pentobarbital on a cortical response evoked during conditioning. *Psychopharmacology* **47**: 119–122.

BRACS, P., JACKSON, D. M. and CHESHER, G. B. (1975) The effect of delta-9-tetrahydrocannabinol on brain amine concentration and turnover in whole rat brain and in various regions of the brain. *J. Pharm. Pharmac.* **27**: 713–715.

BRADY, R. O. and CARBONE, E. (1973) Comparisons of the effects of delta-9-tetrahydrocannabinol, 11-hydroxy-delta-9-tetrahydrocannabinol and ethanol on the electrophysiological activity of the giant axon of the squid. *Neuropharmacology* **12**: 601–605.

BRAESTRUP, C. and SQUIRES, R. F. (1978) Pharmacological characterization of benzodiazepine receptors in the brain. *Eur. J. Pharmac.* **48**: 263–270.

BRITTON, R. S. and MELLORS, A. (1974) Lysis of rat liver lysosomes *in vitro* by delta-9-tetrahydrocannabinol. *Biochem. Pharmac.* **23**: 1342–1344.

BRUGGEMANN, E. P. and MELCHIOR, D. L. (1983) Alterations in the organization of phosphatidylcholine/cholesterol bilayers of tetrahydrocannabinol. *J. Biol. Chem.* **258**: 8298–8303.

BURSTEIN, S. and HUNTER, S. A. (1978) Prostaglandins and cannabis – VI. Release of arachidonic acid from HeLa cells by delta-1-tetrahydrocannabinol and other cannabinoids. *Biochem. Pharmac.* **27**: 1275–1280.

BURSTEIN, S. and HUNTER, S. A. (1981) Prostaglandins and cannabis – VIII. Elevation of phospholipase A_2 activity by cannabinoids in whole cells and subcellular preparations. *J. Clin. Pharmac.* (*Suppl.*) **21**: 240S–248S.

BURSTEIN, S. and HUNTER, S. A. (1984) The role of prostaglandins in the actions of the cannabinoids. In: *The Cannabinoids: Chemical Pharmacologic and Therapeutic Aspects*, pp. 729–738, AGURELL, S., DEWEY, W. L. and WILLETTE, R. E. (eds.) Academic Press, New York.

BURSTEIN, S. and RAZ, A. (1972) Inhibition of prostaglandin E_2 biosynthesis by delta-1-tetrahydrocannabinol. *Prostaglandins* **2**: 369–374.

BURSTEIN, S., LEVIN, E. and VARANELLI, C. (1973) Prostaglandins and cannabis – II. Inhibition of biosynthesis by the naturally occurring cannabinoids. *Biochem. Pharmac.* **22**: 2905–2910.

BURSTEIN, S., HUNTER, S. A. and SHOUPE, T. S. (1978) Inhibition of cholesterol esterases by delta-1-tetrahydrocannabinol. *Life Sci.* **23**: 979–982.

BURSTEIN, S., HUNTER, S. A. and SHOUPE, T. S. (1979a) Cannabinoid inhibition of rat luteal cell progesterone synthesis. *Res. Commun. Chem. Path. Pharmac.* **24**: 413–416.

BURSTEIN, S., HUNTER, S. A. and SHOUPE, T. S. (1979b) Site of inhibition of Leydig cell testosterone synthesis by delta-1-tetrahydrocannabinol. *Mol. Pharmac.* **15**: 633–640.

BURSTEIN, S., HUNTER, S. A. and SHOUPE, T. S. (1980) Cannabinoid inhibition of rat brain cholesterol esterase activity. *Res. Commun. Subst. Abuse* **1**: 125–128.

BURSTEIN, S., HUNTER, S. A., SEDOR, C. and SHULMAN, S. (1982a) Prostaglandins and cannabis—IX. Stimulation of prostaglandin E_2 synthesis in human lung fibroblasts by delta-1-tetrahydrocannabinol. *Biochem. Pharmac.* **31**: 2361–2365.

BURSTEIN, S., OZMAN, K., BURSTEIN, E., PALERMO, N. and SMITH, E. (1982b) Prostaglandins and cannabis—XI. Inhibition of delta-1-tetrahydrocannabinol-induced hypotension by aspirin. *Biochem. Pharmac.* **31**: 591–592.

BURSTEIN, S., HUNTER, S. A. and OZMAN, K. (1983) Prostaglandins and cannabis—XII. The effect of cannabinoid structure on the synthesis of prostaglandins by human lung fibroblasts. *Mol. Pharmac.* **23**: 121–126.

BURSTEIN, S., HUNTER, S. A., OZMAN, K. and RENZULLI, L. (1984) Prostaglandins and cannabis—XIII. Cannabinoid-induced elevation of lipoxygenase products in mouse peritoneal macrophages. *Biochem. Pharmac.* **33**: 2653–2656.

BURSTEIN, S., HUNTER, S. A., OZMAN, K. and RENZULLI, L. (1985a) *In vitro* models of cannabinoid-induced psychoactivity. In: *Marihuana '84*, pp. 399–406, HARVEY, D. J. (ed.) IRL Press, Oxford.

BURSTEIN, S., HUNTER, S. A. and RENZULLI, L. (1985b) Prostaglandins and cannabis—XIV. Tolerance to the stimulatory actions of cannabinoids on arachidonate metabolism. *J. Pharmac. Exp. Ther.* **235**: 87–91.

BURSTEIN, S., HUNTER, S. A., LATHAM, V., MECHOULAM, R., MELCHIOR, D. L., RENZULLI, L. and TEFFT, R. E. (1986a) Prostaglandins and cannabis—XV. Comparison of enantiomeric cannabinoids in stimulating prostaglandin synthesis in fibroblasts. *Life Sci.* **39**: 1813–1823.

BURSTEIN, S., HUNTER, S. A., LATHAM, V. and RENZULLI, L. (1986b) Prostaglandins and cannabis—XVI. Antagonism of delta-1-tetrahydrocannabinol action by its metabolites. *Biochem. Pharmac.* **35**: 2553–2558.

BURSTEIN, S., HUNTER, S. A., LATHAM, V. and RENZULLI, L. (1987) A major metabolite of delta-1-tetrahydrocannabinol reduces its cataleptic effect in mice. *Experientia* **43**: 402–403.

BURSTEIN, S., HUNTER, S. A., LATHAM, V. and RENZULLI, L. (1988) Prostaglandin E_2 mediation of THC-induced catalepsy in the mouse. In: Marijuana: An International Research Report, pp. 371–376, CHESHER, G., CONSROE, P. and MUSTY, R. (eds) Australian Government Publishing Service, Canberra.

BYCK, R. and RITCHIE, J. M. (1973) Delta-9-tetrahydrocannabinol: Effects on mammalian nonmyelinated nerve fibers. *Science* **180**: 84–85.

CAMPBELL, K. A., FOSTER, T. C., HAMPSON, R. E. and DEADWYLER, S. A. (1986a) Delta-9-tetrahydrocannabinol differentially affects sensory-evoked potentials in the rat dentate gyrus. *J. Pharmac. Exp. Ther.* **239**: 936–940.

CAMPBELL, K. A., FOSTER, T. C., HAMPSON, R. E. and DEADWYLER, S. A. (1986b) Effects of delta-9-tetrahydrocannabinol on sensory-evoked discharges of granule cells in the dentate gyrus of behaving rats. *J. Pharmac. Exp. Ther.* **239**: 941–945.

CARNEY, J. M., BALSTER, R. L., MARTIN, B. R. and HARRIS, L. S. (1979) Effects of systemic and intraventricular administration of cannabinoids on schedule-controlled responding in the squirrel monkey. *J. Pharmac. Exp. Ther.* **210**: 399–404.

CHARI-BITRON, A. (1971) Stabilization of rat erythrocyte membrane by delta-1-tetrahydrocannabinol. *Life Sci.* **10**: 1273–1279.

CHARI-BITRON, A. and BINO, T. (1971) Effect of delta-1-tetrahydrocannabinol on ATPase activity of rat liver mitochondria. *Biochem. Pharmac.* **20**: 473–475.

CHARI-BITRON, A. and SHAHAR, A. (1979) Changes in rat erythrocyte membrane induced by delta-1-tetrahydrocannabinol, scanning electron microscope study. *Experientia* **35**: 365–366.

CLARKE, D. E. and JANDHYALA, B. (1977) Acute and chronic effects of tetrahydrocannabinols on monoamine oxidase activity: Possible vehicle/tetrahydrocannabinol interactions. *Res. Commun. Chem. Path. Pharmac.* **17**: 471–480.

COLLINS, F. G. and HAAVIK, C. O. (1979) Effects of cannabinoids on cardiac microsomal CaATPase activity and calcium uptake. *Biochem. Pharmac.* **28**: 2303–2306.

CONSROE, P., BENEDITO, M. A. C., LEITE, J. R., CARLINI, E. A. and MECHOULAM, R. (1982) Effects of cannabidiol on behavioral seizures caused by convulsant drugs or current in mice. *Eur. J. Pharmac.* **83**: 293–298.

CONTI, L. H. and MUSTY, R. E. (1984) The effects of delta-9-tetrahydrocannabinol injections to the nucleus accumbens on the locomotor activity of rats. In: *The Cannabinoids: Chemical, Pharmacologic and Therapeutic Aspects*, pp. 649–655, AGURELL, S., DEWEY, W. L. and WILLETTE, R. E. (eds.) Academic Press, New York.

CORNICELLI, J. A., GILMAN, S. R., KROM, B. A. and KOTTKE, B. A. (1981) Cannabinoids impair the formation of cholesteryl ester in cultured human cells. *Arteriosclerosis* **1**: 449–454.

COSTA, E., CHENEY, D. L. and MURRAY, T. F. (1981) Levonantradol-induced inhibition of acetylcholine turnover in rat hippocampus and striatum. *J. Clin. Pharmac.* (*Suppl.*) **21**: 256S-261S.

COUPAR, I. M. and TAYLOR, D. A. (1982) Alteration in the level of endogenous hypothalamic prostaglandins induced by delta-9-tetrahydrocannabinol in the rat. *Br. J. Pharmac.* **76**: 115–119.

DAGIRMANJIAN, R. and BOYD, E. S. (1962) Some pharmacological effects of two tetrahydrocannabinols. *J. Pharmac. Exp. Ther.* **135**: 25–33.

DALTERIO, S., BARTKE, A., ROBERSON, C., WATSON, D. and BURSTEIN, S. (1978) Direct and pituitary-mediated effects of delta-9-THC and cannabinol on the testis. *Pharmac. Biochem. Behav.* **8**: 673–678.

DALTERIO, S. L., BERNARD, S. A. and ESQUIVEL, C. R. (1987) Acute delta-9-tetrahydrocannabinol exposure alters Ca^{2+}-ATPase activity in neuroendocrine and gonadal tissues in mice. *Eur. J. Pharmac.* **137**: 91–100.

DEVANE, W. A., SPAIN, J. W., COSCIA, C. J. and HOWLETT, A. C. (1986) An assessment of the role of opioid receptors in the response to cannabimimetic drugs. *J. Neurochem.* **46**: 1929–1935.

DEWEY, W. L. (1986) Cannabinoid pharmacology. *Pharmac. Rev.* **38**: 151–178.

DEWEY, W. L., YONCE, L. R., HARRIS, L. S., REAVIS, W. M., GRIFFIN, E. D. and NEWBY, V. E. (1970) Some cardiovascular effects of trans-delta-9-tetrahydrocannabinol (delta-9-THC). *Pharmacologist* **12**: 258.

DIASIO, R. B., ETTINGER, D. S. and SATTERWHITE, B. E. (1981) Oral levonantradol in the treatment of chemotherapy-induced emesis: preliminary observations. *J. Clin. Pharmac.* (*Suppl.*) **21**: 81S–85S.

DOLBY, T. W. and KLEINSMITH, L. J. (1974) Effects of delta-9-tetrahydrocannabinol on the levels of cyclic adenosine 3′,5′-monophosphate in mouse brain. *Biochem. Pharmac.* **23**: 1817–1825.

DOLBY, T. W. and KLEINSMITH, L. J. (1977) Cannabinoid effects on adenylate cyclase and phosphodiesterase activities of mouse brain. *Can. J. Physiol. Pharmac.* **55**: 934–942.

DOMINO, E. F. (1981) Cannabinoids and the cholinergic system. *J. Clin. Pharmac.* (*Suppl.*) **21**: 249S-255S.

DOMINO, E. F. and BARTOLINI, A. (1972) Effects of various psychotomimetic agents on the EEG and acetylcholine release from the cerebral cortex of brain-stem transected cats. *Neuropharmacology* **11**: 703–713.

EDERY, H. and GOTTESFELD, Z. (1975) The gamma-aminobutyric acid system in rat cerebellum during cannabinoid-induced cataleptoid state. *Br. J. Pharmac.* **54**: 406–408.

EDERY, H., GRUNFELD, Y., BEN-ZVI, Z. and MECHOULAM, R. (1971) Structural requirements for cannabinoid activity. *Ann. N.Y. Acad. Sci.* **191**: 40–53.

ENGLERT, L. F., HO, B. T. and TAYLOR, D. (1973) The effects of (−) delta-9-tetrahydrocannabinol on reserpine-induced hypothermia in rats. *Br. J. Pharmac.* **49**: 243–252.

EVANS, A. T., FORMUKONG, E. and EVANS, F. J. (1987a) Activation of phospholipase A_2 by cannabinoids. FEBS Letters **211**: 119–122.

EVANS, A. T., FORMUKONG, E. A. and EVANS, F. J. (1987b) Actions of cannabis constituents on enzymes of arachidonate metabolism: anti-inflammatory potential. *Biochem. Pharmac.* **36**: 2035–2037.

FAIRBAIRN, J. W. and PICKENS, J. T. (1979) The oral activity of delta-1-tetrahydrocannabinol and its dependence on prostaglandin E_2. *Br. J. Pharmac.* **67**: 379–385.

FAIRBAIRN, J. W. and PICKENS, J. T. (1980) The effect of conditions influencing endogenous prostaglandins on the activity of delta-1-tetrahydrocannabinol in mice. *Br. J. Pharmac.* **69**: 491–493.

FEENEY, D. M. (1979) Marihuana and epilepsy: Paradoxical anticonvulsant and convulsant effects. In: *Marihuana: Biological Effects*, pp. 643–657, NAHAS, G. G. and PATON, W. D. M. (eds.) Pergamon Press, Oxford.

FENNESSY, M. R. and TAYLOR, D. A. (1977) The effect of delta-9-tetrahydrocannabinol on both temperature and brain amine concentrations in the rat at different ambient temperatures. *Br. J. Pharmac.* **60**: 65–71.

FENNESSY, M. R., LEWIS, S. J., TAYLOR, D. A. and VERBERNE, A. J. M. (1983) Delta-9-tetrahydrocannabinol reduces brain regional histamine concentrations. *Br. J. Pharmac.* **78**: 452–454.

FILIPOVIC, N. and TRKOVNIK, M. (1980) Effect of single and repeated administration of delta-9-tetrahydrocannabinol on 5-hydroxytryptamine, noradrenaline, dopamine and tryptophan levels in the brain of Wistar rats. *Arch. Hig. Rada. Toksikol.* **31**: 293–297.

FOY, M. R., TEYLER, T. J. and VARDARIS, R. M. (1982) Delta-9-THC and 17-beta-estradiol in hippocampus. *Brain Res. Bull.* **8**: 341–345.

FRIEDMAN, E., HANIN, I. and GERSHON, S. (1976) Effect of tetrahydrocannabinols on ^{3}H-acetylcholine biosynthesis in various rat brain slices. *J. Pharmac. Exp. Ther.* **196**: 339–345.

GALLAGER, D. W., SANDERS-BUSH, E. and SULSER, F. (1971) Dissociation between behavioral effects and changes in metabolism of cerebral serotonin (5HT) following delta-9-tetrahydrocannabinol (THC). *Pharmacologist* **13**: 296.

GALLAGER, D. W., SANDERS-BUSH, E. and SULSER, F. (1972) Dissociation between behavioral effects and changes in metabolism of cerebral serotonin following delta-9-tetrahydrocannabinol. *Psychopharmacologia* **26**: 337–345.

GARRETT, E. R. and HUNT, C. A. (1974) Physicochemical properties, solubility and protein binding of delta-9-tetrahydrocannabinol. *J. Pharm. Sci.* **63**: 1056–1064.

GAWIENOWSKI, A. M., CHATTERJEE, D., ANDERSON, P. J., EPSTEIN, D. L. and GRANT, W. M. (1982) Effect of delta-9-tetrahydrocannabinol on monoamine oxidase activity in bovine eye tissue *in vitro*. *Invest. Ophthalmol. Vis. Sci.* **22**: 482–485.

GILBERT, J. C., PERTWEE, R. G. and WYLLIE, M. G. (1977) Effects of delta-9-tetrahydrocannabinol and cannabidiol on a Mg^{++}-ATPase of synaptic vesicles prepared from rat cerebral cortex. *Br. J. Pharmac.* **59**: 599–601.

GILL, E. W. and JONES, G. (1972) Brain levels of delta-1-tetrahydrocannabinol and its metabolites in mice—Correlation with behaviour and the effect of the metabolic inhibitors SKF 525A and piperonyl butoxide. *Biochem. Pharmac.* **21**: 2237–2248.

GILL, E. W., PATON, W. D. M. and PERTWEE, R. G. (1970) Preliminary experiments on the chemistry and pharmacology of cannabis. *Nature* **228**: 134–136.

GILL, E. W. and LAWRENCE, D. K. (1974) Blood and brain levels of delta-1-tetrahydrocannabinol in mice—The effect of 7-hydroxy-delta-1-tetrahydrocannabinol. *Biochem. Pharmac.* **23**: 1140–1143.

GILL, E. W. and LAWRENCE, D. K. (1976) The physicochemical mode of action of tetrahydrocannabinol on cell membranes. In: *Pharmacology of Marihuana*, Vol. 1, pp. 147–155, BRAUDE, M. C. and SZARA, S. (eds) Raven Press, New York.

GILL, E. W., JONES, G. and LAWRENCE, D. K. (1973) Contribution of the metabolite 7-OH-delta-1-tetrahydrocannabinol towards the pharmacological activity of delta-1-tetrahydrocannabinol in mice. *Biochem. Pharmac.* **22**: 175–184.

GOUGH, A. L. and OLLEY, J. E. (1977) Delta-9-tetrahydrocannabinol and the extrapyramidal system. *Psychopharmacology* **54**: 87–99.

GOUGH, A. L. and OLLEY, J. E. (1978) Catalepsy induced by intrastriatal injection of delta-9-THC and 11-hydroxy-delta-9-THC in the rat. *Neuropharmacology* **17**: 137–144.

GRAHAM, J. D. P., LEWIS, M. J. and WILLIAMS, J. (1974) The effect of delta-1-tetrahydrocannabinol on the noradrenaline and dopamine content of the brain and heart of the rat. *Br. J. Pharmac.* **52**: 446P.

GREENBERG, J. H. and MELLORS, A. (1978) Specific inhibition of an acyltransferase by delta-9-tetrahydrocannabinol. *Biochem. Pharmac.* **27**: 329–333.

GREENBERG, J. H., SAUNDERS, M. E. and MELLORS, A. (1977) Inhibition of a lymphocyte membrane enzyme by delta-9-tetrahydrocannabinol *in vitro. Science* **197**: 475–477.

GREENBERG, J. H., MELLORS, A. and MCGOWAN, J. C. (1978) Molar volume relationships and specific inhibition of a synaptosomal enzyme by psychoactive cannabinoids. *J. Med. Chem.* **21**: 1208-1212.

GREENTREE, S. G. and PERTWEE, R. G. (1987) Flurazepam enhances the ability of delta-9-tetrahydrocannabinol to induce catalepsy in mice. *Br. J. Pharmac.* **92**: 539P.

GRUNFELD, Y. and EDERY, H. (1969) Psychopharmacological activity of the active constituents of hashish and some related cannabinoids. *Psychopharmacology* **14**: 200–210.

GUHA, D. and PRADHAN, S. N. (1974) Effects of mescaline, delta-9-tetrahydrocannabinol and pentobarbital on the auditory evoked responses in the cat. *Neuropharmacology* **13**: 755–762.

HARRIS, R. A. and STOKES, J. A. (1982) Cannabinoids inhibit calcium uptake by brain synaptosomes. *J. Neurosci.* **2**: 443–447.

HARRIS, L. S., CARCHMAN, R. A. and MARTIN, B. R. (1978) Evidence for the existence of specific cannabinoid binding sites. *Life Sci.* **22**: 1131–1138.

HATTENDORF, C., HATTENDORF, M., COPER, H. and FERNANDES, M. (1977) Interaction between delta-9-tetrahydrocannabinol and d-amphetamine. *Psychopharmacology* **54**: 177–182.

HATTORI, T. and MCGEER, P. L. (1977) Electron microscopic autoradiography on delta-8-[^{3}H]tetrahydrocannabinol localization in brain tissue. *Toxicol. Appl. Pharmac.* **39**: 307–311.

HELMREICH, E. J. M. and PFEUFFER, T. (1985) Regulation of signal transduction by beta-adrenergic hormone receptors. *Trends Pharmac. Sci.* **6**: 438–443.

HERSHKOWITZ, M. and SZECHTMAN, H. (1979) Pretreatment with delta-1-tetrahydrocannabinol and psychoactive drugs: Effects on uptake of biogenic amines and on behavior. *Eur. J. Pharmac.* **59**: 267–276.

HERSHKOWITZ, M., GOLDMAN, R. and RAZ, A. (1977) Effect of cannabinoids on neurotransmitter uptake, ATPase activity and morphology of mouse brain synaptosomes. *Biochem. Pharmac.* **26**: 1327–1331.

HILLARD, C. J. and BLOOM, A. S. (1982) Delta-9-tetrahydrocannabinol-induced changes in beta-adrenergic receptor binding in mouse cerebral cortex. *Brain Res.* **235**: 370–377.

HILLARD, C. J. and BLOOM, A. S. (1983) Possible role of prostaglandins in the effects of the cannabinoids on adenylate cyclase activity. *Eur. J. Pharmac.* **91**: 21–27.

HILLARD, C. J., BLOOM, A. S. and HOUSLAY, M. D. (1986) Effects of delta-9-tetrahydrocannabinol on glucagon receptor coupling to adenylate cyclase in rat liver plasma membranes. *Biochem. Pharmac.* **35**: 2797–2803.

HILLARD, C. J. and BLOOM, A. S. (1984) Further studies of the interaction of delta-9-tetrahydrocannabinol with the beta-adrenergic receptor. In: *The Cannabinoids: Chemical, Pharmacologic and Therapeutic Aspects*, pp. 591–602, AGURELL, S., DEWEY, W. L. and WILLETTE, R. E. (eds) Academic Press, New York.

HILLARD, C. J., HARRIS, R. A. and BLOOM, A. S. (1985) Effects of the cannabinoids on physical properties of brain membranes and phospholipid vesicles: Fluorescence studies. *J. Pharmac. Exp. Ther.* **232**: 579–588.

HO, B. T., TAYLOR, D., FRITCHIE, G. E., ENGLERT, L. F. and MCISAAC, W. M. (1972) Neuropharmacological study of delta-9- and delta-8-L-tetrahydrocannabinols in monkeys and mice. *Brain Res.* **38**: 163–170.

HO, B. T., ESTEVEZ, V. S. and ENGLERT, L. F. (1973) The uptake and metabolic fate of cannabinoids in rat brains. *J. Pharm. Pharmac.* **25**: 488–490.

HOEKMAN, T. B., DETTBARN, W.-D. and KLAUSNER, H. A. (1976) Actions of delta-9-tetrahydrocannabinol on neuromuscular transmission in the rat diaphragm. *Neuropharmacology* **15**: 315–319.

HOLLISTER, L. E. (1970) Tetrahydrocannabinol isomers and homologues: Contrasted effects of smoking. *Nature* **227**: 968–969.

HOLLISTER, L. E. (1973) Cannabidiol and cannabinol in man. *Experientia* **29**: 825–826.

HOLLISTER, L. E. (1986) Health aspects of cannabis. *Pharmac. Rev.* **38**: 1–20.

HOLLISTER, L. E. and GILLESPIE, H. K. (1973) Delta-8- and delta-9-tetrahydrocannabinol. *Clin. Pharmac. Ther.* **14**: 353–357.

HOLLISTER, L. E. and GILLESPIE, H. K. (1975) Action of delta-9-tetrahydrocannabinol. An approach to the active metabolite hypothesis. *Clin. Pharmac. Ther.* **18**: 714–719.

HOLLISTER, L. E., GILLESPIE, H. K., MECHOULAM, R. and SREBNIK, M. (1987) Human pharmacology of 1S and 1R enantiomers of delta-3-tetrahydrocannabinol. *Psychopharmacology* **92**: 505–507.

HOLLISTER, L. E., RICHARDS, R. K. and GILLESPIE, H. K. (1968) Comparison of tetrahydrocannabinol and synhexyl in man. *Clin. Pharmac. Ther.* **9**: 783–791.

HOLTZMAN, D., LOVELL, R. A., JAFFE, J. H. and FREEDMAN, D. X. (1969) 1-delta-9-tetrahydrocannabinol: Neurochemical and behavioral effects in the mouse. *Science* **163**: 1464–1467.

HOSKO, M. J., SCHMELING, W. T. and HARDMAN, H. F. (1984) Delta-9-tetrahydrocannabinol: site of action for autonomic effects. In: *The Cannabinoids: Chemical, Pharmacologic and Therapeutic Aspects*, pp. 635–648, AGURELL, S., DEWEY, W. L. and WILLETTE, R. E. (eds) Academic Press, New York.

HOWES, J. and OSGOOD, P. (1974) The effect of delta-9-tetrahydrocannabinol on the uptake and release of ^{14}C-dopamine from crude striatal synaptosomal preparations. *Neuropharmacology* **13**: 1109–1114.

HOWLETT, A. C. (1984) Inhibition of neuroblastoma adenylate cyclase by cannabinoid and nantradol compounds. *Life Sci.* **35**: 1803–1810.

HOWLETT, A. C. (1985) Cannabinoid inhibition of adenylate cyclase. Biochemistry of the response in neuroblastoma cell membranes. *Mol. Pharmac.* **27**: 429–436.

HOWLETT, A. C. (1987) Cannabinoid inhibition of adenylate cyclase: relative activity of constituents and metabolites of marihuana. *Neuropharmacology* **26**: 507–512.

HOWLETT, A. C. and FLEMING, R. M. (1984) Cannabinoid inhibition of adenylate cyclase. Pharmacology of the response in neuroblastoma cell membranes. *Mol. Pharmac.* **26**: 532–538.

HOWLETT, A. C., QUALY, J. M. and KHACHATRIAN, L. L. (1986) Involvement of G_i in the inhibition of adenylate cyclase by cannabimimetic drugs. *Mol. Pharmac.* **29**: 307–313.

Hunter, S. A., Burstein, S. and Renzulli, L. (1986) Effects of cannabinoids on the activities of mouse brain lipases. *Neurochem. Res.* **11**: 1273–1288.

Hunter, S. A., Latham, V., Renzulli, L. and Burstein, S. (1988) *In vivo* effects of delta-1-tetrahydrocannabinol (delta-1-THC) on rat and mouse prostaglandin tissue levels. In: Marijuana: An International Research Report, pp. 399–404, Chesher, G., Consroe, P. and Musty, R. (eds.) Australian Government Publishing Service, Canberra.

Huszar, L. A., Greenberg, J. H. and Mellors, A. (1977) Effects of delta-9-tetrahydrocannabinol on lymphocyte and synaptosomal lysophosphatidylcholine acyltransferase *in vivo*. *Mol. Pharmac.* **13**: 1086–1091.

Isbell, H., Gorodetzsky, C. W., Jasinski, D., Clausen, U., Spulak, F. v. and Korte, F. (1967) Effects of (−) delta-9-trans-tetrahydrocannabinol in man. *Psychopharmacology* **11**: 184–188.

Izquierdo, I. and Nasello, A. G. (1973) Effects of cannabidiol and of diphenylhydantoin on the hippocampus and on learning. *Psychopharmacology* **31**: 167–175.

Izquierdo, I., Orsingher, O. A. and Berardi, A. C. (1973) Effect of cannabidiol and of other Cannabis sativa compounds on hippocampal seizure discharges. *Psychopharmacology* **28**: 95–102.

Jain, M. L., Curtis, B. M. and Bakutis, E. V. (1974) *In vivo* effect of LSD, morphine, ethanol and delta-9-tetrahydrocannabinol on mouse brain adenosine triphosphatase activity. *Res. Commun. Chem. Path. Pharmac.* **7**: 229–232.

Johnson, K. M. and Dewey, W. L. (1978a) The effect of delta-9-tetrahydrocannabinol on the conversion of [^{3}H] tryptophan to 5-[^{3}H] hydroxytryptamine in the mouse brain. *J. Pharmac. Exp. Ther.* **207**: 140–150.

Johnson, K. M. and Dewey, W. L. (1978b) Effects of delta-9-THC on the synaptosomal uptake of ^{3}H-tryptophan and ^{3}H-choline. *Pharmacology* **17**: 83–87.

Johnson, K. M., Dewey, W. L. and Harris, L. S. (1976a) Some structural requirements for inhibition of high-affinity synaptosomal serotonin uptake by cannabinoids. *Mol. Pharmac.* **12**: 345–352.

Johnson, K. M., Ho, B. T. and Dewey, W. L. (1976b) Effects of delta-9-tetrahydrocannabinol on neurotransmitter accumulation and release mechanisms in rat forebrain synaptosomes. *Life Sci.* **19**: 347–356.

Johnson, K. M., Dewey, W. L. and Bloom, A. S. (1981) Adrenalectomy reverses the effects of delta-9-THC on mouse brain 5-hydroxytryptamine turnover. *Pharmacology* **23**: 223–229.

Jones, R. T. (1985) Cardiovascular effects of cannabinoids. In: *Marihuana '84*, pp. 325–334, Harvey, D. J. (ed.) IRL Press, Oxford.

Jordan, V. C. and Castracane, V. D. (1976) The effect of reported prostaglandin synthetase inhibitors on estradiol-stimulated uterine prostaglandin biosynthesis *in vivo* in the ovariectomized rat. *Prostaglandins* **12**: 1073–1081.

Karler, R. and Turkanis, S. A. (1979) Cannabis and epilepsy. In: *Marihuana: Biological Effects*, pp. 619–641, Nahas, G. G. and Paton, W. D. M. (eds.) Pergamon Press, Oxford.

Kataoka, Y., Ohta, H., Fujiwara, M., Oishi, R. and Ueki, S. (1987) Noradrenergic involvement in catalepsy induced by delta-9-tetrahydrocannabinol. *Neuropharmacology* **26**: 55–60.

Kayaalp, S. O., Kaymakcalan, S., Verimer, T., Ilhan, M. and Onur, R. (1974) *In vitro* neuromuscular effects of delta-9-trans-tetrahydrocannabinol (THC). *Arch. Int. Pharmacodyn.* **212**: 67–75.

Kaymakcalan, S., Ercan, Z. S. and Türker, R. K. (1975) The evidence of the release of prostaglandin-like material from rabbit kidney and guinea-pig lung by (−)-trans-delta-9-tetrahydrocannabinol. *J. Pharm. Pharmac.* **27**: 564–568.

Kelly, L. A. and Butcher, R. W. (1973) The effects of delta-1-tetrahydrocannabinol on cyclic AMP levels in W1-38 fibroblasts. *Biochim. Biophys. Acta* **320**: 540–544.

Kelly, L. A. and Butcher, R. W. (1979) Effects of delta-1-tetrahydrocannabinol on cyclic AMP in cultured human diploid fibroblasts. *J. Cyclic Nucleotide Res.* **5**: 303–313.

Kennedy, J. S. and Waddell, W.J. (1972) Whole-body autoradiography of the pregnant mouse after administration of ^{14}C-delta-9-THC. *Toxicol. Appl. Pharmac.* **22**: 252–258.

Klausner, H. A. and Dingell, J. V. (1971) The metabolism and excretion of delta-9-tetrahydrocannabinol in the rat. *Life Sci.* **10**: 49–59.

Koe, B. K. (1981) Levonantradol, a potent cannabinoid-related analgesic, antagonizes haloperidol-induced activation of striatal dopamine synthesis. *Eur. J. Pharmac.* **70**: 231–235.

Koe, B. K. and Weissman, A. (1981) Facilitation of benzodiazepine binding by levonantradol. *J. Clin. Pharmac.* (*Suppl.*) **21**: 397S–405S.

Koe, B. K., Milne, G. M., Weissman, A., Johnson, M. R. and Melvin, L. S. (1985) Enhancement of brain [^{3}H]flunitrazepam binding and analgesic activity of synthetic cannabimimetics. *Eur. J. Pharmac.* **109**: 201–212.

Kujtan, P. W., Carlen, P. L. and Kapur, B. M. (1983) Delta-9-tetrahydrocannabinol and cannabidiol: Dose dependent effects on evoked potentials in the hippocampal slice. *Can. J. Physiol. Pharmac.* **61**: 420–426.

Kumbaraci, N. M. and Nastuk, W. L. (1980) Effects of delta-9-tetrahydrocannabinol on excitable membranes and neuromuscular transmission. *Mol. Pharmac.* **17**: 344–349.

Lapa, A. J., Sampaio, C. A. M., Timo-Iaria, C. and Valle, J. R. (1968) Blocking action of tetrahydrocannabinol upon transmission in the trigeminal system of the cat. *J. Pharm. Pharmac.* **20**: 373–376.

Laszlo, J., Lucas, V. S., Hanson, D. C., Cronin, C. M. and Sallan, S. E. (1981) Levonantradol for chemotherapy-induced emesis: Phase I–II oral administration. *J. Clin. Pharmac.* (*Suppl.*) **21**: 51S–56S.

Laurent, B. and Roy, P. E. (1975) Alteration of membrane integrity by delta-1-tetrahydrocannabinol. *Int. J. Clin. Pharmac.* **12**: 261–266.

Laurent, B., Roy, P. E. and Gailis, L. (1974) Inhibition by delta-1-tetrahydrocannabinol of a Na^+-K^+ transport ATPase from rat ileum. Preliminary report. *Can. J. Physiol. Pharmac.* **52**: 1110–1113.

Lawrence, D. K. and Gill, E. W. (1975) The effects of delta-1-tetrahydrocannabinol and other cannabinoids on spin-labeled liposomes and their relationship to mechanisms of general anesthesia. *Mol. Pharmac.* **11**: 595–602.

Layman, J. M. and Milton, A. S. (1971) Some actions of delta-1-tetrahydrocannabinol and cannabidiol at cholinergic junctions. *Br. J. Pharmac.* **41**: 379P.

LEADER, J. P., KOE, B. K. and WEISSMAN, A. (1981) GABA-like actions of levonantradol. *J. Clin. Pharmac. (Suppl.)* **21**: 262S–270S.

LEE, G. M. and OLMSTED, C. A. (1976) Effects of cannabinoids on synaptic membrane enzymes. II. *In vivo* studies of NaK-ATPase in synaptic membranes isolated from rat brain. *Am. J. Drug Alcohol Abuse* **3**: 629–638.

LEMBERGER, L. (1980) Potential therapeutic usefulness of marijuana. *Annu. Rev. Pharmac. Toxicol.* **20**: 151–172.

LEMBERGER, L. (1985) Clinical evaluation of cannabinoids in the treatment of disease. In: *Marihuana '84*, pp. 673–680, HARVEY, D. J. (ed.) IRL Press, Oxford.

LEMBERGER, L. and ROWE, H. (1975) Clinical pharmacology of nabilone, a cannabinol derivative. *Clin. Pharmac. Ther.* **18**: 720–726.

LEMBERGER, L., CRABTREE, R. E. and ROWE, H. M. (1972) 11-hydroxy-delta-9-tetrahydrocannabinol: Pharmacology, disposition and metabolism of a major metabolite of marihuana in man. *Science* **177**: 62–63.

LEMBERGER, L., MARTZ, R., RODDA, B., FORNEY, R. and ROWE, H. (1973) Comparative pharmacology of delta-9-tetrahydrocannabinol and its metabolite, 11-OH-delta-9-tetrahydrocannabinol. *J. Clin. Invest.* **52**: 2411–2417.

LEMBERGER, L., MCMAHON, R., ARCHER, R., MATSUMOTO, K. and ROWE, H. (1974) Pharmacologic effects and physiologic disposition of delta-6a, 10a-dimethyl heptyl tetrahydrocannabinol (DMHP) in man. *Clin. Pharmac. Ther.* **15**: 380–386.

LEONARD, B. E. (1971) The effect of delta-1, 6-tetrahydrocannabinol on biogenic amines and their amino acid precursors in the rat brain. *Pharmac. Res. Commun.* **3**: 139–145.

LEUSCHNER, J. T. A., WING, D. R., HARVEY, D. J., BRENT, G. A., DEMPSEY, C. E., WATTS, A. and PATON, W. D. M. (1984) The partitioning of delta-1-tetrahydrocannabinol into erythrocyte membranes *in vivo* and its effect on membrane fluidity. *Experientia* **40**: 866–868.

LEW, E. O. H. and RICHARDSON, J. S. (1981) Neurochemical and behavioural correlates of the interaction between amphetamine and delta-9-tetrahydrocannabinol in the rat. *Drug Alcohol Depend.* **8**: 93–101.

LEWIS, S. J., FENNESSY, M. R., VERBERNE, A. J. M., JARROTT, B. and TAYLOR, D. A. (1986) The effects of delta-9-tetrahydrocannabinol (delta-9-THC) on the regional concentrations of spermidine in the rat brain. *Neurochem. Int.* **9**: 99–102.

LI, D. M. F. and NG, C. K. M. (1984) Effects of delta-1- and delta-6-tetrahydrocannabinol on the adenylate cyclase activity in ventricular tissue of the rat heart. *Clin. Exp. Pharmac. Physiol.* **11**: 81–85.

LINDAMOOD, C. and COLASANTI, B. K. (1980) Effects of delta-9-tetrahydrocannabinol and cannabidiol on sodium-dependent high affinity choline uptake in the rat hippocampus. *J. Pharmac. Exp. Ther.* **213**: 216–221.

LINDAMOOD, C. and COLASANTI, B. K. (1981a) Interaction between impulse-flow and delta-9-tetrahydrocannabinol within the septal-hippocampal cholinergic pathway of rat brain. *J. Pharmac. Exp. Ther.* **219**: 580–584.

LINDAMOOD, C. and COLASANTI, B. K. (1981b) Involvement of brain monoamines in the delta-9-tetrahydrocannabinol-induced reduction of hippocampal choline uptake. *J. Neurochem.* **37**: 788–791.

LITTLE, H. J. and WING, D. R. (1983) Alcohol. In: *Psychopharmacology I. Part I: Preclinical Psychopharmacology*, pp. 398–438, GRAHAME-SMITH, D. G. and COWEN, P. J. (eds) Excerpta Medica, Amsterdam.

LITTLETON, J. (1978) Alcohol tolerance and dependence at the cellular level. *Br. J. Addiction* **73**: 347–351.

MACLEAN, K. I. and LITTLETON, J. M. (1977) Environmental stress as a factor in the response of rat brain catecholamine metabolism to delta-8-tetrahydrocannabinol. *Eur. J. Pharmac.* **41**: 171–182.

MAHONEY, J. M. and HARRIS, R. A. (1972) Effect of delta-9-tetrahydrocannabinol on mitochondrial processes. *Biochem. Pharmac.* **21**: 1217–1226.

MAÎTRE, L., STAEHELIN, M. and BEIN, H. J. (1970) Effect of an extract of cannabis and of some cannabinols on catecholamine metabolism in rat brain and heart. *Agents and Actions* **1**: 136–143.

MAÎTRE, L., BAUMANN, P. A. and DELINI-STULA, A. (1972) Neurochemical tolerance to cannabinols. In: *Cannabis and its derivatives*, pp. 101–119. PATON, W. D. M. and CROWN, J. (eds) Oxford University Press, Oxford.

MARTIN, B. R. (1986) Cellular effects of cannabinoids. *Pharmac. Rev.* **38**: 45–74.

MARTIN, B. R., BALSTER, R. L., RAZDAN, R. K., HARRIS, L. S. and DEWEY, W. L. (1981) Behavioral comparisons of the stereoisomers of tetrahydrocannabinols. *Life Sci.* **29**: 565–574.

MARTIN, B. R., HARRIS, L. S. and DEWEY, W. L. (1984a) Pharmacological activity of delta-9-THC metabolites and analogs of CBD, delta-8-THC and delta-9-THC. In: *The Cannabinoids: Chemical, Pharmacologic and Therapeutic Aspects*, pp. 523–544, AGURELL, S., DEWEY, W. L. and WILLETTE, R. E. (eds) Academic Press, New York.

MARTIN, B. R., KALLMAN, M. J., KAEMPF, G. F., HARRIS, L. S., DEWEY, W. L. and RAZDAN, R. K. (1984b) Pharmacological potency of R- and S-3′-hydroxy-delta-9-tetrahydrocannabinol: Additional structural requirement for cannabinoid activity. *Pharmac. Biochem. Behav.* **21**: 61–65.

MAZOR, M., DVILANSKY, A., AHARON, M., LAZAROVITZ, Z. and NATHAN, I. (1982) Effect of cannabinoids on the activity of monoamine oxidase in normal human platelets. *Arch. Int. Physiol. Biochim.* **90**: 15–20.

MECHOULAM, R. (1973) Cannabinoid chemistry. In: *Marihuana. Chemistry, Pharmacology, Metabolism and Clinical Effects*, pp. 1–99, MECHOULAM, R. (ed.) Academic Press, New York.

MECHOULAM, R. (ed.) (1986) *Cannabinoids as Therapeutic Agents*, pp. 1–186, CRC Press, Boca Raton, Florida.

MECHOULAM, R. and EDERY, H. (1973) Structure-activity relationships in the cannabinoid series. In: *Marihuana, Chemistry, Pharmacology, Metabolism and Clinical Effects*, pp. 101–136, MECHOULAM, R. (ed.) Academic Press, New York.

MELLORS, A. (1979) Cannabinoids and membrane-bound enzymes. In: *Marihuana: Biological Effects*, pp. 329–342, NAHAS, G. G. and PATON, W. D. M. (eds) Pergamon Press, Oxford.

MILLER, L. L. (1984) Marijuana: acute effects on the human memory. In: *The Cannabinoids: Chemical, Pharmacologic and Therapeutic Aspects*, pp. 21–46, AGURELL, S., DEWEY, W. L. and WILLETTE, R. E. (eds) Academic Press, New York.

MILLER, L. L. and BRANCONNIER, R. J. (1983) Cannabis: effects on memory and the cholinergic limbic system. *Psychol. Bull.* **93**: 441–456.

MONTGOMERY, S. P., MOSS, D. E. and MANDERSCHIED, P. Z. (1985) Tetrahydrocannabinol and levonantradol effects on extrapyramidal motor behaviors: neuroanatomical location and hypothesis of mechanism. In: *Marihuana '84*, pp. 295–302, HARVEY, D. J. (ed.) IRL Press, Oxford.

MORONI, F., MALTHE-SORENSSEN, D., CHENEY, D. L. and COSTA, E. (1978) Modulation of ACh turnover in the septal-hippocampal pathway by electrical stimulation and lesioning. *Brain Res.* **150**: 333–341.

MORRISON, K. J. and PERTWEE, R. G. (1985) A possible link between delta-9-tetrahydrocannabinol and GABA in mice. *Br. J. Pharmac.* **86**: 684P.

MOSS, D. E., MANDERSCHEID, P. Z., KOBAYASHI, H. and MONTGOMERY, S. P. (1988) Evidence for the nicotinic cholinergic hypothesis of cannabinoid action within the central nervous system: extrapyramidal motor behaviors. In: Marijuana: An International Research Report, pp. 359–364, CHESHER, G., CONSROE, P. and MUSTY, R. (eds.) Australian Government Publishing Service, Canberra.

MOSS, D. E., MCMASTER, S. B. and ROGERS, J. (1981) Tetrahydrocannabinol potentiates reserpine-induced hypokinesia. *Pharmac. Biochem. Behav.* **15**: 779–783.

MOSS, D. E., MONTGOMERY, S. P., SALO, A. A. and STEGER, R. W. (1984) Tetrahydrocannabinol effects on extrapyramidal motor behaviors in an animal model of Parkinson's disease. In: *The Cannabinoids: Chemical, Pharmacologic and Therapeutic Aspects*, pp. 815–828, AGURELL, S., DEWEY, W. L. and WILLETTE, R. E. (eds.) Academic Press, New York.

MOSS, D. E., PECK, P. L. and SALOME, R. (1978) Tetrahydrocannabinol and acetylcholinesterase. *Pharmac. Biochem. Behav.* **8**: 763–765.

MUSTY, R. E. (1984) Possible anxiolytic effects of cannabidiol. In: *The Cannabinoids: Chemical, Pharmacologic and Therapeutic Aspects*, pp. 795–813, AGURELL, S., DEWEY, W. L. and WILLETTE, R. E. (eds) Academic Press, New York.

NIEMI, W. D. (1979) Effect of delta-9-tetrahydrocannabinol on synaptic transmission in the electric eel electroplaque. *Res. Commun. Chem. Path. Pharmac.* **25**: 537–546.

NOVELLI, G. P., PEDUTO, V. A., BERTOL, E., MARI, F. and PIERACCIOLI, E. (1983) Analgesic interaction between nitrous oxide and delta-9-tetrahydrocannabinol in the rat. *Br. J. Anaesth.* **55**: 997–1000.

NOWICKY, A. V., TEYLER, T. J. and VARDARIS, R. M. (1987) The modulation of long-term potentiation by delta-9-tetrahydrocannabinol in the rat hippocampus, *in vitro*. *Brain Res. Bull.* **19**: 663–672.

NYE, J. S., SELTZMAN, H. H., PITT, C. G. and SNYDER, S. H. (1985) High affinity cannabinoid binding sites in brain membranes labeled with [^{3}H]-5′-trimethylammonium delta-8-tetrahydrocannabinol. *J. Pharmac. Exp. Ther.* **234**: 784–791.

OHLSSON, A., AGURELL, S., LEANDER, K., DAHMEN, J., EDERY, H., PORATH, G., LEVY, S. and MECHOULAM, R. (1979) Synthesis and psychotropic activity of side-chain hydroxylated delta-6-tetrahydrocannabinol metabolites. *Acta Pharmac. Suecica* **16**: 21–33.

OHLSSON, A., WIDMAN, M., CARLSSON, S., RYMAN, T. and STRID, C. (1980) Plasma and brain levels of delta-6-THC and seven monooxygenated metabolites correlated to the cataleptic effect in the mouse. *Acta Pharmac. Toxicol.* **47**: 308–317.

OISHI, R., ITOH, Y., NISHIBORI, M. and SAEKI, K. (1985) Delta-9-tetrahydrocannabinol decreases turnover of brain histamine. *J. Pharmac. Exp. Ther.* **232**: 513–518.

OLMSTED, C. A. (1976) Effects of cannabinoids on synaptic membrane enzymes. I. *In vitro* studies on synaptic membranes isolated from rat brain. *Am. J. Drug Alcohol Abuse* **3**: 485–505.

OSGOOD, P. and HOWES, J. (1974) Cannabinoid induced changes in mouse striatal homovanillic and dihydroxyphenylacetic acid: The effects of amphetamine and L-DOPA. *Res. Commun. Chem. Path. Pharmac.* **9**: 621–631.

OUELLET, J., PALAIC, D., ALBERT, J.-M. and TETREAULT, L. (1973) Effect of delta-9-THC on serotonin, MAO and tryptophan hydroxylase in rat brain. *Rev. Can. Biol.* **32**: 213–217.

PANG, K.-Y. Y. and MILLER, K. W. (1978) Cholesterol modulates the effects of membrane perturbers in phospholipid vesicles and biomembranes. *Biochim. Biophys. Acta* **511**: 1–9.

PATON, W. D. M. (1974) Unconventional anaesthetic molecules. In: *Molecular Mechanisms in General Anaesthesia*, pp. 48–64, HALSEY, M. J., MILLAR, R. A. and SUTTON, J. A. (eds) Churchill Livingstone, Edinburgh.

PATON, W. D. M. (1975) Pharmacology of marijuana. *Annu. Rev. Pharmac.* **15**: 191–220.

PATON, W. D. M. and PERTWEE, R. G. (1973a) The pharmacology of cannabis in animals. In: *Marihuana. Chemistry, Pharmacology, Metabolism and Clinical Effects*, pp. 191–285, MECHOULAM R. (ed.) Academic Press, New York.

PATON, W. D. M. and PERTWEE, R. G. (1973b) The actions of cannabis in man. In: *Marihuana. Chemistry, Pharmacology, Metabolism and Clinical Effects*, pp. 287–333, MECHOULAM, R. (ed.) Academic Press, New York.

PATON, W. D. M., PERTWEE, R. G. and TEMPLE, D. (1972) The general pharmacology of cannabinoids. In: *Cannabis and its Derivatives*, pp. 50–75, PATON, W. D. M. and CROWN, J. (eds) Oxford University Press, Oxford.

PATON, W. D. M., PERTWEE, R. G. and TYLDEN, E. (1973) Clinical aspects of cannabis action. In: *Marihuana. Chemistry, Pharmacology, Metabolism and Clinical Effects*, pp. 335–365, MECHOULAM, R. (ed.) Academic Press, New York.

PEREZ REYES, M., TIMMONS, M. C., LIPTON, M. A., DAVIS, K. H. and WALL, M. E. (1972) Intravenous injection in man of delta-9-tetrahydrocannabinol and 11-hydroxy-delta-9-tetrahydrocannabinol. *Science* **177**: 633–634.

PEREZ REYES, M., TIMMONS, M. C., DAVIS, K. H. and WALL, M. E. (1973a) A comparison of the pharmacological activity in man of intravenously administered delta-9-tetrahydrocannabinol, cannabinol and cannabidiol. *Experientia* **29**: 1368–1369.

PEREZ REYES, M., TIMMONS, M. C., LIPTON, M. A., CHRISTENSEN, H. D., DAVIS, K. H. and WALL, M. E. (1973b) A comparison of the pharmacological activity of delta-9-tetrahydrocannabinol and its monohydroxylated metabolites in man. *Experientia* **29**: 1009–1010.

PERTWEE, R. G. (1983) Cannabis. In: *Psychopharmacology 1. Part 1: Preclinical Psychopharmacology*, pp. 377–397, GRAHAME-SMITH, D. G. and COWEN, P. J. (eds.) Excerpta Medica, Amsterdam.

PERTWEE, R. G. (1985a) Effects of cannabinoids on thermoregulation: A brief review. In: *Marihuana '84* pp. 263–277, HARVEY, D. J. (ed.) IRL Press, Oxford.

PERTWEE, R. G. (1985b) Cannabis. In: *Psychopharmacology 2. Part 1: Preclinical Psychopharmacology*, pp. 364–391, GRAHAME-SMITH, D. G. and COWEN, P. J. (eds.) Elsevier, Amsterdam.

PERTWEE, R. G. and GREENTREE, S. G. (1988a) Delta-9-tetrahydrocannabinol-induced catalepsy in mice is enhanced by pretreatment with flurazepam or chlordiazepoxide. *Neuropharmacology* **27**: 485–491.

PERTWEE, R. G. and GREENTREE, S. G. (1988b) Synergistic interactions between delta-9-THC and flurazepam: further studies. In: Marijuana: An International Research Report, pp. 365–370, CHESHER, G., CONSROE, P. and MUSTY, R. (eds.) Australian Government Publishing Service, Canberra.

PERTWEE, R. G., GREENTREE, S. G. and SWIFT, P. A. (1988) Drugs which stimulate or facilitate central GABAergic transmission interact synergistically with delta-9-tetrahydrocannabinol to produce marked catalepsy in mice. *Neuropharmacology* **27**: 1265–1270.

PERTWEE, R. G. and TAVENDALE, R. (1977) Effects of delta-9-tetrahydrocannabinol on the rates of oxygen consumption of mice. *Br. J. Pharmac.* **60**: 559–568.

PODDAR, M. K. and DEWEY, W. L. (1980) Effects of cannabinoids on catecholamine uptake and release in hypothalamic and striatal synaptosomes. *J. Pharmac. Exp. Ther.* **214**: 63–67.

PODDAR, M. K. and GHOSH, J. J. (1976a) Effect of cannabis extract and delta-9-tetrahydrocannabinol on rat brain catecholamines. *Ind. J. Biochem. Biophys.* **13**: 273–277.

PODDAR, M. K. and GHOSH, J. J. (1976b) Effect of cannabis extract and delta-9-tetrahydrocannabinol on brain adenosine triphosphatase activity. *Ind. J. Biochem. Biophys.* **13**: 267–272.

PONTZER, N. J., HOSKO, M. J. and WILKISON, D. M. (1986) Alteration of electrical correlates of sensory processing by tetrahydrocannabinol. *Exper. Neurol.* **91**: 127–135.

PONTZER, N. J. and WILKISON, D. M. (1987) Inhibition of heterosensory thalamocortical evoked potentials by delta-9-tetrahydrocannabinol. *Exper. Neurol.* **97**: 644–652.

PRYOR, G. T., LARSEN, F. F., CARR, J. D. and BRAUDE, M. C. (1977) Interactions of delta-9-tetrahydrocannabinol with phenobarbital, ethanol and chlordiazepoxide. *Pharmac. Biochem. Behav.* **7**: 331–345.

RAFFEL, G., CLARENBACH, P., PESKAR, B. A. and HERTTING, G. (1976) Synthesis and release of prostaglandins by rat brain synaptosomal fractions. *J. Neurochem.* **26**: 493–498.

RAZ, A. and GOLDMAN, R. (1976) Effect of hashish compounds on mouse peritoneal macrophages. *Lab. Invest.* **34**: 69–76.

RAZ, A., SCHURR, A. and LIVNE, A. (1972) The interaction of hashish components with human erythrocytes. *Biochim. Biophys. Acta* **274**: 269–271.

RAZ, A., SCHURR, A., LIVNE, A. and GOLDMAN, R. (1973) Effect of hashish compounds on rat liver lysosomes *in vitro*. *Biochem. Pharmac.* **22**: 3129–3131.

RAZDAN, R. K. (1986) Structure-activity relationships in cannabinoids. *Pharmac. Rev.* **38**: 75–149.

REICH, R., LAUFER, N., LEWYSOHN, O., CORDOVA, T., AYALON, D. and TSAFRIRI, A. (1982) *In vitro* effects of cannabinoids on follicular function in the rat. *Biol. Reprod.* **27**: 223–231.

REICHMAN, M., NEN, W. and HOKIN, L. E. (1987) Effects of delta-9-tetrahydrocannabinol on prostaglandin formation in brain. *Mol. Pharmac.* **32**: 686–690.

REVUELTA, A. V. and CHENEY, D. L. (1981) Simultaneous reduction in the turnover rates of septal gamma-aminobutyric acid and hippocampal acetylcholine following administration of nabilone. *Neuropharmacology* **20**: 1111–1114.

REVUELTA, A. V., MORONI, F., CHENEY, D. L. and COSTA, E. (1978) Effects of cannabinoids on the turnover rate of acetylcholine in rat hippocampus, striatum and cortex. *Naunyn-Schmiedeberg's Arch. Pharmac.* **304**: 107–110.

REVUELTA, A. V., CHENEY, D. L., WOOD, P. L. and COSTA, E. (1979) GABAergic mediation in the inhibition of hippocampal acetylcholine turnover rate elicited by delta-9-tetrahydrocannabinol. *Neuropharmacology* **18**: 525–530.

REVUELTA, A. V., CHENEY, D. L., COSTA, E., LANDER, N. and MECHOULAM, R. (1980) Reduction of hippocampal acetylcholine turnover in rats treated with (−) delta-8-tetrahydrocannabinol and its 1′2′-dimethyl-heptyl homolog. *Brain Res.* **195**: 445–452.

REVUELTA, A. V., CHENEY, D. L. and COSTA, E. (1982) The dimethylheptyl derivative of (−) delta-8-tetrahydrocannabinol reduces the turnover rate of gamma-aminobutyric acid in the septum and nucleus accumbens. *Life Sci.* **30**: 1841–1846.

ROSELL, S. and AGURELL, S. (1975) Effects of 7-hydroxy-delta-6-tetrahydrocannabinol and some related cannabinoids on the guinea-pig isolated ileum. *Acta Physiol. Scand.* **94**: 142–144.

ROSELL, S., AGURELL, S. and MARTIN, B. (1976) Effects of cannabinoids on isolated smooth muscle preparations. In: *Marihuana: Chemistry, Biochemistry and Cellular Effects*, pp. 397–406, NAHAS, G. G. (ed.) Springer Verlag, New York.

ROSELL, S., BJORKROTH, U., AGURELL, S., LEANDER, K., OHLSSON, A., MARTIN, B. and MECHOULAM, R. (1979) Relation between effects of cannabinoid derivatives on the twitch response of the isolated guinea-pig ileum and their psychotropic properties. In: *Marihuana: Biological Effects*, pp. 63–70, NAHAS, G. G. and PATON, W. D. M. (eds.) Pergamon Press, Oxford.

ROSENKRANTZ, H. (1985) Cannabis components and responses of neuroendocrine-reproductive targets: An overview. In: *Marihuana '84*, pp. 457–505, HARVEY, D. J. (ed.), IRL Press, Oxford.

ROTH, S. H. (1978) Stereospecific presynaptic inhibitory effect of delta-9-tetrahydrocannabinol on cholinergic transmission in the myenteric plexus of the guinea-pig. *Can. J. Physiol. Pharmac.* **56**: 968–975.

ROTH, S. H. and WILLIAMS, P. J. (1979) The non-specific membrane binding properties of delta-9-tetrahydrocannabinol and the effects of various solubilizers. *J. Pharm. Pharmac.* **31**: 224–230.

RYRFELDT, A., RAMSAY, C. H., NILSSON, I. M., WIDMAN, M. and AGURELL, S. (1973) Whole-body autoradiography of delta-1-tetrahydrocannabinol and delta-1,6-tetrahydrocannabinol in mouse. *Acta Pharmac. Suecica* **10**: 13–38.

SAKURAI, Y., OHTA, H., SHIMAZOE, T., KATAOKA, T., FUJIWARA, M. and UEKI, S. (1985) Delta-9-tetrahydrocannabinol elicited ipsilateral circling behavior in rats with unilateral nigral lesion. *Life Sci.* **37**: 2181–2185.

Sarkar, C. and Ghosh, J. J. (1975) Effect of delta-9-tetrahydrocannabinol administration on the lipid constituents of rat brain subcellular fractions. *J. Neurochem.* **24**: 381–385.

Sarkar, C. and Ghosh, J. J. (1976) Effect of delta-9-tetrahydrocannabinol on gangliosides and sialoglycoproteins in subcellular fractions of rat brain. *J. Neurochem.* **26**: 721–723.

Scheel-Krüger, J. (1986) Dopamine-GABA interactions: evidence that GABA transmits, modulates and mediates dopaminergic functions in the basal ganglia and the limbic system. *Acta Neurol. Scand.* **73**: (Suppl. 107) 1–54.

Schildkraut, J. J. and Efron, D. H. (1971) The effects of delta-9-tetrahydrocannabinol on the metabolism of norepinephrine in rat brain. *Psychopharmacology* **20**: 191–196.

Schurr, A. and Livne, A. (1976) Differential inhibition of mitochondrial monoamine oxidase from brain by hashish components. *Biochem. Pharmac.* **25**: 1201–1203.

Schurr, A. and Rigor, B. M. (1984) Cannabis extract, but not delta-1-tetrahydrocannabinol, inhibits human brain and liver monoamine oxidase. *Gen. Pharmac.* **15**: 171–174.

Schurr, A., Porath, O., Krup, M. and Livne, A. (1978) The effects of hashish components and their mode of action on monoamine oxidase from the brain. *Biochem. Pharmac.* **27**: 2513–2517.

Seeman, P. (1972) The membrane actions of anesthetics and tranquilizers. *Pharmac. Rev.* **24**: 583–655.

Seeman, P., Chau-Wong, M. and Moyyen, S. (1972) The membrane binding of morphine, diphenylhydantoin and tetrahydrocannabinol. *Can. J. Physiol. Pharmac.* **50**: 1193–1200.

Segal, M. (1978) The effects of SP-111, a water soluble THC derivative, on neuronal activity in the rat brain. *Brain Res.* **139**: 263–275.

Segawa, T., Bando, S. and Hosokawa, M. (1977) Brain serotonin metabolism and delta-9-tetrahydrocannabinol-induced muricide behavior in rats. *Jpn. J. Pharmac.* **27**: 581–582.

Segawa, T., Takeuchi, S. and Nakano, M. (1976) Mechanism for increase of brain 5-hydroxytryptamine and 5-hydroxyindoleacetic acid following delta-9-tetrahydrocannabinol administration to rats. *Jpn. J. Pharmac.* **26**: 377–379.

Shahar, A. and Bino, T. (1974) *In vitro* effects of delta-9-tetrahydrocannabinol (THC) on bull sperm. *Biochem. Pharmac.* **23**: 1341–1342.

Shannon, M. E. and Fried, P. A. (1972) The macro- and microdistribution and polymorphic electroencephalographic effects of delta-9-tetrahydrocannabinol in the rat. *Psychopharmacology* **27**: 141–156.

Shiomi, H., Nakahara, H., Segawa, M. and Takagi, H. (1979) Relationship between delta-9-tetrahydrocannabinol-induced mouse killing behavior on the rat and the metabolism of monoamines in the brain, particularly the olfactory bulb. *Jpn. J. Pharmac.* **29**: 803–806.

Shoupe, T. S., Hunter, S. A., Burstein, S. H. and Hubbard, C. D. (1980) The nature of the inhibition of cholesterol esterase by delta-1-tetrahydrocannabinol. *Enzyme* **25**: 87–91.

Sidell, F. R., Pless, J. E., Neitlich, H., Sussman, P., Copelan, H. W. and Sim, V. M. (1973) Dimethylheptyl-delta-6a-10a-tetrahydrocannabinol: Effects after parenteral administration to man. *Proc. Soc. Exp. Biol. Med.* **142**: 867–873.

Sofia, R. D., Dixit, B. N. and Barry, H. (1971a) The effect of delta-1-tetrahydrocannabinol on serotonin metabolism in the rat brain. *Life Sci.* **10**: 425–436.

Sofia, R. D., Ertel, R. J., Dixit, B. N. and Barry, H. (1971b) The effect of delta-1-tetrahydrocannabinol on the uptake of serotonin by rat brain homogenates. *Eur. J. Pharmac.* **16**: 257–259.

Sofia, R. D., Delgado, C. J. and Douglas, J. F. (1974) The effects of various naturally occurring cannabinoids on hypotonic-hyperthermic lysis of rat erythrocytes. *Eur. J. Pharmac.* **27**: 155–157.

Spronck, H. J. W., Luteijn, J. M., Salemink, C. A. and Nugteren, D. H. (1978) Inhibition of prostaglandin biosynthesis by derivatives of olivetol formed under pyrolysis of cannabidiol. *Biochem. Pharmac.* **27**: 607–608.

Steger, R. W., De Paolo, L., Asch, R. H. and Silverman, A. Y. (1983) Interactions of delta-9-tetrahydrocannabinol (THC) with hypothalamic neurotransmitters controlling luteinizing hormone and prolactin release. *Neuropharmacology* **37**: 361–370.

Strichartz, G. R., Chiu, S. Y. and Ritchie, J. M. (1978) The effect of delta-9-tetrahydrocannabinol on the activation of sodium conductance in node of Ranvier. *J. Pharmac. Exp. Ther.* **207**: 801–809.

Sung, S.-C. and Jakubovic, A. (1987) Interaction of a water-soluble derivative of delta-9-tetrahydrocannabinol with [^{3}H]diazepam and [^{3}H]flunitrazepam binding to rat brain membranes. *Prog. Neuro-Psychopharmac. Biol. Psychiat.* **11**: 335–340.

Tamir, I. and Lichtenberg, D. (1983) Correlation between the psychotropic potency of cannabinoids and their effect on the ^{1}H-NMR spectra of model membranes. *J. Pharm. Sci.* **72**: 458–461.

Taylor, D. A. and Fennessy, M. R. (1977) Biphasic nature of the effect of delta-9-tetrahydrocannabinol on body temperature and brain amines of the rat. *Eur. J. Pharmac.* **46**: 93–99.

Taylor, D. A. and Fennessy, M. R. (1979a) The effect of delta-9-tetrahydrocannabinol (delta-9-THC) on the turnover rate of brain serotonin of the rat. *Clin. Exp. Pharmac. Physiol.* **6**: 327–334.

Taylor, D. A. and Fennessy, M. R. (1979b) The effect of (−) trans-delta-9-tetrahydrocannabinol on regional brain levels and subcellular distribution of monoamines in the rat. *Clin. Exp. Pharmac. Physiol.* **6**: 541–548.

Taylor, D. A., Sitaram, B. R. and Elliot-Baker, S. (1988) Effect of delta-9-tetrahydrocannabinol on the release of dopamine in the corpus striatum of the rat. In: Marijuana: An International Research Report, pp. 405–408, Chesher, G., Consroe, P. and Musty, R. (eds.) Australian Government Publishing Service, Canberra.

Taylor, C. W. and Merritt, J. E. (1986) Receptor coupling to polyphosphoinositide turnover: A parallel with the adenylate cyclase system. *Trends Pharmac. Sci.* **7**: 238–242.

Taylor, K. M. and Snyder, S. H. (1972) Dynamics of the regulation of histamine levels in mouse brain. *J. Neurochem.* **19**: 341–354.

Toro-Goyco, E., Rodriguez, M. B. and Preston, A. M. (1978) On the action of delta-9-tetrahydrocannabinol as an inhibitor of sodium- and potassium-dependent adenosine triphosphatase. *Mol. Pharmac.* **14**: 130–137.

Tramposch, A., Sangdee, C., Franz, D. N., Karler, R. and Turkanis, S. A. (1981) Cannabinoid-induced enhancement and depression of cat monosynaptic reflexes. *Neuropharmacology* **20**: 617–621.

TRIPATHI, H. L., VOCCI, F. J., BRASE, D. A. and DEWEY, W. L. (1987) Effects of cannabinoids on levels of acetylcholine and choline and on turnover rate of acetylcholine in various regions of the mouse brain. *Alcohol Drug Res.* **7**: 525–532.

TURKANIS, S. A. and KARLER, R. (1975) Influence of anticonvulsant cannabinoids on posttetanic potentiation of isolated Bullfrog ganglia. *Life Sci.* **17**: 569–578.

TURKANIS, S. A. and KARLER, R. (1981a) Electrophysiologic properties of the cannabinoids. *J. Clin. Pharmac. (Suppl.)* **21**: 449S–463S.

TURKANIS, S. A. and KARLER, R. (1981b) Excitatory and depressant effects of delta-9-tetrahydrocannabinol and cannabidiol on cortical evoked responses in the conscious rat. *Psychopharmacology* **75**: 294–298.

TURKANIS, S. A. and KARLER, R. (1983) Effects of delta-9-tetrahydrocannabinol on cat spinal motoneurons. *Brain Res.* **288**: 283–287.

TURKANIS, S. A. and KARLER, R. (1986a) Effects of delta-9-tetrahydrocannabinol, 11-hydroxy-delta-9-tetrahydrocannabinol and cannabidiol on neuromuscular transmission in the frog. *Neuropharmacology* **25**: 1273–1278.

TURKANIS, S. A. and KARLER, R. (1986b) Cannabidiol-caused depression of spinal motoneuron responses in cats. *Pharmac. Biochem. Behav.* **25**: 89–94.

VARDARIS, R. M., WEISZ, D. J. and TEYLER, T. J. (1977) Delta-9-tetrahydrocannabinol and the hippocampus: Effects on CA1 field potentials in rats. *Brain Res. Bull.* **2**: 181–187.

VAYSSE, P. J.-J., GARDNER, E. L. and ZUKIN, R. S. (1987) Modulation of rat brain opioid receptors by cannabinoids. *J. Pharmac. Exp. Ther.* **241**: 534–539.

VITEZ, T. S., WAY, W. L., MILLER, R. D. and EGER, E. I. (1973) Effects of delta-9-tetrahydrocannabinol on cyclopropane MAC in the rat. *Anesthesiology* **38**: 525–527.

WEIGANT, V. M., SWEEP, C. G. J. and NIR, I. (1987) Effect of acute administration of delta-1-tetrahydrocannabinol on beta-endorphin levels in plasma and brain tissue of the rat. *Experientia* **43**: 413–415.

WEISZ, D. J., GUNNELL, D. L., TEYLER, T. J. and VARDARIS, R. M. (1982) Changes in hippocampal CA1 population spikes following administration of delta-9-THC. *Brain Res. Bull.* **8**: 155–162.

WELCH, B. L., WELCH, A. S., MESSIHA, F. S. and BERGER, H. J. (1971) Rapid depletion of adrenal epinephrine and elevation of telencephalic serotonin by (−) trans-delta-9-tetrahydrocannabinol in mice. *Res. Commun. Chem. Path. Pharmac.* **2**: 382–391.

WHITE, H. L. and TANSIK, R. L. (1980) Effects of delta-9-tetrahydrocannabinol and cannabidiol on phospholipase and other enzymes regulating arachidonate metabolism. *Prostaglandins and Medicine* **4**: 409–417.

WILKISON, D. M., PONTZER, N. and HOSKO, M. J. (1982) Slowing of cortical somatosensory evoked activity by delta-9-tetrahydrocannabinol and dimethylheptylpyran in alpha-chloralose-anesthetized cats. *Neuropharmacology* **21**: 705–709.

WING, D. R. and PATON, W. D. M. (1979) Effects of acute delta-1-tetrahydrocannabinol treatment, of hypothermia and of ambient temperature on choline incorporation into mouse brain. *Biochem. Pharmac.* **28**: 253–260.

YAGIELA, J. A., MCCARTHY, K. D. and GIBB, J. W. (1974) The effect of hypothermic doses of 1-delta-9-tetrahydrocannabinol on biogenic amine metabolism in selected parts of the rat brain. *Life Sci.* **14**: 2367–2378.

YOSHIMURA, H., FUJIWARA, M. and UEKI, S. (1974) Biochemical correlates in mouse-killing behavior of the rat: Brain acetylcholine and acetylcholinesterase after administration of delta-9-tetrahydrocannabinol. *Brain Res.* **81**: 567–570.

YOUNG, A. M., KATZ, J. L. and WOODS, J. H. (1981) Behavioral effects of levonantradol and nantradol in the rhesus monkey. *J. Clin. Pharmac. (Suppl.)* **21**: 348S-360S.

ZIMMERMAN, S., ZIMMERMAN, A. M. and LAURENCE, H. (1981) Effect of delta-9-tetrahydrocannabinol on cyclic nucleotides in synchronously dividing Tetrahymena. *Can. J. Biochem.* **59**: 489–493.

CHAPTER 13

OCCURRENCE AND TREATMENT OF SOLVENT ABUSE IN CHILDREN AND ADOLESCENTS

H. G. Morton
Department of Child and Family Practice, Ninewells Teaching Hospital and Medical School, Dundee, U.K.

1. INTRODUCTION

Solvent abuse is the intentional inhalation of volatile substances in order to achieve a partial or complete state of intoxication. The terms "volatile substance abuse" (VS abuse) (Ron, 1986) and "inhalant misuse" (Watson, 1986) are often employed to describe the activity, but both have drawbacks; and the widely used term "glue-sniffing" (O'Connor 1979) is insufficiently precise to cover the large range of substances misused in this way. When "glue-sniffing" occurs, it is not the glue itself which is inhaled, but the volatile solvents present in it (Bowers and Sage, 1983). Furthermore, not all solvents which are misused are sniffed; at times they are drunk, for example from a soaked rag (O'Connor, 1983). In this review the term solvent abuse is used throughout except where precise identification of the abuse route is necessary, or the use of an alternative term is more accurate.

It is known that inhalation of intoxicants has gone on at least since classical times. The use of inhalants was recognised in early Greek and other civilizations as an adjunct to mystical experience and religious practice (Black, 1982b). Novak (1980) draws attention to the use of hallucinogenic-like snuffs in ceremonies to mark the rites of passage of the young. The intentional inhalation of volatile substances for recreational purposes was known in the mid-19th century (Nicholi, 1983). Attention was drawn to petrol sniffing in the U.S.A. before World War II. The first epidemic of model aeroplane glue sniffing occurred in the U.S.A. in the mid-1950s, possibly as a result of publicity of a localized episode (Cohen, 1984). By the 1960s the habit had begun to spread, evidently eastwards across the U.S.A. from origins in California. Kupperstein and Susman (1968) cite a report of an arrest of a child for glue sniffing in 1959. Concern about the extent of solvent abuse—essentially a youthful activity, compared to the inhalation of nitrites engaged in more by adults (Cohen, 1984)—has now been indicated from many countries including Mexico, Japan, Sweden, Norway, and West Germany (Nicholi, 1983); South Africa (Moosa and Loening, 1981); South America (Watson, 1984); Hungary and Israel (O'Connor, 1983); Australia (Eastwell, 1983; O'Connor, 1983); Singapore (Devathasan *et al.*, 1984); Canada (Gellman, 1968) and France (Abgrall and Botta, 1983). British reports began in the early 1960s when a case of glue sniffing was reported by Merry and Zachariadis (1962). Solvent abuse was first noted in the West of Scotland in 1970 (Watson, 1986).

This widespread concern at the practice of solvent abuse arises because of the medical significance of the habit—the solvents used are all toxic in some degree, and may be fatally so—and because of the effects of solvent abuse on the behavior of the affected individual. Although these effects may be short-lasting, they can be incapacitating and possibly dangerous and even associated with criminal behavior. There is also the possibility of solvent abuse being associated with other forms of drug taking. Attitudes to solvent abuse tend to be ambiguous as are attitudes to adolescence generally. Black (1982a) sees substance abuse as part of delinquent behavior, yet views the phenomenon as essentially benign and draws attention to low morbidity and mortality rates from solvent abuse, compared to other risk-taking adult behavior. The wide variation in viewpoints regarding solvent abuse and its dangers is also pointed out by Herzberg and Wolkind (1983). O'Connor (1983) highlights the polarity of views; on the one hand, glue sniffing is dangerous and should be stopped; on the other, glue sniffing is not dangerous, and should be ignored. Evans (1982), in a major British text on adolescent psychiatry, mentions solvent abuse only in passing; rather modest attention is paid to the habit in the standard British text on child and adolescent psychiatry (Strang and Connell, 1985; Oppenheimer, 1985).

The purpose of this review is to survey the literature on solvent abuse in children and adolescents with reference to the pharmacology and toxicology of organic solvents, the epidemiology of solvent abuse, the nature of the habit and the individuals affected, and the methods which have evolved, on the one hand for the care of those affected, and on the other for the control of the behavior in the population as a whole.

2. THE ORGANIC SOLVENTS

The organic solvents which are used for their intoxicant effect are hydrocarbons which are volatile or gaseous at room temperature. Any such substance is potentially abuseable (Ives, 1981), but the most frequently employed are acetone, methyl and ethyl ketones, benzene, toluene, xylene, hexane, trichlorethane, trichloroethylene, the Freons, and the volatile nitrites. The substances used include glues and adhesives, paint thinners, paint strippers, rubber cements, aerosol sprays, polystyrene cements, model aeroplane "dope", nail polish removers, typewriter correcting fluid, fire-extinguishing agents, dry cleaning fluids, anti-freeze compounds, hair lacquer and lighter fuel (see Table 1).

In the U.K., the majority of abusers use proprietary brands of glue (Masterton and Sclare, 1978) which generally contain toluene or acetone (Watson, 1982; Sourindhrin and Baird, 1984). A minority, however, make use of the hydrocarbon propellants in aerosol sprays. The propellant in an aerosol allows the product to be released in the form of a mist, spray or foam when a button is pressed (Roberts, 1982), and is usually a liquified halogenated or non-halogenated hydrocarbon gas; different products use from as little as 5% of this (e.g. in shaving cream) to more than 90% (e.g. in pain relief spray). Halogenated hydrocarbon propellants include chloro- and fluoro-methane compounds, at times in the proprietary combination Freon; non-halogenated hydrocarbon propellant is usually butane mixed with propane. In addition to the propellant, an aerosol product may itself have a solvent base.

Petrol is primarily a mixture of medium chain aliphatic hydrocarbons, but it also contains aromatic hydrocarbons including xylene, toluene, benzene, paraffins, and naphthenes in small quantities. The composition of the finished product is very variable depending on the source of the petroleum and the refining method used. At times petrol (gasoline) is chosen for abuse in preference to other solvents. Although reports of this have been widespread, there has been particular concern regarding petrol sniffing in ethnic groups such as American and Canadian Indians, who live in isolated areas (Fortenberry, 1985; Coulehan *et al.*, 1983). Lighter fluid, sniffing of which has been described by Ackerly and Gibson (1964), consists essentially of a mixture of volatile and highly inflammable aliphatic hydrocarbons, primarily naphtha.

TABLE 1. *Agents Used by Solvent Abusers*

Aerosols including hair lacquer, pain killer, etc.	Freons (fluorocarbons), propane, isobutane
Antifreeze	Ethylene glycol
Drycleaning fluids	Trichloroethylene, carbon tetrachloride
Fire extinguishing agents	Bromochlorodifluoromethane
Fingernail polish remover	Acetone, ethyl and amyl acetate
Gas lighter fuel	Butane, propane
Household glues and adhesives	Toluene, acetone, naphtha
Lighter fluid	Various petrol mixtures including naphtha and other aromatic hydrocarbons
Model cements	Methyl and ethyl ketones, *N*-hexane
Paint thinners and paint strippers	Toluene, ethyl acetate, benzene, various alcohols
Petrol	Benzene, naphthenes, xylene
Rubber solution	Benzene, hexane
Typewriter correction fluid	Amyl acetate, dichloroethane trichloroethane

It is likely that ease of use (King, 1982) is important in determining the abuser's choice of substance. Ready availability, low cost, rapid speed of action, and a fairly short-term effect also influence choice (Sourindhrin, 1985). The ease with which a preparation can be stolen is a further factor in some circumstances.

2.1 Pharmacology and Toxicology

Organic solvents and related substances are central nervous system depressants with an initial shortlived excitant effect on inhalation, which is an efficient method for achieving very rapid transport of the active ingredients of a drug to the brain (Novak, 1980). It is a method generally chosen by numerous users of cocaine and heroin as well as the users of volatile substances. Absorption of inhaled solvent is rapid across the large surface area of the alveoli in the lungs into the blood, so that the immediate effect of inhalation is like an intravenous injection of drugs. (Watson, 1982). Organic solvents are fat-soluble and are stored in high concentrations in lipid in the central nervous system. In the brain, there is disruption of function by virtue of the effect on neuromembrane ionic channels, and this accounts for the acute and chronic brain syndromes seen in the more severe and persistent solvent abusers. Toluene, the chief solvent in the commonly available adhesives in the U.K., is a potent and rapidly acting narcotic in rodents (Bruckner and Peterson, 1981). After inhalation, some toluene is eliminated unchanged through the lungs, but the major metabolism takes place in hepatic microsomes by oxidation to benzoic acid which is conjugated with glycine to form hippuric acid, which is excreted by the kidneys. If the concentration of toluene in inhaled air is constant, blood toluene concentration reaches 60% of a maximum after 10–15 min of exposure and the blood concentration curve becomes asymptotic within 30 mins (Ron, 1986).

The precise toxicology of many organic solvents is unclear. Reports from industrial populations exposed to low levels of solvent vapor over long periods may not accurately reflect the situation in solvent abusers in whom the concentration of solvent is high over a relatively short period of time. King (1983) points out that the airborne concentration of solvents to which it is considered workers may be exposed repeatedly without adverse effect may be exceeded several hundredfold by the solvent abuser. Reports from animal studies require cautious interpretation. The pharmacokinetics of volatile solvents following acute sniffing are not well understood (Ramsay and Flanagan, 1982b).

The detection of organic solvent in body fluid is a complex problem. More than 50 commonly abused solvents are reported in the literature (Oliver, 1982) but commercially available products in any case tend to contain mixtures of solvents (Nicholi, 1983), which may have moderating or potentiating effects on each other. Oliver and Watson (1977) reviewed 50 cases of solvent abuse in the first major toxicological study undertaken in the U.K. and confirmed the preference of solvent abusers for substances containing toluene or acetone. Oliver's (1982) account, of analysis of samples of venous blood for the presence of a variety of solvents by gas liquid chromatography, gives details of sampling techniques and of qualitative and quantitative analytic methods, and attempts clinical correlates. Lush *et al.* (1980) found that where toluene was detected and levels measured, it appeared that the common sign below 1 μg/g was a smell of solvent on the breath. Acutely intoxicated patients had levels of around 2.5 μg/g. The study by King (1982) of patients admitted to hospital after toluene abuse found blood toluene concentrations from 0.8 μg/g to 8 μg/g. Ramsay (1983) described the ready detection of toluene 4 days after the last episode of sniffing, by portable mass spectrometry. Garriott and Petty (1980) have shown a half-life of toluene in blood of between one and two hours, when measured within two hours of sniffing. A simple and reliable temperature programme gas chromatographic method for detecting and identifying a range of volatile organic compounds, including those commonly abused, has been developed by Ramsay and Flanagan (1982a). Only small specimens of blood (200 μl) or tissue (200 mg) are required and valuable diagnostic information may be obtained where inhalation abuse of solvents is suspected.

2.2 Toxicity of Organic Solvents

Organic solvents are generally irritating to the eyes, nose, throat and upper respiratory tract. Significant toxicity to other systems occurs mostly with cylic compounds and aerosols, although carbon tetrachloride is hepatotoxic and cardiotoxic. Toxicity of acetone through abuse has not been reported.

2.2.1. *Toluene*

Glaser and Massengale (1962), and Wyse (1973) considered that toluene abuse was free of serious side-effects. However, toluene is known to have effects on the kidney (O'Brien *et al.* 1971; Will and MacLaren, 1981); the heart (Bass, 1970); and the gastrointestinal tract and central nervous system (Streicher *et al.*, 1981). It may alter the metabolism of other solvents (Smyth *et al.*, 1969); and the possibility that supposed toxicity of toluene is actually due to other solvents, present with toluene in greater or lesser quantities, has been raised by Novak (1980). King (1982) considers that toluene abuse may lead to permanent neurological damage.

2.2.2. *Benzene and Related Compounds; Petrol*

Benzene alone is probably not neurotoxic (Prockop, 1979). Myelotoxicity in humans has been reported (Snyder and Kocsis, 1975) although other solvents frequently present with benzene, as in petrol, may be implicated. Naphthalene toxicity resulting from solvent abuse has not been reported. *N*-hexane is almost always associated, as a solvent, with *N*-heptane. It is neurotoxic as an abused solvent (Korobkin *et al.*, 1975) and neuropathy has been reported (Goto *et al.*, 1974, Towfighi *et al.*, 1976). Prockop (1979) reported neurotoxicity from inhalation of lacquer thinner, probably as a result of *N*-heptane.

Petrol is the most important mixed organic solvent. Concern over toxicity of petrol centers on the toxic effects of lead, which is commonly added to petrol as tetraethyl lead as an 'anti-knock' agent, although lead-free petrol is increasingly available following recognition of the danger of accumulation of environmental lead. It is not known whether the amount of tetraethyl lead which is inhaled during a single episode of "petrol sniffing" is sufficient to cause hallucinations and behavioral changes (Fortenberry, 1985); it is possible that tetraethyl lead potentiates short-term effects of other volatile substances in petrol. Chronic leaded petrol inhalation has neurotoxic effects (Seshia *et al.*, 1978) and the blood lead level becomes rapidly elevated in children who sniff leaded petrol only a few times (Kaufman and Weise, 1978). The lead content of 24 hr urine collections is more difficult to correlate with the clinical situation (Fortenberry, 1985).

2.2.3. *Aerosols*

Aerosols irritate the upper respiratory tract, and produce central nervous system depression or anesthesia. Most volatile halogenated hydrocarbons found in aerosols are eliminated unchanged by the lungs, but trichlorethylene is metabolized by the liver and excreted through the kidneys. It has been reported to be associated with cranial nerve damage but the reasons for any cranial nerve selectivity are unknown (King, 1983). The Freons are compounds of low molecular weight which are highly fat soluble; these fluorocarbons do not appear to affect the liver or kidneys. The sudden death which can occur following aerosol abuse (Bass, 1970) is probably due in some cases to cardiotoxicity; the heart is sensitized to adrenaline-induced ventricular arrhythmias by brief inhalation of fluorocarbons especially in the presence of hypercapnia such as is rapidly produced by rebreathing from a bag (Novak, 1980).

3. THE EPIDEMIOLOGY OF SOLVENT ABUSE

The epidemiological study of solvent abuse is peculiarly difficult. The ascertainment of abusers by social work or medical services discloses a different prevalence from that obtained when abusers are ascertained by the police. School surveys may not accurately reflect the true prevalence of solvent abuse in a school-age population, since many users are truants or drop-outs (Crites and Schuckit, 1979). 1,300 new cases of solvent abuse were reported to the police in a secondary school population of about half a million in 1980 (King, 1982). Ramsey (1982) found a point prevalence of 9.8% for boys aged 13 to 15 years attending a Glasgow secondary school. Davies *et al.* (1985) estimated that between 3% and 5% of 15 year olds had sniffed solvents at some point in early adolescence, and that about 10% of these went on to become chronic solvent abusers. Ives (1986) cites a report that 6% of children of secondary school age had experimented with solvent abuse in an English provincial town. However, the prevalence of solvent abuse in the U.K. remains uncertain (Sourindhrin, 1985; Ron, 1986). The position is no clearer in other countries, although it has been reported from the U.S.A. that 8% of high school students and 11% of junior high school students try inhalants at least once (Crites and Schuckit, 1979). In some areas the prevalence may be considerably higher (Novak, 1980).

Solvent abuse is primarily a phenomenon of adolescence. Press and Done (1967) reported from a study carried out in New York and Chicago Police Departments between 1963 and 1965 that significant numbers of children under the age of 10 were found to be abusing solvents. Yet the mean age of affected children was still 14.8 years; and Wyse (1973) gives the mean age as between 14 and 15 years. Certainly the report (Nitsche and Robinson, 1959) of a 12 year old boy who had apparently been seeking out petrol fumes to sniff since eighteen months of age is quite exceptional, although Press and Done (1967) considered that children begin abusing solvents at a younger age in larger cities. Watson (1977) cites a report of a 6 year old sniffing regularly. Barnes (1979) and Crites and Schuckit (1979) found that the habit generally started between the ages of 10 and 15 years. Watson (1982), from a study of 400 cases referred to her between 1975 and 1981, found an age range between 8 and 19 years, with a peak incidence between 13 and 15 years. Similar figures have been quoted elsewhere (*Lancet* editorial, 1982).

Many studies indicate that male solvent abusers considerably outnumber females. Press and Done (1967) felt that boys abused solvents more than girls by a factor of about 10 to 1, and that girls were more likely to be "social" sniffers who rarely become habituated. Ron (1986) asserts that in the U.K., volatile substance abuse appears to be at least twice as common in males as in females. Studies in Glasgow have found solvent abuse to occur mainly in boys (Sourindhrin, 1985). Novak (1980) cast some doubt on the increased male incidence, pointing out that the male:female ratio may vary depending on geographical area, age range, and type of adolescent population studied. However no studies have been reported which throw doubt on the generally accepted male preponderance.

Social factors may be significant in at least partially determining the pattern of solvent abuse in the community. A higher incidence in children from single parent families has been reported, as has an association with paternal unemployment (Sourindhrin, 1985). Black (1982a) drew attention to solvent abuse as affecting deprived youngsters in inner city areas in the U.K., but this association is not well established. Indeed Gay (1981) found no association between solvent abuse, social deprivation and alcohol-related problems in the abuser's family. Solvent abusers reaching medical attention, who often engage in the habit on their own, may be more likely to have a disrupted family life (Masterton and Sclare, 1978; Skuse and Burrell, 1982). Solitary, habitual abusers do not invariably come from a background of urban deprivation or have alcoholic or uncaring parents, however (Watson, 1986).

4. SOLVENT ABUSERS AND THEIR BEHAVIOR

Most authors agree that solvent abuse by children and adolescents is essentially a group activity (Sutherland, 1982; Clements and Simpson, 1978), which may have ritual qualities (Kupperstein and Susman, 1968). Watson's (1975) study of solvent abusers in an area of West Scotland found that the activity occurred mostly in groups of boys, a considerable number of whom had antisocial tendencies. Lone solvent abusers are relatively uncommon and are more likely to use dangerous methods (Herzberg and Wolkind, 1983). For many individuals, solvent abuse can be regarded as part of the normal process of experimentation in adolescence, and not in itself pathological (Watson, 1979c), although it nevertheless has the potential for adversely affecting health. A classification of solvent abusers (based on Ives, 1986) is as follows:

(1) Experimenters, who try solvent abuse as a new experience but do not persist with the habit. They may sample the experience in school holidays or when otherwise bored (Novak, 1980). Such experimentation does not of itself disrupt the abuser's functioning.
(2) Regular abusers, who persist with the habit for a few weeks or months, often in groups. A small percentage of these become habitual long-term abusers.
(3) Long-term abusers, who use solvents for their chemical effects, often as a solitary activity.

Watson (1986) found that 30–40% of solvent abusers were involved on only a few occasions; 40–50% were involved sporadically with their contemporaries over a few weeks or months; and 10% were likely to become habitual abusers. Masterton (1979) divided solvent abusers into a large group, who experiment with solvents as a result of cultural expectation and in whom the activity is socially determined, and a smaller group of abusers who may become psychologically habituated and may be neurotic or affectionless in character. The solvent abuser has no typical personality profile, but O'Connor (1979) considered that "at risk" factors included immaturity, anxiety, emotional deprivation, and inadequate coping skills. He found that solvent abusers were more vulnerable to group pressure than other children, and turned to solvent abuse as an escape from feelings of inadequacy. Watson (1977) reported an association between solvent sniffing, high truancy rates, and low academic performance, tending to confirm earlier U.S. reports (Massengale *et al.*, 1963; Press and Done, 1967). Family disruption may be commoner in habitual solvent abusers. Press and Done (1967) found that absence from the home of the abuser's father, through divorce, death or prolonged institutionalization, was common; even when the father was physically present he had little or no positive relationship with his son. Masterton and Sclare (1978) found that more than half of their sample of solvent abusers had an absent parent due to divorce, separation or death. If parents were together, their relationship was often dysfunctional; the father was often alcoholic and/or unemployed. Skuse and Burrell's (1982) group of solvent abusers seen at a child psychiatric clinic tended to come from disrupted families, and had experienced emotional rejection by their mothers from birth. Massengale *et al.* (1963) found that one or both parents were missing from the homes of three quarters of glue sniffers, about half of whom had one or two alcoholic parents. The antisocial behavior of children and adolescents from such homes is exemplified in a study reporting solvent abusers, in a population of adolescents referred by Courts to three community centers, to be at high risk for the diagnosis of antisocial personality (Crites and Schuckit, 1979). These individuals were more likely than those who were abusing other drugs to have committed offences known to the police, or to have run away from home repeatedly before the age of 16. Robins (1966) has shown how such persons have a high risk of proceeding to criminal behavior.

Barnes (1979) has proposed a causal model of adolescent solvent abuse which attempts to take into account individual, family, neighborhood and cultural factors and which recognizes the role of peer group influences. The model is of interest in drawing together many of the complex strands in the etiology of solvent abuse.

The majority of children and adolescents abusing solvents in the U.K. at the present time use a household glue. This is spread inside a small plastic or paper container, typically an empty potato crisp packet, which is placed over the face prior to inhalation. Alternatively the contents of a can of glue may be inhaled direct from the can. Where liquid solvents are preferred, a rag may be dipped in the solvent and then applied to the face much in the way in which a mask was used in general anesthesia to allow a volatile anesthetic such as ether to flow over the patients' face. Some chemicals used in solvent abuse are very irritant and are therefore kept off the nasal or oral mucosa (Wyse, 1973). An aerosol may be sprayed direct into the mouth (Wyse, 1973), as may gas such as butane lighter fuel. Occasionally a liquid solvent such as lighter fuel is drunk, usually mixed into a fizzy drink such as Coca-Cola (Black, 1982b). Gellman (1968) reported children ingesting nail polish remover in Coca-Cola. Sometimes solvent may be poured on to the clothes and inhaled from there; a wide variety of such techniques is described by O'Connor (1983). Butane "fire-breathing" (Marsh, 1984) is a varient of solvent abuse having more than the usual risks of the activity.

The effects of inhalation probably vary depending on age, physique, personality, type of solvent abused, and duration of abuse (Wyse, 1973). Immediate intoxication lasts for a short period, generally between 20 and 30 min; the effect of this "high" or "buzz" is probably partly determined by the expectations of the abuser. O'Connor (1983) draws a comparison between the effects of breath-holding attacks as seen in young children, the effects pursued during the activity game of "breath-holding" sometimes played by school children, and the element of intoxication induced by the inhalation of solvent. Recovery from inhalation usually follows within about an hour, at times accompanied by amnesia for the episode (Herzberg and Wolkind, 1983). Experienced abusers may be able to maintain a "high" for up to 12 hr by intermittent inhalation (Wyse, 1973).

The subjective experience of many solvent abusers using glue appears to be an initial euphoria, followed by confusion, mild but often increasing excitement, a buzzing noise in the ears, and eventually hallucinations. As the experience develops, there may be feelings of grandiosity, omnipotence even; and a sensation of floating, with distortions of space and time. (Press and Done, 1967). Differing sensations may occur with other solvents; thus Novak (1980) draws attention to the nausea, excess salivation, and sense of drowsiness and weakness, which may be experienced by those inhaling petrol and related substances. The hallucinations of solvent abuse vary from a relatively mild visual perceptual disturbance, through a more severe distortion of reality, to dramatic, generally visual images occasionally having an erotic content. Auditory hallucinations are uncommon (Press and Done, 1967). Barnes (1979) considers the occurrence of hallucinations to be the major difference between the symptoms of drunkenness due to alcohol, and those of intoxication from inhalation of solvents. O'Connor (1983) cites detailed descriptions of experiences after solvent inhalation given by patients attending a counseling clinic. He considers that intoxication as a result of solvent abuse prevents self-awareness, in contrast to the effects of hallucinogenic drugs such as cannabis and lysergic acid diethylamide (LSD), which appear to stimulate awareness of the drug-induced state. There is often no hangover from solvent abuse, or at least only a relatively mild one (Watson, 1982); headache is the hangover symptom most often mentioned (Cohen, 1984).

Habitual solvent abusers may engage in periods of inhalation several times a day. The sites chosen for occasional, as well as persistent solvent abuse, often signify a wish for concealment of the habit from society at large. Deserted areas of parks, derelict property, abandoned cars, public toilets and railway carriages are but a few of those chosen; descriptions of the social environment in which solvent abuse occurs are given by O'Connor (1979) and Sutherland (1982).

The behavioral effects of solvent abuse are numerous. In general terms, intoxicated behavior in children and adolescents is found offensive by society and the public nuisance caused leads to alarm and anger in the community. More specifically, there may be an inability to remember recent events, a tendency to isolation and to act out of character. Abusers may become belligerent, and have inexplicable temper outbursts (O'Connor, 1983), they may take unnecessary, unwarranted or unreasonable risks, or their behavior may become self-destructive (Chapel and Taylor, 1968). Press and Done (1967) found that a number of solvent abusers came to the attention of law enforcement agencies because of their erratic driving while under the influence of solvents. Antisocial behavior including truancy and property damage is widely reported (Wyse, 1973; Skuse and Burrell, 1982; O'Connor, 1983). Burglary and shop-lifting are sometimes committed to obtain solvents (Ackerly and Gibson, 1964). Reed and May (1984), in a controlled study comparing 100 juvenile delinquents identified as chronic inhalant abusers with two groups of other, non-abusing delinquents, found that inhalant abusers were much more likely to be arrested for virtually every type and category of delinquent activity. Watson (1979b) found that police cases of solvent abuse associated for less than 15% of all juvenile cases, however. The rela-

cases of solvent abuse associated for less than 15% of all juvenile cases, however. The relationship between solvent abuse and delinquency remains unclear; studies of solvent abusers in institutional populations of delinquents have not shown them to have markedly different characteristics from non-abusers (Black, 1982a; Morton, unpublished data).

5. THE CLINICAL FEATURES OF SOLVENT ABUSE

Many solvent abusers do not come to medical examination (Herzberg and Wolkind, 1983). Watson (1979a) found from a study of hospital casualty department attendances and in-patient records that only a very small proportion of patients had been involved in solvent abuse. Those who do present may be brought by parents, teacher, social worker, youth and community worker, or police. Concern may be aroused by the discovery of glue patches on the clothes or schoolbag or of empty cans of glue. A smell of solvent may have been noticed on the affected person. Marks of spilt glue may have been found at home, in the bedroom or bathroom particularly. Alternatively suspicion may be aroused by an apparent deterioration in school performance; or by the onset of behavior which is apparently 'out of character.'

The clinical features are protean. There may be erythematous spots around the nose and mouth and occasionally more widely over the face and neck, sometimes termed "gluesniffer's rash." A white powdery ring may be seen around the mouth of less experienced sniffers (Chapel and Taylor, 1968). Examination during the intoxicated state reveals euphoria, blurring of vision, disorientation, slurring of speech and ataxia. Hallucinations are reported by about half of all solvent abusers (Ives, 1986) and a wide variety of other perceptual distortions may occur. There may be abdominal pain, nausea and vomiting. Chest pain and bronchospasm occur in some cases. Impaired judgement, irritability and excitement are frequent, although a full delirium with clouding of consciousness is less common (Sourindhrin, 1985). Convulsions, status epilepticus and coma may occur (Allister *et al.*, 1981; Francis *et al.*, 1982).

In a study of 20 patients aged between 8 and 14 years who were admitted to the Royal Hospital for Sick Children in Glasgow following toluene abuse by glue sniffing, King (1982) found the following presenting features: euphoria (9 cases), drowsiness (7), ataxia (5), coma (5), dysarthria (5), suicidal ideas (4), convulsions (3), headache (3), oral or nasal ulceration (3), visual hallucinations (3), and vomiting (3).

Examination of the habitual abuser in particular may disclose signs of complications. Excessive nasal and lacrimal secretion, poor muscle control, anorexia and weight loss may occur (Black, 1982b). The combination of dizziness, amnesia, inability to concentrate, disorientation, unsteady gait and slurred speech suggests the development of an organic brain syndrome. Fortenberry (1985) considers that an apparently toxic encephalopathy or a movement disorder in a child or adolescent should always raise the possibility of petrol sniffing.

6. THE PHYSICAL COMPLICATIONS OF SOLVENT ABUSE

A number of the physical complications of solvent abuse which have been reported have occurred in young adults, and have developed over a long period of time. They are included here because of their implications for the management of solvent abuse in children and teenagers. It is noteworthy that the majority of solvent abusers do not develop physical complications (Herzberg and Wolkind, 1983); those who do may show evidence of slow deterioration in health rather than acute symptomatology.

Neurological complications have aroused the greatest concern, especially encephalopathy, cerebellar degeneration, and peripheral neuropathy.

6.1 ENCEPHALOPATHY

Ron (1986) has criticized the use of the term 'encephalopathy' in connection with solvent abuse, pointing out that the majority of neurological symptoms present in those abusers who come to medical attention are quickly reversible. Nevertheless, the main toxic impact of toluene is on the central nervous system (King, 1983) and toluene inhalation (through glue-sniffing) does appear to cause a form of encephalopathy in childhood and may lead to permanent neurological damage. Patients in the study of King *et al.* (1981) of 19 toluene inhalers presented with ataxia, hallucinations, behavior disturbance, diplopia, convulsions or coma; 13 recovered completely over the period of follow-up. Schikler *et al.* (1982) reported 6 out of 11 toluene abusers, who had continued the habit for over ten years, to have cerebral cortical atrophy at computerized tomography scan. Seshia *et al.* (1978) found, in their study of 50 children and adolescents who were chronically sniffing leaded petrol that 27 had EEG abnormalities. Boeckx and Coodin (1977) reported lead encephalopathy in two 14 year old boys and a 6 year old girl after chronic inhalation of petrol; in one boy the condition was ultimately fatal. Lead toxicity accompanying gasoline sniffing has also been reported by Coulehan *et al.* (1983). Fortenberry (1985) described an acute or subacute encephalopathy, with hallucinations, disorientation, insomnia, violent behavior and paranoid features, apparently due to tetraethyl lead in petrol; it is not clear whether this ever occurs in children and adolescents.

6.2. Cerebellar Degeneration

Transient cerebellar signs may occur in acute toluene intoxication. More persistent cerebellar dysfunction related to petrol sniffing was reported by Young *et al.* (1977). Seshia *et al.* (1978) found evidence of cerebellar dysfunction in many of their 50 patients who were inhaling leaded petrol, and noted that this group had significantly higher blood lead levels ($\geq$40 μg/dl). Malm and Lying-Tunell (1980) described an 18 year old girl with prolonged and severe cerebellar symptoms due to sniffing pure toluene; the symptoms disappeared fully only after the patient stopped sniffing after becoming pregnant. Takeuchi *et al.* (1981) reported a 19 year old male who had sniffed lacquer thinner containing toluene, ethyl acetate, methyl isobutyl ketone, 3% isopropyl alcohol, and 3% butyl acetate, for 8 months; he had cerebellar dysfunction and visual disorders, which cleared up during a 3 month period of hospital treatment. King (1982) reported a case in which cerebellar signs following toluene abuse persisted over an 18 month follow-up period, despite apparent abstention from the habit. Fornazzari *et al.* (1983) found cerebellar signs, whose presence and severity correlated with computerized tomography findings, in about half of the young adult toluene abusers admitted to a Canadian drug abuse treatment clinic.

6.3. Peripheral Neuropathy

Peripheral neuropathy occurring in association with solvent abuse (Altenkirch *et al.*, 1977) is chiefly attributable to *N*-hexane inhalation (Sourindhrin, 1985; Ron, 1986). The peripheral neuropathy of solvent abuse has been reported as severe and disabling (Goto *et al.*, 1974; Korobkin *et al.*, 1975; King *et al.*, 1985). Seshia *et al.* (1978) reported a peripheral neuropathy which improved slowly after cessation of petrol sniffing. King *et al.* (1985b) found slow peripheral nerve conduction with extensive muscle denervation in 3 young adult males with a long history of glue vapour inhalation. It was considered that a combination of methyl ethyl ketone and methyl butyl ketone in the substances inhaled by their patients might be responsible, possibly because of competition for metabolic pathways. It seems likely that toluene abuse on its own does not carry a great risk of peripheral nerve damage.

6.4 Other Neurological Complications

Irreversible optic atrophy has been described in toluene abusers (Keane, 1978; Fornazzari *et al.*, 1983). Ehyai and Freeman (1983) reported progressive optic neuropathy and severe sensorineural hearing loss in a young man with a 5 year history of glue sniffing. Allister *et al.* (1981) recorded severe status epilepticus in a 15 year old boy, in association with glue sniffing. The outcome in this case was poor; the patient continued to have 1–2 seizures per month and to present major behavioral problems. Parker *et al.* (1984) reported a 12 year old habitual glue sniffer who developed a dense hemiparesis in association with an episode of glue sniffing. Occlusion of the right middle cerebral artery was found on investigation. Prockop and Karampelas (1981) reported a 19 year old male with diffuse, multifocal neurological deficit including dementia, nystagmus, dysarthria, truncal ataxia, extremity dysmetria and pathologically increased tendon reflexes after petrol sniffing; the relative contributions to the symptomatology of lead and volatile hydrocarbons could not be determined.

6.5. Miscellaneous

A number of complications can affect other systems.

(1) *Respiratory.* Respiratory complications ranging from restrictive ventilatory defect and reduced diffusion capacity, to a degree of pulmonary hypertension with cor pulmonale, were found in 13 solvent abusers aged 14 to 18 years by Devathasan *et al.* (1984). Schikler *et al.* (1984) found high residual volumes in inhalers, compared with controls.

(2) *Renal.* Renal damage as a result of solvent abuse appears to range from transient presence of red cells in urine, and proteinuria to apparently reversible acute renal failure (King, 1981; O'Brien, 1981; Russ *et al.*, 1981; Will and McLaren, 1981). Renal calculi may develop (Kroeger *et al.*, 1980).

(3) *Cardiovascular.* Mee and Rite (1980) reported a fatal congestive cardiomyopathy in a young male adult following chronic inhalation of shoe cleaner fluids.

(4) *Haematological.* Two deaths have been attributed to aplastic anemia developing as a toxic effect of solvent abuse (Powars, 1965).

(5) *Hepatic.* Acute hepatic damage is cited by Sourindhrin (1985); Barnes (1979) considers that the risk of liver disease after sniffing solvent is greater in those who have previous hepatic disease and those who simultaneously take alcohol.

(6) *Locomotor.* Kovanen *et al.* (1983) described acute severe recurrent myopathy with myoglobinuria after petrol sniffing. Signs of myotonia were observed by Devathasan *et al.* (1984).

(7) *Genitourinary.* Goodwin *et al.* (1981) drew attention to the possible consequences for intrauterine development and for subsequent parenting, of inhalant abuse during pregnancy. These workers suggested that children exposed to toxic effects of inhalant *in utero*, and then exposed passively during childhood, could develop chronic mental changes by the age of 9. The significance for reproductive function of Prasad's (1984) report of elevated prolactin levels in a small group of late adolescent solvent abusers is unclear.

7. SUDDEN DEATH RESULTING FROM SOLVENT ABUSE

That solvent abuse carries a risk to life is evident from the distressing reports of deaths of young people who abuse, which occasionally feature in the press and on television. Bass (1970) reported 110 sudden deaths from solvent abuse, without asphyxia, which had occurred in the U.S.A. Severe cardiac arrhythmias were regarded as the most likely explanation of sudden death after inhalation of aerosols, with stress or activity or overbreathing as exacerbating factors. The use of a plastic bag placed over the head to administer the solvent is dangerous; re-breathing leads to a rapid increase in p_{CO_2} and a decrease in p_{O_2} in arterial blood, so that any arrhythmogenic tendency which the solvent itself may have is aggravated (Bass, 1970; Taylor and Harris, 1970). A plastic bag may in itself be responsible for death by suffocation if the sniffer becomes unconscious (Press, 1963; Chapel and Taylor, 1968). Death may occur from inhalation of aerosol as a result of laryngeal spasm caused by cold gas sprayed into the mouth (Black, 1982b). Cronk *et al.* (1965) reported respiratory arrest in a 21 year old male after a 6 hr glue sniffing session. Resuscitation was successful in this case, but it is suggested that respiratory arrest may be an important cause of sudden death in solvent abusers. The sudden death of 4 adolescents from inhalation of typewriter correction fluid containing dichlorothane is reported by King *et al.* (1985a). Smeeton and Clark (1985) reported 5 deaths from deliberate inhalation of bromochlorodifluoromethane, a vaporizing liquid fire-extinguishing agent. Sudden death from deliberate inhalation of petrol has been reported but appears rare (Poklis and Burkett, 1977); the risk of severe injury or death from fire is much greater.

Anderson *et al.* (1985) extended previous work (Anderson *et al.*, 1982) to report on 282 deaths from solvent abuse in the U.K. during the period 1971–1983. The annual mortality rate showed an increase towards the end of the period, reaching 80 in 1983. 72% of deaths from solvent abuse in the period occurred in persons under the age of 20; 95% were in males. Rates were highest in Scotland and in urban areas. 51% of deaths were attributed to direct toxicity; 21% to asphyxia as a result of plastic bag use; 18% to inhalation of stomach contents; and 11% to other trauma sustained during solvent abuse. Of the solvents and solvent products implicated, 24% were gas fuels, mostly butane; 17% were aerosols; 27% were glue-based; and 31% were in other categories—fire extinguishing agents, typewriter correction fluid, and various cleaning agents. Deaths associated with glue sniffing appeared more likely to be traumatic. Only 6% of deaths were due to abuse of glues by children under 16. The causes of death from inhalant abuse in the U.S.A. appear similar (Garriott and Petty, 1980). Sourindhrin and Baird (1984) found a low mortality rate in 300 solvent abusers seen at a Glasgow clinic.

8. PSYCHOLOGICAL AND PSYCHIATRIC ASPECTS OF SOLVENT ABUSE

Much attention has been devoted to seeking answers to the question of why children and adolescents abuse solvents. Abusers themselves may reveal information of interest. Thus O'Connor's patients (O'Connor, 1983) reported that (sniffing solvent) was exciting; that parents and teachers did not like it; and that it made them forget. Other reasons almost certainly include relief from boredom (Novak, 1980); response to peer group pressure (Laury, 1972; Clements and Simpson, 1978; Jamieson, 1980); curiosity; and attempts to gain status (Sourindhrin, 1985). O'Connor (1979) viewed the activity as compensatory for low self-esteem and feelings of inadequacy. Kupperstein and Susman (1968) compared the use of glue by children and adolescents to tide them over stress situations with the use of drugs and alcohol by adults in situations of frustration, anxiety or crisis. Alcohol and tobacco are used by adults; solvents have a special use by young people (Ives, 1986).

The family structure of solvent abusers may be important in some cases (Framrose, 1982) but such family dysfunction as may be present may not be specific to solvent abusers (Black, 1982a). It is not known whether family structure is more important in chronic solvent abusers who have emotional or personality problems. Brozovsky and Winkler (1965) drew attention to a group of children who sniffed glue to escape the pain of beating by their parents; they reported complete insensitivity to corporal punishment after sniffing.

However, it is the psychological characteristics of the individual solvent abuser which have received the most scrutiny. Press (1963) considered that children involved in repeated episodes of glue sniffing mostly manifested other social or emotional maladjustment. Clements and Simpson (1978) felt little doubt that psychologically the behavior (glue sniffing) was symptomatic of emotional maladjustment, although the 47 adolescents they studied had all been diagnosed as behaviorally disordered and/or socially maladjusted and were a highly selected sample. Sourindhrin (1985) suggests that solvent abuse should be regarded as "essentially a socialised disturbance of conduct" but such diagnostic categorization may be of dubious value. Ron (1986) asserts that personality disorders of an antisocial type are common in volatile substance abusers especially in those who also abuse other drugs and alcohol. It is likely, though, that solitary and/or habitual abusers, who are more likely to come to psychological or psychiatric assessment, have a substantially higher rate of such personality disorder than, or at least differ in personality characteristics from, the great majority of occasional or "one-off" abusers (Chapel and Taylor, 1968). Masterton (1979) saw the habitual solvent abuser as "the natural product of his subculture" usually demonstrating features of gross social disadvantage including poverty, unemployment, large family, overcrowded housing, family history of antisocial behavior and minor psychiatric illness, and heavy alcohol abuse by the father or father-figure. Gay *et al.* (1982) found that solitary solvent abusers, who made up 13% of their survey of 304 young persons involved in solvent abuse, had multiple and often more fundamental personality and interpersonal relationships problems, and possibly a poorer prognosis than group abusers. Woolfson (1982) investigated 12 glue sniffing boys, comparing them with nonsniffing delinquents in terms of personality variables as assessed on the High School Personality Questionnaire. A small number of significant differences were found suggesting that the glue sniffing children were more outgoing, cheerful and adventurous.

Psychiatric disorder has been reported in association with solvent abuse although the concept of inhalation psychosis (Glaser, 1966) has not been taken up widely. Black (1967) described a 15 year old boy who presented schizophrenia-like symptomatology after 2.5 years of episodic petrol vapor inhalation. Comstock (1978) found that solvent abusers scored lower than other substance abusers on a number of scales of the Hamilton rating scale for depression. Skuse and Burrell (1982) found in their study of a child psychiatric clinic group of solvent abusers that abuse did not appear to be a cause of psychiatric disturbance; nevertheless it occurred in a group of individuals with a high psychiatric morbidity. Mood changes were especially reported by chronic abusers. Lockhart and Lennox (1983) did not detect any significant difference in psychiatric symptomatology between abusers and non-abusers receiving care in conditions of security. There may be a group of solvent abusers in whom the abuse is psychologically determined in the sense that it represents a response to underlying distress or disorder within the individual such as occurs following a bereavement (Masterton, 1979). Finally, there exists the possibility that the persistent visual hallucinations which may occur secondary to chronic glue sniffing (Channer and Stanley, 1983) may cause difficulty in psychiatric diagnosis.

Solvent abuse in a child or adolescent may be suspected because of deterioration in school performance. Dodds and Santostefano (1964) could not demonstrate any permanent effect of solvent abuse on school adjustment and performance yet the association between abuse and low performance has frequently been noted (Press and Done, 1967; Watson, 1977). There are many difficulties in determining whether deteriorating or low academic performance is directly the result of solvent toxicity or whether is it associated with other school or social factors. A number of solvent abusers are truants and it would not be surprising to find their educational achievements at a lower level than their contemporaries. Furthermore, there are considerable difficulties in determining the often subtle neuropsychological sequelae of solvent abuse (King, 1983). Korman *et al.* (1981) found inhalant abusers to perform more poorly than other drug abusers on a number of neuropsychological measures including Wechsler IQ, suggesting deficits in a broad range of cognitive skills as a result of the abuse. Mahmood (1983) found some differences in tests of ability between non-active solvent abusing adolescents and controls, the former performing less well on most tests. Allison and Jerrom (1984) administered a psychological test battery to assess memory, intelligence and attention to 10 delinquent solvent inhalers and 10 matched controls. The solvent abuse group showed significant impairment in tests of memory, non-verbal intelligence, and attention and concentration. The effects of toluene abuse on the visual system have been investigated by Cooper *et al.* (1985) who found small but persistent abnormalities in 12 adolescent subjects. The long-term neurological, intellectual and psychiatric sequelae of solvent abuse have been extensively reviewed by Ron (1986).

Withdrawal symptoms following cessation of solvent inhalation (Glaser and Massengale, 1962) are evidently not severe compared to those which occur following narcotic withdrawal, and may not occur if the duration of abuse has been less than 3 months (Press and Done, 1967). Sourindhrin and Baird (1964) did not find withdrawal symptoms in their study of solvent abusers. Psychological dependence may be seen frequently, however (Novak, 1980), and is manifested by a compelling need to inhale, and anxiety about not being able to gain access to the inhalant. O'Connor (1983) considered that the most serious psychological ill-effect of solvent abuse is the force of the habit itself; the stress-reducing effect of inhalation is such as to reinforce the behavior, and increase the likelihood of its being repeated.

9. THE RELATIONSHIP BETWEEN ABUSE OF SOLVENTS AND ABUSE OF ALCOHOL AND OTHER DRUGS

A significant aspect of public anxiety about solvent abuse lies in the possibility that it may be linked to excessive alcohol consumption or, more seriously, to the taking of drugs including the narcotics. Solvent abuse and the drinking of alcohol were at one time considered to be mutually exclusive activities. This belief has been questioned by Crites and Schuckit (1979) although their study of solvent abusing adolescents was based on a population primarily referred because of "alcohol-related" problems. Novak (1980) considered that if inhalant abuse was persistent, there was usually a combination with alcohol and drugs, especially central nervous system depressants. Cohen (1984) asserted that solvent abusers tended to become alcohol or sedative abusers on reaching adulthood, but continuities and discontinuities in this area are particularly difficult to study. Skuse and Burrell (1982) found in their clinic population that solvent abuse was often associated with the use of alcohol and multiple illicit drugs, and that the effect of solvent abuse could be enhanced by drinking alcohol and smoking cigarettes. Watson (1986), on the other hand, found little relationship between solvent abuse and alcohol consumption. Whitehead *et al.* (1972), in a study of marijuana users in three Canadian cities, found them to be six times as likely to have abused glue as non-users of marijuana.

D'Amanda *et al.* (1977) suggested that heroin addicts who had previously sniffed glue were more likely to attempt suicide than those who had not; a quarter of the participants in a heroin addiction treatment program had histories of sniffing. Other studies in this area were considered by Barnes (1979) who regarded the results as suggestive of a pattern of progression from solvent abuse to opiate abuse. Davies *et al.* (1985) reported 4 glue sniffers who had progressed to using illicit drugs or abusing alcohol or both. All had suffered parental deprivation or rejection in childhood and all had progressed from sniffing glue to inhaling heroin and thence to injecting heroin. The authors speculate that such progression may be commoner than hitherto supposed. The factors determining motivation towards maintaining solvent abuse may be important in relation to possible progression to other drugs (Matthews and Korman, 1981).

10. THE MANAGEMENT OF SOLVENT ABUSE IN CHILDREN AND ADOLESCENTS

Although there would be a general consensus that the management of solvent abuse should consist of early, "minimal non-dramatic, non-alarmist intervention" (Sourindhrin, 1985) there is often uncertainty as to what this intervention should include. It may be disputed whether solvent abuse represents a habit, or a disorder; whether solvent abusers are psychologically disordered or not; and whether services for solvent abusers should be developed, or not, and if they are, what they should provide. Solvent abuse at times appears to present an embarrassment to children's services, rather than a challenge. These ambiguities are sharpened by the difficulty of researching solvent abuse. Watson (1986) has described an attempt to mount a prevalence survey in schools, and its abandonment in the face of adverse publicity. A lack of information about all aspects of solvent abuse makes it very difficult to develop appropriate management strategies; yet a policy of nonintervention, based on the transient nature of much solvent abuse is nevertheless unsatisfactory, even if only because of the ill-effects on the community of a proportion of abusers (O'Connor, 1983). Still more would differing views be expressed over the question of whether young people should be taught how to practise solvent abuse safely (Black, 1982a; Masterton, 1979).

10.1. Management of the Individual Solvent Abuser

10.1.1. *Medical Management*

Acute intoxication with organic solvents can be alleviated adequately with fresh air, and oxygen if required (Chapel and Taylor, 1968). If the affected young person is comatose, or respiration is severely depressed, artificial ventilation may be required. Collapse occasioned by cardiac arrhythmia requires full resuscitative measures. The general health of solvent abusers who come to medical attention should be attended to; O'Connor (1983) draws particular attention to the poor diet of a proportion. Where the physical state is unsatisfactory on recovery from intoxication, or where complications are present, hospital admission for investigation should be advised. Commencement of abstinence from solvent abuse may lead to withdrawal symptoms, necessitating mild sedation (Wyse, 1973) but this is very uncommon. The full medical investigation of solvent abusers should include a neurological examination. It may be useful to estimate the blood concentration of toluene, and the measurement of urinary concentrations of benzoic acid and hippuric acid (metabolites of toluene) and of toluric acid (metabolite of xylene) can be carried out by high performance liquid chromatography. A urinary hippurate to creatinine ratio greater than unity generally indicates exposure to toluene (Ramsay and Flanagan, 1982b). Where petrol sniffing is suspected, the blood lead level should be estimated. The electroencephalogram in solvent abuse is variable (Brozovsky and Winkler, 19865; Press and Done, 1967). Diffuse or focal slow or sharp wave disturbance may occur (King *et al.*, 1981). Wyse (1973) considered that such EEG abnormalities as might be present were transient. They tend not to be present on repeat EEG recording taken after some weeks have elapsed (King, 1982), and in any case are not always evident at first examination. More persistent abnormalities may be present in those who sniff leaded petrol (Seshia *et al*, 1978). Lamont and Adams (1982) described a case in which glue sniffing was associated with a positive radioisotope brain scan.

No specific medical treatment is indicated in the majority of solvent abusers. In petrol sniffers, where the blood lead level is raised and neurological symptoms are present, chelation therapy should be considered (Eastwell *et al.*, 1983) as it is of proven effectiveness (Seshia *et al.*, 1978; Brown, 1983). A suitable treatment schedule including calcium disodium edetate, dimercaprol, and penicillamine has been described (Fortenberry, 1985).

10.1.2. *Psychological and Psychiatric Care*

O'Connor (1983) takes the view that solvent abuse is essentially a psychological problem, approaches to which should provide "a substitute form of loving care and attention imbued with sensible discipline and guidance." While this does not imply the wide use of psychological and psychiatric services, it is wise to consider specialist referral if there is severe intoxication, solitary or prolonged abuse, or employment of dangerous methods (Herzberg and Wolkind, 1983). Psychiatric help is certainly indicated in those solvent abusers who have evidence of a persistent organic brain syndrome (Comstock, 1978). Sourinhdrin and Baird (1984) found 8 of 134 cases to be in need of psychiatric care. De Barona and Simpson (1984) describe the inclusion of inhalant abusers in a general drug abuse prevention programme in the U.S.A., but Strang and Connell (1985) rightly advocate the management of younger solvent abusers within conventional psychiatric and community resources, outwith drug dependence services.

Individual psychiatric or psychological care should be based on assessment (Strang and Connell, 1985), and needs to be combined with approaches to family and school (Black, 1982; Cohen, 1984; Sourindhrin and Baird, 1984). Few cases will require care because of a toxic psychosis; it is to the reduction or elimination of the solvent abuse that most attention will be given. Behavior modification techniques, including aversion methods, have been employed in an attempt to reduce or eliminate solvent sniffing behavior (Lowenstein, 1982; O'Connor, 1983; Sourindhrin and Baird, 1984). O'Connor (1982) also describes the use of suggestion techniques. Hypnosis has been employed in an attempt to reduce glue sniffing (O'Connor, 1982; Bowers and Sage, 1983). Laury (1972) described individual psychotherapy focused on exploring underlying causes, with attempts being made to channel the child's activities in another direction and also to change parental attitudes and behavior. Non-directive, Rogerian psychotherapeutic techniques have also been attempted (O'Connor, 1983).

Rubin and Babbs (1970) compared four management methods, 3 of them Court based, and found that an approach which concentrated on the individual (through counselling), his leisure time, and his family, produced better results than work based solely on the individual abuser. O'Connor (1983) described the work of a counselling clinic in an English city; guidelines for management of their children were given to parents, and use was also made of the teaching of reading to abusers, a number of whom were found to be deficient in reading skills. Masterton (1979) described group therapy run in a Social Work Department "Intermediate Treatment" Center. The technique employed made use of peer group cohesion although it is pointed out that such cohesion may as readily perpetuate solvent abuse as help to terminate it. Indeed, it is recognized that reduction in solvent abuse in a group of adolescents may at times only be achieved by removal from the group of an individual with affectionless personality traits, who may exert a quite disproportionate influence on his contemporaries by his forceful and aggressive behavior.

Considerable stress occurs in a family one of whose members is abusing solvent (Masterton, 1979). The difficulties which arise for the family are well described by Watson (1986), and it has been recognized for some time that involvement of the family in management is important (Chapel and Taylor, 1968; Kaufman, 1981). Particular help may be needed by single parents of solvent abusers (Sourindhrin and Baird, 1984). Framrose (1982) described family therapy with a number of solvent abusers. He identified the way in which glue sniffing in adolescents from families in which the marital relationship was poor, and the fathers often uninvolved and ineffective in their parental role, served the function of allowing the young person some affiliation with a delinquent peer group while at the same time arousing continuing maternal care and concern. Family work may also be required where death has occurred from solvent abuse, when in addition to sorrow there are problems of guilt, recrimination and anger (O'Connor, 1983).

Solvent abuse may occur as a rapidly spreading epidemic in a boarding school or children's home; the waves of abuse, as more and more youngsters try it out, are exceeded only by the waves of panic engendered among staff (Boeckx and Coodin, 1977, 1978). Three quarters of solvent abusers in a community home studied by Pierce (1982) had developed the habit on the premises. In the face of a local epidemic a strategy employing diversion of those affected into other activities, coupled with a calm approach to the abuse itself, and education of staff and young people, will usually bring the outbreak to a close.

The present position of psychological and psychiatric approaches to solvent abuse is unsatisfactory. The management techniques discussed above have not been adequately evaluated, partly because of the difficulty inherent in studying many forms of psychological treatment and partly because of the problem of distinguishing the casual and occasional abuser from the more longterm, habitual abuser who may be more likely to have underlying personality disorders. O'Connor's (1983) assertion that the effectiveness of treatment is conditional on the degree to which the abuser wishes to stop the habit, and experiences a caring relationship with the therapist as a strong healing process, may express a clinical reality; it does not, however, advance the development of therapeutic techniques.

10.2. Community Approaches to the Management of Solvent Abuse

Concern over the prevalence of solvent abuse in the U.K. increased considerably during the 1970s. In 1981 the Department of Health and Social Security in the U.K. examined how the provision of information on solvent abuse to the public could be improved, and advocated community-based approaches via multidisciplinary networks aimed at education and counselling (Blyth, 1982). A threefold approach has been described by Peers (1981); primary prevention, including the provision of education to counteract the development of "problematic behaviour" with the aim of changing attitudes of young people sufficiently early to preempt the development of solvent abuse; secondary prevention, which uses education as an intervention procedure to modify behavior so that it no longer presents a problem; and treatment, which aims to substitute new behavior for problem behavior. Most community approaches to solvent abuse contain elements of the multidisciplinary and threefold intervention models, and in the Strathclyde Region of Scotland, Watson has pioneered the development of services along these lines. She describes (Watson, 1986) the setting up of multidisciplinary solvent abuse committees including general practitioners, psychiatrists, community doctors and nurses, teachers, social workers, health education workers, and police to exchange relevant information, and discuss local problems, with a view to developing suitable intervention strategies.

Control of the development and spread of solvent abuse is difficult but is nevertheless demanded by an anxious public. Publicity regarding solvent abuse and the dangers of organic solvents carries the danger of stimulating the curiosity of young people (Press and Done, 1967; Edwards, 1982). There are plainly risks involved in an approach to solvent abuse emphasizing physical hazards and lethal potential, which may increase the problem by pointing up the attractiveness of the habit as a high risk and therefore a high status activity (Rowell and Wood, 1981). Restriction on sales of solvent products to the age group considered to be at risk has been implemented in a rather uneven fashion in the U.K. The view of the Department of Health and Social Security in 1981 was that such restriction was likely to be impractical, as was any attempt at reformulation of commonly abused solvent products to remove the solvent or substitute a non-toxic agent. Adding deterrent substances to abused solvent products was advocated by Masterton (1979); Benarie (1982) strongly recommended denaturation of solvents susceptible to abuse. These measures have not been taken up to any extent; and there has been recognition that repackaging of solvent products to make them less easily abused is equally impractical (Sourindhrin, 1985). Anderson *et al.* (1985) point out that because of the small proportion of deaths from volatile solvent abuse occurring in children under the age of 16, attempts to limit access to glue by this group of young people were likely to have little impact on mortality.

In the U.S.A., too, the view of Government was that controls on the sale (and abuse) of solvent products would be impractical and unrealistic (Peers, 1981). Persuasion and education were seen as more appropriate. Despite this, 13 states in the U.S.A. had already enacted legislation for the control of glue sniffing by the latter half of the 1960s; the scepticism of Kupperstein and Susman (1968) regarding the value of legislation had not been heeded. They had pointed out that legislation would be likely to be negative in its consequences since it would redefine deviant behavior as delinquent behavior, and transfer a social and psychological problem legislatively to Courts and correctional agencies which had neither the resources nor the competence to effectively manage the treatment and preventive aspects of the problem (Rubin and Babbs, 1970). Specifically, a ban was placed on the manufacture and interstate commerce of aerosol products containing fluorinated hydrocarbons by the Food and Drug Administration and the Environmental Protection Agency of the U.S. Government in 1979.

In the U.K., a number of private Parliamentary Bills to make public sniffing of solvents an offence, or to require manufacturers to add unpleasant odors to their products, have failed. In 1983, however, the Solvent Abuse (Scotland) Act reached the statute book. It allows a child who "has misused a volatile substance by deliberately inhaling other than for medicinal purposes that substance's vapour" to be referred to the Children's Panel (the Scottish forum in which most juvenile justice, care and protection matters are dealt with) as possibly being in need of measures of compulsory care. Two years later, the Intoxicating Substances Supply Act of 1985, applying to England and Wales, made it an offence for a person to supply to someone under the age of 18 substances he or she knows, or has reason to believe, are to be used to achieve intoxication. Criticism of the Scottish act (Craig, 1983; Asquith and Didcott, 1984) has pointed to the legislation's failure to assist in developing appropriate methods for dealing with children who inhale solvents. The immediate aftermath of the legislation has also been discussed by Ashton (1984).

Referrals on account of solvent abuse to Reporters to Children's Panels in Scotland increased from 102 out of 30,100 referrals in 1983 (the year in which legislation was enacted) to 672 out of 31,600 referrals in 1984 (*Glasgow Herald*, 22.4.86). It is not known whether this increase has been sustained. In one Scottish city, 43 children were referred to the Reporter to the Children's Panel primarily on account of episodes of solvent abuse in 1982; nearly 15% of these children had been similarly notified to the Reporter in the previous year. In 1983, 11 children were referred; the number rose to 31 in 1984 but declined again to 27 in 1985 (Meek, personal communication, 1986).

Increased knowledge of the dangers of solvent abuse among retailers of solvent products has led in some areas to the imposition of a voluntary code of conduct regarding marketing and display, which may have had benefit in limiting casual abuse (Sourindhrin and Baird, 1984). Much publicity has occurred when shopkeepers have been prosecuted for selling 'glue sniffing kits'; Willock (1984) discusses the legal implications involved in the conviction of two shopkeepers who received a sentence of 3 years imprisonment. Hindmarsh *et al.* (1983) found that knowledge about solvent abuse was patchy among shopkeepers in a province of Canada.

The police may have solvent abusers brought to their attention because of intoxicated behavior (whether dangerous or not) or because of the theft of solvent products. Knight (1982) pointed out the unacceptability to the police force of any impression that sniffing glue vapor might be officially sanctioned, but emphasized the value of the flexible approach to the problem which was open to the police when their role in working with other agencies, and in conjunction with Health Education personnel, was not constrained by legislation. O'Connor (1983) noted that at times reporting of solvent abuse by the police was variable because they found that referrals to social services rarely led to an effective response.

Rowell and Wood (1981) saw the prevention of solvent abuse as the province of health education. The demonstration that health education used on a routine basis is an effective measure is difficult, however (Press and Done, 1967). Woodcock (1982) reviewed research on health education in the area of solvent abuse and found little evidence that it was effective in preventing experimentation with solvents, but considered that it could be effective in modifying the abuser's choice of substance, and style of use. Ramsay (1982) suggested the introduction of appropriate strategies to define the nature of solvent abuse, reduce the number of abusers, and then assess the effectiveness of the programme. Useful work has been done to produce information literature for professionals, parents, and children and young people. The Scottish Health Education Group's (1982) publication "Solvent Abuse; A Report for Professionals Working in Scotland" includes sections on those solvents which are abused; the characteristics of abusers; the response of society; and the development of strategies by the professions involved. There is a helpful design for a workshop on solvent abuse. The same organization's "Drugs and Young People in Scotland" (1984), which is aimed at teachers and youth workers, contains a short section on glues and solvents. RESOLV (The Society for the Prevention of Solvent and Volatile Substance Abuse) advocates an essentially educational approach to solvent abuse and has contributed to the dissemination of helpful information (Merrill, 1985).

11. CONCLUSION

Solvent abuse is an international phenomenon. Affecting adolescents above all, it provides for the majority a transient intoxicating experience which takes its place beside the other experimentation in which young people engage as they grow up. Peer group pressure may be as important a factor in stopping a youngster abusing solvent, as in starting the habit. For a minority, solvent abuse becomes persistent, in which case it often has a considerable effect on health, education and behavior, and may scarcely even serve as an effective shield against the unpleasant realities of day-to-day life. The mortality rate from solvent abuse is low, but engenders much concern; and the development of strategies for treatment of individual abusers and for the control and prevention of the habit reflect the difficulties inherent in all problems concerned with human development and behavior.

REFERENCES

Abgrall, J.-M. and Botta, A. (1983) Approche psychiatrique d'un fait criminologique; La toxocomanie aux colles et solvents. *Bull. Acad. Natl. Med.* **167**: 849–854.

Ackerly W. C. and Gibson, G. (1964) Lighter fluid 'sniffing'. *Am. J. Psychiat.* **120**: 1056–1061.

Allison, W. M. and Jerrom, D. W. A. (1984) Glue sniffing. A pilot study of the cognitive effects of longterm use. *Int. J. Addict.* **19**: 453–458.

Allister, C., Lush, M., Oliver, J. S. and Watson, J. M. (1981) Status epilepticus caused by solvent abuse. *Br. Med. J.* **283**: 1156.

Altenkirch, H., Mager J., Stoltenburg, G. and Helmbrecht, J. (1977) Toxic polyneuropathies after sniffing a glue thinner. *J. Neurol.* **214**: 137–152.

Anderson, H. R., Dick, B., Macnair, R. S., Palmer, J. C. and Ramsey, J. D. (1982) An investigation of 140 deaths associated with volatile substance abuse in the U.K. (1971–1981). *Hum. Toxicol.* **1**: 207–221.

Anderson, H. R., Macnair, R. S. and Ramsey, J. D. (1985) Deaths from abuse of volatile substances: a national epidemiological study. *Br. Med. J.* **290**: 304–307.

Ashton, M. (1984) Solvents law in Scotland. *I.S.D.D. Druglink Information Letter*: Spring 1984, 1–7.

Asquith, S. and Didcott, P. (1984) The management of solvent abuse—an exploratory study. *Social Work Services Group, Scottish Office, Edinburgh.*

Barnes, G. E. (1979) Solvent abuse: a review. *Int. J. Addict.* **14**: 1–26.

Bass, M. (1970) Sudden sniffing death. *J. Am. Med. Ass.* **212**: 2075–2079.

Benarie, M. (1982) Olfactive and visual labelling of solvents. *Sci. Total Environ.* **25**: 1–2.

Black, D. (1982a) Glue sniffing. *Arch. Dis. Child.* **57**: 893–894.

Black, D. (1982b) Misuse of solvents. *Health Trends* **14**: 27–28.

Black, P. D. (1967) Mental illness due to the voluntary inhalation of petrol vapour. *Med. J. Aust.* **ii**: 70–71.

Blyth, A. M. (1982) Solvent abuse: summary of a paper presented on behalf of the D.H.S.S. *Hum. Toxicol.* **1**: 347–349.

Boeckx, R. L., Postl, B., and Coodin, F. S. (1977) Gasoline sniffing and tetra-ethyl lead poisoning in children. *Pediatrics* **60**: 140–145.

Boeckx, R. L., Postl, B. and Coodin, F. S. (1978) An epidemic of gasoline sniffing. In: *Voluntary Inhalation of Industrial Solvents*, Sharp, C. W. and Carroll, L. T. (eds). Rockville, Maryland.

Bowers, A. J. and Sage, L. R. (1983) Solvent abuse in adolescents: the Who? What? and Why?. *Child Care Health Dev.* **9**: 169–178.

Brown, A. (1983) Petrol sniffing lead encephalopathy. *N.Z. Med. J.* **96**: 421–422.

Brozovsky, M. and Winkler, E. G. (1965) Glue sniffing in children and adolescents. *N.Y. St. J. Med.* **65**: 1984–1989.

Bruckner, J. V. and Peterson, R. G. (1981) Evaluation of toluene and acetone inhalant abuse. I. Pharmacology and pharmacodynamics; II. Model development and toxicology. *Toxic. Appl. Pharmac.* **61**: 27–38; 302–312.

Channer, K. S. and Stanley, S. (1983) Persistent visual hallucinations secondary to chronic solvent encephalopathy: case report and review of the literature. *J. Neurol. Neurosurg. Psychiat.* **46**: 83–86.

Chapel, J. L. and Taylor, D. W. (1968) Glue sniffing. *Missouri Med.* **65**: 288–296.

Clements, J. E. and Simpson, R. (1978) Environmental and behavioural aspects of glue sniffing in a population of emotionally disturbed adolescents. *Int. J. Addict.* **13**: 129–134.

Cohen, S. (1984) The hallucinogens and the inhalants. *Psychiatr. Clin. N. Am.* **7(4)**: 681–688.

Comstock, B. S. (1978) Psychological measurements in long-term chronic inhalant abusers. In: *Voluntary Inhalation of Industrial Solvents*, Sharp, C. W. and Carroll, L. T. (eds) Rockville, Maryland.

Cooper, R., Newton, P. and Reed, M. (1985) Neurophysiological signs of brain damage due to glue sniffing. *Electroenceph. Clin. Neurophysiol.* **60**: 23–26.

Coulehan, J. L., Hirsh, W., Brillman, J., Sanandria, J., Welty, T. K., Colaiaco, P., Koros, A. and Lober, A. (1983) Gasoline sniffing and lead toxicity in Navajo adolescents. *Paediatrics* **71**: 113–117.

Craig, B. J. S. (1983) Stuck with the Act. A psychiatrist's view of the Solvent Abuse (Scotland) Act. 1983. *Scottish Child* **1**: 2–5.

Crites, J. and Schuckit, M. A. (1979) Solvent misuse in adolescents at a community alcohol center. *J. Clin. Psychiat.* **40**: 39–43.

Cronk, S. L., Barkley, D. E. H. and Farrell, M. F. (1985) Respiratory arrest after solvent abuse. *Br. Med. J.* **290**: 897–898.

D'Amanda, C., Plumb, M. M. and Taintor, Z. (1977) Heroin addicts with a history of glue sniffing: A deviant group within a deviant group. *Int. J. Addict* **12**: 255–270.

Davies, B., Thorley, A. and O'Connor, D. (1985) Progression of addiction careers in young solvent misusers. *Br. Med. J.* **290**: 109–110.

De Barona, M. S. and Simpson, D. D. (1984) Inhalant users in drug abuse prevention programs. *Am. J. Drug Alcohol Abuse.* **10**: 503–518.

Devathasan, G., Low, D., Teoh, P. C., Wan, S. H. and Wong, P. K. (1984) Complications of chronic glue toluene abuse in adolescents. *Aust. N. Z. J. Med.* **14**: 39–43.

Dodds, J. and Santostefano, S. (1964) A comparison of the cognitive functioning of glue sniffers and non-sniffers. *J. Pediat.* **64**: 565–570. *Drugs and Young People in Scotland*. 3rd ed, (1986) Scottish Health Education Group, Edinburgh.

Eastwell, H. D., Thomas, B. J. and Thomas, B. W. (1983) Skeletal lead burden in Aborigine petrol sniffing. *Lancet* **ii** 524–525.

Editorial (1982) Solvent abuse. *Lancet* **ii**: 1139–1140.

Edwards, I. R. (1982) Solvent abuse (Leading article) *N.Z. Med. J.* **95**: 879–880.

Ehyai, A. and Freeman, F. R. (1983) Progressive optic neuropathy and sensorineural hearing loss due to chronic glue sniffing. *J. Neurol. Neurosurg. Psychiat.* **46**: 349–351.

Evans, J. (1982) *Adolescent and Pre-Adolescent Psychiatry*. Grune and Stratton, New York.

Fornazzari, L., Wilkinson, D. A., Kapur, B. M. and Carlen, P. L. (1983) Cerebellar cortical and functional impairment in toluene abusers. *Acta Neurol. Scand.* **67**: 319–329.

Fortenberry, J. D. (1985) Gasoline sniffing. *Am. J. Med.* **79**: 740–744.

Framrose, R. (1982) From structure to strategy with the families of solvent abusers. *J. Fam. Ther.* **4**: 43–59.

FRANCIS, J., MURRAY, V. S. G., RUPRAH, M., FLANAGAN, R. J. and RAMSEY, J. D. (1982) Suspected solvent abuse in cases referred to the Poison's Unit, Guy's Hospital, July 1980–June 1981. *Hum. Toxicol.* **1**: 271–280.

GARRIOTT, J. and PETTY, C. S. (1980) Death from inhalant abuse: toxicological and pathological evaluation of 34 cases. *Clin. Toxicol.* **16**: 305–315.

GAY, M. (1981) *The Avon Solvent Monitoring Study*. Solvent misuse workshop, Guy's Hospital. Cited in BLACK, D. (1982b). Misuse of solvents. *Health Trends* **14**: 27–28.

GAY, M., MELLER, R. and STANLEY, S. (1982) Drug abuse monitoring; a survey of solvent abuse in the county of Avon. *Hum. Toxicol.* **1**: 257–263.

GELLMAN, V. (1968) Glue-sniffing among Winnipeg school children. *Can. Med. Ass. J.* **98**: 411–413.

GLASER, F. B. (1966) Inhalation psychosis and related states. *Arch. Gen. Psychiat.* 14: 315–322.

GLASER, H. H. and MASSENGALE, O. N. (1962) Glue sniffing in children. *J. Am. Med. Ass.* **181**: 300–303.

GOODWIN, J. M., GEIL, C., GRODNER, B. and METRICK, S. (1981) Inhalant abuse, pregnancy and neglected children (Letter). *Am. J. Psychiat* **138**: 1126.

GOTO, I., MATSUMURA, M., INOUE, N., MURAI, Y., SHIDA, K., SANTA, T. and KUROIWA, Y. (1974) Toxic polyneuropathy due to glue sniffing. *J. Neurol. Neurosurg. Psychiat.* **37**: 848–853.

HERZBERG, J. L. and WOLKIND, S. N. (1983) Solvent sniffing in perspective. *Br. J. Hosp. Med.* **29**: 72–76.

HINDMARSH, K. W., HENSMAN, L. R., KOLBINSON, C. L. and MUCHA, A. M. (1983) Solvent abuse—attitudes and knowledge among Saskatchewan retailers. *Int. J. Addict.* **18**: 139–142.

IVES, R. (1981) Solvent abuse: a review of research. *Highlight No. 43*. National Children's Bureau, London.

IVES, R. (1986) Solvent misuse. *Highlight No. 72*. National Children's Bureau, London.

JAMIESON, J. H. (1980) All buzzed up. *Community Homes Gazette* **74**: 171–174.

KAUFMAN, A. and WIESE, W. (1978) Gasoline sniffing leading to increased lead absorption in children. *Clin. Pediat.* **17**: 475–477.

KAUFMAN, E. (1981) Family therapy—a treatment approach with substance abusers. In: *Substance Abuse: Clinical Problems and Perspectives*. LOWINSON, J. H. V. and RUIZ, P. (eds) Williams and Wilkins, Baltimore, Maryland.

KEANE, J. R. (1978) Toluene optic neuropathy. *Ann. Neurol.* **4**: 390.

KING, G. S., SMIALEK, J. E. and TROUTMAN, W. G. (1985a) Sudden death in adolescents resulting from the inhalation of typewriter correction fluid. *J. Am. Med. Ass.* **253**: 1604–1606.

KING, P. J. L., MORRIS, J. G. L. and POLLARD, J. D. (1985b) Glue sniffing neuropathy. *Aust. N.Z. J. Med.* **15**: 293–299.

KING, M. D. (1981) Reversible renal damage due to glue sniffing (Letter). *Br. Med. J.* **283**: 919.

KING, M. D., DAY, R. E., OLIVER, J. S., LUSH, M. and WATSON, J. (1981) Solvent encephalopathy. *Br. Med. J.* **283**: 663–665.

KING, M. D. (1982) Neurological sequelae of toluene abuse. *Hum. Toxicol.* **1**: 281–287.

KING, M. D. (1983) Long term neuropsychological effects of solvent abuse. In: *Neuropsychological Effects of Solvent Exposure*, CHERRY, N. and WALDRON, H. A. (eds) The Colt Foundation.

KNIGHT, W. (1982) Solvent abuse—the role of the police. *Toxicology* **1**: 345–346.

KORMAN, J., MATTHEWS, R. W. and LOVITT, R. (1981) Neuropsychological effects of abuse of inhalants. *Percept. Mot. Skills* **53**: 547–553.

KOROBKIN, R., ASBURY, A. K., SUMNER, A. J. and NIELSEN, S. L. (1975) Glue sniffing neuropathy. *Arch. Neurol.* **32**: 158–162.

KOVANEN, J., SOMER, H. and SCHROEDER, P. (1983) Acute myopathy associated with gasoline sniffing. *Neurology* **33**: 629–631.

KROEGER, R. M., MOORE, R. J., LEHMAN, T. H., GIESY, J. D. and SKEETERS, C. E. (1980) Recurrent urinary calculi associated with toluene sniffing. *J. Urol.* **123**: 89–91.

KUPPERSTEIN, L. R. and SUSMAN, R. M. (1968) A bibliography on the inhalation of glue fumes and other toxic vapours—a substance abuse practice among adolescents. *Int. J. Addict.* **3**: 177–197.

LAMONT, C. M. and ADAMS, F. G. (1982) Glue-sniffing as a cause of a positive radio-isotope brain scan. *Eur. J. Nucl. Med.* **7**: 387–388.

LAURY, G. V. (1972) Psychotherapy with glue sniffers. *Int. J. Child Psychother.* **1**: 98–110.

LOCKHART, W. H. and LENNOX, M. (1983) The extent of solvent abuse in a regional secure unit sample. *J. Adolesc.* **6**: 43–55.

LOWENSTEIN, L. F. (1982) Glue sniffing. Background features and treatment by aversion methods and group therapy. *Practitioner* **226**: 1113–1116.

LUSH, M., OLIVER, J. S. and WATSON, J. M. (1980) The analysis of blood in cases of suspected solvent abuse with a review of results during the period October 1977 to July 1979. In: *Forensic Toxicology*, OLIVER, J. S. (ed.) Croom Helm, London.

MAHMOOD, Z. (1983) Cognitive functioning of solvent abusers. *Sc. Med. J.* **28**: 276–280.

MALM, G. and LYING-TUNELL, U. (1980) Cerebellar dysfunction related to toluene sniffing. *Acta. Neurol. Scand.* **62**: 188–190.

MARSH, W. W. (1984) Butane firebreathing in adolescents; a potentially dangerous practice. *J. Adolesc. Health Care.* **5**: 59–60.

MASSENGALE, O. N., GLASER, H. H., LELIEVRE, R. E., DODDS, J. B. and KLOCK, M. E. (1963) Physical and psychological factors in glue sniffing. *New Engl. J. Med.* **269**: 1340–1344.

MASTERTON, G. and SCLARE, A. B. (1978) Solvent abuse. *Health Bull.* (*Edinburgh*) **36**: 305–309.

MASTERTON, G. (1979) The management of solvent abuse. *J. Adolesc.* **2**: 65–75.

MATTHEWS, R. W. and KORMAN, M. (1981) Abuse of inhalants; motivation and consequences. *Psychol. Rep.* **49**: 519–526.

MEE, A. S. and WRIGHT, P. L. (1980) Congestive (dilated) cardiomyopathy in association with solvent abuse. *J. R. Soc. Med.* **73**: 671–672.

MERRILL, E. (1985) *Sniffing Solvents*, Pepar Publications, Birmingham.

MERRY, J. and ZACHARIADIS, N. (1962) Addiction to glue sniffing. *Br. Med. J.* **ii**: 1448.
MOOSA, A. and LOENING, W. E. K. (1981) Solvent abuse in black children in Natal. *S. Afr. Med. J.* **59**: 509–510.
NICHOLI, A. M. (1983). The inhalants: an overview. *Psychosomatics.* **24**: 914–921.
NITSCHE, C. J. and ROBINSON, J. F. (1959) A case of gasoline addiction. *Am. J. Orthopsychiat.* **29**: 417–419.
NOVAK, A. (1980) The deliberate inhalation of volatile substances. *J. Psychedelic Drugs.* **12**: 105–122.
O'BRIEN, E. T., YEOMAN, W. B. and HORBY, J. A. E. (1971) Hepatorenal damage from toluene in a "glue sniffer". *Br. Med. J.* **ii**: 29–30.
O'CONNOR, D. (1979) A profile of solvent abuse in school children. *J. Ch. Psychol. Psychiat.* **20**: 365–368.
O'CONNOR, D. (1982) The use of suggestion techniques with adolescents in the treatment of glue sniffing and solvent abuse. *Hum. Toxicol.* **1**: 313–320.
O'CONNOR, D. (1983). *Glue Sniffing and Volatile Substance Abuse.* Gower Press, England.
OLIVER, J. S. and WATSON, J. M. (1977) Abuse of solvents "for kicks." *Lancet* **i**: 84–86.
OLIVER, J. S. (1982) The analytical diagnosis of solvent abuse. *Hum. Toxicol.* **1**: 293–297.
OPPENHEIMER, E. (1985) Drug taking. In: *Child and Adolescent Psychiatry—Modern Approaches*, RUTTER, M. and HERSOV, L. (eds) Blackwell, Oxford.
PARKER, M. J., TARLOW, M. J. and MILNE ANDERSON, J. (1984) Glue sniffing and cerebral infarction. *Arch. Dis. Ch.* **59**: 675–677.
PEERS, I. S. (1981) A community approach to the problems of solvent abuse. *Health Educ. J.* **40**: 31–40.
PIERCE, J. G. (1982) Glue sniffing in a community home. Unpublished report cited in BOWERS, A. J. and SAGE, L. R. (1983) (op. cit.).
POKLIS, A. and BURKETT, C. D. (1977) Gasoline sniffing: A review. *Clin. Toxicol.* **ii**: 35–41.
POWARS, D. (1965) Aplastic anaemia secondary to glue sniffing. *New Eng. J. Med.* **273**: 700–702.
PRASAD, A. J. (1984) Endocrine abnormalities in solvent sniffers. *Psychoneuroendocrinology* **9**: 315–316.
PRESS, E. (1963) Glue sniffing (Editor's column). *J. Pediat.* **63**: 517–518.
PRESS, E. and DONE, A. K. (1967) Solvent sniffing. Physiological effects and community control measures for intoxication from the intentional inhalation of organic solvents. *Pediatrics* **39**: 451–461, 611–622.
PROCKOP, L. D. (1979) Neurotoxic volatile substances. *Neurology* **29**: 862–865.
PROCKOP, L. D. and KARAMPELAS, D. (1981) Encephalopathy secondary to abusive gasoline inhalation. *J. Fla. Med. Ass.* **68**: 823–824.
RAMSAY, A. W. (1982) Solvent abuse: an educational perspective. *Hum. Toxicol.* **1**: 265–270.
RAMSAY, J. D. and FLANAGAN, R. J. (1982a) Detection and identification of volatile organic compounds in blood by headspace gas chromatography as an aid to the diagnosis of solvent abuse. *J. Chromat.* **240**: 423–444.
RAMSAY, J. D. and FLANAGAN, R. J. (1982b) The role of the laboratory in the investigation of solvent abuse. *Hum. Toxicol.* **1**: 299–311.
RAMSAY, J. D. (1983) The role of the laboratory in the investigation of solvent abuse. *J. Forens. Sci. Sco.* **23**: 245.
REED, B. J. F. and MAY, P. A. (1984) Inhalant abuse and juvenile delinquency. A control study in Albuquerque, New Mexico. *Int. J. Addict.* **19**: 789–803.
ROBERTS, D. J. (1982) Abuse of aerosol products by inhalation. *Hum. Toxicol.* **1**: 231–238.
ROBINS, L. (1966) *Deviant Children Grown Up.* Williams and Wilkins, Baltimore, Maryland.
RON, M. A. (1986) Volatile substance abuse: a review of possible long-term neurological, intellectual and psychiatric sequelae. *Br. J. Psychiat.* **148**: 235–246.
ROWELL, V. and WOOD, P. J. W. (1981) A health education approach to solvent abuse. *Health Educ. J.* **40**: 41–45.
RUBIN, T. and BABBS, J. (1970) The glue sniffer. *Federal Probation.* **34**: 23–28.
RUSS, G., CLARKSON, A. R., WOODROFFE, A. J., SEYMOUR, A. E. and CHENG, I. K. P. (1981) Renal failure from 'glue sniffing.' *Med. J. Aust.* **2**: 121–122.
SCHIKLER, K. N., SEITZ, K., RICE, J. F. and STRADER, T. (1982) Solvent abuse associated cortical atrophy. *J. Adolesc. Health Care* **3**: 37–39.
SCHIKLER, K. N., LANE, E. E., SEITZ, K. and COLLINS, W. M. (1984) Solvent abuse associated pulmonary abnormalities. *Adv. Alcohol Substance Abuse* **3**: 75–81.
SESHIA, S. S., RAJANI, K. R., BOECKX, R. L. and CHOW, P. N. (1978) The neurological manifestations of chronic inhalation of leaded gasoline. *Dev. Med. Child Neurol.* **20**: 323–334.
SKUSE, D. and BURRELL, S. (1982) A review of solvent abusers and their management by a child psychiatric outpatient service. *Hum. Toxicol.* **1**: 321–329.
SMEETON, W. M. I. and CLARK, M. S. (1985) Sudden death resulting from inhalation of fire extinguishers containing bromochlorodifluoromethane. *Med. Sci. Law* **25**: 258–262.
SMYTH, H. F., WEIL, C.S., WEST, J. S. and CARPENTER, C. P. (1969) An exploration of joint toxic action: twenty seven industrial chemicals intubated in rats in all possible pairs. *Toxicol. Appl. Pharmac.* **14**: 340–347.
SNYDER, R. and KOCSIS, J. J. (1975) Current concepts of chronic benzene toxicity. *C. R. C. Crit. Rev. Toxicol.* **3**: 265–288.
Solvent Abuse. A Report for Professionals Working in Scotland (1982) Scottish Health Education Group, Edinburgh, and Intermediate Treatment Resource Centre, Renfrewshire.
SOURINDHRIN, I. and BAIRD, J. A. (1984) Management of solvent misuse. A Glasgow community approach. *Br. J. Addict* **79**: 227–232.
SOURINHDRIN, I. (1985) Solvent misuse. *Br. Med. J.* **290**: 94–95.
STRANG, J. and CONNELL, P. (1985) Clinical aspects of drug and alcohol abuse. In: *Child and Adolescent Psychiatry—Modern Approaches*, RUTTER, M. and HERSHOV, L. (eds) Blackwell, Oxford.
STREICHER, H.Z., GABOW, P. A., MOSS, A. H., KONG, D. and KAEHNY, W. D. (1981) Syndromes of toluene sniffing in adults. *Ann. Intern. Med.* **94**: 758–762.
SUTHERLAND, I. (1982) When yer oan the glue yer mental. *New Soc.* **59**: 196.
TAKEUCHI, Y., HISANAGA, N., ONO, Y., OGAWA, T., HAMAGUCHI, Y. and OKAMOTO, S. (1981) Cerebral dysfunction caused by sniffing of toluene-containing thinner. *Ind. Health* **19**: 163–169.
TAYLOR, G. J. and HARRIS, W. S. (1970) Glue sniffing causes heart block in mice. *Science* **170**: 866–868.

Towfighi, J., Gonatas, N. K., Pleasure, D., Cooper, H. S. and McCree, L. (1976) Glue sniffer's neuropathy. *Neurology* **26**: 238–243.

Watson, J. M. (1975) A study of solvent sniffing in Lanarkshire. *Health Bull.* **23**: 153–155.

Watson, J. M. (1977) 'Glue-sniffing' in profile. *Practitioner* **218**: 255–259.

Watson, J. M. (1979a) Morbidity and Mortality Statistics on Solvent abuse. *Med. Sci. Law* **19(4)**: 246–252.

Watson, J. M. (1979b) Solvent abuse: a retrospective study. *Community Med.* **1**: 153–156.

Watson, J. M. (1979c) Glue sniffing. Two case reports. *Practitioner* **222**: 845–847.

Watson, J. M. (1982) Solvent Abuse: presentation and clinical diagnosis. *Hum. Toxicol.* **1**: 249–256.

Watson, J. M. (1984) Solvent abuse and adolescents. *Practitioner* **228**: 487–490.

Watson, J. M. (1986) *Solvent Abuse. The Adolescent Epidemic?* Croom Helm, London.

Whitehead, P. C., Smart, R. G. and Laforest, L. (1972) Multiple drug use among marijuana smokers in Eastern Canada. *Int. J. Addict.* **7**: 179–190.

Will, A. M. and McLaren, E. H. (1981) Reversible renal damage due to glue sniffing. *Br. Med. J.* **283**: 525–526.

Willock, I. (1984) Some lessons of Khaliq. *Scottish Legal Action Group Bulletin*, No. 96, September 1984, pp. 124–126.

Woodcock, J. (1982) Solvent abuse from a health education perspective. *Hum. Toxicol.* **1**: 331–336.

Woolfson, R. C. (1982) Psychological correlates of solvent abuse. *Br. J. Med. Psychol.* **5**: 63–66.

Wyse, G. (1973) Deliberate inhalation of volatile hydrocarbons: a review. *Can. Med. Ass. J.* **108**: 71–74.

Young, R. S. K., Grzyb, S. E. and Crisman, L. (1977) Recurrent cerebellar dysfunction as related to chronic gasoline sniffing in an adolescent girl. *Clin. Pediat.* **16**: 706–708.

CHAPTER 14

NICOTINE AS THE BASIS OF THE SMOKING HABIT

D. J. K. BALFOUR
Department of Pharmacology & Clinical Pharmacology, University Medical School, Ninewells Hospital, Dundee, DD1 9SY, Scotland, U.K.

1. INTRODUCTION

The general public were first made aware of the association between tobacco smoking and the development of serious diseases of the respiratory and cardiovascular systems by reports of the Royal College of Physicians of England in 1962 and the United States Surgeon General in 1964. These reports have been followed by others (e.g. Surgeon General, 1979; Royal College of Physicians, 1977) which have confirmed and expanded upon the earlier findings. During the period since the first reports, the level of tobacco smoking amongst the adult population, in the western world at least, initially levelled off and then began to decline significantly (Stepney 1984). Nevertheless, in 1981, in excess of 30% of the adults in the United States and approaching 40% of those in the United Kingdom continued to smoke. Thus a large proportion of the population continued to be exposed to the constituents of tobacco smoke.

It is generally believed that many of the people who smoke do so in order to dose themselves with the nicotine (Armitage *et al.*, 1968; Hall and Morrison, 1973; Bättig, 1980, 1981). Nicotine is certainly the most potent psychopharmacologically active component of tobacco smoke. However, as Ashton and Stepney (1982) report in their book on smoking, many other factors also influence the tobacco smoking habit and it would be wrong to assume that smoking behavior is governed entirely by the smoker's desire for nicotine. Nevertheless nicotine does indeed appear to be a major factor in maintaining the habit in many smokers and in this review the evidence supporting this conclusion is examined and mechanisms which could account for the rewarding effects of nicotine are considered.

2. EVIDENCE IMPLICATING NICOTINE IN THE TOBACCO SMOKING HABIT

The approach adopted in many laboratories in experiments designed to implicate nicotine as the reason for smoking has been to study the effects on the desire to smoke by either manipulating the concentration of nicotine in the smoke or pretreatment with nicotine. Other groups have also examined the effects of compounds which might be expected to antagonize the effects of nicotine in the central nervous system.

2.1. STUDIES DIRECTED AT DEMONSTRATING A ROLE FOR NICOTINE

Results reported from a number of laboratories suggest that most smokers alter their smoking habits if they are given cigarettes which contain either more or less nicotine than the brand they normally smoke. Smokers who are given cigarettes containing tobacco with a lower nicotine concentration are reported to increase the number of cigarettes smoked, whereas those given cigarettes with more nicotine reduce the number smoked (Goldfarb *et al.*, 1970; Frith, 1971a; Turner *et al.*, 1974; Forbes *et al.*, 1976; Goldfarb *et al.*, 1976; Jarvik *et al.*, 1978; Stepney, 1980). There is also evidence to suggest that the administration of nicotine, either by intravenous injection or orally in the form of chewing gum, can reduce the number of cigarettes smoked, although the effects of oral nicotine in the craving to smoke remain controversial (Brantmark *et al.*, 1973; Lucchesi *et al.*, 1967; Russell *et al.*, 1977; Schneider *et al.*, 1977; Russell *et al.*, 1980; West *et al.*, 1984a; Hughes *et al.*, 1986;

Nemeth-Coslett and Henningfield, 1986; West *et al.*, 1986). Nicotine-containing chewing gum is now widely used as sole therapy or as an adjunct to other therapies in a number of smoking-cessation clinics (Fee and Stewart, 1982; Hjalmarson, 1984; Jarvis *et al.*, 1982; Russell *et al.*, 1983b). In addition the administration of mecamylamine, an antagonist of the nicotinic acetylcholine receptor of ganglia which crosses the blood/brain barrier, has been shown to increase the number of cigarettes smoked, the number of puffs taken per cigarette, the amount of smoke inhaled and the quantity of nicotine absorbed (Nemeth-Coslett *et al.*, 1986; Stolerman *et al.*, 1973b; Pomerleau *et al.*, 1987). These data have been taken as evidence that many smokers adjust their smoking in order to titrate the plasma nicotine level to the one they are used to and find most rewarding (Ashton and Stepney, 1982; McMorrow and Foxx, 1983; Moss and Prue, 1982). The case for self-regulation of nicotine intake by smokers, however, is not fully established since studies reported by a number of groups have failed to find evidence for it (see review by McMorrow and Foxx, 1983). The efficacy of nicotine-containing chewing gum as an aid during smoking withdrawal has also been questioned by some (Puska *et al.*, 1979; Jamrozik *et al.*, 1984).

One important factor which almost certainly contributes to the wide degree of variation in the results reported is the fact that smokers can adapt their smoking habits in a number of ways which do not necessarily result in a reduction in the number of cigarettes smoked. In particular they may alter significantly the amount of smoke they inhale from each cigarette. Therefore it is important that the methodology used to measure changes in smoking is sufficiently rigorous to be able to detect relatively subtle changes in smoking habits. McMorrow and Foxx (1983) drew attention to the fact that a number of the studies designed to investigate the role of nicotine in tobacco smoking failed to use an appropriate means of measuring the changes in smoking behavior and these authors concluded that this, in part, contributed to the variability of the results reported.

Benowitz and Jacob (1984) have reported that, under controlled conditions in a medical center, the daily intake of nicotine by smokers who were free to smoke their normal brands of cigarettes as they wished, correlated with the number of cigarettes smoked but not with the nicotine yield of the cigarettes measured using a 'smoking' machine. However the correlation coefficient (0.59) indicated that the number of cigarettes smoked could account for only 35% of the total variance in the daily nicotine intake. Thus, even under well-controlled experimental conditions, an estimate of the number of cigarettes smoked per day cannot provide an accurate prediction of the amount of nicotine absorbed by the smoker. In addition it is important to remember that the correlation observed by Benowitz and Jacob may not hold or may be different for smokers who smoke an unfamiliar brand or are pretreated with nicotine before smoking. Many groups who have sought to investigate changes in smoking habits have, therefore, used biochemical measures as a means of providing a quantitative measure of the change. In early studies measurements of either plasma or urinary nicotine were made (e.g. Gritz *et al.*, 1976; Russell *et al.*, 1975; Goldfarb *et al.*, 1976). The plasma half-life of nicotine in humans is only about 2 hr (Isaac and Rand, 1969; Benowitz and Jacob, 1984) and therefore it is necessary to use this parameter as a measure of total nicotine intake with great care. Nevertheless, in their controlled study, Benowitz and Jacob (1984) found that the plasma nicotine level, measured at either noon or 4 pm, correlated well ($r = 0.8$) with nicotine intake. However the correlation with blood nicotine measured at 8 pm was appreciably poorer ($r = 0.56$) although still statistically significant ($P < 0.01$). Urinary nicotine levels appear to be a poor predictor of nicotine intake since the proportion of the drug absorbed which is excreted as unchanged nicotine varies greatly between subjects and can be influenced by many factors including the degree to which the drug metabolizing enzymes in the liver may have been induced, urinary flow and urinary pH (Beckett and Triggs, 1966, 1967; Feyerabend and Russell, 1978; Schievelbein, 1984; Schachter, 1978). It is, therefore, not surprising that nicotine intake does not correlate well with urinary nicotine excretion measured over 24 hr (Benowitz and Jacob, 1984).

In contrast the excretion of cotinine, one of the principal metabolic products of nicotine in man, appears to be much more consistent and not affected significantly by the induction of the drug metabolizing enzymes in the liver although it is influenced by the pH of the urine and urine flow (Beckett and Triggs, 1966; Feyerabend and Russell, 1978; Schievelbein, 1984). As a result the excretion of cotinine, measured over 24 hr, correlates reasonably well ($r = 0.62$) with nicotine intake (Benowitz and Jacob, 1984) and has been used as a measure of nicotine intake in studies of the role of nicotine in tobacco smoking (e.g. Goldfarb *et al.*, 1976; Ashton *et al.*, 1979).

Another approach used in some laboratories is to measure carboxyhemoglobin levels or the amount of carbon monoxide in the expired air (West *et al.*, 1984a; Henningfield and Griffiths, 1979; Russell *et al.*, 1980). These methods are based on the fact that tobacco smoke contains significant quantities of carbon monoxide and, because of its high affinity for hemoglobin, it provides a relatively stable measure of the amount of smoke inhaled by the subject in the preceding hours. Benowitz and Jacob (1984) showed that, in smokers allowed to smoke their normal brand *ad libitum*, carboxyhemoglobin levels measured at any point in the day (8 am, noon or 4 pm) correlated consistently, although not particularly closely ($r = 0.6$) with nicotine intake. However the real value of the carbon monoxide measurement is that it provides an estimate of smoke inhalation which is independent of the amount of nicotine absorbed from the smoke. Thus it can be used to evaluate the effectiveness of nicotine replacement therapy on tobacco smoking (Russell *et al.*, 1980) or to investigate changes in smoking habits associated with changes in the nicotine content of the smoke (McMorrow and Foxx, 1983; West *et al.*, 1984b).

Much of the data relating to the role of nicotine in tobacco smoking has been obtained from studies using subjects attending anti-smoking clinics or who were taking part in a research programme in which they were required to visit the test laboratory at intervals over a period of weeks (see McMorrow and Foxx, 1983 for review). In this type of study it was sometimes possible to make fairly comprehensive measurements of the change in smoking habits which had occurred. However, in a large number of the studies performed in a clinical situation, such as a smoking withdrawal clinic, validation of the changes in smoking habits reported by the subjects was done using samples taken at only one point in the day. In many cases the experimenters took great care to sample in such a way that they minimized that variation in the parameters measured as far as possible (e.g. West *et al.*, 1984b). Nevertheless the correlations between inhalation of tobacco smoke and the biochemical markers used to measure the intake do not appear to be very close or, in the case of nicotine, very stable when measured under controlled experimental conditions in smokers who are, presumably, smoking normally (Benowitz and Jacob, 1984). The validity of these markers as accurate measures of changes in smoking behavior, particularly when used as single time point measures, does not seem to have been considered in detail. Indeed McMorrow and Foxx (1983) have suggested that some of the conflicting results which have been reported concerning the extent to which compensation occurs in smokers pretreated with nicotine or who smoke cigarettes containing a nicotine concentration which is different to their normal cigarettes could be the result of the fact that researchers failed to sample at more than one point in the day.

One of the other factors which almost certainly contributes to the wide variation in the responses to nicotine pretreatment or manipulation of the nicotine content of the cigarettes is the fact that the tobacco smoking population is heterogeneous. Thus there are probably many factors which influence smoking habits. For example most, although not all, smokers smoke unevenly through the day and it seems likely that, for many smokers, external environmental cues may precipitate the desire to smoke (Ashton and Stepney, 1982). The nature of these cues can vary from being simply in the presence of another smoker to being in an environment in which the subject usually smokes (i.e. after a meal or with a drink in the evening). For some smokers at least, exposure to stressful environments is also reported to increase the desire to smoke (Frith, 1971b; Thomas, 1973; Armitage *et al.*, 1968; Hall and Morrison, 1973; Conway *et al.*, 1981). Schachter and his colleagues (1977) have argued that the increased desire to smoke in stressful environments is caused by the fact that the urine becomes acid and the rate of excretion of nicotine is increased. However, Ashton and Stepney (1982) have identified inconsistencies with the hypothesis and

Balfour (1984a) has suggested that other factors could also explain increased smoking in stressful situations. Whatever the reason, these studies draw attention to the fact that smoking is influenced by external factors and, therefore, studies in which smoking habits are examined within the confines of an experimental laboratory may not necessarily give an accurate measure of the changes in smoking habits which would have occurred in the normal environment in which the subject smoked.

The clinical evaluation of nicotine substitution procedures using nicotine-containing chewing gum suggest that it is most efficacious in heavy smokers who appear to be more dependent upon the nicotine content of the smoke (Brantmark *et al.*, 1973; Russell *et al.*, 1980; West *et al.*, 1986). Subjects who smoke in a way which produces little nicotine absorption are thought to benefit to a considerably lesser extent from nicotine substitution therapy and a proportion of these subjects may actually find nicotine-containing chewing gum unpleasant to take. In early studies with the gum little attention seemed to be paid to the selection of suitable subjects and this may have contributed to some of the equivocal results obtained with the material. When the gum is used with greater care and in appropriate subjects, the results are reported to be more consistent (Russell *et al.*, 1980; West *et al.*, 1986). However, one of the major problems associated with identifying the smokers who would benefit most from nicotine-substitution therapy lies in the fact that a smoker's nicotine intake does not correlate well with the nicotine yields predicted by 'machine-smoking' the brand of cigarettes the smoker uses. West *et al.* (1986) reported that the relief obtained by chewing nicotine-containing gum during smoking abstinence correlated best with the carbon monoxide content of expired air measured before cessation. The authors, however, noted that their study was performed with subjects who, on average, smoked more cigarettes per day than the mean for the smoking population as a whole. There is also evidence that the efficacy of the gum may be related to the dose of nicotine taken in from the material (Nemeth-Coslett *et al.*, 1987). However, gums containing high doses of the drug appear to be less acceptable to smokers and there appears to be a significant problem in formulating a preparation which delivers sufficient nicotine to reduce the craving for tobacco smoke to negligible proportions but which abstinent smokers find reasonably pleasant to chew.

In a study with a small number of subjects, Hughes *et al.* (1986) reported that a majority of subjects who were using nicotine-gum as an aid to giving up smoking remained dependent upon nicotine and that the abrupt withdrawal of gum precipitated a withdrawal effect. This study emphasized the point that, for these subjects, dependence had simply been transferred from one nicotine preparation to another and that care was needed during withdrawal from the gum.

The data currently available, therefore, appear consistent with the hypothesis that many, although almost certainly not all, smokers smoke in order to receive a dose of nicotine or to maintain their plasma nicotine levels. They also suggest that a significant proportion of smokers may be dependent upon nicotine. However, it is also clear that a number of other factors also contribute to the tobacco smoking habit and that the pleasure associated with smoking cannot be explained solely in terms of the nicotine content of the smoke.

2.2. Other Factors Which Could Contribute to the Tobacco Smoking Habit

In their study of the effects of nicotine-containing chewing gum on smoking cessation, West and his colleagues (1986) reported that nicotine appeared to be associated with the stimulant effects of smoking and the development of dependence upon tobacco smoke but not with its sedative effects, indulgent (smoking for pleasure) or automatic smoking. These authors suggested that the rewarding effects of tobacco smoking which do not appear to be associated with the nicotine content of the smoke may not be pharmacological in nature. Ashton and Stepney (1982) summarized evidence that, for some, the act of smoking may be a displacement activity which allows them to cope with stressful environmental stimuli.

However, it is important to remember that nicotine is absorbed very rapidly from cigarette smoke inhaled into the lungs whereas its absorption into the plasma via the buccal mucosa from nicotine-containing chewing gum is, in comparison, somewhat slower (Russell *et al.*, 1980). Therefore the failure of nicotine, given in the form of the chewing gum, to mimic all effects of cigarette smoke may, in part, reflect the different pharmacokinetic properties of the two preparations. Certainly in animal studies there is evidence that some of the pharmacological responses observed following the systemic administration of nicotine, which produces a rapid rise in plasma nicotine, are not observed in animals given oral nicotine which elicits a much slower rise in the level of the drug in the plasma (Balfour, 1979). West *et al.* (1986) suggested that some of the pleasurable effects of smoking, most notably indulgent-smoking, may be experienced in response to the nicotine bolus presented to the brain of a subject as he or she smokes a cigarette. Chewing nicotine-containing gum would not, therefore, produce this form of stimulation.

There is also evidence that the taste and throat irritation produced by tobacco smoke can contribute to the pleasure of smoking (Zagona and Zurcher, 1965). More recently, Rose *et al.* (1984) have reported that anesthetization of the upper and lower airways with local anesthetics also reduces the craving to smoke, a finding which, these authors concluded, indicated that effects on sensory systems were an important element in smoking satisfaction. It is, of course, quite possible that the nicotine contributes to the sensory effects of tobacco smoke although it is likely that other components also contribute since most smokers appear to be able to distinguish the smoke of their normal brand of cigarettes from others (Ramond *et al.*, 1950). It is, perhaps, likely that some smokers indulge in the habit solely to experience the effects of the smoke on the sensory terminals of the mouth, nose and throat and that the absorption of nicotine into the plasma and thence into the brain are of no importance. For these smokers, nicotine substitution therapy would be of little benefit.

However, in assessing the role of sensory stimulation in the pleasure associated with tobacco smoking it is important to remember that this form of stimulation could also act as a cue which precedes the arrival of nicotine in the brain. These sensory cues, themselves, could thus become pleasurable because they predict the imminent reward of a dose of nicotine. Therefore the fact that the sensory systems of the mouth and airways appear to be implicated in the pleasure associated with tobacco smoking does not preclude a role for nicotine. Indeed the hypothesis that the pleasures of smoking are multifactorial and involve a number of sensory stimuli could provide one of the reasons for the observation that oral nicotine can apparently relieve some, but not all, of the effects of smoking withdrawal (Hughes *et al.*, 1984; West *et al.*, 1986).

3. STUDIES ON THE EFFECTS OF NICOTINE IN HUMANS

When smokers are canvassed for the reasons why they smoke they give a range of different answers. However, they regularly report that smoking helps them concentrate, particularly when they are performing boring or repetitive tasks (Warburton and Wesnes, 1978; Bättig, 1981) and that smoking also exerts a 'tranquilizing' effect in stressful situations (Gilbert, 1979). Studies designed to investigate the role of nicotine in the tobacco smoking habit have, therefore, focussed on the possibility that the drug is responsible for these effects of tobacco smoke.

3.1. The Effects of Nicotine on Performance, Memory and Information Processing

Although, in experimental animals at least, the acute administration of high doses of nicotine can cause changes in the cerebrocortical electroencephalogram (EEG) similar to those seen in response to depressant drugs (Armitage *et al.*, 1969), the most reproducible effects of nicotine and tobacco smoke on brain EEG patterns are those of a stimulant drug (Gilbert, 1979; Warburton and Wesnes, 1979). Behaviorally both nicotine and tobacco smoke also cause psychomotor stimulation (Wesnes and Warburton, 1984a).

Smoking has been shown to stimulate psychomotor performance in a number of ways. For example Frankenhaeuser *et al.* (1970) found that smokers tested on a prolonged (80 min) simple visual reaction time test showed no decrement in reaction time over the course of the experiment providing they were allowed to smoke. However, when denied cigarettes, a significant decrement in performance was observed as the experiment progressed. More recent studies indicate that smoking attenuates the decline in stimulus sensitivity observed during both visual and auditory vigilance tasks (Wesnes and Warburton, 1978; Mangan and Golding, 1978). There is also evidence that smoking improves rapid visual information processing (Wesnes and Warburton, 1983). Subsequent studies have shown that nicotine alone can exert similar effects to smoking on the performance of vigilance tasks and information processing (Wesnes and Warburton, 1984b; Warburton and Wesnes, 1984; Wesnes *et al.*, 1983) and, therefore, there is little doubt that the nicotine present in tobacco smoke is the agent responsible for the effects of the smoke on these tasks.

The pretrial administration of nicotine, usually in the form of tobacco smoke, has been shown to improve learning in a number of tests whereas post-trial administration appears to have little effect (Warburton and Wesnes, 1984; Wesnes and Warburton, 1984a; Peeke and Peeke, 1984). The mechanisms involved in the effects of nicotine on memory are not yet fully understood although it appears very likely that the raised level of attention and increased rate of information processing evoked by the drug are important factors. Peters and McGee (1982) were among the first to provide clear evidence that the facilitation of learning caused by smoke could result in state-dependent learning. This observation has been supported by subsequent studies (e.g. Warburton *et al.*, 1986). Peeke and Peeke (1984) drew attention to the possibility that, for smokers used to learning information under the influence of the facilitatory effects of the smoke, the sudden loss of this facilitation following smoking withdrawal would contribute significantly to relative loss of cognitive skills and thus to the difficulty in remaining abstinent. It also seems reasonable to suggest that some of the apparent impairments of cognitive function often reported by smokers when they abstain could be the result of a failure to recall information learned under state-dependent conditions when they were smoking.

Nicotine is not invariably reported to enhance information processing and facilitate learning. For example Dunne *et al.* (1986) found that nicotine, taken in the form of nicotine-containing chewing gum, failed to enhance performance of problem solving tasks involving words or numbers and, indeed, found that immediate and delayed recall and recognition were impaired in the nicotine-treated group. The authors concluded that facilitation of cognitive function by nicotine may be task-specific. However they did not consider the possibility that the route of administration of the drug could also influence the results. Nicotine is absorbed rapidly from tobacco smoke whereas its absorption from nicotine-gum is slow (Russell *et al.*, 1980) and it is clearly possible that this could account for the apparent conflict between the studies which report facilitation and those, like that of Dunne *et al.* (1986) which fail to find this effect.

In one of the few studies designed to see if smoking facilitated cognitive function outside the laboratory, Warburton *et al.* (1984) reported that, amongst university students, smokers scored significantly higher marks in examinations and for tutorial assignments than nonsmokers. These data are clearly consistent with the hypothesis that smoking does exert a facilitatory effect on cognitive function, although, of course, they do not provide unequivocal proof of this because there are other explanations for the effect. For example the authors themselves suggest that the data could be explained by the possibility that ambitious students, with a high level of motivation to succeed, may choose to smoke in the belief that it will aid their studies.

3.2. Electroencephalographic Studies

Another means of examining the effects of nicotine in human brain is to study the changes in EEG evoked by administration of the drug alone or in the form of tobacco smoke. At the simplest level there is clear and consistent evidence that both nicotine and tobacco smoke produce shifts in EEG patterns which are consistent with the stimulatory effects of nicotine on attention and psychomotor performance (Edwards and Warburton, 1984; Pickworth *et al.*, 1986). However, many factors influence EEG activity and the interpretation of any changes found is often difficult because little is yet known of the significance of the many subtle changes in electrical activity which occur in the EEG pattern recorded from the scalp.

One approach which has proved particularly useful in the investigation of nicotine is the use of event related potentials (ERPs). ERPs are potentials evoked by exogenous events and, under controlled conditions, it is possible to extract those potentials in the EEG which are evoked by a specific stimulus. This type of experiment has been used to examine the effects of nicotine on the speed of response to a specific stimulus and to determine if the effects of the compound on information processing occur because the sensory information arrives in the cortex more quickly or because it is genuinely processed at a faster rate.

Some of the earliest studies on ERPs examined the effects of nicotine on the contingent negative variation (CNV). The CNV is a small negative potential which appears and builds slowly between a warning signal and an imperative stimulus requiring a response, typically a motor response such as pressing a button. Ashton and her colleagues (1974) found that smoking increased CNV amplitude in seven smokers, decreased the amplitude in eleven smokers and evoked a biphasic response in four. In a subsequent study the administration of nicotine was shown to evoke the same response as tobacco smoke in each of the subjects tested, clearly suggesting that the changes were caused by the nicotine present in the smoke (Ashton *et al.*, 1978b). Studies with other drugs (caffeine and nitrazepam) suggested that an increased CNV amplitude corresponded with the stimulant properties of nicotine whereas a decreased amplitude corresponded with its depressant properties. The precise physiological or behavioral significance of the CNV remains unclear although Ashton *et al.* (1978a) have suggested that the potential arises in the arousal systems of the brain, including particularly the ascending reticular activating system. Edwards and Warburton (1984), however, cast some doubt on the validity of this conclusion. Thus the functional significance of the changes reported by Ashton and her colleagues remains unclear. Measurements of the CNV may have the potential to reveal much about psychopharmacology of nicotine although, to date, this potential has not been fulfilled. The factors which influence the effects of nicotine and of smoking on the CNV appear to be more complex than was originally thought, the effects being influenced by such things as the personality of the smoker and the way in which the cigarette is smoked (Edwards and Warburton, 1984). Therefore, a full understanding of the significance of the changes in the CNV in terms of the role in nicotine in the tobacco smoking habit must await a more careful analysis of the interrelationships between the effects of the drug and these other variables.

In other studies on ERPs, Warburton and his group (Edwards and Warburton, 1984) have reported results which suggest that nicotine can speed up the stimulus evaluation process. These experiments imply that nicotine may not only regulate sensory input into the cortex, but, that it may also enhance information processing in the cerebral cortex, an observation which, Edwards and Warburton suggest, may reflect the improvement in the ability to concentrate often reported by smokers.

3.3. Nicotine as a 'Tranquilizer'

There is evidence that many smokers tend to smoke more heavily in stressful situations (Kissen, 1960; Conway *et al.*, 1981; Frith, 1971b) and that this occurs because smokers perceive tobacco smoke as having a tranquilizing effect when they are subjected to stressful environmental stimuli (Ikard *et al.*, 1969; Poulton, 1977; Wesnes *et al.*, 1984). However, as both Revell *et al.* (1985) and Gilbert (1979) point out this is a paradoxical response since the doses of nicotine absorbed by smokers almost invariably cause cortical arousal whereas the tranquilizing drugs depress cortical activity (cause synchronization of cortical alpha rhythm). Smoking also enhances the increase in heart rate observed in subjects exposed to an environmental stress (Poulton, 1977). In support of the hypothesis that smoking does exert a tranquilizing effect, Nesbitt (1973) reported that smokers behave less emotionally when they are allowed to smoke. The effect was most marked when high-nicotine cigarettes were smoked. Schechter and Rand (1974) also observed that smokers were less aggressive when allowed to smoke. However, neither study was designed sufficiently rigorously to exclude other explanations for the results obtained and, thus, they did not provide unequivocal evidence for a tranquilizing effect of cigarette smoke. Therefore, although many smokers do appear to experience relief of anxiety when they smoke, there is little evidence that this is associated with a tranquilizing property of tobacco smoke similar to that of conventional anxiolytic drugs or, indeed, other sedative drugs (Gilbert, 1979; Revell *et al.*, 1985).

Other theories have sought to show that, under certain circumstances, the stimulant properties of nicotine could, paradoxically, account for the apparent 'tranquilizing' effect of tobacco smoke. For example Schachter (1973) suggested that the cortical arousal caused by smoking was sufficiently similar to that evoked by stress, that a smoker who smokes in a stressful environment attributes the signals of arousal to the tobacco smoke rather than the stress and, as a result, feels more calm. As an alternative explanation he invoked the 'Law of Initial Values' to suggest that the increment in arousal evoked by exposure to a stressful environmental stimulus would be perceived as being less stressful, if the preceding 'resting' level of arousal had been raised by the inhalation of tobacco smoke. These, and other theories, have been reviewed in detail by Gilbert (1979). However, although the data currently available perhaps favor the hypothesis that the apparent 'tranquilizing' effects of tobacco smoke are related, in some way, to the stimulant properties of nicotine, none of the theories proposed thus far have provided a truly convincing explanation.

4. EFFECTS OF NICOTINE ON ANIMAL BEHAVIOR

The behavioral responses to nicotine have been the subject of a number of reviews in recent years (e.g. Hendry and Rosecrans, 1984; Clarke, 1987). This review will, therefore, focus specifically on the contribution behavioral studies have made to our understanding of the role of nicotine in the tobacco smoking habit.

4.1. Spontaneous Behavior

The acute administration of high doses of nicotine to experimental animals usually decreases spontaneous activity. For example both Morrison and Stephenson (1972) and Stolerman *et al.* (1973a) found that acute nicotine reduced both spontaneous locomotor activity and the number of rears the animals made. Acute nicotine has also been shown to decrease the activity of mice (Morrison and Armitage, 1967; Masner, 1972). The acute administration of lower doses (<0.2 mg/kg) to rats causes a more variable response.

Chronic injections of nicotine almost invariably cause tolerance to its depressant effects and in these animals nicotine causes psychomotor simulation (Morrison and Stephenson, 1972; Stolerman *et al.*, 1973b; Keenan and Johnson, 1972). In rats, once tolerance has been established, it is reported to last for at least 90 days after the administration of the last injection (Stolerman *et al.*, 1973a).

The effects of nicotine on spontaneous activity appear to be influenced by a number of factors. For example almost all the early studies were performed with animals which had been given nicotine by either subcutaneous or intraperitoneal injection. The animals therefore received the drug as a series of boli. More recently Cronan *et al.* (1985) examined the effects of sustained intravenous administration from osmotic minipumps implanted subcutaneously in the rats. Under these conditions nicotine initially stimulated locomotor activity (days 1 and 2) but thereafter it had no significant effect. The sex and strain of the rats has also been found to influence the response to nicotine. Female rats are generally more active than males. Studies reported by Bättig and his colleagues (Bättig and Schlatter, 1978, 1979; Bättig *et al.*, 1976) indicate that the stimulatory effects of nicotine on spontaneous activity are more marked in the more active female rats. Some strains of rats are also more active than others and, again, the stimulation of activity evoked by nicotine appears to be greater in the more active strains (Hendry and Rosecrans, 1984; Schlatter and Bättig, 1979; Bättig, 1983). By contrast, Rosecrans (1971) showed that, if rats of the same strain were preselected on the basis of their basal levels of locomotor activity, nicotine consistently stimulated the activity of the low activity rats whereas it was relatively ineffective in the more active rats.

Thus, in summary, the acute administration of low doses of nicotine and the chronic administration of both low and moderately high doses of the drug generally stimulate behavior. However, a number of factors, including particularly the sex and strain of the animals used, influence the response observed.

In the rat, exposure to an aversive stimulus causes suppression of spontaneous activity and behavioral disruption (Nelsen, 1978). The administration of nicotine to rats exposed to such stimuli is reported to ameliorate the behavioral disruption observed and there is some evidence that these effects are more marked in animals which exhibit higher levels of inborn emotionality (Nelsen, 1978). Recent studies in the author's laboratory also suggest that the stimulant properties of nicotine may be greater in aversive environments, in part at least, because nicotine attenuates the reduction in spontaneous locomotor activity which occurs in response to an aversive environment (Vale and Balfour, 1989).

4.2. Effects of Nicotine on Operant Behavior for a Positive Reward

The effects of nicotine on the acquisition and performance of a range of different operant behavioral schedules have been studied in a number of laboratories (see Hendry and Rosecrans, 1984 for review). The responses to the drug appear to depend to a marked extent on the schedule used and, in particular, on the basal rates of activity elicited by the schedules. Thus, in fixed ratio (FR) schedules in which rats were required to press a lever a preset number of times before receiving a reward, low doses of nicotine generally increase response rates whereas higher doses (<0.2 mg/kg s.c.) tend to decrease the number of responses or to have no effect (Morrison, 1967; Morrison and Armitage, 1967; Pradhan, 1970). In rats trained on either fixed (FI) or variable interval (VI) schedules a more consistent stimulation was observed (Pradhan, 1970; Morrison, 1967) although, again, a moderately high dose of the drug (0.4 mg/kg s.c.) initially depressed responding. Schedules using fixed or variable intervals tend to elicit lower pressing rates than ratio schedules and, therefore, the effect of nicotine seems to be governed more by the basal levels of activity rather than the nature of the schedule itself (Hendry and Rosecrans, 1984). This conclusion is supported by the fact that Stitzer *et al.* (1970) found that nicotine, given subcutaneously in a dose range of 0.05 to 0.4 mg/kg tended to decrease response rates in rats trained to lever-press for a water reward. These authors used a fixed interval (99 sec) which was shorter than the FI-120 sec schedule used by Morrison (1967) and, as a result, evoked much faster pressing rats for the saline controls. Stitzer *et al.* (1970) themselves, suggested that this could account for the discrepancy between the two studies.

In summary, therefore, nicotine tends to stimulate lever pressing in operant schedules in which basal pressing rates are low whereas its effects on schedules which elicit high basal pressing rates are less consistent. Interestingly, however, Morrison and Armitage (1967) and Morrison and Stephenson (1973) found that nicotine did not cause a significant increase in lever pressing when the rats were trained on a differential reinforcement of low rate (DRL) schedule. This schedule is very similar to a fixed interval schedule with the exception that a response during the interval postpones the possibility of reinforcement for another complete interval. Thus, in order to receive a reward, the rats must press slowly. Clearly, therefore, the stimulant effect can be suppressed in situations in which it becomes a disadvantage.

4.3. Avoidance and Punished Behavior

In their review Hendry and Rosecrans (1984) drew attention to the wide variation in the reported effects of nicotine on different forms of avoidance behavior and, as a result, no clear pattern of response emerges. However, there is some evidence to suggest that nicotine may enhance acquisition of shock avoidance schedules (Morrison, 1974; Erickson, 1971) although this does not always seem to be the case (Fleming and Broadhurst, 1975). Morrison (1974) also found that rats trained with nicotine avoided more shocks than rats trained with saline. In her study Morrison used a Sidman avoidance schedule with inter-shock (SS) and response next shock (RS) intervals of 30 sec. Very few, if any, of the rats trained with nicotine received more than 20 shocks per session (out of a possible 120), whereas this was not the case for the rats trained with saline. Morrison concluded, therefore, that nicotine appeared to be particularly beneficial to rats which would otherwise have experienced difficulty in learning the task.

In mice nicotine has been shown to enhance acquisition of a passive avoidance task when given subcutaneously at a low dose (0.125 mg/kg) which also caused locomotor stimulation, whereas administration of a higher dose (0.500 mg/kg) which depressed activity had no effect on passive avoidance (Nordberg and Bergh, 1985). The mice given the low dose of nicotine showed significantly greater passive avoidance both when it was measured 24 hr and six days post-trial. The authors concluded that stimulant doses of nicotine improved passive avoidance learning, and particularly, memory consolidation.

Nicotine has also been examined for its effects on unconditioned avoidance. Morrison and Stephenson (1970) investigated the effects of nicotine in rat behavior in an elevated Y-maze in which one arm was an open platform. In this apparatus benzodiazepine and barbiturate anxiolytic drugs caused consistent increases in the relative amount of time spent in the more aversive open arm and increased total activity (total entries into all three arms of the maze). The effects of nicotine on avoidance of the open arm of the maze were not consistent and appeared to depend upon the baseline spontaneous activity of the rats. Nicotine tended to decrease avoidance of the open arm if baseline activity was low but to increase avoidance of the open arm when baseline activity was high. Amphetamine evoked a similar pattern of response although, rather surprisingly, it failed to cause consistent increases in total activity. At a high dose (3.2 mg/kg) amphetamine decreased both total activity and the relative amount of time spent in the open arm.

More recently, Balfour *et al.* (1986b) examined the effects of nicotine in the elevated X-maze test for anxiety. This apparatus consists of two open and two enclosed arms. Benzodiazepine anxiolytic drugs increase the percentage of total time spent in the more aversive open arms and they also increase the percentage of the total entries made into the open arms (Pellow *et al.*, 1985; Balfour *et al.*, 1986b). Neither the acute nor subchronic administration of nicotine (0.4 mg/kg) had any significant effects on avoidance of the open arms (Balfour *et al.*, 1986b). In the apparatus, as in other tests (Keim and Sigg, 1977; Le Fur *et al.*, 1979), diazepam diminished the plasma corticosterone response (Pellow *et al.*, 1985). Subchronic injections of nicotine also caused a significant reduction in plasma corticosterone although the effect was small when compared with that of diazepam (Balfour *et al.*, 1986b). Nicotine also has no effect on the relative number of open arm entries made by rats tested repeatedly in the maze (Vale and Balfour, 1987). Thus, in the elevated X-maze at least, there is no evidence that nicotine can exert an anxiolytic effect.

In rats, anxiolytic drugs characteristically restore lever pressing in conflict tests in which responding for a reward is punished, generally with an electric shock (e.g. Geller and Seifter, 1960; Geller *et al.*, 1962). In this test, nicotine also fails to exhibit anxiolytic properties and, indeed, tends to increase the suppression of lever pressing caused by punishment although not consistently so (Morrison, 1969). In this respect its effects are similar to those of another stimulant drug, amphetamine, which is consistently reported to enhance suppression of lever pressing in conflict tests (Geller and Seifter, 1960; Morrison, 1969). This response to amphetamine is consistent with it having anxiogenic properties and, interestingly, there is other evidence from both passive avoidance experiments (Kumar, 1968) and studies with the elevated X-maze (Pellow *et al.*, 1985) that amphetamine does have the behavioral properties of an anxiogenic compound. Thus, although nicotine does appear to resemble amphetamine to some extent, the data available suggest that, in tests designed to reveal anxiolytic or anxiogenic activity, amphetamine appears to be significantly more anxiogenic than nicotine and there is no good evidence that either drug exhibits classical anxiolytic responses.

4.4. Effects of Nicotine on Aggressive Behavior

Silverman (1971) reported that nicotine caused a consistent reduction of aggressive behavior in rats. More recently Driscoll and Baettig (1981) and Rodgers (1979) have shown that nicotine causes a dose-dependent inhibition of shock-induced fighting in rats. Hutchinson and Emley (1973) found that nicotine also inhibited shock-induced biting in monkeys whereas its withdrawal increased aggressive behavior.

4.5. Behavioral Evidence for Interactions with Ethanol

Ethanol consumption is reported to increase tobacco use in man (Griffiths *et al.*, 1976) and, therefore, studies in a number of laboratories have examined the interaction between the psychopharmacological effects of ethanol and nicotine. These studies have shown that nicotine can potentiate ethanol discrimination (Signs and Schechter, 1986) and increase ethanol consumption (Potthoff *et al.*, 1983) in experimental rats. Studies in humans suggest that nicotine enhances the state-dependent learning properties of alcohol (Lowe, 1986). However, in no case has a clear mechanism for the interactions between nicotine and ethanol been established.

5. MODELS OF NICOTINE DEPENDENCE

5.1. Nicotine Self-Administration

Most of the drugs which cause dependence in humans can act as rewards in self-administration studies with infrahuman species (Johanson, 1978). There is evidence that experimental animals will self-administer nicotine although it has been clear for some years that it is very much more difficult to induce rats to self-inject nicotine than many of the better established drugs of dependence (Battig, 1980; Hanson *et al.*, 1979). Thus, for example, Lang and colleagues (Lang *et al.*, 1977; Smith and Lang, 1980) have shown that rats maintained at their normal body weight do not readily learn to self-inject nicotine whereas rats whose food is restricted in order to keep their weight at only 80% of normal will self-inject the drug. Acquisition of the response was also enhanced under schedule-controlled conditions in which lever-pressing was associated with the presentation of a second reward (a food pellet) (Lang *et al.*, 1977; Singer *et al.*, 1978). However, nicotine self-administration was not contingent on schedule control and the studies provided some evidence for genuine nicotine self-administration although, clearly, additional environmental factors seemed to play an important part in the response. Other studies (Battig, 1980; Hanson *et al.*, 1979) suggest that exposure to a stressful stimulus may increase nicotine self-administration in rats.

Hanson *et al.* (1979) have demonstrated nicotine self-administration in rats in the absence of schedule-control or weight reduction although they found that the response only developed slowly and the response rates were always slow when compared with those seen for rats self-injecting morphine, cocaine or amphetamine. More recently, Cox *et al.* (1984) have also reported that rats can be trained to self-inject nicotine and that acquisition of the response is slow. Interestingly, in this study, the authors reported that almost all the injections occurred during the night and suggested that some of the previous studies had failed to find nicotine self-administration because the experiments were performed during daytime. Thus studies with rats suggest that they will self-inject the drug but that external environmental factors may play a more important role than they do for many other drugs of dependence. These observations led Balfour (1984a) to suggest that nicotine self-administration may, in part at least, reflect negative reinforcement resulting from the ability of the drug to ameliorate the effects of some environmental stressors, such as hunger and, perhaps, other unpleasant stimuli. If this is the case then exposure to such stimuli could be expected to enhance self-administration of the drug whereas a failure to incorporate such a stimulus in the experimental design could explain a failure to observe self-administration.

Nicotine self-administration has also been demonstrated with monkeys. Slifer (1983) reported that rhesus monkeys will exhibit schedule-induced nicotine self-administration. More recently Hutchinson and Emley (1985) have shown that the ingestion of nicotine by squirrel monkeys is increased if they are exposed to an aversive stimula (unavoidable electric shocks) but that the preference for the nicotine solution is lost when the aversive stimulus is removed. There is evidence from studies with human smokers that they, too, find the intravenous administration of nicotine rewarding (Henningfield and Goldberg, 1983; Henningfield *et al.*, 1983). However, in this type of study, the subjects can generally distinguish the presence of active drug from saline in the injection fluid by its local and central effects and may opt for the active preparation because they assume this preparation will be effective. It is also possible to perform a similar study with nicotine-containing chewing gum. In a study in which the subjects knew they were being offered either the nicotine gum or a placebo, they chose to chew significantly more of the gum containing the active material (Hughes *et al.*, 1985). However, if the subjects were told that placebo gum contained active drug in a different formulation which would not produce the same side-effects, the subjects used the two gums in equal quantities. This suggests that the selection of the nicotine-containing gum in the first study may be based, at least in part, on the fact that the subjects could detect its side-effects and thus knew it was the active gum. The second study suggests, therefore, that in these subjects (all ex-smokers tested during the first two weeks of abstinence) the rewarding effects of nicotine *per se* were not that strong. In trying to interpret the results of these experiments it is important to remember that nicotine was being examined for its ability to substitute for tobacco smoke and not for its ability to act as a reinforcer in a subject not previously exposed to the compound.

5.2. Conditioned Place Preference

Another method of studying the rewarding effects of drugs is to use conditioned place preference (CPP). In this procedure drug administration is paired with a distinctive environment and if the drug is rewarding in the drug-free state the animal will opt to spend most time in the environment in which the drug was given. Conversely animals will tend to avoid environments paired with an aversive drug. This procedure has been used to demonstrate the rewarding properties of cocaine (Mucha *et al.*, 1982), opioid drugs (Katz and Gormezano, 1979; Mucha *et al.*, 1982) and amphetamine (Carr and White, 1983; Reicher and Holman, 1977). Fudala *et al.* (1985) used this procedure to show that, in rats, subcutaneous injections of nicotine at doses between 0.1 and 0.8 mg/kg, appeared to exert rewarding effect. However, at a higher dose (1.2 mg/kg) the animals responded in a way which indicated that they found the drug aversive. The effects of nicotine were antagonized by mecamylamine, but not hexamethonium, suggesting that the effects were mediated by central nicotinic receptors. More recently, however, in contrast to the results of Mucha *et al.* (1982), Clarke (1987) has reported that nicotine fails to elicit CPP. Clearly, therefore, further studies are necessary before this property of nicotine is established with certainty.

5.3. The Effects of Nicotine Withdrawal on Rat Behavior

Although there is a very close relationship between the ability of a drug to act as a reward in a self-administration schedule and the potential of the compound to cause dependence in humans, self-administration itself is not a measure of dependence. In his review on drugs of dependence, Johanson (1978) made it clear that a number of studies had shown that animals trained to self-administer morphine were not necessarily physically dependent upon the drug and it is clear that physical dependence upon morphine is not a necessary precondition for the opiate to act as reinforcer. However, the withdrawal of a drug from an individual who is dependent upon the compound invariably does elicit some form of withdrawal effect and it seems reasonable to define an addicted individual as one who exhibits withdrawal symptoms (Balfour, 1984a). In the case of drugs which cause physical dependence, such as the opiates or barbiturates, the abstinence syndrome is easy to observe and is clearly distressing. This is not always the case for drugs which cause only psychological dependence since, although in humans withdrawal can evoke a marked craving for the substance which may be associated with somatic symptoms, the withdrawal effect is often largely emotional in nature and appropriate animal models are difficult to design. This certainly appears to be true for nicotine.

Data reviewed in Section 4.1 indicated that the more consistent response to chronic nicotine administration in experimental animals is locomotor stimulation. Withdrawal of the drug, following periods of chronic treatment ranging between 8 and 40 days resulted in the activity returning to control levels (Stolerman *et al.*, 1973a; Vale and Balfour, 1987). Since there is evidence that nicotine self-administration may also occur predominantly at night (Cox *et al.*, 1984) the data appear consistent with the hypothesis that nicotine dependence may occur more readily during nocturnal hours when the rats are most active. More studies, however, are necessary for this hypothesis to gain widespread acceptance.

In a study designed to investigate the role of stress in the development of nicotine dependence, Morrison (1974) examined the effects of nicotine-withdrawal on the behavior of rats trained to perform an unsignalled Sigman avoidance task. The administration of nicotine prior to each training session improved acquisition of the task. However, once trained, if the injection of nicotine was replaced by one of saline, a marked deterioration of performance was observed, the nicotine-withdrawal rats receiving significantly more shocks than both the rats trained and tested with nicotine and the control rats trained and tested with saline. The results of other studies, particularly with humans, have shown that nicotine can elicit state-dependent learning (Warburton *et al.*, 1986; Peters and McGee, 1982). However Morrison (1974) reported that the effects she had observed did not appear to be the result of state-dependent learning upon the compound since reversing the procedure by giving nicotine to rats trained with saline did not cause disruption of performance. She concluded, therefore, that her study had identified a test which could detect the effects of nicotine withdrawal.

In order to examine further the role of stress in the development of nicotine dependence, Morrison (1974) also investigated the effects of nicotine withdrawal in rats trained with nicotine on less stressful Sidman schedules which used warning or feedback signals. Withdrawal of the drug from rats trained on these schedules did not evoke a significant withdrawal effect despite the fact that improved acquisition of the task was still apparent in the nicotine-treated rats. Thus Morrison concluded that the development of nicotine dependence was related to the degree of stress associated with the test procedure.

In another approach to the problem, Harris *et al.* (1986) used a drug discrimination protocol to investigate the similarities between nicotine withdrawal and the administration of an anxiogenic drug. Their studies showed that, in rats trained to discriminate pentylenetetrazol from saline, nicotine withdrawal evoked a weak response similar to that of pentylenetetrazol which could be reversed by the administration of diazepam. The withdrawal of anxiolytic drugs, such as diazepam has also been reported to evoke pentylenetetrazol-like activity in this test and this has been interpreted as a measure of the anxiety caused by withdrawal of the drug (Emmett-Oglesby *et al.*, 1983). However, the test is by no means specific for anxiolytic drugs since the same group have reported that pentylenetratrazol discrimination also generalizes to the effects of morphine-withdrawal (Emmett-Oglesby *et al.*, 1984) and, indeed, have made it clear that the test does not detect the withdrawal effects of a specific class of drug (Harris *et al.*, 1986). Thus the experiments do not provide evidence that nicotine is an anxiolytic drug.

5.4. The Effects of Nicotine on Plasma Hormone Levels

In unstressed rats, acute injections of nicotine cause an increase in the plasma corticosterone and adrenocorticotrophin (ACTH) concentrations (Balfour *et al.*, 1975; Cam *et al.*, 1979; Sharp *et al.*, 1987). However, the chronic administration of nicotine rapidly induces tolerance to these changes and, in these rats, nicotine withdrawal causes an increase in plasma corticosterone which is statistically significant in rats treated with daily injections of the drug for 40 days (Benwell and Balfour, 1979). The withdrawal of two other drugs of dependence, morphine and ethanol, has also been shown to increase the plasma corticosterone concentration (Kokka *et al.*, 1973; Pohorecky *et al.*, 1978). More recently the administration of a benzodiazepine receptor antagonist to rats treated chronically with diazepam has also been shown to increase plasma corticosterone (Eisenberg, 1987) although this is not the case if diazepam is simply withdrawn from unstressed rats (Copland and Balfour, 1987). These results suggest that the withdrawal or antagonism of a number of drugs of dependence, including nicotine, stimulates corticosterone secretion in unstressed rats. The pharmacological significance of the response remains to be established although it is tempting to suggest that there may be a relationship between the changes in plasma corticosterone and the generalization of pentylenetetrazol discussed in the previous section.

The administration of nicotine to rats made tolerant to the acute effects of the drug on plasma corticosterone has little or no effect on the plasma corticosterone response to a novel or aversive stimuli (Benwell and Balfour, 1982a; Balfour *et al.*, 1986). Nicotine is also reported to be without effect on the ACTH response to stress (Sharp *et al.*, 1987). However, if rats, exposed repeatedly to the stress of an elevated open platform were given nicotine prior to each test session, the reduction in the plasma corticosterone response, observed in the saline-treated controls as they habituate to the procedure is significantly attenuated (Benwell and Balfour, 1982a). In the saline-treated rats, habituation to the procedure is also associated with the development of a significant positive correlation between plasma corticosterone and the concentration of 5-hydroxytryptamine (5-HT) in the hippocampus. By contrast, in the rats given nicotine, a negative correlation between plasma corticosterone and hippocampal 5-HT was observed. These data were taken as evidence that nicotine interacted with the mechanism by which the rats habituated to the aversive stimulus. If nicotine was withdrawn from these rats, the plasma corticosterone concentration remained elevated but the relationship with the hippocampal 5-HT concentration was lost. The psychopharmacological significance of these effects of nicotine on plasma corticosterone in the stress-induced rats remains unclear although Benwell and Balfour (1982a) suggested that the disruption in the relationship between plasma corticosterone and hippocampal 5-HT, observed in the nicotine-withdrawn rats, could be associated with the development of nicotine dependence. In a more recent series of experiments, Copland and Balfour (1987) showed that the withdrawal of diazepam from rats which had been treated with the drug while they habituated to the stress of the elevated platform, also increased plasma corticosterone. The dose of diazepam needed to elicit this effect, however, was large and it was concluded that the response was probably a measure of the development of dependence upon the sedative rather than the anxiolytic properties of the drug.

In addition to their effects on the pituitary-adrenocortical system, many stressors also increase plasma prolactin levels. Sharp and his colleagues (1987) found that both acute and subchronic nicotine depressed this response in rats exposed to restraint stress. This observation appears to be one of the first to show that nicotine can attenuate some physiological responses to stressful stimuli although the possible behavioral significance of the effect remains unclear at present.

6. THE ROLE OF SPECIFIC NEUROTRANSMITTER SYSTEMS

The effects of nicotine on brain neurotransmitter systems have been reviewed in detail elsewhere (Balfour, 1984b). This review, therefore, focuses only on the systems which have been implicated specifically in the behavioral responses to nicotine and the role of the drug in the tobacco smoking habit.

6.1. Acetylcholine

Armitage *et al.* (1968) reported that the intravenous administration of low doses of nicotine to anesthetized cats stimulated the release of acetylcholine (ACh) into a cup placed on the surface of the parietal cortex. At higher doses the drug appeared to decrease ACh release although this was not an entirely consistent observation. Studies *in vitro* have shown that there are nicotinic receptors on the ACh-secreting terminals of the cerebral cortex and that stimulation of these receptors evokes the release of ACh (Rowell and Winkler, 1984; Beani *et al.*, 1985). Thus the release of ACh evoked by nicotine *in vivo* could clearly be mediated by these receptors. However, Warburton and his colleagues believe that the effects of nicotine on ACh release are mediated by receptors located on cells in the mesencephalic reticular formation (Wesnes and Warburton, 1984a).

It is now generally agreed that nicotine exerts most of its effects in the central nervous system by acting upon receptors located on neuronal membranes and the properties of these receptors have been studied in some detail using radioligands. One of the first radioactive ligands to be used for this purpose was the neurotoxin α-bungarotoxin which was found to bind displaceably and with high affinity to mammalian brain membranes (Morley *et al.*, 1979; Morley and Kemp, 1981). However, although nicotine has some affinity for the α-bungarotoxin acceptor site, studies by Romano and Goldstein (1980), using [^{3}H]nicotine as the ligand, showed that the mammalian CNS contained an acceptor site for nicotine which had a high affinity for the ligand (Kd 10 nm). This site bound nicotine stereospecifically, having a higher affinity for the pharmacologically-active (−)-enantiomer, but had little or no affinity for α-bungarotoxin. This, therefore, was clearly not the site labelled with radioactive toxin in the earlier experiments and, indeed, subsequent studies have shown that the properties and distribution of the (−)-nicotine and α-bungarotoxin binding sites within the brain are quite different (Marks *et al.*, 1986; Larsson and Nordberg, 1985; Clarke *et al.*, 1985b; Marks and Collins, 1982). The studies reported by Romano and Goldstein (1980) indicated that compounds which acted as agonists at the nicotine receptor of autonomic ganglia had a relatively high affinity for the binding site, cytisine having an IC_{50} value some threefold lower than (−)-nicotine itself although, with the exception of lobeline, all of the other compounds tested had a much lower (at least 10-fold) affinity for the site when compared with (−)-nicotine. In contrast nicotine antagonists had a low affinity for the site and, indeed, many of them did not displace (−)-nicotine when present at concentrations as high as 1 mM.

Subsequent studies in a number of laboratories (e.g. Benwell and Balfour, 1985; Marks *et al.*, 1986; Marks and Collins, 1982; Costa and Murphy, 1983) have confirmed the presence of the high affinity nicotine binding sites and the initial findings of Romano and Goldstein (1980) concerning its relative affinities for nicotinic agonists and antagonists. Schwartz *et al.* (1982) reported that, if brain membranes were incubated with [^{3}H]ACh in the presence of an inhibitor of acetylcholinesterase and a muscarinic receptor antagonist, displaceable binding to a nicotinic cholinoreceptor could be measured. The properties of this receptor appeared to be very similar to those of the site labelled with (−)-[^{3}H]nicotine including, particularly, the fact that the receptor had a high affinity for nicotinic agonists but little affinity for antagonists and there is now increasing evidence to suggest that [^{3}H]nicotine and [^{3}H]ACh label the same nicotine cholinoreceptor (Marks *et al.*, 1986; Martino-Barrows and Kellar, 1987).

A majority of the research groups who have attempted to characterize the receptor involved in mediating behavioral responses to nicotine have exploited the fact that nicotine can act as a stimulus in a drug discrimination protocol. Using this approach, both Meltzer *et al.* (1980) and Romano *et al.* (1981) have shown that rats trained to discriminate the pharmacologically active (−)-enantiomer of nicotine require a tenfold increase in the dose of the (+)-enantiomer to elicit the same response. Other studies (Romano *et al.*, 1981; Pratt *et al.*, 1983; Stolerman *et al.*, 1984) indicate that the discrimination response to nicotine will generalize to the other ganglionic agonists which compete with nicotine for the high affinity acceptor site on brain membrane preparations. Many other drugs which have no affinity for the nicotinic receptor were found not to generalize the nicotine cue. These observations have been interpreted as evidence that the discriminative response to nicotine is mediated by the nicotinic receptor with high affinity for (−)-nicotine (Romano *et al.*, 1981; Pratt *et al.*, 1983; Stolerman *et al.*, 1984; Rosecrans and Meltzer, 1981). Studies using the intraventricular route of administration have implicated central nicotinic receptors specifically in the response (Romano *et al.*, 1981).

Experiments with antagonists, however, reveal a less clear relationship between the ability to displace (−)-nicotine from nicotinic receptors *in vitro* and the ability to antagonize the effects of nicotine *in vivo*. Mecamylamine, which has a very low affinity for the nicotinic receptor *in vitro* (Romano and Goldstein, 1980; Benwell and Balfour, 1985; Marks and Collins, 1982) antagonizes the discriminative response to nicotine (Romano *et al.*, 1981; Stolerman *et al.*, 1983, 1984). The intraventricular administration of chlorisondamine is also reported to block the nicotine cue (Kumar *et al.*, 1987). The reason for the discrepancies between the *in vivo* and *in vitro* results is not entirely clear although it seems likely that the differences reflect the fact that the antagonists do not act competitively.

In comparison with the drug discrimination studies, relatively little attention has been paid to the role of nicotinic receptors in the other behavioral responses to nicotine. However, Clarke and Kumar (1983) have made some attempt to characterize the receptor which mediates the stimulant properties of the drug. They found the (−)-enantiomer was at least ten times more potent than the (+)-enantiomer and that the response could be blocked by systemic mecamylamine and intraventricular chlorisondamine. Thus there appears to be a clear relationship between the effects of these drugs in the drug discrimination protocols and their effects on locomotor activity. Interestingly, this study also showed that a single bilateral administration of chlorisondamine into the lateral ventricles produced a prolonged blockade (at least 20 days) of the locomotor stimulant response to nicotine. As yet there is no satisfactory explanation for the mechanism underlying the prolonged effects of the drug.

Recent studies (Shimohama *et al.*, 1985; Flynn and Mash, 1986) have confirmed the presence of high affinity (−)-nicotine binding sites in human brain. It seems reasonable to suggest that these receptors mediate at least some of the effects of nicotine inhaled in tobacco smoke although their role has not been established unequivocally for any specific response.

There is evidence from a number of laboratories to suggest that (−)-nicotine also binds to a second site which, relative to the nicotinic site discussed above, has a much lower affinity for the ligand (Romano and Goldstein, 1980; Benwell and Balfour, 1985; Shimohama *et al.*, 1985). However not all groups find this site to be present (Flynn and Mash, 1986; Lippiello and Fernandes 1986). Marks and Collins (1982) and, more recently, Flynn and Mash (1986) have suggested that the low affinity site is detectable if the incubations are performed at 4°C whereas its affinity for nicotine is too low at higher temperatures for the binding to be detected reliably. However, Benwell and Balfour (1985) were able to detect the second site following incubation at 25°C although the results were very inconsistent. Lippiello and Fernandes (1986) suggest that the composition of the incubation medium is the important factor and that the absence of divalent ions and the presence of a protease inhibitor prevents the appearance of the second site. Thus the properties of the site and its possible role in the psychopharmacological responses to nicotine have not been studied in any detail.

Wonnacott (1986) has suggested that the α-bungarotoxin binding site, present in brain tissue, may be the site which is labelled with low affinity by nicotine although experiments in this laboratory (Winch and Balfour unpublished) have failed to confirm this. Nevertheless, Collins *et al.* (1986) have suggested that the effects of nicotine in mice may be mediated by two receptors which differ in their sensitivity to mecamylamine. They found that some responses such as nicotine-induced seizures and the startle response were antagonized by low doses of mecamylamine (IC_{50} value = approx. 0.1 mg/kg) whereas much higher doses (IC_{50} values = approx. 1 mg/kg) were needed to antagonize the effects of nicotine on other responses (respiration, spontaneous activity, heart rate and body temperature). Higher doses of nicotine were required to elicit the effects which were most sensitive to mecamylamine and, therefore, these authors concluded that they were probably mediated by the low affinity site, the other effects being mediated by the high affinity site. By using two strains of mice with different densities of nicotine and α-bungarotoxin binding sites and differing sensitivities to nicotine, the authors also concluded that the low affinity nicotine binding site was the one which could be labelled *in vitro* with radioactive α-bungarotoxin.

The chronic administration of nicotine, either as an infusion or as a series of injections, has been shown to increase the density of high affinity (−)-nicotine binding sites (Marks *et al.*, 1983; Marks and Collins, 1985; Marks *et al.*, 1985; Nordberg *et al.*, 1985). Consistent with the hypothesis that (−)-[^{3}H]nicotine labels the nicotinic cholinoreceptor, chronic nicotine also increases the binding of [^{3}H]ACh to its nicotinic receptors in the brain (Schwartz and Kellar, 1983, 1985). In contrast, chronic inhibition of acetylcholinesterase in the central nervous system decreases the density of [^{3}H]ACh and [^{3}H]nicotine binding sites (Schwartz and Kellar, 1985). Thus, although it has not been established with certainty, it seems reasonable to suggest that the increased density of nicotinic receptors occurs as a result of prolonged or repeated desensitization of the receptors (Wonnacott, 1987).

The behavioral significance of the up-regulation of the nicotinic receptors has not been fully established. Marks *et al.* (1985) have suggested the increased density of sites correlated with the development of tolerance to the effects of nicotine on the activity of mice in a Y-maze (rears and locomotor activity) and on body temperature whereas correlations with its effects on respiration, startle response and heart rate were not significant or inconsistent. The correlations, of course, do not establish a causal relationship between the changes in receptor density and the development of tolerance to nicotine. However, the authors did conclude that although changes in nicotine binding could be implicated in the development of tolerance to some of the effects of nicotine, other mechanisms also appeared to be involved. Studies by Ksir *et al.* (1985) suggest that the enhanced stimulant response to nicotine, observed in rats treated chronically with the drug, also correlated with an increase in the density of nicotinic ACh receptors. Schwartz and Kellar (1985) have also suggested the development of nicotine dependence could be related to the change in receptor density. These conclusions are not supported by studies reported by Benwell and Balfour (1985) which showed that the chronic administration of nicotine, using an injection protocol which had previously been shown to elicit behavioral tolerance to the drug and is also thought to elicit nicotine dependence, failed to change the density of the receptors. Thus the pharmacological significance of the correlations between the changes in receptor density and some of the central responses to nicotine remains to be established with certainty.

Most studies assume that the responses to nicotine which are mediated by central nicotinic receptors reflect stimulation of the receptor. However, if the up-regulation of the receptors occurs because repeated or prolonged nicotine administration causes a persistent desensitization blockage of the receptor complex, more attention should, perhaps, be paid to the pharmacological sequelae of receptor inactivation. Studies with antagonists suggest that the stimulant properties of the drug and its ability to act as a discriminative stimulus are unlikely to reflect inactivation of the receptors (see Clarke, 1987 for review) although the fact that the antagonists generally have a very low affinity for the receptor *in vitro* means that the interpretation of the results of behavioral studies with the antagonists has to remain circumspect. However, recent studies in this laboratory (Benwell, Balfour and Anderson, 1988) have shown that cigarette smoking is associated with an up-regulation of nicotinic receptors similar in magnitude to that observed in experimental animals treated chronically with nicotine. This observation raises the interesting possibility that the rewarding properties of tobacco smoke could be related to the desensitizing effects of nicotine rather than its ability to stimulate nicotinic receptors. In support of this conclusion there is some preliminary evidence that oral mecamylamine may help habitual heavy smokers to stop smoking (Tennant *et al.*, 1983). The study, however, was not well controlled and the results must remain speculative. Nevertheless they raise the interesting possibility, which merits further consideration, that nicotinic receptor antagonists may have a role to play in the treatment of the withdrawal effects observed during smoking cessation.

6.2. Norepinephrine

In the 1970s, experiments reported from a number of laboratories suggested that nicotine might stimulate the secretion of catecholamines in the brain. Studies *in vivo* indicated that both the acute and chronic administration of nicotine increased norepinephrine (NE) turnover in the brain and that the effect could be blocked by mecamylamine (Bhagat, 1970; Fuxe *et al.*, 1977; Lee, 1985; Morgan and Pfeil, 1979). *In vitro* studies have shown that relatively low concentrations of nicotine (10^{-6} M) can stimulate the release of NE from hypothalamic synaptosomes (Balfour, 1973; Yoshida *et al.*, 1980). This effect appears to be Ca^{2+}-dependent and to be mediated by nicotinic receptors located on NE-secreting nerve terminals (Hall and Turner, 1972; Westfall, 1974). *In vivo* experiments in the anesthetized cat have shown that the systemic administration of nicotine also stimulates NE release from the hypothalamus and that the release could also be evoked by injecting small amounts of nicotine directly into the third ventricle (Hall and Turner, 1972).

There are also reports that nicotine can evoke NE release from nerve terminals in other areas of the brain such as the hippocampus (Arqueros *et al.*, 1978; Balfour, 1973), cerebal cortex and cerebellum (Westfall, 1974). However, *in vitro*, the concentrations of nicotine required to elicit this effect are high and it seems unlikely that the increased release evoked by nicotine *in vitro* is relevant to the behavioral responses to nicotine (Balfour, 1984b). Indeed Taube *et al.* (1977) have reported that the NE-secreting nerve terminals of the rat occipital cortex do not appear to have presynaptic nicotine receptors. This does not, of course, preclude an effect of nicotine on NE release in the extra-hypothalamic sites since nicotine could evoke the release of another transmitter which acts presynaptically or stimulates the neurones on the cell soma. The latter is probably the most likely site of action since there is evidence for the presence of nicotinic receptors on the cell soma of NE-secreting cells in the locus coeruleus (Engberg and Svenssen, 1980; Svenssen and Engberg, 1982).

The possible role of brain NE neurones in the responses to nicotine which may be implicated in the tobacco smoking habit remain unclear. Hall *et al.* (1978) reported that intraventricular injections of nicotine in both rats and cats could reduce plasma glucocorticoid levels if the pretreatment levels were high. These authors attributed this effect to increased NE secretion in the hypothalamus which resulted in decreased adrenocorticotrophic hormone (ACTH) secretion from the anterior pituitary. However, there is little evidence that the systemic administration of nicotine reduces plasma glucocorticoid levels in stressed rats (Balfour *et al.*, 1975; Benwell and Balfour, 1982a) although a recent study did find a very small reduction in rats tested in the elevated X-maze test for anxiety following subchronic treatment with nicotine (Balfour *et al.*, 1986b). There is little evidence to date to suggest that NE-secreting neurones play a specific role in any of the behavioral responses to nicotine (see Balfour, 1984b for review).

6.3. Dopamine

Early studies designed to investigate the effects of nicotine on dopamine (DA) secretion tended to investigate the effects of relatively high nicotine concentrations on the release of [^{3}H]DA *in vitro* from slices or synaptosomes pre-incubated with [^{3}H]DA. The results of these studies were equivocal both in terms of the regions of the brain from which nicotine could evoke DA release process and the mechanisms by which the drug evoked this effect (see Balfour, 1984b for review). However, more recent studies have tended to provide clear support for the hypothesis that nicotine can stimulate DA secretion in the brain. For example, Lichtensteiger *et al.* (1982) have reported that the direct iontophoretic administration of the drug directly onto the DA-secreting cells of the substantia nigra caused them to discharge. The stimulatory effects of systemic nicotine on these cells have been confirmed by the more recent study of Clarke *et al.* (1985a) which also showed that the effects of the drug could be antagonized by the systemic administration of mecamylamine but not by the quaternary ganglion blocking drug, chlorisondamine. In another study Clarke and Pert (1985) used an autoradiographic approach to demonstrate the presence of nicotinic receptors on DA neurones in the substantia nigra and ventral tegmental area and on the DA-secreting terminals in the striatum, nucleus accumbens and olfactory tubercle. Thus there appears to be an accumulation of evidence to support the hypothesis that nicotine does stimulate DA secretion in the brain and that it does so by stimulating nicotinic receptors located on the DA-secreting cells.

Experiments *in vivo* in which the effects of nicotine on DA turnover were examined in rats pretreated with an inhibitor of tyrosine hydroxylase indicated that nicotine stimulates DA turnover in both the mesolimbic and nigrostriatal systems (Anderson *et al.*, 1981a,b), results which are clearly in accord with the electrophysiological and receptor studies cited above. However, in a more recent study, Imperato *et al.* (1986) used *in vivo* dialysis to investigate the effects of nicotine on DA release in the striatum and nucleus accumbens of freely moving rats. These experiments suggested that nicotine preferentially stimulated the release of DA in the mesolimbic system, apparently via stimulation of central nicotinic receptors which could be blocked by mecamylamine. The mechanism by which the drug exerts this selective effect remains unclear although the authors draw attention to the fact that both ethanol and the opiates also exhibit a similar preferential effect on the mesolimbic system (see Imperato *et al.*, 1986 for reference).

DA-secreting neurones are thought to play an important role in the 'reward pathways' of the brain, and experimental animals will readily learn to stimulate these neurones either by means of intracranial electrodes located in the DA-secreting fibers or by self-administration of drugs which act on these neurones (Wise, 1980; Wise and Bozarth, 1981). Indeed most, if not all, of the drugs known to stimulate brain DA secretion are drugs of dependence and it is widely assumed that their ability to simulate the proposed 'reward pathways' in the brain is directly related to their potential to cause dependence. There is evidence that the self-administration of both morphine and the psychostimulants amphetamine and cocaine is associated particularly with stimulation of the mesolimbic DA system (Bozarth and Wise, 1981, 1984; Wise and Bozarth, 1981). The psychostimulant properties of amphetamine also appear to be mediated by the mesolimbic DA terminals in the nucleus accumbens (Kelly *et al.*, 1975). The increase in mesolimbic DA secretion, evoked by the local injection of morphine directly into the ventral tegmental area also results in increased locomotor activity (Joyce and Iversen, 1979). Therefore, it seems reasonable to suggest that both the psychostimulant properties of nicotine and the ability of the drug to cause dependence are also related to its effects on brain DA systems and, indeed, this hypothesis has been proposed by Andersson *et al.* (1981a,b), Imperato *et al.* (1986) and Clarke (1987). Direct support for the hypothesis comes from the studies of Pert and Chiueh (1986) who showed that the local administration of the nicotinic agonist, cytisine, into the ventral tegmentum caused increased locomotor activity and from the studies of Singer *et al.* (1982) which showed that lesions of the mesolimbic DA system attenuated nicotine self-administration.

6.4. 5-Hydroxytryptamine

The effects of nicotine on brain 5-HT systems have also been the subject of study in a number of laboratories. For example Balfour *et al.* (1975) showed that 45 min after an acute subcutaneous injection of the drug to unstressed rats, hippocampal 5-HT was decreased, whereas 60 min after the injection, the concentration was increased when compared with controls. Hippocampal 5-hydroxyindoleacetic acid (5-HIAA) was also reduced significantly in rats treated acutely or subchronically with nicotine prior to testing in the elevated X-maze test for anxiety (Balfour *et al.*, 1986b). Rosecrans (1971) has reported that acute nicotine lowers the concentration and turnover of 5-HT in the forebrain of female rats selected for their high levels of spontaneous locomotor activity. In contrast the levels and turnover of 5-HT in the midbrain and hindbrain of rats with low levels of spontaneous activity were decreased by nicotine. Rosecrans concluded that his studies suggested that the inherent basal activity of the rats appeared to be related to brain 5-HT function and that this could be an important factor in the effects of drugs on these systems.

Studies by Benwell and Balfour (1979, 1982b) have shown that the chronic administration of nicotine to unstressed rats causes a regionally-selective decrease in the concentration and biosynthesis of 5-HT in the hippocampus. These data are consistent with the conclusion that nicotine decreases the turnover of 5-HT in this region of the brain. In a more recent post-mortem study, Benwell *et al.* (in press) found the concentration of 5-HT and 5-HIAA in human hippocampus were also reduced, in a regionally selective way when the tissue was taken from the brains of subjects who had been smokers. The density of 5-HT_{1A} receptor sites was increased in the hippocampus of these subjects. These results suggest that a similar decrease in 5-HT turnover in the hippocampus is evoked by smoking tobacco and, clearly, it seems reasonable to suggest that the effect is caused by the nicotine present in the smoke.

The mechanisms by which nicotine might alter 5-HT secretion in the brain remain unclear. *In vitro* studies have shown that nicotine can stimulate the release of [^{14}C]5-HT from synaptosomes or brain slices pre-incubated with the radiolabelled monoamine (Balfour, 1973; Goodman and Weiss, 1973). However, the concentrations of the drug required to evoke this effect were high and it seems unlikely that the effects are related to the changes in 5-HT and 5-HIAA observed in rats treated with pharmacologically sensible doses of nicotine. More recently Westfall *et al.* (1983) investigated the effects of both nicotine and the nicotinic agonist dimethylpiperazinium iodide (DMPP) on the release of both of [^{3}H]5-HT and endogenous 5-HT from rat striatal slices. DMPP evoked a concentration-dependent increase in the release of both tritiated and endogenous 5-HT by a process which was blocked by hexamethonium. The concentrations of DMPP used were also fairly high (up to 500 μM). However, in contrast, nicotine was at least 10 times less potent than DMPP at stimulating 5-HT release and both compounds were found to exert greater effects on DA secretion. In reviewing the topic Balfour (1984b) suggested that the data available at that time were most consistent with the hypothesis that the effects of nicotine on brain 5-HT systems were probably mediated via a second transmitter whose release was altered by nicotine and which acted upon serotonergic neurones. Nothing has been published since that review to alter this conclusion.

The possible role of brain 5-HT systems in behavioral and physiological responses to nicotine have been studied using a range of protocols. Serotonergic neurones do not seem to mediate the ability of nicotine to act as a discriminative stimulus in a drug discrimination protocol (Schechter and Rosecrans, 1972; Stolerman *et al.*, 1983). However the stimulant effect of nicotine on locomotor activity was reduced by pretreating the rats with parachlorophenylalanine (PCPA) to deplete the brain of 5-HT (Fitzgerald *et al.*, 1985). The studies reported by Balfour *et al.*, (1986a) suggest that the serotonergic innervation to the hippocampus was probably not implicated in the effects of PCPA on the psychostimulant properties of nicotine since selective lesions of the pathway did not influence the locomotor response to nicotine. The lesions did, however, attenuate the development of tolerance of the plasma corticosterone response to the drug. Other studies (Benwell and Balfour, 1982a) provide further circumstantial evidence for a role for hippocampal 5-HT in the effects of nicotine on habituation of the plasma corticosterone response to an aversive stimulus. These experiments showed that, in rats given saline, habituation to the stress on an elevated open platform was associated with the development of a positive correlation between the concentrations of corticosterone in the plasma and 5-HT in the hippocampus. In rats given nicotine the correlation was also significant but negative. No significant correlation was apparent in nicotine-withdrawn rats. Benwell and Balfour (1982a) suggested that the changed relationship between hippocampal 5-HT and plasma corticosterone, observed in the rats given nicotine, provided clear evidence for an effect of the drug on the process by which the rats had habituated to the aversive stimulus and that the effects on habituation to stress could be related to the development of dependence upon the drug in stressful environments (see also Balfour, 1984a). However a direct association between the changes in hippocampal 5-HT evoked by nicotine and a behavioral or physiological measure of nicotine-withdrawal remains to be established.

7. MECHANISMS UNDERLYING THE DEVELOPMENT OF NICOTINE DEPENDENCE

In an earlier review, Balfour (1984a) summarized evidence that most of the drugs of dependence exhibited two basic properties:

(1) they could act as rewards in drug self-administration schedules;

(2) their withdrawal following a period of chronic treatment should be associated with the expression of an abstinence syndrome.

Results presented in the preceding sections of this review have shown that nicotine can satisfy both criteria although it is clear that environmental factors play a significant role in the expression of both responses. Exposure to aversive environmental stimuli appears to be precipitating factor in both nicotine self-administration (Hanson *et al.*, 1979; Bättig, 1980) and the behavioral manifestation of nicotine withdrawal (Morrison, 1974). In the earlier review, it was, therefore, suggested that the data available at that time were consistent with the hypothesis that amelioration of the emotional response to aversive environmental stimuli was one of the principal rewarding properties of nicotine. Results published since publication of that review tend to support the conclusion (e.g. Hutchinson and Emley, 1985). The amelioration of stress by nicotine does not appear to reflect an anxiolytic property similar to that of benzodiazepine anti-anxiety drugs (Balfour *et al.*, 1986b). Indeed the studies of Singer and his colleagues (1982) suggest that, like amphetamine and cocaine (Lyness *et al.*, 1979; Pettit *et al.*, 1984) nicotine self-administration depends upon stimulation of the dopaminergic neurones which innervate the nucleus accumbens and frontal cortex. There is clear evidence that nicotine stimulates DA secretion in the mesolimbic system (Imperato *et al.*, 1986) and, therefore, it seems reasonable to suggest that the rewarding properties of the drug may be associated with its ability to act as a stimulant. However there appears to be little, if any, evidence to suggest that the rewarding properties of other drugs such as amphetamine and morphine which also stimulate mesolimbic DA secretion (Kelly *et al.*, 1975; Wise and Bozarth, 1981) are more apparent in aversive environments. Thus the effects of nicotine on this system would not seem to provide an explanation for its reported ability to alleviate the effects of stress (Gilbert, 1979) and the fact that stress seems to enhance the rewarding properties of the drug.

Unlike amphetamine, nicotine also stimulates the secretion of ACh and this effect has been associated with its ability to improve cognitive function (see Section 3.1). It is possible that improved cognitive performance results in an enhanced ability to cope with stressful situations and that this is perceived by the smoker as a 'tranquilizing' effect in spite of the fact that many of the physiological responses to such stimuli may actually be increased by cigarette smoking (Poulton, 1977; Pomerleau and Pomerleau, 1987). In a very elegant study Bozarth and Wise (1984) showed that the rats will self-administer morphine into the ventral tegmental area of the brain where its effect is to stimulate the DA-secreting cells of the mesolimbic system. However the administration of morphine into this area of the brain, even at fairly high doses, never resulted in the development of physical dependence upon the drug. In contrast it proved impossible to train rats to self-administer morphine into the periventricular gray whereas the study provided clear evidence that rats could develop physical dependence to the drug when it was given into this region of the brain. The authors concluded, therefore, that distinct anatomical sites within the brain mediate the rewarding properties of morphine and the expression of the abstinence syndrome following its withdrawal. Thus it would appear that the opiate abstinence syndrome may be totally unrelated to the rewarding properties of these drugs which, in the first instance at least, encourage people to take them. Avoidance of the abstinence syndrome may develop subsequently as a reason for drug taking behavior as the subject becomes physically dependent and, indeed, avoidance of the withdrawal effects may become the principal reason for continuing to take these compounds. The data presently available are probably most consistent with this hypothesis.

It is quite possible that there is a similar anatomical dissociation between the rewarding properties of nicotine and the withdrawal effects observed when it is withdrawn. However, the hypothesis proposed by Balfour (1984a) implies that this is not the case at least as far as its putative anti-stress properties are concerned. The hypothesis suggested that specific pathways within the central nervous system are associated with the mechanism by which animals adapt or habituate to aversive stimuli. If, however, the animal is given a drug which ameliorates the effects of stress then there is diminished requirement for the animal to invoke the normal mechanism used to cope with aversive stimuli. Thus the hypothesis also suggested that the symptoms of nicotine-withdrawal were most marked when the animals were exposed to aversive stimuli from which they had been previously protected by nicotine. Balfour (1984a) went on to argue that the effects on hippocampal 5-HT systems (see Balfour, 1984b for review) reflected its ability to ameliorate the effects of stress and that the effects could be implicated in the behavioral expression of the withdrawal effect (Morrison, 1974). More recent studies (Balfour *et al.*, 1986a; Graham and Balfour, unpublished results) suggest that diminished secretion of 5-HT in the hippocampus is associated with behavioral changes similar to those seen in animals given an anxiogenic drug. There is little evidence, however, that nicotine acts directly on the serotonergic neurones which innervate the hippocampus and it seems reasonable to suggest that the effects of the drug on this system are the result of changes elsewhere in the brain.

One interesting corollary of the hypothesis is that it can offer one explanation for the fact that only a proportion of smokers experience severe withdrawal symptoms when they stop smoking (Gilbert, 1979). Those smokers who cope well with environmental stressors and find tobacco smoking rewarding for other reasons would be less likely to become dependent upon the proposed anti-stress properties of the drug whereas those whose central coping mechanism is not particularly effective would find the anti-stress properties especially rewarding and would experience more severe withdrawal effects.

The possible role of brain nicotinic receptors in the development of dependence remains unclear although Schwartz and Kellar (1985) have been tempted to speculate that the up-regulation of the receptors, evoked by chronic treatment with nicotine, may be implicated in this process. Although the recent studies of Benwell *et al.* (1988) which have shown that the density of the receptors is also increased in the brains of smokers, other animal studies (Benwell and Balfour, 1985) have shown that injection schedules which are reported to cause dependence in experimental rats do not invariably cause up-regulation of the receptors.

8. CONCLUDING REMARKS

The evidence summarized in this review is intended to lead the reader to the conclusion that a majority of people who smoke tobacco do so in order to experience the pleasurable psychopharmacological properties of nicotine. This conclusion implies that procedures directed at either aiding people to abstain from smoking or at making smoking safer should take full account of this fact. The introduction of nicotine-containing chewing gum as a palliative for smokers (see Section 2.1) was based on the assumption that maintenance of the plasma nicotine concentration was the principal objective of tobacco smoking. This is almost certainly a considerable over-simplification of the situation which ignores, for example, the role of environmental factors. As a result the gum was not entirely successful although, clearly, it does have an important role to play in smoking-withdrawal clinics. Future studies may show that other routes of administration, especially those which, like inhaled cigarette smoke, cause a rapid rise in nicotine levels, may prove more beneficial than the gum for some smokers. There has already been some movement towards this idea in the experiments performed with nicotine administered via the nasal route (Russell *et al.*, 1983a).

Interestingly, there seems to have been little movement towards the introduction of cigarettes containing tobacco with raised concentrations of nicotine relative to other constituents of the leaf. This idea, first proposed by Russell in 1975, seems a logical development in the search for a 'safer' cigarette if nicotine is, indeed, the primary rewarding constituent of the smoke. There are a number of possible explanations for the failure of this approach to gain wide acceptance. One reason could be the problem that, for this type of cigarette to gain a significant share of the market, it would be necessary for smokers to change from their existing brand to a new one containing the new tobacco. Initially they may well find the new cigarettes less acceptable because sensory cues associated with inhalation of the smoke may play an important part in the mechanism by which smokers titrate the appropriate quantity of nicotine into their lungs (see Section 2). Inhalation of the smoke from the enhanced nicotine tobacco would yield inappropriate cues and the smoker would, initially at least, inhale an unpleasantly high dose of nicotine. Secondly there are considerable ethical problems associated with advertising such a product which means that it would probably be very difficult to make the smoker aware of the product and, in particular, the reasons for making it available.

REFERENCES

ANDERSSON, K., FLUXE, K. and AGNATI, L. F. (1981a) Effects of single injections of nicotine on the ascending dopamine pathways in the rats. *Acta Physiol. Scand.* **112**: 345–347.

ANDERSSON, K., FLUXE, K., AGNATI, L. F. and ENEROTH, P. (1981b) Effects of acute central and peripheral administration of nicotine on ascending dopamine pathways in the male rat brain. Evidence for nicotine induced increases in dopamine turnover in various telencephalic dopamine nerve terminal systems. *Med. Biol.* **59**: 170–176.

ARMITAGE, A. K., HALL, G. H. and MORRISON, C. F. (1968) Pharmacological basis of the tobacco smoking habit. *Nature* **217**: 331–334.

ARMITAGE, A. K., HALL, G. H. and SELLARS, C. M. (1969) Effects of nicotine on electrocortical activity and acetylcholine release from calf cerebral cortex. *Br. J. Pharmac.* **35**: 152–160.

ARGUEROS, L., NAQUIRA, D. and ZUNINO, E. (1978) Nicotine-induced release of catecholamines from rat hippocampus and striatum. *Biochem. Pharmac.* **27**: 2667–2674.

ASHTON, H. and STEPNEY, R. (1982) *Smoking Psychology and Pharmacology*, Tavistock Publications, London.

ASHTON, H., MILLMAN, J. E., TELFORD, R. and THOMPSON, J. W. (1974) The effect of caffeine, nitrazepam and cigarette smoking on the contingent negative variation in man. *Electroenceph. Clin. Neurophysiol.* **37**: 59–71.

ASHTON, H., MARSH, V. R., MILLMAN, J. E., RAWLINS, M. D., TELFORD, D. R. and THOMPSON, J. W. (1978a) The use of event-related slow potentials of the brain as a means to analyse the effects of cigarette smoking and nicotine in humans. In: *Smoking Behaviour: Physiological and Psychological Influences*, THORNTON, R. E. (ed.) Churchill Livingston, Edinburgh.

ASHTON, H., MILLMAN, J. E., RAWLINS, M. D., TELFORD, D. R. and THOMPSON, J. W. (1978b) The use of event-related slow potentials of the brain in the analysis of effects of cigarette smoking and nicotine in humans. In: *International Workshop on the Behavioural Effects of Nicotine*, pp. 26–37. BATTIG, K. (ed.) Karger, Basel.

ASHTON, H., STEPNEY, R. and THOMPSON, J. W. (1979) Self-titration by cigarette smokers. *Br. Med. J.* **2**: 357–360.

BALFOUR, D. J. K. (1973) The effects of nicotine on the uptake and retention of ^{14}C-noradrenaline and ^{14}C-5-hydroxytryptamine by rat brain homogenates. *Eur. J. Pharmac.* **23**: 19–26.

BALFOUR, D. J. K. (1979) Studies on the biochemical and behavioural effects of oral nicotine. *Archs Int. Pharmacodyn. Thér.* **245**: 95–103.

BALFOUR, D. J. K. (1984a) The pharmacology of nicotine dependence: a working hypothesis. In: *International Encyclopedia of Pharmacology and Therapeutics, Section* 114, *Nicotine and the Tobacco Smoking Habit*, pp. 101–112, BALFOUR, D. J. K. (ed.) Pergamon Press, Oxford.

BALFOUR, D. J. K. (1984b) The effects of nicotine on brain neurotransmitter systems. In: *International Encyclopedia of Pharmacology and Therapeutics, Section* 114, *Nicotine and the Tobacco Smoking Habit*, pp. 61–74. BALFOUR, D. J. K. (ed.) Pergamon Press, Oxford.

BALFOUR, D. J. K., KHULLAR, A. K. and LONGDEN. A. (1975) Effects of nicotine on plasma corticosterone and brain amines in stressed and unstressed rats. *Pharmac. Biochem. Behav.* **3**: 179–184.

BALFOUR, D. J. K., BENWELL, M. E. M., GRAHAM, C. A. and VALE, A. L. (1986a) Behavioural and adrenocortical responses to nicotine measured in rats with selective lesions of the 5-hydroxytryptaminergic fibres innervating the hippocampus. *Br. J. Pharmac.* **89**: 341–347.

BALFOUR, D. J. K., GRAHAM, C. A. and VALE, A. L. (1986b) Studies on the possible role of brain 5-HT systems and adrenocortical activity in behavioural responses to nicotine and diazepam in an elevated x-maze. *Psychopharmacology* **90**: 528–532.

BÄTTIG, K. (1980) The smoking habit and the psychopharmacological effects of nicotine. *Activ. Nerv. Sup.* **22**: 274–288.

BÄTTIG, K. (1981) Smoking and the behavioural effects of nicotine. *TIPS* **3**: 145–147.

BÄTTIG, K. (1983) Spontaneous tunnel maze locomotion in rats. In: *Application of Behavioural Pharmacology in Toxicology*, pp. 15–26, ZBINDEN, G., CUOMO, V., RACAGNI, G. and WEISS, B. (eds) Raven Press, New York.

BÄTTIG, K. and SCHLATTER, J. (1978) Effects of nicotine and amphetamine on maze exploration and on spatial memory by Roman high avoidance and Roman low avoidance rats. In: *International Workshop on Behavioral Effects of Nicotine*, pp. 38–55. BATTIG, K. (ed.) Karger, Basel.

BÄTTIG, K. and SCHLATTER, J. (1979) Effects of sex and strain on exploratory locomotion and development on non-reinforced maze patrolling. *Animal Learn. Behav.* **7**: 99–105.

BÄTTIG, K., DRISCOLL, P., SCHLATTER, J. and USTER, H. (1976) Effects of nicotine on the exploratory locomotion patterns of female Roman high and low avoidance rats. *Psychopharmacology* **4**: 435–439.

BEANI, L., BIANCHI, C., NILSSON, L., NORDBERG, A., ROMANELLI, L. and SIVILOTTI, L. (1985) The effect of nicotine and cytisine on ^{3}H-acetylcholine release for cortical slices and guinea-pig brain. *Archs Pharmac.* **331**: 293–296.

BECKETT, A. and TRIGGS, E. J. (1966) Determination of nicotine and its metabolite cotinine in urine by gas chromatography. *Nature, Lond.* **211**: 1415–1417.

BECKETT, A. and TRIGGS, E. J. (1967) Enzyme induction in man caused by smoking. *Nature, Lond.* **216**: 587.

BENOWITZ, N. L. and JACOB, P. (1984) Daily intake of nicotine during cigarette smoking. *Clin. Pharmac. Ther.* **35**: 499–504.

BENWELL, M. E. M. and BALFOUR, D. J. K. (1979) Effects of nicotine and its withdrawal on plasma corticosterone and brain 5-hydroxyindoles. *Psychopharmacology* **63**: 7-11.

BENWELL, M. E. M. and BALFOUR, D. J. K. (1982a) Effects of chronic nicotine administration on the response and adaptation to stress. *Psychopharmacology* **76**: 160-162.

BENWELL, M. E. M. and BALFOUR, D. J. K. (1982b) Effects of nicotine administration on 5-HT uptake and biosynthesis in rat brain. *Eur. J. Pharmac.* **84**: 71-77.

BENWELL, M. E. M. and BALFOUR, D. J. K. (1985) Nicotine binding to brain tissue from drug-naive and nicotine-treated rats. *J. Pharm. Pharmac.* **37**: 405-409.

BENWELL, M. E. M., BALFOUR, D. J. K. and ANDERSON, J. M. (1988) Evidence that smoking increases the density of nicotine binding sites in human brain. *J. Neurochem.* **50**: 243-247.

BENWELL, M. E. M., BALFOUR, D. J. K. and ANDERSON, J. M. Smoking-associated changes in serotonergic systems of discrete regions of human brain. *Psychopharmacology* (in press).

BHAGAT, B. (1970) Influence of chronic administration of nicotine and the turnover and metabolism of noradrenaline in rat brain. *Psychopharmacologia* **18**: 325-332.

BOZARTH, M. A. and WISE, R. A. (1981) Intracranial self-administration of morphine into the ventral tegmental area in rats. *Life Sci.* **28**: 551-555.

BOZARTH, M. A. and WISE, R. A. (1984) Anatomically distinct opiate receptor fields mediate reward and physical dependence. *Science* **224**: 516-517.

BRANTMARK, B., OHLIN, P. and WESTLING, H. (1973) Nicotine-containing chewing gum as an anti-smoking aid. *Psychopharmacologia* **31**: 191-200.

CAM, G. R., BASSETT, J. R. and CAIRNCROSS, K. D. (1979) The action of nicotine on the pituitary-adrenal cortical axis. *Archs Int. Pharmacodyn. Thér.* **237**: 49-66.

CARR, G. D. and WHITE, N. M. (1983) Conditioned place preference from intra-accumbens but not intra-caudate amphetamine injections. *Life Sci.* **33**: 2551-2557.

CLARKE, P. B. S. (1987) Nicotine and smoking: a perspective from animal studies. *Psychopharmacology* **92**: 135-143.

CLARKE, P. B. S. and KUMAR, R. (1983) Characterization of the locomotor stimulant action of nicotine in tolerant rats. *Br. J. Pharmac.* **80**: 587-594.

CLARKE, P. B. S. and PERT, A. (1985) Autoradiographic evidence for nicotine receptors on nigrostriatal and mesolimbic dopaminergic neurons. *Brain Res.* **348**: 355-358.

CLARKE, P. B. S., HOMMER, D. W., PERT, A. and SKIRBOLL, L. R. (1985a) Electrophysiological actions of nicotine on substantia nigra single units. *Br. J. Pharmac.* **85**: 827-835.

CLARKE, P. B. S., SCHWARTZ, R. D., PAUL, S. M., PERT, C. B. and PERT, A. (1985b) Nicotinic binding in rat brain: autoradiographic comparison of [^{3}H] acetylcholine, [^{3}H] Nicotine and [^{125}I]-α-bungaratoxin. *J. Neurosci.* **5**: 1307-1315.

COLLINS, A. C., EVANS, C. B., MINER, L. L. and MARKS, M. J. (1986) Mecamylamine blockade of nicotine responses: evidence for two brain nicotinic receptors. *Pharmac. Biochem. Behav.* **24**: 1767-1773.

CONWAY, T. L., VICKERS, R. R., WARD, H. W. and RAHE, R. H. (1981) Occupational stress and variation in cigarette, coffee and alcohol consumption. *J. Health Soc. Behav.* **22**: 155-165.

COPLAND, A. M. and BALFOUR, D. J. K. (1987) The effects of diazepam on brain 5-HT and 5-HIAAA in stressed and unstressed rats. *Pharmac. Biochem. Behav.* (in press).

COSTA, L. G. and MURPHY, S. D. (1983) [^{3}H] Nicotine binding in rat brain: alteration after chronic cholinesterase inhibition. *J. Pharmac. Exp. Ther.* **226**: 392-397.

COX, B. M., GOLDSTEIN, A. and NELSON, W. T. (1984) Nicotine self-administration in rats. *Br. J. Pharmac.* **83**: 49-55.

CRONAN, T., CONRAD, J. and BRYSON, R. (1985) Effects of chronically administered nicotine and saline on motor activity in rats. *Psychopharmac. Biochem. Behav.* **22**: 897-899.

DRISCOLL, P. and BÄTTIG, K. (1981) Selective inhibition by nicotine of shock-induced fighting in the rat. *Pharmac. Biochem. Behav.* **14**: 175-179.

DUNNE, M. P., MACDONALD, D. and HARTLEY, L. R. (1986) The effects of nicotine on memory and problem solving performance. *Physiol. Behav.* **37**: 849-854.

EDWARDS, J. A. and WARBURTON, D. M. (1984) Smoking nicotine and electrocortical activity. In: *International Encyclopedia of Pharmacology and Therapeutics, Section* 114, *Nicotine and the Tobacco Smoking Habit*, pp. 113-131, BALFOUR, D. J. K. (ed.) Pergamon Press, Oxford.

EISENBERG, R. M. (1987) Diazepam withdrawal as demonstrated by changes in plasma corticosterone: a role for the hippocampus. *Life Sci.* **40**: 817-825.

EMMETT-OGLESBY, M. W., SPENCER, D. G., LEWIS, M., ELMESALLAMY, F. and LAL, H. (1983) Anxiogenic aspects of diazepam withdrawal can be detected in animals. *Eur. J. Pharmac.* **92**: 127-130.

EMMETT-OGLESBY, M. W., HARRIS, C. M., LANE, J. D. and LAL, H. (1984) Withdrawal from morphine generalizes to pentylene-tetrazol stimulus. *Neuropeptides* **5**: 37-40.

ENGBERG, G. and SVENSSON, T. H. (1980) Pharmacological analysis of a cholinergic receptor mediated regulation of brain norepinephrine neurones. *J. Neural. Transm.* **49**: 137-150.

ERICKSON, C. K. (1971) Studies on the mechanism of avoidance facilitation by nicotine. *Psychopharmacologia* **22**: 357-368.

FEE, W. M. and STEWART, M. J. (1982) A controlled trial of nicotine chewing gum in a smoking withdrawal clinic. *Practitioner* **226**: 148-151.

FEYERABEND, C. and RUSSELL, M. A. H. (1978) Effect of urinary pH and nicotine excretion rate on plasma nicotine during cigarette smoking and chewing nicotine gum. *Br. J. Clin. Pharmac.* **5**: 293-297.

FITZGERALD, R. E., OETTINGER, R. and BATTIG, K. (1985) Reduction of nicotine-induced hyperactivity by pCPA. *Pharmac. Biochem. Behav.* **23**: 279-284.

FLEMING, J. C. and BROADHURST, P. L. (1975) The effects of nicotine on two-way avoidance conditioning in bi-directionally selected strains of rats. *Psychopharmacologia* **14**: 432-438.

FLYNN, D. D. and MASH, D. C. (1986) Characterization of L-[^{3}H] nicotine binding in human cerebral cortex; comparison between Alzheimer's disease and the normal. *J. Neurochem.* **47**: 1948-1954.

FRANKENHAUESER, M., MYRSTENK, K. A-L., POST, B. and JOHANSSON, G. (1971) Behavioural and physiological effects of cigarette smoking in a monstrous situation. *Psychopharmacologia, Berl.* **22**: 1–17.

FRITH, C. D. (1971a) The effect of varying the nicotine content of cigarettes on human smoking behaviour. *Psychopharmacologia* **19**: 188–192.

FRITH, C. D. (1971b) Smoking behaviour and its relation to the smokers' immediate experience. *Br. J. Social Clin. Psychol.* **10**: 73–78.

FUDALA, P. J., TEOH, K. W. and IWAMOTO, E. T. (1985) Pharmacologic characterization of nicotine-induced conditioned place preference. *Pharmac. Biochem. Behav.* **22**: 237–241.

FUXE, K., AGNATI, L., ENEROTH, P., GUSTAFSSON, J-A, HOKFELT, T., LOFSTROM, A., SKETT, B. and SKETT, P. (1977) The effect of nicotine on central catecholamine neurons and gonadotropin secretion. In: Studies in the male rat. *Med. Biol.* **55**: 148–157.

GELLER, I. and SEIFTER, J. (1960) Effects of meprobamate, barbiturates, d-amphetamine and promazine on experimentally induced conflict in the rat. *Psychopharmacologia* **1**: 482–492.

GELLER, I., KULAK, J. T. and SEIFTER, J. (1962) The effect of chlordiazepoxide and chlorpromazine on punished discrimination. *Psychopharmacologia* **3**: 274–385.

GILBERT, D. G. (1979) Paradoxical tranquilizing and emotion-reducing effects of nicotine. *Psychol. Bull.* **86**: 643–661.

GOLDFARB, T. L., JARVIK, M. E. and GUCK, S. D. (1970) Cigarette nicotine content as a determinant of human smoking behavior. *Psychopharmacologia* **17**: 89–93.

GOLDFARB, T. L., GRITZ, E. R., JARVIK, M. E. and STOLERMAN, I. P. (1976) Reactions to cigarettes as a function of nicotine and "tar." *Clin. Pharmac. Ther.* **19**: 767–772.

GOODMAN, F. R. and WEISS, G. B. (1973) Alterations of 5-hydroxytryptamine-^{14}C efflux by nicotine in rat brain area slices. *Neuropharmacology* **12**: 955–965.

GRIFFITHS, R. R., BIGELOW, G. E. and LIEBSON, I. (1976) Facilitation of human tobacco self-administration by ethanol: a behavioral analysis. *J. Exp. Anal. Behav.* **25**: 279–292.

GRITZ, E. R., BAER-WEISS, V. and JARVIK, M. E. (1976) Titration of nicotine intake with full-length and half-length cigarettes. *Clin. Pharmac. Ther.* **20**: 552–556.

HALL, G. H. and MORRISON, C. F. (1973) New evidence for a relationship between tobacco smoking, nicotine dependence and stress. *Nature* **243**: 199–201.

HALL, G. H. and TURNER, D. M. (1972) The effects of nicotine on the release of ^{3}H-noradrenaline from the hypothalamus. *Biochem. Pharmac.* **21**: 1829–1838.

HALL, G. H., FRANCIS, R. L. and MORRISON, C. F. (1978) Nicotine-dependence avoidance behaviour and pituitary-adrenocortical function. In: *International Workshop on Behavioural Effects of Nicotine*, pp. 94–107, BATTIG, K. (ed.) Karger, Basel.

HANSON, H. M., IVESTOR, C. A. and MORTON, B. R. (1979) Nicotine self-administration in rats. In: *Cigarette Smoking as a Dependence Process*, pp. 70–90, KRASNEGOR, N. A. (ed.) NIDA Research Monograph, Rockville.

HARRIS, C. M., EMMETT-OGLESBY, M. W., ROBINSON, N. G. and LAL, H. (1986) Withdrawal from chronic nicotine substitutes partially for the viteroceptive stimulus produced by pentylenetetrazol (PTZ). *Psychopharmacology* **90**: 85–89.

HENDRY, J. S. and ROSECRANS, J. A. (1984) Effects of nicotine on conditioned and unconditioned behaviors in experimental animals. In: *International Encyclopedia of Pharmacology and Therapeutics, Section* 114, *Nicotine and the Tobacco Smoking Habit*, pp. 75–99, BALFOUR, D. J. K. (ed.) Pergamon Press, Oxford.

HENNINGFIELD, J. E. and GOLDBERG, S. R. (1983) Nicotine as a reinforcer in human subjects and laboratory animals. *Pharmac. Biochem. Behav.* **19**: 989–992.

HENNINGFIELD, J. E. and GRIFFITHS, R. R. (1979) A preparation for the experimental analysis of human cigarette smoking. *Behav. Res. Meth. Instr.* **11**: 538–544.

HENNINGFIELD, J. E., MIYASATO, K. and JASINSKI, D. R. (1983) Cigarette smokers self-administer intravenous nicotine. *Pharmac. Biochem. Behav.* **19**: 887–890.

HJALMARSON, A. I. (1984) Effect of nicotine chewing gum in smoking cessation: a randomized, placebo-controlled, double-blind study. *JAMA* **252**: 2835–2838.

HUGHES, J. R., HATSUKAMI, D. K., PICKENS, R. W., KRAHN, D., NALIN, S. and LUKNIC, A. (1984) Effect of nicotine on the tobacco withdrawal syndrome. *Psychopharmacology* **83**: 82–87.

HUGHES, J. R., PICKENS, R. W., SPRING, G. W. and KEENAN, R. M. (1985) Instructions control whether nicotine will serve as a reinforcer. *J. Pharmac. Exp. Ther.* **235**: 106–112.

HUGHES, J. R., HATSUKAMI, D. K. and SKOOG, K. P. (1986) Physical dependence on nicotine gum: placebo substitution trial. *JAMA* **255**: 3277–3279.

HUTCHINSON, R. R. and EMLEY, G. B. (1973) Effects of nicotine on avoidance, conditioned suppression and aggression response measures in animals and man. In: *Smoking Behavior: Motives and Incentives.* DUNN, W. L. (ed.) Winston, Washington, D.C.

HUTCHINSON, R. R. and EMLEY, G. S. (1985) Aversive stimulation produces nicotine ingestion in squirrel monkeys. *Psychol. Rec.* **35**: 491–502.

IKARD, F. F., GREEN, D. E. and HORN, D. (1969) A scale to differentiate between types of smoking as related to the management of affect. *Int. J. Addict.* **4**: 649–659.

IMPERATO, A., MULAS, A. and DI CHIARA, G. (1986) Nicotine preferentially stimulates dopamine release in the limbic system of freely moving rats. *Eur. J. Pharmac.* **132**: 337–338.

ISAAC, P. F. and RAND, M. J. (1969) Blood levels of nicotine and physiological effects after inhalation of tobacco smoke. *Eur. J. Pharmac.* **8**: 269–283.

JAMROZIK, K., FOWLER, G., VESSEY, M. and WALD, N. (1984) Placebo controlled trial of nicotine chewing gum in general practice. *Br. Med. J.* **289**: 794–797.

JARVIK, M. E., POPEK, P., SCHNEIDER, N. G., BAER-WEISS, V. and GRITZ, E. R. (1978) Can cigarette size and nicotine content influence smoking *Psychopharmacology* **58**: 303–306.

JARVIS, M. J., RAW, M., RUSSELL, M. A. H. and FEYERADBEND, C. (1982) Randomised controlled-trial of nicotine chew-gum. *Br. Med. J.* **285**: 537–540.

Johanson, C. E. (1978) Drugs as reinforcers. In: *Contemporary Research in Behavioural Pharmacology*, pp. 325–390, Blackman, D. E. and Sanger, D. J. (eds) Plenum, New York, London.
Joyce, E. M. and Iversen, S. D. (1979) The effect of morphine applied locally to mesencephalic dopamine cell bodies on spontaneous motor activity in the rat. *Neurosci. Lett.* **14**: 207–212.
Katz, R. J. and Gormezano, G. (1979) A rapid and inexpensive technique for assessing the reinforcing effects of opiate drugs. *Pharmac. Biochem. behav.* **11**: 232–233.
Keenan, A. and Johnson, F. N. (1972) Development of behavioral tolerance to nicotine in the rat. *Experientia* **28**: 428–429.
Keim, K. L. and Sigg, E. B. (1977) Plasma corticosterone and brain catecholamines in stress: effect of psychotropic drugs. *Pharmac. Biochem. Behav.* **6**: 79–85.
Kelly, P. H., Seviour, P. W. and Iversen, S. D. (1975) Amphetamine and apomorphine response in the rat following 6-OHDA lesions of the nucleus accumbens septi and corpus striatum. *Brain Res.* **94**: 507–522.
Kissen, D. M. (1960) Psycho-social factors in cigarette smoking motivation. *Med. Offr.* **104**: 365–372.
Kokka, N., Garcia, J. F. and Elliott, H. W. (1973) Effects of acute and chronic administration of narcotic analgesics on growth hormone and corticotrophine (ACTH) secretion in rat. *Prog. Brain Res.* **39**: 347–360.
Ksir, C., Hakan, R., Hall, D. P. and Kellar, K. J. (1985) Exposure to nicotine enhances the behavioural stimulant effect of nicotine and increases binding of [^{3}H]acetylcholine to nicotinsic receptors. *Neuropharmacology* **24**: 527–531.
Kumar, R. (1968) Psycho-active drugs exploratory activity and fear. *Nature* **218**: 665–667.
Kumar, R., Reavill, C. and Stolerman, I. P. (1987) Nicotine cue in rats: effects of central administration of ganglion blocking drugs. *Br. J. Pharmac.* **90**: 239–246.
Lang, W. J., Latiff, A. A., McQueen, A. and Singer, G. (1977) Self-administration of nicotine with and without a food delivery schedule. *Pharmac. Biochem. Behav.* **7**: 65–70.
Larsson, C. and Nordberg, A. (1985) Comparative analysis of nicotine-like receptor-ligand interactions in rodent brain homogenate. *J. Neurochem.* **45**: 24–31.
Lee, E. H. Y. (1985) Effects of nicotine on exploratory behavior in rats: correlation with regional brain monoamine levels. *Behav. Brain. Res.* **17**: 59–66.
Le Fur, G., Guilloux, F., Mitrani, N., Mizoule, J. and Uzan, A. (1979) Relationships between plasma corticosterone and benzodiazepines in stress. *J. Pharmac. Exp. Ther.* **211**: 305–308.
Lichtensteiger, W., Hefti, F., Felix, D., Huwyler, T., Melamed, E. and Schlumpf, M. (1982) Stimulation of nigrostriatal dopamine neurons by nicotine. *Neuropharmacology* **21**: 963–968.
Lippiello, P. M. and Fernandes, K. G. (1986) The binding of L-[^{3}H]nicotine to a single class of high affinity sites in rat brain membranes. *Molec. Pharmac.* **29**: 448–454.
Lowe, G. (1986) State-dependent learning effects with a combination of alcohol and nicotine. *Psychopharmacology* **89**: 105–107.
Lucchesi, B. R., Schuster, C. R. and Emley, G. S. (1967) The role of nicotine as a determinant of cigarette smoking frequency in man with observations of certain cardiovascular effects associated with tobacco. *Clin. Pharmac. Ther.* **8**: 789–796.
Lyness, W. H., Friedle, N. M. and Moore, K. E. (1979) Destruction of dopaminergic nerve terminals in nucleus accumbens: effects on d-amphetamine self-stimulation. *Pharmac. Biochem. Behav.* **11**: 553–556.
Mangan, G. L. and Golding, J. (1978) An 'enhancement' model of smoking maintenance? In: *Smoking Behaviour: Physiological and Psychological Influences*, pp. 87–113, Thornton, R. E. (ed.) Churchill Livingston, London.
Marks, M. J. and Collins, A. C. (1982) Characterization of nicotine binding in mouse brain and comparison with the binding of α-bungarotoxin and quinuclidinyl benzilate. *Molec. Pharmac.* **22**: 554–564.
Marks, M. J. and Collins, A. C. (1985) Tolerance, cross-tolerance and receptors after chronic nicotine or oxotremorine. *Pharmac. Biochem. Behav.* **22**: 283–291.
Marks, M. J., Burch, J. B. and Collins, A. C. (1983) Effects of chronic nicotine infusion on tolerance development and nicotinic receptors. *J. Pharmac. Exp. Ther.* **226**: 817–825.
Marks, M.J., Stitzel, J. A. and Collins, A. C. (1985) Time course study of the effects of chronic nicotine infusion on drug response and brain receptors. *J. Pharmac. Exp. Ther.* **235**: 619–628.
Marks, M. J., Stitzel, J. A., Romm, E., Wehner, J. M. and Collins, A. C. (1986) Nicotinic binding sites in rat and mouse brain: comparison of acetylcholine, nicotine and α-bungarotoxin. *Molec. Pharmac.* **30**: 427–436.
Martino-Barrow, A. M. and Kellar, K. J. (1987) [^{3}H]acetylcholine and [^{3}H](−)nicotine label the same recognition site in rat brain. *Molec. Pharmac.* **31**: 169–174.
McMorrow, M. J. and Foxx, R. M. (1983) Nicotine's role in smoking: an analysis of nicotine regulation. *Psychol. Bull.* **93**: 302–327.
Meltzer, L. T., Rosecrans, J. A., Aceto, M. D. and Harris, L. S. (1980) Discriminative stimulus properties of the optical isomers of nicotine. *Psychopharmacology* **68**: 283–286.
Morgan, W. W. and Pfeil, K. A. (1979) Mecamylamine blockade of nicotine enhanced noradrenaline turnover in rat brain. *Life Sci.* **24**: 417–420.
Morley, B. J. and Kemp. G. E. (1981) Characterization of a putative nicotinic acetylcholine receptor in mammalian brain. *Brain Res. Rev.* **3**: 81–101.
Morley, B. J., Kemp, G. E. and Salvaterra, P. M. (1979) α-bungarotoxin binding sites in the CNS. *Life Sci.* **24**: 859–872.
Morrison, C. F. (1967) Effects of nicotine on operant behavior of rats. *Neuropharmacology* **6**: 229–240.
Morrison, C. F. (1969) The effects of nicotine on punished behaviour. *Psychopharmacologia* **14**: 221–232.
Morrison, C. F. (1974) Effects of nicotine and its withdrawal on the performance of rats on signalled and unsignalled avoidance schedules. *Psychopharmacologia* **38**: 25–35.
Morrison, C. F. and Armitage, A. K. (1967) Effects of nicotine upon the free operant behavior of rats and spontaneous motor activity of mice. *Ann. N.Y. Acad. Sci.* **142**: 268–276.
Morrison, C. F. and Stephenson, J. A. (1970) Drugs effects on a measure of unconditioned avoidance in the rat. *Psychopharmacologia* **18**: 133–143.

MORRISON, C. F. and STEPHENSON, J. A. (1972) The occurrence of tolerance to a central depressant effect of nicotine. *Br. J. Pharmac.* **46**: 151–156.

MORRISON, C. F. and STEPHENSON, J. A. (1973) Effects of stimulants on observed behaviour of rats on six operant schedules. *Neuropharmacology* **12**: 297–310.

MOSS, R. A. and PRUE, D. M. (1982) Research on nicotine regulation. *Behav. Ther.* **13**: 31–46.

MUCHA, R. F., VANDER KOOY, D., O'SHAUGHNESSY, M. and BUCENIEKS, P. (1982) Drug reinforcement studied by the use of place conditioning in rat. *Brain Res.* **243**: 91–105.

NELSEN, J. M. (1978) Psychobiological consequences of chronic nicotinization. In: *International Workshop on Behavioural Effects of Nicotine*, pp. 1–17, BATTIG, K. (ed.) Karger, Basel.

NEMETH-COSLETT, R. and HENNINGFIELD, J. E. (1986) Effects of nicotine chewing gum on cigarette smoking and subjective physiological effects. *Clin. Pharmac. Ther.* **39**: 625–630.

NEMETH-COSLETT, R., HENNINGFIELD, J. E., O'KEEFFE, M. K. and GRIFFITHS, R. R. (1986) Effects of mecamylamine on human cigarette smoking and subjective ratings. *Psychopharmacology* **88**: 420–425.

NEMETH-COSLETT, R., HENNINGFIELD, J. E., O'KEEFFE, M. K. and GRIFFITHS, R. R. (1987) Nicotine gum: dose-related effects on cigarette smoking and subjective ratings. *Psychopharmacology* **92**: 424–430.

NESBITT, P. D. (1973) Smoking, physiological arousal and emotional response. *J. Personal. Soc. Psychol.* **25**: 137–144.

NORDBERG, A. and BERGH, C. (1985) Effect of nicotine on passive avoidance behaviour and motoric activity in mice. *Acta Pharmac. Toxicol.* **56**: 337–341.

NORDBERG, A., WAHLSROM, G., ARNELO, V. and LARSSON, C. (1985) Effect of long-term nicotine treatment on [^{3}H] nicotine binding sites in the rat brain. *Drug Alcohol Dep.* **16**: 9–17.

PEEKE, S. C. and PEEKE, H. V. S. (1984) Attention, memory and cigarette smoking. *Psychopharmacology* **84**: 205–216.

PELLOW, S., CHOPIN, P., FILE, S. E. and BRILEY, M. (1985) Validation of open:closed arm entries in an elevated plus-maze as a measure of anxiety in the rat. *J. Neurosci. Meth.* **14**: 149–167.

PERT, A. and CHIUEH, C. C. (1986) Effects of intracerebral nicotinic agonists on locomotor activity: involvement of mesolimbic dopamine. *Soc. Neurosci. Abstr.* **12**: 250.4.

PETERS, R. and MCGEE, R. (1982) Cigarette smoking and stale-dependent memory. *Psychopharmacology* **76**: 232–235.

PETTIT, H. O., ETTENBERG, A., BLOOM, F. E. and KOOB, G. F. (1984) Destruction of dopamine in the nucleus accumbens attenuates cocaine but not heroin self-administration in rat. *Psychopharmacology* **84**: 167–173.

PICKWORTH, W. B., HERNING, R. I. and HENNINGFIELD, J. E. (1986) Electro-encephalagraphic effects of nicotine chewing gum in humans. *Pharmac. Biochem. behav.* **25**: 879–882.

POHORECHY, L. A., NEWMAN, B., SUN, J. and BAILEY, W. H. (1978) Acute and chronic ethanol ingestion and serotonin metabolism in rat brain. *J. Pharmac. Exp. Ther.* **104**: 424–432.

POMERLEAU, C. S. and POMERLEAU, O. F. (1987) The effects of a psychological stressor on cigarette smoking and subsequent behavioural and psychological responses. *Psychophysiology* **24**: 278–285.

POMERLEAU, C. S., POMERLEAU, O. F. and MAJCHRZAK, M. J. (1987) Mecamylamine pretreatment increases subsequent nicotine self-administration as indicated by changes in plasma nicotine level. *Psychopharmacology* **91**: 391–393.

POTTHOFF, A. D., ELLISON, G. and NELSON, L. (1983) Ethanol intake increases during continuous administration of amphetamine and nicotine, but not several other drugs. *Pharmac. Biochem. Behav.* **18**: 489–493.

POULTON, P. (1977) The combination of smoking with psychological and physiological stress. *Ergonomics* **20**: 665–670.

PRADHAN, S. N. (1970) Effects of nicotine on several schedules of behavior in rats. *Archs Int. Pharmacodyn. Thér.* **183**: 127–138.

PRATT, J. A., STOLERMAN, I. P., GARCHA, H. S., GIARDINI, V. and FEYERABEND, C. (1983) Discriminative stimulus properties of nicotine further evidence for mediation at a cholinergic receptor. *Psychopharmacology* **81**: 54–60.

PUSKA, P., BJORKQUIST, S. and KOSKELA, K. (1979) Nicotine-containing chewing gum in smoking cessation: a double-blind trial with half-year follow-up. *Addict. Behav.* **4**: 141–146.

RAMOND, C. K., RACHAL, L. H. and MARKS, M. R. (1950) Brand discrimination among cigarette smokers. *J. Appl. Psychol.* **34**: 282–284.

REICHER, M. A. and HOLMAN, E. W. (1977) Location preference and flavor aversion reinforced by amphetamine in rats. *Anim. Learn. Behav.* **5**: 333–346.

REVELL, A. D., WARBURTON, D. M. and WESNES, K. (1985) Smoking as a coping strategy. *Addict. Behav.* **10**: 209–224.

RODGERS, R. J. (1979) Effects of nicotine, mecamylamine and hexamethonium on shock-induced fighting, pain reactivity and locomotor behaviour in rats. *Psychopharmacology* **66**: 93–98.

ROMANO, C. and GOLDSTEIN, A. (1980) Stereospecific nicotine receptors in rat brain membranes. *Science* **210**: 647–650.

ROMANO, C., GOLDSTEIN, A. and JEWELL, N. P. (1981) Characterization of the receptor mediating the nicotine discriminative stimulus. *Psychopharmacology* **74**: 310–315.

ROSE, J. E., ZINSER, M. C., TASHKIN, D. P., NEWCOMBE, R. and ERTLE, A. (1984) Subjective response to cigarette smoking following airway anesthetized. *Addict Behav.* **9**: 211–215.

ROSECRANS, J. A. (1971) Effects of nicotine on brain area 5-hydroxytryptamine function in female rats selected for differences in activity. *Eur. J. Pharmac.* **14**: 29–37.

ROSECRANS, J. A. and MELTZER, L. T. (1981) Central sites and mechanisms of action of nicotine. *Neurosci. Biobehav. Rev.* **5**: 497–501.

ROWELL, P. P. and WINKLER, D. L. (1984) Nicotinic stimulation of [^{3}H]acetylcholine release from mouse cortical synaptosomes. *J. Neurochem.* **43**: 1593–1598.

ROYAL COLLEGE OF PHYSICIANS (1977) *Smoking or Health.* Pitman Medical, London.

RUSSELL, M. A. H. (1975) Safer cigarettes. *Br. Med. J.* **3**: 41.

RUSSELL, M. A. H., JARVIS, M. J., FEYERABEND, C. and FERNO, O. (1983a) Nasal nicotine solution: a potential aid to giving up smoking. *Br. Med. J.* **286**: 683–684.

Russell, M. A. H., Merriman, R., Stapleton, J. and Taylor, W. (1983b) Effect of nicotine chewing gum as an adjunct to general practitioners advice against smoking. *Br. Med. J.* **287**: 1782–1785.

Russell, M. A. H., Raw, M. and Jarvis, M. J. (1980) Clinical use of nicotine chewing-gum. *Br. Med. J.* 1599–1602.

Russell, M. A. H., Wilson, C., Patel, V. A., Feyerabend, C. and Cole, P. V. (1975) Plasma nicotine levels after smoking cigarettes with high, medium and low nicotine yields. *Br. Med. J.* **2**: 414–416.

Russell, M. A. H., Sutton, S. R., Feyerabend, C., Cole, P. V. and Saloojee, Y. (1977) Nicotine chewing gum as a substitute for smoking. *Br. Med. J.* **280**: 1599–1602.

Schachter, S. (1973) Nesbitt's paradox. In: *Smoking Behaviour: Motives and Incentives*, pp. 142–155, Dunn, W. L. (ed.) V. H. Winston, Washington, D.C.

Schachter, S. (1978) Pharmacological and physiological determinants of smoking. In: *Smoking Behaviour*, pp. 208–228, Churchill Livingston, London.

Schachter, S., Silverstein, B., Kozlowski, L. T., Herman, C. P. and Leibling, B. (1977) Effects of stress on cigarette smoking and urinary pH. *J. Exp. Psychol.* **106**: 24–30.

Schechter, M. D. and Rand, M. J. (1974) Effect of acute deprivation of smoking on aggression and hostility. *Psychopharmacologia, Berl.* **35**: 19–28.

Schechter, M. D. and Rosecrans, J. A. (1972) Nicotine as a discriminative stimulus in rats depleted of norepinephrine or 5-hydroxytryptamine. *Psychopharmacologia, Berl.* **24**: 417–429.

Schievelbein, H. (1984) Nicotine resorption and fate. In: *International Encyclopedia of Pharmacology and Therapeutics, Section* 114, *Nicotine and the Tobacco Smoking Habit*, pp. 1–15, Balfour, D. J. K. (ed.) Pergamon Press, Oxford.

Schlatter, J. and Bättig, K. (1979) Differential effects of nicotine and amphetamine on locomotor activity and maze exploration in two rat lines. *Psychopharmacology* **64**: 155–161.

Schneider, N. G., Popek, P., Jarvik, M. E. and Gritz, E. R. (1977) The use of nicotine chewing gum during cessation of smoking. *Am. J. Psychiat.* **134**: 439–440.

Schwartz, R. D. and Kellar, K. J. (1983) Nicotinic cholinergic receptor binding sites in the brain: regulation *in vivo*. *Science* **220**: 214–216.

Schwartz, R. D. and Kellar, K. J. (1985) *In vivo* regulation of [^{3}H]acetylcholine recognition sites in brain by nicotinic cholinergic drugs. *J. Neurochem.* **45**: 427–433.

Schwartz, R. D., McGee, R. Jr. and Kellar, K. J. (1982) Nicotinic cholinergic receptors labelled by [^{3}H]acetylcholine in rat brain. *Molec. Pharmac.* **22**: 56–62.

Sharp, B. M., Beyer, S., Levine, A. S., Morley, J. E. and McAllen, K. M. (1987) Attenuation of the plasma prolactin response to restraint stress after acute and chronic administration of nicotine to rats. *J. Pharmac. Exp. Ther.* **241**: 438–442.

Shimohama, S., Taniguchi, T., Fujiwara, M. and Kameyama, M. (1985) Biochemical characterization of the nicotinic cholinergic receptors in human brain: binding of (−)-[^{3}H] nicotine. *J. Neurochem.* **45**: 604–610.

Signs, S. A. and Schechter, M. D. (1986) Nicotine-induced potentiation of ethanol discrimination. *Pharmac. Biochem. Behav.* **24**: 769–771.

Singer, G., Simpson, F. and Lang, W. J. (1978) Schedule induced self-injections of nicotine with recovered body weight. *Pharmac. Biochem. Behav.* **9**: 387–389.

Singer, G., Wallace, M. and Hall, R. (1982) Effects of dopaminergic nucleus accumben lesions on the acquisition of schedule induced self-injection of nicotine in the rat. *Pharmac. Biochem. Behav.* **17**: 579–581.

Slifer, B. C. (1983) Schedule-induction of nicotine self-administration. *Pharmac. Biochem. behav.* **19**: 1005–1009.

Smith, L. A. and Lang, W. J. (1980) Changes occurring in self-administration of nicotine by rats over a 28-day period. *Pharmac. Biochem. Behav.* **13**: 215–220.

Stepney, R. (1980) Cigarette consumption and nicotine delivery. *Br. J. Addict.* **75**: 81–88.

Stepney, R. (1984) Human smoking behaviour and the development of dependence on tobacco smoking. In: *International Encyclopedia of Pharmacology and Therapeutics Section* 114, *Nicotine and the Tobacco Smoking Habit*, pp. 153–176, Balfour, D. J. K. (ed.) Pergamon Press, Oxford.

Stitzer, M., Morrison, J. and Domino, E. F. (1970) Effects of nicotine on fixed-interval behavior and their modification by cholinergic antagonists. *J. Pharmac. Exp. Ther.* **171**: 166–177.

Stolerman, I. P., Fink, R. and Jarvik, M. E. (1973a) Acute and chronic tolerance to nicotine measured by activity in rats. *Psychopharmacologia* **30**: 329–342.

Stolerman, I. P., Goldfarb, B. T., Fink, R. and Jarvik, M. E. (1973b) Influencing cigarette smoking with nicotine antagonists. *Psychopharmacologia* **28**: 247–259.

Stolerman, I. P., Pratt, J. A., Garcha, H. S., Giardini, V. and Kumar, R. (1983) Nicotine cue in rats analysed with drugs acting on cholinergic and 5-hydroxytryptamine mechanisms. *Neuropharmacology* **22**: 1029–1037.

Stolerman, I. P., Garcha, H. S., Pratt, J. A. and Kumar, R. (1984) Role of training dose in discrimination of nicotine and related compounds. *Psychopharmacology* **84**: 413–419.

Surgeon General (1979) *Smoking and Health.* US Department of Health, Education and Welfare, Washington.

Svensson, T. H. and Engberg, G. (1982) Effect of nicotine on single cell activity in the noradrenergic locus coeruleus. *Acta Physiol. Scand.* (suppl.) **479**: 31–34.

Taube, H. D., Starke, K. and Borowski, E. (1977) Presynaptic receptor systems on the noradrenergic neurones of the rat brain. *Nauyn Schmederbergs Arch. Pharmac.* **299**: 123–141.

Tennant, F. S., Tarver, A. L. and Rawson, R. A. (1983) Clinical evaluation of mecamylamine for withdrawal from nicotine dependence. *NIDA. Monog. Ser.* **49**: 239–246.

Thomas, C. B. (1973) The relationship of smoking and habits of nervous tension. In: *Smoking Behavior: Motives and Incentives*, pp. 157–170, Dunn, W. L. (ed.) Winston, Washington.

Turner, J. A. M., Sillett, R. W. and Ball, K. P. (1974) Some effects of changing to low-tar and low-nicotine cigarettes. *Lancet* **ii**: 737–739.

Vale, A. L. and Balfour, D. J. K. (1987) The role of hippocampal 5-HT in the effects of nicotine on habituation to an x-maze. *Eur. J. Pharmac.* **41**: 313–317.

VALE, A. L. and BALFOUR, D. J. K. (1989) Aversive environmental stimuli as a factor in the psychostimulant response to nicotine. *Pharmacol. Biochem. Behav.* **32**: 857–860.

WARBURTON, D. M. and WESNES, K. (1978) Individual differences in smoking and attentional performance. In: *Smoking Behaviour: Physiological and Psychological Influences*, pp. 19–144, THORNTON, R. E. (ed.) Churchill Livingston, London.

WARBURTON, D. M. and WESNES, K. (1979) The role of electrocortical arousal in the smoking habit. In: *Electrophysiological Effects of Nicotine*, pp. 183–199, REDMOND, A. and IZARD, C. (eds) Elsevier, Amsterdam.

WARBURTON, D. M. and WESNES, K. (1984) Drugs as research tools in psychology: cholinergic drugs and information processing. *Neuropsychology* **11**: 121–132.

WARBURTON, D. M., WESNES, K. and REVELL, A. (1984) Smoking and academic performance. *Curr. Psychol. Res. Rev.* **3**: 25–31.

WARBURTON, D. M., WESNES, K., SHERGOLD, K. and JAMES, M. (1986) Facilitation of learning and state dependency with nicotine. *Psychopharmacology* **89**: 55–59.

WESNES, K. and WARBURTON, D. M. (1978) The effects of cigarette smoking and nicotine tables on human attention. In: *Smoking Behaviour: Physiological and Psychological Influences*, pp. 131–147, THORNTON, R. E. (ed.) Churchill Livingston, London.

WESNES, K. and WARBURTON, D. M. (1983) Effects of smoking on rapid information processing performance.

WESNES, K. and WARBURTON, D. M. (1984) Smoking nicotine and human performance. In: *International Encyclopedia of Pharmacology and Therapeutics, Section* 114, *Nicotine and the Tobacco Smoking Habit*, pp. 133–152, BALFOUR, D. J. K. (ed.) Pergamon Press, Oxford.

WESNES, K. and WARBURTON, D. M. (1984b) The effects of cigarettes of varying yield on rapid information processing performance. *Psychopharmacology* **82**: 338–342.

WESNES, K., WARBURTON, D. M. and MATZ, B. (1983) Effects of nicotine on stimulus sensitivity and response bias in visual vigilance task. *Neuropsychobiology* **9**: 41–44.

WESNES, K., REVELL, A. and WARBURTON, D. M. (1984) Work and stress as motives for smoking. In: *Smoking and the Lung*, pp. 233–248, CUMMING, G. and BONSIGNORE, G. (eds) Plenum, New York.

WEST, R. J., JARVIS, M., RUSSELL, M., CARRUTHERS, M. and FEYERABEND, C. (1984a) Effect of nicotine replacement on the cigarette withdrawal syndrome. *Br. J. Addict.* **79**: 215–219.

WEST, R. J., RUSSELL, M. A. H., JARVIS, M. J. and FEYERABEND, C. (1984b) Dose switching to an ultra-low nicotine cigarette induce nicotine withdrawal effects. *Psychopharmacology* **84**: 12–123.

WEST, R. J., HAJEK, P. and BELCHER, M. (1986) Which smokers report most relief from craving when using nicotine chewing gum. *Psychopharmacology* **89**: 189–191.

WESTFALL, T. C. (1974) Effect of nicotine and other drugs on the release of ^{3}H-norepinephrine and ^{3}H-dopamine from rat brain slices. *Neuropharmacology* **13**: 693–700.

WESTFALL, T. C., GRANT, H. and PERRY, H. (1983) Release of dopamine and 5-hydroxytryptamine from rat striatal slices following activation of nicotine cholinergic receptors. *Gen. Pharmac.* **14**: 321–325.

WISE, R. A. (1980) The dopamine synapse and the notion of 'pleasure centers' in the brain. *TINS* **3**: 91–95.

WISE, R. A. and BOZARTH, M. A. (1981) Brain substrates for reinforcement and drug self-administration. *Prog. Neuro-Psychopharmac.* **5**: 467–474.

WONNACOTT, S. (1986) α-Bungarotoxin binds to low-affinity nicotine binding sites in rat brain. *J. Neurochem.* **47**: 1706–1712.

WONNACOTT, S. (1987) Brain nicotine binding sites. *Human Toxicol.* **6**: 343–353.

YOSHIDA, K., KATO, Y. and IMURA, H. (1980) Nicotine-induced release of noradrenaline from hypothalamic synaptosomes. *Brain Res.* **182**: 361–368.

ZAGONA, S. V. and ZURCHER, L. A. (1965) An analysis of some psychosocial variables associated with smoking behavior in a college sample. *Psychol. Rep.* **17**: 967–978.

INDEX

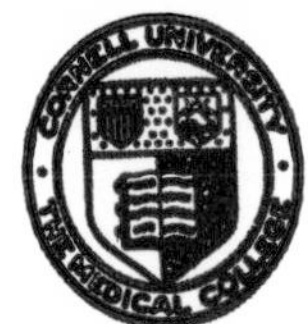
CORNELL UNIVERSITY
THE MEDICAL COLLEGE